PATHOLOGY

BY

Peter A. Herbut, M.D.

Professor of Pathology, Jefferson Medical College and Director of Clinical Laboratories,
Jefferson Medical College Hospital, Philadelphia, Pennsylvania

Second Edition, Thoroughly Revised
1506 Illustrations on 758 Figures and 6 Color Plates

Lea & Febiger

PHILADELPHIA   1959

CONTRIBUTORS

Except as indicated, all contributors are connected with the Jefferson Medical College, Philadelphia, Pennsylvania.

Bernard J. Alpers, M.D., Sc.D.
Professor of Neurology and Head of the Department.

Eugene Aserinsky, Ph.D.
Assistant Professor of Physiology.

Gordon O. Bain, M.D.
Assistant Professor of Pathology, Faculty of Medicine, University of Alberta, Edmonton, Alberta, Canada.

Robert T. Carroll, B.S., M.D.
Head Section on Blood Transfusion, Charlotte Drake Cardeza Foundation, and Assistant in Medicine.

Richard T. Cathcart, B.A., M.D.
Assistant Professor of Medicine.

Anthony F. DePalma, M.D.
James Edwards Professor of Orthopedic Surgery and Head of the Department.

John E. C. Dorchester, B.A., M.A., Ph.D.
Assistant Professor of Physiology.

Willard M. Drake, Jr., A.B., M.D.
Associate in Urology.

M. H. F. Friedman, B.Sc., M.A., Ph.D.
Professor of Physiology and Head of the Department.

Franz Goldstein, M.D.
Instructor in Medicine.

Fred Harbert, A.B., M.D., M.Sc., D.Sc.
Professor of Oto-Rhino-Laryngology and Broncho-Esophagology and Head of the Department.

W. Paul Havens, Jr., A.B., M.D.
Professor of Medicine and Professor of Clinical Microbiology.

Hans G. Keitel, B.S., M.D.
Professor of Pediatrics and Head of the Department.

Joseph F. McCloskey, B.S., M.D.
Associate Professor of Pathology.

(3)

121070

William V. McDonnell, A.B., M.D.
Associate Professor of Pathology.

Francis A. McKeon, Jr., B.S., M.D.
Instructor in Pathology.

Abraham E. Rakoff, A.B., M.D.
Clinical Professor of Obstetric and Gynecologic Endocrinology.

Joseph J. Rupp, B.S., M.D.
Assistant Professor of Clinical Medicine.

William A. Sodeman, B.S., M.D.
Dean and Professor of Medicine.

Leandro M. Tocantins, M.D.
Professor of Clinical and Experimental Medicine and Director Charlotte
Drake Cardeza Foundation.

Frederick B. Wagner, Jr., A.B., M.D.
Clinical Professor of Surgery.

PREFACE TO THE SECOND EDITION

In this second edition of Pathology your author has endeavored to correct some of the defects in the first edition that have been so kindly and so constructively pointed out by both colleagues and medical students alike. This, of necessity, has added 288 pages and 213 photographs to the book but still, it is hoped, keeps it within usable bounds.

In the first section on general pathologic processes material pertaining to the following subject matter has been added, extended, or completely rewritten, in most instances with greater emphasis on mechanisms and pathophysiologic aspects: names of more recently deceased pathologists of note, laws concerning disposal of bodies after death, atrophy, fibrinoid degeneration, amyloidosis, mucus, carbohydrate metabolism, lipid metabolism, iron and iron metabolism, hemoglobin, bilirubin, vitamins, porphyrins, melanin, inflammation, allergic inflammations, viral inflammations, rickettsial inflammations, fungous inflammations, parasitic inflammations, tuberculous inflammation, syphilitic inflammation, fluid balance, shock, thrombosis, embolism, heat exhaustion, heat stroke, chilblains, hypothermia, electricity, and irradiation.

The greatest change effected in the remainder of the book on systemic pathology has been the addition of a section on pathologic physiology at the beginning of each chapter and concerned with the organ or system therein discussed. Where possible, the material included consists of (1) brief summary of the normal physiology, (2) a discussion of the deviations from normal referring to specific disease states or groups of diseases in which such deviations occur, (3) an explanation, as far as possible, on morphologic grounds of the reasons for the altered physiology, and (4) a brief discussion of the various laboratory tests by which altered physiologic function can be discerned. This rather formidable task was accomplished by twenty of your author's colleagues at Jefferson. To these contributors your author is most grateful. Some of the remaining revisions and additions in connection with systemic pathology are concerned with hypopotassemia, myxedema heart, Fiedler's myocarditis, transaminase, heart failure, cardiac arrest, mechanism of arteriosclerosis, dissecting aneurysm, glomus jugulare tumors, malignant granuloma of the face, mucocele of the sinuses, eosinophilic granuloma of the lungs, pulmonary hemosiderosis, tumors of the nasopharynx, pulmonary edema, pulmonary microlithiasis, cretinism with goiter, intestinal polyposis and mucocutaneous pigmentation, syndrome of malignant carcinoid, barium sulfate granuloma, subphrenic abscess, nephrocalcinosis, fibromatosis, discoid lupus erythematosus, reticulohistiocytic granuloma, and keratoacanthoma.

Finally, this second edition would not have been possible without the continued interest and encouragement of Lea & Febiger in publishing the book, the aid of Mr. Robert T. Lenz and his library staff in providing medical journals, and the loyalty and perseverance of Miss Lucille S. Holmes in the adroitness of the secretarial work. To all of these your author wishes to express sincere thanks.

Peter A. Herbut, M.D.

Philadelphia, Pa.

PREFACE TO THE FIRST EDITION

THIS book on Pathology is intended for the student of medicine—be he undergraduate or postgraduate. It consists of a general dissertation on both medical and surgical diseases and represents an attempt to reduce an encyclopedic amount of information to the confines of a single volume. To achieve this end a rather rigid pattern is necessarily followed throughout the text and the material is presented with little if any adornment.

The first Chapter is concerned with orientation. It contains a delineation of pathology and its various subdivisions, a sketchy outline of the evolution of pathology as a separate specialty in medicine, and brief mention of some of the great names and contributions of the past. The second Chapter deals with the all-important but often neglected topic of The Autopsy. It encompasses a brief account of the ownership of the body, permission for autopsy, equipment necessary for performance of an autopsy, actual procedure involved, medicolegal autopsy, and weights and measurements of normal organs. The next five Chapters are devoted successively to general discussions of the basic pathologic processes of Congenital Anomalies, Degenerations, Inflammations, Physical Disturbances, and Tumors. This division sets the pattern for the majority of the remaining Chapters wherein the diseases of most of the organs are classified into the five major categories just listed. In addition, whenever a disease receives more than passing comment, its characteristics are usually presented in the following sequence: definition, incidence, cause, gross appearance, microscopic appearance, spread (in the case of tumors), complications, clinicopathologic correlation, diagnosis, treatment, and prognosis. In each instance, while the pathologic anatomy is stressed, an attempt has been made to include enough of the other aspects to give the reader a bird's-eye view of the disease as a whole.

Much of the incentive for undertaking the writing of the book has come from association with enthusiastic and inquisitive medical students. To them, your author wishes to voice genuine appreciation. He also wishes to express sincere gratitude to Doctor Bernard J. Alpers for contributing the Chapter on the Central Nervous System, to the Staff Members of the Department of Pathology and Clinical Laboratories for their helpful suggestions and aid in preparing material for photography, to Doctor William V. McDonnell for the monotonous and unrewarding task of reading the manuscript, to Miss Lucille S. Holmes for excellent secretarial performance, to Mr. Robert T. Lentz and the library personnel for their co-operation, and to Mr. Allen F. Hancock for the photography. The photographs of parasites were made from slides purchased from Ward's Natural Science Estab., Inc., Rochester, N. Y. and Tropical Biologicals, San Juan, Puerto Rico.

PETER A. HERBUT, M.D.

PHILADELPHIA, PA.

Contents

PATHOLOGY

Chapter

1

Orientation

DEFINITIONS

In order to better understand the meaning of pathology, one must first know what is meant by disease and this, in turn, requires an understanding of the meaning of health. *Health* (AS. = whole) may be defined as a normal state of the body or as the condition of the body when it exists in complete harmony with its surroundings. *Disease* (Fr. = negative + ease) is any departure from a state of health or the state of the body when it exists in discord with its surroundings. It is a disordered condition of the mind or body.

Pathology (Gr. = disease + discourse) may be defined as a study of disease or as that fundamental branch of medicine that is concerned with the study of the causes, nature, and evolution of disease and the changes in anatomy, physiology, and chemistry resulting therefrom. The study of the causation of disease is spoken of as *etiology* (Gr. = cause + discourse). The precise etiological or causative agents are known in many diseases but in others they are as yet obscure. Some of the more common causes of disease are bacteria, rickettsia, viruses, fungi, parasites, chemicals, heat, cold, light, electricity, irradiation, foreign bodies, and trauma. The *nature* of a disease may be defined as its essential character or its distinguishing quality. Fundamentally, diseases may be divided into the following five groups: congenital anomalies, degenerations, inflammations, physical disturbances, and tumors. The *evolution* of a disease, known as *pathogenesis* (Gr. = disease + origin), is its unfolding or development. Changes in anatomy connote morphologic alterations and are grouped under the designation of *pathologic anatomy*. This branch is further subdivided into gross, microscopic, general, and special pathology. *Gross* (or macroscopic) pathology means the study of alterations in organs and tissues as seen with the naked eye. *Microscopic* (or histologic) pathology concerns changes in organs, tissues, and cells as visualized with the aid of a microscope. *General* pathology encompasses fundamental processes which are usually common to more than one tissue or organ and which often eventuate from more than one etiologic agent. An example is parenchymatous degeneration which affects the liver, kidneys, and other organs and results from the action of bacteria, chemicals, and other agents. The term *special* pathology is reserved for the study of diseases peculiar to certain organs or systems. Thus, one speaks of *surgical* pathology (those conditions that come within the field of surgery), *genito-urinary* pathology (changes confined to the genital and urinary systems), *gynecological* and *obstetrical* pathology (disorders of the female generative system), *neuropathology* (alterations in nerve tissue), pathology in *internal medicine* (those conditions that come within the scope of the internist), etc. Changes in physiology consequent to disease are referred to as *pathologic physiology*, and changes in chemistry are called *pathologic chemistry*. *Clinical pathology* is that branch of pathology that is usually practiced in a hospital. It is a hybrid that is closely connected with clinical medicine and encompasses chemistry, parasitology, hematology, serology, bacteriology, and pathologic anatomy. *Experimental pathology* is the study of disease willfully produced in animals. *Comparative pathology* is that branch of pathology wherein diseases of lower animals are compared with those in man.

EVOLUTION OF PATHOLOGY

It is apparent, from the above definitions, that pathology is intimately associated with disease and it is not surprising, therefore, that it did not emerge as a basic and more or less separate science until relatively recently.

In *ancient times* theology dominated the practice of healing. The diseased visited the temples of the gods for relief from their miseries. As a token of their appreciation, some of those who were cured left rewards of sculptured or modeled forms which have from time to time been unearthed by archeologists. A few of the disorders thus represented are varicose veins, ulcers, hernias, obesity, and breast tumors. Aside from these, the earliest records of disease date to ancient Egypt. Here, too, theology dominated the scene. Demons caused disease and the art of healing was relegated to priests who drove out the evil spirits. By 1550 B. C. there was some knowledge concerning intestinal parasites, castration, circumcision, bone injuries, ulcerating masses, and trachoma.

Around the *time of Christ* there were five men that made a lasting imprint on medicine. *Hippocrates* (460–370 B. C.) was the first to break away from the demonistic doctrines. He propounded the theory that disease was caused by disturbances in body fluids or humors, and so was born *humoral pathology*. According to Hippocrates, the body contained four humors— blood which came from the heart, phlegm from the brain, yellow bile from the liver, and black bile from the spleen. He described suppuration and introduced the terms cancer and scirrhous. *Aristotle* (384–322 B. C.), through extensive animal dissections, originated the science of Zoology. At Alexandria, he founded the first university and it was here that dissection of the human body (on a large scale) was first practiced. *Herophilus*, born in 300 B. C., held that life was based on the following four factors: nourishment which originated from the liver and the digestive tract, warmth which came from the heart, mental activity which was associated with the brain, and sensations derived from the nerves. *Cornelius Celsus* (30 B. C.–38 A. D.) was the first to write a text on special pathology. Among other things, he propounded the cardinal signs of inflammation: rubor (redness), tumor (swelling), calor (heat), and dolor (pain). Finally, there was *Galen* (129–201 A. D.) who expanded the humoral pathology of Hippocrates and, through his writings, dominated thinking in medicine for centuries to come. With the Christian era, dissection of human bodies practically ceased. Galen, therefore, turned to the dissection of animals and projected his findings to man. He explained disease on two factors—presentation and adhesion. If proper amount of material was presented to a part, it adhered and was utilized; otherwise, it was discarded. He wrote more than five textbooks on pathology.

Following Galen there was little progress in medicine until the *Renaissance* (14th to 16th centuries) when *pathologic anatomy* emerged as a separate science. *Antonio Benivieni* (1440–1502) was the first to ask relatives for postmortems on obscure cases. *Fracastoro* (early 1500) likened fermentation of wine to infection and spoke for the first time of a transmissible virus. He gave an excellent account of the clinical course of syphilis and both recognized and emphasized its venereal origin. *Jean Fernel* (born in 1497) wrote extensively on syphilis and suggested that aneurysms were of syphilitic origin.

The seventeenth century produced several great men in medicine. *William Harvey* (1578–1657) discovered the circulation. *Marco Aurelio Severino* (1580–1656) wrote extensively on tumors of the genital organs. *Thomas Bartholin* (1616–1656) organized the first medical journal. *Johann Jakob Wepfer* (1620–1695) discovered the relationship of cerebral hemorrhage to apoplexy. *Marcello Malpighi* (1628–1694) introduced the microscope into pathology and, among other things, described the histology of the kidneys, lungs and spleen. *Georgio Baglivi* (1669–1707) looked upon the body as a complicated machine, placed diseases in the solid portions of the body rather than in the humors, and thus was the first to break away from the humoral pathology of Hippocrates and Galen. Also born in the 17th century, but really a product of the 18th century, was *Giovanni Battista Morgagni* (1682–1771). In his great work, the "Seat and Causes of Disease," he was the first to correlate organic changes found at postmortem with clinical symptoms. Thus, it was with him that modern pathology began.

Gradually the great centers of medicine, and therefore pathology, shifted from the Mediterranean area to central and western Europe and then to America. *France* produced several notables. *Raymond de Vieusseus* (1641–1716) recognized aortic insufficiency and gave a lucid description of its effect upon the pulse. *Bichat* (1771–1802) was aware of the need of histologic methods for the further advancement of pathology. He contended that the body was made of textures or tissues and that diseases of organs were in reality diseases of tissues. By means of fine dissection and subjection of organs to action of heat and chemicals he recognized twenty-one different tissues in the body. *Laennec* (1781–1826) contributed greatly to the knowledge of pulmonary tuberculosis, bronchiectasis, emphysema, and lobar pneumonia and also invented the stethoscope. *Jean Cruveilheir* (1791–1873) was made Professor of Pathologic Anatomy at Hotel Dieu in Paris (the first to occupy such a position anywhere) and produced a lithographed atlas on pathologic anatomy. *Philip Record* (1799–1889) separated gonorrhea from syphilis, and *Jean Martin Charcot* (1825–1893) excelled in pathology of the nervous system. Although best known for his work on a destructive type of arthritis he also contributed to multiple sclerosis, amyotropic lateral sclerosis, and locomotor ataxia.

In *England* there were at least six men who distinguished themselves. *John Hunter* (1728–1793) wrote extensively on the treatment of battle wounds to which he was exposed during the Seven Years' War, discovered collateral circulation, and recognized the usefulness of the clotting of blood. *Mathew Baillie* (1761–1823) wrote the first textbook devoted exclusively to pathology. *Richard Bright* (1789–1858) correlated albuminuria, kidney disease, and dropsy. *Thomas Addison* (1793–1860) described a refractory type of anemia and tuberculous disease of the adrenal cortex, both of which bear his name. *James Paget* (1814–1899) described an eczema of the nipple and a lesion of bones which are now known respectively as Paget's disease of the nipple and Paget's disease of bone (osteitis deformans). The sixth man was *Jonathan Hutchinson* (1828–1913) who is remembered for his work on congenital syphilis.

In *Vienna* the greatest single figure of all time in the field of pathology was *Carl Rokitansky* (1804–1878). He insisted upon a careful examination of the entire body at postmortem and not only correlated these findings with clinical manifestations but was also interested in their etiology and evolution. At the time of his retirement, he had available 70,000 protocols of autopsies performed under his directorship.

In the last century *Germany*, too, produced a brilliant and colorful array of students in pathology. Their father was *Johannes Muller* (1801–1858). To him can be credited two achievements that stand apart from other successes—(1) the routine use of the microscope in analyzing tissues and (2) the training of three pupils—Henle, Schwann, and Virchow. *Jacob Henle* (1809–1885) was the first to classify tissues histologically. *Theodore Schwann* (1810–1882) established the fact that all animal tissue was cellular. The most flamboyant, however, was *Rudolph Virchow* (1821–1902). He wrote voluminously on many topics including inflammation, pyemia, embolism, and thrombosis. He divided leukemias into two types—one in which the cells were like those in lymph nodes and the other in which they resembled those in the spleen. In 1847, he started a medical journal which is now known as Virchow's Archives. Other men of import in Germany were (1) *Recklinghausen* (1833–1910) known for his work on neurofibromatosis and osteitis fibrosa cystica, (2) *Klebs* (1834–1913) remembered for linking bacteriology with pathology, (3) *Julius Cohnheim* (1839–1884) noted for explaining the origin of tumors from misplaced rests of tissues, and (4) *Carl Weigert* (1834–1904) known for his work on tissue degeneration, necrosis and repair, and innovations in histologic technique.

Gradually but inexorably the center of interest in pathology (and indeed in medicine as a whole) began to shift from Europe to America where it is now focused. Some Americans of the past who have contributed to the field of pathology are: *Samuel D. Gross* (1805–1884) gave the first course in pathology in the United States and, in 1839, wrote a textbook on pathology; *William Pepper* (1843–1898) separated pseudoleukemia from leukemia and described the changes in the bone marrow in pernicious anemia; *Francis Delafield* (1841–1915) and *Mitchell Prudden* (1849–1924), in 1885, wrote the second textbook on pathology in America; *William Osler* (1849–1919) did much to correlate clinical medicine and pathology; *William Henry Welsh* (1850–1934) advanced more than anyone else the field of experimental pathology and bacteriology; *Frank Burr Mallory* (1862–1941) developed and perfected numerous tissue stains, especially emphasized the demonstration of collagen, myoglia, and neuroglia fibrils, and wrote a book on Pathological Technique which, although out of print today, still remains a classic; *William George MacCallum* (1874–1944) worked on parasites, demonstrated that the lymphatic system is a closed system, discovered that calcium metabolism is controlled by the parathyroid glands, showed that carbohydrate metabolism is regulated by the islets of Langerhans in the pancreas, and wrote a textbook on pathology that was used in medical schools for thirty years; *James Ewing* (1866–1943) who can best be described as the father of oncology in America. He will be remembered (1) for his treatise on Neoplastic Diseases which has been used as a reference book for decades, and (2) for championing the use of roentgen rays and radium in the treatment of cancer; *Tracy Burr Mallory* (1896–1951) developed the clinicopathologic conference into one of the most important teaching conferences in medicine; and *Ludwig Hektoen* (1863–1951) contributed notably to our understanding of immunology and infectious disease.

Other, more recently deceased, pathologists of note were: *Balduin Lucke* (1889–1954) who discovered that an adenocarcinoma of the kidney of the leopard frog (*Rana pipiens*) was due to a filter-passing virus and that it was easily transplantable into the anterior chamber of the eye and who enhanced our knowledge of such disorders as influenza, viral hepatitis, and the renal changes in shock; *Horst Ortel* (1873–1956) who contributed much to our understanding of renal diseases and who insisted that pathology be studied from strictly causative and logically observed aspects; *Carl Vernon Weller* (1887–1956) who, among other things, pioneered in the study of cancer of the lung and who was Editor-in-Chief of the American Journal of Pathology from 1941–1956; and *G. Lyman Duff* (1904–1956) who approached pathology from an experimental point of view and who concentrated on elucidating the pathogenesis of arteriosclerosis.

Thus, after a rather prolonged evolution, pathology has at length emerged as a fundamental branch of medicine that not only holds its own with other specialties but that serves as a hub around which medical practice is built. In a modern institution the pathologist always holds a key position. He is the "silent partner"—the "father confessor"—who hears, weighs, and advises on the many problems that perplex the practicing physician. Without his aid the road for the clinician would indeed be rough and the outcome for the patient would often be disastrous.

REFERENCES

Krumbhaar, E. B.: *Pathology* (Volume 19 of Clio Medica), New York, Paul B. Hoeber, Inc. 1937.

Long, E. R.: *History of Pathology*, Baltimore, The Williams & Wilkins Co., 1928.

Chapter

2

The Autopsy

DEFINITION AND PURPOSE

AN external and internal examination of the body after death is *known* as a *postmortem* (L. = after death), an *autopsy* (Gr. = self + view), a *necropsy* (Gr. = dead + view), or *necroscopy* (Gr. = corpse + to view). The procedure is a scientific investigation of tissues, organs, and body fluids. It consists primarily of an anatomic examination (first with the naked eye and then with the aid of a microscope) and secondarily of other types of examinations including bacteriologic studies and chemical determinations. Its *purposes* are twofold—first, to ascertain the cause of death and second, to gather knowledge regarding the nature, extent, and evolution of a disease.

THE BODY

The body of a deceased is special property—property that cannot be bought or sold and property that must be suitably disposed of by law. While there are no specific laws in many of the States relative to *property rights* in the body, American courts have gradually established a precedent giving such rights "to the surviving relative in the *order of inheritance of property.*" In practice, this means the surviving spouse, the surviving parent, oldest adult child in the case of a lone parent, oldest surviving sibling in the case of an unmarried person, etc. In the absence of a relative, the property right in the body passes to a *friend* and in the absence of a friend, statuary laws in most of the United States provide for the *disposal* of dead human bodies by *Anatomic Acts*. These usually state that all dead bodies not claimed by relatives or friends become the property of the Anatomic Board. In the absence of such Anatomic Acts the responsibility for custody and property disposal of the body is placed by *common law* on the *owner or tenant* of the *building* housing the body, or the *administrator* of a *hospital* or *institution* where death occurred. In most States there are also no specific laws that bear directly on the point of whether or not a person can dispose of his own body after death as he sees fit by *will* during his lifetime. In these States a precedent has been established and followed that the dead body is not part of the estate of the deceased and that it, therefore, cannot be disposed of by will. In other words, regardless of the will, the property right passes to the next of kin. A few States, however, such as California, Louisiana, Minnesota, New York, North Carolina, Pennsylvania, North Dakota, South Dakota, and Washington, do have laws giving every person the right to direct the manner in which his body will be disposed of after death. Thus, since it is apparent that precedents and laws vary from locality to locality, it behooves every physician to become thoroughly familiar with the accepted procedures in the State in which he is practicing— lest he run afoul of the courts.

(14)

PERMISSION FOR AUTOPSY

In order that a pathologist may legally perform an autopsy, permission for such an operation must first be secured. Failure to do so is grounds for civil suit for damages and may even be a violation of the criminal code. Depending upon circumstances, permission may be obtained from (1) the next of *kin* or a *friend*, (2) the *Coroner* or *Medical Examiner*, or (3) the *Anatomic Board*. Permission from the Anatomic Board is required in all cases where the body is unclaimed by a relative or a friend. Permission from the *Coroner* or *Medical Examiner* is required in all cases that come under the jurisdiction of these offices. Although *statuary regulations* vary from State to State, a Coroner's or Medical Examiner's case is generally one in which (1) death occurs under suspicious circumstances, (2) there is a possibility of a crime having been committed, or (3) the health of the public may be affected if the nature of the disease is unknown. The Coroner or Medical Examiner does not require consent for the performance of an autopsy from the next of kin. For all cases that do not come under the Anatomic Board or the Coroner or Medical Examiner, the pathologist performing an autopsy must get permission from the next of kin or, in the absence of relatives, from a friend.

In order to avoid future litigation, *authorization* to perform an autopsy should always be obtained *in writing*. The form is not standard and need not be elaborate. Basically it should include the following information: name of deceased, place, date and time of death, name of attending physician, clinical diagnosis, extent of the examination to be performed (chest, abdomen, neck, brain, spinal cord, and any special tissues or organs as extremities, eyes, etc.), space for any specific instructions to the pathologist, a note to the effect that the pathologist may retain such tissues and organs as are necessary for further examination or for educational or research purposes, signature and address of the grantor and his relation to the deceased, signature of the person obtaining the permission, and the name of the funeral director to whom the body is to be released together with the promised time of release.

It cannot be overemphasized that proper consent from the proper authority must be obtained in every case. Otherwise, the doctor performing the autopsy, the doctor or person connected in any way with the ordering of the examination, and the institution in which the autopsy is made are liable for damages.

EQUIPMENT

The *autopsy room* should be made of material that can be easily and thoroughly cleaned. It should be provided with good refrigeration, an adequate and easily cleanable autopsy table, illuminating gas, running water adequate fluorescent lighting, and a sensitive balance. The *instruments* need not be particularly varied but they must, at all times, be *sharp*. As a minimum, one should have each of the following: stout blade autopsy knife, long blade knife, rat-tooth forceps, osteotome, hemostat or similar clamp, probe, grooved director, scalpel, spatula, scissors with the tip of one blade blunt and that of the other sharp, enterotomy scissors, orthopedic mallet, bone chisel, saw, cutting edge suture needle, and store string for suturing. Although there are many adequate solutions for fixing tissues for microscopic examination, 10 per cent formalin is the cheapest and best for all-around purposes. A pint Mason jar three-quarters full of fluid is generally sufficient for the usual number of sections from one cadaver.

PERFORMANCE OF THE AUTOPSY

Before the pathologist proceeds with the autopsy he should be familiar with an abstract of the *history* and *clinical findings* for this knowledge is invaluable in determining the proper approach to the dissection of the diseased organs. The examination itself is comparable in part to an ordinary physical examination in that *close inspection* and *gentle palpation* are of the essence. It may be divided into two parts—external and internal.

External examination of the body should be methodical. It should start with the scalp and end with the soles of the feet and it should include detailed inspection and palpation of structures such as ears, eyes, nose, mouth, umbilicus, urethral opening, scrotum, vagina, and anus. In general, it may be stated that any changes in shape, size, color, texture, or anatomical relationships of any component parts of the body should be noted. Two items to be determined first are (1) has death occurred and (2) when did it occur? The *signs* of *death* may be divided into physiologic and anatomic.

Physiologic signs of *death* may be listed as follows: (1) cessation of *pulse beat* (elicited by palpating the radial artery at the wrist), (2) cessation of *heart beat* (elicited by palpating or auscultating the precordial area), (3) cessation of *respiration* (elicited by observing lack of movement of the thoracic cage or by noting absence of clouding of a cold mirror held adjacent to the nostrils or mouth), (4) cessation of *body movements* (elicited by observation), and (5) *algor mortis* (L. = coldness + of death)—gradual drop in body temperature to equal that of the surrounding atmosphere (elicited by actual oral, rectal, axillary, or perineal thermometric readings).

Anatomic signs of *death* appear at varying intervals after cessation of physiologic activities and depend upon the nature of death, the condition of the body prior to death, and the nature of the surrounding medium. They consist of desiccation of the cornea, livor mortis, rigor mortis, and decomposition.

Desiccation or drying of the cornea is one of the earliest of anatomic changes. In fact, depending upon the atmospheric humidity and temperature, it may even become apparent before death actually occurs. It is evident as a milky opacity of that part of the cornea that is not covered by the eyelids and is due to evaporation of fluid from the superficial cells.

Livor mortis (L. = lividity + of death) is a mottled pink, red to bluish discoloration of the skin of the dependent portions of the body (Fig. 1). It is due to gravitation of blood in vessels, usually appears within two hours after death, is accompanied by blanching upon change of body position or digital pressure for the first twelve hours after death, and becomes permanent in position or fixed thereafter (Moritz and Lund).

Rigor mortis (L. = rigidity + of death) is rigidity or stiffness of the striated muscles of the body (Fig. 1). It becomes apparent first in the muscles of the face about two hours after death, involves progressively the rest of the body, is complete within four to twelve hours, and disappears spontaneously in the order in which it appeared in from ten to forty-eight hours. It appears sooner and is of greater intensity in the presence of a previously healthy body, is accelerated by heat, and is delayed by cold. The process represents a coagulation of protein—a transformation of myosinogen into myosin. Once it is forcibly broken or spontaneously disappears (due to the action of autolytic enzymes) it does not recur.

Decomposition (L. = negative + put together) may be defined as separation of the complex molecules of cells and tissues into their constituent parts or elements. The term is synonymous with *decay* (L. = down + to fall). Actually, decomposition of the body is brought about by two usually inseparable fundamental processes—autolysis and putrefaction. *Autolysis*

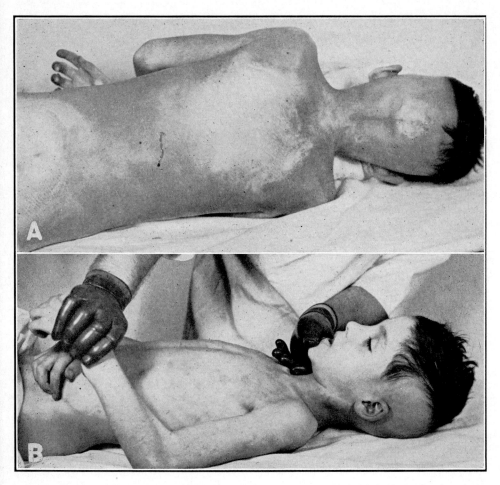

FIG. 1.—Demonstrating two anatomic signs of death. Liver mortis (*A*) is indicated by a mottled appearance of the skin of the back except at pressure points over the occiput, thorax, and buttocks where it is blanched. A small incision in the low thoracic area resulted in a trickle of blood. Rigor mortis (*B*) is demonstrated by the tenseness of the muscles of the jaw and left forearm upon manual exertion of pressure in the corresponding areas.

(Gr. = self + solution) signifies disintegration of cells or tissues by the action of their own autogenous enzymes. Two examples of postmortem autolysis are digestion and even perforation of the stomach wall by gastric juice, and softening and disintegration of the pancreas by pancreatic juice. *Putrefaction* (L. = render putrid) connotes disintegration of animal cells and tissues by microorganisms with the production of solids, fluids, and gases, some of which have a foul odor. In man the microorganisms most commonly involved in putrefaction are bacilli of the colon and gas gangrene groups. They gain entrance from the intestinal tract shortly before or shortly after death. Some of the intermediary products of putrefaction are amino acids, fatty acids, and ptomaines and these finally are broken down into ammonia, ammonium compounds, hydrogen, sulfurated hydrogen, mercaptans, nitrogen, carbon dioxide, methane, and water. Tissues under-going decomposition vary in appearance depending upon the degree and rapidity of disintegration and this, in turn, depends upon the condition of the body before death and the nature of the surrounding medium after death. Generally they possess a foul odor (due especially to mercaptans) and pass progressively through the stages of softening, swelling, discolora-tion, fluidification, and finally complete disintegration.

Internal examination must likewise be carried out methodically. The usual *order* of *examination* is (1) thorax, neck, and oral cavity, (2) abdomen, (3) head, (4) spinal cord, and (5) peripheral portions of the body. Regard-less of the area of the body under consideration, certain *guiding principles* that should be abided by are (1) incisions should be clean-cut and sweeping but yet precise, (2) the organs, serosal cavities, body, instruments, autopsy table, and the operator must at *all times* be *cleaned* of free *blood* and other body fluids, (3) the anatomic relationships of the various tissues and organs must always be ascertained before they are disturbed, (4) special care must be taken not to disfigure in any way exposed portions of the body or vessels leading to these areas which may prohibit the embalmer from performing his duty skillfully, (5) the procedure of dissection should be altered locally whenever such a change will better expose the disease process, and (6) at least one piece of tissue not more than 4 mm. thick and 15 mm. square should be taken from each organ for microscopic examination. In general, each *system* and each *organ* should be examined with the following points in mind: (1) changes in topographic anatomic relationships, (2) variations in shape, (3) increase or decrease in size and weight, (4) alterations in color, (5) decrease or increase in consistency, and (6) changes in minute anatomic structure on cut surface or on further dissection.

The *thorax* is exposed by two cutaneous incisions. The first is semicir-cular extending from one acromioclavicular joint to the other and encom-passing the lateral and inferior borders of each breast. The skin flaps so created and the underlying tissues are then dissected free of the bony cage from below up. The second incision is midline in position, is placed just to the left of the umbilicus, and serves also to expose the abdominal organs. It extends from the first incision as it crosses the midline of the sternum to the symphysis pubis. The thorax is entered by cutting across the cartilages just medial to the chondrocostal junctions and through the sternoclavicular joints and by lifting off the sternal plate. The *thymus* is then identified and dissected.

The *pericardial cavity* is opened by an inverted Y-shaped incision and the upper limb of the incision is then carried superiorly to expose the *arch* of the *aorta* and the *great vessels*. The latter are tied and severed just above the arch. The *heart* is removed by lifting the apex and severing, from below up, the vessels as they enter and leave the various cardiac chambers. The heart is dissected with scissors by following the course of the blood stream from right to left. The superior and inferior vena cava are joined laterally and the incision is continued to the apex of the right ventricle. From the inferior point it is extended out through the pulmonic valve to the pulmonary artery. The procedure is the same on the left side where the pulmonary

veins are joined as they enter the left atrium. The incision is carried laterally to the apex of the left ventricle and the cut is then made through the
anterior portion of the left ventricle through the aortic valve to the aorta.
The *coronary arteries* are opened from their origins in the sinuses of Valsalva to their termination in the myocardium.

The *rest* of the *thoracic structures* together with the upper portion of the
trachea, larynx, thyroid gland, parathyroid glands, upper portion of the
esophagus, pharynx, tongue, tonsils, and soft palate may be removed together. This is accomplished by carefully dissecting away the skin of the
neck, from below up, and freeing the structures of the neck mentioned by
keeping the knife's edge *close* to these tissues. The tongue is freed by incising the floor of the mouth (from below) and the soft palate and tonsils
are freed by sweeping the tip of the blade of the knife circumferentially. By
exerting traction upon the tongue (which is pulled down over the larynx
beneath the skin of the neck) all the structures mentioned are dissected
free of the vertebræ. At the level of the diaphragm the esophagus and aorta
are severed and the thoracic contents are then removed all together. The
thyroid and *parathyroid glands* are identified and removed. The *thoracic
aorta* is opened longitudinally and dissected away. The *pharynx* and
esophagus are opened posteriorly and are then dissected from the larynx,
trachea, and lower mediastinal structures. The *larynx, trachea,* and *bronchi*
are opened posteriorly after which each lung is sectioned in several planes
from the periphery to the hilum. The *mediastinal lymph nodes, soft tissues,*
and other structures are then examined carefully. The *thoracic duct* should
be examined (when desirable) after the heart is removed. It is located in
the posterior mediastinum between the aorta and azygos vein and is most
readily demonstrated by flipping the right lung over the mediastinum into
the left side of the thorax.

The *abdomen* is best examined by incising the diaphragm and allowing
the structures to ascend into the thorax. The *omentum, mesentery,* and
mesenteric structures (vessels, lymph nodes, and lymphatics) are examined
first. After doubly ligating the duodenojejunal junction and cutting between the ligatures, the entire intestinal tract (to the rectum) is removed
from above down by severing the mesentery at its junction with the bowel
wall. The intestinal tract is opened longitudinally, using the enterotomy
scissors. The *spleen* is removed by severing the hilar structures. The
adrenals are then located and removed. Generally it is desirable to remove
the mesentery, stomach, duodenum, pancreas, extrahepatic biliary system, and
liver together. The *stomach* is opened along the greater curvature with the
incision being swung anteriorly at the pylorus and then along the greater
curvature of the *duodenum.* The *Ampulla of Vater* is identified and the
pancreatic duct, extrahepatic ducts, and *gallbladder* are opened from below
up. Dissecting this group of organs from the posterior aspect, the *splenic
artery* and *vein,* the *superior mesenteric vein,* and the *portal vein* are opened
longitudinally. The pancreas is cut into numerous slices either longitudinally or transversely. The *liver* is detached by severing its hilar attachments and is also sectioned into numerous slices in a plane exposing the
greatest surface area. Returning to the *abdomen* the remaining portion of
the *aorta* and the *renal* and *iliac arteries* are opened *in situ.* After inspecting
and dissecting the *ureters* free, each *kidney* is removed and sectioned longitudinally from the lateral border to the hilum. The *bladder, urethra,
generative tract,* and *rectum* are removed together. In the female the *urethra*
may be removed in its entirety with the incision cutting across the distal

portion of the vagina and the anorectal junction. In the male the urethra is usually severed retropubically, just distal to the prostate and the incision is carried across the anorectal junction. When desirable, the entire urethra may be removed along with the penis by carrying the retropubic dissection beneath the skin of the penis to the corona. The urethra is opened anteriorly and the incision is then carried to the dome of the *bladder* along the midline anteriorly. The *rectum* is opened longitudinally along its posterior border. The *female generative system* is dissected from below up. After the bladder is removed the vagina, cervix, and uterus are opened anteriorly. At the fundus of the uterus the incision is carried laterally to the entrance of each fallopian tube. The tubes are opened longitudinally and the ovaries are sectioned in slices to present the greatest possible surface area. The *male generative system* may be removed intact but usually the testes and spermatic cords are examined separately by introducing them into the abdomen by way of the inguinal canals. Each testis is cut longitudinally from the periphery to the hilum. The prostate and seminal vesicles are sectioned into thin slices transversely in a postero-anterior direction. Routine examination of the *bone marrow* consists of sawing a thin slice of the bodies of the thoracic and lumbar vertebræ. When desired, the sternum and ribs may be sectioned longitudinally and the bones of the pelvis may also be entered from the pelvic cavity.

The portion of the *head* not already investigated is examined almost exclusively by way of a single incision of the scalp that extends over the vertex from ear to ear just above the hair line. The skull is entered by two semicircular saw incisions that join each other just above the ear. The anterior incision extends through the temporal, parietal, and frontal bones and should be far enough posteriorly so as not to produce a ridge across the forehead upon reconstruction. The posterior incision involves the temporal, parietal, and occipital bones. Upon removal of the skull plate, the dura is cut at the same level as the bones. The superior sagittal sinus is examined and the falx cerebri is cut anteriorly and lifted back. The *brain* is then removed by cutting its attachments to the base of the skull in consecutive order from before back, by incising the tentorium cerebelli laterally, and by severing the cord just distal to the medulla. The brain is best sectioned in thin slices coronally after it has been fixed in 10 per cent formalin for about a week. The *pituitary* gland is removed by chiselling away the clinoid processes. Before peeling off the remainder of the dura, the rest of the *venous sinuses* are examined. The inner ear and mastoid are entered by chiselling through the petrous portion of the temporal bone. The *frontal sinuses, ethmoid sinuses, nasal cavity, orbital fossæ,* and *eyes* are all exposed from inside the cranium by removing, with a chisel, the bones overlying these structures. The *maxillary sinuses* are entered through the maxillary bones from below by way of incisions through the mucosa, just inferior to the prominences of the zygomatic bones.

The *spinal cord* is removed by making a midline incision over the summit of the spine from the base of the skull to the sacrum with the body in the prone position, by cutting the lamina on each side of the spinous processes and removing the detached bony covering, and by cutting the nerves extradurally just before they leave the spinal canal. The removed cord is then fixed in 10 per cent formalin for about a week and sectioned transversely at varying intervals.

The *peripheral portions* of the *body* include the extremities and areas of the head that cannot be reached from the inside. The approach to these structures is direct and, of course, varies with the area to be examined. In the procedure, two thoughts should be kept in mind—specific permission for the examination should be obtained and incisions should be such as to leave the least possible evidence of disturbance.

In addition to the routine examination just outlined, *special examinations* are often necessary. They include bacteriological, immunological, and chemical studies.

Bacteriological studies should always be carried out in cases of suspected infection. In order that they may be performed intelligently and satisfactorily, the pathologist must anticipate the type of disease present. To this end a knowledge of the clinical findings and diagnosis is mandatory. In performing bacteriological studies on cadavers, the same technique should prevail as in performing them on living persons. In culturing for ordinary pyogenic organisms (in order to prevent external contamination) the surface of the area to be cultured should be seared with a heated spatula and then punctured with a scalpel that has been sterilized in the flame. Next, a sterile, cotton-tipped applicator is inserted into the puncture wound. Blood to be cultured may be obtained from either ventricle by similarly puncturing the wall and drawing the blood in a pipet or in a syringe. For other organisms such as tubercle bacilli, gas gangrene bacilli, tetanus bacilli, viruses, fungi, etc., tissues from the various lesions and organs should be secured. Since the areas involved differ to some extent, the pathologist must be familiar with what material to collect and, if the examination cannot be carried out immediately, he should also be familiar with how it should be preserved.

Immunological studies may be carried out on serum separated from blood obtained from the heart. For this purpose, about 25 cc. of blood will suffice. It should be removed from the body as soon as possible.

Chemical studies must be carried out whenever poisoning (be it intentional, accidental, or occupational) is suspected. The *history* regarding (1) the type of drug or chemical in question, (2) the symptoms and signs, and (3) the duration of illness are invaluable in determining the tissues or fluids to be analyzed. If this information is not immediately available, the following materials should be saved in separate containers for the following respective examinations (The Autopsy—Armed Forces Institute of Pathology): (1) brain—500 gm.—alcohols, chloroform, ether, alkaloids, barbiturates, and benzene, (2) liver—500 gm.—metals, barbiturates, fluorides, and oxalates, (3) blood—500 gm.—all gaseous poisons, (4) urine—all available—barbiturates, sulfonal, and metals, (5) kidney—one—metals, particularly mercury, (6) lung—one—inhaled poisons, (7) hair—10 gm.—arsenic, (8) contents gastrointestinal tract—all—any poison taken by mouth, and (9) bone—lead, arsenic, and radium.

One of the most common causes of death to be determined is that from *drowning*. The specimens to be collected are about 10 cc. of blood from each ventricle—each to be put in a separate container and labeled "left heart" and "right heart." A specimen of water in which the body was found should also be obtained. Each of the three specimens should then be examined for chloride content. In cases of drowning in sea water, the chloride content in the blood from the "left heart" is greater than in the blood from the "right heart." In cases of drowning in fresh water, the reverse is true. An even simpler procedure is the determination of the specific gravity of plasma from the atria of the heart (Durlacher). In nondrowning deaths the specific gravity of plasma from the left atrium is higher than that from the right atrium. In drowning cases, due to absorption of water by the pulmonary venous circulation, the reverse is true—regardless of the salinity of the inahled water.

MEDICOLEGAL AUTOPSY

Medicolegal autopsy should be witnessed by one or more persons and the names of the witnesses should be made part of the record. Aside from scientific objectives, its main purpose is administration of justice.

The actual performance of the autopsy is similar to that outlined above. In addition to being a physician and a pathologist, the operator must also be somewhat of a detective. Before the body is moved, or for that matter even touched, the exact position and appearance of all surrounding objects must be carefully noted. Ordinarily this is best accomplished by working hand in hand with the police and there is no better way of obtaining permanent records than by photography.

Of *special importance*, from a medicolegal point of view, are the following (Moritz and Lund): (1) Identification of *remains* as *human*. This is easy when the body has been dead a short while but is more difficult when it has disintegrated. If putrefactive changes are not too advanced, precipitin tests are of value. Later identification by skeletal remains can almost always be made. (2) *Identification* of the *body*. Among others this can be accomplished by an examination of the belongings on the person, clothes, laundry marks, photographs, finger prints, sex by contour of pelvis or skull size, age by epiphysis and teeth, stature from length of long bones, and known diseases by various organs. (3) Determination of *time* of *death*. Contrary to lay belief, the determination of the exact time of death is well nigh impossible. The approximate time of death may be determined by considering the physiologic and anatomic signs of death already listed. Of additional value are (*a*) the condition of shrubs and plants adjacent to and beneath the body, (*b*) presence of insects, eggs, and larvæ, (*c*) degree of dilution and putrefaction of blood stains, (*d*) degree of digestion of last meal, (*e*) volume of urine in bladder in a person found dead in bed, and (*f*) dates on letters or stoppage of a watch. (4) Determination of *place* of *fatal injury*. Did the injury take place where the body was found or was the body moved thereafter? (5) *Reconstruction* of *injury*. One should determine whether the injury was single or multiple, its location, direction of the blow, time of injury, type of weapon used, and number of assailants. One should also look for traces of assailant on victim (bullet, empty shell case, pattern of automobile tire, blood stains, hair in dead persons hand, etc.) and for traces of victim on the suspected assailant (particularly blood stains).

RESTORATION OF BODY

Basically the two most important items in reconstructing the body are (1) leaving the peripheral vascular supply intact with long sutures tied to the proximal ends of the severed vessels, and (2) sponging away all free blood and leaving the skin spotlessly clean. Organs or portions of organs used for further examination or museum purposes only should be kept. Others should be returned to the body. Whether the calvarium is to be filled with plaster of Paris and all incisions tightly sewed, or whether the calvarium be left empty and only periodic interrupted sutures be placed in the incision varies with the mortician. The pathologist should become acquainted with his likes and dislikes and proceed accordingly. Finally, the body should be properly wrapped and tagged.

RECORDS

A complete detailed description of the entire autopsy should be made at the autopsy table or, at most, immediately after completion of the examination. Both positive and pertinent negative data should be recorded.

Weights and Measurements of Normal Adult Organs

(Adapted from The Autopsy, AFIP)

Organ	Weight	Measurements
Brain	1250–1400 gm.	16.5 × 12.5 cm.
Spinal cord	27– 28 gm.	length 45 cm.
Pituitary gland	610 mg.	
Pineal gland	140– 170 mg.	
Parotid gland	30 gm.	
Submaxillary gland	17 gm.	
Thymus	19– 23 gm.	
Heart	275– 325 gm.	L. V. 8–10 mm.
		R. V. 2–3 mm.
Thyroid gland	40 gm.	2 × 3.5 × 5.5 cm.
Parathyroid glands (4)	115– 130 mg.	
Right lung	375– 550 gm.	
Left lung	325– 450 gm.	
Liver	1500–1700 gm.	27 × 20 × 8 cm.
Spleen	125– 175 gm.	3.5 × 8.5 × 13 cm.
Pancreas	90– 120 gm.	3.8 × 4.5 × 23 cm.
Kidney	140– 160 gm.	3.5 × 5.5 × 11.5 cm.
Testis and epididymis	17– 27 gm.	2.5 × 3 × 4.5 cm.
Prostate	14– 16 gm.	2.7 × 3.6 × 1.9 cm.
Adrenal gland	5.7 gm.	0.5 × 3 × 4.5 cm.
Esophagus (length)		25 cm.
Stomach (length)		25–30 cm.
Duodenum (length)		30 cm.
Small intestine (length)		550–660 cm.
Large intestine (length)		150–170 cm.
Nulliparous uterus	40– 60 gm.	
Parous uterus	75– 125 gm.	
Ovary	8– 12 gm.	

Weights of Normal Organs of the Newborn at Term (3439.0 Gm.)

(Adapted from Potter)

Organ	Weight	Organ	Weight
Thyroid	2.4 gm.	Spleen	11.1 gm.
Thymus	10.8 gm.	Pancreas	3.6 gm.
Heart	21.7 gm.	Kidneys	26.6 gm.
Lungs	59.4 gm.	Adrenals	9.3 gm.
Liver	151.5 gm.	Brain	429.6 gm.

REFERENCES

DURLACHER, S. H. et al.: A.M.A. Arch. Path., 56, 454, 1953 (Drowning).

MORITZ, A. R., and LUND, H.: Medicolegal Autopsy. See Reference No. 5.

POTTER, E. L.: Pathology of the Fetus and the Newborn, Chicago, The Year Book Publishers, Inc., 1952.

REGAN, L. J.: Legal Authorization for Autopsy, R. B. H. Gradwohl, Legal Medicine, St. Louis, C. V. Mosby Co., 1954, p. 68.

The Autopsy, Armed Forces Institute of Pathology, Washington, D. C., 1951.

The Doctor and the Law; Wrongful Autopsies, Volume 6, No. 2, Law Department of the Medical Protective Company of Fort Wayne, Indiana, Wheaton, Illinois, 1939.

Chapter

3

Congenital Anomalies

GENERAL CONSIDERATIONS

DISEASE processes in man are generally dividable into several groups. The first of these may be considered in a broad sense under heading of Congenital Anomalies or Congenital Abnormalities. Upon superficial examination it might appear that this category is not only small but that it comprises rare or, at most, uncommon disorders. Upon closer analysis, however, it becomes apparent that congenital aberrations form the basis of disease and that they are the all-important determiners of life itself. Fundamentally, an individual's destiny is established at the time of inception. Whether the fertilized ovum will develop into an embryo or will die and be aborted; whether the newborn infant will succumb to an abnormality of development or an infectious disease, or whether an adult will survive the expected "three score years and ten" or die at an earlier age of some degenerative, inflammatory, or neoplastic disorder depends primarily upon the quality of his particular cells and tissues. This quality, in turn, depends upon the genes carried in the parental germ cells that brought about his very existence.

The caption *congenital* (L. = born together) *anomaly* connotes an abnormality born with a person. While it is generally reserved to designate an obvious failure of embryonic development, as for example absence of an ear, in a broader sense it also includes subtle defects in the germ plasm which may become apparent in that particular individual or which may appear only in the next or subsequent generations. *Heredity* (L. = heirship) or *inheritance* concerns itself with the transmission from parent to offspring of normal characteristics such as stature, facies, color and type of hair, color of eyes, etc., and also of abnormal characteristics which become manifested as disease. A *hereditary disease* may be defined as one which is derived from ancestry and which can be traced from generation to generation. Although often used in a different sense, a *familial disease* is actually a hereditary disease. It, too, is derived from ancestry but because it skips one, two, or more generations it is more difficult to trace. Another term that looms forth in connection with heredity is *constitution*. It may be defined as "that aggregate of hereditarial characters influenced more or less by environment which determines the individual's reaction successful or unsuccessful to the stress of environment" (Draper). It represents "the sum total of an individual's characteristics as they are potentially determined at the time of fertilization" (Bauer) and comprises physical, physiological, and mental traits which are both visible and invisible.

In discussing *obvious failures* of *embryonic development* there are certain general terms that are in constant usage. *Agenesis* (Gr. = privation + generation) and *aplasia* (Gr. = privation + formation) are used synonymously to indicate incomplete or defective development of an organ or a

(24)

tissue. *Hypoplasia* (Gr. = under + formation) means underdevelopment of an organ. The individual constituents of an organ are qualitatively normal but are defective in number and size. *Stenosis* (Gr. = narrow) connotes narrowing of a canal or opening. *Atresia* (Gr. = negative + boring) implies imperforation, absence, or closure of a normal opening. *Ectopia* (Gr. = displaced) and *dystopia* (Gr. = ill + placement) denote displacement or malposition of an organ. *Heterotopia* (Gr. = other + place) signifies the presence of tissue in abnormal locations, such as pancreas in the small intestine. A *fissure* (L. = to split) means a cleft, split, or groove made by a parting of tissues. A *sinus* (L. = bent surface or curved) connotes a blindly ending tract that extends from the mucosa of a hollow viscus or from the surface of the body or an organ into adjacent tissues. A *fistula* (L. = music pipe) indicates a tract connecting a hollow organ with another cavity or the exterior of the body.

MECHANISM OF HEREDITY

As already stated in the preceding section, heredity is possible because the various traits are transmitted from parent to offspring by *genes* (Macklin). Genes are located in *chromosomes* and chromosomes, in turn, are paired structures derived from nuclear chromatin and seen in the cell when it is in the process of mitosis. In man, each cell contains 48 chromosomes arranged in 24 pairs. One of each pair comes from the mother and the other comes from the father. In the process of ordinary cell division, each chromosome splits longitudinally, resulting in the maintenance of 48 chromosomes in each of the offspring cells. In addition to ordinary cell division, the *germ cells* undergo a process of *maturation* in which each pair of chromosomes actually separates with only one of the pair going to the mature germ cell. Thus, the resulting mature germ cell contains either the maternal or paternal chromosomes of the pair and only one-half (24) of the total number of chromosomes. Such a germ cell (from the male or the female) is ready for fertilization and when it unites with another mature germ cell from the opposite sex (female or male) the original number of chromosomes (48) is again restored.

Each member of a pair of chromosomes carries the same developmental traits. Each will thus possess genes for color of the hair, color of the eyes, stature, etc., but each of the pair may not necessarily be the same. When both the father and the mother furnish identical genes the resulting individual is pure for that particular trait and is referred to as a *homozygote*. When they furnish genes of a different quality the resulting individual is referred to as a *heterozygote* or *hybrid*. As far as any specific quality is concerned, maturation of germ cells from a homozygote results in the formation of germ cells of only one type, while maturation of germ cells from a heterozygote can result in the production of mature cells of two types. If, as an example, the quality in question happens to be the color of eyes, a homozygote with brown eyes will produce germ cells that will carry genes for brown eyes only, but a heterozygote with brown eyes will produce germ cells that will carry genes for both brown eyes and blue (or other colored) eyes. The eyes are brown, however, because the quality brown surpasses the quality blue. Brown, in this instance, is known as *dominant* and is represented by the letter D. Conversely, the quality blue is suppressed by the quality brown. Blue, in this instance, is known as a *recessive* and is represented by the letter R. A dominant quality always dominates and becomes apparent in both a homozygous individual (DD + DD = 4 DD) and a heterozygous individual (DD + DR = 2 DD and 2 DR). A recessive quality is always superseded by a dominant quality (DD + DR = 2 DD and 2 DR) and becomes apparent only in a homozygous individual (DR + DR = DD, 2 DR and RR). It may thus be carried silently from generation to generation and its presence will not become known until its gene meets up with another gene carrying the same recessive characteristic.

Sex, like other characteristics, is also hereditary for it is propagated by the germ plasm. In each germ cell one of the twenty-four pairs of chromosomes determines sex and its two component units are known as the *sex chromosome*. In the *female*, each of the sex chromosomes is identical with the other and each is represented by the letter X. Since there are two sex chromosomes the pair is designated as XX and since they are alike, each mature ovum contains one of these—the other being eliminated in the process of reduction. In the *male*, one of the pair of sex chromosomes is identical with that in the female and is designated as X. The other is dissimilar, is designated as Y, and contains no known genes for transmission of traits. Thus, following maturation, the resulting spermatazoöns will be of two types—one carrying the X chromosome and the other the Y chromosome. Hence, the possibilities upon fertilization are female X and X + male X and Y = XX, XX (two females) and XY, XY (two males).

Just as normal characteristics are passed from generation to generation by way of genes so are *disease processes* transmitted from parent to offspring through the medium of genes. The behavior is similar to that outlined above. Disorders that are propagated in ordinary chromosomes and dominate are referred to as *simple dominant;* those that are passed in ordinary chromosomes and are superseded by other disorders are called *simple recessive*, while those transmitted by sex chromosomes are known as *sex-linked*. A sex-linked disease is always recessive. The disorder may or may not become apparent in the female since she has two X chromosomes but it always becomes manifest in the male since he has only one X chromosome.

ROLE OF CONSTITUTION IN DISEASE

As already indicated in the opening paragraphs of this section, constitution is inherited and comprises the aggregation of an individual's physical, physiological, and mental qualities. Many centuries ago, long before bacteria were discovered, constitution was deemed as playing the all-important role in causation of disease. With the discovery of bacteria, rickettsia, viruses, fungi, parasites, and other agents, its importance was more or less minimized by these more tangible factors. In recent decades, however, interest in its behalf has again been renewed to the point where, at present, it is generally recognized to form the basis of disease.

It is well known that a short, stocky, plump person with a wide substernal angle and a pleasing disposition is likely to develop gout, gallbladder disease, diabetes, hypertension, or heart disease. It is also well known that a tall, lean individual with a narrow subcostal angle, narrow facies, and evidence of hyperactivity of the sympathetic nervous system is prone to develop ulcers of the stomach and duodenum. In general, *males* are more commonly affected with diseases of the digestive tract, respiratory tract, urinary tract, bones, and certain disorders (infarction) of the heart (Allen). *Females*, on the other hand, are more frequently the victims of gallbladder disease, varicose veins, and functional nervous disorders such as Raynaud's

disease, migraine, and hyperthyroidism.   Certain diseases of metabolism
have a predilection for specific *races* as, for example, Gaucher's disease for
Jewish people.   *Cancer* is more common in some races than others and in
any particular race the incidence of cancer of one particular organ dominates over cancer of other organs.   An example is carcinoma of the liver in
Chinese people which is not only more common than carcinoma of the liver
in other races but also more common than carcinoma of other organs in
the Chinese themselves.   In the white race, carcinoma of the stomach is
much more common in males than in females and carcinoma of the breast
is more frequent in females than it is in males.   Then there are so-called
cancer families where males or females for several generations have developed cancer of the same organ at approximately the same period of life.
Even in connection with *infectious disease*, constitution plays an all-important role.   It appears to explain why the incidence of tuberculosis and
syphilis is so high in the Negro population, why the death rate of lobar
pneumonia is much greater in some families than in others, why rheumatic
fever will cripple several members of one family and not affect the neighbors or
even other members of the same family, and why allergic diseases are
familial in distribution.   In *summary*, it may be stated that constitution
may bring about a predisposition for a disease or make the soil right for a
disease to develop provided the environment is correct.   By the same token,
it may bring about a certain resistance which will prevent a disease from
developing regardless of the environment.

METHODS OF STUDYING HEREDITY

Heredity is best studied in *experimental animals* where mating can be controlled and where the life span of the species is short.   Unfortunately the
findings in experimental animals are not necessarily directly applicable to
man and it is, therefore, virtually mandatory to obtain data from a study
of *man* himself.   This is best accomplished by the following means (Macklin): (1) tracing the incidence of certain disorders in consanguineous mar-
riages, (2) observing disease processes in identical (monozygotic) twins
(Margolis and Eisenstein), (3) investigating the family history (pedigree
method) for evidences of the disease in question (especially applicable in
cases of obvious deformities such as absence of phalanges, extra digits, etc.),
and (4) comparing the frequency of diseases in related persons with the
frequency in the general population.

HEREDITARY DISEASES

In general, obvious *failures* of *embryonic development* will be discussed in
succeeding chapters under the heading of *Congenital Anomalies*.   They
will, therefore, not be considered at this time.   A few of the more common
but more subtle *hereditary disease processes* and *hereditary traits* may be
noted as follows (Macklin): (1) *Dominant*—achylia gastrica, sickle cell
anemia, infantile anemia, arthritis, asthma, blood groups, loose joints,
diabetes insipidus, telangiectasia, dimples, baldness, hypertrichosis, xanthoma, glaucoma, Huntington's chorea, migraine, and neurofibromatosis,
(2) *Recessive*—alkaptonuria, deaf-mutism, Gaucher's disease, hemophilia,
lefthandedness, Niemann-Pick's disease, fragilitas osseum, polycythemia,
thromboangiitis obliterans, torticollis, twinning, amaurotic family idiocy,

color-blindness, word-blindness, and paralysis agitans, and (3) *Dominant and/or Recessive*—Addison's disease, diabetes mellitus, dwarfism, obesity, pernicious anemia, purpura haemorrhagica, tumors, albinism, hypotrichosis, feeblemindedness, muscular dystrophy, and peroneal atrophy.

REFERENCES

ALLEN, E. V.: Ann. Int. Med., 7, 1000, 1934, (Sex and Disease).

BAUER, J.: *Constitution and Disease*, 2nd Ed., New York, Grune & Stratton, 1945.

DRAPER, G.: *Human Constitution. A Consideration of Its Relationship to Disease*, Philadelphia, W. B. Saunders Co , 1924.

KEMP, T.: *Genetics and Disease*, Copenhagen, Ejnar Munksgaard, 1951.

MACKLIN, M. T.: Medicine, *14*, 1, 1935, (Heredity in Disease).

MARGOLIS, H. M., and EISENSTEIN, V. W.: Ann. Int. Med., *6*, 1489, 1933, (Twins and Constitution).

SNYDER, L. H.: *Medical Genetics*, Durham, N. C., Duke University Press, 1941.

Chapter

4

Degeneration

GENERAL CONSIDERATIONS

MEDICALLY speaking, *degeneration* (L. = to degenerate) may be looked upon as a deterioration of tissues or organs accompanied by a reduction in both vitality and physiologic activity. The term connotes a fundamental pathologic process that, in one way or another, becomes manifested in all diseases. Conversely, diseases characterized predominantly by degenerative processes are referred to simply as *degenerations* or as *degenerative diseases*. The final *cause* of degenerative processes is interference in the normal metabolism of cells. This is usually due to lack of proper oxygenation and is mediated through the action of intracellular enzymes. A few of the many causes of improper oxygenation (anoxia) are bacteria, rickettsia, viruses, fungi, parasites, chemicals, split tissue proteins, failure of circulation, and decreased number of circulating erythrocytes (anemia).

While there are many *types* of *degenerations*, it is well to keep in mind (1) that several processes usually occur in the same cell at the same time, (2) that a simple degenerative process may pass progressively into a more severe degenerative process until the cell dies and completely disintegrates, and (3) that the cell may, upon removal of the injurious agent, revert to normal provided the degeneration has not progressed beyond a certain point. The process is generally referred to as *reversible* when the cell is restorable to normal and *irreversible* when it is not restorable to normal. Anatomically, degenerative changes occur both in the *cytoplasm* and in the *nucleus*. As far as life for a particular cell is concerned, the nuclear changes are by far the more important for as long as they remain reversible the cell will not die regardless of the degree of cytoplasmic alterations.

In the *remaining paragraphs*, the following degenerations will be discussed in the order mentioned: atrophy, parenchymatous degeneration, hydropic degeneration, hyaline droplet degeneration, hyaline degeneration, Zenker's degeneration, amyloidosis, mucoid degeneration, disturbances of carbohydrate metabolism, disturbances of lipid metabolism, disturbances of calcium metabolism, pathologic ossification, pathologic pigmentation, necrosis, gangrene, and avitaminosis.

ATROPHY

The term *atrophy* (L. or Gr. = not + to nourish) means a wasting away or diminution in bulk from want of nourishment. It is an acquired state and presupposes a reduction in size of a tissue, organ, or part after it has reached normal proportions. This decrease in mass results from a reduction in size and, to a lesser extent, from an actual disappearance of the component cells. The *causes* of lack of nourishment are many but generally they may be attributed to a relative or an absolute decrease in the flow of blood.

Grossly the involved part *usually* discloses the following: decrease in size and weight, wrinkling of the surface, decrease in consistency, deepening of color, diminution in the amount of blood, and maintenance of the anatomical markings. *Histologically*, as stated in the definition, the cells are decreased in both size and number. The cell borders are distinct; the cytoplasm is condensed and deeply staining, and the nuclei are smaller and more basophilic. The spaces between the cells may be filled with connective tissue, fat cells, edema fluid, or other substances.

While atrophy may be divided into many different types a completely satisfactory *classification* is wanting not only because the precise etiologic factor in each instance may be difficult to determine but also because several causative agents often operate simultaneously. Nevertheless the following grouping may be presented: (1) *Nutritional*. Although, by definition, lack of nutrition forms the subtle basis of all atrophy, there are a number of instances where it is obviously the determinant of the retrogressive change. Generally, a lack of proper assimilation of food leads to a diminution of bulk and atrophy of all the tissues and organs of the body. This lack of assimilation may be due to unavailability of food as in a famine, to lack of its digestion and absorption by the gastrointestinal tract from organic or psychosomatic diseases of this system, or to its failure to reach the gastrointestinal tract as a result of obstructive or other diseases of the mouth and esophagus. Locally, any tissue or organ gradually deprived of an adequate arterial blood supply may undergo atrophy. This is especially true of organs such as the brain, heart, and kidneys where the collateral circulation is poor. Although the causative arterial disorders are many, the most common is hardening of the arteries (arteriosclerosis). In such a lesion the lumen is gradually encroached upon, the amount of blood entering the organ is progressively diminished, and the cells gradually decrease in size and disappear. Concomitantly, of course, the physiologic activity of the involved organ is progressively diminished. (2) *Disuse*. Cells that are not continuously exercised are vulnerable to retrogressive changes and atrophy. While the ultimate cause again is local diminution in nutrition this is brought about by lack of physiologic stimulation. The best example of disuse atrophy is perhaps the striated muscles of an extremity that has been confined to a cast for a prolonged period. In such an instance not only do the muscle fibers decrease in size and disappear but they are also replaced with fibrous tissue and, if care is not taken, full physiologic function of the muscles may never be restored. (3) *Overuse*. Although overuse as an eventual precursor to atrophy has been questioned by some, it is your author's opinion that such a sequence of events may take place. A good example is the myocardium in patients with long-continued high blood pressure (hypertension). In such cases, there is an increased resistance of the flow of blood through the vascular system necessitating increased work by the myocardium. The latter responds by an increase in size of the individual myocardial fibers. Since the increased peripheral resistance continues, the myocardial enlargement must also continue in order for the heart to compensate. The heart is capable of doing so, however, only as long as its coronary blood supply is adequate. Once this becomes disproportionately low the myocardial fibers not only undergo atrophy but, in focal areas, also complete disappearance. (4) *Pressure*. Pressure as an ultimate cause of atrophy produces the retrogressive tissue change either by interfering with the main blood supply to the area or by direct compression of the cells in question. The main arterial supply to an area may be interfered with as a result of pressure from any space-taking mass such as tumor, blood clot, local dilatation of a vessel (aneurysm), etc. The consequent atrophy thus actually falls under local nutritional atrophy as described above. Direct compression of tissue leading to its decrease in bulk and decrease in numbers of cells is seen in cases of pressure on the skin over bony prominences when a patient is confined to bed for a prolonged period (bed sores). It is also seen in many hollow organs such as the biliary tree, the pancreas, the gastrointestinal tract, and the urinary tract. In such cases the contents of the lumens of these systems accumulate and, pressing upon the wall, produce atrophy of the cells and thinning of the wall itself to only a fraction of its normal thickness. (5) *Physiologic.* During intra-uterine life the lungs of the fetus are not aerated so that there is no need for the blood to circulate through the pulmonary

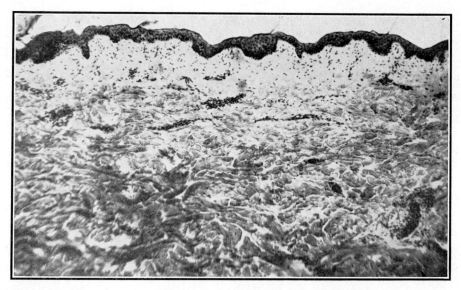

FIG. 2.—Senile atrophy of the skin showing thinning of the epidermis, absorption of the rete pegs, virtual disappearance of the epidermal appendages and condensation of the tissue of the dermis. × 50.

circulation. It is thus by-passed from the pulmonary artery to the aorta by way of the ductus arteriosus. After birth there is no further use for this shunt and the ductus arteriosus hence undergoes physiologic atrophy. An even more vivd example of such atrophy is seen in the female reproductive organs. Each month, as a result of hormonal stimulation, functioning cells of the lobules of the breast undergo an increase in number and an increase in size just prior to menstruation. Upon completion of the menstrual period the same cells undergo a decrease in size and a decrease in number. This cycle is repeated as long as menstruation occurs. In such instances the atrophy is a normal physiological process. If the increase in size and number continued and the atrophy would not follow it would not take long before the breasts would assume monstrous proportions. Another good example in this category is enlargement of the uterus during pregnancy and its decrease in size (involution) after pregnancy has terminated. (6) *Senile.* A withering away of the body with advancing age is a familiar sight to all (Fig. 27). This is known as senile atrophy. The epidermis becomes thinned, the rete pegs are flattened, and the dermis is reduced to only a fraction of its normal thickness (Fig. 2). This, along with loss of elasticity and disappearance of the subcutaneous fat, is responsible for the wrinkles that become so evident. In the same person, atrophy of the cells of the bony skeleton accounts for a decrease in stature and atrophy of the cells of organs such as the liver, kidneys, heart, brain, etc. accounts for a diminution in size of these structures. Although the precise mechanism in senile atrophy is complicated, two factors playing a decisive role are hardening of the arteries

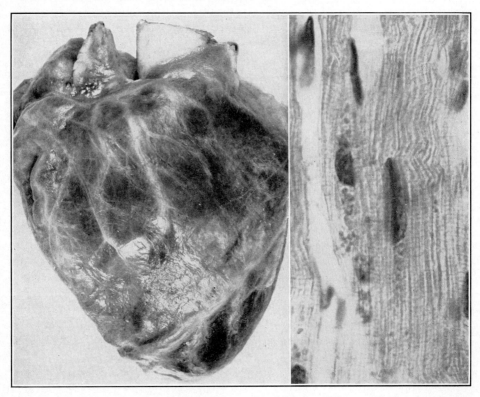

Fig. 3.—Brown atrophy of the heart showing, to the left, a small heart with deep brown myocardium and conspicuous coronary vessels and, to the right, bipolar deposition of brown granules within myocardial fibers. × 1350.

(arteriosclerosis) and hormonal changes. (7) *Neurotrophic.* In order for cells of the body to maintain their normal physiologic activity they must receive proper nerve stimulation. When the reflex arc is disrupted, as it is in poliomyelitis, the striated muscle supplied by the involved arc becomes paralyzed and undergoes a decrease in size and number of its cells. Such a change is referred to as neurotrophic atrophy. (8) *Toxic.* The term toxic atrophy is reserved for the retrogressive changes that occur in all tissues, but especially in fat and muscle, in patients with long continued fevers from whatever cause. In such instances the causative factors consist of the toxins responsible for the fever in the first place, the increased metabolism of the body, and failure of body intake and assimilation of proper nutrition.

In addition, three *special types* of *atrophy* may be mentioned, namely, (1) *Brown atrophy* of the *heart*. This is usually seen in old people of small stature and poor nutrition. The heart is small; the myocardium is thin, deep brown and soft, and the coronary arteries (because of decrease in size of the heart) are tortuous and conspicuous (Fig. 3). Histologically the myocardial fibers are decreased in size and disclose cytoplasmic accumulations of brown pigment near the oples of the nuclei. (2) *Irradiation atrophy*. When sufficient roentgen or radium irradiation is administered the target tissues undergo atrophy due to decrease in size and disappearance in number of cells. The effect is mediated directly through the action of the rays on the tissue cells and indirectly by way of vascular occlusion. (3) *Serous atrophy*. This term is applied to the condition when fat cells, in areas such as the pericardium and bone marrow, disappear rapidly and extensively and their interstices become filled with serous fluid (Fig. 4).

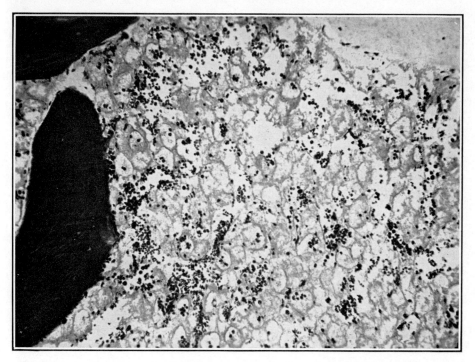

FIG. 4.—Serous atrophy of the bone marrow showing the framework of former fat cells filled with granular, protein precipitate. × 100.

PARENCHYMATOUS DEGENERATION

Parenchymatous degeneration, also known as *albuminous degeneration* (because it is the protein or albumin of the cells that is affected) and *cloudy swelling* (because of the cloudy and swollen appearance of the organ), is the commonest of all retrograde processes. It may be defined as the basic degenerative change in the cytoplasmic protein of the functioning (parenchymatous) cells of an organ. It is seen, to a greater or lesser degree, in most autopsies but is particularly prevalent in cases of gradual death and in cases of overwhelming infection or intoxication. Because of alterations in cellular metabolism the osmotic pressure within the cell increases and the

cell absorbs fluid from the surrounding tissue spaces. As a consequence the
cell enlarges, the borders become indistinct and may even burst, and the
cytoplasm (including mitochondria and the Golgi apparatus) becomes granular (Fig. 5A). The nuclei either remain unchanged or become slightly
enlarged and light-staining. The latter nuclear changes correlate well with
changes in their desoxyribonucleic and ribonucleic acid contents for, by

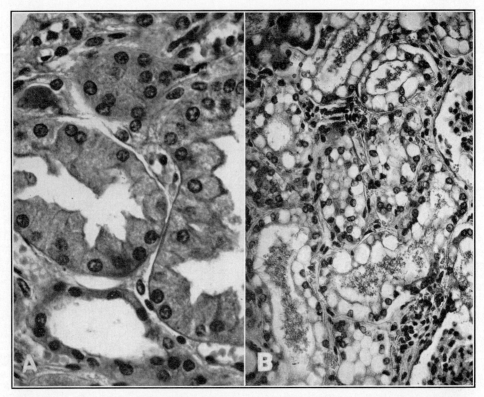

FIG. 5.—A, Parenchymatous degeneration in the epithelium of the proximal convoluted tubules
of the kidney. The cells are swollen; the borders are indistinct or completely effaced, and the
cytoplasm is granular. × 400. B, Hydropic degeneration also in renal tubular epithelium. The
cells are distorted and even ruptured by varisized vacuoles which, with appropriate staining, are
negative for glycogen and fat. × 200.

histochemical and chemical methods, it has been shown that both of these
acids are diminished in the affected cells (Fonnesu and Severi). Grossly, the
organ is enlarged, appears swollen, and presents a dull, "cloudy" surface.
In practice, pathologists generally pay little or no attention to minor degrees
of parenchymatous degeneration, not only because the change is extremely
common but also because it is indistinguishable from postmortem atuolysis.

HYDROPIC DEGENERATION

Hydropic (also called *vacuolic*) *degeneration* represents a progression of
parenchymatous degeneration. It, therefore, occurs under similar circumstances, appears the same grossly (except in extreme cases where actual
"blisters" may be seen), and differs microscopically in that the cells are

filled with vacuoles (Fig. 5B). These vacuoles are distinguished from glycogen and fat droplets in that they fail to take the specific stains for these substances.

HYALINE DROPLET DEGENERATION

Hyaline droplet degeneration is likewise intimately associated with parenchymatous degeneration. It consists of the presence of varisized, single or multiple, round, homogeneously eosinophilic, intracytoplasmic collections of "protein" material (Fig. 6). The process is best visualized in the epithe-

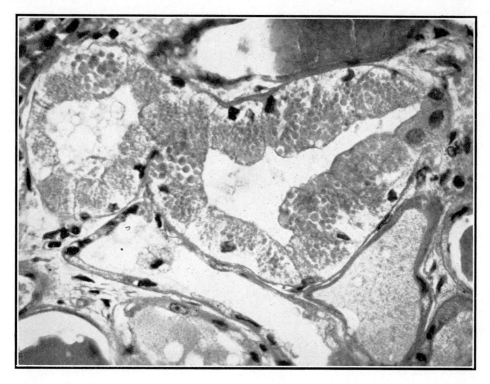

Fig. 6.—Hyaline droplet degeneration showing epithelial cells of the proximal convoluted tubules of a kidney filled with small to large, round, homogeneously eosinophilic structures. × 400.

lium of the proximal convoluted tubules in certain inflammations of the kidney (subacute diffuse glomerulonephritis), in hepatic cells in patients addicted to chronic alcoholism, and in plasma cells (Russell's bodies) in some chronic infections. In the kidney, histochemical studies (Govan) have shown that the bodies do not contain free polysaccharide or lipid but that they do contain a carbohydrate radicle (because they give a positive per—iodic acid—Schiff reaction), protein (because they show marked affinity for orange G), and probably nucleic acid (because they give a positive Feulgen reaction). Whether the glycoprotein is derived from filtered plasma protein (globulins) or whether it results from a breakdown of the epithelial basement membrane of the glomeruli has as yet not been determined.

FIBRINOID DEGENERATION

The term *fibrinoid* (Gr. = fibrin+form) has, from its inception, been used to indicate a change in collagen fibers characterized by the assumption of structural and tinctorial qualities of fibrin (Klemperer) and the phrase *fibrinoid degeneration* has been employed to describe the retrogressive process involved. Because fibrinoid degeneration affects many organs and sites of the body and is present in a variety of conditions, disorders bearing this alteration as a common denominator are often loosely grouped under the

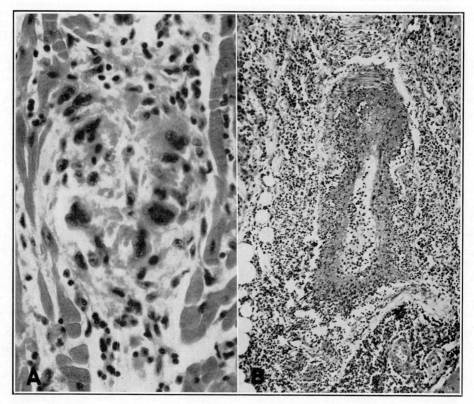

FIG. 7.—Fibrinoid degeneration in (*A*) a rheumatic nodule of the myocardium. × 400 and (*B*) an arteriole in peri-arteritis nodosa. × 100.

heading of *collagen diseases*. Some of the diseases so categorized are rheumatic fever, rheumatoid arthritis, periarteritis nodosa, dermatomyositis, scleroderma, lupus erythematosus, and thrombotic cytopenic purpura (Altshuler and Brunsen). Other lesions in which fibrinoid degeneration occurs are arterioles in malignant hypertension, arteries in arteriosclerosis, inflammations of allergic or other origins, tumors, and even the floor of peptic ulcers.

In *microscopic* sections stained by the ordinary hematoxylin and eosin method, fibrinoid is composed of loosely or tightly bound eosinophilic fibrillar or sometimes more granular material that has a tendency to smudging (Fig. 7). It may affect the connective tissue throughout the body but has a special predilection for groups of organs or sites depending upon the disease it represents. Thus, for example, in rehumatic fever it involves principally the heart, in rheumatoid arthritis the joints, and in periarteritis nodosa the smaller arteries. *Histochemically* fibrinoid has the following rather specific staining characteristics: toluidine blue—on occasion metachromatic; crystal violet—purple; phosphotungstic acid hematoxylin—yellow to orange with occasionally a superimposed blue fibrillar material; van Gieson's stain —yellow to orange to red; periodic acid luekofuchsin—red, and Sakaguchi— yellow orange (Altshuler). Aside from fibrinoid itself, the degenerative change is sooner or later accompanied by varying degrees of inflammatory reaction. Such alterations, however, are of secondary importance (Brunson).

The *nature* of *fibrinoid* has been the subject of much investigation (Klemperer). Because it is a connective tissue alteration seen in allergic reactions some consider any disease disclosing the change to be of allergic origin. This contention has recently been strengthened somewhat by the disclosure of Vazquez and Dixon that the lesions do contain an excessive deposition of gamma globulins—a circumstance consistent with an antigen-antibody reaction. Gitlin, on the other hand, proved to his satisfaction, by studying the lesions with fluorescein-labeled rabbit antisera against human fibrin, albumin, and gamma globulin, that fibrinoid represents a local deposition of fibrin. In the same vein, Movat and More, as a result of observations from morphologic, tinctorial, histochemical, and histo-enzymatic studies, were of the opinion that fibrinoid is derived from exuded plasma proteins, particularly fibrin. Altshuler and Angevine, by histochemical means, concluded that fibrinoid is formed by a precipitation of acid mucopolysaccharide of the ground substance of the connective tissue and that the precipitant is an alkaline protein derived from tissue necrosis or the interaction of the tissue with a damaging agent. The protein moiety is digested by trypsin, contains tyrosine, and could be a globulin. Since, however, fibrinoid is seen in many disorders, other investigators hold that the change simply represents the limitation of connective tissue response—a necrosis of collagen or a coagulation of ground substance. To this, it must be added that the source or nature of fibrinoid may not be the same in all instances. While most investigators have been concerned with connective tissue fibrinoid, Muirhead has demonstrated that vascular fibrinoid is derived mainly from altered smooth muscle of the media. He has further demonstrated that it is composed of fats, fatty acids, phospholipids, aldehyde groups of polysaccharide origin, free potassium, free carbonyl groups, sulfuric ester of mucopolysaccharide origin, and protein-bound sulfhydryl groups. Thus, as is quite apparent, the last word has by no means been said.

Experimentally fibrinoid has been readily produced in connective tissue and in vessels in a variety of animals by many methods (Klemperer, Altshuler, and Gamble). Some of these are as follows: (1) trivial mechanical injury, such as squeezing the skin of a rat, (2) hypersensitivity to protein, such as rabbits sensitized to horse serum, (3) in vessels in experimental hypertension, (4) visceral arterioles of dogs after large doses of adrenalin, (5) acute bacterial infection, (6) prolonged passive hyperemia. (7) large doses dexoxycorticosterone, (8) meningococcal endotoxin, (9) combs of newborn chicks treated with testosterone, and (10) thyroidectomized guinea pigs treated with thyrotropic hormone.

HYALINE DEGENERATION

The term *hyalin* (Gr. = glass) is purely descriptive and denotes nothing more than a homogeneously glassy substance that is eosinophilic. The

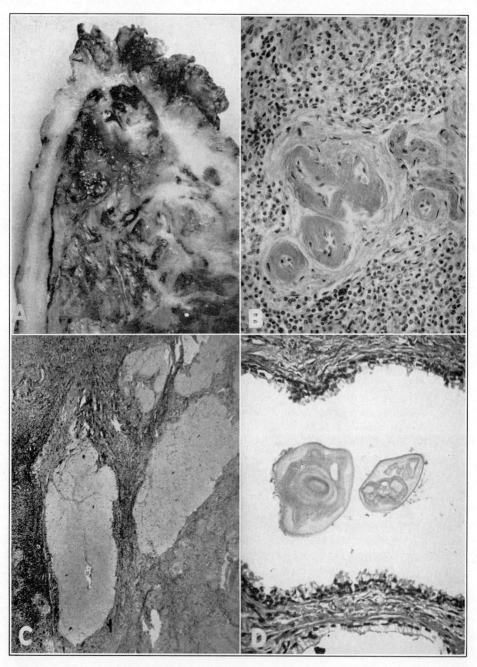

FIG. 8.—Hyalin in different forms showing *A*, a greatly thickened, white, firm, unyielding pleura, *B*, several arterioles with deposition of hyalin in the intima and media. × 200, *C*, old corpora albicantia of the ovary composed of hyalin. × 25, and *D*, corpora amylacea of the prostate also composed of hyalin. × 100.

caption *hyaline degeneration* or *hyalinosis* thus connotes a retrograde process characterized by the deposition of hyalin. Chemically, hyalin is diversely constituted and pathologically it encompasses many processes. *Hyaline droplet degeneration*, considered in the preceding paragraph, is a form of hyaline degeneration. Similarly, *corpora amylacea* (L. = bodies + starch) that are found in the normal prostate, in the senescent brain, in certain inflammations of the lung, and in some tumors also constitute a form of hyalin (Fig. 8). While the composition of even corpora amylacea probably varies from organ to organ, it has been shown by histochemical methods that the structures in the brain are composed of glycoprotein-like material which is not of nuclear origin and that they are devoid of lipid and mineral constituents (Wagner).

Of greater importance, perhaps, is hyalin that is formed in *connective tissue*. Normally, connective tissue is variously divided according to the fibers it contains in its intercellular substance but all types show collagenous or white fibers as their most characteristic element (Maximow and Bloom). In loose connective tissue the fibers are few in number and are composed of threads or ribbons. In dense connective tissue they are more abundant and are more closely applied to each other. Collagen fibers consist of extremely fine, longitudinally arranged, cross striated fibrils held together by a cement substance. Collagen itself may be looked upon as normal hyalin. When its deposition is within physiological limits for that particular tissue the tissue is said to be normal. When, however, its deposition is in excessive amount, the tissue is said to undergo hyaline degeneration. As such, the collagen bundles fuse with each other to form large areas of dense, homogeneously eosinophilic, structureless material in which all cellular outlines and fibrillar details are effaced (Fig. 8). Grossly, the tissue is gray, glassy, firm, and unyielding. A few of the diverse sites exhibiting hyaline degeneration are intima and media of the arteries in hardening of the arteries (arteriosclerosis), old inflammations of the pleura and other mesothelial surfaces, scar from whatever cause, some tumors of mesodermal origin, stroma of other tumors, and old corpora albicantia of the ovary.

ZENKER'S DEGENERATION

Zenker's degeneration (named after a German pathologist, Frederick Albert Zenker, 1825–1898) or *waxy degeneration* is hyaline degeneration occurring in striated muscle. Although it usually accompanies severe infectious diseases, such as pneumonia and typhoid fever, it is also found in cases of death from anaphylaxis (Wells). The condition is seen best in the rectus abdominis muscle and the muscles of respiration, especially the diaphragm. *Grossly,* the muscle is swollen and glassy and, as a result of rupture, may disclose foci of hemorrhage. *Histologically,* the affected muscle fibers are broadened, stain homogeneously eosinophilic, and disclose loss of striations (Fig. 9). *Clinically,* Zenker's degeneration may be responsible for respiratory failure.

AMYLOIDOSIS

Amyloid (Gr. = starch + to form) is a hyalin that, in some of its reactions, resembles starch. It has been separated from other hyalins because it can be identified by special staining (grossly deep brown with Lugol's iodine, grossly blue with Lugol's iodine followed by sulphuric acid, grossly and microscopically red with congo red, microscopically violet red with

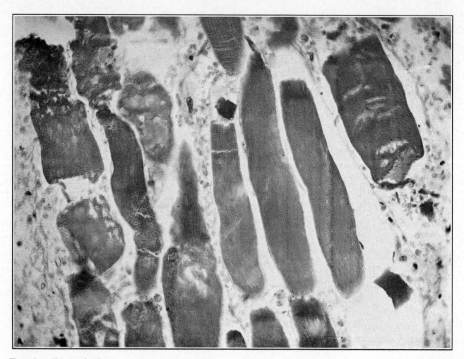

FIG. 9.—Zenker's degeneration. Parts of three of the smaller muscle fibers are of normal width and disclose cross striations.   The rest of two of these fibers and other fibers in the field are broad, homogeneously eosinophilic, and devoid of all cross striations.   × 200.

crystal, methyl, or gentian violet).   The substance is doubtlessly a glyco-protein that consists of a combination of a mucopolysaccharide and a globulin (Teilum).   The exact *mechanism* of its *formation* has not been agreed upon.   Among others, it has been considered to arise as a result of (1) an antigen-antibody reaction in the presence of a relative excess of antigen over antibody, (2) a disturbance in the protein-producing cellular system, (3) perverted fibroblastic activity in which case it has been suggested that excessive breakdown of connective tissue might release soluble components of ground substance into the blood stream which could then be precipitated elsewhere as amyloid, (4) an alteration of the mucopolysaccharide response of the reticulo-endothelial system, (5) a faulty production of a pathological protein by normal or abnormal plasma cells, and (6) the general adaptation syndrome of Selye wherein stress of any variety stimulates the adrenal medulla to produce adrenalin.   This stimulates the anterior pituitary to produce ACTH (adrenocorticotropic hormone) which in turn stimulates adrenal cortical hormone production with resulting destruction of lympho-cytes, leukopenia, atrophy of lymphoid tissue, and increase in serum beta and gamma globulin.   The globulin in turn combines with mucopolysac-charide and forms amyloid (Jackson, Rukavina, Symmers, and Teilum).

In *experimental animals*, amyloidosis has been produced (1) by prolonged immunization of horses with diphtheria toxins, (2) by subjecting rabbits to repeated staphylococcus infections or to subcutaneous injections of pus, (3) by injecting rabbits subcutaneously with sodium ribonucleate, (4) by sub-cutaneous injections of sodium caseinate in mice, and (5) by subjecting mice to a cheese diet.

In *man*, amyloidosis may be divided into three essential categories—secondary amyloidosis, primary amyloidosis, and amyloid tumors. Regardless of its distribution, however, amyloid *grossly* is a waxy, glassy, translucent substance and *histologically* (in hematoxylin and eosin preparations) it stains homogeneously and brightly eosinophilic.

Secondary amyloidosis is by far the commonest of the three but, with better control of chronic diseases, its incidence in recent years has dropped considerably. The condition usually occurs as an *accompaniment* of long-continued pus-producing *infections* such as tuberculosis, osteomyelitis, certain types of syphilis, and loculations of pus within body cavities. It is also seen secondary to rheumatoid arthritis and idiopathic ulcerative colitis and has been recorded following nitrogen mustard therapy and, in acute disseminated lupus erythematosus, following treatment with ACTH and cortisone. Rarely it is found in conjunction with cancers—especially with cancer of bone marrow cells called multiple myeloma. In secondary amyloidosis the amyloid is *deposited* primarily in *connective tissue* and, although any organ of the body may be affected, the most common sites of involvement are spleen, liver, kidneys, adrenals, and arterioles. The *spleen* is generally enlarged and firm. The capsule is tense and the edges are relatively sharp. Cut surfaces more commonly present a mottled appearance (sago spleen) and less commonly a diffusely glassy appearance (bacony spleen). The former is due to deposition of the amyloid within and about the arterioles of the lymphoid follicles while the latter is due to its deposition in the connective tissue of the pulp (Fig. 10). The *liver*, too, is usually diffusely enlarged and firm. Histologically it discloses a deposition of amyloid between the sinusoidal endothelium and the hepatic cells. As the amyloid accumulates it bulges into the sinusoids and, in the opposite direction, produces pressure atrophy of the hepatic cells. The *kidneys* may be normal in size or they may be enlarged. Microscopically they reveal deposition of the hyaline material within the glomerular tufts, in the tubular basement membrane, in the interstitial connective tissue, and in the intima and media of arterioles. The *adrenals* may be normal in size or enlarged. The amyloid is deposited in the supporting connective tissue and when it becomes abundant it produces atrophy of the parenchymatous cells. In the *arterioles* amyloid accumulates in the inner portion of the media, in the connective tissue of the intima, and sometimes in the connective tissue of the adventitia. When it is present in appreciable amounts it encroaches upon and even obliterates the vascular lumen.

Primary amyloidosis differs from secondary amyloidosis in that (1) it is not preceded or accompanied by another known pathologic process and (2) its chief deposition is in the muscles of the body, especially the heart and tongue. Its precise site of accumulation, however, is the connective tissue between the muscle fibers and not within the muscle fibers themselves. Primary amyloidosis is considerably less common than secondary amyloidosis.

Amyloid tumors are rare. They are usually found in the larynx and other portions of the upper respiratory tract. They are probably connective tissue tumors that later become permeated with amyloid.

Clinically the diagnosis of amyloidosis may be difficult. Of importance are (1) a history of a chronic suppurative infection in the presence of hyperglobulinemia, reversal of the albumin/globulin ratio of the blood, albuminuria, hepatomegaly, and splenomegaly, (2) aspiration biopsy of the liver or spleen, and (3) removal of more than 60 per cent of congo red from the

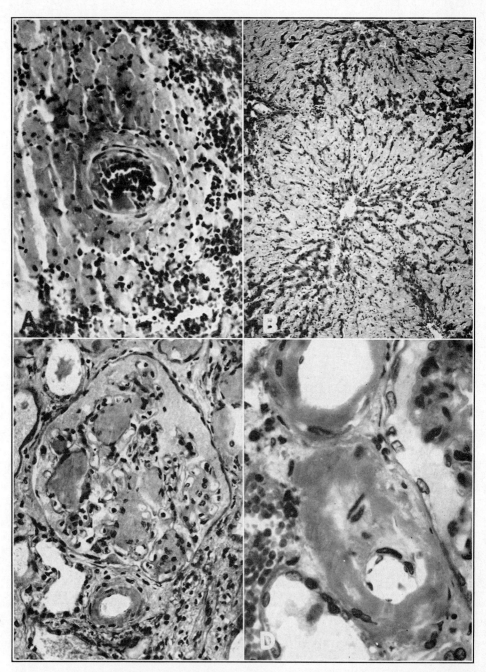

FIG. 10.—Amyloidosis showing the material deposited *A*, within and about a splenic arteriole *B*, between hepatic cells, *C*, within a glomerulus, and *D*, within two renal arterioles.   Note the coexisting atrophy of the hepatic cells.

blood stream within one hour after the dye is injected intravenously (Bero, Perasalo, and Jackson).   Amyloidosis is reversible when it occurs in the presence of another disease and when this disease is eradicated.   Due to pressure effects of the amyloid deposits on parenchymatous cells, the functioning cells of an organ may become atrophic and destroyed.   Thus, depending upon which organ is affected, the patient may exhibit hepatic, adrenal, renal, or cardiac failure.

MUCOID DEGENERATION

Before proceeding with the discussion of mucoid degeneration it may be in order to define several of a group of confusing terms.   *Mucus* is a clear, viscid, slimy substance that is normally secreted by the lining cells of the respiratory tract, gastro-intestinal tract, and portions of the genital tract. It is also found normally in the umbilical cord, synovial cavities, and bursas. It is thus formed by certain epithelial cells and certain connective tissue cells of the body.   The terms *mucous* and *mucoid* are adjectives (although mucoid is sometimes used as a noun) that connote pertaining to or resembling mucus.   *Mucin* is a mucopolysaccharide or glucoprotein and represents the chief constituent of mucus.   Being acid, it precipitates with dilute acetic acid and stains with basic dyes.   *Mucinous* and *mucinoid* are adjectives that denote a substance resembling mucin and, since mucin is the chief constituent of mucus, they are used synonymously with mucous and mucoid.   *Pseudomucin* is a substance that physically resembles mucus (mucin) but that differs from mucus chemically in that, being alkaline, it does not precipitate with dilute acetic acid and it stains with acid dyes. *Pseudomucinous* is an adjective meaning pertaining to or like pseudomucin.

Wherever it is formed, one of the chief *physiologic* properties of mucus is its lubricant action.   This is certainly true in connection with *joints* and *bursas* and in connection with the gastrointestinal tract.   In the *stomach* it is secreted in response to local (traumatic), nervous, and hormonal stimuli (Florey).   By adherence to the mucosa it prevents gastric juices from contacting and destroying the surface cells; by its lubricant action it protects the mucosa from mechanical trauma, and by the concomitant secretion of bicarbonate it indirectly helps to neutralize the gastric hydrochloric acid and lessen the action of pepsin.   In the *intestine* mucus entraps bacteria and food particles and thus expedites their forward movement.   Since it does not prevent diffusion of small particles it does not interfere with absorption of food.   In the *respiratory tract* mucus entraps bacteria, virus, and other particles thus not only preventing them from contacting the underlying mucosa but also removing them entirely from the tracheobronchial tree. It also serves to dilute microbial toxins thus making them less irritating. In addition, it forms a protective film over the mucosa separating the latter from noxious gases, chemicals, etc. that may be inhaled.   Respiratory mucus has not been shown to contain antibacterial and antiviral properties against pathogenic organism but it has been shown to contain a lysozyme which dissolves or inhibits growth of saprophytic organisms.

When mucus (or mucin or pseudomucin) is formed within physiologic limits the cells and tissues are said to be normal.   When, however, it is formed in abnormal amounts the cells become distorted, undergo retrogressive changes, and may be even completely destroyed.   Such a chain of events is referred to as *mucoid* (mucous, mucinous, mucinoid, or pseudomucinous) *degeneration*.   *Grossly* the involved tissues and organs become

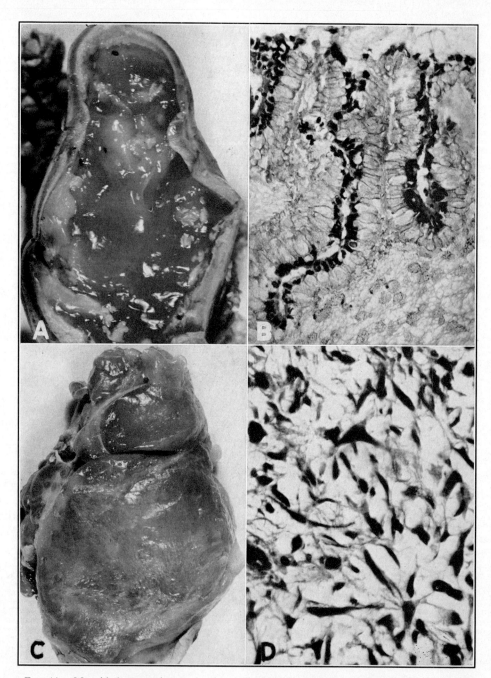

FIG. 11.—Mucoid degeneration: A, obstruction of appendix (mucocele) showing the lumen filled with clear, gelatinous material, B, cyst of an ovary (pseudomucinous) illustrating mucoid material in degenerating epithelial cells and free in the lumen of the cyst. × 200, C, tumor of connective tissue (myxoma) disclosing a gelatinous appearance, D, similar tumor showing stellate cells separated by mucoid material. × 400.

covered, filled, or permeated (as the case may be) with clear, colorless, viscid, slimy material (Fig. 11). *Histologically*, affected *epithelial cells* become distended with and distorted by mucoid material until ultimately the cell membranes burst, the mucoid material, escapes, and the cells disintegrate. Affected *connective tissue cells* become elongated and stellate in outline with the mucoid material filling the intercellular spaces. A few examples of *mucoid degeneration* of *epithelium* are: common cold, inflammation of the trachea and bronchi, bronchial asthma, inflammation of the gastrointestinal tract, obstruction of the appendix (mucocele), and certain cancers (mucinous) of the gastrointestinal tract and breast. Examples of mucoid degeneration of *connective tissue* are: certain tumors (myxoma and myxosarcoma), cystic swelling of a tendon sheath (ganglion), tendons overriding bony prominences, and the dermis in myxedema (condition caused by thyroid deficiency).

Mucoid degeneration is significant *clinically* because, as already listed, it predisposes to or is associated with a variety of disturbances. In the gastrointestinal tract, for example, a destruction of the mucous secreting cells ultimately decreases the flow of mucus and this in turn allows the mucosa to become vulnerable not only to trauma but also to the action of its own juices. Obstruction of the base of the appendix, in the presence of excessive secretion of mucus followed by mucoid degeneration of the mucosa, leads to accumulation of mucus within the appendiceal lumen and ultimately to inflammation of the organ or to rupture with spilling of the contents into the peritoneal cavity. Excessive secretion of mucus by the respiratory mucosal cells may lead to obstruction of the bronchial or bronchiolar lumens with secondary infection and inflammation distal to the obstruction or it may be followed by local degeneration and disappearance of the mucosal cells and local infection and inflammation. The mucoid degeneration present in tumors is of significance only in that the accumulation of such material is space taking and adds to the compressive manifestations of the growths.

DISTURBANCES OF CARBOHYDRATE METABOLISM

Francis A. McKeon, Jr.

Recent physiological advances in the knowledge of enzyme systems and the hormonal influences on these systems have elucidated many pathways in *metabolism* in general. A knowledge of these is a prerequistie for a true understanding of the *pathologic physiology*, the *morphologic changes*, and *rational therapy* of metabolic disturbances which may result from specific "biochemical" defects.

The metabolic pathways of carbohydrate, lipid, and protein metabolism are intimately related so that defects of one aspect of metabolism may secondarily and significantly influence other metabolic reactions. Normally, in *carbohydrate metabolism*, the monosaccharides, (glucose, galactose, fructose, pentoses, etc.) produced after hydrolysis and enzymatic degradation of ingested carbohydrate, are passively and/or actively absorbed chiefly by the small intestine and thereby pass into the blood. Intestinal diseases such as sprue, other functional and anatomical disturbances, and hypothyroidism result in decreased absorption. Thyroid hormone, as is evidenced in hyperthyroidism, facilitates absorption. Vitamins also play a role in glucose absorption.

Once in the blood stream, the hexoses are transported to the cells where, in the presence of specific enzymes, they are phosphorylated and stored intracellularly in a colloidal state in the form of glycogen. Glucose is phosphorylated by glucokinase (*hexokinase*) to glucose-6-phosphate and may proceed to glycogen by way of glucose-1-phosphate through the action of phosphoglucomutace, phosphorylase, and a "branching" enzyme. In some cases of glycogen storage disease, a defect in the latter has been implicated. Hexoses other than glucose are rapidly converted to glycogen or glucose-6-phosphate in the normal liver and the delayed conversion of galactose is the basis for the galactose tolerance test for liver dysfunction.

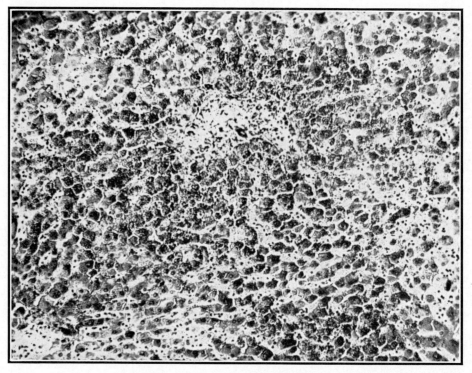

FIG. 12.—Liver showing numerous intracytoplasmic glycogen
granules. Best's carmine stain. × 100.

Although *glycogen* is present in almost all tissues, it is stored principally in the liver (5%) and muscle (0.5%). The process of glycogen formation (glycogenesis) is facilitated by insulin and inhibited by the anterior pituitary and adreno-cortical hormones. The amount of glycogen in the otherwise normal liver is quite variable and is influenced by many factors (nutrition, anesthesia, etc.). It may be readily demonstrated in hepatic cells (Fig. 12) as bright red intracytoplasmic granules when the tissue is fixed in absolute alcohol, Carnoy's fluid, alcoholic formalin, aqueous formalin or any non sublimate-containing fixative and stained with Best's carmine. It may also be demonstrated histochemically by "aldehyde reactions" as with Schiff's reagent (fuchsin sulfurous acid) after prior oxidation with chromic acid (Bauer's method) or periodic acid (Hotchkiss-McManus method) or after controlled acid hydrolysis (Fuelgen reaction). Glycogen may be differenti-ated from other Schiff positive substances by prior treatment with *diastase* (amylase) which removes glycogen and starch (Gomori). The morphology of glycogen will vary with the different methods of fixation from coarse droplets (alcoholic or acid-containing fixatives) to fine uniform granules (formalin bichromate or simple formalin). Glycogen is normally found in the post-ovulatory endometrium (Fig. 13) and local increases are found in inflammation, dead tissue, and certain tumors of the kidney, heart, and adrenal cortex.

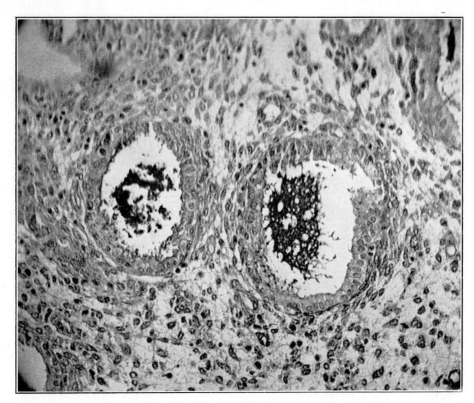

Fig. 13.—Endometrium in the late secretory phase revealing dark staining glycogen within the acinar lumens and minute fine granules near the luminal borders of the lining epithelial cells. Aqueous formalin fixation and staining with Periodic-acid Schiff (PAS). × 200.

Fructose is not insulin dependent and apparently bypasses a defect in hepatic glucose uptake (Moorhouse). The deficiency of a specific *transferase* prevents the utilization of galactose resulting in the condition known as *galactosemia* (Isselbacher). *Blood glucose* is maintained by the breakdown of liver glycogen (glycogenolysis) by way of glucose-6-phosphatase and a specific phosphatase whose enzymatic action as facilitated by *glycogenolytic* hormones such as *adrenalin* and *glucagon*. This enzyme is normally absent in muscle and abnormally deficient in von Gierke's (glycogen storage) disease.

In the *intermediate metabolism* of *carbohydrate*, glucose obtained from glycogen is enzymatically degraded (*glycolysis*) to pyruvate by way of the anaerobic (Embden-Meyerhoff) scheme, whereas the aerobic oxidation of pyruvate to carbon dioxide and water proceeds through the tricarboxylic (Krebs) cycle. An "alternate oxidative" phosphogluconate pathway exists and the production of pentose as a precursor of pentose nucleic acid probably depends on this pathway (Bondy).

The free *energy* obtained from the oxidation of glucose is invested and stored in "energy rich" phosphate bonds in such compounds as adenosine triphosphate (ATP) which may later yield this energy to do "biochemical" work. The demonstration of coenzyme A (CoA) and its acetyl-complex (acetyl-CoA) in relation to the Krebs Cycle and to the transfer of *"active acetate"* has established the "final common pathway" of glucose metabolism. The "active acetate" is reversably linked with the formation of *cholesterol, steroid hormones, phospholipids, fatty acids, ketone bodies,* and *acetylated compounds* such as hyaluronic acid and chondroitin.

The synthesis of glucose from noncarbohydrate sources, such as from certain amino acids, is known as *gluconeogenesis.* Such a transformation displays one of many possibilities along the "final common pathway" and brings one to a closer understanding of the dynamic relationship that exists between carbohydrate, protein, and fat metabolism.

Disturbances of *carbohydrate metabolism* may be briefly discussed under two main categories—(1) enzymatic defects and (2) hormonal disturbances.

One of the best known examples of an *enzyme defect* is *glycogen storage disease* (von Gierke's disease). In this condition, the enzymatic lesion is a deficiency or absence of *glucose-6-phosphatase* resulting in the storage of abnormal amounts of glycogen in the liver (hepatic type), heart (myocardial type), and skeletal muscle (muscular type). Routine laboratory tests for carbohydrate metabolism are usually normal in the cardiac and muscular types, but are abnormal in the hepatic type. In other types of glycogen storage disease, which primarily involve the heart, muscle, kidneys and leukocytes, there is an abnormality in the structure of glycogen which sometimes resembles *corn starch* (Najjar) and a disturbance or deficiency in various *"branching"* and *"debranching"* enzymes is implicated. The clinical manifestations of glycogen storage disease (hepatomegaly, acidosis, keto is and convulsions) are the result of increased deposition of unavailable glycogen resulting in *hypoglycemia,* increased fatty acid breakdown, and *ketosis.* Administration of epinephrine fails to elevate the blood sugar. Histologically, the increased deposition of glycogen is evidenced by vacuolization cf the cells and fibers of the involed organs and may be demonstrated by the appropriate staining techniques for glycogen. Therapy consists of a high protein diet (to promote gluconeogenesis). Corticotrophin has been used with success in some cases but, since spontaneous remission of the disease has been reported after puberty, its efficacy remains in doubt.

A second example of an enzyme defect is *galactosemia.* This is an inborn error in metabolism in which there is a specific inability to convert galactose to glucose. It is due to a *deficiency* of a specific enzyme *phospho-galactose uridyl transferase.* The disorder occurs in infants and is characterized by increased levels of galactose (a reducing but nonfermentable sugar) in the blood (galactosemia) and urine (galactosuria). The disorder is also characterized by cataracts, mental deficiency, proteinuria, possibly amino aciduria—all of which result from the toxic effect of either the increased galactose or metabolic intermediates. The diagnosis is made on the above findings and the presence of a decreased galactose tolerance test. Therapy consists of the exclusion of galactose from the diet. This produces a reversal and often complete disappearance of symptoms. Otherwise, death may occur.

A third example of an enzymatic defect is *fructosemia.* In this disorder, the defect is one affecting the enzyme *fructokinase*. Since, however, fructose is excreted rapidly in the urine (fructosuria), the patients are symptom free. A fourth example of an enzymatic defect is *pentosuria*. In this condition, the metabolic abnormality is unknown.

Hormonal disturbances are both common and important. The homeostatic hormonal mechanisms which regulate, within relatively narrow limits regardless of diet, the level of blood glucose are dependent upon the finely balanced functional integration of many organs and glands, notably, the pancreas, adrenals, pituitary, liver, thyroid, and kidneys, as well as the central and autonomic nervous systems. Since protein and fat metabolism are dependent for their normal course upon unaltered glucose metabolism, any disturbance in glucose metabolism may be accompanied by corresponding disturbances in protein and fat metabolism. It should thus be evident that the etiology and metabolic manifestations of *hyperglycemia* (increased blood sugar) and *hypoglycemia* (decreased blood sugar) and the pathologic physiology involved are variable and complex.

Hormones directly or indirectly influencing the level of *blood glucose* may be listed as follows: (1) *insulin* from the beta cells of the islets of Langerhans, (2) *anterior pituitary fractions* independent of adrenocortico-trophic hormone (ACTH), which act by way of stimulation of the adrenal complex, (3) *adrenocortical* hormones, (4) *epinephrine*, (5) *thyroid* hormone and (6) *hyperglycemic* factor (glucagon) produced by the alpha cells of the gastrointestinal mucosa. The net effect of insulin is the production of hypoglycemia while the effect of the remainder is to promote hyperglycemia. Conversely, relative or absolute deficiencies of the hormones will produce a reverse effect. While all the hormones mentioned play a role, a major portion of the control in maintaining blood sugar is commanded by the effect of insulin on the one hand and adrenocortical and pituitary hormones on the other.

Disturbances in *carbohydrate metabolism* may be present for some time and may be quite severe before they are reflected in the fasting blood glucose which ordinarily is maintained within narrow limits (60–100 mg/100 ml) by compensatory mechanisms. Because of this, the clinical magnitude of the hormonal imbalance is best measured by *glucose* and/or *insulin tolerance* tests.

The condition most frequently associated with either latent or overt hyperglycemia is *diabetes mellitus*. Undoubtedly, there are many causes and forms of diabetes but whatever the cause, the condition is commonly associated with a relative or absolute deficiency of insulin with or without characteristic lesions of the islet cells being observed (Najjar). Although several theories, based on experiments, have been purported to explain the action of insulin, none explains the entire metabolic defect in diabetes mellitus (Stadie). The most consistent morphological changes associated with diabetes mellitus are (1) hyalinization of islets of Langerhans (less than 50% of cases), (2) hyaline degeneration of the renal glomeruli (intercapillary or diabetic glomerulosclerosis), (3) associated vascular involvement (arteriosclerosis) and (4) glycogen degeneration of the epithelial cells of the terminal portions of the proximal convoluted tubules of the kidneys (Armanni-Ebstein cells). In ordinary hematoxylin- and eosinstained sections, these cells appear greatly ballooned and distorted by empty intracytoplasmic spaces (Fig. 14). In sections appropriately stained for glycogen they are filled with glycogen-positive granules. Diabetes mellitus is discussed further in the section on the Pancreas (page 874).

Other causes of *hyperglycemia* (forms of diabetes) are noted in excessive

4

secretion and hyperplasia or functioning neoplasia of the (1) pituitary gland (acromegaly, Cushing's disease), (2) adrenal cortex (Cushing's syndrome), and (3) alpha cells of the pancreas or argentophilic cells of the gastrointestinal mucosa (glucagon). Epinephrine has the same net hyperglycemic effect as glucagon and the hyperglycemia noted in intracranial disorders (tumors, hemorrhage, *etc.*) and emotional states probably results from increased secretion of epinephrine.

When the blood sugar decreases to below 50 mg. per 100 ml., the condition is referred to as *hypoglycemia*. Depending not only on the blood sugar level but also on the rate of decline and duration of hypoglycemia, symptoms vary

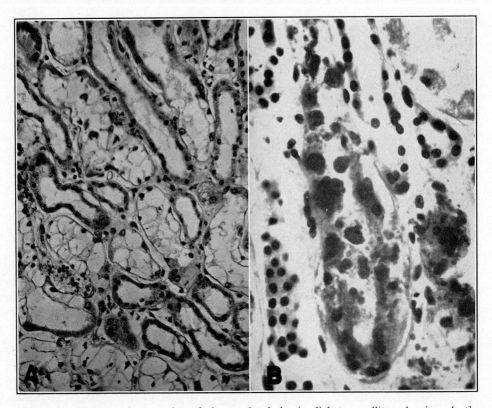

FIG. 14.—Glycogen degeneration of the renal tubules in diabetes mellitus showing *A*, the epithelial cells ballooned and distorted by intracytoplasmic vacuoles. Hematoxylin and eosin. × 200, and *B*, the epithelial cells filled with bright red intracytoplasmic granules. Best's carmine. × 400.

from weakness, pallor, epigastric discomfort, diaphoresis, disorientation, and syncope to severe manifestations of cerebral dysfunction with convulsions and deep coma. In this condition, glucose can be utilized but is not available and the tissue is starved as it is in diabetes. The metabolic defects are similar, except that convulsions commonly occur. In hypoglycemia, the brain probably reflects the only constant changes found. They consist of congestion, hemorrhages, and irreversible degenerative changes of the ganglion cells (Jones).

Other causes of hypoglycemia, which is encountered less frequently than hyperglycemia, may be (1) hyperinsulinism (functioning hyperplasia or neoplasia of the islets of Langerhans), (2) functional hyperinsulinism (hypersensitivity and responsiveness of histologically normal islet cells, manifesting itself after food intake), (3) hepatic diseases (infection, toxicity, tumor, or glycogen storage disease), (4) hypofunction of the anterior lobe of the pituitary, (5) hypofunction of the adrenal cortex (tuberculosis, histoplasmosis, Waterhouse-Friderichsen syndrome, *etc.*), (6) lesions of the hypothalamus or brain stem, (7) hypothyroidism (myxedema or cretinism), and (8) hypofunction of the alpha cells of the islets of Langerhans. The last mentioned has been proclaimed by some to account for the condition called "idiopathic infantile hypoglycemia."

In *summary*, the factors which tend to lower blood sugar are the opposite of those that produce hyperglycemia and, of the entire group, organic and functional hyperinsulinism and hepatogenic hypoglycemia account for a majority of cases.

DISTURBANCES OF LIPID METABOLISM

Francis A. Mc. Keon, Jr.

The general "group of naturally occurring substances consisting of the higher fatty acids, their naturally occurring compounds, and substances found naturally in chemical association with them are known as lipids" (Bloor). *Lipids* are insoluble in water but soluble in "fat solvents" such as ether, chloroform, and benzene.

Lipids of *physiological importance* in man may be classified into three major groups as follows: (1) *Simple lipids*. These are triglycerides (fatty acid esters) of glycerol (neutral fats and oils) or of higher alcohols (waxes). (2) *Complex lipids* or *lipoids*. These are compounds which contain other groups in addition to fatty acids and alcohols. They may be subgrouped into (*a*) phospholipids (lecithin, cephalin, and sphingomyelin), and (*b*) glycolipids (cerebrosides and gangliosides). (3) *Substances derived* from or *associated* with *lipids* such as fatty acids, alcohols, bases, steroids, carotenoids, tocopherols, and K vitamins. Cholesterol is the most important steroid. The specific functions of many of these substances in the human organism have not been convincingly elucidated. Undoubtedly, fatty acids serve as a source of energy and cholesterol probably serves as a source of various steriod hormones and bile acids.

Normally, ingested fat is either partially (partition hypothesis) or completely (lipolytic hypothesis) hydrolyzed by digestive enzymes (lipases) and the degraded products enter the intestinal cell. Here the fatty acids combine with glycerol to form neutral fats or are phosphorylated to phospholipids, either directly or by replacing endogenous fatty acids and phospholipids already present within the cell. Fatty acids may also combine with cholesterol and be absorbed as cholesterol esters, while phosphotides may be absorbed as such. The digestion and absorption of fats is facilitated by the emulsifying actions of bile salts. Absorption of fats is most active in the upper intestine, primarily by way of the lymphatics, and the absorbed constituents appear largely in the form of neutral fat as minute fat droplets (chylomicra) or as collodial phospholipids (hydrophilic) and cholesterol esters (hydrophobic). Almost all of the lipid in the blood stream is carried in the form of lipoprotein complexes, while some free fatty acids are associated with the albumin fraction and are taken up primarily by the fat cells in adipose tissue and secondarily by those in the liver. On the basis of their chemical and physcial characteristics *serum* or *plasma lipoproteins* may be separated into two major groups—(1) the low density or beta lipoprotiens and (2) the high density or alpha lipoproteins. They contain (1) neutral fat, (2) free and esterified cholesterol, (3) phospholipids, and (4) traces of fat soluble vitamins and steroid hormones. Ordinarily, the phospholipids-cholesterol ratio is 1 (one) and turbidity of the plasma may result from ratios below certain critical values. Males generally have higher serum lipid levels than females up to the age of 60 years, after which the reverse is the case (Lawry).

The *blood lipid level* is the resultant of the rates of *storage, synthesis, utilization*, and *mobilization*. The regulatory mechanisms, however, are not as clearly understood as those, for instance, of glucose in carohydrate metabolism. *Storage* of lipids occurs in specialized (adipose) tissue and is not simply deposited in connective tissue. Body fat, which represents about 20 per cent of the total body weight, consists mainly of (1) neutral fats and oils (triglycerides of long chain fatty acids), (2) phospholipids (lecithin, cephalin, sphingomylein, etc.), and (3) steroids (particularly cholesterol). Within certain limits, the quality and quantity of stored fat may be altered by the diet.

True (neutral) fats are stored primarily in *adipose tissue* which is an "active organ" and participates in lipogenesis, whereas phospholipids and cholesterol are present in almost every cell. The ability to store fat is a specific property of this tissue, as is evidenced by the continued storage of fat by grafted abdominal skin to other areas normally devoid of fat. Actually, adipose tissue may be considered as part of the reticuloendothelial system with definite functions. In addition to synthesis and storage of fat, it can store vital dyes, participates in the formation of antibodies and, under certain conditions, may resume its primitive blood forming function (Gelvin). The chief source of stored (neutral) fat is carbohydrate, while a secondary source is dietary fat.

The *intracellular distribution* of the various lipids is complex and not well understood. As already stated, neutral fat is largely confined to the fat depots (adipose tissue). Phospholipids (lecithin and cephalin) are found in practically all tissues, while a major amount of glycolipids (cerebrosides and gangliosides) is present in nerve tissue. Sphingomyelin is present mainly in the lungs and brain. Significant amounts of free cholesterol are present in brain tissue; its ester predominates in the adrenal cortex, and both are found in the liver and plasma. Representatives of every class are encountered in the liver, which commands a central position in lipid metabolism (Cantarow).

The utilization, synthesis, and mobilization of the diversity of compounds encompassed by the term "lipids" is not well understood and is best discussed by following the *intermediate metabolism* of the *fatty acids*. Fatty acids produced by intracellular hydrolization of fat are enzymatically degraded by oxidation to two carbon fragments (acetyl CoA), the same acetyl fragments encountered in glucose and amino acid catabolism. Most of these enter the "metabolic furnace" of the Krebs cycle while the remainder normally produces small amounts of ketone bodies and steroids or is used in acetylating reactions. Normal carbohydrate metabolism is essential for the complete oxidation of fatty acids, a concept embodied in the often quoted "fat burns in the flame of carbohydrate metabolism." In the presence of abnormal carbohydrate metabolism (diabetes mellitus, storage disease, *etc.*), there is compensatory catabolism of fatty acids. This overloads the Krebs cycle, resulting in the production of abnormal amounts of ketone bodies (ketosis) and possibly also cholesterol—both of which may be abnormally elevated in the plasma (ketonemia and hypercholesterolemia). Because the production of acetyl CoA from pyruvate in glucose catabolism is not reversible, there normally is no conversion of fatty acids to carbohydrate, although the glycerol moiety of neutral fat and certain amino acids may be converted to carbohydrate (gluconeogenesis). *Synthesis* of fat is a direct reversal of the catabolic pathway and carbohydrate is the major raw material for synthesis. Neutral fat is synthesized primarily in the liver and adipose tissue. In animals, the ratio of saturated to unsaturated fatty acids in neutral fat is 1:2. Certain unsaturated fatty acids are essential (oleic, linoleic, and arachidonic) in the diet, although some may be synthesized to a limited extent. A high carbohydrate diet results in the synthesis of fat with a higher melting point. In sclerema neonatorum, the nature of the fat appears altered, resulting in a higher melting point (p. 1327). The mammary gland synthesizes "milk-fat" from glucose. The intermediate metabolism and significance of *waxes* is obscure. They may, however, be important in contributing to the pliability and waterproofing of the skin. The *hormonal influence* of insulin, adrenocortical, and pituitary factors on fat metabolism is probably indirectly due to disturbances of carbohydrate metabolism, while the specific action of the sex hormones (estrogen, testosterone) remains obscure. The synthesis, but not the degradation, of *fatty acids* is dependent on insulin. The direct action of the thyroid hormone in regards to fat metabolism is unknown. *Cholesterol* and probably other steroids are synthesized from smaller fragments probably by way of a common precursor. Cholesterol is esterified in the intestinal mucosa and liver. Although the liver is the major site of cholesterol synthesis, it can also be synthesized by the arterial wall. Cholesterol in the blood is present in both the alpha and beta lipoprotein fractions, and normally 60 to 80 per cent is esterified. In cholesterol catabolism, a major portion (80–90%) is converted to bile acids and excreted by way of bile into the intestines. Some is excreted as neutral sterols. Biliary and exogenous cholesterol appears to be used only as a carrier during the absorption of lipids and is subsequently degraded in the reticulo-endothelial system. The half life (50% turnover rate) of serum cholesterol is 8 days, while that of neutral fat varies, being shortest in liver and intestinal mucosa (1 to 3 days) and longest in the brain (15 days). Certain sterols in the skin are transformed under the influence of ultraviolet light to vitamin D_3.

It is interesting that substances with the properties of phospholipids are believed to function in *blood coagulation*. Heparin exerts a *clearing action* on turbid (hyperlipemic) plasma and its action is correlated with an enzyme "*lipoprotein lipase.*" The phospholipid-cholesterol ratio appears to be related to the particle size or aggregation of lipoproteins. Although the specific function and metabolism of the glycolipids and phospholipids is unknown, the latter may promote fat mobilization. Such substances that promote clearance of lipid from the liver are termed *lipotrophic agents* (choline, inositol, and lipocaic).

Lipids that are synthesized or stored in one tissue may, in response to physiological demands, be *transported* to another site. The methods of transport (lipoproteins) and the regulatory mechanisms for control of plasma and cellular lipid metabolism are at present under intense investigation. This is especially true with regards to arteriosclerosis and metabolic disturbances that manifest a disturbance in lipid metabolism.

The *pathologic lesions* resulting from disturbances of lipid metabolism are difficult to classify because (1) of the diversity of compounds involved, (2 abnormalities may occur at any level in lipid metabolism (diet, absorption, intermediate metabolism, and excretion), and (3) the manifestations may be local and/or systemic in nature. Of the many lipids involved in pathologic processes, the following are of importance: (1) neutral fat (triglycerides), (2) complex lipids (phospholipids and glycolipids), and (3) cholesterol. Disturbances of deposition of fat include (1) emaciation, (2) obesity, and (3) fatty metamorphosis.

Emaciation (L. = to become lean) connotes an abnormal loss of body weight which may result from a variety of causes. There is marked decrease in tissue bulk because catabolism of carbohydrates, fats, and proteins exceed anabolism. The ultimate cause is a relative or absolute deficiency of food intake, absorption, or utilization. *Malabsorptive syndromes* (pancreatic disease, celiac disease, intestinal lipodystrophy, severe liver disease, sprue, *etc.*) exhibit striking defects in absorption of fat and fat soluble substances (Volwiler). They may be accompanied by rancid, bulky, pale stools with increased fecal fat (steatorrhea) (see Chapter 18, p. 698).

Obesity may be defined as an increase in weight (in excess of 10 per cent of the optimum weight of an individual) due to an accumulation of adipose tissue (Gelvin). Using this criterion, it is estimated that 5 million persons in the United States are overweight. The essential types of obesity are three—(1) *android* type where the obesity is primarily concentrated on the upper half of the body and secondarily on the abdomen, (2) *gynoid* type where the fat is present predominantly at the level of the hips, (3) *buffalo* or *bullfrog* type where the distribution may be localized about the head and neck, and (4) *generalized* type where the fat is evenly distributed over the trunk and extremities. The generalized type is the most common. Although heredity, endocrine disorders, central nervous system lesions, and psychosomatic factors may play a role in its development, the *cause* of obesity is generally considered to be a relative excess of caloric intake over caloric expenditure (Conn and Barach). Obesity in children probably does not differ from that observed in adults. The increased incidence of diabetes, gallbladder disease, and abnormalities of the cardiovascular system in association with obesity is of importance, and statistics clearly indicate that life expectancy is considerably shortened under such circumstances.

Fatty metamorphosis is a noncommittal term used to indicate a degenerative change in parenchymal cells characterized by the presence of fat droplets. It includes *fatty degeneration* (unmasking of or accumulation of fat within injured or dying cells) and *fatty infiltration* (accumulation of fat within or between parenchymal cells as the manifestation of obesity or as a primary disorder of fat metabolism). Although this basic distinction, originally introduced by Virchow, may not apply in all disturbances of lipid metabolism (because in the functioning cells of an organ fat accumulates by both methods), both terms are still retainable.

Fatty infiltration is encountered in cases of obesity and is best exhibited in the pancreas or heart. These organs become enlarged and are permeated with fat that merges with the surrounding accumulations. Histologically, there is a separation and resultant atrophy of the parenchymal cells by the fat tissue (Fig. 15).

Fatty degeneration may occur in any cell or organ undergoing degeneration or necrosis, including neoplasms. The accumulations of stainable fat, as well as cholesterol, is considered secondary to the causes of necrosis, which are many. Once cellular death supervenes and the process persists, there is eventual replacement by granulation and scar tissue. The same end result may, however, also occur in disorders of fat metabolism. As an example of the latter, liver cells with deficiency of lipotrophic factors undergo a fatty change. When the excessive accumulation of lipids is sufficiently great, the cells rupture and are eventually replaced by scar tissue. Therefore, in considering pathologic lesions associated with abnormal deposits of stainable lipids, it should be determined whether the presence of the abnormal lipid represents a primary defect in lipid metabolism or whether it is secondary to some other cause of cell injury (Hartroft).

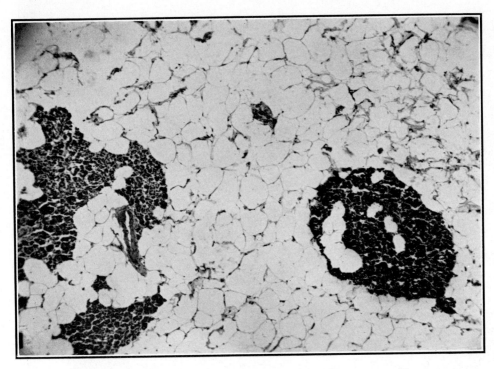

Fig. 15.—Fatty infiltration of the pancreas in an obese person. The pancreatic tissue is separated widely by fat tissue. × 50.

Fatty metamorphosis is best seen in the liver, heart, and kidneys. The *liver* is large and moderately firm and the sectioned surfaces may appear greasy and light yellowish brown (Fig. 16). The presence of fat can actually be demonstrated by scraping the surface with a knife, emersing the knife in water, and observing the fat droplets on the surface. Histologically, fat droplets of varying sizes appear in hepatic cells with no particular predilection for any portion of the hepatic lobule. When the accumulation is great enough, the hapatic cells completely disappear and eventually may even become replaced with fibrous tissue. It is possible that any one or many of the following basic factors may result in a "fatty liver:" (1) oversynthesis of lipids, (2) undermobilization of lipids from the liver to the storage depots, (3) underutilization or overmobilization of lipids from storage depots to the liver, and (4) overfeeding of lipids. Despite the variety of mechanisms that may be implicated, the histological picture is invariably the same. The

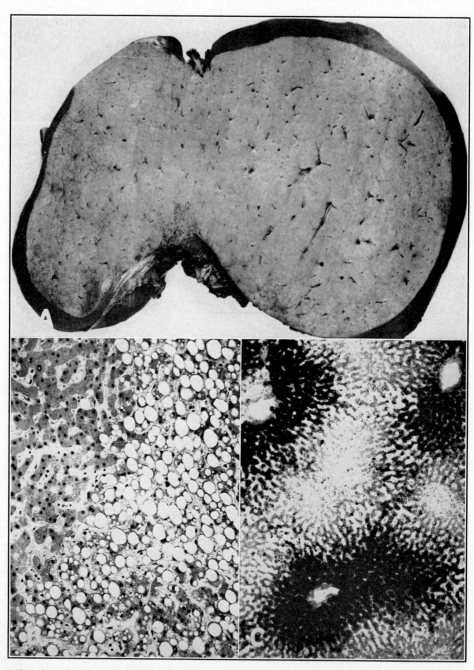

Fɪɢ. 16.—Fatty metamorphosis of the liver showing *A*, a light yellowish-brown cut surface, *B*, vacuoles in the cytoplasm of hepatic cells. Hematoxylin and eosin. × 100, and *C*, hepatic cells filled with fat that stains black. Osmic acid. × 50.

heart, especially the inner portion of the left ventricle, discloses a distinct orange, yellow, and brown mottling and is thus referred to as the "tabby cat" or "tigroid" heart (Fig. 17). Histologically, fat droplets are deposited within the myocardial fibers between the myofibrils. The *kidneys* are enlarged and the cortices are extremely pale and yellowish brown. Histologically, fat droplets are first visible at the base of the epithelial cells of the

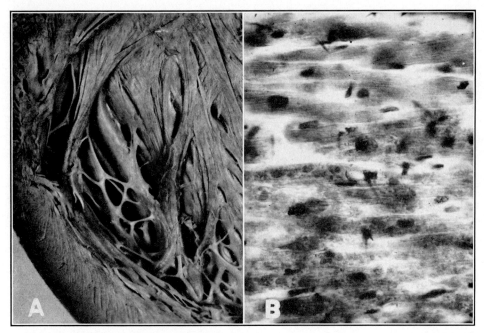

Fig. 17.—Fatty metamorphosis of the heart showing *A*, the inner surface of the left ventricle presenting a mottled appearance and *B*, fat positive droplets within the myocardial fibrils. Sudan III. × 400.

proximal convoluted tubules (Fig. 18). Later, as they extend they have no characteristic distribution and, in extreme cases, they may completely destroy the cells. Usually, other degenerative changes (parenchymatous, hydropic, and hyaline droplet) are also present in the affected cells.

A sharp *histochemical separation* of many of the individual *lipids* is practically impossible at the present time. Some may, however, be demonstrated by (1) physical methods, that is, staining by oil soluble dyes, fluorescence, and polarization microscopy, and (2) chemical methods, that is, certain dyes, osmic acid, or specific chemical reactions such as demonstrated by the Liebermann-Burchardt test for cholesterol. In practice, the method of making frozen sections of formalin fixed tissue and *staining* them with dyes is generally used. The staining of lipids by fat soluble dyes is affected mostly by (1) melting point, and (2) presence or absence of hydrophilic groups in the lipid, especially when aqueous solutions of dyes are used (Gomari). Fat soluble dyes such as Sudan III, Sudan IV, and Oil red O stain triglycerides, fatty acids, and to a certain extent phospholipids red, while Sudan black B stains them bluish black. The latter dye is good for the demonstration of phospholipids and may also be used to differentiate petrolatum, which stains clear violet, from animal lipids which stain bluish black. The kerasin in Gaucher cells is sudanophilic only after breaking the kerasin protein complex by prior boiling at pH 4. Nile blue stains triglycerides (neutral fat) red (provided the temperature is not below the melting point of the fat) and fatty acids and phospholipids (acidic lipids) blue. Obviously, admixtures of these lipids will produce intermediate shades. *Fluorescence* with ultraviolet light is displayed by many lipid substances (ceroid, oxidized products of cholesterol and unsaturated fatty acids, vitamin A, *etc.*) and the conspicuous double refractileness (birefringence) of cholesterol may be observed with polarized light. Cholesterol and its esters may also be demonstrated as bluish green deposits by the histochemical application of the Liebermann-Burchardt reaction (Schultz's method).

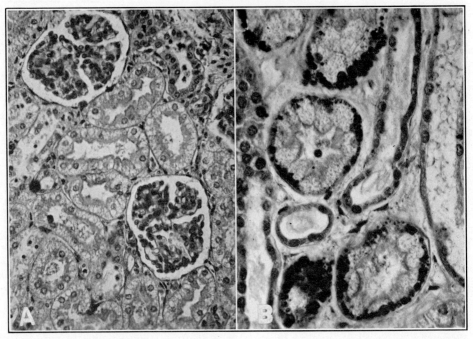

FIG. 18.—Fatty metamorphosis of the kidney showing *A*, vacuoles located basally in the epithelial cells of the proximal convoluted tubules. Hematoxylin and eosin. × 100, and *B*, black-staining droplets in the same location. Osmic acid. × 400.

Osmic acid renders phospholipids, cholesterol esters, and unsaturated fatty acids black but will not stain petrolatum. *Dichromate* methods oxidize unsaturated lipids to compounds stainable with Sudan dyes. Lipogenous pigments (ceroid, hemofuscin, lipofuscin, and wear and tear pigment) are iron free brownish pigments in unstained sections and probably represent various oxidized polymerized unsaturated fatty acids. Their other properties include staining by basic aniline dyes, metachromasia with methyl green, a positive Schiff reaction after periodate oxidation (PAS), and brownish fluorescence. Some are acid fast (ceroid) and reduce silver (lipofuscin).

Complex lipids include (1) phospholipids found in almost all cells and consisting of lecithins, cephalins, sphingomyelins (especially abundant in the lungs and brain), plasmalogens, and phosphatidic acids, and (2) glycolipids composed of cerebrosides and gangliosides and found respectively in large amounts in white and gray matter of nerve and brain tissue. As previously stated, representatives of every class of complex lipids are found to some extent in the liver. Known *disturbances* of *metabolism* with regards to these lipids include (1) *Niemann-Pick's disease* in which mainly sphingo-myelin and lesser amounts of lecithin, cephalin, and gangliosides are present in abnormal amounts in the spleen, liver, lymph nodes, bone marrow, and central nervous system, (2) *Gaucher's disease* where cerebrosides, especially kerasin is present in large amounts in the spleen, liver, lymph nodes, and bones, (3) *Tay-Sach's disease* where gangliosides and lesser amounts of. sphingomyelin are increased in the brain and spleen, (4) *cephalin-lipoidosis*, recently described as a lipid storage disease involving the reticulo-endothelial system with identification of the lipid as inosamine phosphatide (Baar), and (5) possibly also *gargoylism* (Hunter-Hurler's disease) in which there is, among other things, intracellular deposition of stainable lipid granules in the brain. Niemann-Pick's, Gaucher's, and Hand-Schüller-Christian's (eosinophilic granuloma, Letterer-Siwe) diseases are usually collectively referred to as *lipoid storage diseases*, *lipoidoses*, or *primary xanthomatoses* However, Hand-Schüller-Christian's disease, in which there is deposition of cholesterol and its esters in tissue, should not generally be considered to be a primary disturbance of lipid metabolism. These are considered further in Chapter 24, page 913.

Hyperlipemia and *hypercholesterolemia* refer respectively to an abnormal increase in blood lipid and cholesterol concentrations. Transient elevations of these may normally occur following ingestion of foods high in lipid content. As previously stated, neutral and complex lipids as well as cholesterol are transported in the plasma as lipoproteins. Generally, an elevation in the neutral lipids is accompanied by a concomitant rise in phospholipid concentration, and often by an elevation in the total cholesterol. Two apparently primary disorders in lipid metabolism manifested as such are (1) *familial* or *essential hypercholesterolemic xanthomatosis*—of unknown cause and characterized by hypercholesterolemia often with a clear serum, arteriosclerosis, and deposition of cholesterol in the skin, tendons and around joints (Wheeler), and (2) *idiopathic familial lipemia*—characterized by a marked increase in neutral fats of the blood to a lesser extent an increase in phospholipids and total cholesterol with a turbid serum, hepatomegaly, splenomegaly, recurrent attacks of abdominal pain and xanthomas of the skin. The cause of this condition is also unknown but the disturbance has been correlated with decreased plasma *lipoprotein lipase* activity. The latter enzyme catalyses the hydrolysis of triglycerides and its activity is increased by heparin resulting in a "clearing" of the serum both *in vivo* and *in vitro*. Impairment of liver function affecting heparin metabolism may be a factor in this disorder (Najjar).

Diabetes mellitus, hepatic disease (biliary cirrhosis, storage disease), severe malnutrition, or other conditions which secondarily affect lipid metabolism may result in an *accumulation* of *circulating lipids*. Hyperlipemia, especially hypercholesterolemia, in (1) hypothyroidism, (2) lipoid nephrosis (a degenerative condition of the kidneys), (3) glomerulonephritis, and (4) obstructive jaundice without cellular injury, is probably secondary to depression of liver function (Najjar). Severe parenchymatous disease of the liver (hepatitis, *etc.*) is usually attended by a decrease in plasma phospholipids and a marked depression of cholesterol esters with a normal or low total cholesterol. When, however, obstruction of the biliary passages occurs (intra- or extrahepatic), the plasma lipids rise, particularly phospholipids and free cholesterol.

Local manifestations of *disturbances* of *cholesterol metabolism* may be either primary (familial xanthomatosis) or secondary to some other cause (anything that will produce degeneration or necrosis of cells). Often, the deposition of cholesterol in tissue is accompanied by deposition of varying amounts of other lipids such as phospholipids and even neutral fat and lipogenous pigments (ceroid). The histological picture varies according to the relative quantity of each. Deposition of cholesterol in tissue is characterized by the presence of elongated crystals or rhomboid plates (each with a notched corner) of cholesterol or of granules of cholesterol esters in large phagocytic (foam) cells (Fig. 19). Surrounding such areas, there is frequently an inflam-

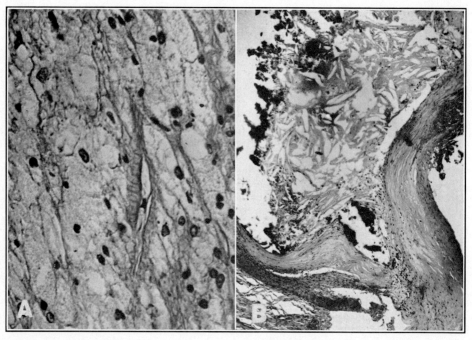

Fig. 19.—Lipoid degeneration showing *A*, cholesterol esters deposited in foam cells in the intima of an arteriosclerotic aorta. × 400, and *B*, cholesterol crystals deposited in the intima of an arteriosclerotic coronary artery. Some of the dead tissue about the periphery (black areas) has been calcified. × 50.

matory reaction. Some conditions, exhibiting cholesterol ester deposition, are degenerating or necrotic tissue, hydrocele fluid, gall stones, inflammation of the gallbladder, cysts lined by squamous epithelium, xanthomas, and the intima in arteriosclerosis.

The relationship between diet, sex (hormones), and both primary and secondary disturbances in lipid metabolism in relation to *atherosclerosis* (primary lipid concept of atherogenesis) is a problem yet to be solved. The most that can currently be stated is that persistent elevation of the plasma cholesterol and lipoproteins, especially the low density beta lipoproteins predisposes to atherosclerosis, although this tendency may not be realized in any given individual. In general, the phospholipids are thought to keep cholesterol in solution in plasma and their ratio with cholesterol is also deemed important. It appears that the major factor in dietary fats which produces depressions of elevated serum cholesterol and phospholipids is the total mean unsaturation of the dietary fat, that is, the number of double bonds (Ahrens). Ironically, the specific metabolic role of unsaturated fatty acids is unknown. There is recent evidence to suggest that atheroma may be due to the laying down of fibrin (fibrin concept of atherogenesis) on the endothelium which proliferates and overgrows the fibrin. The resultant focal thickening in the subintima is thought to interfere with the metabolic exchanges within the vessel wall leading to depositions of lipid. This concept has been fortified by the association of hypercoagulability of the blood and the inhibition of fibrinolysis by hyperlipemia (Grieg). The "clearing action" of heparin on hyperlipemic serum and its relationship to arteriosclerosis and hepatic disease is intriguing. The histological picture is compatible with both theories. The combined efforts of the nutritionist, biochemist, clinician, and pathologist appear to be essential to solve the riddle of lipid metabolism and possibly of atherosclerosis.

DISTURBANCES OF CALCIUM METABOLISM

Man's chief *sources* of *calcium* are milk, cheese, butter, eggs, green vegetables, and nuts (Hunter). In food, calcium consists of the organic and inorganic forms but by the process of digestion it is changed to inorganic form and is absorbed as partly or completely ionized calcium salts. The daily requirement for a normal adult varies between 0.4 and 1.0 gram. In the body, calcium has a remarkably constant *distribution*. It exists in blood serum at levels of 9 to 11.5 mg. per cent, in soft tissues in comparable amounts, and in bone (mostly as calcium phosphate but also as calcium carbonate) at an approximate level of 10,000 mg. per cent. It is excreted from the body mainly by the large intestine (both as unabsorbed and as re-excreted calcium) and to a lesser degree by the kidneys. The chief *functions* of calcium are: (1) formation of bone (which in turn serves as a reservoir), (2) lessening the irritability of tissues and thereby aiding in the control of heartbeat, contractility of muscles, and transfer of impulses at the neuromuscular junction, and (3) aiding in the coagulation of shed blood (Hunter). The *blood level* (and metabolism) of calcium is directly proportionate to (1) the availability of vitamin D and (2) the secretion of parathormone (hormone of the parathyroid gland). It is inversely proportionate to the blood level of phosphorus.

Disturbances of calcium metabolism may be conveniently divided into (1) disturbances of calcium levels of the blood and (2) its deposition in other than normal sites.

An increase in the blood level of calcium over 11.5 mg. per cent is known as *calcemia* or *hypercalcemia*. It may be due to (1) *Hyperparathyroidism*. When the parathyroid glands become enlarged (hyperplasia or tumor) they secrete an excess amount of parathormone. This causes mobilization of calcium from bones which, in turn, results in (*a*) flooding of the blood and tissues with calcium, (*b*) weakness and lethargy due to excessive amounts of calcium, (*c*) cystic swellings, softenings, and deformities of bones (osteitis fibrosa cystica), and (*d*) deposition of calcium in the kidneys and other soft tissues of the body. Similar changes occur in experimental animals treated with excessive amounts of parathormone (Thomson and Collip). (2) *Hypervitaminosis D*. Both in man and experimental animals, administration of excessive amounts of vitamin D has resulted not only in simple hypercalcemia but also in untoward effects consisting of loss of appetite, loss of weight, nausea, vomiting, abdominal pain, diarrhea, muscle weakness, headaches, excessive urination, excessive thirst, and (in animals) coma followed by death (Tumulty and Howard). (3) *Renal failure.* Prolonged primary renal insufficiency results in improper excretion of phosphate ions which upsets the calcium phosphorus ratio and produces a secondary hypertrophy of the parathyroid glands. This, in turn, causes hypercalcemia. (4) *Dietary.* Prolonged ingestion of large amounts of milk, calcium, and alkalies in the treatment of peptic ulcer may not only produce elevation of serum calcium but also a syndrome characterized by elevation of serum phosphorous, metastatic calcinosis, keratitis, hypocalcinuria, mild alkalosis, and anemia with normal alkaline phosphatase levels (Snapper). (5) *Bone lesions.* Aside from osseous changes in hyperparathyroidism complete immobilization of young persons (as for broken bones, paralysis, *etc.*) and widespread bone-destroying cancer of the skeleton are accompanied by demineralization of bones and this in turn results in increased calcium levels in the bood (Snapper).

A decrease in the blood calcium below 9 mg. per cent is known as *hypocalcemia.* It may occur under the following circumstances: (1) *Decreased calcium assimilation.* This may be due to lack of calcium in the diet or to decreased absorption by the intestine on chronic conditions such as steatorrhea. (2) *Increased calcium needs.* This occurs during pregnancy and lactation. (3) *Increased calcium excretion.* Renal excretion of calcium is enhanced by an acid-forming diet or by administration of large doses of ammonium chloride. (4) *Hypovitaminosis D.* In addition to hypocalcemia, a deficient amount of vitamin D results in a disturbance in the normal process of ossification in children (rickets) and in softening and deformity of bones in adults (osteomalacia). (5) *Hypoparathyroidism.* A deficient secretion of parathormone (usually due to destruction or removal of the parathyroid glands) results in deficiency of calcium which brings about hyperirritability of the nerve muscle system and tetany. Other causes of hypocalcemic tetany are loss of hydrochloric acid by vomiting, loss of carbon dioxide by pulmonary overventilation, and ingestion of large amounts of sodium bicarbonate.

Deposition of calcium in other than normal sites is referred to as *pathologic calcification.* *Grossly,* deposits of calcium, when in sufficient amounts, appear as white granules, clumps, or large plaques of extremely firm, gritty, uncuttable material. *Histologically* they consist of irregular granules or clumps that stain deep blue with hematoxylin and black with silver nitrate (Figs. 19*B* and 20). *Chemically* areas of pathologic calcification are similar, both qualitatively and quantitatively, to normal bone (Meeker and Kesten). Pathologic calcification may be divided into (1) dystrophic calcification, (2) metastatic calcification, and (3) calcinosis.

Dystrophic (Gr. = ill + to nourish) *calcification* may be defined as calcification in degenerating, dying, or dead tissue without regard to the concentration of calcium in the blood stream. It is the most common type of pathologic calcification. A few of the numerous examples in this category are: old tuberculous tissues, intima in hardening of the arteries (arteriosclerosis), media of the large arteries, cartilages of the ribs and trachea in old age, animal parasites, healed venous thrombi (phleboliths), psammoma bodies (circumscribed structures found in a variety of retrograde processes), epithelium in the convoluted tubules of the kidney in mercury bichloride poisoning, heart valves in healed inflammations, some forms of inflammation of the pericardium (pericarditis), some tumors (thyroid adenoma and dystrophic calcification is not well understood. There are at least two factors

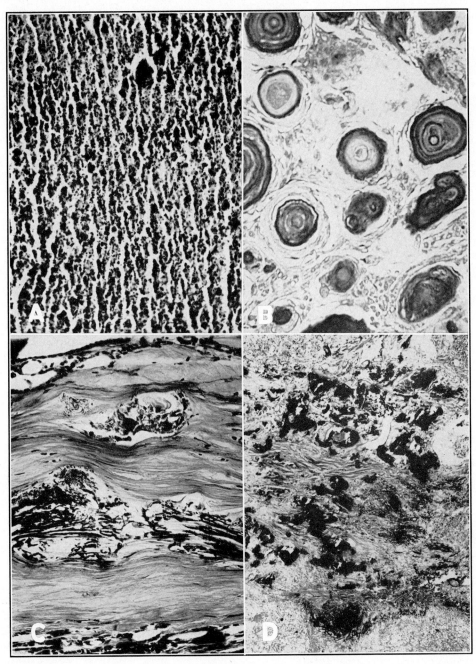

FIG. 20.—Dystrophic calcification illustrating deposition of dark-staining calcium granules in
A, the center of an old, caseous, tuberculous mass, B, psammoma bodies in a tumor of the
meninges, C, the capsule of a tumor (benign adenoma) of the thyroid, and D, the periphery of
dead tissue in the spleen. × 100.

that are concerned—local increase of alkaline phosphatase and local decrease of carbon dioxide (McLean).   Normally *alkaline phosphatase* has been seen in osteoblasts, periosteum, and endosteum while abnormally it is demonstrable locally in certain types of injured tissues.   Under the latter circumstances its presence increases the production of calcium and phosphate ions locally, beyond their solubility, thus resulting in calcification.   It is a known fact that *alkalinity* augments calcium deposition.   It is also known that carbon dioxide production is low or absent in necrosis, degeneration (especially of elastic tissue), chronic inflammation, scars, and infarcts.   Under such circumstances, therefore, the medium becomes alkaline and deposition of calcium and phosphate ions is favored.

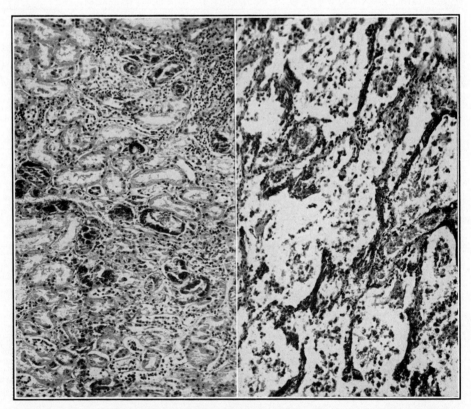

Fig. 21.—Metastatic calcification showing calcium deposits in the renal tubules (left) and pulmonary alveolar walls (right).   × 100.

Metastatic calcification may be defined as the deposition of calcium in tissues previously normal but with a tendency to alkalinity (Mulligan).   The condition occurs exclusively in conjunction with hypercalcemia (see previous section) and the deposits are characteristically found in the lungs (alveolar walls and pulmonary vessels), kidneys (tubular epithelium, lumens, and basement membranes), mucosa of the fundus of the stomach, and myocardium of the left ventricle (Fig. 21).   The precise mechanism of metastatic calcification is unknown.   Supersaturation of the serum with calcium (and phosphate) ions is definitely a factor.   Other contributing factors probably consist of local reduction of tissue concentration of hydrogen ions and local activity of alkaline phosphatase.

Calcinosis may be defined as an abnormal deposition of calcium salts in various portions of the body unassociated with detectable disturbances in calcium metabolism and unaccompanied by preceding (at least demonstrable) local changes. The condition is generally divided into a circumscribed and a universal variety (Lutz and Rosenberg), although some authors (Rothstein and Welt) maintain that such a division is artificial and unnecessary. *Circumscribed calcinosis* is usually seen in women beyond forty years of age and consists of a deposition of calcium in subcutaneous tissues, particularly about the joints of the hands and feet. Clinically it is of little significance. *Universal calcinosis* is often encountered in children but occurs at all ages. It consists of a deposition of calcium in subcutaneous tissues (sometimes skipping the hands and feet), in muscles, and occasionally along nerve trunks (especially of the extremities) (Fig. 22). Clinically the deposits may be extensive enough to interfere with locomotion.

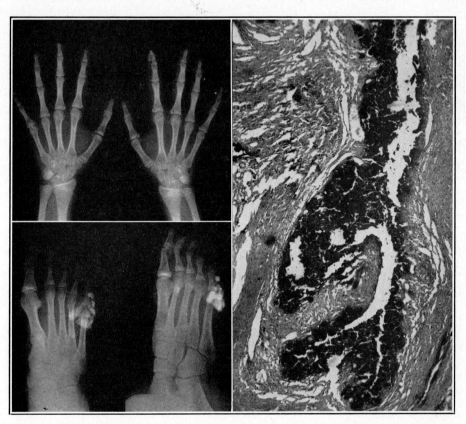

FIG. 22.—Universal calcinosis disclosing roentgenograms of calcium deposits about the digits (left) and a photomicrograph of similar deposits about the peri-articular tissues. × 50. (Films and tissue submitted by Dr. H. T. Tamaki).

PATHOLOGIC OSSIFICATION

Pathologic ossification consists of the formation of true bone in other than normal sites. It usually represents a sequel of old calcification. *Histologically* the deposits consist of adult bone with the usual lamellæ, lacunæ, and even bone marrow (Fig. 23). The bone arises from osteoblasts

5

which, in turn, probably originate from primitive mesenchymal (reticulum) cells.

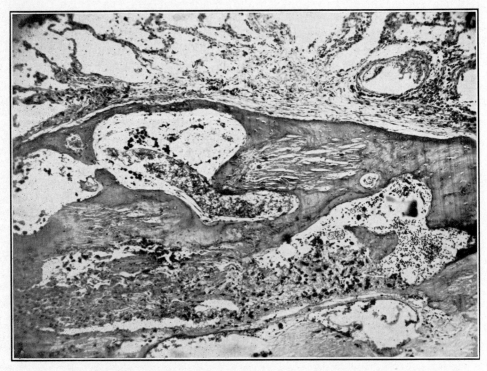

FIG. 23.—Pathologic ossification showing the formation of bone and bone marrow in an old tuberculous focus in the apex of a lung. × 50.

PATHOLOGIC PIGMENTATION

Under this heading may be included disorders characterized by the presence of colored compounds that are of heterogenous origin, that are not necessarily related chemically, and that have in common the physical property of being pigmented. Body pigments may be classified into two broad groups—endogenous and exogenous. *Endogenous* (Gr. = within + to produce) are pigments that are formed within the body. *Exogenous* (Gr. = out + to produce) are pigments that are formed outside of the body and are deposited within tissues and organs in more or less unaltered state.

ENDOGENOUS PIGMENTATION

Although endogenous pigments are quite varied, they may be divided into three broad groups—blood pigments, lipochromes, and melanin.

BLOOD PIGMENTS

For practical purposes, the important blood pigments consist of hemoglobin and its derivatives. Some of the more important members of the group are: hemoglobin itself, iron (hemosiderin), hematoidin, bilirubin, urobilinogen, malarial pigment, hematin, porphyrins, and pigment in chloroma.

PLATE I

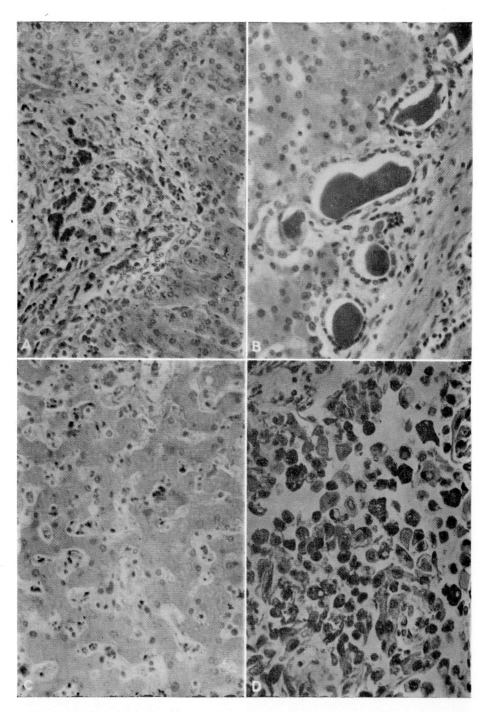

Pathologic pigmentation showing *A*, golden brown hemosiderin granules in hepatic cells and periportal fibrous tissue from a case of hemochromatosis, *B*, bilirubin in the form of bile casts within bile ducts from a case of obstructive jaundice, *C*, deep brown to black malarial pigment in reticulo-endothelial (Kupffer's) cells of the liver. and *D*, black melanin granules in tumor cells from a case of melanoblastoma (malignant melanoma). × 200.

HEMOGLOBIN

Leandro M. Tocantins

Hemoglobin is the oxygen-carrying *pigment* of red blood cells. It has a molecular weight of 68,000 and is made up of a protein component (globin), which is colorless, with four small groups of heme molecules distributed over it. It is the *heme* portion of the hemoglobin molecule which gives it the red color. The heme itself is a metal complex made up of a porphyrin (protoporphyrin) structure with an iron atom. *Globin* has a molecular weight of 66,000 and is a complex of the amino acids leucine, valine, aspartic acid, alanine, lysine, histidine, phenylalanine, glutamic acid, threonine, proline, glycine, serine, tyrosine, arginine, tryptophane, methionine, and cystine.

The individual *human red cell* contains an average of 29 micrograms of hemoglobin within a mean corpuscular volume of 85 cubic microns. Hemoglobin makes up approximately 33 per cent of the contents of the red cell. When hemoglobin is destroyed, the iron is split off and the globin is liberated. This process apparently takes place in the reticulo-endothelial system, giving rise to *biliverdin* which is later reduced to the compound *bilirubin*. The *iron* remains bound to the protein in the tissues and from there goes, through the blood, to either the bone marrow, where it is used to make new hemoglobin, or to storage depots. The *free globin* is broken down and joins the general body pool of amino acids. Bilirubin is transported to the liver through the blood, bound principally to albumin and to the alpha and beta globulins. The protein bound bilirubin, as it passes through the liver cells, loses its protein. The free bilirubin passes in the bile and is secreted through the bile ducts into the duodenum.

A *normal adult man* has approximately 750 grams of hemoglobin and since the span of red cells is approximately 120 days, and a certain number are destroyed every day, this destruction requires the production of 6.25 grams of hemoglobin per day to maintain the hemoglobin level. The destruction of this amount of hemoglobin leads to the liberation of 21 milligrams of bilirubin daily. The iron is kept within the body and used over again, but the bilirubin is a waste product and is excreted in the bile.

Abnormalities of hemoglobin may be divided into two groups—those due to disturbances in the heme moiety and those due to disturbances in the globin moiety. *Hemoglobinopathies* due to an abnormal *heme moiety* are concerned with reduced hemoglobin, carboxyhemoglobin, methemoglobin, sulfhemoglobin, and porphyria. Certain forms of deep cyanosis in cardiac or pulmonary diseases accompanied by severe dyspnea are due to the presence of large amounts of *reduced hemoglobin*. *Carboxyhemoglobin* results from the combination of carbon monoxide and hemoglobin. The affinity of carbon monoxide for human hemoglobin is two hundred and ten times that of oxygen. It, therefore, will displace oxygen and remain attached to the hemoglobin, rendering it unavailable for carrying oxygen. *Methemoglobin* is a form of hemoglobin in which the ferrous prophyrin complex has been changed to the ferric form and, as such, is unavailable for combination with oxygen, and is of no value for respiration. Methemoglobin can be reduced to hemoglobin through the action of agents such as ascorbic acid and glutathione. Methemoglobinemia may be observed in a congenital or familial form, or may be acquired through exposure to industrial chemical compounds and certain therapeutic agents. Some of the toxic agents are anilin, phenacetin, acetanilid, nitrobenzene, and sulfanilamide. The congenital or hereditary forms of methemoglobinemia are relatively rare, the majority of them having been observed in Greeks. *Sulfhemoglobin* results from a combination of hemoglobin with soluble inorganic sulfides and nitrites. It has been observed after the prolonged use of acetanilid in the form of Bromo-Seltzer, but phenacetin in other drug combinations has also been a common offender. Enterogenous methemoglobinemia and sulfahemoglobinemia have been attributed to the absorption of nitrates and sulfides from the intestine as a result of disturbed intestinal function. *Porphyria* is a disturbance of porphyrin metabolism and is considered on page 75.

When looking for *abnormal hemoglobin pigments*, it is well to observe if the plasma is clear, to eliminate hemolysis and abnormal plasma pigments. The whole blood may be then shaken and if it assumes a bright red color the presence of abnormal intracellular pigments is unlikely. If the blood remains dark after being shaken, such pigments must be considered. If the

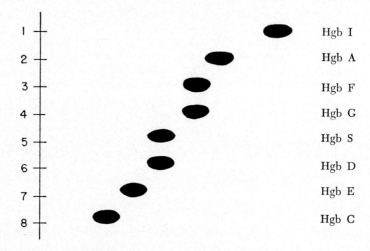

Fig. 24.—Schematic representation of hemoglobin patterns as demonstrated by paper electrophoresis. Whatman No. 3-MM filter paper with barhtal buffer at pH 8.8 and ionic strength 0.06. Run carried out for eight to ten hours at 350 volts (direction of anode to right). Chernoff, courtesy of New England J. Med.

blood is cherry red even before shaking, the presence of carboxyhemoglobin must be suspected. Methemoglobin in high concentration produces a chocolate brown and sulfhemoglobinemia produces a lavender color.

Hemoglobinopathies due to an abnormal *globin moiety* have really come to the forefront only recently. Within the last ten years it has been shown in different species that while the heme structure of the hemoglobin does not vary, the globin moiety may differ as to iso-electric point and amino acid composition. An *adult* (A) and *fetal* (F) forms of hemoglobin have been recognized for some time. It has been shown that a peculiar sickling of certain red cells is due to the presence in these cells of an abnormal *hemoglobin* (S), which, upon deoxygenation, twists itself into long rigid rods. It has since been established that this same hemoglobin under certain conditions moves at an electrophoretic velocity much slower than normal. At least *ten different types* of hemoglobin, labeled according to letters of the alphabet and differentiated by various physiochemical criteria, have been described.

TABLE 1.—SUMMARY OF USUAL FINDINGS IN ABNORMAL HEMOGLOBINOPATHIES AND THALASSEMIA. (Wintrobe's Clinical Hematology).

Condition	Hgb Types[1]	Sickling	Microcytosis	Hypochromia	Target Cells[2] Per cent	Hemolytic Anemia[3]	Splenomegaly
None—adult	AA	0	0	0	0	0	0
None—newborn	AF	0	0	0	0	0	0
Traits:							
Sickle cell trait[4]	AS	+	0	0	4	0	0
Hgb C trait[4]	AC	0	0	+	0-40	0	0
Hgb D trait	AD	0	0	0	?	0	0
Hgb E trait	AE	0	0	0	2	0	0
Hgb G trait[4]	AG	0	0	0	0	0	0
Hgb H trait (?)	AH	0	+	0	+	++	++
Hgb I trait	AI	0	0	0	<2	0	0
Diseases:							
Sickle cell anemia[4]	SS	++	0	0,+	5-30	++++	0
Homozygous Hgb C[4]	CC	0	±	+	40-100	++	++
" Hgb E	EE	0	++	0	25-60	+[7]	±
" Hgb G[4]	GG	0	0	0	0	0	0
Sickle cell-Hgb C[4,5]	SC	++	±	+	20-85	++	++
Sickle cell-Hgb D[6]	SD	+	+	0	±	++	++
Sickle cell-Hgb G	SG	+	0	0*	+	0	0
Thalassemia minor	AA	0	±	±,+*	+	0[7]	±
Thalassemia major	AF	0	++	++*	10-35	++	+++
Sickle cell-thalassemia[6]	SF	+	++	±*	20-40	++	++
Hgb C-thalassemia[4]	CA	0	+++	+*	+++	0	0
Hgb E-thalassemia	EF	0	+++	+*	10-40	++	++
Hgb G-thalassemia (?)	GF	0	+++	+	++	++	0
Sickle cell-hereditary spherocytosis	SA	+	+	0	++	++	++

[1] The major hemoglobin component is shown first. In sickle cell anemia especially, there may also be a substantial proportion of Hgb F

[2] Osmotic fragility is reduced more or less proportionately to the number of target cells

[3] Mechanical fragility and RBC survival correspond as a rule to the presence and degree of hemolytic anemia

[4] Chiefly in Negroes

[5] Cases of sickle cell anemia intermediate in severity between sickle cell trait and sickle cell anemia

[6] Sickle cell disease in Caucasians

[7] Or polycythemia with microcytosis

* Basophilic stippling of the red corpuscles

These criteria are based on the behavior of these hemoglobins upon electro-phoresis, alkaline denaturation, solubility in water, and immunological testing. Human fetal hemoglobin is more resistant to denaturation by alkali than adult hemoglobin. The variations in solubility of hemoglobin in cer-tain solutions have made it possible to distinguish adult hemoglobin from the fetal type and particularly from sickle hemoglobin which has the lowest solubility. Hemoglobin D which has an electrophoretic mobility like hemo-globin S can be distinguished from the latter because it has a normal solubil-ity. In Figure 23 are represented schematically the relative location of the hemoglobin spots as observed by paper electrophoresis of solutions of various types of hemoglobin.

Clinically, the principal *hemoglobinopathies* are represented by sickle cell anemia and thalassemia. The sickling defect is found principally in Negroes. In Table 1 are listed the hematological characteristics of the various forms of hemoglobinopathy. Combinations of these abnormal hemoglobins pro-duce a wide variety of clinical manifestations which have been, and still are, a source of confusion. The differentiation of the hemoglobinopathies by the methods above mentioned have helped us to recognize these combina-tions, and to identify the relative proportions of each hemoglobin in them.

IRON AND IRON METABOLISM

Francis A. McKeon, Jr.

The average daily diet contains 10–15 mg. of iron. In the normal person 10 per cent of this, in the *ionizable* form, is absorbed principally in the stom-ach and proximal portion of the small intestine. *Ferrous* (reduced) iron is preferentially absorbed to ferric (oxidized) iron.

Substances that form insoluble compounds or complexes (phosphates and phytic acid) decrease available *absorbable* iron and, conversely, substances that favor *reduction* (ascorbic acid and sulfhydril compounds) or ionization (hydrochloric acid) increase available absorbable iron. Calcium in moderate amounts removes the inhibition of phosphates and phytic acid.

The amount of absorbable iron that actually penetrates the gastro-intestinal tract depends on a more complex transfer mechanism present within the mucosal cell and referred to as the *mucosal barrier*. According to this concept of *"selective iron absorption"* the mucosal cell contains a protein acceptor (apoferritin) which is synthesized according to need and which accepts iron in the ferric form to become *ferritin*. The ferrous iron which passes into the mucosal cell is in equilibrium with the ferric iron of ferritin which also has been found to have vasodepressor (VDM) and anti-diuretic properties.

A "mucosal block" is said to occur when all of the acceptor is utilized and no more iron can transgress the cell until some acceptor is made avail-able by the removal of the ferrous iron directly into the blood stream. It is oxidized to the ferric form in the plasma which is the chief medium of *iron transport*. It then unites *in vivo* and *in vitro* with a specific B_1 globulin to form a complex (*siderophilin, metal binding globulin, transferrin*) which is salmon pink with maximal light absorption at 520 millimicrons (the basis for measuring available serum or plasma *iron-binding-capacity*). The *normal serum* iron is 110 micrograms/100 ml. in females and 129 micrograms/100 ml. in males, while the *total serum binding capacity of iron* is 300 to 350 micro-grams/100 ml. of serum, representing approximately 33 per cent saturation of the B_1 globulin. Although the serum iron (0.1% of the circulating iron) and the B_1 globulin (3% of serum proteins) appear quantitatively minor, they are sensitive "barometers" of iron metabolism. Clinically, these reflect the balance that exists as a resultant of absorption, utilization, storage, excretion, and reutilizable iron (blood destruction). Exact *homeostatic* mechanisms are not known but the regulation of iron absorption appears to be closely correlated with body requirements and storage of iron. Excretion plays a minor role in homeostasis and the combined loss by all routes (urine, sweat, feces, desquamated cells) amounts to 0.5 to 1.5 mg/day with additional average menstrual loss of 1 mg/day. In certain disorders there may be a marked iron loss in the urine (hemosiderinuria) as occurs in paroxymal hemoglobinuria (Wintrobe). In nephrosis the renal loss may be as much as 1.5 mg. of iron per day, as the B_1 globulin complex.

The *partition* of iron is of unique importance in mammalian physiology but a detailed discussion of the various components is beyond the scope of this discussion.

The *normal total body iron* (4-5 grams) exists principally either in a *chelated form* as blood hemoglobin (60 to 70%), myoglobin (5%), and heme enzymes (0.2%), or in combination with a protein (transferrin (0.1%), ferritin (15 to 20%), and hemosiderin. Hemoglobin breakdown contributes 20 to 25 mg. of iron per day but this joins the circulating iron pool and is reutilized in hemoglobin synthesis.

Storage of iron occurs chiefly in the liver, spleen, and bone marrow as *ferritin* and *hemosiderin*. Normally, both forms are present but only with increased storage can hemosiderin be detected by staining methods. The mechanism appears similar to that in the mucosal cell but, when the ability to synthesize apoferritin is exceeded, the iron is stored as hemosiderin (Granick). The amount of hemosiderin in bone marrow aspirates and in liver biopsies has been used as a rough index of the iron stores in the body.

Hemosiderin (Gr. = blood+iron) microscopically in *unstained* sections occurs as discrete yellow brown granules (Plate 1*A*). Ferritin consists of ferric hydroxide and a protein moiety (apoferritin) and is water soluble, whereas hemosiderin consists of ferric hydroxide stabilized by protein and is realtively insoluble. This difference in solubility has been utilized in separating these two forms of storage of iron.

In alcohol or formalin fixed tissue, most of the ferritin is lost and the iron in hemosiderin may be liberated with dilute solutions of strong acids and demonstrated as blue granules by (1) the formation of *Prussian blue* (ferriferrocyanide) after the addition of potassium ferrocyanide or (2) the formation of *Turnbull's blue* (ferrous ferricyanide) by addition of potassium ferricyanide with previous reduction of iron by ammonium sulfide. Other iron containing pigments (malarial pigment, hemoglobin, and formalin pigment) are negative by this method and are iron positive *only* after destroying the organic portion of the composite. *Hemofuscin* and *lipofuscin* are iron free lipogenous pigments while *cytosiderin* appears to be a mixture of hemosiderin and lipogenous pigment (Gomori). *In vivo* deposition of hemosiderin in the skin may be demonstrated (Prussian blue) by the intradermal injection of a small amount of equal parts of 0.5 per cent potassium ferrocyanide and N/100 hydrochloric acid (Fishback reagent).

As may be deduced from what has been said, *iron balance* is precarious, particularly in women and children. The normal daily requirements that have been recommended are: infants and children, 1 mg. and 0.6 mg. per kilogram of body weight respectively; adult males, a total of 10 mg.; adult female, a total of 12 to 20 mg., depending on menses and pregnancy.

By present standards, anemias in general are common and *iron deficiency anemia* is the most common of all. *Disturbances* in *iron metabolism* principally involve disturbances in *absorption* and/or *storage* of iron. Intestinal dysfunction and disease may be the cause of decreased absorption. "Selective iron absorption" eventuates in a variety of conditions (hemolytic and pernicious anemias and pysidoxine defficiency) and there is increased absorption of iron even when the storage of iron is known to be adequate or excessive. The toxicity of excessive deposits of iron in the tissues is a moot question. Toxic reactions, even fatalities, have followed the accidental ingestion of massive amounts of ferrous sulphate by children. As previously noted, the determination of serum iron, iron binding capacity, and hemosiderin deposition in bone marrow aspirates and liver biopsy is utilized as an index of disturbed metabolism.

In cases of *iron deficiency anemia*, whether due to decreased intake or absorption or to increased loss (hemorrhage), the total serum capacity to bind iron increases while the per cent saturation with iron decreases. Both these factors (total binding capacity and per cent saturation) are decreased in conditions such as infection and cancer.

In conditions in which there is a *plethora* of *iron* in the storage depots (liver, spleen, and bone marrow), there is a decreased total binding capacity with a marked increase in the per cent saturation (up to 100%). When the iron transport system is overloaded, the excess iron is deposited in body tissues as hemosiderin. In the unstained state, it exists as coarse, golden brown granules that are found (as the case may be) free in tissue spaces and within phagocytes, reticulo-endothelial cells, and occasionally in hepatic and renal tubular cells (Plate 1*A*).

Since iron is valuable, it is *utilized*, upon liberation from hemosiderin, in the resynthesis of hemoglobin, so that normally only occasional cells of the reticulo-endothelial system or its derivatives exhibit this pigment. *Local accumulations* of hemosiderin may be found in the vicinity of old hemorrhages, in phagocytic cells (heart failure cells) in the lungs in cases of chronic passive congestion, and even in early arteriosclerotic plaques (Paterson).

When, as a result of multiple blood transfusions, nutritional disorders (exogenous), hemolytic disease, or due to inborn errors in iron metabolism (endogenous), the dissemination of hemosiderin is more widespread and involves the reticulo-endothelial cells of organs such as the liver, spleen, bone marrow, pancreas, *etc.*, the condition is referred to as *hemosiderosis*. When there is, in addition, pigmentation of the skin, fibrous tissue replacement of the hepatic cells (cirrhosis), increase of fibrous tissue in the pancreas, and diabetes mellitus, the disorder is referred to as *hemochromatosis* (p. 804). In both of these states, the heart plays an important role.

Heart failure is the major cause of death in 15 to 20% of the cases of hemochromatosis. In cardiac hemosiderosis, there is associated cardiomegaly and iron pigment deposition in the fibers which reveal degeneration but no fibrosis. On the other hand, in nutritional disease associated with generalized hemosiderin, as reported in the South African Bantu, there is no hemosiderin in the heart (Higginson). Apart from this, the exact reason for an *associated fibrosis* in some cases of hemosiderosis is not known.

HEMATOIDIN

Hematoidin contains no iron, does not give a positive Prussian blue reaction, and is identified in areas of old hemorrhage as brown, rhombic plates or fine, axially-crossed needles. It may also be seen free and within phagocytic cells as fine, deep brown, amorphous granules. Ordinarily, however, it remains in solution in the blood and tissue juices. Unlike hemosiderin, hematoidin is expendable and normally is excreted in the bile as bilirubin.

BILIRUBIN

Francis A. McKeon, Jr.

Bilirubin (L=bile+red) is the pigment in bile and, as just stated, is closely related to or identical with hematoidin. It is formed by reticulo-endothelial cells from the breakdown of hemoglobin and is transported in the plasma to the liver where it is excreted in the bile. In the intestines, bilirubin is reduced by bacteria to stercobilinogen (urobilinogen) and a variable amount of the latter undergoes spontaneous oxidation to stercobilin (urobilin) and is excreted as the brown pigment in the stool. Some is reabsorbed with (1) most removed from the blood by the liver and (2) a small portion entering the systemic circulation, being excreted by the kidneys.

The bilirubin in the blood stream is altered by the liver in the process of excretion into the bile. This alteration, dependent on an enzyme glucuronyl transferase, results in conjugated glucoronide derivatives (water soluble and readily oxidized pigments I and II) and possibly other nonglucuronide derivatives, the presence of which is detected by a *direct* or prompt diazo reaction (van den Bergh). There apparently also exists an extra hepatic mechanism for the production of conjugated bilirubin (direct reacting). The unaltered bilirubin (lipid soluble, relatively stable) reacts with the diazo reagent to produce an *indirect* or delayed (van den Bergh) reaction (Billing). Both bilirubin and its conjugated derivative are transported in the blood attached to plasma albumin and normally the processed or conjugated derivative is present in minute amounts (less than 0.25 mg./100 ml.). Normally, the total bilirubin (direct and indirect reacting) content of the blood is low (0.8 mg./100 ml.) and, since its excretion keeps pace with its formation, it produces no alteration in the color of the tissues. However, whenever there is a relative or absolute decrease of its excretion as compared with its formation, the blood, tissues and organs become flooded with bilirubin (bilirubinemia), and the patient develops *jaundice* or *icterus*. This condition is manifested clinically (among other things) by a yellowish discoloration of the sclera, skin, and mucous membranes. Autopsy may reveal most organs and tissues to be similarly discolored. If such organs are left exposed to the atmosphere, the bilirubin is oxidized to biliverdin and the color changes from yellow to green. Similar demonstration of bilirubin as the emerald green *biliverdin* in frozen sections of tissue may be accomplished by oxidation with potassium dichromate (Glenner). Because of its solubility, it normally cannot be identified in routine histological preparations: however it may be seen as a homogeneous yellowish deposit where it accumulates in large quantities as a result of stasis, for example, in bile ducts in cases of biliary obstruction (Plate 1*B*), or in the renal tubules.

Clinically jaundice may be *classified* under the following categories:
   (1) Pre-hepatic: *i.e.*, increased destruction or hemolysis of erythrocytes.
   (2) Hepatic, such as congenital or acquired hepato-cellular disturbances.
   (3) Post-hepatic, which is caused by obstruction to the flow of bile (intrinsic or extrinsic).

In hemolytic disease which characterizes a *retention* or prehepatic type jaundice, there is often a low bilirubin ratio, *i.e.*, ratio of direct reacting to indirect (conjugated) is low. While a majority of patients with jaundice due to primary hepatic disease have bilirubin ratios in the same general range as is found in cases of biliary obstruction (45% to 80%), there is a significant segment of cases with hepatic disease in which ratios below 40 per cent are encountered. When the bilirubin ratio is below 35 per cent there is little likelihood of confusion with obstructive type jaundice (Watson). Needless to say, there is a great deal of overlapping, and the number of liver function tests verifies this statement.

Two recently described disorders of bilirubin excretion are worthy of note:

(1) *Constitutional hepatic dysfunction* (congenital hepatic dysfunction, familial non-hemolytic icterus, Gilbert's disease) is a benign familial disease characterized by intermittent or chronic icterus with onset in infancy, childhood, or early adulthood. Exacerbations may be induced by strenuous excercise. There is no hepatomegaly and the liver is normal both grossly and histologically. The defect consists in a deficiency of an enzyme (glucuronyl transferase) in the hepatic cells (Arias), which is essential in the production of the conjugated bilirubin derivative (direct reacting type). Therefore, the total which is usually less than 5 mg/100 ml consists mainly of the "indirect type" with a bilirubin ratio less than 29 per cent. The indirect (non-water soluble) is not excreted by the kidneys. During remission, the only abnormality is delayed bilirubin excretion as manifested by the "bilirubin excretion test."

(2) *Chronic idiopathic jaundice* (Dubin-Johnson syndrome, Nelson-Sprintz disease) is a benign familial uncommon disorder which is more common in males (38 males of 47 cases reported). The onset and clinical picture with recurrent icterus and symptoms of fatigue, dyspepsia, aggravation by intercurrent disease and life long course resembles "constitutional hepatic dysfunction." However, it differs from the latter by the presence of dark urine (bilirubinuria) and a major portion (60%) of the serum bilirubin is in the form of conjugated (direct) bilirubin (Dubin). Since the liver cell is able to conjugate the bilirubin, it appears that there is inability to excrete the latter into the bile at the *normal rate* with subsequent regurgitation into the blood and excretion in the urine. Bromsulphalein excretion, which is normal in "constitutional hepatic dysfunction," is impaired and the gallbladder *characteristically* is not visualized on oral cholecystography, even in the absence of jaundice. *Grossly*, hepatomegaly may be present and the otherwise normal liver is discolored "dark brown," "slate blue" to "green black" to "black." *Microscopically*, the liver is normal except for the presence of a granular, brown, lipochrome-like pigment which tends to be confined to the hepatic cells around the central vein and becomes less dense toward the periphery of the lobule. This pigment, thought to be related to lipofuscin, is relatively insoluble, gives a positive Periodic acid-Schiff (PAS) reaction, and is darkly stained by Sudan black B in paraffin sections. There is no evidence of progressive hepatic damage and the disorder is compatible with long life.

MALARIAL PIGMENT

Malarial pigment is formed within erythrocytes by the action of malarial parasites on hemoglobin. Upon disintegration of the erythrocytes, both the parasites and the pigment are liberated and the latter is engulfed by the reticuloendothelial cells of especially the liver and spleen (Plate IC).

The pigment is finely granular and dark brown.   It contains iron but does not give a positive Prussian blue reaction.

HEMATIN

Hematin arises from hemoglobin as a result of the action of acids or alkalis. It is seen in old hemorrhage of the gastrointestinal and urinary tracts and is sometimes present in tissues.   Morphologically it exists as fine, dark brown granules but it is better identified spectroscopically.   Although it contains iron it fails to give a positive Prussian blue reaction.

PORPHYRINS

The term *porphyrin* (Gr. = purple) was first used to designate the iron-free compound obtained when blood is treated with concentrated sulfuric acid (Watson).   Since this was derived from blood the particular porphyrin was referred to as *hematoporphyrin*.   Actually, today the term porphyrin is used to encompass a group of iron-free or magnesium-free pyrrole derivatives which occur universally in protoplasm, which form the basis of the respiratory pigments of both plants and animals, and which may be obtained from chlorophyll or hemoglobin.   Porphyrin complexes are fundamental structural components of compounds which play important roles in a variety of vital metabolic processes, the knowledge of which has been revolutionized in recent years by the use of isotopic tracer techniques (Aldrich and Sunderman).   By utilizing the green magnesium porphyrin chlorophyll, plants (by means of a process known as photosynthesis) are capable of converting carbon dioxide, water, and solar energy into oxygen and organic compounds commonly called food.   The product of photosynthesis—food, on the other hand, is a most essential source of energy for animals and the release of this is dependent upon iron protoporphyrin structures.   Included in the latter group are hemoglobin and myoglobin and such enzymes as catalases, oxidases, peroxidases, and cytochromes.

In the *laboratory* four etioporphyrins were originally synthesized.   They are referred to as series I, II, III, and IV.   Of these, only I and III have thus far been found in nature.   Of these two, series III porphyrins are normally produced in *man* in relatively large proportions and are important in metabolism while series I porphyrins are normally produced in relatively minute amounts and have not yet been shown to possess any important metabolic function.   The actual naturally occurring porphyrins in man are (1) uroporphyrins (I and III) originally identified in urine, (2) coproporphyrins (I and III) originally identified in feces, and (3) protoporphyrins (III) found in hemoglobin. The relationship and metabolic pathway of the group III porphyrins may be as follows (Aldrich and Sunderman). Two molecules of delta aminolevulinic acid (a succinyl derivative of glycine or acetate) condense forming a pyrrole compound called porphobilinogen. Four molecules of porphobilinogen condense to form uroporphyrin III. According to one concept decarboxylation of the acetyl groups of uroporphyrin III results in the formation of coproporphyrin III.   According to another concept porphobilinogen may be transformed directly into coproporphyrin III without passing through an intermediary uroporphyrin III stage.   At any rate coproporphyrin III is then transformed into protoporphyrin III.   This, in turn, unites with ferrous iron to form heme which is a main constituent of hemoglobin, myoglobin, and catalase. The metabolic pathway for series I porphyrins is similar, with this series being formed as a by-product of series III.

Pathologically defective synthesis of porphyrins in man brings about metabolic diseases referred to as porphyria and porphyrinuria. *Porphyria* encompasses those disorders in which relatively large amounts of uroporphyrins and their precursor, porphobilinogen, appear in the urine. *Porphyrinuria* embraces those disturbances in which abnormally large amounts of porphyrins other than uroporphyrins (usually coproporphyrins) appear in the urine.

While there are many *classifications* of *porphyria* the following one proposed by the Sundermans appears to be quite satisfactory: (1) erythropoietic porphyria and (2) hepatic porphyria with subdivisions (*a*) paroxysmal hepatic porphyria, (*b*) photosensitive hepatic porphyria, and (*c*) combined paroxysmal and photosensitive hepatic porphyria.

Erythropoietic porphyria is a rare disorder arising as a result of a genetic enzymatic defect in the synthesis of hemoglobin. It is usually discovered in infancy or early childhood, predominates in males, and is characterized by (1) sensitivity of the skin to sunlight with development of bullæ, vesicles, melanosis, and hypertrichosis in exposed areas, (2) susceptibility of the skin to trauma, (3) hemolytic anemia, (4) splenomegaly, (5) red teeth and skeleton due to deposition of uroporphyrin I, and (6) burgundy-red colored urine which deepens on standing. This red color is due to the presence of large amounts of uroporphyrin I and coproporphyrin I in the free state. Examination of bone marrow by ultra-fluorescent microscopy discloses abnormal deposits of porphyrins within normoblasts. The course of erythropoietic porphyria is protracted, with death occurring after a period of years from secondary infection or anemia. Some patients are benefited by splenectomy.

Hepatic porphyria is the most common variety of porphyria observed clinically. It occurs as a result of genetically or chemically induced disturbance of porphyrin metabolism in the liver with the fault residing primarily in the enzyme catalase. *Paroxysmal hepatic porphyria* (also called acute porphyria) arises in the third and fourth decades of life and affects women more frequently than men. The clinical manifestations may be (1) gastrointestinal consisting of pain, vomiting, constipation, and diarrhea, (2) neurologic consisting of motor weakness, hyporeflexes, muscle pain, and sensory loss, (3) mental consisting of irritability, psychosis, and delerium, and (4) miscellaneous consisting of tachycardia, hypertension, fever, pigmentation, red urine, and hepatic dysfunction. Photosensitivity is absent. The diagnosis is made on finding excessive amounts of (1) porphobilinogen in urine, (2) uroporphyrin I and III and coproporphyrins I and III in the urine and feces, and (3) porphobilinogen and uroporphyrin in a biopsy of the liver. Treatment is unsatisfactory. *Photosensitive hepatic porphyria* (also called porphyria cutanea tarda) occurs after the second decade and is more common in men. It is a disturbance of hepatic porphyrin metabolism associated with hepatic insufficiency, alcoholism, diabetes, or syphilis. It is characterized by cutaneous photosensitivity, susceptibility of the skin to trauma, hypertrichosis, brown discoloration of the skin, abdominal colic, hypertension, psychosis, neuritis, and red urine. The diagnosis is made upon finding excessive amounts of (1) uroporphyrin I and III and coproporphyrin I and III in the urine and feces, and (2) uroporphyrin in a biopsy of the liver. Treatment consists of a high protein diet, vitamin B_{12} and abstinence from alcohol and barbiturates. The prognosis is good. *Combined paroxysmal and photosensitive hepatic porphyria* includes those cases of hepatic porphyria in which abdominal pain and neurologic manifestations are combined with photosensitivity.

Porphyrinuria occurs secondary to (1) chemical toxicity, (2) hypermetabolism as in fevers, thyrotoxicosis, and exercise, (3) hepatic disease as cirrhosis, hepatitis, and cancer, (4) hematologic conditions as pernicious anemia, hemolytic anemias, hemochromatosis, and lymphoblastoma, (5) hypovitaminosis, and (6) no detectable preceding condition. Of these, the chemical toxicity group is especially important for it includes various metals (lead, arsenic, mercury, bismuth, *etc.*), sedatives, sulfonamides, alcohol, and industrial compounds as TNT, methyl chloride, and carbon tetrachloride. The diagnosis of porphyrinuria is established by demonstrating abnormally large amounts of ether-soluble porphyrins (chiefly coproporphyrins) in the urine.

In *animals*, other than man, spontaneous porphyria resembling the erythropoietic type in man occurs in cattle and pigs while physiologic porphyria resembling the hepatic porphyria in man occurs in the fox squirrel (Aldrich). *Experimentally* rabbits treated with various combinations of lead, phenylhydrazine, Rose Bengal dye, and ultraviolet light develop porphyria that resembles mostly the erythropoietic type but also with features of the hepatic type in man. Experimentally also rabbits, rats, and chickens treated with allylisopropylacetylcarbamide or allylisopropylacetamide develop porphyria resembling paroxysmal hepatic (intermittent acute) porphyria in man. In this group the liver catalase activity is reduced to low levels due to impaired synthesis of this enzyme. In porphyric chick embryos there is an excellent correlation between a reduction in uric acid excretion and a simultaneous increase in porphyrin excretion. This indicates a derangement in purine metabolism and is explained by the fact that both purines and porphyrins use delta aminolevulinic acid in their formation. Thus, while all the answers are not yet known, the use of appropriate drugs in the production of experimental porphyria shows promise for future enhancement of our knowledge of porphyrin metabolism.

CHLOROMA

Chloroma is a rare type of myeloid leukemia characterized by the formation of greenish colored tumor masses. Experimentally, a green-pigment-producing myelogenous leukemia has been produced in Wistar rats by gastric instillation of methylcholanthrene (Shay). An analysis of the pigment in this experimental chloroma has shown it to be due to a variety of porphyrins but consisting chiefly of protoporphyrins and to a lesser extent of coproporphyrins (Schultz). At one time it was thought that the accumulation of the pigment in chloroma tissue may have been due to (1) result of abnormal hemoglobin catabolism, (2) blood already present in the tissue, or (3) to affinity of chloroma tissue for porphyrins produced in large amounts in nontumor tissue. Because the ratio of protoporphyrins to coproporphyrins is the same in chloroma tissue as it is in normal liver, erythrocytes, and bone marrow it is more probable, however, that excessive amounts of porphyrins are produced directly by the chloroma tissue rather than absorbed by it as a result of catabolic processes elsewhere. Furthermore, this excessive production may be due to a verdoperoxidase which has been demonstrated in unusually large amounts in the chloroma tissue itself.

LIPOCHROMES

Lipochromes (Gr. = fat + pigment) are fat-soluble, weakly fat-positive, hydrocarbon pigments that are found both in the animal and plant kingdoms. They are also known as *chromolipoids* and *carotinoids*. Morphologically the pigments exist as fine, yellow intracytoplasmic granules. In *man*, lipochrome pigment has been identified in practically every tissue of the body but is especially prevalent in heart muscle in brown atrophy (Fig. 3 p. 32), adrenal cortex, corpus luteum of the ovary, seminal vesicles, interstitial cells of Leydig, nerve ganglion cells, and even the stratum corneum where it is one of the pigments responsible for the normal color of the skin (Cohen). Lipochromes are also found in products of animal origin such as eggs, butter, milk, and cheese (Bickoff). Regardless of the animal tissues or animal products in which they are found, the sources of animal lipochromes are exogenous (ingested vegetables) or endogenous (animal tissue metabolites). In *plants*, lipochromes are generally referred to as carotinoids and consist of a number of pigments that include both carotenes and xanthophylls. All green plant tissue contains carotinoids in which the chief component is beta carotene. Yellow plant tissue such as corn, carrots, sweet potatoes, and yams are especially rich in carotinoids. Aside from rendering color to animal tissue, carotene is of even greater importance in that it is a precursor of vitamin A, with the conversion occurring in the wall of the intestine (Morton). An excessive amount of lipochrome pigmentation in man is referred to as *carotenemia*. In this condition the skin assumes a yellowish discoloration due to an overabundant accumulation of carotinoids in the stratum corneum. The pigmentation is especially marked in the palms and soles. In most instances, carotenemia is alimentary in origin, that is, arises on the basis of eating large amounts of vegetables rich in carotene over a prolonged period. In other instances, however, it may be secondary to diabetes mellitus, hypothyroidism, nephritis, or disorders of the liver. Carotenemia as such is harmless but it is important to recognize the disorder for it may be readily mistaken for a much more serious condition—jaundice.

Ceroid is a pigment that may be related to lipochrome. It develops from cells containing fat and was first identified as light greenish-yellow globules of variable size and shape in periportal fibrous tissue in experimental dietary cirrhosis in rats (Popper). It is insoluble in fat solvents, takes a positive fat stain, and is fluorescent. In man, the pigment is found (1) in the liver, heart muscle, and other tissues in nutritional disorders in which there is impairment of intestinal absorption, (2) in cirrhosis of the liver, (3) in hemochromatosis, and (4) in focal degenerative lesions (Pappenheimer and Victor). The pigmentation is probably related to vitamin E deficiency.

MELANIN

Melanin (Gr. = black) is an amorphous pigment that normally is responsible for the color in the hair, skin, adrenals, choroid, and pia. Grossly it appears dark brown, bluish, or black while microscopically it consists of fine, deep brown, intracellular and extracellular granules (Plate ID). Cells containing the pigment are of two varieties—those that simply carry the pigment and those that form it. Cells that carry the pigment are derived from the reticulo-endothelial system, are purely phagocytic, and are called *melanophages* or *melanophores*. Cells that form the pigment are derived from the neural crest, are thus neuro-ectodermal in origin, and are called *melanoblasts* when they are immature and *melanocytes* when they are mature. Melanocytes can be identified morphologically by staining with silver, gold, or methylene blue and histochemically by the *dopa* (3–4 dihydroxyphenyla-lanine) reaction. In the skin, melanocytes are located in the basal layer of the epidermis, in the hair bulbs, and in lesions called nevi (p 1393). The cells are continually renewed and in this process the pigment is eliminated about every three weeks either by shedding through the skin surface or with the stratum corneum or by being absorbed by the lymphatics (Lerner).

The *formation* of *melanin* is a complicated enzymatic chain reaction which in essence consists of the oxidation of the amino acid tyrosine by the enzyme tyrosinase to produce the brown pigment. Tyrosinase is a copper enzyme complex (with the copper ions playing a vital role in the reaction) located in the mitochondrial elements in the cytoplasm of melanocytes. More specifically, as a result of hormonal or sympathetic nervous stimulation, the enzyme tyrosinase by an oxidation process converts tyrosine to dopa. Dopa in turn is oxidized to produce a dopa quinone in which the nitrogen undergoes ring closure resulting in the formation of a leucocompound. The leucocompound is oxidized to form indole, 5, 6—quinone which is oxidized and polymerized to form melanin. From this it is apparent that the forma-tion of melanin depends upon the availability of (1) the enzyme tyrosinase, (2) the substrate tyrosine, and (3) molecular oxygen. The absence of any one of these will result in a decrease in melanin formation and, conversely, the overabundance of each of these will result in an increase in melanin formation.

The *rate* of *melanin formation* is *controlled* by (1) temperature, (2) reduc-tion-oxidation potential within the cell, (3) agents affecting the copper ions of tyrosinase, (4) hormones, and (5) neurogenic impulses.

Temperature is an important factor in the rate and amount of pigment formation. *In vitro* studies indicate that the reaction proceeds slowly at 25 °C, that it becomes more rapid at 37 °C, and that it ceases above 50 °C due to destruction of the enzyme. *In vivo*, a normal increase in temperature in body folds and mucous membranes results in hyperpigmentation, and abnormal increase in temperature caused by exposure to a hot water bottle, burning fireplace, or hot stove results in similar deposition of pigment in affected areas.

The *reduction-oxidation* (redox) *potential* near the location of tyrosinase in the melanocyte is important in tyrosinase activity which in turn is the all important first step in the chain reaction in melanin formation. Hyper-pigmentation is usually a sequel of ionizing irradiation. The mechanism of excessive pigment formation in this connection may be that the ionizing irradiation produces a reduction-oxidation potential more favorable to tyrosinase thus increasing its activity and increasing the output of the pigment.

As already stated, the *copper ions* of *tyrosinase* play a vital role in the chain reaction leading to melanin formation. Thus, anything that combines and inactivates the copper ions will also inhibit the action of tyrosinase and this, of course, will decrease the formation of melanin. The sulfhydryl groups act in this capacity. Conversely, anything that oxidizes, combines with, or destroys sulfhydryl groups will favor the activity of tyrosinase and the formation of melanin. This is probably the mechanism in the increased pigmentation seen after exposure to ultraviolet light and ionizing irradiation, treatment with arsenic, and inflammation.

There are many *hormones* that have a direct or indirect bearing on the amount of melanin produced by the body. The intermediate lobe of the *pituitary* produces two melanocyte-stimulating hormones referred to as alpha and beta MSH. Administration of MSH to man results in increased generalized pigmentation that resembles Addison's disease and in an increase in pigmentation of cutaneous nevi. The changes, incidentally, are more striking in dark-colored than in light-colored people. Such pigmentation, however, is only temporary for the skin returns to normal a few weeks after MSH is discontinued. Further evidence of the importance of MSH in melanin formation is gleaned from the fact that (1) the blood and urine levels of MSH are increased during pregnancy, in Addison's disease, and in alopecia areata, (2) MSH was absent in the urine of a hypophysectomized man, (3) there is an increase of pigmentation and of excretion of MSH in man after bilateral adrenalectomy and prevention of pigmentation together with decreased MSH excretion upon treatment with cortisone and hydrocortisone, and (4) there is darkening of isolated frog skin upon exposure to MSH and prevention of darkening by adding small quantities of adrenalin or noradrenalin to the solution. *Steroid hormones* of various types also affect melanin production. *In vitro*, progesterone darkens frog skin. In pregnancy there is an increase in progesterone, MSH, and pigmentation. Estrogens applied to nipples of guinea pigs result in both an enlargement and a darkening of these structures. Diethylstilbesterol administered to a hypo-ovarian woman produced darkening of the nipples, linea alba, and pigmented nevi. Chronic liver disease is attended by an increase of circulating estrogens and darkening of the skin. Eunuchoid males will not acquire a suntan unless they are treated with testosterone. Finally, as already stated, cortisone and hydrocortisone decrease pigmentation by interfering with release of MSH. The *thyroid gland* plays a role in pigmentation but the exact mechanism is unknown. It is a fact, for example, that patients with hypothyroidism tend to have vitiligo. In fowl, thyroxin is needed for normal pigmentation of feathers of both male and female brown leghorn chickens. In fish, administration of crude thyroid extract to rainbow trout results in blanching of the skin. *Other drugs* also have an effect on pigmentation. Mesantoin (an anti-convulsant) given over a prolonged period produces hyperpigmentation that is similar to Addison's disease. It also has an MSH-like action on the isolated frog skin. Chloroquin, used in the treatment of lupus erythematosus, has lightened the color of hair in children. Whether these drugs act through hormonal, neurogenic, or enzymatic processes is not known.

Melanocytes are subjected to *neurogenic control*. This should not be surprising in view of the fact (1) that melanocytes arise from neural crests, (2) that they resemble nerve cells in that they are dendritic in shape, (3) that they produce dopa which is similar chemically to noradrenalin produced by adrenal medulla—an organ that is also of nerve tissue origin, and (4) that they give use to tumors which are resistant to irradiation to a degree comparable to other neurogenic tumors. In fish, severing the nerve to a fin results in darkening of the color. As the nerve regenerates the fin becomes lighter. Faradic stimulation of the intact nerve is accompanied by a blanching of the color of the fin. In man, most cases of neurofibromatosis (tumors of peripheral nerves) are accompanied by pigmented (café au lait spots) cutaneous areas, and vitiligo (areas of depigmentation) is said to be due to an increase in activity of the sympathetic nervous system at the nerve endings. Finally, the two hormones—adrenalin and noradrenalin, both produced by nerve tissue, inhibit the darkening action of MSH on isolated frog skin.

In *man*, there is *normally* considerable *variation* in the *pigmentation* of the skin, hair, and eyes which runs the gamut from white to black. This variation is due to the pigment producing capacities of melanocytes and the amount of pigment in a melanocyte is determined by a balance of enzymatic, hormonal, and neurogenic factors. The albino, white man, and Negro have the same number of melanocytes in any one location and excrete the same quantity of MSH in the urine. In the albino, however, there is a genetic absence of tyrosinase so that melanin cannot be formed. In darker skinned races (1) the total amount of tyrosinase may be increased, (2) the normal inhibitors of tyrosinase may be decreased, or (3) the reduction-oxidation potential in melanocytes may be more favorable for tyrosinase action. At *birth* the skin is light colored and is usually free from pigmentary lesions. Shortly *thereafter* nevi and freckles appear and the nevi grow and darken in color for the first three decades of life. During the first two decades the skin, hair, and eyes darken in color. About the latter one-half of the fourth decade the hair lightens and eventually turns gray. In *all age groups* hyperpigmentation occurs (1) in exposed areas due to increased numbers of melanocytes and repeated exposure to ultraviolet light, (2) in body folds due to increased numbers of melanocytes and to increased temperature, and (3) at sites of pressure and trauma due to increased temperature from accelerated blood flow or direct effect of pressure.

Variations in pigment formation, either *hyperpigmentation* or *hypopigmentation*, are many. They have already been mentioned and discussed in the preceding paragraphs and are again referred to under the various diseases as they are discussed throughout the text. At this point, therefore, they need only be enumerated under the following nine etiologic headings (Lerner): (1) *Genetic*—hyperpigmentation consisting of racial, freckles, pigmented nevi, and senile lentigines, and hypopigmentation consisting of albinism and premature graying of hair, (2) *Physical*—hyperpigmentation consisting of ionizing irradiation and heat, and hypopigmentation consisting of severe thermal burns and severe trauma, (3) *Chemical*—hyperpigmentation consisting of heavy metal intoxication (arsenic, silver, and bismuth) and photosensitization (psoralen derivatives), and hypopigmentation consisting of hydroquinone derivatives and chemical burns, (4) *Endocrine*—hyperpigmentation consisting of Addison's disease, ACTH therapy, hyperthyroidism, acromegaly, pregnancy, estrogen or androgen therapy, and chronic hepatic insufficiency, and hypopigmentation consisting of panhypopituitarism, (5) *Neurogenic*—hyperpigmentation consisting of café au lait spots (pigmented areas associated with neurofibromatosis) and lines of demarcation, and hypopigmentation consisting of vitiligo and alopecia areata, (6) *Nutritional*—hyperpigmentation consisting of malnutrition and pellagra and hypopigmentation consiting of pantothenic acid and para-aminobenzoic acid deficiency, (7) *Inflammatory*—hyperpigmentation consisting of chronic systemic infection (as tuberculosis) and chronic dermatoses and hypopigmentation consisting of leprosy and pinta, (8) *Neoplastic*—hyperpigmentation consisting of chronic illness with any tumor, acanthoiss nigricans, and melanoblastoma, and (9) *Unclassified*—hyperpigmentation consisting of scleroderma, hemochromatosis, skin graft, polyostotic fibrous dysplasia, melanosis coli, and intestinal polyposis, and hypopigmentation consisting of scleroderma and skin graft.

Melanosis coli is an innocuous brown to black pigmentation of the mucosa

6

of the large intestine and appendix characterized by the presence of melanin granules, both free and in melanophores (Fig. 25). The condition is usually seen in people beyond forty years of age, is associated with chronic constipation, and results from a conversion of protein disintegration products into melanin by intestinal ferments.

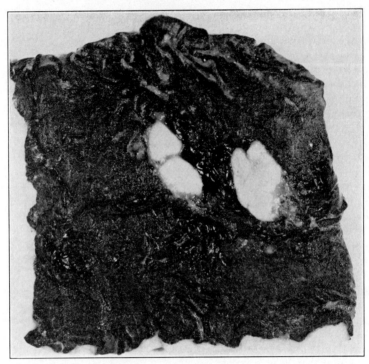

Fig. 25.—Melanosis coli showing dark pigmentation of the mucosa of a segment of the large bowel. The two white areas represent cut surfaces of two tumor nodules that are unrelated to the melanosis.

Hereditary ochronosis is an hereditary disease representing an inborn error of phenylalanine and tyrosine intermediary metabolism (Lichtenstein and Cooper). Normally a certain gene controls the enzyme which makes possible the breakdown of the benzene ring of homogentisic acid (an intermediary metabolite of the amino acids phenylalanine and tyrosine) by way of aceto-acetic acid to carbon dioxide and water. In ochronosis this gene and dependent enzyme are lacking. As a result, the homogentisic acid cannot be metabolized and is excreted in the urine and deposited in the tissues. Under these circumstances, therefore, it is not surprising that a diet rich in phenylalanine and tyrosine augments the formation of homogentisic acid and, conversely, a diet poor in these amino acids decreases its formation. *Experimentally* white rats fed a diet rich in phenylalanine and guinea pigs fed a diet deficient in vitamin C excrete homogentisic acid in the urine. *Clinically* hereditary ochronosis is carried as a mendelian recessive in about one out of every 500 persons, appears as a disease in about one out of 1,000,000 persons, and starts in early life. The two most obvious *manifestations* are a dark urine and gray-blue to black discoloration of the skin. The urinary change is referred to as *alkaptonuria*—the presence of alkaptone or homogentisic acid in the urine. If the urine is acid, upon excretion, it is of normal color but if it is alkaline, or is made so upon standing or addition of ammonium hydroxide, it becomes dark brown to black (Jensen). The cutaneous changes are due to *pathologic* deposition of homogentisic acid within endothelial cells of blood vessels, macrophages, sweat glands, and sebaceous glands. Similar pigment is deposited throughout the body in cartilage, intima and media of blood vessels, normal or pathologic dense connective tissue, tendons, cardiac valves, epithelial cells of the proximal convoluted tubules of the kidneys, and endocrine glands such as the islet cells of the pancreas, pineal gland, and pituitary gland. Far from harmless, hereditary ochronosis may *ultimately eventuate in* disabling osteo-arthritis and spondylitis, cardiac lesions such as aortic stenosis, severe arteriosclerosis, ochronitic nephrosis, and urinary calculi.

Exogenous ochronosis consists of a deposition of a brown pigment in areas similar to that in hereditary ochronosis but due to prolonged use of phenol-containing compounds (carbolic and picric acid) as in dressings for cutaneous ulcers (Lichtenstein). Actually, the designation is a misnomer for the pigment in urine and in tissues is 2, 5-dihydroxyphenyl-acetic acid and not homogentisic acid. Also, unlike hereditary ochronosis, the disturbance ceases upon discontinuation of use of the phenol-containing compounds.

EXOGENOUS PIGMENTATION

Exogenous pigments reach the body by one of the following three routes: (1) skin—*tattoo*, (2) respiratory tract—various *dusts*, producing lesions that are collectively called *pneumoconioses*, and (3) gastrointestinal tract—*plumbism* and *argyria*. Of these, the *pneumoconioses* will be omitted from discussion for they are considered in conjunction with the Lower Respiratory System, Chapter 12, page 462.

TATTOO

Tattoo (Polynesian = puncturation) is a form of body marking accomplished nowadays by introducing various pigments into the dermis with an electric needle. Three chief *pigments* used are (1) India ink, giving a blue or black color, (2) mercuric sulfide, imparting a red color, and (3) kurkuma, producing a yellow color. Following the completion of the procedure, the skin becomes swollen, hot, and crusted but in a week the crusts fall off and the *design* (unlimited in variance) becomes apparent (Fig. 26). *Histologically* the pigment is seen deposited between the connective tissue cells of the dermis. Of the three pigments, mercuric sulfide is the most irritating and it may produce not only local inflammation and excessive fibrous tissue formation but also changes (hyperkeratosis and acanthosis) in the epidermis.

PLUMBISM

Plumbism (L. = lead) is lead intoxication or poisoning. The condition occurs mostly in industry, especially in connection with manufacture of storage batteries (Belknap). The *routes* of lead absorption are the gastrointestinal and respiratory tracts. Clinically a distinction is usually made between lead absorption and lead intoxication. *Lead absorption* simply means excessive uptake of lead by the system and its presence in the body.

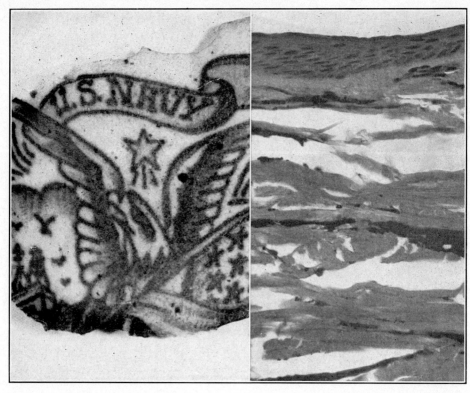

FIG. 26.—Tattoo illustrating, to the left, a well-defined gross design and, to the right, deposition of strands of black pigment between collagenous connective tissue cells. (The separation of the fibers represents an artifact.) × 400.

One of its chief manifestations is the presence of a fine line of blue-black lead sulfide deposited in the submucosal papillæ of the gums at their junction with the teeth. Other evidences of lead absorption are basophilic stippling of erythrocytes and elevated lead levels in the urine and blood. *Lead intoxication* is lead absorption of sufficient degree to produce (in addition to the above) a variety of clinical manifestations, among which are (1) anemia (due to destruction of erythrocytes), (2) intestinal colic (due to spasm of smooth muscle), (3) palsy (especially wrist drop—due to degeneration of axis cylinders of nerves), and (4) lead encephalopathy (due to edema and to ganglion cell loss consequent to vascular occlusion from endothelial proliferation).

ARGYRIA

Argyria (Gr. = silver) is a condition of permanent ashen-gray discoloration of the skin, mucous membranes, and internal organs brought about by the prolonged use of silver salts (Fig. 27). The disorder usually occurs in patients beyond forty years of age and generally takes from two to three years to develop. The silver gains *entrance* into the body by way of the gastrointestinal tract (pills or capsules), respiratory tract (sprays, nose drops, or paints), and other mucous membranes (irrigations). *Histologically*, brilliantly illuminated granules of silver are readily identifiable under dark field illumination in the following cutaneous structures: (1) elastic fibers of the corium, (2) basement membranes of the sweat glands, sebaceous glands, and hair follicles, (3) vessels, (4) muscles, and (5) nerves (Hill and Montgomery). In general, it may be stated that silver granules (whichever organ is involved) are found between connective tissue and elastic fibers and, less often, within phagocytes (Gettler).

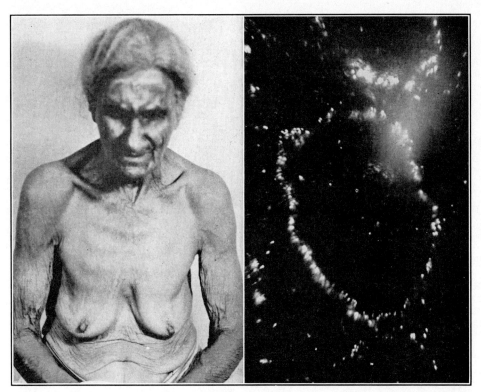

FIG. 27.—Argyria in a white woman showing, to the left, the typical ashen-gray discoloration of the skin and, to the right, brilliantly illuminated silver granules in the skin. Dark field. × 100.

NECROSIS

Necrosis (Gr. = deadness) connotes local death of tissue. The term is really synonymous with *necrobiosis* (Gr. = dead body + life) although the latter is often used to indicate physiologic death of cells as, for example, the continuous death of the superficial cells of the epidermis. The *causes* of death of tissue are the same as the causes of disease and, in general, may be listed as bacteria, rickettsia, viruses, fungi, parasites, chemicals, heat, cold, light, electricity, irradiation, foreign bodies, and trauma.

The *morphologic* changes observed in the cells actually occur as a result of enzymatic action after the cells have died. They are both nuclear and cytoplasmic. Of the two, the *nuclear* changes are more significant. They consist of (1) *karyorrhexis* (Gr. = nut + to split) in which the nuclear membrane breaks and the chromatin material is dispersed in the form of irregular, deeply staining, intensely basophilic granules, (2) *karyolysis* (Gr. = nut + loosening) or *chromatolysis* (Gr. = color + loosening) in which the nucleus enlarges, becomes lighter staining or watery, and gradually fades from view, and (3) *pyknosis* (Gr. = condensation) in which the nucleus decreases in size and the chromatin condenses into a solid, densely basophilic, structureless mass (Fig. 28). In any case, the retrograde process continues until ultimately the nucleus and its remnants completely disappear. The *cytoplasmic* changes are those of degeneration. In some instances, the cytoplasm from the onset becomes more and more watery and lighter staining. In other instances it becomes more and more condensed and more intensely eosinophilic. In either case, the cell membrane ultimately ruptures and the cytoplasm disintegrates and disperses.

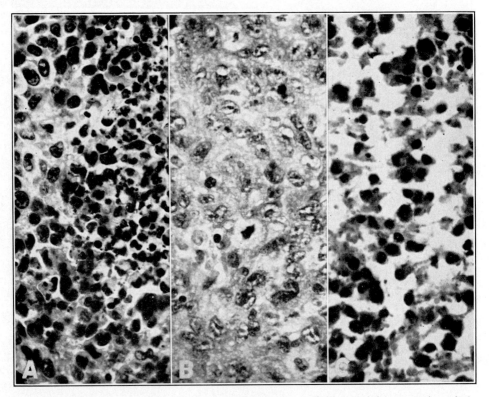

Fig. 28.—Necrosis showing *A*, normal cells about the periphery and fragmentation of the nuclei (karyorrhexis) centrally and to the right, *B*, ballooning and gradual fading of the nuclei (karyolysis), and *C*, shrinking and condensation of the nuclei (pyknosis).

Grossly necrosis may be divided into several types depending upon the tissue involved and the causative agent (Figs. 29 and 30). *Coagulation* (L. = clotting or gelling) *necrosis* is best seen following arteriolar occlusiod in organs as the spleen and kidneys where the arteries are more or less enn arteries and the anastomosis is poor. The involved area is grayish-white, peripherally located, solid, and firm. Histologically the structural pattern of the affected tissue can still be discerned but the cellular details are lost. *Caseation* (L. = cheese) *necrosis* is the type of tissue death occurring in tuberculosis. The affected area is grayish-white, dry, and crumbly. Histologically the architecture is completely lost and the cells are replaced with fine, amorphous, eosinophilic granules. *Liquefaction* or *colliquative necrosis* is tissue death attended by fluidification of the involved area. It is best seen in the central nervous system following arterial occlusion but is also encountered in other tissues, especially when the area is invaded by bacteria. Grossly, the center of the lesion is replaced with varicolored fluid while the periphery consists of soft, gray, friable tissue. Histologically the former exists as an empty space or, at most, as precipitated protein while the latter shows tissue in various stages of disintegration. *Fat necrosis*

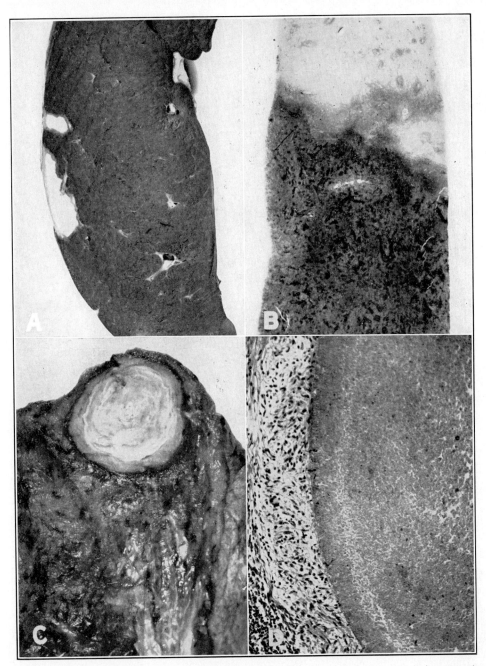

Fig. 29.—Necrosis showing *A* and *B*, gross and microscopic appearance of coagulation necrosis of the spleen and *C* and *D*, gross and microscopic appearance of caseation necrosis of the lung.

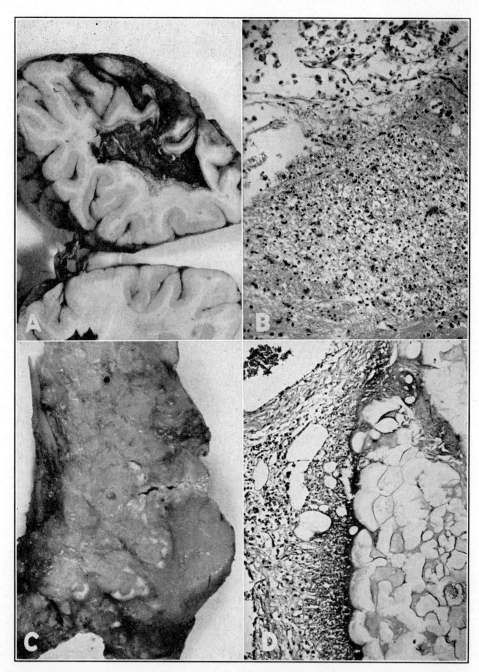

Fig. 30.—Necrosis showing *A* and *B*, gross and microscopic appearance of liquefaction necrosis of the brain and *C* and *D*, gross and microscopic appearance of fat necrosis of the pancreas.

means simply necrosis of fat tissue. Usually it is brought about by lipases released upon disintegration of pancreatic tissue or rupture of the pancreatic ducts, but occasionally the lesion results from direct trauma. The fat is split into glycerol and fatty acids and the latter react with calcium to form a calcium soap. Grossly, the lesion is characterized by sharply circumscribed, firm, chalk-like areas. Histologically the affected fat cells are filled with opaque, granular material. At the junction with normal tissue there is a zone of granular, bluish-staining material (calcium soap) and beyond this, a zone of inflammation.

The *fate* of necrotic tissue is variable. It may (1) extend to produce larger areas of necrosis (gangrene) and cause death of the patient, (2) become liquefied and absorbed with restoration to normal by regeneration of tissue similar to the original, (3) extend to the surface and become transformed into an ulcer, (4) be completely replaced by fibrous tissue, (5) remain in its necrotic state (when large) but become walled off by a fibrous tissue capsule, or (6) ultimately become calcified or even ossified.

GANGRENE

Gangrene may be *defined* as massive death of tissue with addition of saprophytic organisms. It *affects* both the exposed and the internal portions of the body although the former are generally considered as typifying the process because they are more readily apparent. The fundamental *cause* of gangrene is interference in circulation. As a rule, this is relegated to *arterial obstruction* and, among others, consists of (1) congenital anomalies (weakness of the wall with rupture and hemorrhage), (2) degenerations (senile or diabetic arteriosclerosis obliterans), (3) inflammations (thromboangiitis obliterans and acute inflammations), (4) physical disturbances (consisting of (*a*) spasm as seen in trench foot, immersion foot, frostbite, ergotism, and Raynaud's disease, (*b*) plugging of the lumen with a blood clot, (*c*) simple prolonged pressure, and (*d*) severance), and (5) tumors (causing compression from the outside). Sometimes gangrene results primarily from *venous obstruction* (ligation of femoral veins, inflammation, or occlusion by pressure from the outside). Once the tissue is destroyed, *saprophytic organisms* are added (1) from the skin—consisting of *B. subtilis*, staphylococci, streptococci, and diphtheroids, (2) from the gastrointestinal tract—consisting of streptococci, colon bacilli, *B. lactis aerogenes*, and *Cl. welchii*, or (3) from the respiratory tract—consisting of diphtheroids, streptococci, staphylococci, pneumococci, spirochetes and fusiform bacilli, and *M. tetragenous*. *Microscopically* gangrene discloses all the changes seen in necrosis. When the process is fully developed, however, it reveals complete replacement of all cellular structures with stringy or granular debris. *Grossly* gangrene is generally conveniently divided into three types—dry, moist, and gas gangrene.

Dry gangrene, as the term indicates, is gangrene unattended by moisture. It is the type usually seen in a lower extremity in old age and diabetes mellitus. It results from a gradual occlusion of arterial supply in the presence of relatively good venous drainage. The portion of the limb furthest away from the heart becomes affected first. Initially it becomes pale, cold, clammy, and pulseless. The actual necrotic changes generally begin in the great toe adjacent to the nail bed or over a callus. They consist of a livid, black to green discoloration (due to disintegration products of erythrocytes) attended by drying, shrinkage, mummification, and a peculiar

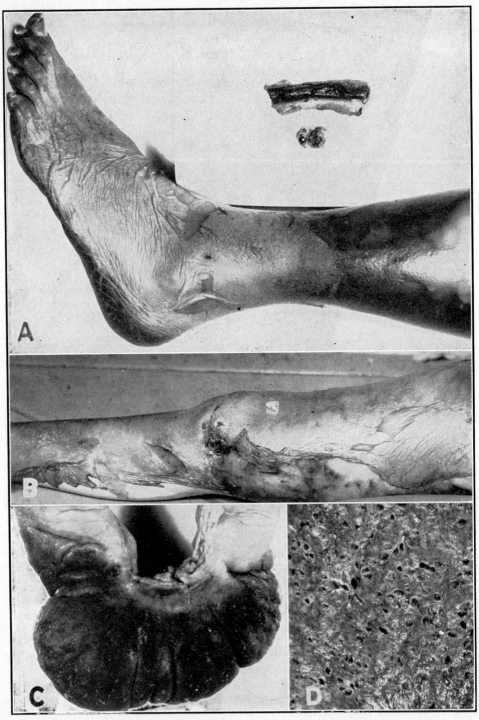

FIG. 31.—Gangrene. *A*, early dry gangrene of a lower extremity due to occlusion of the femoral artery (inset) by a blood clot. *B*, moist gangrene showing swelling and mottling of the extremity as a whole and blistering and sloughing of the epidermis. *C*, moist gangrene of a segment of small elbow revealing intense discoloration. *D*, gas gangrene of the liver disclosing numerous small gas bubbles.

musty (due to disintegration products of proteins) odor (Fig. 31*A*). Gradually the process extends proximally until it reaches a level where the blood supply is adequate. At this point the affected tissue is sharply demarcated from the viable tissue and the latter discloses a zone of inflammatory reaction of varying width and intensity. Although saprophytic organisms are present in dry gangrene they do not flourish because lack of moisture and decrease in temperature are not conducive to their multiplication.

Moist gangrene is massive death of tissue maintained in a wet state and accompanied by overwhelming proliferation of saprophytic organisms It is the type usually seen in internal organs such as the bowel, lungs, ovarian tumors, etc., and is occasionally encountered in an extremity (Figs. 31*B* and 31*C*). It results from a more or less rapid occlusion of arterial supply in the presence of relatively poor venous drainage or, rarely, from rapid venous occlusion alone. In contrast to dry gangrene, the process spreads rapidly and is not as sharply demarcated. The part becomes varicolored, swollen, tense, and malodorous. If an extremity is affected the epidermis may blister and slough. Because of rapid formation and absorption of tissue and bacterial protein split products, patients with moist gangrene frequently reveal profound clinical manifestations and, if not treated properly, die from the overwhelming toxemia.

Gas gangrene is moist gangrene abounding in gas-producing, anaerobic organisms. Chief among these is *Clostridium welchii*—a gram-positive, nonmotile, spore-bearing organism that is normally found in the gastrointestinal tract and soil. This type of gangrene is thus encountered in massive necrosis of the intestinal tract and in wounds (war casualties) contaminated with feces or soil. Because the organisms are gas-producing the affected tissues, especially muscle which contains an abundance of glycogen, become filled with bubbles of gas which can be both seen and felt. Sooner or later, the organisms gain entrance into the general circulation where they produce an overwhelming systemic reaction and frequently death. In such cases the liver is found to be riddled with varisized gas bubbles (Fig. 31*D*).

VITAMINS

Joseph F. McCloskey

Vitamins (L. = life + amine) may be defined as a group of unrelated organic compounds occurring usually in small amounts in many foods and being essential for normal metabolic function and nutrition of the body. *Avitaminosis* is any disease resulting from a deficiency of vitamins. The deficiency may be due to a lack of the compound in the diet, to a lack of assimilation, or to a lack of proper utilization by the animal host. Many, if not all vitamins, play an active role in the intracellular enzyme systems. The *nomenclature* used in connection with vitamins is still quite confusing. Originally, they were given names according to the letters of the alphabet or according to the deficiency disease produced. However, as their chemical formulæ were discovered, an attempt was made to standardize the nomenclature accordingly. Presently, most authors have reverted to using the alphabetical letters to indicate the major groups and to using the chemical name to designate the subgroups.

VITAMIN A

Vitamin A, the anti-xerophthalmic or anti-infective vitamin, is found in both plants and animals. In *plants* it exists as a group of red or yellow, fat soluble, plant pigments known as *carotenes*, the most important of which is beta carotene. These pigments, *found* in green leafy vegetables such as spinach, green peas, and cabbage and in yellow or red vegetables such as carrots and corn, must be converted into vitamin A within the wall of the intestinal tract. The most important source of *animal* vitamin A is in fish liver oils where it is usually found in the form of esters or bound to a protein molecule. Saponification of these oils is necessary for the liberation of the pure vitamin. Vitamin A is now produced synthetically and is marketed as an acetate or the palmitate ester. These esters, synthetic or naturally occurring, are hydrolized by enzymes of the intestinal tract and absorbed in the upper portion of the small intestine in the form of an alcohol. *Chemically*, vitamin A is a high molecular primary aliphatic alcohol which occurs in several forms. Some of these are mere stereoisomers while others result from the hydrogenation, oxidation, or dehydration of vitamin A_1 (axerophthol). All of the various compounds have similar actions and can be regarded as one. Vitamin A is *essential* to the *health* and *growth* of all vertebræ. It participates in the formation of *visual purple* (rhodopsin) and maintains the health of epithelial cells. A *deficiency* of vitamin A in animals causes severe retardation of skeletal growth. In man, the deficiency results in night blindness (nyctalopia) and changes in epithelium, particularly of the secretory type. First there is manifest atrophy. This is followed by a reactive hyperplasia of the basal cells resulting in replacement by keratinizing stratified squamous epithelium. These changes occur in the conjunctival, corneal, and lacrimal gland epithelium and result in *xerophthalmia*. In this condition, the scleræ become inflamed and may ulcerate. Secondary infection through this ulceration results in panophthalmitis. Similar changes in the respiratory epithelium result in atelectasis, pneumonia, and bronchiectasis. Metaplastic changes occur also in the epithelium of the renal pelves, uterus, salivary gland ducts, and sebaceous gland ducts. *Cortical hyperostosis*, especially of the ulna and metatarsal bones, occurs in chronic vitamin A poisoning both in man and animals due to the ingestion of massive amounts of the vitamin.

VITAMIN B COMPLEX

In 1911 Funk published a series of papers describing the isolation from rice polishings of a substance (vitamin B) capable of curing beri-beri. In 1920 Emmett and Luros, basing their contention on finding a difference in the susceptibility to heat between an anti-neuritic factor and a growth promoting factor, suggested that vitamin B was not a single entity. In 1926 Smith and Hendrick isolated the two distinct factors, a thermal labile anti-neuritic factor and a thermal stable growth-promoting factor. Subsequent work did show the original vitamin described by Funk to contain multiple factors. Currently, the following are considered members of this group: thiamine, riboflavine, nicotinic acid and niacin, pyridoxine, biotin, pantothenic acid, choline, inositol, para-aminobenzoic acid, folic acid complex, and vitamin B_{12}. Several other compounds have been discovered and are being currently investigated.

Thiamine (Vitamin B₁)

Thiamine is also known as the anti-neuritic or anti-beri-beri vitamin. It is a pyrimidine-thiazole compound that is water soluble and heat labile and

that is *found* in yeast, grain, and cereals. It is vitally concerned with carbohydrate metabolism, being involved in the utilization of pyruvic acid. It is
also necessary in the transmission of peripheral nerve impulses by augment-
ing the activity of acetylcholine through the inhibition of the formation of
cholinesterase. A *deficiency* of vitamin B_1 leads to *beri-beri*, characterized
by polyneuritis, muscular atrophy, cardiovascular changes, serous effusions, and anasarca. When the nervous system is chiefly involved the condition is called *dry beri-beri* whereas when the cardiovascular symptoms

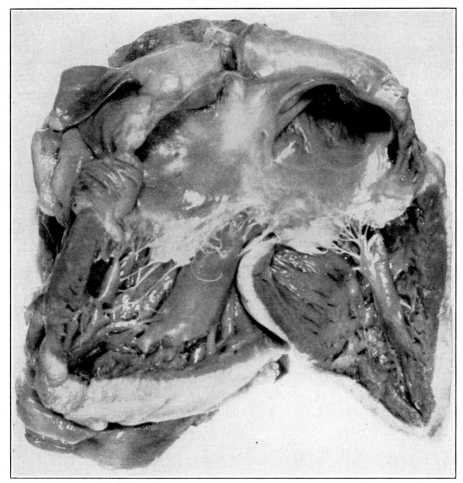

Fig. 32.—Hypertrophy of the right side of the heart in beri-beri.

with edema predominate it is known as *wet beri-beri*. The patients die of
acute cardiac failure or intercurrent infections. Those dying of heart failure
show a dilatation and hypertrophy of the right side of the heart (Fig. 32).
Histologically, the myocardium shows parenchymatous, hydropic, and
fatty degeneration and the supporting tissue reveals edema, slight infiltration with lymphocytes and later fibrosis (Fig. 33). The nerves show
degeneration of the myelin sheath, hydropic degeneration of the cells of
Schwamm, and fragmentation of the axis cylinder. Ganglion cells in the
medulla and pons also show degenerative changes.

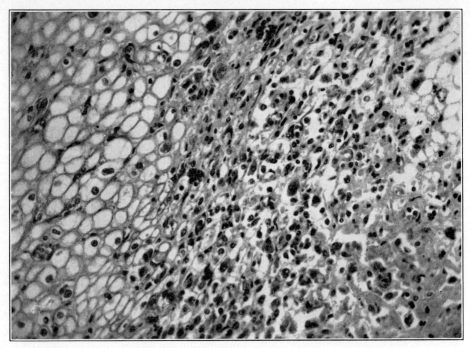

Fig. 33.—Myocardium of the right ventricle in beri-beri showing hydropic
degeneration and lymphocytic infiltration. × 200.

Riboflavin (Vitamin B₂ or Vitamin G)

Riboflavin is a complex, water-soluble, heat-stabile pigment *found* in
yeast, milk, growing leafy vegetables, kidney, liver, and heart. It combines
in the body with phosphoric acid and/or a protein to form a complex system
of enzymes which regulates the oxidation reaction within the cells and which
plays some part in the metabolism of carbohydrates. The vitamin is
essential for growth and normal health in all animals. A *deficiency* results
in (1) cessation of growth, (2) seborrheic type of dermatitis of the nose, ears,
and eyes, (3) conjunctivitis, (4) keratitis, and (5) vascularization with subsequent opacity of the cornea. There also occurs about the mouth an
angular stomatitis, fissures, cheilosis, vertical fissuring of the vermillion
border of the lips, and crusting and desquamation of the mucous membrane.

Nicotinic acid and Niacin

Nicotinic acid is beta-pyridine carboxylic acid. *Niacin* is the amide form
of nicotinic acid. Niacin was shown by Warburg to be the active group of
Codehydrogenase I and II, an enzyme system concerned with the hydrogen
transport in the living cell. The amide is soluble in water and heat stabile
and *occurs* in all living cells, particularly in the liver, kidney, and yeast.
It is essential for the metabolism of carbohydrate and for proper nutrition
in animals. A *deficiency* in man causes *pellegra*, manifested by dermatitis,
diarrhea, delirium, and death. Dermatitis occurs on the skin exposed to
sunlight and friction and consists of a bright red erythema resembling
sunburn. In the later stages, the skin becomes atrophic and shows excess
pigmentation. Diarrhea results from severe acute enterocolitis and is often

accompanied by glossitis, pharyngitis, esophagitis, proctitis, and vaginitis. The central nervous system symptoms range from weakness and lassitude to acute delirium and psychoses. Histologically, one sees scattered degeneration of the axis cylinder of the cortical pyramidal cells and degeneration of the myelin sheaths of the spinal cord and peripheral nerves.

Pyridoxine (Vitamin B₆)

Pyridoxine is a pyridine derivative which participates in a wide variety of enzyme systems having to do with the metabolic utilization and transformation of amino acids. It is *found* in yeast, liver, cereal polishings, cereals, and fish. In animals, a *deficiency* causes dermatitis, lesions in the blood vessels resembling atherosclerosis as seen in man, fatty metamorphosis and cirrhosis of the liver, and an anemia resembling Mediterranean anemia (thalassemia). Although a clear-cut deficiency disease due to vitamin B_6 is probably not seen in man, human volunteers in whom an experimental vitamin B_6 deficiency is produced develop a seborrheic-like dermatitis about the eyes, nose, and mouth.

Biotin (Vitamin H, Co-Enzyme R)

A *deficiency* of biotin produced in human volunteers manifests itself as a scaly dermatitis, atrophy of the lingual papillæ, mild depression, muscle pains, nausea and vomiting, local paresthesias, anemia, and a striking increase in the bile pigments and cholesterol in the blood.

Pantothenic Acid

Co-enzyme A which is concerned with acetylation is derived from *pantothenic acid*. Pantothenic acid is essential for adequate nutrition in certain animals such as the monkey, dog, rat, and mouse but it is still not known whether it is essential for human nutrition. A *deficiency* in animals is manifested by achromotrichia (graying of the hair), anemia, lack of growth, gastroenteritis, and adrenal hemorrhage and necrosis. No known deficiency syndrome has been shown in man.

Choline

There is still some question as to whether *choline* should be included in the vitamin B complex group. It is a lipotrophic factor and is *found* in wheat germ, peas, spinach, soya beans, liver, kidneys, and egg yolk. A *deficiency* in animals produces a diffuse nodular cirrhosis, degeneration of renal cortex, and a hemorrhagic tendency manifested especially in the kidneys and eye. In the rat, choline protects the liver against hepatotoxic agents such as chloroform and carbon tetrachoride and prevents the formation of fatty liver in animals fed a high diet. Probably no deficiency syndrome occurs in man since abundant amount of choline is available as part of lecithin.

Inositol

A *deficiency* in mice and rats produces alopecia and loss of weight and, in dogs, gastrointestinal hypertonicity and hypomotility. The status in human nutrition is still unknown and no deficiency state has been produced.

Para-Aminobenzoic Acid

It is doubtful whether *para-aminobenzoic acid* should be included in the category of a vitamin and yet it is an integral part of folic acid and is essential to animal nutrition and possibly to human nutrition. It definitely inhibits the growth of *Mycobacterium tuberculosis* in vitro. It has been *used* with success in the *treatment* of certain of the rickettsial diseases as Rocky Mountain spotted fever, typhus, and tsutsugamushi fever. It has also been used with some success in the treatment of myeloid leukemia where continued use of para-aminobenzoic acid results in a striking lowering of myeloid cells. It is doubtful that a deficiency state exists in animals or man.

Folic Acid Complex

The *folic acid complex*, known collectively as simply *folic acid*, is a group of similar compounds differing in the number of the glutamic acid radicals attached to the pteroyl group. They are *found* in fresh green leafy vegetables, liver, cauliflower, kidneys, and wheat cereals. In aminals, a *deficiency* produces an anemia, leukopenia, diarrhea, and atrophy of the intestinal tract. In man, it has been found that folic acid produces a hematopoietic response in many types of megaloblastic anemias, including Addison's pernicious anemia, pernicious anemia of pregnancy, and the anemia of sprue and pellegra. It converts a megaloblastic bone marrow to a normoblastic one but does not prevent the spinal cord degeneration that occurs in Addison's pernicious anemia. Certain chemicals interfere with the synthesis or utilization of folic acid and are known as *folic acid antagonists*, an example of which is aminopterin (aminopteroyl glutamic acid). These compounds inhibit mitoses of normal and malignant cells and have been used in the treatment of leukemia.

Vitamin B$_{12}$

In 1948 Smith and Rickes and his associates independently crystallized an antipernicious anemia factor, known as vitamin B$_{12}$, from liver concentrates. It is *found* in small amounts in meat, milk, cheese, eggs, and fish, and in high concentrations in liver extracts and in the culture broth used in the production of certain antibiotics such as Streptomycin, Aureomycin, and Terramycin. This chemical controls all manifestations of pernicious anemia including the transformation of a megaloblastic marrow to a normoblastic one and the simultaneous prevention of the postero-lateral degeneration of the spinal cord. In animals, the *deficiency* has a deleterious effect on growth and a case of a deficiency in a human infant has been reported, the child manifesting a failure to gain weight.

VITAMIN C

Vitamin C, the antiscorbutic vitamin, is ascorbic (cevitamic) acid. It is water soluble, heat labile, and a powerful reducing agent. It is *found* in all living tissues, both plants and animals, and is particularly concentrated in berries, citrus fruits, green leafy vegetalbes, potatoes, cabbages, and turnips. A *deficiency* results in the failure of formation and maintenance of intercellular cement substance and the deficiency in man is known as *scurvy*. This disorder is manifested by hemorrhages, loosening of the teeth, failure of wounds to heal, and, in the infant, extensive subperiostial hemorrhages and separation of the epiphysis of long bones. The hemorrhages are particularly prominent in the skin, in the gingivae, and in joints causing swelling, pain, local heat, and tenderness. The bleeding is said to be due to abnormal capillary fragility. It has been suggested that the increased fragility is due to defects in the substance binding the capillary endothelium or in the pericapillary connective tissue, although no definite morphologic changes have yet been demonstrated. The loosening of the teeth results from lesions in the tooth pulp and dentine and subsequent resoprtion of alveolar bone. Failure of wounds to heal is said to be due to a lack of intercellular substance and capillary formation. Fibroblastic proliferation does occur but there is no elaboration of intercellular material and blood vessels do not penetrate

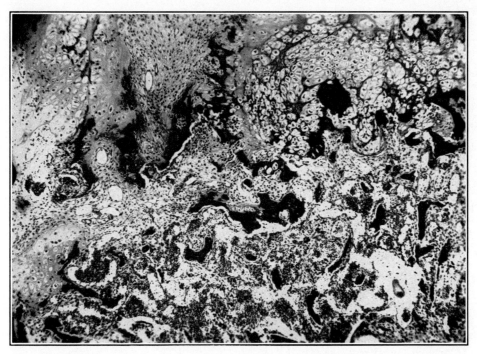

Fig. 34.—Bone in scurvy showing irregularity of epiphyseal cartilage, lack of osteoid formation, hemorrhage, fibrous tissue replacement, and scattered fragments of calcified cartilage. × 50.

this poorly developed granulation tissue. Since ascrobic acid is essential for the formation of bone and cartilage, osseous changes are particularly prominent in children. The lesions are most common in the costochondral junction and the ends of the long bones. Histologically, the various changes are seen in the osteoblasts which lose their shape tending to resemble fibroblasts, leave the trabeculae, and migrate toward the diaphysis. Such matrix as is produced appears as loose connective tissue which does not ossify. Later, there is present at the epiphyseal end of the shaft a dense zone of provisional calcification distal to which is a zone of connective tissue in which are embedded fragments of old calcified cartilaginous matrix devoid of osteoid formation (Fig. 34). The normal hematopoietic marrow previously formed becomes converted into a loose connective tissue showing a few cells and much ground substance. Simultaneously, with the changes at the ends of the long bones, there continues an abnormal periosteal growth. Trabecular instead of compact bone is formed and within this poor bone hemorrhages develop leading to the stripping of the periostium from the bony surfaces.

VITAMIN D

Vitamin D, the anti-rachitic or calcifying vitamin, is derived from the irradiation of certain sterols, the two most important being ergosterol and 7-dehydro-cholesterol. *Ergosterol* is *found* in plants, molds, and yeast and, when irradiated, is converted into viosterol. *Viosterol*, which has been purified and crystallized, is known as calcificerol or vitamin D_2. *7-dehydrocholesterol*, formed from animal fat by dehydrogenation in the wall of the small intestine, is converted by irradiation into vitamin D_3. At the present time there are at least 20 other forms of vitamin D, none of which as yet appears to be important clinically. *Calciferol*, the most important and probably the one produced in greatest abundance, is the compound usually referred to as vitamin D. *Man* is supplied with vitamin D by (1) irradiation of the skin and (2) ingestion of preformed vitamin from fish liver oils or synthetically produced products. Vitamin D *regulates* the *metabolism* of calcium and phosphorus. The exact mechanism of this regulation is still unknown but is probably best explained by considering the action as being primarily that of phosphorus metabolism, essentially by activation of alkaline phosphatases which liberate inorganic phosphorus from the phosphoric acid esters. Vitamin D is also related to the action of the *parathyroid glands* and to growth, decreased amounts resulting in impairment of growth and excessive amounts increase in growth. The *deficiency* syndrome in man is entirely related to the skeleton. In children, it produces the disease known as *rickets* and in adults *osteoporosis* when the deficiency is moderate and *osteomalacia* when the deficiency is severe. In the deficiency state, there is a lowered concentration of phosphorus in the blood, an increase in alkaline phosphatase, an improper relation of phosphorus and calcium salts due mainly to lack of precipitation of calcium phosphate, and failure of calcification of osteoid. This failure to mineralize new osteoid and cartilage in children results in a destruction of the orderly processes of bone formation and eventuates in bony deformities referred to as *rickets*. Normally, bones grow in length by an orderly production and calcification of the cartilage present between the diaphysis and epiphysis. New cartilage is constantly being laid down on the epiphyseal side and, synchronously, the cartilage on the diaphysial side undergoes degeneration, subsequent invasion with capillaries and osteoblasts, and simultaneous calcification of the degenerated cartilage. *Pathologically*, in rickets, the cartilaginous growth goes on as usual but degeneration ceases. Capillaries and osteoblasts appear as usual to form osteoid but the osteoid remains uncalcified. As a result, the cartilaginous zone increases in size and the metaphysis enlarges. Cut surfaces of the bone in this area reveal an irregular, thick, bluish, translucent mass of cartilage instead of the ordinary narrow straight line of calcified osteoid (Fig. 35). Similar changes occur beneath the periosteum and, concomitantly, the trabeculæ of the cancellous portions of the bone undergo reactive resorption. All these result in a softened bone which, when subjected to the various stresses and strains, becomes bent and fractured. *Clinically*, rickets is manifested by flattening of the occipital bones, formation of bossæ and circumscribed areas of decalcification and thinning (craniotabes) in the skull, pigeon breast (protrusion of sternum with depressions of the anteriolateral portion of the ribs), beading of the ribs (rackitic rosary), compression of the lungs due to loss of thoracic rigidity, kyphosis and scoliosis, and bowing of the extremities. In *adults*, the endochrondial ossification having ceased, a deficiency in vitamin D is manifested by a withdrawal of calcium from bones (*osteoporosis*) with deposition of osteoid beneath the periostium and around the trabeculæ. In extreme cases, the bones become exceedingly soft (*osteomalacia*) and, as in infants and chidren, fractures and deformities occur.

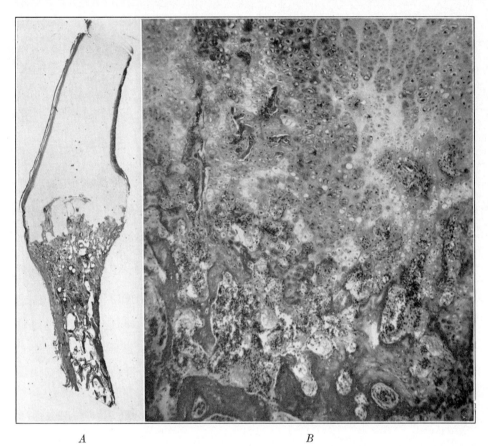

A   B

FIG. 35.—Bone in rickets illustrating *A*, semigross appearance of a longitudinal section of the costochondral junction. The cartilage is overabundant, bulging, and irregular at its junction with the bone, and *B*, overabundance and irregularity of the cartilaginous zone, old bony trabeculæ with surrounding new bone formation, and fibrous tissue replacement of the marrow. × 50.

Excessive ingestion of vitamin D results in *poisoning*. In acute cases, the patients may die of uremia and dehydration. In chronic cases, the patients exhibit *metastatic calcification*, that is, withdrawal of calcium from the bones with its subsequent deposition in the tubules of the kidney, media of the blood vessels, lungs, heart, stomach, joints, synovial membranes, skin, and eyes. The changes in the kidney may result in death from uremia.

VITAMIN E

Vitamin E, the antisterility or antidystrophic vitamin, occurs as *tocopherol*. Of the various forms, the Alpha form is the most biologically active. Vitamin E is an oil and is, therefore, soluble in fat solvents. It is *found* in wheat germ, brown rice, oatmeal, green vegetables, sardines, and eggs. The usual forms used today have been synthesized. The vitamin has an anti-oxidant action protecting vitamin A, carotene, biotin, and vitamin B complex from destruction in the lumen of the gastrointestinal tract by rancid, unsaturated fatty acid. Its exact function in cells is still unknown but apparently it is mostly concerned with cell maturation and differentiation. The *deficiency* state has been studied mostly in rats. In the male rat there is produced a degeneration of the spermatozoa and in the female rat a degeneration of the placental and fetal tissues about midway through gestation. There also occurs dystrophy of striated muscle accompanied by degenerative changes in the central nervous system, especially the spinal cord ganglion cells. The status of a deficiency disease in man is controversial. The vitamin has been used with some success in certain cases of habitual abortion, certain cases of toxemia of pregnancy, and some cases of muscular dystrophy.

VITAMIN F

A group of essential fatty acids have been designated as *vitamin F*. The important members of this group are linoleic and linolenic acids, which are of vegetable origin, and arachidonic acid, which is found only in animal lipids. These fatty acids are important because they became rancid quite easily by oxidation when exposed to air and the products of the rancidity are in themselves toxic. The rancid oils produce an anemia and, when present in food, lead to oxidation and destruction of other substances, such as vitamins A, E, and B complex. They are thus capable of converting a diet adequate in these substances into one that is deficient. A *deficiency* of vitamin F in animals results in changes in the skin manifested by dermatitis and alopecia and in the kidney by areas of calcification and necrosis. Although no definite deficiency syndromes have been described in man, the administration of the unsaturated fatty acids to patients with eczema causes healing of the lesions.

VITAMIN K

Vitamin K is basically a naphthoquinone which is fat soluble, alkaline labile, and easily inactivated by light. The compound first isolated from alfalfa has been called vitamin K_1 while that isolated from fish meal has been designated as vitamin K_2. Presently, many vitamin K compounds are being synthesized, one of which is water-soluble phthicol. Vitamin K is *found* in large amounts in green plants (especially alfalfa), spinach, cauliflower, cabbage, carrot tops, tomatoes, *etc.* It is also formed by activity of bacteria and, therefore, a certain amount is produced in the intestine of man by the action of *E. coli*. Vitamin K is essential for normal blood coagulation. It partakes in the production of *prothrombin* in the liver by acting in the enzyme system synthesizing prothrombin. A *deficiency* is manifested by a lowering of blood prothrombin and this results in hemorrhages of various sizes in all locations of the body. A deficiency may result not only from lack of inadequate intake but also from inadequate absorption and as a result of various diseases of the liver.

VITAMIN P

Vitamin P, also called citrin, is a flavon or flavon glucoside. Since other flavons, such as hesperidin and rutin, have the same effect, vitamin P is probably not a single entity. The compound is said to control capillary resistance and permeability and *deficiency*, therefore, results in petechial hemorrhages.

REFERENCES

Atrophy

BRADLEY, H. C.: Physiol. Rev., *18*, 173, 1938 (Atrophy).

Parenchymatous Degeneration

BELL, E. T.: J. A. M. A., *61*, 455, 1913 (Cloudy Swelling).
FONNESU, A., and SEVERI, C.: Br. J. Exper. Path., *34*, 341, 1953 (Nucleic Acids).
LUCKÉ, B., and McCUTCHEON, M.: A. M. A. Arch. Path., *2*, 846, 1926 (Reversible and Irreversible Changes).
OGILVIE, R. F.: J. Path. & Bact., *35*, 743, 1932 (Early Phases Degeneration).
SHANNON, W. R.: J. Lab. & Clin. Med., *1*, 541, 1916 (Experimental).

Hydropic Degeneration

ANDERSON, W. A. D., and BETHEA, W. R., JR.: J. A. M. A., *114*, 1983, 1940 (Sucrose).
GEILING, E. N. K., and CANNON, P. R.: J. A. M. A., *111*, 919, 1938 (Sulfanilamide).
LUCKÉ, B., and McCUTCHEON, M.: A. M. A. Arch. Path., *10*, 662, 1930 (Injury and Cell Permeability).

Hyaline Droplet Degeneration

GOVAN, A. D. T.: J. Path. and Bact., *68*, 642, 1954 (Hyaline Droplets).
SMETANA, H., and JOHNSON, F. R.: Am. J. Path., *18*, 1029, 1942 (Renal Tubules).

Fibrinoid Degeneration

ALTSHULER, C. H. and ANGEVINE, D. M.: Am. J. Path., *25*, 1061, 1949 (Histochemical Studies).
BRUNSON, J. G., and DAVIS, R. L.: A.M.A. Arch. Path., *60*, 593, 1955 (Systemic).
GAMBLE, C. N., and BRUNSON, J. G.: A.M.A. Arch. Path., *60*, 583, 1955 (Experimental in Rabbits).
GITLIN, D., *et al.*: Am. J. Path., *33*, 55, 1957 (Nature).
KLEMPERER, PAUL: Am. J. Path., *26*, 505, 1950 (Concept Collagen Diseases).
MOVAT, H. Z., and MORE, R. H.: Am. J. Clin. Path., *28*, 331, 1957 (Nature).
MUIRHEAD, *et al.*: A.M.A. Arch. Path., *63*, 213, 1957 (Muscle).
VAZQUEZ, J. J., and DIXON, F. L., Jr.: Lab. Investig., *6*, 205, 1957 (Immunohistologic Study).

Hyaline Degeneration

MAXIMOW, A. L., and BLOOM, W.: *A Textbook of Histology*, Philadelphia, W. B. Saunders Co., 1957, p. 62 (Collagen).
WAGNER, B. M., *et al.*: Lab. Investig., *6*, 259, 1957 (Cerebral Corpora Amylacea).

Zenker's Degeneration

WELSS, H. G.: A. M. A. Arch. Path., *4*, 681, 1927 (Diaphragm Causing Death).

Amyloidosis

ATLAS, H., *et al.*: Am. J. Clin. Path., *20*, 371, 1950 (Primary).
AUERBACH, O., and STEMMERMAN, M.: Am. J. M. Sci., *208*, 305, 1944 (Congo Red Test).
BALLINGER, J.: Am. J. M. Sci., *217*, 308, 1949 (Heart Disease).
BERO, G. L.: Ann. Int. Med., *46*, 931, 1957 (Clinical and Pathological).
CRACOVANER, D. J., *et al.*: U. S. Armed Forces M. J., *2*, 707, 1951 (Symposium).
DAHLIN, D. C.: Am. J. Path., *25*, 105, 1949 (Primary).
————: Ann. Int. Med., *31*, 105, 1949 (Secondary).
HIGGINS, W. H., and HIGGINS, W. H., JR.: Am. J. M. Sci., *220*, 610, 1950 (Primary).
JACKSON, A.: A.M.A. Arch. Int. Med., *93*, 494, 1954 (Etiology).
JONES, R. S., and FRAZIER, D. B.: A. M. A. Arch. Path., *50*, 366, 1950 (Primary).

PERASALO, O., and LATVALAHTI, V.:   Acta Path. Microb., *34*, 208, 1954 (Clinical and Experimental).

RICHTER, G. W.:   Am. J. Path., *30*, 239, 1954 (Resorption).

RUKAVINA, J. G., *et al.*:   Medicine, *35*, 239, 1956 (Review Primary).

SPAIN, D. M., and BARRETT, R. C.: A. M. A. Arch. Path., *38*, 203, 1944 (Atypical Sites).

SYMMERS, W. ST. C.:   J. Clin. Path., *9*, 187, 1956 (Etiology: Primary).

TEILUM, G.:   Am. J. Path., *32*, 945, 1956 (Glycoproteins and Reticular Cells).

TIBER, A. M., *et al.*:   A. M. A. Arch. Int. Med., *68*, 309, 1941 (Hepatic Function).

Mucous Degeneration

FLOREY, H.:   Proceed. Royal Sec. London, *143*, 147, 1955 (Function Mucin).

Disturbances of Carbohydrate Metabolism

BONDY, P. K.:   Am. J. Med., *24*, 428, 1958 (Metabolism Liver Disease).

BROH-KAHN, R. H., and MIRSKY, I. A.:   Science, *106*, 148, 1947 (Hexokinase and Diabetes).

CANTAROW, A., and SCHEPARTZ, B.:   *Biochemistry*, Philadelphia, W. B. Saunders, 1954.

GOMORI, G.:   *Microscopic Histochemistry*, Chicago, University of Chicago Press, 1952, pp. 61 to 68

HENNEMAN, D. H., and BUNKER, J. D.:   Am. J. Med., *23*, 34, 1957 (Intermediary Carbohydrate Metabolism in Cushing's Syndrome).

HOLZEL, A. *et al.*:   Am. J. Med., *22*, 703, 1957 (Galactosemia).

IS SELBACHER, K. J. *et al.*:   Science, *123*, 635, 1956 (Congenital Galactosemia).

JONES, G. M.:   Am. J. M. Sc., *213*, 206, 1947 (Posthypoglycemic Encephalopathy).

LEVINE, R. *et al.*:   Am. J. Physiol., *163*, 70, 1950 ("Permeability" of Cells to Free Hexoses).

MOORHOUSE, J., and KARK, R.:   Am. J. Med., *23*, 46, 1957 (Fructose and Diabetes).

MOSCHCOWITZ, E.:   A.M.A. Arch. Path., *61*, 136, 1956 (Hyalinization of Islets of Langerhans).

NAJJAR, V. A.:   Ped., *15*, 444, 1955 (Review Metabolism of Carbohydrates, Fats and Bile Pigments by the Liver).

RALLI, E. P., and DUMM, M. E.: N. York State J. Med., *54*, 341, 1954 (Endocrine Control Carbohydrate Metabolism).

STADIE, W. C.:   Physiol. Rev., *34*, 52, 1954 (Action of Insulin).

WOOD, H. G.: Physiol. Rev., *35*, 841, 1955 (Pathways Glucose Metabolism).

ZELIWEGER, H. *et al.*:   Ped., *15*, 715, 1955 (Glycogen Disease Skeletal Muscle).

Disturbances of Lipid Metabolism

AHRENS, E. H.:   Am. J. Med., *23*, 928, 1957 (Nutritional Factors and Serum Lipid Levels).

BAAR, H. W., and HICKMANS, E. M.:   Acta Med. Scandinav., *155*, 49, 1956 (Cephalin Lipoidosis).

BARACH, J. H.:   Am. J. Digest. Dis., *19*, 37, 1952 (Obesity).

BISHTON, R. L., *et al.*:   J. Clin. Path., *9*, 305, 1956 (Gargoylism).

BLOOR, W. R.:   *Biochemistry of Fatty Acids*, New York, Reinhold Publishing Corp., 1943.

CANTAROW, A., and SCHEPARTZ, B.:   *Biochemistry*, Philadelphia, W. B. Saunders Co., 1954, pp. 438 to 484.

CONN, J. W.: Physiol. Rev., *24*, 31, 1944 (Obesity).

EDER, H. A.: Am. J. Med., *23*, 269, 1957 (Serum Lipoproteins).

GELVIN, E. P., and McGAVACK, T. H.: *Obesity; Its Cause, Classification and Care*, New York, Medical Book Department of Harper and Brothers, 1957.

GOFMAN, J. W., *et al.*:   Science, *3*, 166, 1950 (Lipids and Lipoproteins in Atherosclerosis).

GOMORI, G.: *Microscopic Histochemistry*, Chicago, University of Chicago Press, 1952, pp. 91 to 135.

GRIEG, H. B. W.: Lancet, *2*, 16, 1956 (Lipemia and Fibrinolysis).

HARTROFT, W. S., and THOMAS, W. A.:   J.A.M.A., *164*, 1899, 1957 (Pathological Lesions in Disturbances of Lipid Metabolism).

KEYS, A.:   Conference on Atherosclerosis and Coronary Heart Disease, N. Y. Heart Assoc. Inc., January 15, 1957.

LAWRY, E. Y., *et al.*: Am. J. Med., *22*, 605, 1957 (Serum Lipids and Coronary Artery Disease).

NAJJAR, V. A.:   Ped., *15*, 444, 1955 (Review Metabolism of Carbohydrates, Fats and Bile Pigments by the Liver).

SODEMAN, W. A.:   *Pathologic Physiology; Mechanisms of Disease*, Philadelphia, W. B. Saunders Co., 1956, pp. 647 to 652.

VERCHURE, J. C. N.: Clin. Chem., *3*, 577, 1957 (Clinical Chemistry and Lipoproteins).

VOLWILER, W.: Am. J. Med., *23*, 251, 1957 (Malabsorptive Syndromes).
WHEELER, E. O.: Am. J. Med., *23*, 653, 1957 (Genetic Aspects of Atherosclerosis).
ZILVERSMIT, D. B.: Am. J. Med., *23*, 120, 1957 (Current Concepts of Lipid Metabolism).

Disturbances of Calcium Metabolism

BARR, D. P.: Physiol. Rev., *12*, 624, 1932 (Pathologic Calcification).
HUNTER, D.: Quart. J. Med., *24*, 393, 1931 (Parathyroids and Calcium).
LUTZ, J. F.: Ann. Int. Med., *14*, 1270, 1941 (Universal Calcinosis).
MCLEAN, L. D.: So. Med. J., *48*, 354, 1955 (Mechanisms Calcification).
MEEKER, D. R., and KESTEN, H. D.: J. Biol. Chem., *113*, 289, 1936 (Composition Calcium Deposits).
MULLIGAN, R. M.: A. M. A. Arch. Path., *43*, 177, 1947 (Metastatic Calcification).
ROSENBERG, E. F.: J. A. M. A., *115*, 1791, 1940 (Calcinosis).
ROTHSTEIN, J. L., and WELT, S.: A. M. A. Am. J. Dis. Child., *52*, 368, 1936 (Calcinosis).
SNAPPER, I.: A.M.A. Arch. Int. Med., *93*, 807, 1954 (Hypercalcemia and Metastatic Calcification).
THOMSON, D. L., and COLLIP, J. B.: Physiol. Rev., *12*, 309, 1932 (Parathyroids).
TUMULTY, P. A., and HOWARD, J. E.: J. A. M. A., *119*, 233, 1942 (Irradiated Ergosterol).

Pathologic Pigmentation

ALDRICH, R. A., *et al.*: Am. J. Med. Sc., *230*, 675, 1955 (Porphyrins).
ARIAS, I. M., and LONDON, I. M.: Science, *126*, 563, 1957 (Gilbert's Disease, Congenital Hepatic Dysfunction).
BELKNAP, E. L.: J.A.M.A., *139*, 818, 1949 (Lead Poisoning).
BICKOFF, E. M.: Methods Biochem. Anal., *4*, 1, 1957 (Carotene).
BILLING, B. H., and LATHE, G. H.: Am. J. Med., *24*, 111, 1958 (Bilirubin Metabolism in Jaundice).
BLOCH, B.: Am. J. M. Sci., *77*, 609, 1929 (Melanin).
CHERNOFF, A. I.: New England J. Med., *253*, 332, 1955 (Hematological Studies of Hemoglobin).
COHEN, E. L.: Br. J. Derm., *69*, 101, 1957 (Carotenemia).
COOPER, J. A., and MORAN, T. J.: A.M.A. Arch. Path., *64*, 46, 1957 (Ochronosis).
DUBIN, I. M.: Am. J. Clin. Path., *25*, 514, 1955 (Iron Metabolism).
DUBIN, I. N.: Am. J. Med., *24*, 268, 1958 (Chronic Idiopathic Jaundice).
EDITORIAL: Ann. Int. Med., *42*, 458, 1955 (Iron Metabolism).
FINCH, C. A., *et al.*: Blood, *5*, 593, 1950 (Pathophysiology of Iron Storage).
GETTLER, A. O., *et al.*: Am. J. Path., *3*, 631, 1927 (Argyria).
GLENNER, G. G.: Am. J. Path., *27*, 1, 1957 (Pigments in Tissue Sections).
GOMORI, G.: *Microscopic Histochemistry; Principles and Practice*, Chicago, University of Chicago Press, 1952, pp. 134 to 136; 149 to 151.
GRANICK, S.: Bull. N. Y. Acad. Med., *30*, 81, 1954 (Iron Metabolism).
GUBLER, C. J.: Science, *123*, 87, 1956 (Iron Metabolism).
HAHN, P. F.: Medicine, *16*, 249, 1937 (Iron Metabolism).
HIGGINSON, J., *et al.*: Brit. Heart J., *17*, 337, 1955 (Chronic Malnutrition).
HILL, W. R., and MONTGOMERY, H.: A.M.A. Arch. Dermat. & Syph., *44*, 588, 1941 (Argyria).
HUMBLE, J. G.: Quart. J. Med., *15*, 299, 1946 (Chloroma).
JACOBSEN, V. C., and KLINCK, G. H., Jr.: A.M.A. Arch. Path., *17*, 141, 1934 (Melanin).
JENSEN, B.: Acta Med. Scand., *153*, 383, 1956 (Ochronosis).
LAIDLAW, G. F.: Am. J. Path., *8*, 477, 1932 (Melanin).
LAWRENCE, R. D.: Lancet, *1*, 736, 1949 (Haemochromatosis).
LERNER, A. B.: Am. J. Med., *19*, 902, 1955 (Review Melanin).
LEWIS, H. P.: Am. J. Med. Sc., *227*, 544, 1954 (Heart in Hemochromatosis).
LICHTENSTEIN, L., and KALAN, L.: Am. J. Path., *30*, 99, 1954 (Ochronosis).
MORRISON, D. B., and ANDERSON, W. A. D.: Pub. Health Rep., *57*, 90, and 161, 1942 (Malarial Pigment).
MORTON, R. A., and GOODWIN, T. W.: Br. Med. Bull., *12*, 37, 1956 (Carotinoids).
MUIR, R., and NIVIN, J. S. F.: J. Path. & Bact., *41*, 183, 1935 (Blood Pigments).
MUIRHEAD, E. E., *et al.*: A. M. A. Arch. Int. Med., *83*, 477, 1949 (Hemosiderosis).
PAPPENHEIMER, A. M., and VICTOR, J.: Am. J. Path., *22*, 395, 1946 (Ceroid).
PATEK, A. J., JR., and HEATH, C. W.: J. A. M. A., *106*, 1463, 1936 (Chlorosis).
PATERSON, J. D., *et al.*: A.M.A. Arch. Path., *61*, 496, 1956 (Hemosiderin Deposition in Arteriosclerosis).
POPPER, H., *et al.*: A. M. A. Arch. Path., *37*, 161, 1944 (Ceroid).
RUKSTINAT, G. J.: A. M. A. Arch. Path., *31*, 640, 1941 (Tattoos).

SCHULTZ, J., *et al.*: Cancer Research, *16*, 569, 1956 (Chloroma).
SCHULTZ, J., and SCHWARTZ, S.: Cancer Research, *16*, 565, 1956 (Chloroma).
SCHWARTZ, S. O., and BLUMENTHAL, S. A.: Blood, *3*, 617, 1948 (Hemochromatosis).
SCHWARTZ, S. S.: Am. J. Clin. Path., *26*, 744, 1956 (Exogenous Hemochromatosis).
SHAY, H., *et al.*: Blood, *7*, 613, 1952 (Experimental Chloroma).
STEWART, M. J., and HICKMAN, E. M.: J. Path. & Bact., *34*, 61, 1931 (Melanosis Coli).
SUNDERMAN, F. W., JR., and SUNDERMAN, F. W.: Am. J. Clin. Path., *25*, 1231, 1955 (Porphyrins).
WATSON, C. J.: Advances Int. Med., *6*, 235, 1954 (Porphyrins).
WATSON, C. J.: Ann. Int. Med., *45*, 351, 1956 (Fractional Serum Bilirubin).
WATSON, C. J.: Blood, *1*, 99, 1946 (Hemoglobin Derivatives).
——————: New England J. Med., *227*, 665, and 705, 1942 (Bile Pigments).
WINTROBE, M. M.: *Clinical Hematology*, 4th Ed., Philadelphia, Lea & Febiger, 1956, pp. 132 to 138).

Gangrene

BELL, E. T.: A. M. A. Arch. Path., *49*, 469, 1950 (Gangrene Extremities).
HAIMOVICI, H.: Circulation, *1*, 225, 1950 (Gangrene Venous Origin).
ORR, K. D., and FAINER, D. C.: U. S. Armed Forces M. J., *3*, 95, 1952 (Frostbite).
SARNOFF, J.: New York State J. Med., *48*, 1480, 1948 (Gangrene Venous Origin).
WARTHEN, H. J.: Ann. Surg., *115*, 609, 1942 (Gas Gangrene).

Vitamins

General

BECKNELL, F., and PRESCOTT, F.: *The Vitamins in Medicine*, New York, Grune and Stratton, 1953.
CLARK, G. W.: *A Vitamin Digest*, Springfield, Charles C Thomas, 1953.
EDDY, W. H.: *Vitaminology*, Baltimore, Williams & Wilkins Co., 1949.
ROBINSON, F. A.: *The Vitamin B Complex*, New York, John Wiley & Sons, Inc., 1951.
ROSENBERG, H. R.: *Chemistry and Physiology of the Vitamins*, New York, Interscrena Publishers, Inc., 1942.
SEBRELL, W. H., JR., and HARRIS, R. S.: *The Vitamins. Chemistry, Physiology and Pathology.* Three Volumes, New York, Academic Press, Inc., 1954.
WOLBACH, S. B., and BESSEY, O. A.: Physiol. Rev., *22*, 233, 1942 (Tissue Changes in Avitaminosis).
YOUMANS, J. B.: *Nutritional Deficiencies*, Philadelphia, J. B. Lippincott, 1941.

Vitamin A

MASON, K. E.: Sebrell and Harris' *The Vitamins*, Vol. I, p. 137 (Vitamin A Deficiency in Human Beings).
MILAS, N. A.: Sebrell and Harris' *The Vitamins*, Vol. I, p. 4 (Chemistry of Vitamin A and Carotenes).
WOLBACH, S. B.: Sebrell and Harris' *The Vitamins*, Vol. I, p. 106 (Vitamin A Deficiency and Hypervitaminosis A in Animals).

Vitamin B Complex

HOWITT, M. K.: Sebrell and Harris' *The Vitamins*, Vol. III, p. 380 (Riboflavin Deficiency in Animals).
——————: Sebrell and Harris' *The Vitamins*, Vol. III, p. 387 (Riboflavin Deffciency in Man).
HUNDLEY, J. M.: Sebrell and Harris' *The Vitamins*, Vol. II, p. 551 (Niacin Deficiency in Man).
WUEST, H. W.: Sebrell and Harris' *The Vitamins*, Vol. I, p. 417 (Industrial Preparation of Vitamin B_{12}).

Vitamin C

HARRIS, R. S.: Sebrell and Harris' *The Vitamins*, Vol. I, p. 177 (Nomenclature and Formulas of Ascorbic Acid).
VILTER, R. W.: Sebrell and Harris' *The Vitamins*, Vol. I, p. 347 (Ascorbic Acid Deficiencies in Human Beings).

Vitamin D

BILLS, C. E.: Sebrell and Harris' *The Vitamins*, Vol. II, p. 132 (Chemistry of Vitamin D).
HARRIS, R. S.: Sebrell and Harris' *The Vitamins*, Vol. II, p. 132 (Nomenclature and Formulas of Vitamin D).
KRAMER, B., and KANOF, A.: Sebrell and Harris' *The Vitamins*, Vol. II, p. 232 (Vital Deficiency in Pathology of Human Beings).

Vitamin F

HANSEN, A. E., and WRESE, H. F.: Sebrell and Harris' *The Vitamins*, Vol. II, p. 300 (Essential Fatty Acids Deficiency in Human Beings).
HARRIS, R. S.: Sebrell and Harris' *The Vitamins*, Vol. II, p. 268 (Nomenclature and Formulas of Essential Fatty Acids).
HOLMAN, R. T.: Sebrell and Harris' *The Vitamins*, Vol. II, p. 292 (Essential Fatty Acids Deficiency in Animals and Insects).

Inflammations

GENERAL CONSIDERATIONS

Inflammation (L. = to set on fire) is the reaction of tissue to injury. It is the sum total of all the changes that take place in tissue from the moment of application of an irritant to the time of its expulsion or neutralization and repair of the damage. An *irritant* is any substance, compound, or agent that produces undue stimulation, undue sensitization, or undue excitation of tissues. *Infection* is more limited in scope. It connotes inflammation caused by pathogenic organisms. In general, inflammation is *designated* by the suffix -*itis* added to the name of the tissue or organ as, for example, dermatitis (inflammation of the skin or derma), appendicitis (inflammation of the appendix), salpingitis (inflammation of the salpinx), colitis (inflammation of the colon), etc.

Inflammation constitutes a *fundamental process* in pathology and, primarily or secondarily, is associated with almost every disease. The *causes* of inflammation are, therefore, the causes of disease and the more common of these may be listed as bacteria, rickettsia, viruses, fungi, parasites, chemicals, heat, cold, light, electricity, irradiation, foreign bodies, and trauma. Although, at first glance, the multitude of these heterologous etiologic agents may suggest diverse trigger *mechanisms*, such actually is not the case for, upon closer scrutiny, it becomes apparent that one common denominator in all inflammatory processes, regardless of their origins, is destruction of tissue. Carrying the reasoning a step further, it is quite possible that the destroyed tissue, either directly or by way of a disintegration product, then acts upon the remaining viable tissues to put into effect the inflammatory response. Actually, most investigators do agree that the ultimate initiating agent is a *tissue degeneration product* but they do not agree upon its precise nature. In 1924, Lewis postulated that the tissue product was *histamine* or at least a substance so closely related to histamine that he called it a *histamine-like* or *H-substance*. This conclusion was based not on the isolation of the histamine-like substance, which he was unable to do, but on the observation that the reaction induced was indistinguishable from that produced by histamine itself. Thus, because his hypothesis was strengthened by analogy only, it did not meet with universal approval. Reinvestigating the problem in 1936, Menkin showed that the fluid recovered from the site of inflammation contains a factor that is capable of inducing an increase in capillary permeability—one of the most important and first steps in an inflammatory reaction. Chemical extraction yielded a nonprotein, crystalline-like material which he called *leukotaxine*. It might be added, at this point, that others have since confirmed this finding. Leukotaxine possesses an alpha amino group and an indole nucleus, appears to be a chemical entity, is probably a polypeptide, and has none of the properties of histamine. The increase in capillary permeability induced by leukotaxine can be counteracted only by extracts (cortisone and hydrocortisone) of the adrenal cortex. More recently Menkin, in extending his studies, has shown that leukotaxine has yet a second fundamental property—that of being concerned with the migration of neutrophils (and later mononuclear phago- cytes) to the site of the injury. That this is a positive attraction (chemo- taxis) can be readily demonstrated *in vivo* by injecting leukotaxine into tissues and noting the migration of neutrophils through the capillary wall to the point of injection and *in vitro* by noting a clumping of neutrophils about particles of leukotaxine when the latter are covered with a drop of exudate. Thus, the fundamental trigger mechanism and sequence of events in any inflammatory process, regardless of the initial inciting agent, appear to be irritant—destruction of tissue—release of leukotaxine—increased capil- lary permeability—changes characteristic of inflammation.

Once inflammation is initiated, its subsequent *course* depends upon (1) the nature, concentration, and abundance of the causative agent, (2) the tissue affected, and (3) the resistance susceptibility, and recuperative powers of the host. Since *agents* that *cause* inflammation are quite diverse it is obvi- ously impossible at this point to discuss their variations in any detail. Hence, the citing of an example or two will suffice. If the irritant is, say hydrochloric acid, and a drop of a concentrated solution is placed on the forearm, it may well burn a hole through the skin into the subcutaneous tissues. A large quantity, say 1 ml., will surely cause wider and deeper damage while a quantity transportable on a pinhead may produce simply a local irritation. If this hydrochloric acid is successively diluted by larger and larger quantities of water, a point of concentration will ultimately be reached where the original drop or the original 1 ml. will possess not even an irritating effect upon the skin. The same reasoning may also be applied to microorganisms. When available in large numbers and in maximum concentrations they may elicit severe inflammatory reactions. Contrarily, when they are present in small numbers and in high dilutions they may rpo- duce no response whatsoever. In the case of microorganisms, however, inherent factors such as type, strain, and virulence loom forth as of extreme importance. It is obvious that certain organisms possess slow pathogenicity while others possess a high degree of infectivity and it is also obvious that these characteristics vary from strain to strain in the same type of organism.

The course of inflammation is also determined by the *tissue affected*. Some tissues are resistant to some irritants while others are susceptible. The hydrochloric acid mentioned in the preceding paragraph is more irritating to the mucosa of the mouth than it is to the skin and elicits an even greater inflammatory response when applied to the conjunctiva of the eye than it does in either of the other two locations. Talcum powder applied to the skin produces no irritating effect; when inhaled it may elicit a mild pulmonary reaction; but when dropped into the peritoneal cavity it results in a severe inflammatory response that is accompanied by extensive adhesion formation. In the intestinal tract colon bacilli are normally present in large numbers and produce no disturbance but transplant them into the peritoneal cavity and they elicit a severe inflammation. Gonococci inoculated into the urethra eventuate in a severe infection and inflammation but when applied to the skin in similar numbers they will not produce even a local irritation. Tu- bercle bacilli have a predilection for lymphoid structures, typhoid bacilli for the reticulo-endothelial system, rickettsia for endothelial cells, and viruses for the liver, central nervous system, skin, *etc.*

Factors determining the *resistance, susceptibility*, and *recuperative powers* of the host are somewhat more nebulous and thus more difficult to evaluate. They are concerned, of course, mostly with infection. Resistance may be defined as the ability of a person to combat infection (Harrell). Susceptibility is the reverse, that is, it represents lack of security against or inability of a person to combat infection. Susceptibility varies in reverse ratio to resistance. A few of the many factors concerned with resistance may be outlined as follows: (1) *Race*. Race is, of course, hereditarily determined and the latter plays a definite role in some infections. For example, the Negro and the American Indian are susceptible to tuberculosis while the white person is relatively resistant. Conversely white people are more susceptible to vivax malaria than are Negroes. (2) *Sex*. Tuberculosis reaches a peak in adolescent girls at an earlier age than in males. Urinary tract infections are more common in girls than in boys, especially with pleuropneumonia group of organisms. Pregnancy has a retarding effect on the spread of syphilis in the mother. (3) *Age*. The newborn infant is resistant to exanthemata of all types due to possession of immune bodies transmitted by the mother. The ovaries and testes of children are resistant to mumps virus while those of adults are susceptible. The child's vagina is susceptible to gonococci whereas that of the adult is more resistant. Infants and old people are susceptible to pneumonia and older men are more prone to re-activation or reinfection with tuberculosis. (4) *Diet*. The type and amount of food one eats plays an important role in resistance and susceptibility to infection. Tuberculosis follows malnutrition and, conversely, a dietary regime is all important in treating this disease. Epidemics of many types go hand in hand with famine. Uncontrolled diabetics, in whom there is improper assimilation of food, are subjected to many infections, especially staphylococcic and streptococcic. Avitaminoses of various kinds lead to degenerative changes in tissues making them more susceptible to bacterial infection. (5) *Rest*. Lack of proper rest decreases ones resistance to such infections as the common cold, pneumococcic pneumonia, and, when stretched over a long period, tuberculosis. (6) *Exposure*. Chilling of the body is an important factor in contraction of infection by the virus of the common cold and this paves the way for secondary bacterial invasion. It is also a common predisposing factor for pneumonia developing in alcoholics. Exposure to high humidity, especially in areas where clothing rubs, predisposes to bacterial and fungus infections of the skin. Sunlight and wind produce drying of the mucocutaneous junction of the lips and thus predispose to infection with the virus of herpes simplex. (7) *Emotions*. Emotional swings have a definite bearing on disease. Depression appears to be accompanied by decrease in resistance while elation or euphoria have an opposite effect. While not directly concerned with the problem of infection, emotional swings have been known to precipitate leukemia and hyperthyroidism and to worsen the condition of the diabetic. (8) *Seasons*. The seasons of the year influence some diseases. Peptic ulcer, for example, is more common in the spring. Pneumonia is more prevalent in the winter. Exanthemata occur in epidemics in late winter and early spring. (9) *Intercurrent Disease*. One disease may lower the patient's resistance and predispose to the acquisition of another disease. Nephrosis is commonly complicated by pneumococcic peritonitis. Diabetes and leukemia are frequently discovered following crops of furuncles and carbuncles. Malaria increases the susceptibility to a variety of infections. (10) *Impairment Nervous Function*. Organs and tissues with an intact nerve circuit are resistant to infection and inflammation.   Once the circuit is broken, however, this resistance is dissipated.   Two examples that may be given are inflammation of the urinary bladder following spinal cord injury and paralysis and inflammation of a joint following degeneration consequent to tabes dorsalis. (11) *Acquired Immunity*.   As the term indicates, acquired immunity is a protective mechanism that develops in the body after birth.   It is specific and develops in response to specific antigens.   The degree of immunity fluctuates with the inciting agent and the time following exposure.   It may be *cellular*, that is, fixed to the cells or *humoral*, that is, due to substances circulating in the blood stream.   In the latter category may be mentioned such antibodies as agglutinins, antitoxins, bacteriolysins, precipitins, and opsonins.   (12) *Natural Immunity*.   In attempting to isolate one of the components of complement, Pillemer, in 1954 reported the discovery of a new serum protein—a euglobulin which he called *properdin* (Clough).   This substance occurs naturally, is a normal constituent of serum, and is an important factor in innate immunity.   It acts only in the presence of complement and Mg^{++} and is characterized by a low order of specificity as exemplified by the fact that it (a) requires no prior antigenic stimuli for its formation, (b) destroys bacteria, (c) neutralizes viruses, (d) produces lysis of certain abnormal erythrocytes, (e) is destroyed in animals by total-body irradiation, and (f) combines with many high molecular weight polysaccharides or polysaccharide complexes.

There are many *classifications* of inflammation and, as is so often the case under such circumstances, none is entirely satsifactory.   As in any other group of diseases, so in inflammation, an etiologic categorization is the best. This, however, is not completely satisfactory because the precise cause of any given inflammation is not always known and because frequently the causative agents are mixed.   For this reason, and because it suits the purposes of a general discussion on inflammation, a classification based on the duration of the process and the type of tissue reaction, as acute, subacute, and chronic appears to be quite satisfactory.   *Acute inflammation* is explosive, usually happens within a short period of time, and is attended principally by a neutrophilic response (examples—pimple, boil, carbuncle, etc.). *Subacute inflammation* is less explosive, less intense, happens over a longer period of time, and is attended principally by an eosinophilic response (examples—certain bacterial infections of the skin, certain inflammations of the appendix, some inflammations of the nose and sinuses, etc.).   *Chronic inflammation* is gradual in its development, spreads over a considerable interval of time, and is attended principally by a plasma cell, lymphocytic, and monocytic response (examples—tertiary syphilis, inflammation about a foreign body, late stages of burns, etc.).

Regardless of the type of inflammation, the fundamental *pathophysiologic changes* are the same.   They are, however, best *studied* in conjunction with *acute inflammation* because all the steps here are accelerated and increased in degree as compared with those in subacute and chronic inflammation. Thus, in the succeeding paragraphs most of the remarks (unless otherwise stated) apply to acute inflammation.   Many of the physiologic changes can actually be visualized by the time-tested experiment of placing the omentum or web of a foot of a curarized, live frog over the stage of a microscope, focusing on the vessels, and then gingerly applying a weak acid.   The morphologic changes are best observed by inducing an acute inflammatory response in the experimental animals, sacrificing the animals at regular intervals, and studying the affected tissue (after proper preparation)

microscopically. Although the alterations in inflammations proceed con-
cimitantly, overlapping, and progressively, they may nevertheless, for the
sake of description, be divided into the following categories: vascular
response, cellular response and exudation, fate, and complications. Finally,
a few separate words about subacute and chronic inflammations and concise
general descriptions of some of the more important groups of inflammations
will be presented.

VASCULAR RESPONSE IN INFLAMMATION

Normally the *vascular bed* of a given area is not used to capacity. In
fact, the majority of the capillaries are by-passed, bloodless, and virtually
invisible. When the tissue is exposed to an *irritant*, the first change noted
is a fleeting *constriction* of vessels probably due to the action of the noxious
agent directly on the vascular wall. This change, however, is only temporary, being followed rapidly by *dilatation* of the arterioles, venules, and
capillaries in the order mentioned. While axone reflexes may play a part
in vascular dilatation, the most important factor in bringing about this
change is doubtlessly paralysis of the wall itself due to the direct action of
the irritant and histamine, histamine-like (H) substance, or leukotaxine
(depending upon which theory is accepted). As a result of vascular dilatation, the resting capillary bed is opened and becomes conspicuously filled
with blood (Fig. 36*A*). Concomitantly, the affected part discloses the

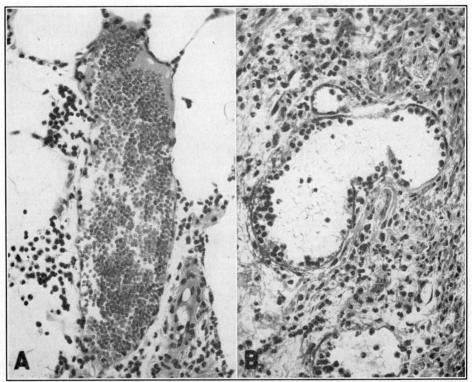

Fig. 36.—Vascular response in inflammation showing *A*, dilatation and engorgement of a
capillary with erythrocytes, and *B*, alinement (margination) of leukocytes along the capillary
endothelium. × 200.

following: (1) swelling or *tumor* (first due to increase in volume of blood but later aggravated by escape of fluid), (2) red discoloration or *rubor* (due to increase in number of erythrocytes), (3) increase in temperature or *calor* (due to a more rapid flow of blood from inside the body), and (4) pain or *dolor* (due to pressure on nerve endings). These, as we have seen, are the *cardinal signs* and *symptoms* of inflammation propounded by Celsus some 2000 years ago.

With initial dilatation of the vessels there is an *acceleration* of flow of the *bloodstream.* This is made possible because of the larger caliber of the vessels which, in turn, enables the arterial pressure to be transmitted more directly. As the pressure becomes equalized, however, the rate of *flow of blood decreases* progressively until, in unusual instances, it may cease flowing entirely and result in clotting of the blood. As a rule, though, deceleration stops before this point is reached. Retardation of the flow of blood is brought about by at least three factors—(1) swelling of the vascular endothelium and formed elements of the blood due to imbibition of water. This results from increased permeability of the cellular membranes which, in turn, is brought about by the action of the irritant and products of metabolism, (2) increased viscosity of the blood consequent to outpouring of plasma and increase in size of blood elements, and (3) increased resistance brought about by the alinement of leukocytes along the endothelium (see succeeding paragraph). Normally, because of the existence of an eddying force, blood flows through a vessel in two zones—a *central* or *axial zone* consisting of the formed elements of the blood and a *peripheral clear zone* consisting of plasma only. As the rate of blood flow diminishes, the eddying force decreases and the zonal separation becomes less and less distinct. The first change to occur is an outpouring of *plasma proteins*—albumin, globulins, and fibrinogen—from the vessels into the injured area. As already noted the single most important initiating factor in the escape of fluid from the capillaries is the increase in permeability of the capillary wall due to the direct action of *leukotaxine* (if Menkin's studies are accepted). At this point, it might be added that this is the mechanism in the early stages of inflammation when the medium of the injured area is alkaline. In the later stages, however, when the medium becomes acid leukotaxine is no longer active being replaced with another chemical factor that also increases capillary permeability called *exudin.* This factor too is liberated by injured cells and is contained in the pseudoglobulin-albumin fraction of the exudate. Also present in acid exudates is another even more powerful injury factor called *necrosin.* This substance is found in the euglobulin fraction of the exudate, produces extensive tissue destruction and local inflammation, and is absorbed into the blood stream whereby it produces a profound toxic effect on the body as a whole. Aside from these specific substances, the outpouring of plasma proteins from the vessels is also aided by the increased intraluminal pressure already referred to and by an increase in extravascular osmotic pressure due to protein breakdown products. The first *formed elements* to fall by the wayside are the *leukocytes.* One by one they enter the clear zone and edge their way peripherally. Then they stumble along the capillary endothelium slower and slower until they come to a halt and aline themselves along the inner surface of the vessel (Fig. 36*B*). This phenomenon of alinement is referred to as *margination* or *pavementing* of leukocytes. Almost as soon as they halt they begin to insinuate themselves (by way of ameboid movement) through the capillary wall until ultimately they come to lie free in the extravascular spaces. While the margination of leukocytes is in part a simple mechanical phenomenon wherein they enter the clear zone due to a decrease in the eddying force, it is also in part an active process brought about by an attraction of the leukocytes by leukotaxine which, as we have seen, eventuates from injured tissue cells. Gradually the *erythrocytes*, too, flow into the cytoplasmic zone, become attached to the endothelium, and then escape through the vascular wall to lie free in the extravascular tissue spaces. The process of escape of formed elements in the blood through intact capillaries is referred to as *emigration* or *diapedesis* (Gr. = through ÷ to leap). Diapedesis is active (ameboid) in the case of leukocytes but passive in the case of erythrocytes.

CELLULAR RESPONSE IN INFLAMMATION AND EXUDATION

Cellular response in inflammation encompasses activity on the part of both free (circulating or wandering) and fixed (tissue) cells and, as already indicated, is also accompanied by the escape of fluid from the vessels. The outpouring of an adventitious substance in or on tissues is known as *exudation* (L. = out + to sweat) and the product of exudation is referred to as an *exudate*. In general, an exudate has three essential components — fluid, cells, and necrotic material.

The *fluid* of an exudate comes mostly, as already pointed out, from the lumens of the vessels and is thus composed essentially of plasma (serum), albeit in a slightly altered form. As such, it is composed of the usual plasma proteins and may be rich in *fibrinogen*. The latter, being away from its normal habitat, unites with thrombin (which had previously been formed from the interaction of other blood constituents) to form *fibrin*. The precipitation of fibrin occurs not only between the cells throughout the injured area but, perhaps even more importantly, also within lymphatic channels and later capillaries where it forms fibrin plugs or thrombi. These, in turn, produce a true lymphatic (and later capillary) block which looms forth as an important factor in localizing the irritant. To some extent, this localization is also accomplished by entangling bacteria and other noxious agents and by causing apposition of surfaces when the inflammation reaches the surface. Later it acts as a framework upon which new tissue forms. The fibrin first exists as a meshwork of fine threads but as it ages it clumps and congeals to form masses of hyaline material. Later still, as a result of enzymatic activity, it again fluidifies. Other sources of fluid in an exudate are (1) disintegration of dead cells (brought about chiefly by enzyme activity) and (2) secretion of cuboidal or columnar epithelial cells. The latter occurs only in inflammations of mucous membranes such as those of the respiratory, gastrointestinal, and urogenital tracts and the material secreted is *mucus*. The main *functions* of the *fluid* of an *exudate* are (1) to dilute the original irritant and the noxious tissue metabolites, (2) to bring in various types of immune bodies, and (3) to help evacuate the waste products by washing them into the lympathics.

The *cells* of an *exudate* are derived in part from the bloodstream and in part from the tissues. The former escape from the vessels by the process of diapedesis and the force which causes both them and cells of tissue origin to migrate is called *chemotaxis* (Gr. = chemistry + arrangement). Chemotaxis is accomplished by ameboid movement. It is referred to as positive when cells are attracted to, and negative when they are repelled from, certain other cells or substances. Although the mechanism of chemotaxis is doubtlessly based on physicochemical changes it is as yet poorly undertsood. The initiating factor is leukotaxine which may act by way of electric charges or which, dissolved along with tissue disintegration products, forms a concentration gradient about the cell. The resulting alteration in surrounding tissue fluid produces a change in both the surface tension and the cytoplasm (gel to sol and reverse) of the cell and these, in turn, bring about its movement in one direction or another. The main purpose of chemotaxis is to bring in cells that will combat the irritant and aid in re- solving the inflammation. One of the functions of some of the cells of the exudate is *phagocytosis*. This phenomenon may be defined as the engulfing of bacteria, cells, and other substances by *phagocytes* (Gr. = to eat + cell), that is, by fixed or free cells that possess properties of ingestion. The precise mechanism of phagocytosis, like that of chemotaxis, is not clearly under- stood. It is presumed that when the particle to be engulfed contacts the cell it produces a change in the surface tension of the cell, which in turn, allows the cytoplasm to flow around the particle. Once the particle is within the cell it is acted upon by cytoplasmic enzymes and, depending upon its nature, it may (1) be destroyed, (2) remain in an insoluble state and later be extruded, or (3) destroy the cell and be liberated.

Morphologically the cellular response in inflammation is divided into that occurring in free cells and that occurring in fixed cells. *Free cells* are the cells of the exudate proper and consist of neutrophils, eosinophils, baso- phils, monocytes, lymphocytes, plasma cells, erythrocytes, platelets, and giant cells. *Fixed cells* are the cells of the tissues and comprise reticulum cells, loose connective tissue cells, endothelial cells, epithelioid cells, and foam cells.

Neutrophils (polymorphonuclear leukocytes, polymorphs, or granulocytes) arise from myeloid cells. In the human embryo they first appear in the liver in the second lunar month during the hepatic period of hematopoiesis (Sieracki). At the 9 cm. stage they appear in the spleen and after the fourth lunar month they are manufactured in the bone marrow. In normal adults, the latter is the only source of neutrophils. Factors governing the *maturation* and release of neutrophils from the marrow into the blood stream are not clearly understood. The spleen apparently does play a role, for splenectomy is followed by hyperplasia of the marrow cells and shielding the spleen from irradiation, or the intraperitoneal implantation of splenic tissue, in experi- mental animals, not only prevents total bone marrow aplasia and death from irradiation but also eventuates in a more rapid return of hematopoiesis to normal. Another stimulant is nucleoproteins in general and nucleopro- teins from dying neutrophils in particular. Both of these factors are said to produce maturation of neutrophils and their rhythmic hourly accession to the peripheral blood. Other factors governing the release of mature forms into the blood stream are (1) osmotic concentration of extracellular fluids, (2) diet, (3) destroyed tissue caused by infections, chemicals, neoplasms, thrombi, operations, *etc.*, (4) physical factors such as strenuous exercise, repeated vomiting, tachycardia, vitamins, *etc.*, and (5) hormones such as ACTH, growth hormone of the pituitary, adrenalin, and adrenal cortical extracts (Gordon). The *normal* life span of neutrophils has been determined as varying between 10 to 14 days. In normal adults, neutrophils comprise from 55 to 75 per cent of the leukocytes of the circulating blood. Because of this high percentage, an appreciable increase in their numbers brings about an increase in the total (over 10,000) leukocytic count of the blood— a state known as *leukocytosis* or *neutrophilia* while an appreciable decrease in their numbers brings about a decrease in the total (below 5,000) leukocytic count of the blood—a state known as *leukopenia* or *neutropenia*. While leukocytosis and leukopenia may occur in a variety of conditions they are generally manifestations of infection and in this connection the *mechanisms* involved are fundamental processes that remain constant regardless of the type of infection or inflammation. Leukocytosis is due to two factors—

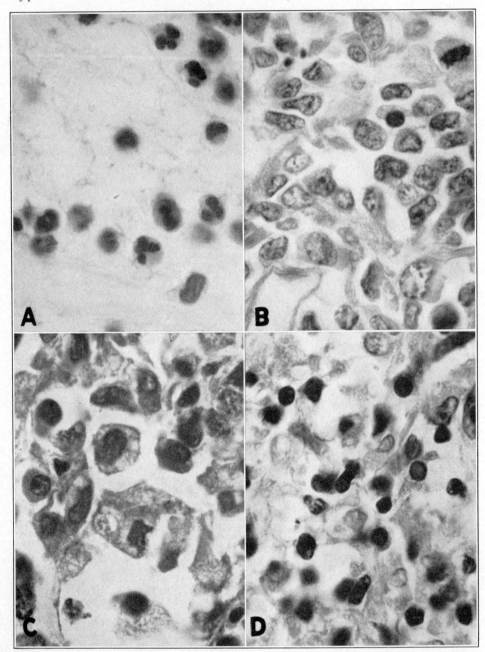

Fig. 37.—Cellular response in inflammation illustrating *A*, neutrophils, *B*, monocytes, *C*, monocytes containing ingested "fatty" material and (one cell in the center) cellular fragments, and *D*, lymphocytes (the dark staining cells). × 1350.

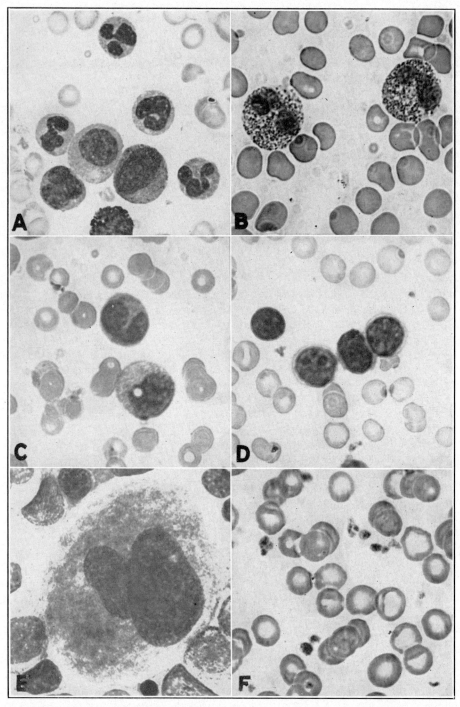

FIG. 38.—Blood smears of cells in inflammation showing *A*, neutrophils, *B*, eosinophils, *C*, monocytes, *D*, lymphocytes, *E*, a megakaryocyte, and *F*, platelets. × 1380.

(1) a thermolabile leukocytosis promoting factor (LPF) present in the exudate of the initial alkaline stage of inflammation and distributed between the alpha$_1$ and alpha$_2$ globulins and (2) a thermostable leukocytosis factor present in older acid exudate and associated with the euglobulin fraction (Menkin). Leukopenia is also due to two factors—(1) leukopenin associated with the pseudoglobulin fraction of alkaline exudates and (2) a leukopenic factor associated with the euglobulin fraction of acid exudates. *Morphologically* neutrophils are round, measure about 10 microns in diameter, possess a moderate amount of cytoplasm containing small neutrophilic granules, and disclose a multilobulated (2 to 5 lobes) nucleus with the lobes connected by threads of chromatin material (Fig. 37A). The details of the cells are less distinct in sections of tissue than they are in smears of peripheral blood stained by the Wright's or similar method (Fig. 38A). Many histochemical and other techniques have been used to study the more detailed constituents of neutrophils. One of these, the *peroxidase* reaction, is quite important in distinguishing neutrophils and eosinophils from other series of cells when their maturation has not been quite completed. Both neutrophils and eosinophils disclose positive blue-black cytoplasmic granules when the cells are treated with peroxidase, copper sulfate, and benzidine. The reaction is due to the presence of an oxidizing enzyme in these myeloid cells. Since this enzyme is absent in basophils, lymphocytes, plasma cells, and nucleated red cells, such cells do not disclose the blue-black granules. Monocytes sometimes give a positive and sometimes a negative reaction. The ordinary neutrophilic granules, when studied with the *electron microscope*, appear as round, oval, or rod-shaped vacuolic structures in air-dried preparations and as homogeneous dense structures with a clearly defined membrane and granular and filamentous mitrochondria in sectioned preparations. Some of the *physical properties* of mature neutrophils are (1) specific gravity 1.065, (2) migration to anode, (3) cataphoretic velocity slower than that of lymphocytes, (4) fragility inversely proportionate to vitamin C content, (5) maintenance of integrity in isotonic or slightly hypertonic solutions, (6) water content of 80 per cent, and (7) possession of an electrical change which by some is said to govern their emigration to inflammation, ameboid movement, phagocytic power, and a tendency to aggregate. The *enyzmatic* activity of neutrophils is quite varied. Among others, they disclose beta glucuronidase, phosphatases, diastase, proteolytic enzymes, lipase, and carbohydrate enzymes. *Neutrophils* are the first to arrive on the scene in any inflammation and are followed later by monocytes (macrophages). While the neutrophilic state may be intense and long in inflammations such as those caused by staphylococcus and quite the converse in those caused say by tubercle bacilli, the sequence of neutrophils followed by monocytes is always the same. This phenomenon is entriely nonspecific and is referable only to the local acidosis (Menkin). As already pointed out, once fibrinogen is transformed to fibrin the local circulation in an area of inflammation is impaired and the area is walled off or isolated. It develops its own hydrogen-ion concentration, circulation, and metabolism and, as a result, varies in its degree of acidity or alkalinity. It has further been established that neutrophils cannot survive at a pH below 7.0 while monocytes appear normal at a pH as low as 6.8. Thus, the cellular response will be dictated by the local situation. Since the initial stage of any inflammation is alkaline in reaction, neutrophils are the first cells to arrive on the scene. They are particularly abundant in acute inflammation caused by pyogenic bacteria. As already stated, they leave the blood vessels by diapedesis and enter the field by ameboid move-

ment. Their primary *function* is phagocytic against bacteria and, to a lesser extent, against other small, foreign particles. Later, as they disintegrate, they liberate enzymes which liquefy dead material and they may yield thromboplastin which aids in the coagulation of the blood.

Eosinophils, like neutrophils, arise from myeloid cells of the bone marrow. The eosinophilic granules, which give the cells their name, make their appearance in the metamyelocyte stage, following which the cells progress through the staff to the mature eosinophilic stage. The control of their *production* and *release* from the bone marrow is probably similar to that governing neutrophils, namely, (1) chemotaxis by way of nucleic acid and nucleoproteins of dying cells, (2) leukocytosis promoting factors, (3) splenic factor, and (4) endocrine glands (Cope). *Normally* eosinophils constitute from 1 to 4 per cent of the circulating leukocytes and number from 100 to 400 per cubic mm. of blood. An increase in number over 500 per cubic mm. or 5 per cent of the circulating white cells is referred to as *eosinophilia* while a decrease below 100 per cubic mm. or 1 per cent of circulating cells is called *eosinopenia*. *Eosinophilia* is seen in many diseases and pathologic states, some of which may be listed as follows: (1) parasitic infections—especially with helminths, (2) allergies—asthma, Loeffler's syndrome, tropical eosinophilia, food sensitivity, hay fever, urticaria, *etc.*, (3) skin conditions—of many types both inflammatory and degenerative such as pemphigus, eczema, *etc.*, (4) acute infections—scarlet fever and rheumatic fever especially during convalescence, (5) drugs and (6) miscellaneous—periarteritis nodosa, Hodgkin's disease, malignant tumors, ulcerative colitis, irradiation, and eosinophilic leukemia (Cope and Spiers). *Locally* an increase in eosinophils is noted in any subacute inflammation, in waning acute inflammation, in allergic inflammations, around parasites lodged in tissues, in hemorrhagic pleural fluids, in sputum of asthmatics, in nasal secretions in allergic rhinitis, in intestinal blood and mucus in bacillary dysentery, *etc.* *Eosinopenia* is also seen in a variety of pathologic states. It occurs, for example, as an accompaniment of hemorrhage, cold, shock, poisons, operative procedures, and a wide variety of infections. In other words, eosinopenia is a common manifestation of *stress phenomenon* of any type. The mechanism of eosinopenia is as follows. Injury or stress of any type is transmitted by nerve impulses through the peripheral nerves and spinal cord to the hypothalamus. The hypothalamus stimulates the anterior pituitary gland to produce ACTH (adrenocorticotropic hormone) which stimulates the adrenal cortex to produce corticoids and these in turn act upon the eosinophils to produce eosinopenia. The corticoids having the most profound effect are cortisone and compound E, that is, 11-17 oxysteroids (Thorn). Corticosterone (compound B) and dehydrocorticosterone (compound A) produce mild eosinopenia while 11-desoxycorticosterone, 11-desoxy-17-hydrocorticosterone (compound S), dehydroisoandosterone, and adrenosterone have no effect. Administration of cortisone or hydrocortisone to man either orally or intravenously is accompanied by a progressive eosinopenia ending in complete disappearance of eosinophils from the blood. This pehnomenon is made use of in establishing the integrity of the adrenal cortex in conditions such as Addison's disease or in determining the adequacy of bilateral adrenalectomy. In the test, referred to as the *Thorn test*, the administration of 25 mg. of ACTH intramuscularly produces a drop of 50 per cent in the eosinophilic count in the peripheral blood in a normal person as a result of stimulation of the adrenal cortex with production of adrenal cortical steroids. When adrenal cortex is not present, administration of ACTH will have no effect upon the eosinophilic count. Before leaving the adrenal gland it must also be stated that adrenalin alone will produce eosinopenia. It, however, produces its effect independent of the adrenal cortex. *Eosinopenia* is *produced* as a result of (1) lysis of eosinophils, (2) sequestration out of the blood stream into the tissues of the body especially reticulo-endothelial cells, intestines, lungs, and salivary glands, and (3) blocking of the bone marrow, that is, hyperplasia of the cells without maturation and release into the blood stream. *Morphologically* eosinophils are similar to neutrophils except that they disclose large intensely eosinophilic intracytoplasmic granules (Fig. 38*B*). These granules are insoluble in fat solvents as well as unheated acetic acid and dilute alkalies, are soluble in strong acids and alkalies, contain iron and phospholipids, stain with sudan III and Nile blue sulphate, and are not affected by trypsin or autolytic enzymes (Rebuck). Eosinophils give a positive oxidase and peroxidase reaction, show no phosphatase activity and, while they possess ameboid motion, their locomotion is less active and slower than that of neutrophils. Aside from indicating a staisfactory response of the organism to an illness the only other possible functions of eosinophils are that they may serve as a source of histamine and that they are concerned in some way with antigen-antibody reaction.

Basophilic cells are of two varieties—basophils of the circulating blood and mast cells of tissues. *Basophils* of the circulating blood, like neutrophils and eosinophils, arise from the myeloid cells of the bone marrow. Morphologically they appear similar to neutrophils except that they contain large coarse, varisized, metachromatic, purplish or bluish, water-soluble granules that frequently obscure the nucleus (Spiers). Most observers maintain that the granules are peroxidase negative while only a few have found that they are peroxidase positive (Rebuck). The *functions* of basophils have as yet been poorly elucidated. Since some amphibia have large numbers of such cells in their circulating blood, it has been suggested that they represent a functionless evolutionary state in man (Wintrobe). Against this, however, is the fact that, along with tissue mast cells, they appear in great numbers in healing inflammation and in various chronic inflammations. They are not phagocytic. They disappear from the blood after oral cortisone, during acute inflammation, and during stress. They contain histamine and their granules are rich in the anticoagulant—heparin. The latter property may facilitate resolution of an inflammation by preventing clotting of blood in capillaries and lymphatic channels in the late stages of the process. *Mast cells* develop *in situ* in tissues. They are larger than basophils and show no ameboid movement but are chemotaxic. Their granules are large, coarse, varying sudanophilic, phosphatase positive, and less water soluble than those of circulating basophils. The granules or cytoplasm lack nucleic acid lipase, peroxidase, free iron, and glycogen. In tissue culture the cells are quite active, vary tremendously in size, and when young possess fine granules and when old coarse granules. *Functionally*, mast cells disintegrate and disappear following stress or cortisone injections, are rich in heparin, and, showing a plasma clearing effect on lipemic blood, may be important in lipoprotein metabolism (Sjoredsma). Mast cells in mast cell tumors of mice and dogs and in the skin of man in urticaria pigmentosa are rich in histamine and mast cells from the skin and intraperitoneal washings of rats as well as mast cell tumors of mice abound in seratonin. Thus, they appear to have a species specificity as far as their histamine and seratonin containing properties are concerned.

Monocytes have a twofold origin, namely, (1) the bone marrow from a series of cells that is probably separate from the myeloid or other series and (2) throughout the body from the reticulum cells of the reticulo-endothelial system. In the latter instances, reticulum cells are said to give rise to a common free primitive round cell which then may differentiate into a monocyte or a lymphocyte. A third possibility, occurring under some circumstances, is that monocytes develop from lymphocytes in the process of becoming phagocytic (Tompkins). Normally, monocytes constitute from 3 to 6 per cent of the leukocytes of the circulating blood. In *tissues*, mono-cytic cells are known as macrophages, large mononuclears, mononuclear phagocytes, polyblasts, clasmatocytes, splenocytes, adventitial cells, resting wandering cells, endothelial leukocytes, and (in the brain) Gitter cells. Tissue macrophages develop from maturation of monocytes or directly from reticulum cells. Monocytes and tissue macrophages thus are normal in-habitants of all tissues that contain cells of the reticuloendothelial system and hence predominate in lymph nodes, spleen, bone marrow, and loose connective tissue. *Morphologically*, in blood smears, monocytes are larger than neutrophils, measuring baout 15 microns in diameter (Fig. 38C). Because the cells are mobile, their shape depends upon their movement. Generally, however, the contour is rounded, the cytoplasm is abundant, grayish-blue, and ground glass like, and the nucleus is large, indented, and central or eccentric (Wintrobe). The cytoplasm contains varisized vacuoles that stain supravitally with neutral red. The vacuoles are either scattered throughout the cytoplasm or are clustered in a rosette fashion in the area of the centriole. In addition, the cytoplasm contains neutral red granules which, however, are not specific for monocytes because they are present in other cells derived from the reticulo-endothelial system. In tissues, the cells are rounded; the cytoplasm is sharply defined, dense, and agranular, and the nucleus is round, elongated, or indented, and discloses uniformly distributed chromatin (Fig. 37 B and C). *Functionally*, monocytes are chemotaxic in tissues, are motile, and although actively phagocytic for a variety of sub-stances they are less so than tissue macrophages (Rebuck). In tissue cul-tures and in areas of inflammation they are rapidly transformed into tissue macrophages. In either case, they possess enzymes which doubtelssly aid in their phagocytic ability. Some of these are oxidases, proteolytic enzymes, peroxidases, and phosphatases. Other substances present are nucleic acid, lipids, phospholipids, and ribonucleoprotein. Aside from their phagocytic property, both monocytes and tissue macrophages are considreed cytologic sites for production of antibodies, with shedding of their cytoplasm being the mechanism by which this is accomplished. Two other sources of ma-terial added to the organism are the vacuoles of the cells and disintegration of monocytes themselves as a result of adrenal cortical activity such as occurs in the stress phenomenon. *Pathologically*, monocytes in the lungs have a particular propensity for ingesting carbon pigment and hemosiderin. When they contain the latter they are referred to as *heart failure cells* because they are especially numerous in cases of cardiac failure. Monocytes are present in acute, subacute, and chronic inflammations. In ordinary acute inflammations they appear late in the process but in some inflammations, such as viral infections and typhoid fever, they appear early and dominate the scene.

Lymphocytes are formed in lymphatic tissues throughout the body and are thus produced mostly in lymph nodes, Peyer's patches of the small intestine, spleen, tonsils, and thymus. To a lesser extent, they are also formed in bone marrow and connective tissue. In a *normal adult* they constitute from approximately 25 to 33 per cent and from 1,500 to 3,000 of all the luekocytes in the circulating blood (Wintrobe). In infants this number may be doubled. Numbers in excess of the maximum are referred to as *lymphocytosis* while numbers below the minimum are called *lymphopenia*. Some of the *causes* of *lymphocytosis* are (1) acute infections such as pertussis, infectious mononucleosis, and infectious lymphocytosis, (2) exanthemata such as mumps and German measles, (3) chronic infections such as tuberculosis, syphilis, undulant fever, and infectious hepatitis, (4) convalescence from acute infection, (5) endocrine disturbance such as thyrotoxicosis, (6) degenerations such as rickets and malnutrition, (7) tumors such as leukemia, and (8) relative such as in neutropenia. *Lymphopenia* is generally seen in conjunction with leukopenia—when all circulatory white blood cells are decreased in number. In addition, it may be encountered in Hodgkin's disease, cardiac failure, uremia, and cholemia. As has already been noted, it also follows the administration of ACTH or adrenal cortical hormones and is an accompaniment of the stress phenomenon. *Morphologically* small cells are usually considered to be mature lymphoid cells and are referred to as lymphocytes while larger cells are generally thought to represent immature lymphoid cells and are called lymphoblasts. Under normal circumstances, lymphocytes only are present in the circulating blood. Stained by Wright's method they are round and measure about 10 microns in diameter (Fig. 38*D*). The ctyoplasm is scanty or moderately abundant, sky blue, and forms a fine rim around the nucleus. Occasionally it contains bright red (azurophil) granules that are peroxidase negative. It also contains mitochondria that stain well with Janus green and appear as short thick rods arranged in clumps or encircling the nucleus. The nucleus is round or slightly indented and eccentric in position. Its margins are sharp and its nucleus is deep blue and contains dense aggregations of chromatin. In tissue sections lymphocytes are round, measure about 7.5 microns in diameter, reveal a scanty amount of almost imperceptible cytoplams and contain a round, deeply stained nucleus with uniformly dispersed cytoplasm (Fig. 37*D*). Based primarily on *tissue culture* techniques evidence has been presented that lymphocytes or their immediate precursors do transform into monocytes, macrophages, and plasma cells and that they may also be capable of transforming into neutrophils, epithelioid cells, giant cells, fibroblasts, and even erthryocytes. In changing to macrophages they disclose an increase in cytoplasm, phagocytic activity for bacteria as well as cellular debris and vital dyes, size of nucleus, parachromatin, number of neutral red cytoplasmic vacuoles, and depolarization locomotion (Rebuck). *Functionally*, lymphocytes are phagocytic for vital dyes, show no chemotaxis, and are motile. As a result of a tremendous amount of experimental work in recent years, there is much to indicate that cells in lymph nodes, including those destined for circulation, are capable of antibody formation (Sundberg). It has been shown, for example, that typhoid vaccine injected into the foot pad of rabbits is followed by an outpouring of lymphocytes from the popliteal lymph node and an increase in antibodies in popliteal lymph. Initially the node shows diffuse hyperplasia and secondarily it develops large germinal centers. It has also been demonstrate that mice treated with ACTH or adrenal cortical extracts disclose a decrease of lymphocytes in lymph nodes along with lymphopenia and at the same time they reveal an increase in serum proteins. Histologically the lymph nodes showed degenerative changes within 6 hours, reparative changes with mitoses of reticulum cells and maturation of lymphocytes within 9 hours, and restoration of the architecture to normal within

24 hours. ACTH administered to adrenalectomized animals produces no effect. Such experiments would tend to indicate that lymphocytes are concerned in the production of serum proteins and antibodies and that the mechanism may be under the control of the pituitary and adrenal glands. Finally, along similar lines, rabbits given 250 r. total-body irradiation develop lymphopenia. If they are injected with antigens 8 hours after exposure they reveal an extremely poor antibody response. This also presumably indicates that lymphocytes are concerned with antibody formation. The *enzymatic* content of lymphocyte varies (Rebuck). Lymphocytes in rabbits contain cathepsin, nuclease, amylase, lipase, lysozyme, and adenosinase. In man, circulating lymphocytes do not contain phosphatases but those present in lymph nodes, spleen, and bone marrow do. Adenosinase is also present in lymphocytes in man, and because of this, lymphocytes are said to be important in splitting toxic products of protein metabolism. Possibly as expressions of all the activities mentioned, lymphocytes are present locally in the late stages of acute, in subacute, and in chronic inflammations.

Plasma cells arise from lymphocytes and directly from reticulum cells. The most important sites of manufacture in the body, therefore, are lymphoid structures and to a lesser extent bone marrow. Normally, plasma cells are not present in the *circulation*. Abnormally, however, they may be seen in the peripheral blood in large numbers in serum sickness, German measles, and infectious hepatitis in which instances they are generally associated with a lymphocytosis. They may also be seen in the blood in smaller numbers in infectious mononucleosis, conditions associated with eosinophilia, hemolytic anemia, septicemia, agranulocytosis, and aplastic anemia (Sundberg). Both plasma cells and their precursors are present in the peripheral blood in plasma cell myeloma and leukemic reticulo-endotheliosis. *Morphologically*, plasma cells in tissues are readily identifiable. They measure from 8 to 20 microns in diameter, are rounded or oval, possess a moderate to abundant amount of lightly basophilic cytoplasm, and disclose a round, eccentrically placed or overhanging nucleus (Fig. 39). The nuclear chromatin is often clumped in small masses about the periphery rendering what is referred to as a cartwheel-like appearance. In smears of *peripheral blood* the cells are somewhat larger and are spherical or ellipsoidal (Fig. 40). The cytoplasm is abundant and deep blue (Wintrobe). Occasionally it contains colorless to pale pink granules in the perinuclear region and, when stained supravitally, discloses numerous mitochondria. Vacuoles are commonly present. The nucleus is round or oval and contains large dense masses of chromatin which may be arranged in a cartwheel-like fashion. *Functionally*, plasma cells are not remarkably phagocytic although immature forms do ingest erythrocytes, hemosiderin, crystals, and typhoid bacilli (Sundberg). Because plasmacytosis is attended by hyperglobulinemia and because antibodies are present in the globulins of the serum, plasma cells have long been considered as a source of antibodies (Sundberg). In recent years, numerous fruitful experiments have been conducted to illustrate this all important property. Rabbits treated with antigens consisting of such diversified materials as egg white, pneumococci, horse serum, and typhoid-paratyphoid vaccine have shown increases in plasma cells in bone marrow, spleen, and adipose tissue of the renal sinus and such increases have concomitantly been accompanied by measurable increases of antibodies in the serum. Children with rehumatic fever, chorea, and streptococcic pharyngitis show a plasmacytosis of the bone marrow and a simultaneous increase in serum gamma globulins. Most myeloma proteins, which are

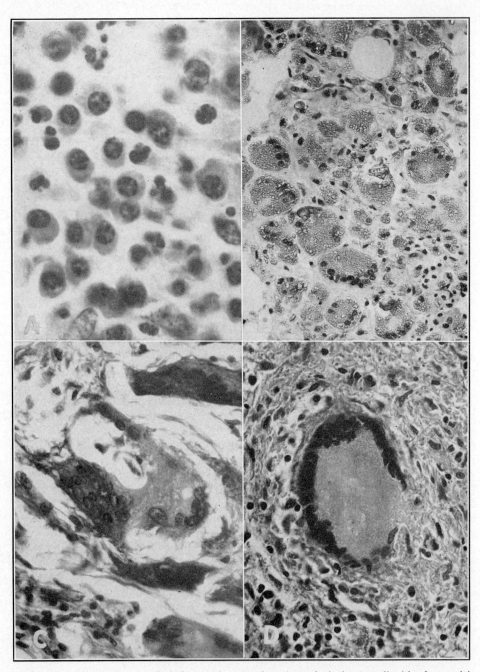

Fig. 39.—Cellular response in inflammation showing *A*, typical plasma cells (the few multi-nucleated cells are neutrophils). × 1350, *B*, multinucleated foreign body giant cells containing numerous intracytoplasmic talc granules. × 200, *C*, a multinucleated foreign body giant cell containing a fragment of a suture. × 400, and *D*, a typical Langhans' giant cell. × 400.

produced by the plasma cells of the myeloma, are immunologically related
to a portion of normal gamma globulin. Cases in humans have been recorded in whom there are no measurable gamma globulins, no evidence of
tissue or serum antibody formation, and no iso-agglutinins against heterologous blood groups. In such people, intense antigenic stimulation results
in no antibody titer or appearance of gamma globulins in their plasma.
They likewise disclsoe an absence of plasma cells in their bone marrow and
intense antigenic stimulation is not accompanied by plasmacytosis either in
the bone marrow or lymph nodes. Using the fluorescent antibody technique,
the administration of DPT (diphtheria, pertussin, and tetanus) and typhoid-
paratyphoid vaccine to normal children results in (1) an increase of medullary cells and prominence of well-defined follicles with active germinal

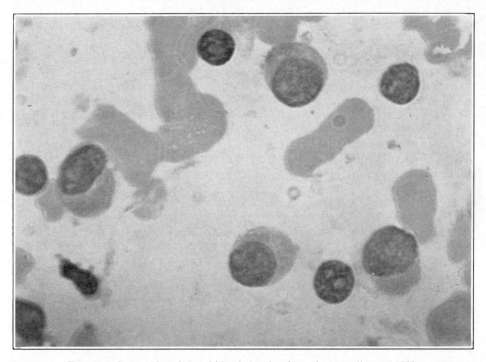

FIG. 40.—Smear of peripheral blood showing four plasma cells. × 1380.

centers in lymph nodes, (2) presence of plasma and preplasma cells in the
cortex of lymph nodes, (3) gamma globulin in cells of the interstitial fluid,
(4) pertussis antigen in reticulo-endothelial cells, and (5) antibodies against
diphtheria and tetanus toxins in plasma cells. Administration of these
vaccines to children with agammaglobulinemia discloses (1) narrow cortices
and absence of germinal centers and plasma cells in lymph nodes, and (2)
presence of the antigens but absence of both specific antibodies and gamma
globulins in the cells of the nodes. In other words, in agammaglobulinemia
there is a deficiency of cells (plasma cells) responsible for antibody formation.
From these, and other studies, it may be concluded that young plasma cells
or their precursors are favored as formers of antibodies because these cells
contain large amounts of antibody. Conversely, when plasma cells and
their precursors are absent antibody production is not possible. The fact

that with antibody formation there is usually also an increase in lymphocytes and a hyperplasia of lymph nodes may be explained by possible
transformation of young lymphocytes into immature plasma cells.

Erythrocytes, also known as *red blood cells* and *rubricytes*, first appear in
the human embryo in the liver in the second lunar month during the hepatic
period of hematopoiesis, in the spleen at the 9 cm. stage, and in the bone
marrow after the fourth lunar month (Sieracki). Normally, in adults, they
are manufactured only by the bone marrow. Abnormally, however, not only
the spleen and liver but also other organs of the reticulo-endothelial system,
such as lymph nodes, may take over their formation. In normal adults they
number from 4.5 to 5.8 million per c. mm. and by vloume constitute from
37 to 54 cc. per 100 cc. of circulating blood (Wintrobe). Also in normal
adults the total blood volume is about 75 cc. per kilogram of body weight,
the plasma volume is about 45 cc. per kilogram of body weight, and the red
blood cell volume is about 30 cc. per kilogram of body weight. A *decrease*
in blood volume due to a decrease in erythrocytes is known as *anemia*
(Gr. = negative + blood), *erythroctyopenia* (Gr. = red cell + poverty),
erythropenia (Gr. = red + poverty), or *oligemia* (Gr. = little + blood).
A decrease in blood volume due to a decrease in its fluid component or serum
is known as *anhydremia* (Gr. = negative + water + blood). When this is
accompanied by a depletion of fluid in the tissues the condition is referred
to as *dehydration* (L. or Gr. = away + water). An *increase* in blood volume
in general is referred to as plethora (Gr. = fullness), while an increase in its
serum component is called *hydremia* (Gr. = water + blood) and an increase
in its erythrocytic component is known as *polycythemia* (Gr. = many +
cells + blood). These and other related conditions are discussed more fully
in the succeeding sections in connection with Circulatory Disturbances,
page 188 and the Blood, Chapter 25, page 928. *Morphologically* erythrocytes
are circular, measure about 7.7 microns in diameter, possess no nucleus, and
exist as biconcave discs (Figs. 36*A* and 38—*A*, *B*, *C*, *D*, and *F*). Their main
function is the carrying of oxygen by way of the hemoglobin content. They
arrive on the inflammatory scene by passing through either intact (by
diapedesis) or ruptured (by rhexis) vessels.

Platelets, also known as *thrombocytes* (Gr. = clot + cell), have, at one time
or another, been considered to arise from plasma, vascular endothelium,
erythrocytes, nuclei of primitive red blood cells, nuclei of leukocytes, and
reticulo-endothelial cells (Wintrobe). Today, however, it is generally accepted that they stem from megakaryocytes of the bone marrow and
represent pinched-off portions of megakaryocytic cytoplasm. Evidence in
favor of a megakaryocytic origin consists of (1) platelets appear in the
embryo at the same time that megakaryocytes make their appearance,
(2) increasing the platelet count by repeated hemorrhages, by injection of
hemolytic substances, or by blocking the reticulo-endothelial system is
associated with an increase in megakaryocytes, (3) changes in megakaryocytes *in vitro* appear to mimic those thought to take place in the production
of platelets *in vivo*, (4) there is a close chemical similarity in the composition
of the cytoplasm of platelets and of megakaryocytes, and (5) the granules
in platelets are similar to the granules in megakaryocytes. The *rate* of
production of platelets has been estimated to be about 100,000 per c. mm.
per day. It has also been determined that all the platelets may be replaced
within 3 to 4 days and that after splenectomy for thrombocytopenic purpura
the count may reach 1,000,000 or more per c. mm. within 24 hours. The
life span of platelets is about 8 to 9 days. An accurate *enumeration* of plate-

lets is difficult because they are so labile. Nevertheless the normal number in newborn infants, by most accepted methods, ranges between 150,000 to 250,000 per c. mm. of blood. Wihtin three months this number reaches the normal adult range of 140,000 to 340,000 per c. mm. of blood. Physiologically, the number drops to as low as 25 per cent of normal during the first day of menstruation but by the third day of menstruation the number begins to increase again. An increase in platelet count is also noted after exercise, living at high altitudes, and after injection of adrenalin or histamine. *Pathologically* a temporary *increase* occurs as a result of trauma (especially fracture or surgical operation), asphyxia, acute blood loss, and acute infection such as rheumatic fever and suppuration of any kind. A more persistent increase is seen in chronic myeloid leukemia, erythremia, Hodgkin's disease, splenic atrophy, and after splenectomy. Occasionally the number may be elevated in carcinoma, Boeck's sarcoid, hyperadrenalism, splenic vein thrombosis, and idiopathically. A *decrease* in the number of circulating platelets is known as *thrombocytopenia* and may be seen idiopathically or following chronic blood loss. It may also occur as a result of the action of myelo-suppressive chemicals such as the nitrogen mustards, urethane, TEM, myleran, and benzol or as a result of agents to which the patient may be sensitive such as organic arsenicals, sulfonamides, quinidine, quinine, salicylates, antipyrine, phenobarbital, digitoxin, and mercurials. Other conditions causing or accompanied by thrombocytopenia are irradiation, ingestion of certain foods or orris root, animal products such as snake venoms and insect bites, disorders of the hematopoietic system such as leukemias and anemias as well as any of the splenomegalies, infections such as septicemia and bacterial endocarditis, and blood transfusions. *Morphologically*, the appearance of platelets is affected by the nature of the contacting surface, the anticoagulant, the thickness and moisture of the preparation, etc. Thus, many of the described variations are artefacts. Despite these limitations, however, platelets are colorless, moderately refractile, spherical, oval, and less commonly rod-shaped, nuclear-free structures that measure 2 to 4 microns in diameter and 7 to 8 c. microns in volume (Fig. 38*F*). Special staining (Romanowsky method) discloses azure granules in a hyaline light blue cytoplasm. Even with other stains these granules may be seen to be packed closely together rendering a mass that may be mistaken for a nucleus. Ordinarily the cytoplasm is lightly and diffusely eosinophilic. When the cytoplasm is basophilic it is said to represent young forms and when it contains vacuoles it is said to represent degenerating forms. Also younger platelets are larger than 4 microns in diameter and they are usually more irregular (dumbbell, comma, club, *etc.*) in appearance. Dark field illumination of adult platelets discloses translucent immobile granules in the center and electron microscopy reveals the internal structure to be composed of reticulated fibers. *Chemically* platelets consist principally of protein with lesser amounts of lipid and polysaccharide added. Some of the enzymes that have been demonstrated are peptidase, nucleotidase, acid phosphatase, oxidase, catalase, esterase, glycuronidase, dehydrogenase, pyrophosphatase, and acetylcholinesterase. The *functions* of platelets are concerned mainly with coagulation of blood. Because they agglutinate readily they tend to seal directly the injured vessel. Their agglutinative capacity is favored by colloid solutions such as gelatin, peptone, and lecithin and prevented by oxalate, citrate, and heparin. Platelets are also extremely important in initiating and enhancing clot formation as a result of liberation of thromboplastinogenase upon their disintegration. In addition, they possess a factor which neutralizes the action of heparin, a factor which possesses antifibrino-lytic activity, a factor which produces clot retraction, and seratonin which results in vasoconstriction.

Giant cells, as the term implies, are large cells that usually contain two or more nuclei. In general, they may be divided into those that are asso-ciated with inflammation or reaction to endogenous or exogenous foreign material of one type or another and those that represent rapidly proliferating and bizarre tumor cells. Here we are concerned only with the former. One of the first and classical papers devoted to the origin and description of the giant cells seen in tuberculosis was by Langhans in 1868 (Haythorn). His observations were most accurate and still hold good today (Fig. 39*B*, *C*, and *D*). He worked entirely with fresh tissue derived from miliary tubercles from the pleura and peritoneum. These he teased out or crushed and examined in salt solution, serum, or glycerine or in chromic or acetic acid. He discovered that the cells varied greatly in shape, size, and number of nuclei. They were round, oval, sausage shaped, elliptical, stellate, or irreg-ular. Some were sharp, others were ill defined. In size, some were small while others measured as much as 0.3 mm. in diameter. The nuclei varied from 2 to 100 or more. They were round or oval and sharply defined and generally contained nucleoli and central vacuoles. While the nuclei were usually arranged about the periphery with their long axis at right angles to the cell wall, some were bipolarly disposed and others were more diffusely scattered throughout the cell. The cytoplasm was abundant, pale, and homogeneous or finely granular. The center was clear or contained a fine fibrillar network. Since he worked with tubercular tissue, the designation *Langhans' giant cells* has since been applied to the giant cells seen in this disease. What he described, however, were giant cells that are seen not only in tuberculosis but are present in conjunction with reaction to any foreign material, that is, *foreign body giant cells*. If there is a difference between the two it exists in the distribution of the nuclei. In tuberculous giant cells the nuclei are usually, but not always, distributed about the periphery, while in foreign body giant cells they are usually, but not always, distributed diffusely or centrally. The *origin* of giant cells has elicited a great deal of investigation. At one time or another they have been considered to arise from connective tissue, epithelium, endothelium, muscle, nerves, fat cells, leukocytes, mesothelial cells, and endothelial cells. Today, however, most observers generally agree that monocytes and macrophages or their progen-itors—the reticulum cells—are the most important sources of giant cells. As to their mode of origin, some believe they arise as a result of amititoc nuclear division without corresponding cytoplasmic division while others believe they arise as a result of fusion of single cells. Since observations of tumor tissue supports the former and observations of tissue culture supports the latter, it is entirely likely that both modes are possible, depending upon particular circumstances. There is virtually complete agreement among all observers that the main *function* of giant cells is phagocytosis and that their formation is called forth in the presence of any foreign or insoluble substances in tissues that cannot be disposed of by neutrophils, monocytes, or macro-phages. In general, these substances consist of necrotic material, crystals, organisms such as tubercle bacilli or fungi and yeast, or anything that is insoluble or deleterious to tissue. Once the material is ingested intracellular enzymes act upon it and destroy it. If the material is inert it is extruded or liberated upon death of the cell. In the latter respect, giant cells may also help to spread infection rather than contain it. Once formed, giant cells may (1) fibrillate, split, and divide into mononuclear cells or (2) disintegrate and undergo absorption like all other cells. Among other sites, giant cells may be *seen* in (1) granulation tissue, (2) areas of degeneration about deposits of amyloid, hyalin, colloid, cholesterol, *etc.* or foci of necrosis including bone, (3) foreign bodies such as fats, oils, sutures, talcum powder, splinters, *etc.*, (4) infections such as tuberculosis, syphilis, fungous inflammations, *etc.*, (5) about animal parasites, and (6) miscellaneous granulomas.

Reticulum (reticular) *cells* are the primitive cells of the reticulo-endothelial system and as such are found in most tissues and organs of the body. In the quiescent state they are elongated, ill-defined, and inconspicuous. The cytoplasm is moderate in amount and eosinophilic and the nuclei are oval or elongated, relatively large, and evenly stained. When stimulated to proliferation the cells become bulkier and polygonal or rounded and measure 20 to 30 microns in diameter (Fig. 41 *A* and *B*). The cytoplasm becomes more dense and more eosinophilic while the nuclei become more rounded. In either case special (reticulum) stains show cytoplasmic processes of the cells connected directly with the underlying reticulum framework. Reticulum cells are actively phagocytic and are concerned with antibody formation. In addition, they are the primitive cells from which most, if not all, of the other mesenchymal (including hematological) cells of the body are derived. More specifically, they are the progenitors, either directly or indirectly of neutrophils, eosinophils, basophils, tissue mast cells, monocytes, macrophages, lymphocytes, plasma cells, erythrocytes, platelets, giant cells, connective tissue cells, endothelial cells, epithelioid cells, and foam cells. They are thus important in the genesis of all the cells that are concerned with inflammation. Since reticulum cells form an integral part of the reticuloendothelial system they are discussed further in Chapter 24, page 911.

Loose connective tissue cells arise from the mesenchyme which remains after other connective tissues of the body have been formed (Maximow and Bloom). Loose connective tissue is, however, still primitive and does give rise to other types of connective tissue. It exists as a white sticky mass and forms, as its main normal *function*, the supporting structure or framework of all organs, allowing safe movement of the connected parts in relation to each other. Normally, too, it is important in nutrition of tissues, for all substances to and from parenchymatous cells must pass through its layers. Under abnormal circumstances it forms the stage for the entire process of inflammation and is thus of extreme importance in connection with the topic at hand. Loose connective tissue is composed of cells and intercellular substance. The main *cells* consist of fibroblasts, undifferentiated mesenchymal cells, as well as varying numbers of macrophages and leukocytes already referred to in the preceding paragraphs. *Fibroblasts* are large, elongated spindle or star-shaped cells with a moderate amount of ill-defined eosinophilic cytoplasm that ends in two or more pointed processes (Fig. 41 *C*). Normally, the cytoplasm contains occasional small fat droplets, remains colorless when neutral red is applied supravitally, and discloses, near the nucleus, rod-shaped mitochondria, a diplosome, and a Golgi apparatus. The nuclei are oval or elongated, have a thin delineating membrane, contain fine chromatin, and disclose one or more nucleoli. Some investigators believe that fibroblasts are differentiated end cells which do not give rise to other cells of connective tissue, while other workers hold that they can revert to more primitive cells and thus produce not only other types of connective tissue cells but even such cells as osteoblasts. On occasion, they are slightly phagocytic and, while ameboid pseudopodia have not been demonstrated,

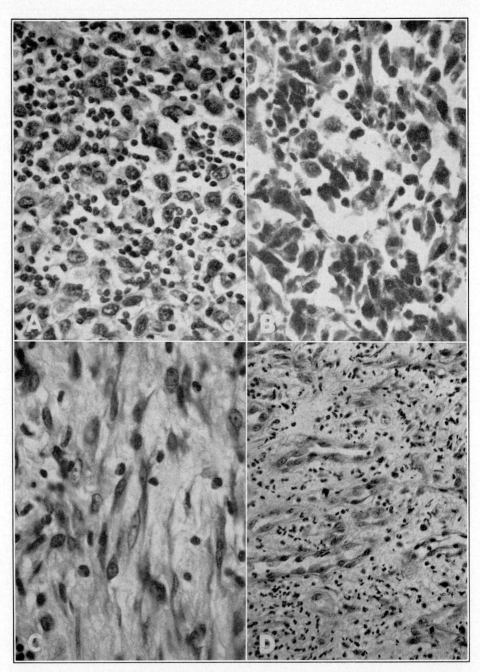

FIG. 41.—Cellular response in inflammation illustrating *A*, faintly staining but large, polyhedral reticulum cells. $\times$ 400, *B*, angular reticulum cells with long cytoplasmic processes. $\times$ 400, *C*, typical fibroblasts. $\times$ 400, and *D*, granulation tissue composed of leukocytes, fibroblasts, and prominent capillaries lined by conspicuous endothelial cells. $\times$ 200.

fibroblasts do move with a gliding motion. *Undifferentiated mesenchymal cells*, precursors of fibroblasts and probably identical with primitive reticulum cells, are scattered through loose connective tissue. The cells actually are similar to fibroblasts but are smaller and are particularly prevalent along capillaries. When stimulated, as in tissue cultures, inflammation, or by injection of toxins, they rapidly proliferate to produce new types of connective tissue cells. While the cells mentioned occupy a vital position in loose connective tissue, the main mass of such tissue is formed by *intercellular substance* which forms from condensation or crystallization of material secreted by the cells and which consists of collagenous, elastic, and reticulum fibers and ground substance. *Collagenous fibers* are long, branching, intertwining, straight or wavy threads or ribbons that measure 1 to 12 microns across. They are colorless and longitudinally striated and are composed of parallel fibrils held together and covered with a protein cement substance. Collagen fibers are flexible but are greatly resistant. They possess no specific staining reactions although they do stain sharply with acid aniline dyes, such as acid fuchsin and aniline blue—especially after mordants have been used. Collagen fibers are important in the healing phase of inflammation in scar formation. *Elastic fibers* are few in number in loose connective tissue. They exist as long, highly refractile, cylindrical, homogeneous, branching threads or flat ribbons that form a loose network, and that stain specifically with orcein or resorcin fuchsin. They yield readily to stretching but, upon release, they return to their former length. They contain a characteristic albuminoid element—elastin—which is resistant to boiling water, acids, and alkalies. *Reticulum fibers*, readily demonstrated with silver stains, are seen as fine thread-like structures that are continuous with collagen fibers. They are especially abundant where connective tissue meets other tissues such as epithelium, and they form networks around blood vessels and capillaries, muscle fibers, nerve fibers, fat cells, and respiratory portions of lungs. *Ground substance* is the homogeneous, metachromatically staining material that contains both the fibers and the cells of the loose connective tissue. It is composed of a mixture of proteins, carbohydrate, lipids, and water and is closely associated with fluid from blood plasma. Its viscosity varies from fluid to gel and is affected by spreading factors such as hyaluronidase and by hormones such as relaxin, ACTH, and cortisone. Thus its state may be an important factor, as the case may be, in either localization or spread of infection.

Endothelial cells, of course, form the inner lining of the entire cardiovascular system. While in other portions of the system there are other components of the wall, in capillaries the endothelial cells alone constitute the enclosing membrane. In inflammation, as already indicated, it is the capillary component of the cardiovascular tree that is all important. Under normal circumstances also, it is the capillaries that finally distribute the nutritive material, oxygen, and hormones to the tissues and in return collect the waste products of metabolism for transmission to the excretory organs. In the *living animal*, such as the omentum or the web of the tongue or foot of the frog or as observed through a special chamber in the ear of a rabbit, endothelial nuclei can be seen scattered along the capillary outlines (Maximow and Bloom). In *fixed tissues* the capillary wall is seen as a thin homogeneous membrane containing endothelial cells at varying distances. Injection of silver nitrate discloses the membrane to consist of a single layer of sharply defined, elongated endothelial cells. While at one time it was thought that these cells were discontinuous, electron microscopy has shown

9

that, with the possible exception of the capillaries in the intestinal villi and renal glomeruli, the endothelial cells form an intact membrane that completely surrounds the lumen. Thus, the exchange of fluid between the capillaries and the tissues is through the cytoplasm of capillary endothelium. *Morphologically*, endothelial cells are similar to fibroblasts (into which they can be transformed) and actually can only be recognized as endothelial cells when they form or attempt to form vascular channels (Fig. 41*D*). They possess tapering ends and are stretched along the axis of the capillaries. They are longer and fewer in number in the narrow capillaries and shorter and greater in number in the wider ones. The nuclei are elongated or oval, possess fine dust-like chromatin particles but no nucleoli, and disclose a delicate membrane that may be longitudinally folded. Wherever they go, capillaries are accompanied by (1) connective tissue cells (often loosely referred to as perithelium) in which are present fixed macrophages, undifferentiated mesenchymal cells, and nerve cells, and (2) collagen and reticulum fibers. The latter form a sheath that separates the endothelium from adjacent tissues. In nonmammals the pericapillary cells form a branching network which surrounds the capillaries and has the property of contraction. In mammals the endothelial cells themselves disclose this phenomenon. Capillaries *develop from* primitive mesenchymal cells or from previously existing capillaries. They are not only important in the initial stages of inflammation but also play a vital role in the reparative stages.

Epithelioid cells are derived from primitive connective tissue cells, reticulum cells, monocytes, and macrophages. They are called thus because they have a superficial resemblance to epithelial cells. They arise in a variety of inflammatory processes as a result of stimulation by a variety of *agents*. Some of the latter are (1) bacteria such as tubercle bacilli, lepra bacilli, typhoid bacilli, organisms of tularemia, gonococci, *etc.*, (2) viruses such as those producing lymphogranuloma venereum, (3) fungi and yeast-like organisms, (4) disintegration products of tumors, and (5) foreign body reactions such as iron filings, silica, nonspecific lipoid material, and even gases such as oxygen, nitrogen, and carbon dioxide (Wright). Epithelioid cell formation is thus a nonspecific reaction. Since, however, the cells form such a characteristic pattern in tuberculosis they have been extensively studied in connection with this disease. Using chemical extracts of cultures of human tubercle bacilli, Sabin demonstrated that epithelioid cells form as a result of the action of the *phosphatide fraction* and that the active principle in this is *phthioic acid*. When these materials are injected intraperitoneally into rabbits or guinea pigs the primitive cells of the omentum respond in characteristic fashion. Within 3 to 4 days they increase in number and in size and disclose within their cytoplasm large vacuoles that vary considerably in shape and size. Within 5 to 7 days their cytoplasm is filled with many coarse vacuoles of uniform size giving it a foamy appearance. By the second week the vacuoles become so fine and tiny that the cytoplasm in fixed cells appears dense and uniform. At this stage the cells attain the typical epithelioid *appearance*. As such, they are large, elongated, and single or clumped (Fig. 42*A*). They disclose ill-defined margins and contain a moderate to abundant amount of lightly eosinophilic ctyoplasm. The nuclei are usually elongated, rather delicately delineated, and lightly stained. The chromatin is finely clumped and often peripherally distributed. After the tenth day, Sabin demonstrated that the epithelioid cells become arranged in circumscribed clusters which are referred to as tubercles. These, as we shall see, are present in tuberculosis and other infections.

Foam cells are derived from reticulum or reticulo-endothelial cells and may thus be looked upon as phagocytic cells that have ingested an abundant amount of fatty material. They are rounded or polyhedral and measure from 20 to 200 microns in diameter (Fig. 42B). The cell borders are fine and distinct; the cytoplasm is abundant and finely granular, lacelike, or even somewhat (but minutely) vacuolated, and the nuclei are relatively small, round, evenly stained, and centrally placed. Foam cells are seen in a variety of nonspecific inflammations wherever fatty material is present such as bronchiectasis, inflammation of subcutaneous tissues, inflammations

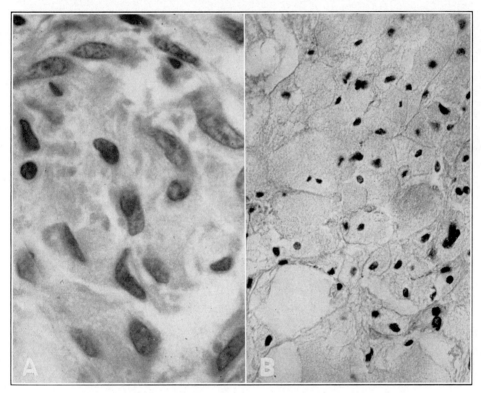

Fig. 42.—Cellular response in inflammation showing *A*, epithelioid
cells. × 900, and *B*, foam cells. × 400.

of the breast, *etc.* In other instances, however, such as in leprosy and scleroma, they form a highly characteristic part of the pathologic change.

The third component of an exudate consists of *necrotic material*. It is composed of (1) nuclear and cytoplasmic fragments derived from both free and fixed cells, (2) dead and disintegrating bacteria, and (3) any other material that may be added from extraneous sources.

Thus, since an exudate consists of fluid, cells, and debris, its appearance varies with the proportion of each of its component parts. Accordingly, *exudates* may be *classified* as follows: (1) catarrhal—when it is rich in mucus (Fig. 43), (2) serous—when it is thin, watery, relatively clear, and composed mostly of altered plasma (Figs. 44 and 45A), (3) fibrinous—when it is rich in fibrin that appears clumped or stringy (Fig. 45B and C), (4) *membranous* —when the fibrin entangles cells, bacteria, and necrotic material to form a

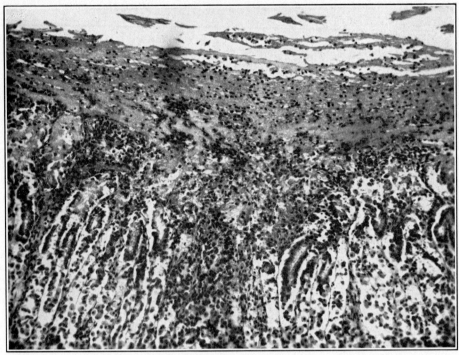

FIG. 43.—Catarrhal inflammation of the stomach disclosing hypersecretion of the gastric cells with outpouring of mucus over the surface.   × 100.

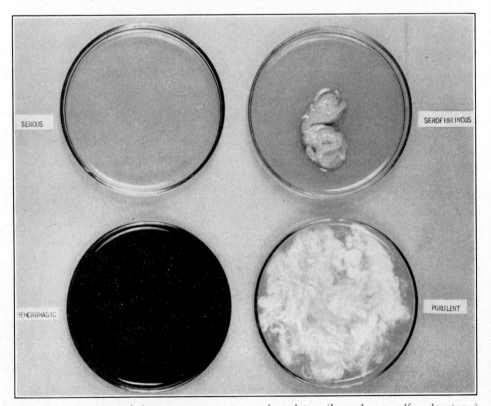

FIG. 44.—Appearance of the more common types of exudates. (Legends are self-explanatory.)

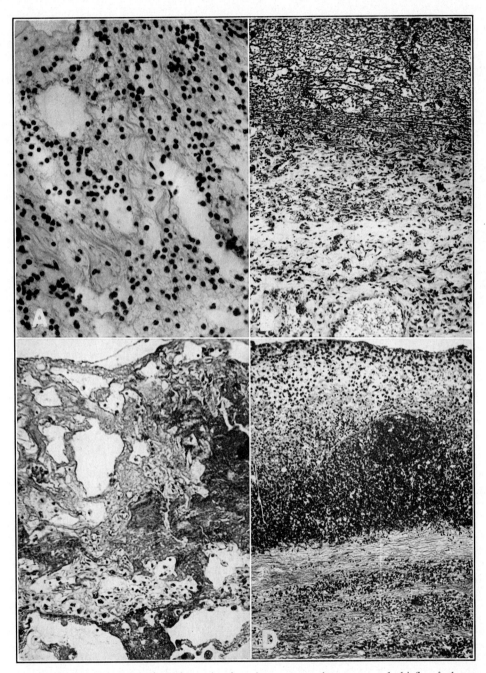

FIG. 45.—Various types of exudates showing *A*, serous exudate composed chiefly of plasma (serum) with scattered leukocytes added. × 200, *B*, fibrinous exudate with the fibrin deposited in the form of fine threads. × 100, *C*, fibrinous exudate with the fibrin deposited in the form of large hyaline clumps. × 100, and *D*, purulent exudate composed principally of fluid, neutrophils, and cellular fragments. × 100.

flat membranous covering, (5) *serofibrinous*—when it is partly serous and partly fibrinous (Fig. 44), (6) *hemorrhagic*—when it abounds in erythrocytes and appears red (Fig. 44), and (7) *purulent*—(pyogenic or suppurative) when it is rich in leukocytes and necrotic material and appears thick and creamy (Fig. 44 and 45*D*).   This type of exudate is also referred to simply as *pus*.

FATE OF INFLAMMATION

The *purpose of inflammation* is to rid the body of the noxious agent and to restore the tissue to normal or to as nearly normal as possible.   Thus, as soon as a particular portion of the body is exposed to an irritant certain defense processes are mobilized.   These, as we have seen, consist essentially of vascular and cellular responses.   If the irritant is not too powerful or abundant and the vascular and cellular responses are sufficient to adequately dispose of the noxious agent before there is extensive local death of cells, the debris is removed, the vessels return to normal, the newly arrived cells die or wander off, and the tissue is restored to normal.   This process is referred to as *resolution*.   It is accomplished essentially by phagocytosis of detritus by monocytes, by liquefaction of the remaining dead cells and debris by means of liberated cellular enzymes, and by absorption of the fluidified material by the lymphatics.

If, however, the irritant is too powerful and too abundant to be neutralized in a short period of time it may prolong the inflammation from acute to subacute or chronic or it may, in addition, bring about extensive destruction of tissue.   In either case, the tissue changes are exaggerated, healing is delayed, and the tissue may not be restored to normal.   When resolution is delayed or when excessive amounts of tissue are destroyed, *granulation tissue* forms to repair the injury.   In ordinary inflammation this consists of an abundance of fibroblasts and newly formed capillaries and a permeation with varying numbers of neutrophils, eosinophils, basophils, monocytes, lymphocytes, and plasma cells (Fig. 41*D*).   The granulation tissue forms from normal tissue at its junction with inflammatory or necrotic tissue and gradually creeps in to replace the latter.   The stimulus for its formation is a growth promoting factor in the exudate.   Eventually the granulation tissue may also disappear.   This is accomplished by liquefaction or wandering away of the leukocytes and by shrinkage and absorption of the capillaries and fibroblasts.   If the area of destruction and granulation tissue formation has not been great and if the tissue affected has good regenerative capacity, the granulation tissue may ultimately be virtually completely resorbed and the area restored to near normal.   Such is the case in clean-cut operations where the edges of the incision are closely applied.   Under these circumstances, healing is said to occur by *first intention* or *primary union* (Menkin).   When, however, the wound is open or suppurates, when *regeneration* of local tissue is slower, and when granulation tissue forms in greater amounts, ultimate resorption is less complete, restoration to normal does not take place, and the site of inflammation is replaced with an overabundance of fibrous tissue formation or *scar*.   This process is referred to as *healing* by *replacement* or *organization*.   Occasionally the tissue, upon regeneration, changes in appearance as for example a transformation of columnar to squamous epithelium.   This process is known as *metaplasia* (Gr. = after + to form).   Tissues that have good regenerative capacities are epithelium, mesothelium, endothelium, connective tissue, fat tissue, bone, bone marrow, cartilage, neuroglia, and nerve fibers; those that have limited regenerative capacity are striated muscle, smooth, muscle, and cardiac muscle, while tissue that has no regenerative capacity is functioning brain tissue (ganglion cells).

COMPLICATIONS OF INFLAMMATION

As already indicated, the purposes of the vascular and cellular responses in inflammation are, first, to localize the process and, second, to rid the body of the noxious agent before irreparable damage is done. If these aims cannot be accomplished, certain complications may accompany or follow the inflammation. Some of these are as follows: (1) *Cellulitis*. Although cellulitis usually means inflammation of cells actually it connotes a

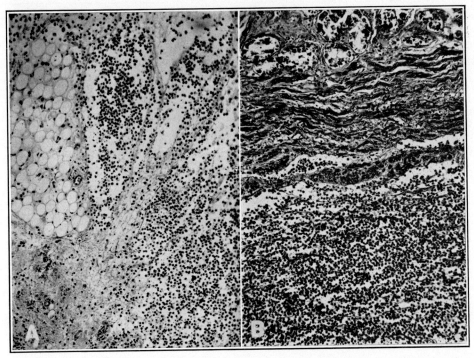

Fig. 46.—Complications of inflammation showing *A*, cellulitis of the loose, subcutaneous connective tissue with neutrophils diffusely permeating the tissue. × 100, and *B*, plegmon of the wall of the stomach with intense neutrophilic infiltration and early breakdown of tissue. × 50.

spreading, purulent inflammation of the loose, subcutaneous, connective tissue (Fig. 46*A*). (2) *Phlegmon*. This results from failure of localization of inflammation of connective tissue and means spread of the process with ultimate breakdown of tissue (Fig. 46*B*). (3) *Abscess*. An abscess (L. = a going away) may be defined as localized collection of broken down tissues and cells (pus) contained in a cavity formed by disintegration of the tissue. It may be acute or chronic. An acute abscess is one that develops over a short period of time and discloses from within out pus, necrotic material, and recent granulation tissue (Fig. 47*A*). A chronic abscess develops over a longer period of time and usually differs from an acute abscess in that the pus is more sharply separated from the wall and the latter is composed of old granulation tissue or dense fibrous tissue (Fig. 47B).   (4) *Ulcer*.   An ulcer is a circumscribed area of destroyed tissue located on a cutaneous or mucous surface (Fig. 48A).   Structurally, it is similar to the wall of an abscess (Fig. 48B).   (5) *Fissure*.   A fissure is a split or groove lined by necrotic and granulation tissue.   (6) *Sinus*.   A sinus is a blindly ending tract also lined by necrotic and granulation tissue.   (7) *Fistula*.   A fistula is similar to a sinus except that the tract connects a hollow organ with another cavity or the exterior of the body (Fig. 48C).   (8) *Subacute inflammation* (see below). (9) *Chronic inflammation* (see below).

Aside from local complications of acute inflammation, *infections* of *bacterial origin* may sometimes extend into the *systemic* circulation and thus be distributed throughout the body.   Intoxication due to the dissemination

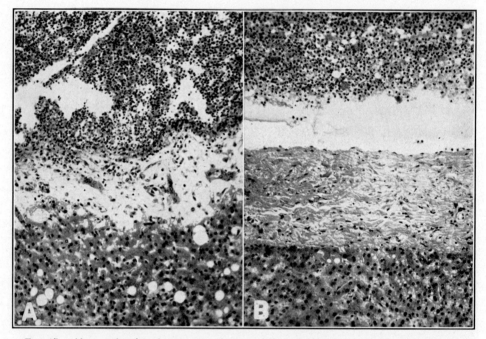

FIG. 47.—Abscess showing *A*, an acute abscess with the lumen containing neutrophils, cellular fragments, and fluid and the wall composed of recent granulation tissue, and *B*, a chronic abscess with the pus in the lumen sharply demarcated from a dense, fibrous tissue wall.   × 100.

of products of saprophytic organisms is referred to as *sapremia* (Gr. = rotten + blood).   The presence of bacteria in the blood without accompanying clinical manifestations is called *bacteremia* (Gr. = rod + blood). Intoxication due to the absorption of bacterial toxins formed at a local site of inflammation is known as *toxemia* (Gr. = poison + blood).   Intoxication due to the presence of pathogenic bacteria and their toxins in the blood is referred to as *septicemia* (Gr. = putrid + blood), *sepsis* (Gr. = decay), or *septic infection*.   Finally, septicemia due to pyogenic organisms and characterized by the presence of multiple abscesses throughout the body is called *pyemia* (Gr. = pus + blood).   Thus, in all these conditions except bacteremia there are general clinical manifestations.   In essence, these consist of fever, chills, sweating, tachycardia, and prostration.   *Fever* is seen in conjunction with local inflammation when the products of inflammation are

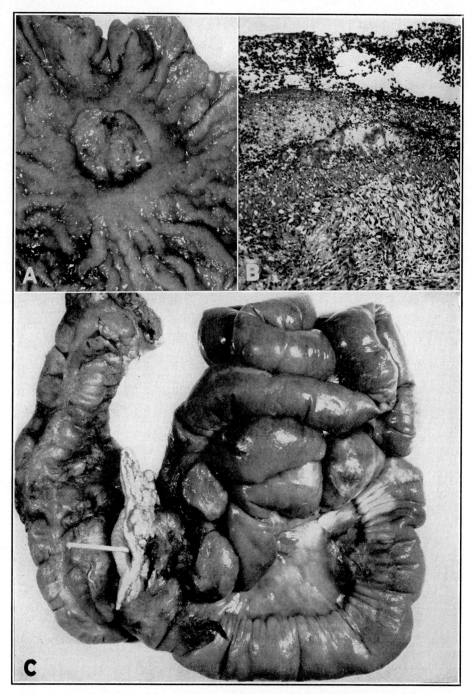

Fig. 48.—Complications of inflammation showing *A*, the gross appearance of an ulcer of the stomach, *B*, the microscopic appearance of an ulcer of the stomach illustrating from above down nuclear fragments, fibrin and neutrophils, and granulation tissue.   × 100, and *C*, ileocutaneous fistula consequent to regional ileitis illustrating an applicator protruding from the cutaneous opening.

absorbed into the blood stream or in conjunction with invasion of the blood stream by the organisms themselves (Harrell). More specifically, in cases of exudation, Menkin has isolated a fever-producing substance which he called *pyrexin*. This is present in the euglobulin fraction of exudates, arises as a protein split product from cellular injury, is a polypeptide to which a carbohydrate group seems to be attached, and has been isolated in crystalline state. At any rate, the absorbed products of inflammation, the organisms themselves, or pyrexin produce an increase in general metabolism of the body which in turn results in consumption of additional calories and generation of additional heat. These have a twofold effect. Unless the consumed calories are supplied in the diet, the body stores of carbohydrate, fat, and protein are depleted resulting in a wasting away of the body as a whole. Unless the increased heat is dissipated, the temperature of the body increases and fever results. Aside from infection, fever may also be seen in conjunction with (1) physiologic processes such as menstruation, (2) interference in evaporation from the skin as a result of increased environmental temperature and humidity or as a result of congenital defects of the skin such as ichthyosis or ectodermal dysplasia, (3) interference in the heat regulating mechanism of the hypothalamus, and (4) absorption of toxic products from degeneration of tumors. *Chills* are seen at the onset of infections and date the invasion of the blood stream by organisms. At this time, the liberation of foreign proteins results in an antigen-antibody reaction which produces constriction of the peripheral arterioles of the skin. The consequent diminution in the flow of blood to the skin causes local chilling. The shivering and shaking which follows represents a reflex increase in muscular activity in an attempt to raise the internal temperature to compensate for the decreased cutaneous temperature. *Sweating* is a mechanism brought into play to lower the temperature of the body by increasing evaporation from the skin. *Tachycardia* (increased heart rate), together with the inevitable concomitant increase in pulse rate, occurs as the temperature rises and represents an attempt to increase the blood flow to the skin in order to increase heat dissipation by radiation. *Prostration* is a manifestation of generalized peripheral vascular collapse which is seen not only in severe local or general infections but also in many other conditions. It is discussed under the heading of Shock, Chapter 6, page 205.

SUBACUTE INFLAMMATION

As already stated in the *definition*, subacute inflammation as compared with acute inflammation is less explosive, less intense, happens within a longer period of time, and is attended principally by an eosinophilic response. The condition is between acute inflammation on the one hand and chronic inflammation on the other. It thus exhibits stigmas of both acute and chronic inflammation, and since there is usually gradation from one to the other, most authors prefer to omit it altogether and speak instead of only acute and chronic inflammation. Subacute inflammation results from prolongation of an acute inflammation or, when conditions are correct, may start as such from the beginning. The *pathogenesis* is exactly the same as that in acute inflammation. *Clinically* the cardinal symptoms and signs of inflammation (swelling, red discoloration, increased temperature, and pain) although present are usually less distinct than in acute inflammation. *Histologically* there is generally less intense leukocytic infiltration, fewer numbers of neutrophils, moderate numbers of plasma cells, lymphocytes, and monocytes, increased numbers of eosinophils, less disintegration of tissue, and greater numbers of capillaries and fibroblasts (Fig. 49). The *fate* and *complications* are similar to those in acute inflammation.

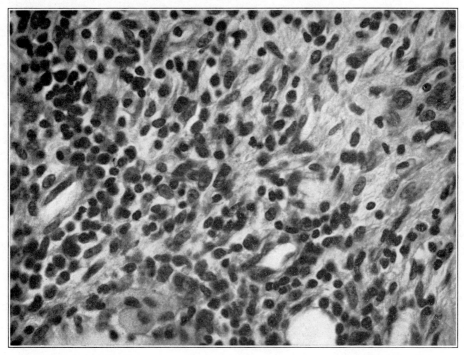

FIG. 49.—Subacute inflammation disclosing a stroma of fibroblasts containing scattered capillaries and permeated with moderate numbers of eosinophils (not recognizable as such in the black and white prints), neutrophils, plasma cells, lymphocytes, and monocytes. × 400.

CHRONIC INFLAMMATION

Chronic inflammation, as compared with acute inflammation, is gradual in development, consumes more time, and is attended principally by a plasma cell, lymphocytic, and monocytic response. It may result from a prolongation of an acute or a subacute inflammation or, when the nature of the irritant as compared with tissue resistance is of a certain quality, it may be chronic from the start. Although more subtle, the pathogenesis is exactly the same as that in acute inflammation. *Clinically*, swelling and pain are generally present but increased temperature and a red discoloration are frequently wanting. *Pathologically*, in comparison with acute inflammation, neutrophils and eosinophils are superseded in number by plasma cells, lymphocytes, and monocytes, fibroblasts are more abundant and more mature, and the capillaries usually have thicker walls (Fig. 50). The *fate* and *complications* are similar to those in acute inflammation but, as a rule, resolution is less complete, regeneration of tissue is less frequent, and healing by fibrous tissue replacement is more common.

BROAD GROUPS OF INFLAMMATIONS

This discussion will be limited to the more common groups of inflammations and, in two instances, to specific inflammations. The considerations

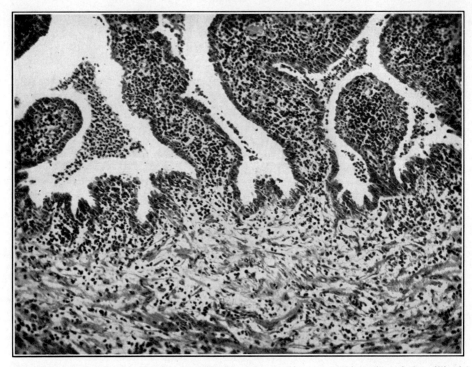

Fig. 50.—Chronic inflammation of a fallopian tube showing great thickening of the villi with plasma cells, lymphocytes, monocytes, and fewer numbers of neutrophils, and granulation tissue in the subepithelial layer. × 100.

will be general, for the various diseases in each group as they are found in the different tissues and organs of the body are taken up in greater detail in appropriate places in subsequent portions of the text. The inflammations to be considered here are allergic, viral, rickettsial, fungous, parasitic, foreign body, granulomatous, tuberculous, and syphilitic.

ALLERGIC INFLAMMATIONS

Allergic inflammation is simply a tissue response developing on the basis of allergy. *Allergy* (Gr. = other + energy) may be defined as a condition of unusual susceptibility to a substance which is harmless in similar amounts to other members of the same species. *Hypersensitivity* or *hypersensitiveness* is a state of altered reactivity in which the body reacts to a foreign agent more strongly than normally. *Idiosyncrasy* (Gr. = own + mixture or temperament) was first employed to indicate an individual and peculiar susceptibility to a drug. Now the term encompasses, in addition, susceptibility to proteins and other agents. In practice, the terms allergy, hypersensitivity, and even idiosyncrasy are used synonymously (Tuft). *Atopy* is still another term in common usage. It was first used by Coca in 1922 in connection with the clinical forms of human hypersensitivity that do not occur in lower animals and that are hereditarily transmitted. It included asthma, hay fever, and atopic dermatitis. Today the term is used to differentiate all familial or hereditary human allergic diseases from artificially induced hypersensitive states (Sheldon). *Anaphylaxis* (Gr. = backward + protection) indicates an exaggerated reaction of an organism to foreing protein or other substances. The designation was originally restricted to sensitization in laboratory animals but more recently it is also widely used in connection with humans.

The *basis* of an *allergic inflammation* is generally regarded as an antigen-antibody reaction. In the latter connection also, there are many confusing words employed which should be defined. An *antigen* (Gr. = antibody + to form) is any substance which when introduced into the blood or tissues incites the formation of an antibody. The designation is most often used in connection with proteins but also includes certain polysaccharides. It encompasses such substances as toxins, ferments, precipitogens, agglutinogens, opsogens, lysogens, and venins. An *antibody* is a specific substance produced in an animal in response to an antigen with which it reacts specifically. Antibodies are specific proteins usually found in the globulin fraction of blood plasma. Some of the more common antibodies are amboceptors, agglutinins, anti-enzymes, antitoxins, bacteriolysins, cytotoxins, hemolysins, opsonins, and precipitins. In *allergy* the respective antigen and antibody are termed *allergen* and *allergin*, in *atopy*—*atopen* and *reagin*, and in *anaphy-laxis*—*anaphylactogen* and *anaphylactin* or *anaphylactic antibody*. Despite these delineations, the terms allergin and reagin are also used synonymously and, in fact, the designation reagin has more or less replaced the word allergin. Finally, a *blocking* or *neutralizing antibody* is an antibody which blocks or inhibits the usual agglutination phenomenon. It competes with reagin (allergin) for the allergen and reacts with it in an innocuous manner. Blocking antibodies are formed in the process of hyposensitization or desensitization.

Referring to allergy in its broadest sense, there are many *types* of *antigens* or *allergens* that are responsible for a hypersensitive state. A few of these may be categorized as follows: (1) *microbes*—including most if not all bacteria, viruses, fungi, and spirochetes, (2) *parasites*—especially the round worm group, (3) *food*—almost any food with the commonest being wheat, egg, milk, potato, beans, tomato, and chocolate (Withers), (4) *animal products*—especially serum, dander, hair, and feathers, (5) *plants* particularly *pollens*—from trees, grasses, flowers, and weeds including especially poison oak, ragweed, and timothy, and (6) *drugs*—such as (*a*) alkaloids—from opium, quinine bark, belladonna leaves, stramonium, and hyoscyanus as well as the cocaine group, (*b*) essential oils and balsams—sandalwood oil and turpentine, (*c*) metals—mercury, arsenic, iron, gold, and nickel, (*d*) halogens —bromides and iodides, (*e*) coal tar—benzol and methane derivatives as antipyrine, iodoform, salicylic acid (aspirin), creosote, and salol, (*f*) endocrine products—insulin, estrogens, and extracts of thyroid, pituitary, liver, pancreas, *etc.*, (*g*) antibiotics and chemotherapeutic agents—penicillin, streptomycin, and similar compounds as well as sulfonamides, and (*h*) miscellaneous—phenolphthalein, barbiturates, certain vitamins, *etc.* (Tuft). The amounts of any of the substances listed necessary to elicit an allergic state vary greatly and the routes of entrance into the body may be inhalation, ingestion, cutaneous, or parenteral.

The *antibodies* produced in response to the many antigens or allergens listed, and to others not listed, are extremely varied and, as already noted, are *variously called*. It is, however, generally accepted that a single antibody is produced for each single determinant in the antigen (Burrage). While the antibodies vary in particle size, molecular weight, electrophoretic mobility, possible valency, firmness of union with antigen, avidity for union with

antigen, avidity for union with complement, *etc.* there is really no evidence
to indicate that all of the named antibodies are actually different.   For
example, it has been shown that agglutinin and precipitin to Type I pneumococcus are identical.   It follows, therefore, that precipitins, agglutinins,
opsonins, and antitoxins in general may be one and the same and that the
apparent differences may be due only to variations in external circumstances
and methods of testing.

Regarding the *formation* of *antibodies*, there are in essence two theories in
vogue currently.   One theory holds that antibodies are globulins and that
their antibody properties are due to adaptation of their shape to that of the
determinant group of the antigen.   This theory requires the continued
presence of antigen for antibody formation.   The second theory holds that
antigen must be present to start antibody formation but once the process is
under way antigen is not necessary for the continued presence of antibody,
for this function is imparted on a permanent basis to subsequent daughter
cells (Burrage).   Since antibody is considered to be protein and since most
living cells produce protein it is theoretically possible for most cells coming
in contact with antigen to be the *site* of *antibody formation.*   In practice,
however, it has been conclusively shown that this site is located in progeny
of the reticulo-endothelial cells, namely, macrophages, lymphocytes, and
plasma cells (Blatt).   Although some evidence favoring these cells has already been presented in preceding sections in connection with the cells of
the exudate, highlights may be briefly summarized here for the sake of
convenience.   *Macrophages* are considered capable of antibody formation
because (1) they are actively phagocytic and are thus capable of ingesting
many types of foreign material including antigen, (2) blockade of macrophages, as by injection of india ink, results in suppression of antibody formation, (3) they reveal the phenomenon of shedding of cytoplasm—a mechanism considered to exist in antibody formation, and (4) they appear to be
capable of manufacturing globulin when grown on culture medium.   *Lymphocytes* are held responsible for antibody formation because (1) small lymphocytes from lymph nodes of vaccinated animals injected into irradiated
animals transfer to these animals the ability to form specific antibodies
against the original vaccine, (2) there is a higher antibody titer in the cell
sediment, which is composed of 99 per cent lymphocytes, than in the lymph
plasma from nodes in the region of a single injection of antigen, (3) lymphocytes from the thoracic duct lymph from animals injected with bacterial
antigens form antibodies *in vitro*, and (4) immune responses to foreign
proteins can be transferred from animal to animal in cells from lymph nodes
which consist of more than 95 per cent lymphocytes.   *Plasma cells* are held
responsible for antibody formation because (1) rabbits immunized intensively with pneumococci show more antibody in extracts of fat of renal
pelvis, which contains mostly plasma cells, than in extracts of other tissues,
(2) antibody is produced *in vitro* by fragments of red pulp (reticulum and
plasma cells) but not of white pulp (lymphocytes) obtained from spleens of
animals given secondary injections of bacteria, and (3) examination of
tissues of vaccinated animals by tracer techniques (fluorescent-stained)
show antibody residing in plasma cells.

Currently there are two *basic concepts* concerning the *mechanism* of *sensitization* (Blatt).   Bela Schick holds that there are two forms of allergy.   One
is physiologic and thus beneficial.   It functions best in the presence of bacteria that produce exotoxins and leads to immunity.   By this mechanism the
host is able to ward off and fight diseases caused by invading pathogenic

microorganisms. The second form of allergy develops following the invasion of any foreign protein (including bacterial) which, because it is an alien substance, must be eliminated. Although the mechanism of formation of this type of allergy is similar to the physiologic type, it results in hypersensitivity which is harmful and pathologic. The second basic concept regarding the mechanism of sensitization is that proposed by Sevog. According to him, the genesis of all allergic manifestations is traced to a single process. In his opinion, any foreign reactive substance entering the animal system and not being immediately destroyed alters cell proteins to make them antigenic, thus causing reactions associated with hypersensitization. In other words, the injured proteins of cells are directly and chemically responsible for the manifestations the patient presents. Antibody formation is secondary and the various antibodies are toxic products produced by the host's metabolic system against the foreign agents. The appearance of antibodies requires a latent period of 10 to 14 days and during this the mechanism of hypersensitivity becomes established. The latter outlasts the antibody response, remains as a potentially active mechanism, responds immediately to secondary antigenic stimuli, does not require a latent preparatory period, affords a defense against infectious agents upon re-exposure, and is called into play when restimulated by allergic agents. Locally, it is accompanied by an accelerated inflammatory response because of previous contact with antigen. The phenomenon of *immunity*, according to Sevog, is intimately related to the hypersensitive mechanism and develops along with it. It results from foreign proteins combining with the host's enzyme system and synthesizing altered globulins or antibodies.

The simplest, and for this reason, the best, *clinical classification* of the *hypersensitive* or *allergic reactions* is the early response and the delayed response (Lawrence). The designation *early response* is employed in connection with those reactions attended by macroscopic manifestations of inflammation within a matter of minutes after the deposition of or contact with the sensitizing agent. This response in addition is characterized by the presence of measurable serum antibody and the passive transfer of the response by means of serum. Furthermore, the antigens evoking this response *in vivo* are not cytotoxic for explanted tissues of the sensitive host, and the inflammatory response requires the presence of vessels or smooth muscle to be manifest, as indicated by the fact that because it does not occur in the cornea. The early response encompasses such conditions as hay fever, asthma, serum sickness, systemic anaphylactic shock, and Arthus phenomenon and is brought about by such sensitizing materials as pollens, soluble proteins, and carbohydrates. The designation *delayed response* is employed in connection with those reactions attended by a maximum macroscopic appearance of inflammatory response in from 18 to 48 hours after the application of the test antigen. The spread of this time interval depends upon the degree of sensitivity of the host and the amount of antigen used. Although it parallels the events in the immune responses in general, the delayed allergy (1) has no relation to serum antibody for specific antibodies are not found in the serum, (2) cannot be passively transferred in serum but can be so transferred by leukocytic cells, (3) discloses a cytotoxic effect of its antigen on explanted cells of the sensitive host in tissue culture, and (4) is characterized by exerting its noxious effects without mediation of blood vessels or smooth muscle, inasmuch as it produces a reaction in the avascular cornea. The delayed response is seen in such conditions as tuberculosis, brucellosis, typhoid, tularemia, lymphogranuloma venereum, histoplasmosis, syphilis, poison ivy, and many others and is brought about by such diverse sensitizing agents as bacteria, viruses, fungi, spirochetes, parasites, plant materials, and simple chemicals. The delayed reaction thus occurs in man in conjunction with many diseases.

The *mechanism* in the *early* or *immediate* type of inflammatory *response* has been explained by two theories, both of which probably operate under certain circumstances (Burdon). The first of these is the *cellular histamine* theory. This theory holds that the early response is the result of antigen-antibody reaction occurring on or in the cells that have removed the antibody from the blood and fixed it to themselves. The response (anaphylactic) is thus associated with fixed antibody and not with circulating antibody. The immune state, on the other hand, is associated with the presence of circulating antibody in sufficient amounts to protect the fixed antibody also present. Thus, the difference between the anaphylactic and immune states is qualitative and depends upon the balance between fixed and circulating antibody. In initiating the early inflammatory reaction the cells containing the antigen are specially injured releasing histamine, histamine-like substances, and other metabolites including heparin and acetylcholine. These, in turn, produce contraction of smooth muscle, changes in capillary permeability, and other changes characteristic of the early response. The second theory is the *humoral* one. It holds that union of antigen with antibody in the blood or body fluids of hypersensitive people produces powerful anaphylactogenic poisons called anaphylatoxins which, in turn, are responsible for the reaction. This theory is supported by two easily reproduced experiments. In the first of these, place an antigen (such as erythrocytes) in a test tube along with homologous antiserum (such as amboceptor) and complement and incubate for a short time until just before the onset of hemolysis. Centrifuge the mixture and inject the supernatant fluid intravenously into a rabbit. The rabbit will die in anaphylaxis. In another experiment, mixing antigens and specific antisera *in vitro* results in the formation of a precipitate. Wash the precipitate, add to it normal guinea pig serum, incubate the mixture briefly, and inject the supernatant into a normal guinea pig. The animal will show marked toxicity and anaphylaxis.

Since the *delayed response* occurs most frequently in conjunction with living organisms the *mechanism* of its inflammatory reaction will be related as it concerns microbes with the understanding that it is probably the same in connection with other sensitizing agents. For this reaction, the entire microbial cell is necessary as the sensitizing agent. It may in addition, though, also bring about the early response. Contrarily, soluble components of microbes or soluble proteins alone produce only the early response. In other words, relatively simple antigens produce the early response while it takes complex antigens to bring about the delayed response. The latter may readily be shown in connection with tubercle bacilli. Ether, alcohol, and chloroform extract (lipopolysaccharide) of tubercle bacilli will not elicit a delayed sensitivity to tuberculin, although serum antibodies and anaphylactic sensitivity to bacillary protein are readily demonstrable. Restoring the soluble lipid extract, which was removed by the extraction, to the bacillary protein produces a mixture that once again regains its capacity to induce tuberculin sensitivity. When either egg albumin or picryl chloride are substituted for the bacillary protein and to these is added the original lipid extract, each mixture will induce delayed hypersensitivity to egg albumin and picryl chloride respectively. This would indicate that the specific antigen in the tubercle bacillus producing the delayed allergy is tubercle bacillary protein while the lipid is nonantigenic and simply directs the host's response to the protein. Lipoidal fractions with similar activity have been found in connection with hemolytic streptococci and vaccinia virus and it is probable that other organisms also possess these fractions. If they do not, however, the necessary lipoidal fractions may be supplied by the host. Before closing this section it must be pointed out that a prerequisite for microbial allergy of the delayed type is prolonged focal contact between considerable numbers of intact microbes and the tissues of the host. It must also be pointed out that the time for development of sensitization is from 10 to 14 days following infection or contact—the same time necessary to form antibodies to known antigens.

Because there are so many disorders that are allergic in nature, it is impossible to describe the *pathologic changes* that take place in them individually at this time. In a general manner, however, there are essentially four different types of patterns, namely, anaphylactoid, necrotizing, granulomatous, and fibrinoid or hyalinoid (Hartman). The *anaphylactoid* lesion is the type seen in allergic rhinitis, bronchial asthma, atopic eczema, urticaria, angioneurotic edema, anaphylactic shock, *etc*. It is characterized by edema and exudation and the amount of each varies greatly from case to case (Fig. 51*A*). Edema is evidenced by separation of the cells or structures of the organ. If it is rich in protein, it will stain eosinophilic. If it is poor in protein its location in the histologic section will be represented only by an empty space. The exudate will be serous, fibrinous, hemorrhagic, purulent, or combinations of these depending upon the proportion of elements present. Among the various leukocytic cells eosinophils are usually prominent. The *necrotizing* lesion is, as the term indicates, associated with necrosis. It may be limited to specific cells such as neutrophils, thrombocytes (platelets), or erythrocytes and may be seen in such conditions as Rh sensitization, transfusion hemolysis, hemolytic or aplastic anemia, thrombocytopenic purpura, and granulocytopenia or it may involve tissues as a whole and be seen in such conditions as diffuse cortical necrosis of the kidney, acute dermal necrosis, acute pancreatic necrosis, acute hepatic necrosis, acute necrotizing appendicitis, acute necrotizing cholecystitis, *etc*. Morphologically the basic pattern is that of extensive and complete necrosis of the tissue that does not differ in any way from any other necrosis (Fig. 51*B*). Aside from this, the junction of the destroyed and viable tissue discloses varying degrees of congestion, vascular thrombosis, edema, and leukocytic infiltration. The leukocytic cells consist mostly of neutrophils, with varying numbers of eosinophils added. Included in this group are the Arthus and Shwartzman phenomena. *Arthus phenomenon*, discovered in 1903, consists of a violent necrotizing local tissue reaction taking place at the site of injection of a protein (serum) in an animal (rabbit) previously sensitized to the same protein (Fig. 52). The sensitizing protein is administered subcutaneously at about 6 day intervals and at least 2 injections are necessary. Sensitization occurs from 2 to 10 days after the last injection (Tuft). The reaction is due to the union of antigen with antibody in the local tissue and its severity depends upon the degree of hypersensitivity. *Shwartzman phenomenon*, discovered in 1928, also consists of a severe necrotizing reaction elicited at the primary site of injection of a bacteria-free filtrate when such an injection is followed in 24 hours by an intravenous injection of a similar filtrate. This reaction thus requires a skin preparatory factor and a reacting factor. Since 1928 it has been demonstrated that the skin preparatory factory may be from one bacterium, as for example, typhoid filtrate and the reacting factor from another bacterium, as for example streptococcus. The phenomenon has thus far been

10

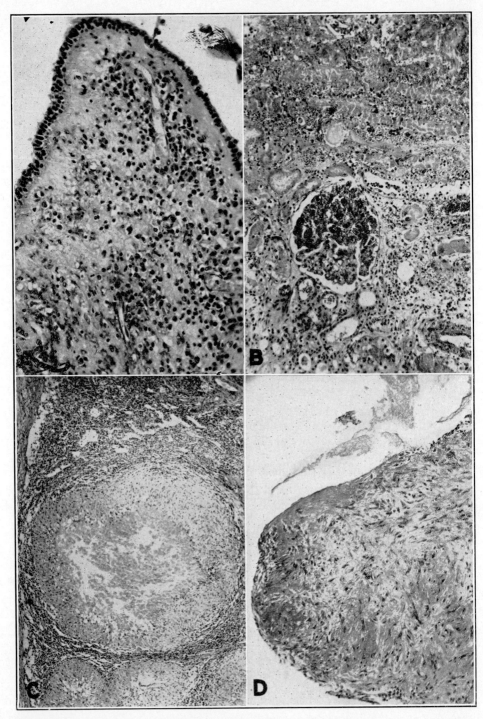

Fig. 51.—Allergic inflammations showing *A*, anaphylactoid type reaction in allergic rhinitis with congestion, edema, and eosinophilic infiltration. × 200, *B*, necrotizing type reaction in diffuse cortical necrosis of the kidney with complete destruction of the tissue in the upper half of the photomicrograph. × 100, *C*, granulomatous type reaction in tuberculosis with central necrosis and peripheral epithelioid cell reaction. × 50, and *D*, fibrinoid type reaction in Libman-Sack's disease with fibrinoid change in a mitral verruca. × 100.

produced by culture filtrates of many pathogenic bacteria as well as with certain viruses and malignant tumors and is apparently dependent upon the presence of a true toxin (Tuft). The *granulomatous* lesion is the type seen in tuberculosis, coccidioidomycosis, sporotrichosis, histoplasmosis, tularemia, brucellosis, berylliosis, *etc.* It is characterized by the presence of a central area of caseation necrosis surrounded by proliferated epitheloid cells that may assume a radial, pallisade arrangement (Fig. 51*C*). Giant cells of the Langhans' or foreign body type may or may not be present. The *fibrinoid* or *hyalinoid* lesion is the type seen in severe serum sickness, periarteritis nodosa, disseminated lupus erythematosus (including Libman-Sacks syndrome), dermatomyositis, rheumatic fever, rheumatoid arthritis, *etc.* It is characterized by the presence of loosely or tightly bound eosinophilic fibrillar

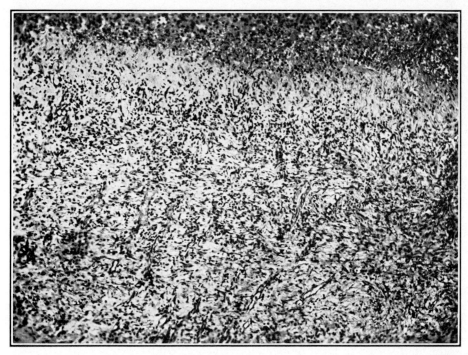

FIG. 52.—Arthus phenomenon, elicited by a subcutaneous injection of horse serum in a rabbit previously sensitized to horse serum, disclosing from above down an area of necrosis merging with edematous connective tissue that is densely permeated with eosinophils. × 100.

or sometimes more granular material that tends to smudge (Fig. 51*D*). About the periphery, such foci are surrounded by various leukocytic cells, among which eosinophils are often numerous.

Complications associated with allergic inflammation, are similar to those mentioned in connection with inflammations in general (page 135). Since the locations of the particular lesions vary greatly from disease to disease it is impossible to list or discuss them at this time. They are, of course, taken up in conjunction with the different disorders in various places in the text. One complication which deserves special mention, however, is the *generalized anaphylactoid reaction*. This usually follows intravenous therapy in susceptible persons and is attended by a rapid onset of sneezing, retching, dyspnea, rapid respiration, accelleration of heart rate, cyanosis, increased reflex excitability, jerky spasms, expulsion of urine, pupillary relaxation, convulsions, and (when severe) death (Tuft). The *clinical manifestations* in allergic inflammation will depend upon the site and extent of tissue involvement, the rapidity and severity of development of the process, and the complications that arise. The *diagnosis* is arrived at from a consideration of the history, onset and initial attack, clinical course, physical examination, skin tests with various allergens, special tests, and results of therapeutic trials. *Treatment*, in principle, consists of elimination or avoidance of etiologic factors, desensitization or hyposensitization, administration of antihistamines, specific and nonspecific drug therapy, symptomatic therapy, and prophylaxis, especially in the immediate post natal period. The *prognosis* depends upon the nature, severity, and location of the inflammatory process. While the mortality, in proportion to the number of cases, is low, the morbidity, contrarily, is high.

VIRAL INFLAMMATIONS

Viral inflammations are tissue reactions caused by viruses. *Viruses* constitute a heterogeneous group of filter-passing infectious agents that are smaller than bacteria and that require susceptible host cells for multiplication and activity (Rivers). Although proof regarding the *origin* of viruses is lacking and although many theories have been expressed, it has been proposed that viruses may represent (1) retrograde forms of free living-ultramicrobes evolving from visible but now extinct microbes or (2) autocatalytic proteins with reproduction of molecules similar to that postulated for genes. Viruses *inhabit* the plant, bacterial (bacteriophages), and animal kingdoms and have the following *properties* in common: (1) are readily destroyed by heat, as for example, 60° C. for 30 minutes, (2) survive for prolonged periods when stored in the frozen (carbon dioxide snow at −60° C.) state, (3) have maximum infectivity over a pH range around neutral, (4) show variable resistance to dessication, (5) are destroyed by brief exposure to ultraviolet light and by the same disinfectants that destroy bacteria, (6) are resistant to glycerol, in which they can be stored for prolonged periods at ordinary refrigerator (+4° C.) temperatures, and (7) with the exception of the psittacosis-lymphogranuloma-pneumonitis group, are insensitive to antibiotics and chemotherapeutic agents (Rhodes and van Rooyen).

The more *specific* morphologic, physical, chemical, and other *properties* are difficult to determine because viruses are bound closely to host cells in which they grow and complete separation of the two is often uncertain. Nevertheless the *size* of viruses, as determined by filtration, centrifugalization, diffusion, and direct light or electron microscopic techniques, has been quite accurately determined and has been shown to vary from 10 to 400 millimicrons. There is likewise no uniformity in *shape*, for the configuration varies from square to rectangular, spherical, ovoid, and irregular. Comparing the *density* of bacteria at 1.10 and protein molecules at 1.33 with that of viruses which varies from 1.10 to 1.30, it is apparent that viruses are similar on the one hand to bacteria and on the other hand to protein molecules. The *chemical composition* of many of the viruses has been determined. Plant viruses, such as the tobacco mosaic, cucumber, and potato, are the simplest, being composed essentially of nucleoprotein and ribose nucleic acid. Bacterial virus are in a similar category being composed of protein and desoxyribonucleic acid. Animal viruses, on the other hand, are much more complex. Vaccinia, for example, is composed of lipids, carbohydrates, thymonucleic acid, several proteins, copper, biotin, and riboflavin. Equine encephalomyelitis virus contains ribonucleic acid, carbohydrate, phospholipid, cholesterol, and fatty acid. Influenza virus consists of a liponucleoprotein complex containing ribonucleic and thymonucleic acids. As another example still, rabbit papilloma virus is composed of 90 per cent protein and 8.7 per cent desoxypentose nucleic acid.

As already stated, viruses grow only in the presence of living cells. They may thus be *cultivated* in tissue cultures, fertile chick embryos, and laboratory animals. The reasons for such selectivity of medium are not apparent. It is theorized, however, that since viruses do not possess an enzyme system or metabolic processes essential for growth or multiplication, these must be supplied by host cells. As to the precise mechanism of reproduction, most workers consider this to be by the conventional means of growth and division. Once the end point is reached, the cell ruptures, the organisms are liberated, and the viruses are free to attack other cells. In the process of reproduction, *mutations* do occur and the mutants reproduce their own kind thereby indefinitely producing strains that are different from the original parent organism. Such a change is explained in some of the larger bacterial viruses, at least, by the fact that they contain as many as 50 genes—the location where mutations occur. Examples of mutations are 17D strain of yellow fever virus, dengue virus passed through mice producing a strain usable for vaccination, and a fibroma virus transformed into a myxoma virus.

The natural *habitat* of virus is considered to be insects and mammals. Infection in *man* is, more or less, accidental. As an example, it may be pointed out that yellow fever virus is normally present in monkeys and mosquitos and that man becomes infected simply because he happens to be in the vicinity. In man the means of *transmission* may be listed as follows: (1) contact by way of the genital organs such as lymphogranuloma venereum, genital warts, and genital herpes, and by way of skin such as warts and molluscum contagiosum, (2) droplets in air such as the common cold, influenza, atypical pneumonia, measles, rubella, varicella, mumps, small pox, and poliomyelitis, (3) wounds such as rabies, (4) arthropod vectors including such insects as mosquitos, mites, fleas, and ticks and carrying virus-producing diseases such as dengue, Rift Valley fever, sand fly fever, and yellow fever, and (5) ingestion of water and food encompassing epidemic hepatitis and poliomyelitis. As a result of the methods of transmission outlined, viral diseases occur endemically, epidemically, and pandemically. The seriousness of the latter two will depend upon the species and strain of virus. Frequently too, the virulence of the organism increases as the epidemic gains momentum.

Viral diseases, as many other infections, are attended by three types of *immunity*—natural, active acquired, and passive. *Natural immunity* is a state of resistance not dependent upon previous contact with the virus or its antibody. Along nonspecific lines, this type of immunity is dependent upon species of virus (certain tissues are resistant while others are susceptible to certain viruses), age of person, sex, state of nutrition, genetic background, and climatic conditions. These factors are difficult to evaluate because escape from disease may represent nothing more than lack of exposure and have nothing to do with susceptibility or immunity. Along the same vein, health is not always a guarantee against contraction of a viral disease for measles, influenza, chickenpox, and smallpox are generally contracted by healthy persons. Contrarily, it has been repeatedly demonstrated that unhealthy laboratory animals are often resistant to certain viral infections. Probably more important than any of the factors already mentioned, is the role of the properdin system in natural immunity against viral diseases, for Pillemer has demonstrated that properdin in the presence of complement and Mg++ offers definite protection against certain viruses. *Actie acquired immunity* is a state of resistance developed as a result of a spontaneous or wilfully produced viral disease or as a result of vaccination. With the exception of the common cold, herpes, and influenza, most viral diseases are followed by a lasting, often lifetime, immunity. Such immunity, as in poliomyelitis and measles, may result from repeated contact with active agents, while in others, such as yellow fever, it may be due to persistence of the virus in the host. Lack of immunity, contrarily, is explanable by the inability of the virus to establish itself permanently in the cells of the host. Active immunity can be produced artificially by the introduction of fully virulent viruses but is not carried out in practice for fear of producing the disease and starting epidemics. For these reasons, attenuated viruses are sometimes used and have been successfully employed in such diseases as rabies, yellow fever, dengue, cattle plague, and poliomyelitis. In most instances, active immunity is associated with demonstrable humoral antibodies consisting of complement fixing antibodies, precipitins, agglutinins, and neutralizing antibodies. The first three of these are probably one and the same but the neutralizing antibodies are different. They are the ones responsible for protection but the exact mechanism of this protection is unknown. *Passive immunity,* as in bacterial infections, is produced by parenteral administration of serum from actively immuned persons or animals containing neutralizing antibodies. Such immunity is, of course, important in prophylaxis and treatment of viral diseases. The mechanism involved is unknown although it is thought that the antibodies protect susceptible cells against entry of viruses, act upon viruses to prevent production of disease, or enhance destruction of viruses by phagocytic cells.

Tropism of viruses for certain tissues is well known. On this basis, viruses may be classified as follows: (1) dermotropic—having an affinity for the skin and conjunctiva and encompassing such conditions as warts, animal tumors, pock group, and molluscum contagiosum, (2) neurotropic—having an affinity for the brain or spinal cord and consisting of epidemic encephalomyelitis, poliomyelitis, rabies, Russian encephalitis, and louping ill, (3) pneumotropic —having an affinity for the lungs and including psittacosis, atypical pneumonia, common cold, and influenza, and (4) hepatotropic—having an affinity for the liver and encompassing yellow fever, Rift Valley fever, and infectious jaundice.

Pathologically, the gross lesions vary greatly, depending upon the organ affected and the virus involved. In the skin, for example, the exanthemata vary from papules, to vesicles, to pustules while the wart and molluscum contagiosum form small tumor nodules. In the brain there may be congestion, edema, and disappearance of the smooth glistening sheen of the meninges or there may be no gross alterations. In the lungs, the areas of pneumonitis may be patchy and extensive or they may be indicated only by a diffuse increase in resistance. In the liver, the acute and severe disease is characterized by a diffuse necrosis while the chronic and more protracted condition is attended by firmness and fibrosis.

Histologically, since all viruses multiply or reproduce within cells, it is within the cells that they are detectable. This may be accomplished morphologically by the identification of elementary and inclusion bodies. The *elementary bodies* probably represent the virus particles themselves. Some of these are large enough to be visible in properly stained preparations by the ordinary or the dark field microscope, while others are detectable only with the aid of the electron microscope. The size and appearance vary greatly and have already been discussed in the opening paragraphs of this section. Some elementary bodies, such as those in psittacosis, lympho-granuloma venereum, and trachoma are almost as large and complex as rickettsiæ and are probably living agents. Others, such as those causing the pock diseases are considerably smaller but are still looked upon as living agents. *Inclusion bodies* are produced by many but not by all viruses. They are, however, not always indicative of viral infection for they are sometimes present in diseases not caused by viruses. Inclusion bodies are best demonstrated by Mann's eosin methylene blue or by Giemsa's stain and exist usually as rounded, single or multiple, intranuclear or intracytoplasmic structures of varying sizes. Intranuclear inclusion bodies are found in herpes simplex, chickenpox, herpes zoster, yellow fever, poliomyelitis, and Rift Valley fever. They are eosinophilic, occupy a good portion or most of the nucleus, are surrounded by a clear zone or halo, and displace the basophilic chromatin of the nucleus peripherally to line the nuclear membrane. Intracytoplasmic inclusion bodies are found in vaccinia (Guarnieri bodies), fowl pox (Bollinger bodies), rabies (Negri bodies), and molluscum contagiosum (Fig. 53A). They are usually eosinophilic, large, and somewhat granular but in some infections they are basophilic, quite small, and distinctly granular. Both intranuclear and intracytoplasmic bodies are found in small pox and paravaccinia. While the nature of all inclusion bodies is unknown, some of the intracytoplasmic inclusion bodies (Guarnieri and Bollinger) are considered to consist of a membrane and substance derived from the cell of of the host in which are embedded elementary bodies or virus particles.

After the entrance of viruses into the cells, the changes that follow may be divided into two types—cellular and inflammatory. The sequence of *cellular changes* is generally *proliferation* followed by degeneration—although the degree of each varies from infection to infection. For obvious reasons, the changes are best followed experimentally and for this the study of the rabbits' cornea inoculated with vaccine virus affords easily traceable alterations. In 3 to 6 hours after inoculation the epithelial cells enlarge, stain less intensely, disclose mitoses, and exhibit amitotic giant cell formation. In 6 to 24 hours Guarnieri bodies appear in affected cells. In 24 to 48 hours small nodules due to epithelial hypertrophy and hyperplasia appear on the surface. After 48 hours, the cells degenerate and disappear. Proliferative changes develop when the action of the virus is not explosive or rapid and when the susceptible cells are capable of proliferation. In humans such changes are particularly manifested in the common wart (Fig. 53B) and to a lesser extent in molluscum contagiosum. In animals their acme is reached in the Rous sarcoma of chickens and the Shope's papilloma virus of rabbits—both of which are true tumors. Following hyperplasia, there is usually *degeneration* and *necrosis*. The degenerative changes consisting of parenchymatous, fatty, hydropic, and other degenerations are similar to those in any inflammatory or retrograde process (page 33). The same is also true for necrosis where pycnosis, karyorrhexis, and karyolysis are the dominant nuclear changes (page 85). Both of these lead ultimately to complete destruction and liquefaction of tissue (Fig. 53C). In some instances, when the action of the virus is explosive and rapid or the susceptible cells are incapable of proliferation, degeneration and necrosis occur from the

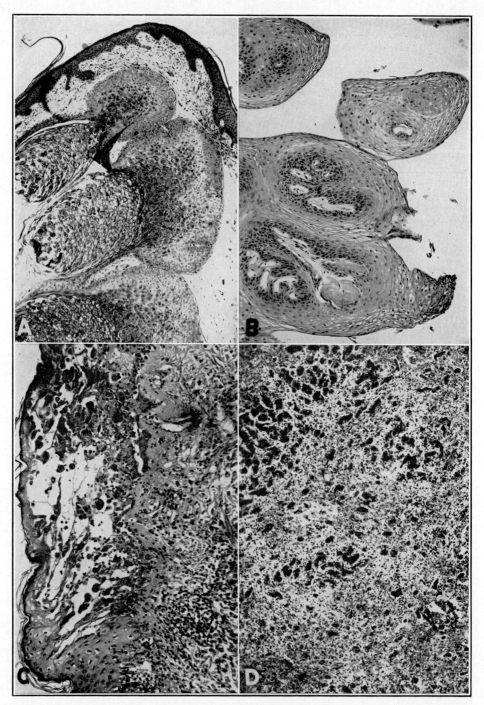

FIG. 53.—Viral inflammations showing *A*, molluscum contagiosum with proliferation of epithelium and numerous, eosinophilic, intracytoplasmic inclusion bodies. × 50, *B*, papilloma with proliferation of squamous epithelium. × 50, *C*, varicella (chickenpox) with degeneration, necrosis, and liquefaction of epithelium following the proliferative phase. × 100, and *D*, infectious hepatitis with almost complete destruction of the hepatic cells. × 50.

onset and are not preceded by proliferation. Such changes are seen in infections of the central nervous system as, for example, rabies, poliomyelitis, and louping ill. They also occur in explosive infections of the liver as Rift Valley fever, yellow fever, and infectious hepatitis (Fig. 53D) where there is no time for hyperplasia to take place. *Inflammatory changes*, in greater or lesser degree, develop in almost every viral disease as a consequence to degeneration. They are, in essence, similar to inflammatory changes caused by bacteria with but a few modifications. The cellular response, for example, is usually mononuclear and rarely neutrophilic. The cells diffusely permeate the tissues or, as in central nervous system lesions, frequently become arranged perivascularly. Edema, as in influenza, is sometimes severe while frank pus does not occur except in lesions secondarily infected with bacteria. Finally, granulomatous lesions are infrequent although, as in lymphogranuloma venereum, they are occasionally encountered.

The *clinical manifestations* of viral infections will vary tremendously from case to case, because of the protean nature of the diseases. They are considered under the specific diseases in various places in the text. The clinical *diagnosis* is frequently established on the basis of a careful history, physical examination including gross appearance of any visible lesions, and, when practical, histologic examination of smears or tissues from the lesions. A more precise diagnosis is made by (1) recovering and identifying the causative agent by inoculating tissue cultures, fertile chick embryos, or susceptible laboratory animals with infected material, (2) demonstrating an antibody response which bears a distinct time relationship to the clinical picture, and (3) identification of a specific antigen in material from the lesion. Generally, *prevention* and *treatment* of viral infections consists of (1) quarantine, which is usually considered to be of doubtful value, (2) control of vectors and reservoirs, (3) vaccination, (4) administration of immune sera which should be carried out after exposure and before the appearance of clinical manifestations, and (5) drugs. So far, drugs have not been too successful in controlling viral infections. Sulfonamides and penicillin are only somewhat efficacious in the psittacosis-lymphogranuloma-trachoma group of infections and chloromycetin and aureomycin are of benefit in psittacosis. The *prognosis* varies with the type and strain of infective agent.

RICKETTSIAL INFLAMMATIONS

Rickettsial inflammations are tissue responses engendered by microorganisms called *rickettsiæ*. These organisms, named after an American pathologist H. T. Ricketts (1871–1910), are intermediate in position in the microbial kingdom being smaller than bacteria and longer than viruses. *Biologically*, they resemble viruses in that they multiply and propagate only in living (endothelial and mesothelial) cells while *morphologically*, they resemble bacteria in that they are gram-negative, are readily visible microscopically, are removed by bacteria tight filters, and are coccobacillary in appearance. In the last respect they are also somewhat similar to the larger viruses of the psittacosis, pneumonitis, lymphogranuloma, and trachoma group (Rodes and van Rooyen). Rickettsia are readily stained by the Giemsa's and Macchiavello's techniques. In endothelial or mesothelial cells (peritoneal or tunica vaginalis of inoculated mice or guinea pigs) they appear in clumps or masses. In exudates or fluids they appear as pleomorphic structures that measure up to 0.35×0.25 microns, that show bipolarity of staining, and that appear singly, in pairs, in short chains, or even filamentous.

Chemically, the composition of some of the organisms has been determined and has been shown to consist of carbohydrate-protein complexes, nucleic acids, and lipids. Rickettsiæ may be *preserved* in tissues stored in glycerol but are best kept alive by quick freezing in an alochol—dry ice mixture, sealed in an ampule, and refrigerated at −70° C. Conversely, they are relatively *labile*, being readily killed by antiseptics such as formalin, phenol, and merthiolate and by temperatures above 56° C. for 30 minutes (Rivers).

In general, rickettsiæ are easily *isolated* by inoculating the peritoneal cavity of susceptible laboratory animals (guinea pigs, mice, and rats) with infected material or with blood clot from febrile patients emulsified in saline. They can also be isolated or further propagated by inoculating the yolk sac of 6 to 7 day old chick embryos with exudate or tissue from the experimental animals, with emulsified human blood clot, or with emulsified anthropod vectors. *Serologically*, highly specific complement fixation reactions have been developed using as antigens, rickettsiæ cultivated in the yolk sac of embryomated eggs. Such reactions are useful in differentiating closely allied infections. Along similar lines, humans infected with different species of rickettsiæ develop specific agglutinins which are also useful in identification. Weil and Felix (who lived at the turn of the century) isolated a strain of *B. proteus* (× 19) from the urine of a patient with epidemic typhus which was agglutinated with high dilutions of serum from typhus patients. It was later shown that strains X2 and XK react similarly and that the best results are obtained using the "O" (OX19, OX2, or OXK) antigens of *B. proteus* Because the proteus organism does not cause typhus, and because it does not belong to the rickettsial group of organisms, this reaction was puzzling until it was determined that the antigenic factor common to both organisms was a heat-stable polysaccharide. Today, the Weil-Felix reaction is used routinely as an easily available and dependable laboratory test for the diagnosis of typhus fever, Rocky Mountain spotted fever, and other rickettsial diseases. Further differentiation of the two is carried out by animal inoculation, complement fixation, and specific agglutination reactions.

Epidemiologically, most rickettsial infections are perpetuated by animal-vector cycles in which man is not essential. The animals generally involved are squirrel, rabbit, chipmunk, rat, mouse, weasel, and other rodents and the vectors are the louse, mite, flea, and tick. Man becomes infected by being bitten by a vector or by contacting its excreta. The only known exception to the animal-anthropod vector-animal cycle cited, as far as man is concerned, is in epidemic typhus and trench fever where the cycle is man-louse-man. *Clinically*, the manifestations vary from case to case and from infection to infection, with some types of infections being attended by mild and others by severe symptoms and signs. In general, the incubation period varies from 10 to 14 days. Prodromal manifestations may consist of headache, lassitude, weakness, and slight fever. These are followed by an abrupt onset of malaises, chills or chilliness, headache, weakness, cough, generalized aches and pains, and a sustained fever. Most diseases are attended by a cutaneous eruption that usually appears about the latter one half of the first week. Initially the rash may be a blotchy erythema but later it forms circumscribed macules or maculopapules that appear pink, red, or hemorrhagic and that measure 2 to 4 mm. in diameter (Fig. 54*A*). The origin and distribution of the rash vary from disease to disease with, in most, the extremities and trunk sooner or later involved. Physical examination varies with the severity and type of infection but in the more profound illnesses may show low blood pressure, rapid pulse, increased respiration, photophobia, flushed face, and even mental dullness, stupor, or delirium.   The ultimate course is either rapid recovery or coma, uremia, shock, and death.

The gross *pathologic* changes are minimal.   In essence, they consist of the skin rash already referred to and small hemorrhages, together with petechiæ, of the viscera and, in some instances perhaps, pneumonia.   The microscopic changes are confined to the capillaries and smaller vessels (Fig. 54B and C).

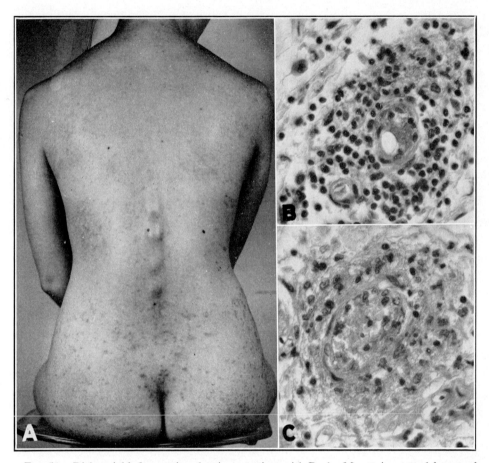

Fig. 54.—Rickettsial inflammation showing a patient with Rocky Mountain spotted fever and illustrating *A*, the typical rash, *B*, a capillary with endothelial proliferation and monocytic and lymphocytic infiltration.   × 400, and *C*, a capillary with thrombosis, necrosis, and hemorrhagic extravasation.   × 400.

Pathogenetically, the rickettsiæ upon deposition in the skin seek out the endothelium of the smaller vascular channels.   Here they multiply and, at the same time, stimulate the proliferation of the endothelial cells.   Ultimately, the latter degenerate and liberate the organisms into the blood stream where they are picked up by other endothelial cells to repeat the process.   Locally, as a result of the proliferation and degeneration, there is vascular thrombosis and, because of the vascular occlusion, focal hemorrhage. Secondarily, the vascular and perivascular tissues are permeated with monocytes, lymphocytes, and fewer neutrophils.

The *diagnosis* of rickettsial infections is made from a consideration of the clinical features, epidemiological data, and serological reactions. *Prevention* and *treatment* is directed toward controlling vectors, vaccination, administration of immune sera after exposure and before the appearance of clinical manifestations, and use of drugs such as chloromycetin and aureomycin. The *prognosis* depends upon the type and severity of the infection, with the mortality ranging from zero in trench fever to as high as 20 per cent in epidemic typhus fever.

On the basis of clinical features, epidermiological aspects, and serological and immunological reactions *rickettsial diseases* in man may be *divided* into the following five groups: (1) typhus, (2) spotted fever, (3) scrub typhus, (4) Q fever, and (5) trench fever (Rivers). The *typhus group* includes epidemic typhus, Brills disease, and murine typhus. The term typhus (Gr. = smoky or hazy) means a confused state of intellect with a tendency to stupor. *Epidemic typhus* is world wide in distribution, has always been associated with wars and famines, and has been one of the major epidemic diseases of all times. It is caused by *R. prowazeki*, possesses a (head or body) louse-man-louse cycle, needs no other animals in its propagation, is pathogenic for the guinea pig, grows in the yolk sac of the chick embryo, and is attended by positive complement fixation, agglutination, and OX19 serologic tests (Rhodes and van Rooyen). *Brills disease*, also known as sporadic typhus, constitutes a recrudescence of epidemic louse-borne typhus in mild form years after the primary attack. *Murine typhus*, also known as endemic typhus, is world wide in distribution, is caused by *R. mooseri*, normally possesses a flea-rat-flea cycle, is transmitted to man by the rat flea, is pathogenic for the guniea pig where it produces scrotal swelling and is demonstrable in its tissues, grows in the yolk sac of chick embryos, and is attended by positive complement fixation, agglutination, and OX19 serologic reactions. The *spotted fever group* in the United States consists of Rocky Mountain spotted fever, rickettsial pox, and maculatum disease, in the Mediterranean area of boutonneuse fever, in Africa of tick-borne typhus, in Brazil of Brazilian spotted fever, in Colombia of Tobia fever, in Mexico of pinta fever, in North Queensland of tick typhus, and in India and Russia of tick-borne rickettsioses. *Rocky Mountain spotted fever* occurs in the Rocky Mountain area of the United States, is caused by *R. rickettsii*, normally possesses a tick-rodent-tick cycle, is transmitted to man by the tick, is pathogenic for the guinea pig where it produces scrotal swelling and is demonstrable in its tissues, grows in the yolk sac of chick embryos, and is attended by positive complement fixation, agglutination, OX19, and OX2 serologic reactions. *Scrub typhus*, also known as Tsutsugamushi fever, occurs in Japan and the Orient, is caused by *R. tsutsugamushi*, normally possesses a mite-rodent-mite cycle, is pathogenic for the mouse and guinea pig where it does not produce scrotal swelling but can be seen in tissues, grows in the yolk sac of chick embryos, and is attended by a positive OXK serologic reaction. *Q fever* is world wide in distribution, is caused by *R. burneti*, normally possesses a tick-cattle or wild animal-tick cycle, is transmitted to man by the tick or by contact (inhalation, handling, swallowing) of infected material, is pathogenic for the guinea pig and mouse when the organisms are found in tissues, grows in yolk sac of chick embryo, and is attended by positive complement fixation and agglutination but negative Weil-Felix reactions. It differs from other rickettsial diseases in that there is no rash and the clinical and pathologic manifestations are similar to those of a typical pneumonia. *Trench fever* is European in distribution, is caused by *R. quintana*, possesses a louse-man-louse cycle, needs no other animal in its propagation, has not been successfully inoculated in experimental animals or in yolk sac of chick embryos, and is attended by a negative Weil-Felix reaction.

FUNGOUS INFLAMMATIONS

Fungous inflammations are tissue reactions produced by fungi. Fungi (L. = mushroom) are microscopic members of the plant kingdom that normally inhabit the soil (Lewis and Moss). They are included in the Phylum Thallophyta which embodies those showing no differentiation into roots, stems, or leaves. The phylum is further divided into Algae—containing chlorophyll and Fungaceae not containing chlorophyll. Fungaceae are divided into Schizomycetes or bacteria (which includes *Actinomyces* and *Nocardia*), Myxomycetes or slime molds, and Eumycetes or true fungi. Finally, Eumycetes are divided into four subclasses of which Hypomycetes or fungi imperfecta (not possessing sexual spores) are the most important for they include most of the fungi that are pathogenic to man.

In general, fungi *exist* in the vegetative or spore form (Fig. 55*A* and *B*). Occasionally the vegetative forms consist of budding cells but more commonly, as in the case of all pathogenic fungi, they display hyphæ. These are filamentous irregularly segmented structures that vary from species to species and that represent the form found in the body. Spore forms are rarely present in tissues, are usually found in artificial media, and are more specific because they are generally used for identification purposes.

Growth of fungi varies with conditions. When these are optimal the vegetative form is produced but when they are adverse the more resistant spore forms are formed. Some of the many artificial media in use are Lithman oxgall agar, Sabouraud glucose agar, corn meal agar, chlamydospore agar, blood agar, and brain heart infusion agar. The addition of antibiotics to these reduces the incidence of contaminants. The usual time of growth on such media varies from 3 to 21 days. More specifically, most pathogenic fungi grow well at room (20° C.) but even better at body (37° C.) temperature. While the water requirements for growth vary, most pathogenic fungi thrive better in moist areas of the body and, artificially, in solid or semisolid media. Excluding *Actinomyces bovis*, virtually all pathogenic fungi require oxygen for multiplication. While ultraviolet light has some inhibitory effect upon growth, it is not lethal, and light in general does not seem to have too much influence on propagation. Some of the specific nutritional requirements are nitrogen, carbohydrates, ammonium, potassium, calcium, magnesium, zinc, iron, coper, manganese, phosphorous, and sulfur, with thiamine and biotin stimulating growth. The usual optimum pH range is 5 to 7. Pigment formation, so characteristic for some fungi, is a product of metabolism that appears to depend on the presence of certain monosaccharides and amount and kinds of minerals. The *appearance* of the *colonies* on culture media varies greatly from species to species, for each of which, however, it is quite specific (Fig. 55*C* and *D*). The color may be white, gray, tan, cream, brown, rose, red, purple, black, *etc.*; the appearance many be moist or dry; the consistency may be downy, feathery, waxy, felty, wooly, *etc.*; the surface may be smooth, rough, pebbled, grooved, furrowed, *etc.*, and the configuration may be rounded, globular, irregular, flat, centrally elevated, centrally depressed, *etc.*

Ordinarily, *man* is quite resistant to fungous infections (see immunity below). What breaks down this resistance and allows the organisms to gain a foothold and flourish is not always determinable. On occasion, however,

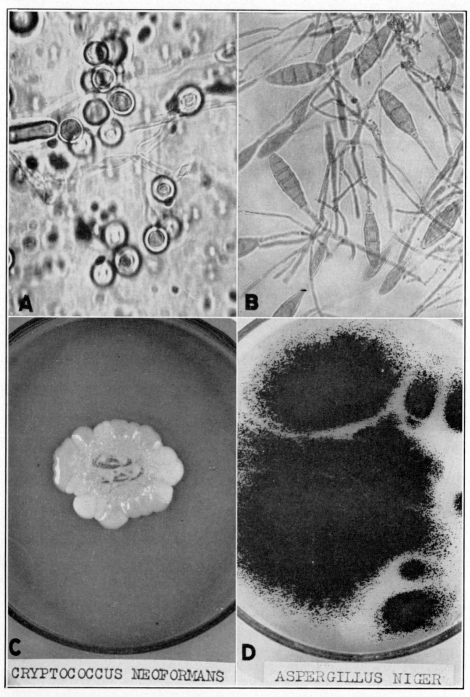

FIG. 55.—Fungi showing *A*, chlamydospores of *Candida albicans*. × 900, *B*, septate hyphæ and macroconidia of Microsporium canis. × 400, *C*, colony of *Cryptococcus neoformans*, and *D*, several colonies of *Aspergillus Niger*.

it is obvious that an intercurrent disease, as for example, uncontrolled diabetes mellitus, may increase one's susceptibility to fungous infections. In recent years, the administration of antibiotics and chemotherapeutic agents has been attended by a notable increase in fungous infections, especially of the superficial type such as that caused by *Candida albicans* (Toreck). Whether this results from some change in the infecting agent or from a change in the resistance of the host has not been determined. The *routes* of infection are usually the skin, sometimes the respiratory tract, and, except for superficial infections, rarely the gastrointestinal tract. Once within the body the infection spreads locally by direct extension to surrounding tissues and systemically by permeation of lymphatic channels and by invasion of the blood stream. The more important *deep infections* of man along with their respective causative agents are: actinomycosis—*Actinomyces (israeli) bovis* (page 515); nocardiosis—*Nocardia asteroides* (page 516); maduromycosis—fungi of the genus Nocarida (page 516); cryptococcosis or torulosis—*Cryptococcus neoformans* (page 515); North American blastomycosis—*Blastomyces dermatitidis* (page 514); South American blastomycosis or paracoccidioidal granuloma—*Blastomyces brasiliensis;* sporotrichosis —*Sporotrichium schenkii* (page 1340); coccidioidomycosis—*Coccidioides immitis* (page 514); histoplasmosis—*Histoplasma capsulatum* (page 513); and rhinosporidiosis—*Rhinosporidium seeberi.* The more important *"superficial infections"* are: moniliasis—*Candida albicans* (page 516); trichomycosis axillaris—*Nocardia tenius;* otomycosis and occasionally pulmonary infection —*Geotrichum, Aspergillus, Penicillium,* or *Mucor mucedo;* chromomycosis or chromoblastomycosis—*Hormodendrum pedrosoi, Homodendrum compactum,* or *Phialophora verrucosa;* tinea versicolor—*Malassezia furfur* (page 1340); and a variety of dermatomycoses or tineas involving the head, face, body, groin, nails, feet, and hands—over 40 different organisms (page 1338).

Concerned with resistance and susceptibility in man and, once the infection is established, with the acuteness or chronicity of the process are immunity and hypersensitivity. *Immunity* may be divided into natural and acquired (Beamer). *Natural immunity* is present in greater or lesser extent in all humans but the degree varies with the race, strain, social-economic conditions, and individual. Some of this resistance may be due to (1) tissues acting as mechanical barriers, (2) elaboration of substances that neutralize or destroy the organisms before they spread into adjacent tissues, (3) cellular (leukocytic or tissue) response of the host, (4) humoral substances including fibrin, complement, and perhaps even natural antibodies such as properdin, (5) increased flow of body fluids, such as blood and lymph, to dilute the invading organisms and their products, and (6) unsuitable environmental factors for the organisms, such as temperature, oxygen and nitrogen tension, improper availability of minerals, and excessive amounts of metabolites. Immunity from, or susceptibility to, infection is also determined by the virulence and numbers of organisms, fomites or other means of transmission, vectors, age of host, nutritional status, fatigue, and, as already mentioned, intercurrent disease and the use of antibiotics and chemotherapeutic agents. *Acquired immunity* results from a recognized or unrecognized attack of the disease. While agglutinins, precipitins, opsonins, and complement-fixing antibodies are formed against many fungi, the demonstration of such antibodies is not absolute evidence of immunity. Even if immunity is present, the degree of resistance is not great and its duration is not long. *Hypersensitivity* develops in fungous infections just as it does in bacterial infections (page 140). The *early response* is associated with demonstrable humoral antibodies and the intense local and general reaction results from the union of antigen with antibody. The *delayed response* is elicited by complex antigens of fungous origin. In this, however, specific antibodies are not demonstrable in the serum of the host, although the reaction is considered to result from an antigen-antibody union within cells.

The *pathologic changes* in tissues vary greatly from infection to infection. *Superficial infections*, such as moniliasis and aspergillosis, do not present any specific gross appearance. They are either superimposed upon a previous cavity or ulcer or produce nonspecific superficial erosions or ulcerations of varying sizes and configurations. Their floors are generally covered with necrotic material and their bases are not indurated. Generally, the first indication of the nature of the lesion is its histologic appearance. The most characteristic feature of this is the presence of the organism itself—almost always in the vegetative or hyphæ stage (Fig. 56*A* and *B*). While these fungi, as almost all others, can be identified in routine hematoxylin and eosin preparations, they are best visualized by the Hotchkiss-McManus, Brown-Brenn, Gridley, or acid-fast stains (Kade). The tissue response of the host to such infections is minimal. There is generally some congestion, edema, and fibroblastic and capillary proliferation but these changes are inconspicuous. Luekocytic response, consisting chiefly of neutrophils, plasma cells, lymphocytes, and monocytes, is limited to the immediate vicinity of the organisms and is likewise sparse. *Deep infections* are likewise variable. The best way to describe their gross appearance, perhaps, is to liken them to those in tuberculosis. The lesions may be multiple or single and they may be so small as to be hardly perceptible to the naked eye or they may measure many centimeters in diameter. The larger infections generally consist of ill-defined, firm, gray or grayish-white swellings that undergo central caseous or liquefaction necrosis (Fig. 56*C*). When the contents reach the surface (either internally or externally) they are discharged and either ulcers or cavities are formed. The histologic structure varies from infection to infection, with always the most characteristic and pathognomonic feature being the organism itself. Usually it exists as hyphæ but occasionally, especially in the yeast-like group, it may also be present in the form of spherules or spore-like structures. The former are invariably found in tissue spaces while the latter may be present either free in tissue spaces or engulfed in monocytes or giant cells. The tissue often responds in a granulomatous reaction with the formation of tubercles that are indistinguishable from those in tuberculosis (Fig. 56*D*). They may consist of central epithelioid cells along with scattered giant cells of foreign body type. Beyond this, there are varying numbers of plasma cells, lymphocytes, and monocytes. Some infections, however, do not elicit a granulomatous reaction. In these, the inflammation is nonspecific. When acute, it abounds in neutrophils and when chronic it contains mostly plasma cells, lymphocytes, and monocytes. The remaining changes, consisting of capillary and connective tissue proliferations, do not form any specific patterns. Although healing of fungous inflammations may occur by resolution, tissue destruction is usually too great and necessitates replacement with or encasement by fibrous tissue. Ultimately the necrotic area may be permeated with calcium salts.

The *clinical manifestations* in fungous infections vary with the organism, the tissue or organ infected, the extent of the process, the acuteness or chronicity of the infection, the complications that arise, *etc.* The cutaneous lesions generally produce only local manifestations, although these may sometimes be most exasperating. They may be associated with discomfort,

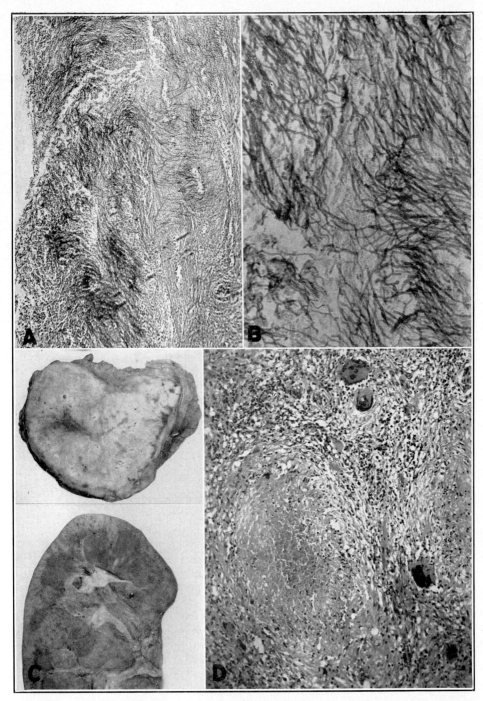

Fig. 56.—Fungous inflammation showing *A*, the microscopic appearance of a superficial infection infection of the esophagus caused by *Aspergillus*. × 50, *B*, the hyphæ of the same lesion shown in *A*. 200, C, gross appearance of histoplasmosis involving the adrenal by a caseous mass and the upper pole of the kidney by small tubercles, and *D*, the same lesion shown in *C*, ilustrating tubercles and giant cells. × 100.

pain, swelling, discharge, itching, bleeding, *etc.* Deep infections may be associated with general manifestations of fever, anorexia, loss of weight, *etc.* as well as local symptoms and signs pertaining to the lungs, mouth, gastro-intestinal tract, *etc.* as the case may be. *Complications* may be many and varied. The *diagnosis* of fungous infections is suspected from a consideration of the history, clinical findings, and cutaneous sensitivity tests but is finally established by (1) identifying the organisms in direct smears of pus or tissue secured from the lesion, (2) isolating and growing the organisms on artificial media, (3) producing the disease in experimental animals, (4) histologic examination of tissues secured from the lesions, and (5) serologic reactions using the patient's serum. The *prognosis* varies with the infection.

PARASITIC INFLAMMATIONS

Parasitic inflammations are tissue reactions induced by parasites. *Parasites* (Gr. = beside + focal) are organisms that live on or within hosts from which they derive protection and nourishment. They may belong to the plant or the animal kingdom. Of concern in this section are the latter. The organism that harbors a parasite is called a *host* (Sawitz). A host is referred to as *definitive* when harboring the adult or sexual stage of the parasite and *intermediate* when harboring the larval or asexual stage. A *carrier* is one who harbors a parasite and may serve as a source of infection but who discloses no apparent clinical manifestations relative to the parasite.

Medically important parasites are *classified* into sub-kingdoms Protozoa and Metazoa. *Protozoa* are unicellular organisms consisting of a nucleus or of nuclei and of cytoplasm. The nucleus is either a mass of chromatin or a well-defined structure with a delineating nuclear membrane and an intra-nuclear karyosome. The cytoplasm is generally divided into (1) an inner endoplasm which is concerned with nutrition and contains ingested material, vacuoles, *etc.* and (2) a dense outer ectoplasm which not only serves as a protective covering but also provides ectoplasmic organelles (pseudopodia, flagella, or cilia) for locomotion, a "buccal" opening for ingestion of food, and means for excretion of waste material. Protozoa that are parasitic in man may be *divided* as follows: (1) *intestinal*—including *Endamoeba histolytica* (page 769), *Endamoeba coli* (page 771), *Giardia lamblia* (page 714), *Chilomastix mesneli* (page 714), and *Balantidium coli* (page 771), (2) *atrial* (mouth, vagina, and urethra)—including *Endamoeba gingivalis, Trichomonas buccalis,* and *Trichomonas vaginalis* (page 1154), and (3) hematological—including *Leishmania tropica, brasiliensis,* and *donovani* (page 923), *Typanosoma gambiense—rhodesiense,* and *cruzi* (page 924), *Plasmodium ovale, vivax malariae,* and *falciparum* (page 946), and *Toxoplasma gondii* (page 518).

Metazoa are divided into two major groups—Helminths and Arthropoda. *Helminths* (worms) are subdivided into two groups Nemathelminths and Platyhelminths. *Nemathelminths* belong to the class *Nematoda* or *round worms.* These parasites have a long, round, cylindrical body with a digestive tract (including mouth and anus) and male or female sex organs. Their motion is that of a snake. From without in they are composed of (1) cuticula or hyaline outer covering, (2) subcuticula consisting of a syncitium of nuclei and fibers, (3) dermomuscular layer consisting of longitudinal muscles, (4) body cavity filled with clear fluid that functions as blood, and (5) viscera (digestive, excretory, and reproductive organs) suspended in the body cavity. Each end possesses papillæ with sensory functions. The digestive tract consists of mouth, buccal capsule, esophagus, intestine, and anus. The excretory system is composed of tubules that lead to excretory pores. In the male, the reproductive system is composed of convoluted tubules ending in an ejaculatory duct. In some, the accessory sex organs are composed of spicules located on a coiled tail. A copulatory bursa is present in some round worms. In the female, the reproductive system is composed of tubular ovaries that connect with a vagina which is located near the middle of the body. Nematodes pass through a cycle that includes (1) the egg, (2) the rhabditiform larva—the feeding, noninfective larva possessing an open mouth and esophageal bulb, (3) the filariform larva—nonfeeding, infective larva possessing a closed mouth and slender esophagus, and (4) the adult. Nematodes of *medical importance* are (1) intestinal which include *Enterobius vermicularis* (page 772), *Trichocephalus trichiurus* (page 774), *Ascaris lumbricoides* (page 715), *Necator americanus* (page 716), *Ancylostoma duodenale* (page 718), *Strongyloides stercoralis* (page 718), and *Trichinella spiralis* (page 1302), and (2) tissue which include *Wuchereria bancrofti* (page 379) and *Onchocerca voluvlus* (page 1341).

Platyhelminths or *flatworms*, as the name implies, are flat and bilaterally symmetrical and lack a body cavity. They are divided into two groups—Cestoda and Trematoda. *Cestoda* or *tapeworms* are ribbon-shaped with the body composed of varying numbers of duplicated segments called proglottids. The *adult* worm is composed of a scolex, neck, and chains of segments. The scolex or head is globular or oval and possesses suckers or grooves for attachment to the intestinal mucosa. The neck is a budding zone of germinative tissue from the posterior portion of which segments are formed. The first segments are immature. These are followed by mature segments possessing male and female reproductive organs and then by gravid proglottids possessing a uterus filled with eggs. The body of the adult worm is covered with a homogeneous, elastic cuticle. Beneath this there is a muscular system composed of an outer layer of circular and an inner layer of longitudinal muscles. These enclose the excretory system which consists of simple tubules and the reproductive organs. Tapeworms have two types of reproductive systems. In one, there is an absence of the uterine pore. As a result, the eggs remain in the uterus and are released only upon disintegration of the proglottids. In the other, the eggs are laid by way of a uterine pore. Tapeworms of *medical importance* are *Taenia saginata* (page 720), *Taenia solium* (page 721), *Diphyllobothrium latum* (page 722), *Hymenolepis nana* (page 719), and *Echinococcus granulosis* (page 828).

Trematoda or *flukes* are leaf-shaped worms that possess two muscular suckers—an anterior or oral that serves as a mouth and means of attachment and a posterior or ventral that functions only as a means of attachment. The body is covered by a noncellular cuticle. Beneath this this are three layers of muscle—outer circular, middle oblique, inner longitudinal. Flukes possess (1) a digestive system composed of a mouth pharynx, esophagus, and two blind ceca, (2) an excretory system composed of flame cells, collecting tubules, excretory bladder, and excretory pore, and (3) a reproductive system with either separate sexes or both male and female organs in the same worm, that is, hermaphroditic. Flukes of *medical importance* are *Schistosoma mansoni* (p. 775), *Schistosoma haematobium* (p. 776), *Schistosoma japonicum* (p. 776), *Fasciola hepatica* (p. 826), *Clonorchis sinensis* (p. 827), and *Paragonimus westermani* (p. 518).

Arthropoda (Gr. = joint + foot) are bilaterally symmetrical animals covered with a chitinous exoskeleton and provided with jointed limbs arranged in pairs. The phylum includes centipedes, crustacea, spiders, ticks, mice, lice, mosquitoes, etc. While there are many organisms in this group, only a relative few are of medical significance to man. They are effective by (1) being pests — causing mechanical trauma, producing lesions that are secondarily infected, or injecting substances that produce severe reactions because of previous sensitivity — examples, bedbug and louse (p. 1340), (2) injecting poisons — example, black widow spider (p. 1342), (3) invading the skin — example, the itch mite (p. 1152), and (4) conveying disease either by microorganisms entering the arthropod where they may or may not undergo a developmental cycle such as plasmodia and filaria in mosquitoes, plague in fleas, rickettsiæ in mites, etc. or by microorganisms simply being carried as contaminants such as typhoid by the common housefly.

The *life cycles* of parasites may be simple or complex (Faust and Russell). In many instances, they require only one host. This host may be specific for a particular parasite or may be only one of several satisfactory hosts. In a great many instances, domestic or wild animals serve as reservoirs for the parasite and man is only incidentally involved because he happens to inhabit the area. The life cycles of the various parasites are outlined in connection with the different diseases as they are discussed in the text and need not be repeated at this time. The *sources* of *exposure* are (1) contaminated soil, water, or food, (2) biting insects possessing the parasite, (3) animals infected with or harboring the parasite, and (4) man himself infected with or contaminated with the parasite. The *portal* of *entry* into the body may be (1) through the mouth as in the case of *Ascaris lumbricoides*, *Enterobius vermicularis*, *Trichimella spiralis*, *Taenia solium*, *Taenia saginata*, etc. (2) through the skin as in the case of *Necator americanus*, *Strongyloides stercoralis*, *Schistosoma mansoni*, etc. as well as the many deposited by blood-sucking arthropods, (3) inhalation of ova as in the case of *Enterobius vermicularis* and *Ascaris lumbricoides*, (4) transplacental as in the case of *Toxoplasma gondii*, and occasionally malarial organisms and blood flukes, and (5) by way of sexual intercourse as in the case of *Trichomonas vaginalis*. *Geographically* parasitic diseases are most common in the tropics and subtropics where individual and group sanitation is at a low level and where warm climatic conditions favor the propagation of parasites and their vectors. The temperate and colder climates, however, are not excluded, especially in those diseases that develop on a person to person basis.

Pathologically, changes in tissues result from traumatic damage, lytic necrosis, stimulation of tissue reactions of host, toxic and allergic phenomenon, and secondary infection (Faust and Russell). *Traumatic damage* results from penetration of the skin as in the case of scabies, fly maggots, tick punctures, mosquito bite, and entrance of flukes. Once in the body, migration of parasites, as in the case of helminths, may result in rupture of capillaries and hemorrhages in tissues such as the lungs, eye, brain, etc. Escape of ova of *Schistosoma* may also be attended by hemorrhages into the urinary bladder or intestinal canal. Intestinal hemorrhages also result from attachment of hook worms to the mucosa. *Wuchereria bancrofti* produce mechanical damage by lodging in and obstructing lymphatic channels (Fig. 57, *A*). Larger worms, such as *Ascaris* and *Taenia*, may by sheer bulk produce intestinal obstruction or by entrance into smaller channels obstruction of the appendix or bile ducts. *Lytic changes* in tissues of the host are produced by liberation of enzymes by the parasites. Actually this is performed for the dual purpose of supplying food for the parasite itself and facilitating its penetration into the tissues. One of the best examples in this category is

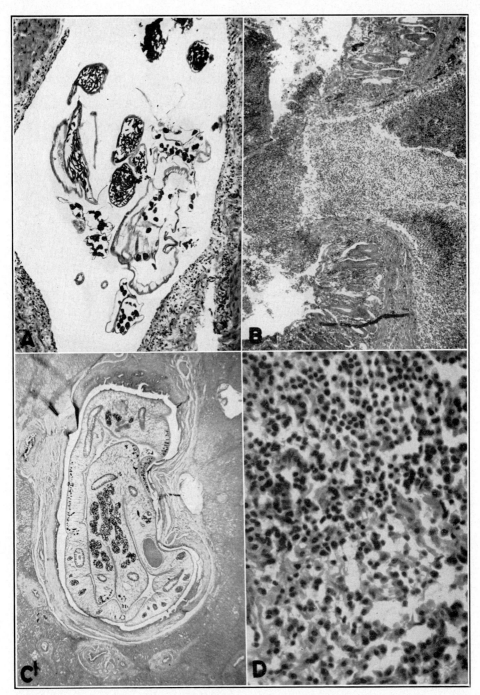

Fig. 57.—Parasitic inflammation showing *A, Wuchereria bancrofti* lodging within and obstructing a lymphatic channel. × 100, *B,* flask-like, lytic ulcer of the colon in amebiasis secondarily infected with bacteria. × 10, *C, Clonorchis sinensis* encapsulated in the liver. × 50, and *D,* eosinophilic, lymphocytic, and plasma cell permeation of tissues in the vincinity of *Wuchereria bancrofti.* × 400.

Endamoeba histolytica (Fig. 57, *B*). Other examples are malarial organisms, leishmania parasites, trypanosome group, and flukes.

Stimulation of *tissue reactions* of the host occurs in response to practically all animal parasites. Whenever a parasite enters the tissues of a host the first reaction is a local proliferation of the tissues in an effort to wall off and destroy the organism (Fig. 57, *C*). If the parasite is lodged in connective tissue, the reaction is fibroblastic while if it is lodged in natural passages such as bile ducts (*Fasciola hepatica*) or lymphatic channels (*Wuchereria bancrofti*) the proliferation is of bile ducts or lymphatic endothelium respectively. Even in the latter instance, though, the connective tissue is secondarily stimulated to produce a fibrous encapsulation. Secondarily also there is a varying degree of proliferation of capillaries and infiltration with neutrophils, plasma cells, lymphocytes, monocytes, and eosinophils (Fig. 57, *D*). Sometimes there is also an epithelioid and giant cell reaction. Hematologically, many parasitic infections are characterized by eosinophilia and those attended by loss of blood (destruction or hemorrhage) may reveal compensatory hyperplasia of the bone marrow. Occasionally the reparative reaction to the parasite may overstep its normal limits and result in the development of neoplasms. While examples of this reaction in man are not common, the following have been recorded: carcinoma of the colon in amebiasis, pathologic picture resembling leukemia in visceral leishmaniasis, carcinoma of the liver in hepatic infections with flukes and *Schistosoma*, and carcinoma of the bladder in infection with *Schistosoma haematobium*.

Toxic and *allergic phenomenon* vary with the parasite. Some arthropods, such as spiders, ticks, scorpions, bees, wasps, and bettles possess powerful toxins which, when injected, result in severe local or general reactions. Others in similar groups bring about little or no ill effects. Proteins and other metabolites of parasites, introduced into the body by any route, may may act as antigens producing specific antibodies so that subsequent introduction of similar substances may result in violent local or systemic (anaphylactic) hypersensitivity reactions. Unlike in the microbial kingdom, immunity of any significant or lasting degree does not occur. Pathologically, the hypersensitivity reactions are similar in all respects to those already described in connection with allergic inflammations (p. 140).

Secondary infection in connection with parasitic invasion is common although the degree of manifestations varies. "Ground itch" at the point of invasion of the hookworm larvas is due to pyogenic bacteria. *Endamoeba histolytica* produces a lytic reaction only. The inflammation that accompanies such as infection is due entirely to secondary bacterial invasion (Fig. 57, *B*). Other cutaneous and intestinal injuries are also accompanied by secondary bacterial infection, albeit in minor degrees. Finally, it is possible that parasites may carry viruses with them into the tissues of the body.

Clinical manifestations in parasitic disease, as would be expected from the protean nature of such infections, vary tremendously from case to case. Locally, there may be symptoms and signs of inflammation with the usual sites being either skin or muscle. Other localizing manifestations may pertain to the gastrointestinal tract such as diarrhea and hemorrhage in amebiasis or to the lungs such as cough, expectoration, etc. in ascariasis. Systemically, there may be fever, loss of weight, anemia, lethargy, leukocytosis, neutropenia, eosinophilia, *etc.* Because of the variability encountered it is hardly possible to discuss clinical manifestations in general. They are, however, considered in connection with descriptions of the individual diseases in the various portions of the text. The *diagnosis* of parasitic infection is made from (1) a consideration of the symptoms and signs, (2) identification of the parasite or its ova in proper preparations of the blood, sputum, feces, urine, fluids, or tissues from the body, and (3) specific immunologic (serologic, cutaneous sensitivity, *etc.*) tests. *Treatment* depends upon the type of infection. It may consist of (1) chemotherapy, as in the case of malaria, amebiasis, trypanosomiasis, oxyuriasis, and filariasis, (2) vermifuges, as in the case of intestinal worms, (3) desensitization, as in the case of bee stings, (4) surgical, as in the case of echinococcosis and intestinal obstruction caused by worms, and (5) local and general supportive therapy. Prevention by appropriate public health measures is of course all important. The *prognosis* varies with the disease.

FOREIGN BODY INFLAMMATIONS

Foreign body inflammations are those caused by the presence of foreign bodies. The latter may be of exogenous (any substance from without the body such as talcum powder, silica, splinters, etc.) or of endogenous (substances originating within the body such as calcified material) origin. The inflammation generally is of a chronic variety, although the initial reaction may be quite acute. *Grossly* the lesions are multifarious in appearance. Some resemble reactions of infectious (fungous, tuberculous, etc.) origin; others appear like ordinary abscesses, and others still are mistaken for neoplasms. *Histologically*, too, the appearance varies. Some are characterized by a diffuse nonspecific leukocytic reaction, while others form tubercles that are virtually indistinguishable from those in tuberculous or fungous infections. One characteristic, however, which is almost always identifiable is the presence of foreign body giant cells grouped around or engulfing the foreign material (Fig. 39B and C, p. 122).

GRANULOMATOUS INFLAMMATIONS

Granulomatous inflammations or *granulomas* are inflammations characterized by the presence of granulation tissue. Literally, therefore, the terms are synonymous with any chronic inflammation since the most outstanding histologic feature of chronic inflammation is granulation tissue. Actually, however, the captions are reserved for chronic inflammation disclosing a cellular proliferation and pattern sufficiently distinctive to allow (in most instances) an etiologic diagnosis (such as syphilis, tuberculosis, histoplasmosis, etc.).

TUBERCULOUS INFLAMMATION

Tuberculous inflammation is commonly referred to and generally known simply as *tuberculosis* (L. = tubercle or nodule + disease). This term was apparently first used by Schonlein in 1839 (Myers). The disease, however, was prevalent many centuries before this, for examination of bones and other human and animal remains indicates that it existed in prehistoric times on the plains of the Ganges, in the land of Moses, and in Babylon, Egypt, and China as early as 6000 B. C. Hippocrates named it *phthisis* (Gr. = consume); the English referred to it as *consumption* (L. = consume or waste), and others have called it the "*Captain of the men of death*," and the "*great white plague.*" Some of the other names relative to tuberculosis of different regions of the body are as follows: *scrofula* (L. = brood sow), king's evil, or struma referring to infection of cervical lymph nodes; *lupus* (L. = wolf) referring to infection of the skin; *tabes* (L. = wasting) *mesentericus* referring to infection of the mesenteric lymph nodes; *Pott's disease* or hunchback referring to infection of the spine; *white swelling* referring to infection of the joints, and *Addison's disease* referring to infection of the adrenal glands.

The *cause* of tuberculosis is the *Mycobacterium tuberculosis*, commonly referred to as *Kock's bacillus* (who discovered the organism in 1882) and simply as the *tubercle bacillus* (Wilson and Miles). Soon after the discovery

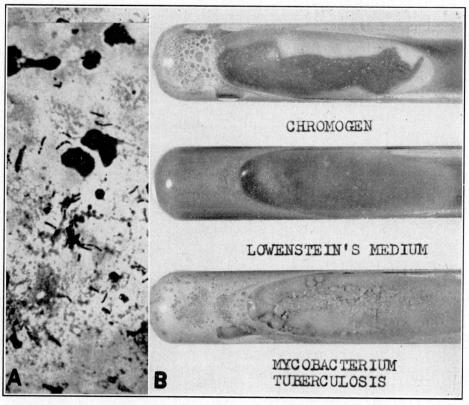

CHROMOGEN

LOWENSTEIN'S MEDIUM

MYCOBACTERIUM
TUBERCULOSIS

A.   B

FIG. 58.—*Mycobacterium tuberculosis* showing *A*, typical organisms in a smear. × 1350, and *B*, the appearance of colonies on artificial media.

of the organism it was shown that there are two types of mammalian tubercle bacilli—human and bovine, both of which produce disease in man. Other types of tubercle bacilli are avian—which produces disease in fowl and rarely in man and cold-blooded which produces disease in cold-blooded animals only. While there are *morphologic* differences between the human and bovine strains, these are too inconstant to be of definitive practical significance. The tubercle bacilli pathogenic for man are rod-shaped, straight or slightly curved organisms with parallel sides and rounded ends that measure from 1 to 4 microns in length and 0.3 to 0.6 microns in width (Fig. 58, *A*). Generally, they are longer and more slender when obtained from animal tissues than they are when obtained from cultures. On artificial media they may present as filamentous, branched, or even clubbed-shaped structures. They are gam-positive and acid fast. While many stains have been developed to demonstrate acid fastness, the most popular still appears to be the Ziehl-Neelsen stain employing carbol-fuchsin as the crucial agent. The acid fastness is probably due to (1) the presence in the bacillus of an unsaponifiable wax—an acid alcohol containing free hydroxyl groups and known as mycolic acid and (2) the existence around the organism of a semipermeable membrane that allows fuchsin to diffuse in but not out. The question as to whether the tubercle bacillus passes through a granular and viral *cycle* has engendered much discussion which is even yet not completely settled. In 1907, Much demonstrated that under certain conditions the bacilli might be present in tissues in the form of nonacid-fast granules— structures later referred to as *Much's granules*. He held that in tuberculous organs granules may be the only stainable form of organism, that they may be accompanied by rods that are not acid fast, and that granular forms are virulent. While most subsequent observers considered these granules as artefacts, Mudd demonstrated oxidative-reductive enzymatic activity within them and considered them as representing mitochondria. To complete the cycle, Fonte's (in 1910), and others since, claimed to have demonstrated filter-passing forms (virus) of tubercle bacilli that possess a low degree of pathogenicity for the guinea pig. This, too, has not been accepted by most workers.

The *chemical composition* of tubercle bacilli has been accurately determined by extraction of large quantities of organisms grown on artificial media. The components fall into three categories—lipids, polysaccharides or carbohydrates, and proteins. The *lipids* consist of (1) phospholipids such as palmitic, oleic, and phthioic acids, (2) waxes such as mycolic acid, phthiocerol, and mycocerosic acid, and (3) acetone soluble fats such as aldol and phthiocol. The lipids account for the acid fastness and the monocytic, epithelioid, giant cell, and tubercle response. The *polysaccharides* on hydrolysis yield mannose, inositol, d-arabinose, galactose, and d-glucose. The polysaccharides are responsible for bacterial virulence and host immunity. The *proteins* are complex and soluble in water. They are responsible for the tissue damage, the tuberculin reaction, and the constitutional symptoms in the hypersensitive or allergic patient.

Culturally, tubercle bacilli vary in the ease with which they grow on artificial media but generally it takes 2 weeks or more for organisms pathogenic for man to produce a visible growth. While many media have been developed, the most satisfactory solid ones contain inspissated serum, coagulated egg, or potato with glycerine added. A good fluid medium (Dubos) consists of an enzymic digest of casein containing asparagin along with salts of iron, copper, magnesium, calcium, and zinc. Regardless of the medium, the growth is usually thick, wrinkled, and dry or moderately moist (Fig. 58, *B*) and possesses a sweet, rather fruity odor. Yellowish or orange pigment is often produced by the human strain of organism. While there are cultural differences which aid in differentiating the tubercle bacilli that produce disease in man, the best way of identifying the species is by *animal inoculation*. The human type is pathogenic for the guinea pig, slightly pathogenic for the rabbit, and nonpathogenic for the calf and fowl. The bovine type is pathogenic for the guinea pig, rabbit, and calf but not for fowl. The avian type is pathogenic for the fowl and rabbit, slightly pathogenic for the calf, and nonpathogenic for the guinea pig. Finally, it should be pointed out that there are a number of *saprophytic acid-fast organisms* found in water, dust, butter, grass, manure, smegma, and soil that are not pathogenic for man, that may be confused with pathogenic organisms morphologically, and that can generally be easily separated from pathogenic organisms in that they grow readily on ordinary culture media in 2 to 3 days.

The problem of *immunity* and *hypersensitivity* or allergy in tuberculosis has been much discussed and confused. Despite statements to the contrary, there is no doubt that man has a great capacity to develop resistance to the tubercle bacillus (Rosenthal). That *native resistance* to this organism does exist is clearly demonstrated by the act that the human strain of tubercle bacillus is most virulent for man, the bovine strain for cattle, and the avian strain for fowl. Although there is cross infection, there is no doubt that species specifity is strong. Within the same species, however, native resistance varies. In man, for example, the Eskimo, American Indian, and Negro are much less resistant than the Caucasian white race. Carrying the point a little further, some individuals of the same, albeit susceptible, race are more resistant to infection than others. While the mechanism of this native resistance is unknown, the following are thought to be significant: inheritance, socio-economic conditions, hormones, and physiologic functions as related to the response of the host to stress stimuli. *Resistance* may be *acquired* by *natural means.* Even before the tubercle bacillus was discovered it was demonstrated that animals inoculated with treated sputum from tuberculous patients developed resistance to subsequent injection of untreated tuberculous sputum. This formed the basis of what is referred to as *Koch's phenomenon.* Briefly, the phenomenon is as follows. Cutaneous injection of tubercle bacilli into the guinea pig for the first time is followed in 2 to 3 weeks by a focal reaction around the injection site. A subsequent cutaneous injection is followed by localization of the organisms at the site of injection, by a severe focal reaction attended by formation of a slough, and by prolongation of the life of the animal. Pathologically, the second reaction is characterized by less exudation and more proliferation and fibrous tissue reaction. As early as 1886 Marfan observed that a similar phenomenon occurred in man in that those who had tuberculous lymphadenitis which healed before adolescence (Ghon complex, p. 494) were less likely to develop pulmonary tuberculosis than were adults who were infected for the first time. Subsequently, this has been proved over and over again in medical students and student nurses. Briefly, people in each of these categories who have had a primary infection, as evidenced by a positive reaction to tuberculin (protein from tubercle bacilli) are more resistant to infection from contact with tuberculous patients than are those who have had no previous exposure. Furthermore, not only is the incidence of infection reduced in those who recovered from a primary infection but if reinfection does occur, the process is more apt to remain localized to the lungs, to be more proliferative and fibrotic, and to offer a better prognosis. It follows, therefore, that *artificial immunization* in those who have not been exposed to previous infection, as demonstrated by a negative tuberculin reaction, is desirable. To this end the *BCG* (bacillus of Calmette and Guérin) vaccine has been developed and used in millions of human inoculations. The BCG is a strain of bovine tubercle bacillus which was isolated by Calmette and Guérin, which was once virulent but now has become attenuated as a result of prolonged cultivation on glycerol potato-bile medium, and which has lost its pathogenicity for the guinea pig, rabbit, calf, and man. Although the use of this vaccine has created a great deal of controversy, it appears to be the concensus that it is the best vaccine available, that it does not produce progressive disease in man or animals, that it does increase the resistance of the body to tuberculous infection, and that vaccination by its use is safer than exposure to virulent organisms such as occurs in primary infections. Without belaboring the desirability of the use of BCG, it may be briefly stated that the vaccination has been generally accepted abroad but that it has met with a great deal of opposition in the United States. Currently, its use on a limited scale has been recommended by the United States Public Health Service, the Council on Chemistry and Pharmacy of the American Medical Association, and the American Trudeau Society. To *summarize*, resistance, either innate or acquired, to tubercle bacilli is a reality as manifested by (1) localization and destruction of organisms at the site of inoculation, (2) inhibition of spread of organisms throughout the body, (3) limitation of multiplication of organisms in distant organs, (4) response of tissues with a productive rather than an exudative reaction, and (5) prolongation of life.

The *mechanism* of *immunity* and *allergy* in tuberculosis is not well understood despite thousands of publications to the contrary. The problems here are essentially the same as those in connection with other bacterial infections. Since they have already been discussed in a general fashion in connection with Allergic Inflammations (p. 140) they will only be touched upon at this time. Despite occasional claims to the contrary, there is no evidence to indicate that *humoral antibodies* (antibodies present in the serum or lymph) develop, in either immunized or actively infected animals, that inhibit the growth of tubercle bacilli on artificial media or that protect the animal against active infection. The *role* of *cells* in *immunity* to tuberculosis, on the other hand, has been amply demonstrated, with the cells in question being *monocytes*. Lurie, for example, inoculated rabbits' corneas with monocytes from immunized and nonimmunized animals containing phagocytosed tubercle bacilli. Quantitative cultural and histologic studies 10 to 20 days later disclosed multiplication of tubercle bacilli in cells from normal animals as compared with a reduction in number in cells from immunized animals. Along similar lines, Suter demonstrated that phagocytes from guinea pigs immunized with BCG inhibited the growth of tubercle bacilli in tissue cultures. Also on the positive side, BCG vaccination is followed by general stimulation of the reticulo-endothelial system—the producer of monocytes, as well as an actual increase in monocytes of the circulating blood. Thus, monocytes appear to play an important role in immunity to tuberculosis. They act by phagocytosis and by actual destruction of the bacilli or prevention of their multiplication. *Tissue environmental factors* may also play a role in immunity. In experimental animals, various organs show a marked difference of infection to tubercle bacilli. In the guinea pig, for example, the kidney, unlike most other organs, is highly resistant. Upon chemical analysis the kidney is found to contain a high concentration of spermine phosphate which is thought to account for the difference in susceptibility. Because oxygen deficiency has a bacteriostatic effect on tubercle bacilli, the oxygen tension of tissue is thought to have some effect on resistance and susceptibility. Variations in organic acids, especially lactic acid, may also play a role.

In tuberculosis, much controversy has arisen concerning the relationship of *allergy* to immunity. Rich considers the allergic state as separate from the immune state while others believe that the allergic state develops concomittantly with the immune state. Regardless of these divergent views, there is no doubt that a delayed allergic response (p. 143) does occur in connection with infection with tubercle bacilli and it is believed that localization of the organisms at the site of entrance is primarily a function of the hypersensitive state. The specific antigen in the tubercle bacilllus responsible for this is tubercle bacillary protein.

Experimentally, many animals have been used to study the pathogenesis of tuberculosis, with the guinea pig and the rabbit heading the list. Of these two, the *rabbit* has been used more extensively, because it has been found that by intravenous injection of bovine tubercle bacilli most of the features of pulmonary lesions encountered in man can be developed in this animal with relative ease and regularly (Medlar). Intravenous inoculation of virulent bacilli into rabbits not previously infected discloses the first *gross* manifestations of disease in the lungs in the form of diffusely scattered white foci by the tenth day. In time, the foci grow larger, coalesce, and form large nodules. Death usually occurs in from 6 weeks to 3 months. At this time, the lesions are firm and on section disclose a light yellowish gray center without softening or cavitation. *Histologically*, at 2 days the alveolar walls show foci of congestion with accumulations of monocytes and neutrophils while adjacent alveolar spaces contain neutrophils. At 5 days the foci in the alveolar walls become larger and are composed mostly of neutrophils while the adjacent alveoli are filled with similar cells. By the end of the second week, the alveolar foci coalesce, with their centers packed with neutrophils but without abscess formation and, for the first time, are loaded with tubercle bacilli. About the periphery, monocytes are present and both scattered monocytes and neutrophils contain phagocytosed organisms. By the end of the fourth week and progressing until death of the animal, increasing necrosis occurs in the central areas of the foci and nodules, identification of tubercle bacilli becomes more and more difficult, and there is a conspicuous ack of proliferation of connective tissue. Classical tubercle formation does not occur. Testing the animals to tuberculin discloses a positive reaction after the third week — at a time when large numbers of tubercle bacilli are being destroyed in the tissues. Decreasing the *number* of *tubercle bacilli* injected changes the lesions quantitatively but not qualitatively. Decreasing the *virulence* of the *organisms*, by using a BCG strain, results in a maximal infiltration of the lungs with small gray foci by 4 weeks and subsequent disappearance and complete resolution by 6 months. Early histologic lesions are similar to those formed by virulent organisms but with a slower tempo. After one week the foci enlarge but the infiltrating cells are mostly monocytes and lymphocytes. Necrosis does not occur. By 3 months many foci resolve and those that remain are composed mostly of monocytes and occasional giant cells or of lymphocytes only. At 6 months the only evidences of infection are scattered scars and scattered collections of lymphocytes. Testing the animals to tuberculin discloses a positive reaction in the majority after 2 months, thus indicating the development of an *allergic state*. Because the rabbits make a complete recovery, they provide excellent hosts for studying reinfection. Inoculating such rabbits with virulent organisms results in chronic progressive pulmonary disease with death of animals between 8 and 18 months. Animals sacrificed at 2 weeks show varying degrees of acute pneumonic consolidation. Histologic sections reveal the foci to consist mostly of monocytes, lymphocytes, and neutrophils with occasional abscesses and occasional foci of necrosis. Animals sacrificed at one month disclose scattered gray foci 1 to 2 mm. in

diameter. Histologically these consist mostly of monocytes and lymphocytes with occasional epithelioid tubercles and giant cells. Animals dying
from reinfection disease show varisized, bilateral, chronic, cavitary lesions
with and without bronchial communications. Histologically the foci consist of an outer zone of fibrous tissue and an inner zone of necrotic tissue
abounding in neutrophils and containing varying numbers of tubercle
bacilli. Noncavitary lesions consist essentially of central foci of necrosis
surrounded by varying amounts of fibrous tissue. In general, therefore,
it may be stated that the inflammatory response in reinfection tuberculosis
is more vigorous and more intense, that it is attended by necrosis and cavitation, that it forms tubercles, and that it elicits a fibrous tissue response.

In *man*, infected for the first time, the *source* of human tubercle bacilli is
man himself, either as a result of direct personal contact or as a result of contact with infected material discharged by such a person (Rich). The latter is
especially dangerous for tubercle bacilli may survive weeks outside the
human body. The source of infection with bovine tubercle bacilli is generally unpasteurized milk or improperly cooked infected meat. In *reinfection*
tuberculosis the source of the organisms is either the same as that of primary
infection or is the original "healed" or "arrested" primary focus in the body
itself that has broken down and released the bacilli. The usual *route* of
infection is pulmonary by inhalation, while the more uncommon route these
days is the gastrointestinal tract by ingestion. Rarely, may the organisms
be transmitted by way of the placenta from an infected mother to her baby.
Finally, inoculation of bacilli through the conjunctiva or through the skin
(as in ritual circumcision) is possible but occurs so rarely that it need scarcely
be mentioned. *Epidemiologically* the overall *incidence* in males is greater
than in females but the incidence in different age periods varies. Up to
puberty, the incidence in the two sexes is about the same. From puberty
to the age of about 30 years the incidence in females is higher than in males.
After this, however, the incidence in females drops and continues to be lower
than in males through the remainder of the life span. The *mortality* varies
with the age. It is highest during the first year of life, is somewhat lower
from 1 to 5 years, is the lowest of any period between 5 to 14 years, increases
sharply from 14 to 25 years, is maintained at a high level for the next
several decades, and increases in rate as old age is approached. *Race*, as
already mentioned, is important in epidemiology for it is common knowledge
that the Eskimo, American Indian, and Negro are much more susceptible
than is the white person. Finally, the *socioeconomic* state is also important
in the spread and contraction of tuberculosis for over-crowding and poor
nutrition predispose to infection.

The *pathologic* changes in man parallel those just described in connection
with the experimentally produced disease in rabbits. *Primary infection*,
that is infection for the first time, usually occurs in infancy or childhood
but may occur in adulthood. It usually affects the lung and thoracic lymph
nodes but, on occasion, may be present in the tonsils and cervical lymph
nodes, or the ileocecal area of the intestines and mesenteric lymph nodes.
Generally, as in experimental animals, such an infection remains localized
and only rarely does it spread and become disseminated. In the lungs the
primary lesion, also called the *Ghon lesion*, is usually single, sharply circumscribed, and located beneath the pleura (Fig. 59, *A* and *B*). It is grayish
white, has a caseous center and only slightly fibrous periphery, and measures
1 to 2 cm. in diameter. The lymph nodes draining the area (especially
those at the hilum of the lung) are involved by a similar process and the

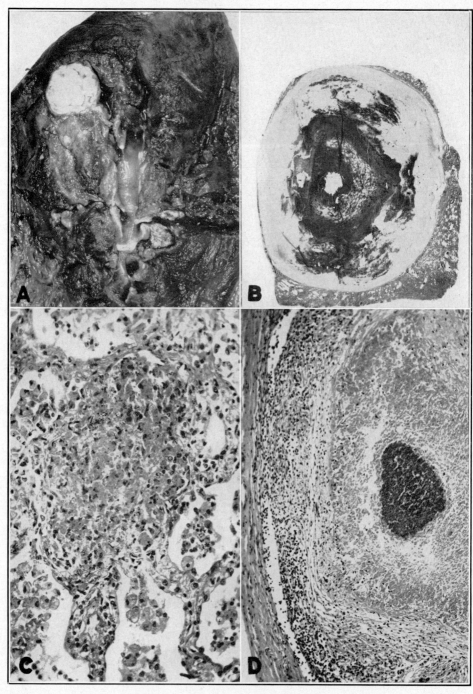

FIG. 59.—Primary tuberculosis showing *A*, a Ghon complex with a circumscribed nodule at the periphery of the lung and a similar nodule in a hilar lymph node, *B*, central calcification of a pulmonary focus.   × 5, *C*, an early focus in a lung composed of central neutrophils and necrotic material and peripheral mononuclear cells.   × 200, and *D*, a Ghon lesion with central caseation necrosis and calcification and peripheral mononuclear and epithelioid cell reaction.   × 100.

combination of the pulmonary and lymph node lesions is called the *primary tuberculous* or *Ghon complex*. Primary lesions are not attended by cavitation or extensive fibrosis. *Histologically* the earliest lesion consists of focal neutrophilic infiltration. This is followed by necrosis and about the periphery mononuclear cell infiltration (Fig. 59, *C*). Eventually the central area becomes caseous and, by coalescence with adjacent areas, enlarges until ultimately it reaches a diameter of 1 to 2 cm. already mentioned (Fig. 59, *D*). It continues to be surrounded by mononuclear cells with the addition of epithelioid cells. Langhans' giant cells are few in number. When the primary infection is small it may ultimately be completely resorbed. When it is larger the central area remains caseous and often calcifies, while the periphery consists of a mantle of epithelioid cells that ultimately are replaced by a band of connective tissue cells.

Secondary infection, commonly referred to as *reinfection tuberculosis*, usually occurs in adults but may also be found in children. Most often the process starts in the lungs and is generally located in the subapical areas. Because the patient has already been sensitized to the protein of the tubercle bacillus, he reacts much more violently to the infection than when exposed for the first time. This reaction consists of necrosis, cavitation, and extensive inflammation. Contrarily, also because the patient was previously exposed, he simultaneously develops a certain degree of immunity or resistance. This reaction is characterized by fibrous tissue proliferation. The resultant of the two, that is destruction on the one hand and repair on the other, determines the ultimate gross and microscopic appearance of reinfection tuberculosis. Grossly, such lesions therefore vary tremendously from tiny, barely perceptible, gray foci to huge areas of caseation, necrosis, fibrosis, and cavitation (Fig. 60, *A*). Histologically, the characteristic unit is the *tubercle* (L. = lump or nodule). At this point, it must be stressed that while the tubercle is characteristic of tuberculosis it is not pathognomonic for this disease for many other diseases (notably fungous infections) are also characterized by the formation of tubercles. In reinfection tuberculosis, tubercles may be of two types—hard and soft. A hard tubercle is composed of a central mass of epithelioid cells fringed by scattered Langhans' giant cells and surrounded by plasma cells, lymphocytes, and monocytes (Fig. 60, *C* and 61*A*). In some instances, the centralmost epithelioid cells undergo caseation necrosis. A soft tubercle resembles more the tubercle seen in primary infection. Early it is composed mostly of neutrophils with but a few monocytes and inconspicuous epithelioid cells added (Fig. 60, *B*). Later it discloses a central area of acute necrosis surrounded by scanty numbers of poorly formed epithelioid cells and more peripherally by plasma cells, lymphocytes, and monocytes (Fig. 61, *B*). Sometimes the center is composed of loosely arranged epithelioid cells rather than of a necrotic focus. Giant cells are only rarely seen in connection with soft tubercles. As the processes age in reinfection tuberculosis and depending upon the resistance of the person, there is in addition to the tubercles a varying degree of fibrous tissue proliferation which of course alters the microscopic appearance. Finally, some lesions are represented by *tuberculous granulation tissue* (Fig. 62). This occurs in the wall of a tuberculous lesion where the center has been converted into an abscess or in those inflammations that reach a free surface and discharge their contents therefrom. From within out it consists of caseous material, fibroblasts and epithelioid cells intermingled with monocytes and other leukocytes, and non-

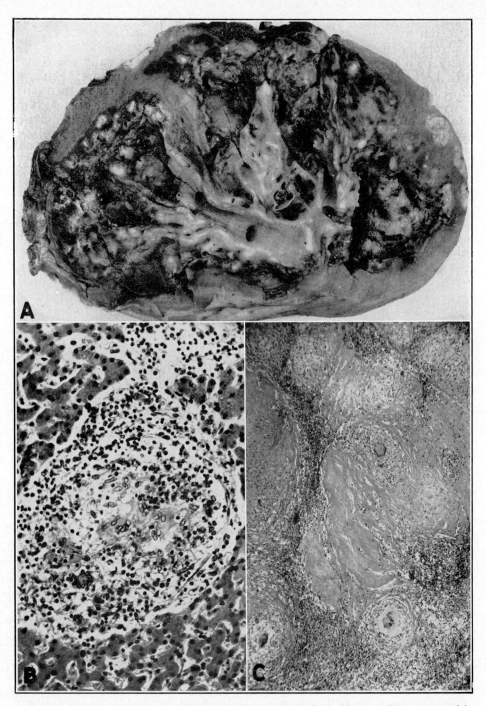

Fɪɢ. 60.—Secondary tuberculosis showing *A*, many nodules of caseation as well as many cavities in a lung, *B*, an early tubercle composed mostly of neutrophils and only a few monocytes and epithelioid cells. $\times$ 200, and *C*, hard tubercles composed of epithelioid cells and Langhans' giant cells surrounded by plasma cells and lymphocytes. $\times$ 50.

specific chronic inflammation.   Giant cells are sparse and attempts at
tubercle formation are poor.

The most important *complications* of tuberculosis are extension of the
process to adjacent organs and widespread dissemination throughout the
body.   The *clinical manifestations* pertain to disturbances of function of
the organ or organs involved.   In addition, absorption of protein products

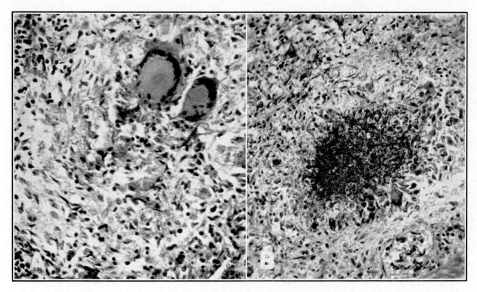

Fig. 61.—Tuberculosis showing *A*, a hard tubercle composed of epithelioid cells, early central
breakdown of cells, two Langhans' giant cells, and plasma cells and lymphocytes about the periphery, and *B*, a soft tubercle composed of central necrotic material surrounded by epithelioid cells,
spurious Langhans' giant cells, and (peripherally) leukocytes.   × 100.

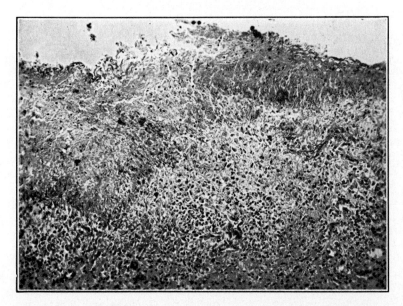

Fig. 62.—Tuberculous granulation tissue disclosing from above down caseation necrosis merging
with a zone of epithelioid cells and fibroblasts.   × 100.   (Herbut, *Urological Pathology*, Lea &
Febiger.)

12

from dead bacteria and destroyed tissues result in general manifestations of weakness, fatigue, anorexia, loss of weight, fever, night sweats, and general wasting away.   The *diagnosis* of tuberculosis is made from the clinical manifestations, endoscopic and roentgen visualizations of the organs or systems in question, microscopic examination of tissue removed by various procedures, and isolation of *Mycobacterium tuberculosis* from secretions or tissues of the body by way of smears, cultures, or animal inoculation.   A positive cutaneous reaction to *tuberculin* (protein from tubercle bacilli) means that a person has had or has tuberculosis.   A negative reaction means that a person has never had tuberculosis or that he now possesses an overwhelming tuberculous or other infection.   *Treatment* consists of proper nutrition, rest, symptomatic relief of manifestations, antibiotic and chemotherapy, and various surgical procedures depending upon the system affected and the extent and severity of the infection.   The *prognosis* depends upon the age, race, sex, type of lesion (primary or secondary), extent of process, organ or organs involved, etc.

Before terminating this general discussion on tuberculosis, it should be pointed out that the disease is considered again in the following portions of the text in connection with the different systems: heart, pages 319 and 324, vessels, page 378; upper respiratory system, page 413; larynx, page 441; lungs, page 492; thyroid, page 571; mouth, page 609; esophagus, page 638; stomach, page 669; small and large intestine, page 712; appendix, page 747; liver, page 814; peritoneum, page 898; spleen, page 969; lymph nodes, page 990; adrenals, page 1004; urethra, page 1025; bladder, page 1033; ureters, page 1042; kidneys, page 1091; penis, page 1112; prostate, page 1119; epididymis, page 1127; testis, page 1130; vulva, page 1149; endometrium, page 1164; fallopian tubes, page 1178; breast, page 1209; bones, page 1234; joints, page 1276; skin, page 1331; and brain, pages 1412 and 1445.

SYPHILITIC INFLAMMATION

Syphilitic inflammation is commonly known simply as syphilis or lues. The term *syphilis* apparently originated in a poem by Fracastorius in 1530 (Shaffer).   According to one version it stems from use in connection with a shepherd inflicted with the disease, while according to another version it is derived from a Greek word meaning together and to love.   The latter connotation would imply venereal contraction.   The term *lues* (L. = plague) simply means a pestilential disease.   Originally the term *lues venerea* was used to indicate syphilis but gradually venerea was dropped and lues alone is now often employed.   Syphilis is an *ancient disease* for the Chinese and Hindus were acquainted with it and even used mercury in its treatment 2000 years ago (Cole).   The disease was recognized in Japan since 800 A. D. and is known to have existed in North and South America since at least 1200 A. D.   Apparently the sailors of Columbus contracted the infection during their visit to the New World and upon their return to Europe were responsible for a virulent epidemic which spread through the Old World about 1500 (Shaffer).

Syphilis may be *defined* as a contagious and infectious disease caused by the *Treponema pallidum*.   Often termed the *Great Imitator*, because it can mimic almost any other disease, it is of worldwide *distribution*.   Its *incidence* increases with a decrease in social conditions, thus making it more prevalent among the poorer than the better-to-do classes.   For obvious reasons, it is more common among the urban than the rural population.   It affects males more often than females and is more frequent in Negroes than in whites. In the United States the all time peak incidence was reached in 1946. Since then, there has been a steady decline, probably due, in part a least, to the widespread use of antibiotics and chemotherapeutic agents for nonsyphilitic conditions.

Epidemiologically, acquired syphilis is transmitted directly from person to person usually by sexual intercourse, occasionally by kissing, and less frequently by biting or abnormal sex practices. Transmission by way of infected articles rarely occurs because the causative organism is quite vulnerable to conditions outside of the body. Not withstanding public opinion to the contrary, infectious lesions are more or less limited to the early stages of the disease, namely the chancre and moist lesions of secondary syphilis. Tertiary lesions are not infective and any form of the disease is rarely transmissible after 5 years. Treatment controls infectiousness, for it has been demonstrated that spirochetes in superficial lesions are destroyed within 24 hours after the first adequate dose of arsenic. Congenitally, syphilis may be transmitted from an infected mother to her baby in the uterus. This too is an infection, however, and not a transmission by way of the genes of the parents. Man does not possess natural *immunity* against syphilis and can acquire immunity only by contracting the infection itself. Injection of dead organisms, in attempts to produce this phenomenon, has not been successful. Ordinarily, it takes about 90 days for immunity to develop against infection but once it occurs it persists throughout life. For some unknown reason, this immunity exists against new organisms from the outside but not against organisms already within the body. Reinfection, however, can occur, provided the organisms are introduced before immunity develops. It is thus possible, for example, for a person to develop a second chancre if he is reinfected before the first one appears. Objectively, protective serum *antibodies* have been demonstrated in low titer in syphilitic infections in man and rabbit and these have been potent enough to make virulent spirochetes noninfective for rabbits (Wilson and Miles). These antibodies appear to be the same as those that account for the immobilization of *Treponema pallidum in vitro* (see section on Diagnosis).

As already stated, the *cause* of syphilis is a spirochete called the *Treponema pallidum.* This organism was discovered by Schandinn and Hoffman in 1905. It is a tightly coiled thread-like organism that possesses 8 to 14 primary coils each about 1 micron long and that measures in the overall about 8 to 14 microns in length and 0.25 to 0.3 microns in width. The organism is readily visible in dark-field preparations of fluids from lesions and in silver impregnations of tissues (Fig. 309C). Electronmicroscopy discloses 4 flagella in a tuft near one end. In the fresh state, *Treponema pallidum* are actively motile. In this process they disclose secondary curves that appear and disappear in rapid succession. Movement is backwards and forwards by rotation around the long axis and by flexion of the whole body. Syphilitic spirochetes are delicate organisms for they are readily destroyed by heat and they die rapidly in stored blood and when exposed outside of the body. The question of *cultivation* of *Treponema pallidum* on artificial medium has engendered controversy ever since success was recorded in 1909. Some workers claim to have grown the organisms on media composed of agar containing animal tissue, hydrocele fluid, or ascitic fluid. Other workers have failed in similar attempts and claim that the organisms grown are contaminants. From this it is gathered that at best cultivation of *Treponema pallidum* is most difficult. *Experimentally,* syphilitic lesions are reproducible in a variety of animals. The rabbit, for example, is susceptible to ocular and testicular infection. From the latter the disease may spread throughout the body. The monkey, especially the chimpanzee, is susceptible to genital infection and reveals in addition secondary lesions. The guinea pig is more resistant but does develop local lesions upon intracutaneous inoculation.

The *gross pathologic* changes vary greatly with the tissues and organs affected, the stage of the infection, and the type of the infection. For practical purposes, syphilis may be divided into two types—acquired and congenital. *Acquired syphilis* is that which is contracted after birth. It may be divided into primary, secondary, and tertiary stages or into early and late syphilis. *Early syphilis* encompasses all forms of the disease that develop within the first four years after inoculation. It thus includes the primary, secondary, and even some of the tertiary lesions of the alternate classification. *Late syphilis* encompasses all lesions that develop beyond the first four years after inoculation. It, therefore, includes only lesions of the tertiary stage. *Congenital syphilis* is that which is contracted by the unborn infant and is manifested either at or after birth.

Primary acquired syphilis is characterized by the *chancre* (L. = crab), also known as the *primary sore* and the *Huntarian chancre* after Jonathan Hunter who produced the lesion by self-inoculation in 1767 (Shaffer). It is the first manifestation of the disease and probably occurs in all infections although, especially in women, it is overlooked in as high as one third of all cases. It is not present, of course, when the disease is contracted by way of parenterally administered blood or serum. It develops in 7 to 42 with an average of 21 days after contraction of the infection at the point of inoculation of the spirochetes. Long before the lesion is apparent, however, the organisms are disseminated throughout the body by way of the lymphatics and blood vessels. Some indication of the rapidity of such dissemination is provided by experiments in which spirochetes have been isolated from regional lymph nodes as early as 5 minutes after cutaneous inoculation of the scrotum of guinea pigs. Because syphilis is usually contracted by sexual intercourse, the chancre is most commonly seen on the external genitals. Extragenital chancres, however, are sometimes encountered on the lips, tongue, tonsils, other areas of the mouth, nose, face, eyelids, nipples, anus, and fingers. In its typical form the primary lesion consists of a painless, indurated, superficially ulcerated mass that measures 1 to 2 cm. in diameter (Fig. 544*A*). The borders are sharply circumscribed and the surface is generally covered with a serous exudate. The draining lymph nodes are large, firm, and nontender. The chancre heals slowly and spontaneously in from 2 to 8 weeks, leaving in its wake only a thin scar.

Secondary acquired syphilis is a systemic disease that becomes manifest up to 3 months with an average of 6 weeks after the beginning of the primary sore (Kierland). While the chief changes occur in the skin, mucous membranes, and lymph nodes other regions of the body such as the eyes, central nervous system, periostium, liver, and even kidneys may at times be affected. The cutaneous lesions are often referred to as *syphiloderma* or *syphilids* (page 1333). They are multiple and varied, and may simulate almost any cutaneous disorder. Usually, they are symmetrical and generalized, involving even the palms and soles. Syphilids may be divided into macules, papules, nodules, vesicles, and pustules. *Macules* (L. = stain or spot) are round, oval, or irregular, nonelevated, light rosy to dark reddish brown patches of varying sizes that occur as the earliest secondary lesion in about

80 per cent of cases. *Papules* (L. = pimple) are basic lesions that arise as such or that develop from macules. As the term suggests they are flat or pointed cutaneous protrusions that generally measure only a few millimeters in greatest diameter (Fig. 63, *A*). They may be few or many in number and they may be single in distribution or clumped. Their surface is smooth or scaly. *Nodules* develop as progressions of papules. As the term suggests, they are nodular lesions that measure as much as 2 cm. in diameter. Usually they are smooth and glossy but they may be covered with scales and they vary in color from light to brownish red. *Vesicles* (L. = bladder or blister) are small, elevated, usually discrete elevations filled at their apex with clear fluid. They are rare. *Pustules* (L. = small elevation filled with pus) are varisized papular lesions capped with pus and covered with crust.

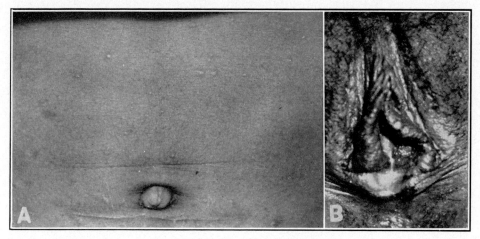

FIG. 63.—Secondary syphilis showing *A*, papules distributed over the skin of the anterior portion of the abdomen and *B*, mucous patches of the vulva and vagina.

They develop as a progression of papules or vesicles, are rare, and generally occur in cachetic people. Other cutaneous manifestations of secondary syphilis are condyloma latum and alopecia. *Condyloma latum* (Gr. = wart + broad or flat) consists of raised, flat, pale, soggy, coalescing, papules or plaques disposed about the genitals and anus. Heat and moisture are responsible for this alteration in the basic appearance of what ordinarily are papules. Condyloma latum abounds in spirochetes. *Alopecia* (Gr. = mange of foxes) is a loss of the hair on the scalp or baldness that occurs in about 7 per cent of cases. The baldness is patchy rather than complete and is temporary inasmuch as growth of hair returns when the local process subsides. The lesions in the *mucous membranes* are referred to as *mucous patches* because they often appear as patches of mucus covering mucous membranes (Fig. 63, *B*). Basically, they are papules that have been altered in their appearance because of moisture and warmth. They are generally seen on the lips, tongue, tonsils, pharynx, larynx, and external genitals. They are irregular in configuration, slightly raised, moist, grayish white or rosy, covered with mucus or a thin gray membrane, and surrounded by an erythematous base. Mucous patches swarm with spirochetes and are thus highly infectious. The *lymph nodes* in secondary syphilis are enlarged, discrete, and nontender. Those most noticeably affected are inguinal, epitrochlear, axillary, and cervical. Secondary lesions like the primary sore are temporary, for they usually disappear spontaneously in from 1 to 6 months.

Tertiary acquired syphilis is protean in nature, occurs from 1 to 40 years after the primary infection, and may affect any tissue or organ of the body with the cutaneous (p. 1333), cardiovascular (pp. 319 and 375), osseous (pp. 1234 and 1276), and central nervous (pp. 1414 and 1419) systems heading the list. The *cutaneous lesions* are solitary, infiltrative, smooth or ulcerating, and nodular. They may measure from a few millimeters to many centimeters in diameter and may mimic almost any other cutaneous disease. They heal centrally and marginally by resolution or granulation tissue and fibrosis, thus producing an arciform configuration. *Vascular* lesions of syphilis are fundamental for, as will be seen under the microscopic description, such changes occur in every stage of syphilitic infection. They consist primarily of endothelial proliferation and leukocytic infiltration. In small vessels the end result is thickening of the wall and vascular occlusion (Fig. 733). In larger vessels, such as the aorta, the vasa vasorum are affected, the walls of the vessels are weakened, and aneurysms are formed. *Cardiac* lesions of syphilis are of two types—most commonly atrophic and fibrotic myocardial due to occlusion of the coronary ostia and rarely focal myocardial infection with gumma formation (Fig. 149). *Gummas* (L. = gum) are circumscribed, gray, rubbery, areas of caseation necrosis that measure from microscopic to many centimeters in diabmeter (Fig. 391, *B*). In acquired syphilis they are always confined to the tertiary stage, probably represent hypersensitivity on the part of the patient, and may be found in any organ of the body. The *osseous* lesions of syphilis consist in essence of osteomyelitis with destruction of bone and deformity (Figs. 520 and 521). The latter occurs especially in the nose where the septum is destroyed and the nose collapses producing what is referred to as a saddle nose. Syphilitic lesions of the *central nervous system* exist in the form of meningitis, vasculitis, gumma, and encephalitis. Involvement of the brain tissue itself (encephalitis) results in general paresis.

Congenital syphilis, as already stated, is acquired by the infant from the mother after the fifth month of pregnancy. If infection occurs before this period abortion usually results. In the child the disease becomes apparent either at birth or during childhood. In essence, the lesions duplicate those of acquired syphilis with the exception that the chancre does not occur. Most *cutaneous* lesions are maculopapular in appearance but nodular manifestations similar to those in tertiary syphilis are also seen. *Nasal* infection usually becomes apparent in from 2 to 6 weeks after birth (p. 413). It consists of mucosal ulcerations attended by abundant secretion resulting in what is usually referred to as snuffles (Fig. 64). Gummatous inflammation of the nasal septum with later collapse of the nose may also occur but generally does not become apparent until about puberty. The most obvious and earliest *buccal* lesions consist of linear fissures and cracks at the mucocutaneous junction of the lips arranged at right angle to the mouth itself (Fig. 64). They are generally called *rhagades* (Gr. = rent). Later, as a result of improper development of the premaxilla, malocclusion of the jaw becomes apparent and *Hutchinson's triad* may be seen (p. 608). This consists of (1) inflammation of the eyes, (2) deafness from paralysis of the eighth cranial nerve, and (3) hypoplastic, peg-shaped, centrally notched permanent incisors. Most *visceral* changes in congenital syphilis consist of an arrest of development. In the *lungs* this results in what is called *pneumonia alba* and consists of unexpanded or poorly expanded alveoli (p. 503).

In the *spleen* the sinusoids are dilated and lined with prominent endothelial cells and hematopoietic foci are present (p. 971).   In the *liver* the cords fail to radiate in their usual pattern and hematopoietic foci are also numerous (p. 818).   In addition, interstitial hepatitis and gummatous infiltration may also be encountered (Fig. 390).   The *thymus* may disclose diffuse fibrosis, gummas, and Dubois abscesses (p. 994). *Osseous* changes may consist of inflammation of the joints (p. 1276) and inflammation of the bone itself in the form of osteochondritis, osteomyelitis, and periostitis (p. 1234).

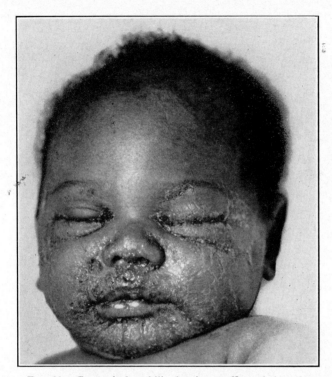

FIG. 64.—Congenital syphilis showing snuffle and rhagades.

Microscopically the fundamental pathologic lesion in syphilis, regardless of the stage of infection, is a *vasculitis* (Fig. 65, *A*).   The spirochetes possess a tropism for all smaller vessels be they arteries, veins, or lymphatics. When larger channels such as the aorta are affected, the primary change occurs in the vasa vasorum and this in turn leads to destruction and finally weakening of the wall with consequent dilatation and even rupture. Upon inoculation, the *Treponema pallidum* seeks out the vessels and produces two types of changes.   One is an evanescent perivascular infiltration with neutrophils which is rapidly replaced with more lasting mantles of lympho- cytes and later plasma cells.   These cells, proceeding from without in, soon permeate the entire vascular wall.   The other change is a concentric prolifer- ation of the vascular endothelium to such a degree that the lumen may be completely obliterated.   Consequent to endothelium damage, the lumens of the vessels may be further occluded by thrombi.   The blood supply to the overlying tissues is thus impaired, nutrition is diminished, and degeneration, necrosis, and ulceration follow.   Meanwhile, the stroma becomes permeated with leukocytes and this, together with concomitant edema further reduces the blood flow and contributes to the retrogressive changes. As the lesion ages, it ultimately heals by resolution or by granulation tissue formation and fibrosis. The *gumma*, histologically, represents a more intense local reaction in a hypersensitive or allergic patient and is actually comparable to the delayed reaction in tuberculosis. It, too, is primarily a vasculitis — but a vasculitis which is so intense and complete that it results in a complete casseous type of necrosis (Fig. 65). This necrosis occupies the central portion of the gumma — be it microscopic or macroscopic in size. This necrosis, however, is not quite as destructive as that seen in tuberculosis for elastic

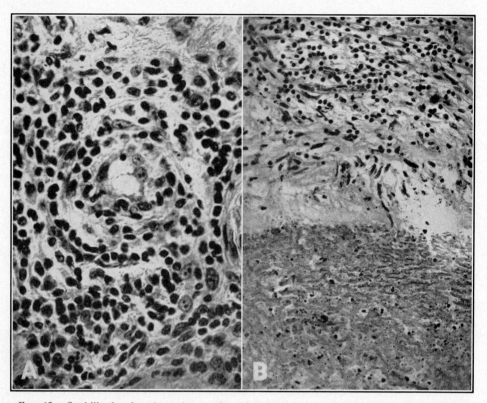

Fig. 65.—Syphilis showing *A*, a chancre in which there is marked endothelial proliferation of an arteriole and a dense peri-arteriolar and arteriolar infiltration with plasma cells, lymphocytes, and monocytes. × 400, and *B*, gumma with the center composed of necrotic material and the periphery consisting of fibroblasts, epithelioid cells, plasma cells, and lymphocytes. × 200.

tissue stains still reveal elastic fibers intact and thereby outlining the configuration of the vascular channels. About the periphery of the necrotic focus are seen epithelioid cells and occasional giant cells and, as the lesion gets older, an ever increasing number of fibroblasts. Gradually, the latter encroach upon the necrotic area and either completely replace it if it is small or permanently encase it by a capsule if it is large.

The *complications* of syphilis are as diverse as the lesions themselves. They may pertain to any organ and are consequent either to the inflammation as such or to the vascular occlusion, with secondary degenerative and retrogressive alterations in the affected areas. The *clinical manifestations* too are extremely varied. In about one quarter to one third of all cases, the patients may be completely unaware of any disturbances. In the others, the symptoms and signs depend upon the type and severity of infection and organs affected. In *acquired syphilis* the *primary stage* is represented simply by a sore and even this may be unnoticed in as many as one third of all infections. The *secondary stage* may be attended by any combination of cutaneous and mucosal lesions, sore throat, anorexia, malaise, slight fever, anemia, headache, meningismus, pains in the bones and joints, and, on occasion, even hepatic and renal impairment. The *tertiary stage* is attended by manifestations pointing to the cutaneous, cardiovascular, osseous, central nervous, or other systems. The more common symptoms and signs in *congenital syphilis* are cutaneous and mucosal lesions, snuffles, malnutrition from interference in feeding, enlarged spleen, and a cracked-pot type of cry due to laryngitis. Later, deformities of the jaw, teeth, nose, and bones make their appearance.

The *diagnosis* of syphilis is made from the history, appearance of the cutaneous and mucosal lesions, roentgenographic studies especially of the bones, endoscopic (laryngeal) examination, biopsy of accessible lesions, demonstration of spirochetes in dark field preparations of serum from the lesions, and *serologic tests.* The routinely performed serologic tests are the complement fixation and flocculation or precipitation reactions. The complement fixation reaction is the *Wassermann* reaction of 1906 or some modification of it. In principle, it consists of the union of antibody with antigen in the presence of complement. The antibody is that found in the serum of a syphilitic patient which develops consequent to infection with *Treponema pallidum.* The antigen usually used is an alcoholic (lipid) extract of beef heart from which the acetone soluble extract has been removed. The complement is supplied by guinea pig serum. To demonstrate the utilization of complement an indicator system is used. This consists of sheep erythrocytes together with their specific hemolytic antibody. The *flocculation* or *precipitation* reactions go under the names of the Kahn, Kline, Eagle, Hinton, VDRL (Venereal Disease Research Laboratory), etc. They depend upon the presence of flocculation or precipitation when the patient's serum containing syphilitic antibody is combined with an antigen. The antigen usually consists of an ether-alcohol extract of beef muscle with cholesterol added. At one time, it was thought that the above serologic tests were 100 per cent diagnostic of syphilis. Recently, it has been shown that *false positive* reactions occur in about 7 per cent of all tests performed in a diagnostic laboratory and that *false negative* reactions occur in about 50 per cent of all syphilitics (Shaffer). A few of the many causes of false positive reactions are alcohol, anesthesia, food rich in cholesterol, vaccination, jaundice, infectious mononucleosis, undulant fever, malaria, leprosy, pneumonia, tuberculosis, infectious hepatitis, lupus erythematosus, exanthemata, arthritis, diabetes mellitus, myocardial infarction, periarteritis nodosa, etc. (Miller). A more specific test for the diagnosis of syphilis is the *TPI* or *Treponema pallidum Immobilization Test.* Its premise is that serum from a patient having immunity to syphilis immobilizes a suspension of *Treponema pallidum* from an early primary lesion of a rabbit's testis when incubated with complement for from 18 to 24 hours (Shaffer). The test, unfortunately, is not practical for routine laboratory use because of technical difficulties, one of which is lack of a good method for cultivating *Treponema pallidum.* It can and should be used, however, to eliminate false positive reactions (Ledbetter). Along the same line, a modified and less expensive procedure is the *TPIA* or *Treponema pallidum Immune Adherence Test* where dead *Treponema pallidum* is used as antigen (Miller). The principle here is that *Treponema pallidum* sensitized by specific antibody present in the patient's serum adheres to the surface of human erythrocytes in the presence of complement. It does not adhere in the presence of normal serum and complement.

Treatment of syphilis is twofold — prophylaxis by preventing infection and eradication of the disease once it has occurred. For decades the standard treatment was arsenic in the form of Salversan discovered by Ehrlich in 1909 and bismuth dicovered by Levaditi in 1922. Today both of these have been largely replaced with penicillin given in large doses in rapid succession. In patients sensitive to penicillin, other antibiotics such as oxytetracycline hydrochloride, chlortetracycline hydrochloride, erythromycin or carbomycin may be used (Thomas). The *prognosis* varies with the stage of disease, organ involved, severity and extent of infection, etc. In general, cutaneous and mucosal lesions of early syphilis respond quickly and completely to treatment. In fact, from one quarter to one third of patients with acquired disease undergo spontaneous cure without any treatment. The prognosis in late syphilis with lesions in the central nervous and cardiovascular systems, on the other hand, is guarded for the damage is permanent and may be serious.

REFERENCES

Inflammation

ADAMI, J. G.: Inflammations. *An Introduction to the Study of Pathology*, 4th Ed., London, The Macmillan Co., 1909.

BERMAN, L.: A. M. A. Arch. Path., *33*, 295, 1942 (Lymphocytes, Macrophages, etc.).

CAPE, R. D. T.: Edin. Med. J., *59*, 374, 1952 (Eosinophils).

CLOUGH, P. W.: Ann. Int. Med., *47*, 599, 1957 (Properdin).

FRIED, B. M.: A. M. A. Arch. Path., *26*, 700, 1938 (Metchnikoff's Contribution).

HARRELL, G. T., JR.: Sodeman's *Pathologic Physiology*, 2nd Ed., Philadelphia, W. B. Saunders Co., 1956, pp. 153 and 169 (Resistance and Effects).

HAYTHORN, S. R.: A. M. A. Arch. Path., *7*, 651, 1929 (Multinucleated Giant Cells).

HERTZOG, A. J.: Am. J. Path., *14*, 595, 1938 (Phagocytic Activity of Leukocytes).

LEWIS, T.: *Blood Vessels of the Human Skin and their Responses*, London, Shaw and Sons, Ltd., 1927 (Histamine).

MAXIMOW, A. A., and BLOOM, W.: *A Textbook of Histology*, 7th Ed., Philadelphia, W. B. Saunders Co., 1957.

McCUTCHEON, M.: A. M. A. Arch. Path., *34*, 167, 1942 (Chemotaxis).

————: Physiol. Rev., *26*, 319, 1946 (Chemotaxis).

McCUTCHEON, M., *et al.*: A. M. A. Arch. Path., *17*, 607, 1934 (Chemotropism of Leukocytes).

————: A.M.A. Arch. Path., *36*, 269, 1943 (Basic Pattern of Inflammation).

————:*Dynamics of Inflammation*, New York, The Macmillan Co., 1940.

MENKIN, V.: Science, *123*, 527, 1956 (Dynamics).

REBUCK, J. W.: Am. J. Cl. Path., *17*, 614, 1947 (Functions Leukocytes).

RICH, A. R.: A. M. A. Arch. Path., *22*, 228, 1936 (Review).

SABIN, F. R.: Physiol. Rev., *12*, 141, 1932 (Reaction to Fractions Tubercle Bacilli).

SJOERDSMA, A., *et al.*: Science, *125*, 1202, 1957 (Mast Cells).

SPIERS, R. S.: Ann. N. Y. Acad. Sc., *59*, 706. 1955 (Eosinophils and Basophils).

SUNDBERG, R. D.: Ann. N. Y. Acad. Sc., *59*, 671, 1955 (Lymphocytes and Plasma Cells).

THORN, G. W.: Am. J. Med., *14*, 139, 1953 (Eosinophils and Stress).

TOMPKINS, E. H.: Ann. N. Y. Acad. Sc., *59*, 732, 1955 (Monocytes).

WINTROBE, M. W.: Clinical Hematology, 4th Ed., Philadelphia, Lea & Febiger, 1956.

WRIGHT, R. W.: Am. J. Path., *6*, 87, 1930 (Epithelioid Reaction to Gas).

Allergic Inflammations

BLATT, H.: Quart. Rev. Allergy, *10*, 496, 1956 (Review Microbes and Allergy).

BURDON, K. L.: J. Ped., *48*, 372, 1956 (Cellular and Humoral Theories).

BURRAGE, W. S., *et al.*: New England J. Med., *255*, 79, 1956 (General Allergy).
HARTMAN, M. M.: Am. J. Med., *21*, 85, 1956 (Clinical and Pathologic).
LAWRENCE, H. S.: Am. J. Med., *20*, 428, 1956 (Delayed Allergy).
SHELDON, J. M., *et al.*: A Manual of Clinical Allergy, Philadelphia, W. B. Saunders Co., 1953 (Definitions and General).
TUFT, L.: Clinical Allergy, Philadelphia, Lea & Febiger, 1949 (Definitions and General).
WITHERS, O. R., and HALE, R.: Ann. Allergy, *14*, 384, 1956 (Food).

Viral and Rickettsial Inflammations

RHODES, A. J., and VAN ROOYEN, C. E.: *Textbook of Virology*, 2nd Ed., Baltimore, Williams & Wilkins Co., 1953.
RIVERS, T. M.: *Viral and Rickettsial Infections of Man*, 2nd Ed., Philadelphia, J. B. Lippincott Co., 1952.

Fungous Inflammations

BEAMER, P. R.: Am. J. Path., *25*, 66, 1955 (Immunity).
KADE, H., and KAPLAN, L.: A.M.A. Arch. Path., *59*, 571, 1955 (Staining).
LEWIS, G. M., and HOPPER, M. E.: *An Introduction to Medical Mycology*, 3rd Ed., Chicago, Year Book Publishers, 1948.
MOSS, E. S., *et al.*: A.M.A. Arch. Path., *59*, 105, 1955 (General).
MOSS, E. S., and McQUOWN, A. L.: *Atlas of Medical Mycology*, Baltimore, Williams & Wilkins Co., 1953.
TORACK, R. M.: Am. J. Med., *22*, 872, 1957 (After Antibiotic Therapy).

Parasitic Inflammation

FAUST, E. C., and RUSSELL, P. F.: Craig and Faust's *Clinical Parasitology*, 6th Ed., Philadelphia, Lea & Febiger, 1957.
SAWITZ, W. G.: *Medical Parasitology*, 2nd Ed., New York, McGraw-Hill Book Co., Inc., 1956.

Tuberculous Inflammation

MEDLAR, E. M.: Am. Rev. Ruber., *71*, Part II, 1, 1955 (Pulmonary Lesions).
MYERS, J. A.: *Tuberculosis*, Springfield, Charles C Thomas, 1957.
RICH, A. R.: *The Pathogenesis of Tuberculosis*, 2nd Ed., Springfield, Charles C Thomas, 1951.
ROSENTHAL, S. R.: *BCG Vaccination against Tuberculosis*, Boston, Little, Brown & Co., 1957.
WILSON, G. S., and MILES, A. A.: Topley and Wilson's *Principles of Bacteriology and Immunity*, Baltimore, Williams & Wilkins Co., 1955.

Syphilitic Inflammations

COLE, H. N.: A.M.A. Arch. Derm., *73*, 425, 1956 (Historical).
KIERLAND, R. R.: Ormsby and Montgomery's *Diseases of the Skin*, 8th Ed., Philadelphia, Lea & Febiger, 1954, p. 1021.
LEDBETTER, R. K.: J.A.M.A., *160*, 1397, 1956 (TPI Test).
MILLER, J. L., and HILL, J. H.: J.A.M.A., *164*, 1461, 1957 (False Positive Reactions).
MILLER, J. N., *et al.*: J.A.M.A., *163*, 112, 1957 (TPIA Test).
SHAFFER, L. W.: Top's *Communicable Diseases*, 3rd Ed., St. Louis, C. V. Mosby Co., 1955, p. 957.
THOMAS, E. W.: J.A.M.A., *162*, 1536, 1956 (Treatment).
WILSON, G. S., and MILES, A. A.: Topley and Wilson's *Principles of Bacteriology and Immunity*, 4th Ed., Baltimore, Williams & Wilkins Co., 1955, Vol. I, p. 1040 and Vol. II, p. 2027.

6

Physical Disturbances

GENERAL CONSIDERATIONS

THE fourth broad category of general disease processes may be designated as *Physical Disturbances*. Within its confines may be included a variety of unrelated conditions characterized more or less by outright mechanical alterations or by direct injury or trauma to the cells, tissues, and organs of the body. For purposes of general discussion, the group may be divided into the following: circulatory disturbances, trauma, obstruction of hollow organs, foreign bodies, hernias, thermal disturbances, light, electricity, irradiation, and chemicals.

CIRCULATORY DISTURBANCES

Although the maintenance of a normal circulation is dependent upon the proper co-ordination of many factors, the three most outstanding determinants are the heart, the vessels, and the blood. It is obvious that there are many *disorders* that may affect each of these portions of the circulatory system. It is equally obvious that the effects of such disorders will be evident either locally or generally depending upon the location, nature, and extent of the disturbance. Thus, for example, a 2-centimeter stab wound of an extremity may result in perforation of but a few capillaries with an inconsequential local extravasation of blood, while a similar stab wound entering the left ventricle of the heart or the aorta will usually result in massive bleeding and prompt death of the patient. Because of their multiplicity and their varied nature, specific disease processes that affect the heart, the vessels, and the blood are discussed in appropriate places in the text. There are, however, certain general principles and general conditions pertaining to *circulatory disturbances* that may be considered collectively under the following headings: general hemic disorders, ischemia, infarction, hyperemia, hemorrhage, disturbance of fluid balance, edema, shock, thrombosis, and embolism.

General Hemic Disorders.—Since the bulk of the formed elements of the blood consists of erythrocytes, the blood volume (for practical purposes) is made up essentially of plasma and red blood cells. *Normally* the *total blood volume* in healthy adults amounts to approximately 7 per cent of body weight, 2,735 cc. per sq. m. of body surface, or 75 cc. per kg. of body weight. The corresponding *plasma volume* amounts to approximately 45 cc. per kg. of body weight leaving a *red blood cell volume* of approximately 30 cc. per kg. of body weight. The normal *erythrocytic count* of the circulating blood in adult females varies from 4.5 to 5.1 millions per c. mm. and in adult males from 5.0 to 5.8 millions per c. mm. (Wintrobe). *Abnormally*, changes in bulk of plasma or erythrocytes or changes in both are responsible for certain hemic disorders that may briefly be considered together. They may be divided into two broad groups—increase in bulk and decrease in bulk. The former comprises such conditions as plethora, hydremia, and polycythemia while the latter encompasses such disturbances as anhydremia, dehydration, and anemia.

Plethora (Gr. = fullness) signifies simply an increase in blood volume without specification as to whether the fluid or formed elements or both are involved. Clinically, the vessels are distended with blood; the pulse is full; the face is flushed, and there is a feeling of tenseness in the head. Because of its general connotation, the term as such is inadequate and is better supplanted by the terms hydremia and polycythemia. *Hydremia* (Gr. = water + blood) means an increase in blood volume due to an increase in its fluid (serum) component. It occurs as a result of relative decrease of fluid excretion over fluid intake or as a result of relative increase of the hydroscopic pressure of the blood. Among other conditions, hydremia is encountered in cardiac failure, renal insufficiency, pregnancy (physiologically), hemorrhage, and intravenous administration of fluids. *Polycythemia* (G. = many + cells + blood) indicates an increase in blood volume as a result of an increase in its formed element (erythrocytic) component. Polycythemia is dividable into primary and secondary types. *Primary polycythemia* (also known as polycythemia vera, polycythemia rubra, erythrocythemia, and erythremia) is persistent and results from an excessive formation of erythrocytes by the bone marrow due to some unknown stimulus. It is discussed further in connection with diseases of the Blood, Chapter 25, page 926. *Secondary polycythemia* (also known as erythrocytosis) is a physiologic increase of erythrocytes in the circulating blood due essentially to deficiency in oxygenation. Most commonly it is seen in people living at high altitudes, in fibrosing processes of the lungs, and in cardiac disease.

Anhydremia (Gr. = negative + water + blood) implies a decrease in blood volume due to a decrease in its fluid (serum) component. The best example of the condition is hemoconcentration which is seen in shock and which eventuates from an escape of intravascular fluid into the tissues. *Dehydration* (L. and Gr. = away + water) denotes a decrease in blood volume due to a decrease in its fluid (serum) component together with a depletion of fluid in the tissues of the body. It comes about as a result of a relatively decreased fluid intake as compared with fluid output and is usually seen when there is excessive loss of either water or salt from the body. More specifically, it may be noted in the presence of excessive perspiration, vomiting, diarrhea, polyuria, high fever, adrenal insufficiency, and diabetic coma. *Anemia* (Gr. = negative + blood) connotes a decrease in blood volume due to a decrease in its formed element (erythrocytic) component. It comes about as a result of (1) decreased erythrocytic production, (2) increased erythrocytic destruction, or (3) loss of erythrocytes (hemorrhage) from the body. Since the term anemia literally means without blood it would be more accurate to supplant it by the terms *erythrocytopenia* (Gr. = red cell + poverty), *erythropenia* (Gr. = red + poverty), or *oligemia* (Gr. = little + blood). The subject is discussed further in connection with diseases of the Blood, Chapter 25, page 926.

Ischemia.—The term ischemia (Gr. = to hold back + blood) means a ocal deficiency of blood to a part of the body or simply local anemia. It is *due to* encroachment upon the lumen of the artery supplying the area. Some of the many *causes* of arterial occlusion are (1) *congenital anomalies* in the form of hypersensitivity resulting in spasm as in Raynaud's disease, (2) *degeneration* especially intimal as in arteriosclerosis, (3) *inflammation* as in periarteritis nodosa or thromboangiitis obliterans, (4) *physical disturbances* as in thrombosis, embolism, pressure from the outside (tourniquet, bedsores, distention of hollow organ, ligation, etc.), and spasm (ergot poisoning, application of cold, application of adrenalin, etc.), and (5) *tumors* either by compression from the outside or growing into the lumen of the artery. The *results* of ischemia depend upon (1) the rapidity of occlusion, (2) the extent of occlusion (partial or complete), and (3) the adequacy of the collateral circulation. When the occlusion is gradual in onset and partial, and the collateral circulation is moderately good but still inadequate, the affected area may reveal blanching, diminished arterial pulsation, various degenerative changes, atrophy, and ultimately fibrous tissue replacement. The ischemia may also be attended by intermittent cramps (claudications). When, on the other hand, the occlusion is rapid in onset and more or less complete, and the collateral circulation is totally inadequate, the affected area will usually reveal a mottled appearance and absence of arterial pulsation, and will be followed rapidly by infarction, necrosis, or gangrene.

Infarction.—The term *infarction* (L. = to stuff in) connotes the formation of an infarct and an *infarct* is an area of necrosis brought about by ischemia. The usual *mechanism* back of infarction is arterial occlusion in the absence of an adequate collateral circulation although occasionally venous obstruction (as in the small intestine) will also produce the disturbance. The *causes* of *arterial occlusion* are similar to those listed in connection with ischemia (see preceding paragraph) with thrombosis, embolism, and arteriosclerosis being the most frequent.

The *pathogenesis* of infarction was elucidated by Karsner several decades ago. The initial change in the affected area is *redness* or *hyperemia*. This is due to engorgement and dilatation of the capillaries. The engorgement results from an inflow of erythrocytes from collateral vessels and veins, while the dilatation is due to paralysis of the walls from anoxia. Some of the blood escapes into the tissues by diapedesis and rhexis. *Decolorization* of the infarct starts soon after its formation. It begins in the center, progresses to the periphery, and is often complete in from twenty-four to forty-eight hours. The change in color is due to laking of the erythrocytes with subsequent removal of the pigment by diffusion and, to a lesser extent, by phagocytosis. *Degenerative changes* in the affected tissue appear in about two hours and progress to culminate in complete necrosis in from forty-eight to seventy-two hours. The necrosis is usually of the coagulation type with outlines of structures remaining for varying periods of time but with cellular details wanting from the start (Fig. 66). Occasionally, however, as in infarcts of the brain, it is of a liquefaction variety. At the junction of the viable with the necrotic tissue (and in the mesothelial covering) there appears a *peripheral zone* of *hyperemia*. This represents an acute inflammatory reaction and is caused by the irritating action of split protein products arising in the necrotic tissue. Gradually, the zone of inflammation is succeeded by granulation tissue and fibroblasts, and the latter creep in to replace the destroyed tissue. If the area of necrosis is small it is ultimately completely replaced with scar tissue but if the area is larger the fibrous tissue simply forms a surrounding capsule.

Grossly, infarcts may be single or multiple and measure from a few millimeters to several centimeters in diameter (Fig. 67). They are usually roughly triangular in outline with the base directed peripherally. Initially, all infarcts are *red* or *hemorrhagic*. If they contain an abundant amount of blood (as in the lungs and liver where there is a dual blood supply or in the small intestine where the collateral circulation is relatively good) they remain hemorrhagic, but if they contain a scanty amount of blood (as in the spleen, kidneys, and heart where there is no dual blood supply and the collateral circulation is poor) they blanch within twenty-four to forty-eight hours and are then referred to as pale, white, or anemic. Initially,

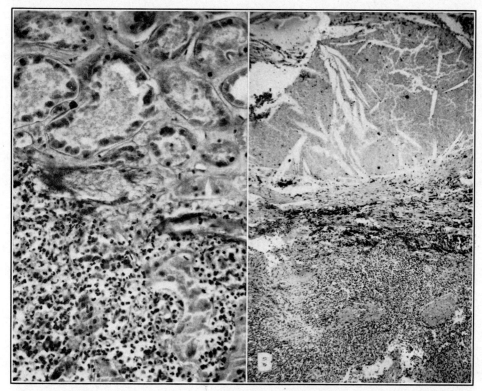

FIG. 66.—Infarction showing *A*, the kidney with coagulation necrosis (above) and extensive leukocytic infiltration (below). × 200, and *B*, the spleen with complete old necrosis (above) separated from normal splenic tissue (below) by a capsule of fibrous tissue. × 50.

chiefly as a result of congestion and edema, the affected area is swollen and protrudes above the surface. As the fluid, erythrocytes, and necrotic tissue are removed the area contracts and becomes depressed beneath the surface of the adjacent parenchyma.

Hyperemia.—The term *hyperemia* (Gr. = over + blood) is synonymous with the term *congestion* (L. = heap together) and connotes an excessive accumulation of blood in any tissue of the body. The condition is generally divided into two groups—active hyperemia and passive hyperemia.

Active hyperemia is that due to an increased inflow of blood to a part. It is brought about by an *active dilatation* of both the arterioles and capillaries. The dilatation results partly from nerve stimuli and, in the case of capillaries, also from the action of noxious agents directly on the vascular walls. Active hyperemia due to nerve stimulation occurs in the following: blush-

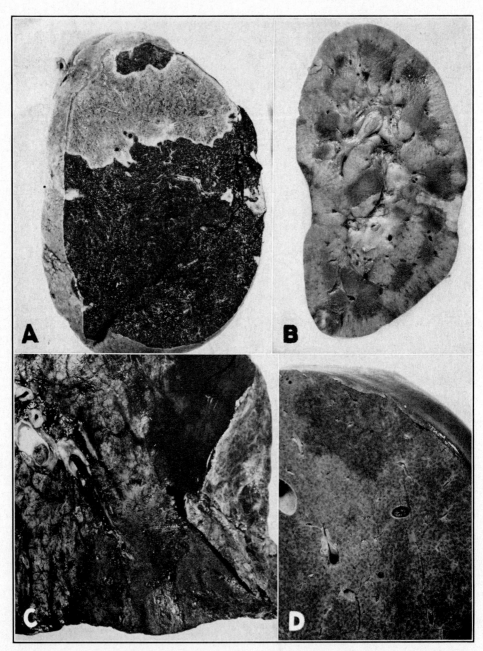

Fig. 67.—Infarction showing *A*, recent pale infarcts in a spleen, *B*, old pale infarct in a kidney, *C*, triangular hemorrhagic infarct in a lung (lower portion), fibrinous pleuritis (to the right), and an arterial thrombus supplying the area of the lung, and *D*, an irregular hemorrhagic infarct of the liver.

ing, flushing in response to heat, gastric mucosa during digestion, muscle during work, and the uterus during pregnancy. Examples of active hyperemia due to nerve stimulation and the action of noxious agents on the vascular wall are to be found in acute inflammation. Although the initial noxious agents are many, the final causative factors may be reduced to anoxia and tissue metabolites. Because there is an increased amount and rate of flow of blood to the part in active hyperemia, oxygenation is increased and, as a consequence, *functional activity* is stepped up. *Pathologically* the area is discolored red or bluish-red and is usually swollen. Histologically the capillaries are dilated and engorged and the extracapillary tissues are permeated with edema fluid and erythrocytes.

Passive hyperemia or *congestion* is that due to a decreased outflow of blood from a part. Since it represents an accumulation of blood in the venous side of the circulation the condition is also known as *venous hyperemia* or *venous congestion*. *Hypostatic congestion* is venous congestion occurring in the lowest or dependent part of an organ and is due to gravity in the presence of a feeble circulation. *Bier's hyperemia* is venous hyperemia induced wilfully by obstructing the venous circulation with a tourniquet. Passive hyperemia may be divided into two broad groups—generalized and localized.

Generalized passive hyperemia is that which occurs in most tissues and organs of the body as a result of failure or obstruction in areas of the body through which all blood must pass, namely, the heart and/or the lungs. It is *acute* when it develops rapidly and persists for only a short period and *chronic* when it develops gradually and persists for a long period. The best *example* of *acute* generalized passive hyperemia is that which occurs just before death when the heart as a whole is failing rapidly. It is manifested *pathologically* by engorgement of the venules with or without escape of plasma and erythrocytes. Grossly, the organs (especially the lungs) are enlarged, deep red, or bluish-red and, when incised, allow a free flow of bloody fluid from the cut surfaces.

Chronic generalized passive hyperemia usually results from gradual, long-standing, cardiac failure. This may be due to chronic valvular disease (stenosis or insufficiency) or to myocardial disease (usually fibrosis). Less often the obstruction to the flow of blood is in the *lungs* and is caused by narrowing of the vessels as in emphysema, diffuse fibrosis, or Ayerza's disease. *Pathologically* the changes are fundamentally the same as they are in the acute form. Because, however, the process is chronic the extravasated erythrocytes tend to break down and liberate hemosiderin pigment, and the concomitant anoxia tends to produce degeneration and necrosis of parenchymatous cells with ultimate fibrous tissue replacement. While these changes are present more or less in all organs, the alterations in the lungs and liver deserve special mention. The *lungs* are enlarged, dark red to brown, subcrepitant, and firmer than normal (Fig. 68). Histologically the alveolar walls are thickened; the alveolar vessels are dilated; the alveoli are often lined with a single layer of cuboidal cells, and the alveolar spaces are filled with erythrocytes, fibrin, edema fluid, and macrophages laden with hemosiderin. These are so often found in cases of cardiac decompensation that they are frequently called "heart failure cells." The *liver* is initially enlarged but later may be decreased in size. It is deep red or brown and firm (Fig. 69). On sectioning, it presents somewhat of a mosaic pattern with the centers of the hepatic lobules deep red and the peripheries light brown or yellowish (nutmeg appearance because it resembles a nutmeg). Histologically the central veins and their tributaries are dilated and

13

engorged; the central hepatic cells show degeneration and necrosis (due chiefly to anoxia); erythrocytes are scattered throughout the area, and the peripheral cells show a fatty change. As the destruction of hepatic tissue progresses the supporting framework in the center of the lobules condenses and fibrous tissue is deposited periportally producing what is known as *cardiac cirrhosis* of the *liver*. *Clinically* chronic generalized passive hyper-

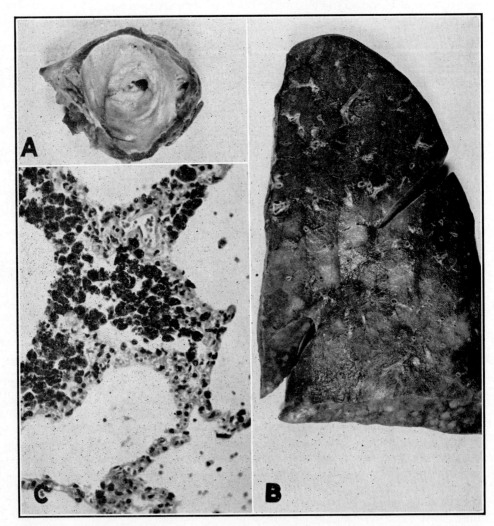

Fig. 68.—Chronic passive hyperemia (congestion) of the lung showing *A*, the causative factor, namely, stenosis of the mitral valve of the heart, *B*, diffusely deep brown discoloration of a lung, and *C*, thickened alveoli containing numerous macrophages laden with hemosiderin. × 200.

emia is attended by (1) *dyspnea* (difficulty in breathing) due to anoxia which, in turn, results from decreased ventilation of blood in the lungs, (2) *cyanosis* due to an increase of reduced hemoglobin in the blood resulting from slow movement of blood in the capillaries, and (3) *increase* in *body weight* and *effusions* (pericardial, pleural, and peritoneal) all due to escape of fluid from the vessels. This is brought about because of damage to the capillary walls and increase in intracapillary pressure.

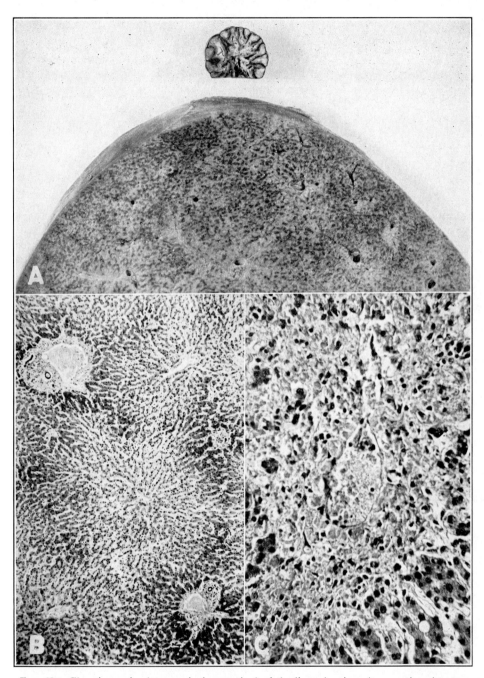

Fig. 69.—Chronic passive hyperemia (congestion) of the liver showing *A*, a sectioned nutmeg at the top and a cut surface of a liver below to illustrate the similarity in appearance, *B*, photomicrograph illustrating involvement of the central portions of hepatic lobules. × 50, and *C*, higher magnification of the central portion of a hepatic lobule disclosing engorgement of the vessels, extravasation of erythrocytes, and degeneration and necrosis of the hepatic cells. × 200.

Localized passive hyperemia is that which occurs in an organ or a part as a result of obstruction of the venous return from this area. The process may be acute or chronic. *Acute localized passive hyperemia* results from sudden occlusion of the venous lumen such as is seen in thrombosis, ligature, or pressure from the outside (hernia, volvulus, hematoma, crushing injury, constricting bands, etc.). Grossly the affected part becomes enlarged, swollen, and deep red to black. Histologically it reveals engorgement of the venules, escapes of fluid into the tissues, extravasation of erythrocytes, and, if the occlusion is complete, acute necrosis of tissue (infarction). *Chronic localized passive hyperemia* results from gradual venous occlusion and may be due to the following changes in the veins: partial thrombosis, compression or invasion by tumor, compression by enlarged lymph nodes, or simply the effect of gravity. *Pathologically* the affected part discloses changes identical with those seen in the various tissues and organs in chronic generalized passive hyperemia. *Anatomically* the veins most commonly affected are the saphenous, femoral, iliac, superior mesenteric, portal, inferior vena cava, superior vena cava, pulmonary, subclavian, and axillary.

Hemorrhage.—The term *hemorrhage* (Gr. = blood + burst forth) is synonymous with *bleeding* and indicates a copious escape of blood from vessels (arteries, veins, or capillaries) or from the heart. It may *come about* as a result of (1) *changes* in *constituents* or *clotting mechanism* of the *blood* (see sections on Thrombosis, page 211 and on Hemorrhagic Diseases, page 943), or (2) *changes* in the *wall* of the cardiovascular tree. These changes may bring about a weakening of the wall to such a degree that even the normal intraluminal pressure is sufficient to produce rupture or they may of themselves eventuate in complete dissolution of the wall. Hemorrhage of this sort is referred to as bleeding by *rhexis*. In the case of capillaries the walls may be injured by various noxious agents (see section on Inflammation, page 106) to a degree sufficient to allow escape of erythrocytes while still remaining intact. Hemorrhage of this sort is referred to as bleeding by *diapedesis*. Usually bleeding of arterial origin is by rhexis. Some of the causes of *rupture* of vessels are: (1) *Congenital Anomalies*—defects in the muscle and/or internal elastic lamina, (2) *Degenerations*—arteriosclerosis and mucoid degeneration of the media, (3) *Inflammation*—perivascular inflammation or abscess, mycotic aneurysm, periarteritis nodosa, ulceration (as in stomach), and syphilitic aneurysm, (4) *Physical Disturbances*—accidental trauma (cuts, tears, bruises, stab wounds, gunshot wounds, etc.), surgical severance, and increased intraluminal pressure (arterial in hypertension and capillary and venous in passive hyperemia), and (5) *Tumors*—by way of ulceration and erosion.

Hemorrhage may be variously *classified*. According to whether it is visible or invisible it is referred to as *concealed* or *internal* when it is hidden within the body and *apparent* or *external* when it escapes from the body or is seen upon external examination. According to the organ involved it is referred to as *cerebral, pulmonary, bronchial, gastrointestinal, uterine*, etc. According to its relation to other conditions it is referred to as *postoperative* —after operation, *postextractional*—after extraction of a tooth, *postpartum*— after delivery, *antepartum*—before delivery, etc. According to the size of the hemorrhage and/or the sites of the body, hemorrhagic extravasations are referred to as *petechiæ* (L. = spots)—pinpoint extravasations of blood, especially in the skin, mucous membranes, and mesothelial surfaces, *purpuric spots* (L. = purple)—larger extravasations, *ecchymoses* (Gr. = out + juice)—still larger extravasations, *hematomas* (Gr. = blood + tumor)

—extravasations of blood of sufficient degree to produce a sizable swelling, *epistaxis* (Gr. = above + to drop)—bleeding from the nose, *hemoptysis* (Gr. = blood + to spit)—spitting or coughing up of blood, *hematemesis* (Gr. = blood + vomiting)—vomiting of blood, *melena* (Gr. = black bile)—passage of dark blood with the stool, *hematuria* (Gr. = blood + urine)—passage of blood in the urine, *hematocolpos* (Gr. = blood + vagina)—collection of blood in the vagina, *menorrhagia* (Gr. = month + burst forth)—abnormal amount of bleeding during menstruation, *metrorrhagia* (Gr. = uterus + burst forth)—bleeding between menstrual periods, *menometrorrhagia*—abnormal amount of bleeding during menstruation and bleeding between menstrual periods, *hematosalpinx* (Gr. = blood + tube)—accumulation of blood in a salpinx (fallopian tube), *hematocele* (Gr. = blood + tumor)—escape of blood into a cavity especially the tunica vaginalis of the testis, *hemothorax* (Gr. = blood + chest)—accumulation of blood in the pleural cavity, *hemopericardium* (Gr. = blood + pericardium)—collection of blood in the pericardial cavity, *hemoperitoneum* (Gr. = blood + peritoneum)—accumulation of blood in the peritoneal cavity, and *apoplexy* (Gr. = from + to strike)—copious bleeding into any organ especially the brain.

Pathologically hemorrhage may have a general or a local effect upon the body. *General effects* are due entirely to blood loss. When blood is *lost rapidly* and in *large amounts* (over 1000 cc.) there is a reduction in blood volume, a rapid drop in blood pressure, and a reduction in blood flow (Moon). This sequence of events brings about generalized anoxia together with depression of the vital centers of the body and, if the blood volume is not restored rapidly, may result in shock or even death of the patient. Within certain limits the blood lost is compensated for physiologically by stimulation of the myocardium, by peripheral vasoconstriction, by discharge of reservoir blood into the systemic circulation (especially contraction of the spleen), and by intravascular absorption of fluid from the tissues. Beyond this it must be restored by artificial means. When the blood is *lost slowly*, but in adequate amounts, there develops a general reduction in circulating erythrocytes or anemia and, when this is severe enough, there is degeneration of the various organs throughout the body. *Locally*, because the blood volume and number of circulating erythrocytes are diminished, there is ischemia of all the organs resulting in decrease in weight, paleness, and dryness. This appearance, however, is altered when shock is secondarily superimposed. At the site of hemorrhage the parenchyma of the affected organ (brain, kidney, liver, etc.) may be destroyed by the bleeding, the organ or structure may be compressed upon from the outside by the extravasated blood (heart in hemopericardium, lung in hemothorax, etc.) or the lumen of a hollow organ (tracheobronchial tree, urinary tract, etc.) may be obstructed by the accumulated blood (Fig. 70). In small hemorrhages the erythrocytes and their disintegration products are completely removed by diffusion and by phagocytoses and the area is usually restored to normal. In large hemorrhages the erythrocytes disintegrate in greater numbers. The resulting hematoidin is absorbed, transformed into bilirubin, and excreted in the bile or it is deposited locally in the form of granules and rhombic plates. The hemosiderin is absorbed and reused or remains deposited locally in the form of golden brown granules. As a result of local irritation of disintegration protein and other products, there is a nonspecific inflammatory reaction which ultimately may result in fibrosis and even calcification (Fig. 70, *D*).

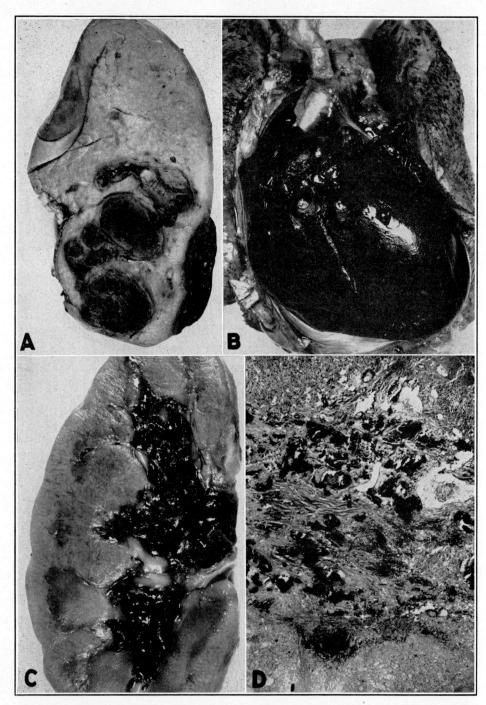

Fig. 70.—Hemorrhage showing *A*, rupture of a spleen with disruption of the parenchyma by massive blood clots, *B*, blood clot in the pericardial cavity compressing the heart, *C*, blood filling the pelvis of a kidney, and *D*, old hemorrhage in a spleen revealing fibrosis, hemosiderin, and calcification. × 50.

DISTURBANCE OF FLUID BALANCE

Hans G. Keitel

In *general*, fluid, for biological purposes, consists of water in which are dissolved solutes. The solutes include (1) the electrolytes, which comprise the cations (sodium, potassium, calcium, magnesium, and hydrogen), and the anions (chloride, phosphates, bicarbonates, sulfates, and proteinates), and (2) the nonelectrolytes (glucose, urea, CO_2, etc.). An abnormality in the distribution or volume of water, or in the ionic content or concentration of any of the body fluid phases, results in a disturbance in body fluid balance.

Physiologically, each separate group of cells (muscle, brain, red cells, etc.) constitutes a separate fluid phase. The various extracellular phases tend to have a similar electrolyte concentration, the small differences that exist being accounted for by Gibbs-Donnan equilibrium. The extra-cellular components have a high concentration of sodium and chloride and a low concentration of potassium in contradistinction to most cells which have a low concentration of sodium and chloride and a high concentration of potassium.

TABLE 2.—The Concentration of Ions in Plasma of Normal Man*

	Adults		Infants†	
	Mean Value	Standard Deviation	Mean Value	Standard Deviation
Sodium, mEq/L plasma	140	2.5	137	(2)
Potassium, " "	4.2	0.25	5.2	0.3
Calcium, " "	5	(0.25)	5	(0.25)
Magnesium, " "	2	(0.2)	(2)	(0.2)
Chloride, " "	102	2.0	107	(3.0)
CO_2, "	26	2	22	2
Phosphorus, mM/L plasma	0.7	(0.1)	1.2	(0.2)
pH	7.43	0.3	7.33	0.4
Glucose, mg%	85	(10)	85	(10)

*These data represent the average of many published data obtained from fasting normal subjects. The values in parenthesis are an estimate of the standard deviation.

†Adult values are found within 3–6 months of life except for the phosphorus concentration which remains elevated until puberty.

The extracellular phase itself is composed of many separate functional divisions, the intravascular phase (plasma volume) and the interstitial phase being the two chief subdivisions. Certain ions (sodium, potassium, glucose, and calcium) when injected intravenously are initially primarily distributed in the extracellular phase. The functional barrier to the free diffusion of these ions from the extracellular phase into the intracellular phase constitutes one of the important reasons for the separation of body fluid phases into cellular and extracellular phases.

Pathophysiologically, many fluid disturbances are recognized by determining blood electrolyte concentrations. Ionic disturbances must be diagnosed during life and cannot be diagnosed after the patient dies because post mortem changes obscure the findings. A list of the ion concentrations found in normal man, the type of ionic alterations that are found in certain conditions or diseases, and the level at which disturbances in ion concentrations of plasma may result in severe clinical symptoms are shown in the accompanying Tables 2 and 3. Marked ionic alterations can result in clinical symptoms because of (1) a direct effect on nerve conduction, (2) an effect on the distribution of water between cells and plasma, and (3) a disturbance in enzyme and high energy transfer mechanisms which are dependent on normal ion concentrations.

Hyponatremia (a low concentration of sodium per liter of plasma or serum) is one of the most commonly observed ionic disturbances and occurs for the following three basic reasons: (1) an "internal" loss of sodium from plasma into cells or an "external" loss in urine, stool, or sweat, (2) retention of water, or (3) the presence in plasma of a high concentration of lipids. Hyperlipemic hyponatremia should be differentiated from 'true' hyponatremia, which results from the loss of sodium from plasma and from the rentention of water. Patients with renal, hepatic, thyroid, or certain other metabolic diseases may have from five to twenty per cent of their plasma as

TABLE 3.—THE RANGE OF CONCENTRATIONS OF IONS IN PLASMA WHICH MAY RESULT IN CLINICAL SYMPTOMS*

	Elevated Values Severity of Symptom		Reduced Values Severity of Symptom	
	Moderate	Severe	Moderate	Severe
Sodium, mEq/L	155–170	170 and above	120–130	120 and below
Potassium, mEq/L	7–9	9 and above	2.2–3.0	2.2 and below
Calcium, mEq/L (if protein and hydroxyl conc's are normal)	6–7	7 and above	3–4	3 and below
Magnesium, mEq/L	?5, and above	?10, and above	?1, and below	?1, and below
pH	7.5–7.6	7.6, and above	7.0–7.15	7.0, and below
Glucose, mg%	?1000, or above		40–60	40
Protein, gm%	(?)	(?)	3–4.5	3, and below

*Patients with ion concentration listed as being "severe" may be asymptomatic and patients with ion concentration listed as "moderate" may have severe symptoms. The values are those which not uncommonly result in symptoms of the degree listed.

lipid and have a corresponding decrease in the plasma sodium concentration per liter of plasma. Since the sodium to water ratio is normal in patients with uncomplicated "hyperlipemic" hyponatremia, the ionic activity (electrical and osmotic) of sodium is unimpaired. Consequently, a change in the distribution of water between cells and extracellular fluid and nerve conduction defects are not present. Patients with edema secondary to cardiac, hepatic, or renal disease who have a low sodium concentration of plasma may, in fact, have an increased total body sodium content since they retain both water and sodium but tend relatively to retain more water than sodium.

Examples of *ionic concentration defects* of *plasma* in various diseases are shown in the accompanying Table 4. The ionic defects listed are not always found in these diseases because the duration and severity of fasting, thirsting, vomiting, diarrhea, sweating, hyperpnea, acidosis, and ketosis which tend to occur in these diseases must be considered in addition to the basic

TABLE 4.—THE RANGE OF LABORATORY FINDINGS FREQUENTLY SEEN IN PATIENTS WITH VARIOUS DISEASES OR CONDITIONS†
(The values with an asterisk (*) are found in the majority of untreated patients)

Plasma	Vomiting Gastric Alkalosis	Diarrhea Acute 1-3 day	Diarrhea Chronic 4-100 day	Uremia (Chronic)	Diabetes Mellitus & Acidosis	Diabetes Insipidus with Hypohydration	Adrenal Insufficiency
Sodium, mEq/L	125–140	120–140	130–150	105*–135	115*–135	150*–190	100*–130
Potassium, "	2*–3.5	3.5–6	2–5	5*–12	2–6	3.5–6	4*–8
Calcium, "	4.5–5.5	9–11	9–11	3–4	4.5–5.5	4.5–6	4.5–5.5
Magnesium, "	2	2	2	2–10	2*	2	2
CO₂, "	30*–45	7–25	15–30	8*–20	4*–15	15–30	10–20
Chloride, "	75*–95	80–130	90–110	75*–105	80*–95	110*–160	70*–90
Phosphorus, mg%	2–6	2–6	2–6	5*–20	3–6	3–6	3–6
Blood							
Glucose, mg%	60–100	60–100	60–100	60–100	250*–1500	60–100	60–100
pH	7.4*–7.6	6.9–7.4	7.3–7.5	6.9*–7.4	6.7*–7.2	7.3–7.5	7.1*–7.3
Urea nit. mg%	10–40	10–40	10–20	30*–500	20*–80	25*–90	30*–90
Alb/Glob, gm%	4-5/2-4	4-5/2-4	2-5/2-5	1-3*/1-4	4-5/2-4	4-5/2-4	3-5/2-5
Cholesterol, mg%	100–250	100–250	100–250	100–400	100–500	100–250	100–250
Hemoglobin, gm%	12–18	12–18	8–18	5*–12	12–18	12–18	9–18

†Great variability in the chemical findings are seen because varying degrees of vomiting, thirsting, and impaired renal function are frequently present in each of the conditions listed.

disease process. For example, patients with diabetes mellitus who are deprived of insulin may develop protracted vomiting which may result in loss of large amounts of chloride. This may protect them from severe acidosis which they otherwise might have as a result of the accumulation of ketonic acids.

Marked *alterations* (both reduced and increased) in the *plasma concentration* of *potassium* result in neurologic and cardiac abnormalities, including paresthesias and paralysis, leading to cardiac and respiratory collapse and death. Death due to hyper- or hypokalemia cannot be diagnosed at autopsy. It must be suspected by the clinician and diagnosed by determining the plasma potassium concentration.

Generalized potassium deficiency, if chronic and severe and associated with loss of potassium from cells, results in necrosis of renal, cardiac, and skeletal muscle cells. There is evidence that the high content of sodium of cells which usually occurs in association with potassium deficiency may also be important in accounting for these changes.

Complex fluid balance disturbances are found in patients with far advanced renal, cardiac, or liver disease. Retention of water and sodium and deficiency or excess of potassium are frequently present, depending on the status of renal function and the occurrence of vomiting, diarrhea, etc. In these patients, a deficiency in blood volume may occur as a result of hypoproteinemia and the loss of oncotic pressure, as well as from anemia. Hypovolemia and hypotension tend to result in retention by the kidney of water and sodium due to (1) a decrease in renal blood flow and (2) secretion of antidiuretic hormone and of adrenal steroids of the aldosterone type which result in the retention water and of sodium chloride, respectively. If renal function is normal, potassium will tend to be lost. Expansion of the extracellular fluid is found in these patients, as a result of these multiple mechanisms. If, on the other hand, patients fail to ingest water or sodium and chloride, they may not be able to form edema fluid.

An increase in the water content of the body, or *hyperhydration*, results from a larger intake of water than is excreted, as might occur as a result of psychogenic polydipsea, the intravenous infusion of an excess amount of water, or renal failure. An excess in the body water content can occur in patients who have severe renal impairment and inability to excrete water, even if the intake of water is normal. Since there is osmotic equilibrium between all fluid phases of the body (with the exception of certain renal and skin cells which facilitate the production of hypotonic or hypertonic urine and hypotonic sweat), "pure" water retention results in expansion of all fluid phases proportionately. Patients with *water intoxication* (excessive hyperhydration) may manifest slight edema, particularly of the skin, but edema due to acute retention of "pure" water is difficult to diagnose clinically or pathologically, since only relatively little solute free water can be retained before serious symptoms, including convulsion and coma, occur. Pathologically, the brain cells of patients with water intoxication are found to be swollen and the ventricular spaces of the central nervous system are compressed.

The accumulation of water in association with the retention of sodium, if extensive, results in *edema*, that is, the retention of water in the extracellular phase. An increase of about 5 per cent in body weight is necessary before edema is manifested clinically (see succeeding section on Edema).

Cell hyperhydration occurs as a result of "pure" water excess (vide supra) and in association with cell death when there is breakdown (autolysis) of large cell molecules (proteins and organic phosphates) into smaller, more numerous ions (polypeptides, inorganic phosphates, etc.).

Generalized hypohydration, or dehydration, can result from loss of "pure" water consequent to an abnormal rate of loss of water, as found in patients with diabetes insipidus and those with hyperpnea and sweating. The concentration of ions in all body fluid compartments is increased when primary water deficiency is present. "Pure" water loss, like that of "pure" water retention, if severe, results in central nervous system symptoms, including convulsion, coma, and finally death. The chief clinical finding is loss of skin turgor and loss of turgor of all tissues. Thrombosis of many veins, including renal and cerebral veins, occurs in severe cases.

Loss of water in association with extracellular solutes (sodium and chloride) in the ratio found in normal subjects results in *hypohydration* of the extracellular phase alone. In such patients, loss of skin turgor and, in severe cases, shock occurs. The tissues of such patients may appear to be slightly dehydrated because the extracellular phase is contracted but the size of the cells will be normal since their water content is normal.

Cell hypohydration due to loss of cell solutes and shift of cell water to the extracellular phase occurs in red cells during alkalosis as a result of the chloride shift. The loss of potassium from cells is usually associated with an equimolar gain in cell sodium content. Therefore, cell dehydration does not usually result from the loss of potassium from cells.

Edema.—The term *edema* (Gr. = swelling) signifies excessive amounts of fluid in the cells and intercellular spaces of the body and the process of its formation is referred to as *effusion* (L. = pouring out). Initially, the fluid is confined to the tissues but, when these become overburdened, it also accumulates in the body cavities. Such a state is then referred to as *dropsy* (Gr. = water) or *anasarca* (Gr. = throughout + flesh). Further, an accumulation of thin, watery or yellowish, relatively clear fluid in the pleural cavity is referred to as *hydrothorax*, in the pericardial cavity as *hydropericardium*, and in the peritoneal cavity as *hydroperitoneum* or *ascites* (Gr. = bag). Also, fluid that develops in response to inflammation is known as an *exudate* (Chapter 5, p. 112) while fluid that is of other than inflammatory origin is called a *transudate* (L. = through + to sweat).

Edema may be confined to a specific organ or area of the body (localized) or may affect most or all of the tissues (generalized). Although all of the factors concerning its *development* are not known, it is generally accepted that the following play an important role: (1) increased permeability of capillary endothelium, (2) variations in osmotic pressure between plasma and tissue fluids, and (3) elevation of capillary blood pressure (Moon). Normally, *capillary endothelium* is pervious to water and crystalloids but is impervious to colloids. When it is *injured*, however, its imperviousness is lost and it allows colloids to escape into the extravascular tissues. This increases the extravascular osmotic pressure and, as a result, more fluid is withdrawn from the vascular lumens. Thus, a vicious cycle is set into operation. Some of the many causes of injury to capillary endothelium are anoxia, bacteria and bacterial toxins, chemicals, protein degeneration products of tissues, and agents such as heat, light, electricity, rays, etc. Normally the colloidal osmotic pressure (due to albumin and globulin) within capillaries is greater than that in tissues and thus tends to draw fluid from the tissues into the capillaries. This advantage is overcome in part by the blood pressure within the capillary lumens and, under physiological conditions, a balance is thus maintained. It is obvious that a *decrease* in *plasma colloids* (below 3 to 4 gm./100 cc. plasma) lowers the intraluminal osmotic pressure, allows fluid to escape into the tissues, and produces edema. The causes of depletion of plasma colloids are deficient production of protein as seen in cases of insufficient intake in the food and excessive loss of protein as seen in renal disease, removal of copious amounts of ascitic or other fluid, and prolonged bleeding. It is also obvious that an *increase* in *capillary blood pressure* tends to force fluid out of the capillaries into the tissue spaces and thus to produce edema. Although capillary blood pressure is sometimes increased actively, as in cases of inflammation, it is usually increased passively by way of venous hyperemia, as seen (generally) in cardiac failure, and (locally) in venous obstruction. In addition to increase in capillary pressure, obstruction of lymphatic channels (due to parasites such as *Wuchereria bancrofti* and nonspecific inflammation) prevents fluid (lymph) from returning to the venous circulation and thus causes its accumulation in the tissues. This type of edema, however, is in a class by itself and is referred to as *lymphedema*.

Edema is usually classified on an etiological basis as follows: (1) *Alimentary* (also called nutritional, famine, hunger, war, and prison)—resulting from an insufficient intake of protein in the food, (2) *Angioneurotic*—occurring in connection with an allergic state, (3) *Cardiac*—seen in cardiac failure, (4) *Hepatic*—brought about by diseases of the liver, (5) *Hereditary*—eventuating as a result of inheritance, (6) *Hydremic*—found in conjunction with hydremia, (7) *Inflammatory*—resulting from inflammation, (8) *Insulin*—occurring after the injection of insulin, (9) *Milroy's*—hereditary and confined to the lower extremities, (10) *Mucous*—seen in conjunction with myxedema, (11) *Neonatorum*—present in the newborn, (12) *Nephrotic*—brought about by a degenerative or an inflammatory change in the kidneys, and (13) *Noninflammatory*—occurring on other than an inflammatory basis and unattended by redness.

The first *indication* of the development of generalized edema is a rapid increase in body weight—an increase that far exceeds that which can be accounted for on a physiologic basis. This is followed by a swelling of the *subcutaneous tissues*. This swelling occurs first in the most dependent portions of the body and thus usually affects the ankles. Later it involves the connective tissue throughout the body. The areas affected increase in size; the crevices and wrinkles are effaced; the covering becomes stretched, thinned, and tense, and, since the fluid is mostly in the tissue spaces, digital pressure permits it to be pushed aside leaving a depression or pit (pitting edema). Cut surfaces of an affected area disclose the connective tissue to be gray, soft, boggy, and gelatinous. Histologically the connective tissue cells are spread apart by the edema fluid and the cytoplasm is drawn out into long processes (Fig. 71*A*). When the protein content is high, the edema fluid stains as a pink precipitate but when it is low its presence is represented by clear, empty spaces. As far as specific *organs* of the body are concerned, the changes consist of an increase in size and weight, increase in firmness, stretching of the capsule or covering, dilution of the original color, and the presence of an excess of clear fluid that often drips freely from the cut surface. Histologically the changes in the stroma are the same as those in the subcutaneous connective tissue. In addition, the parenchymatous cells may show vacuoles or hydropic degeneration. Of all the organs, the *lungs* are of special interest because they almost always reveal edema as a terminal event. Microscopically, pulmonary edema is evidenced by the presence of pink-staining precipitate within the alveolar spaces when the protein content is high and of more watery material when it is low (Fig. 71*B*). Finally, edema fluid also accumulates in *mesothelial-lined cavities* especially pleural, pericardial, and peritoneal. The fluid is usually clear, watery, or straw-colored. Its specific gravity and coagulability vary with its protein content and thus attempts to use these as criteria for differentiating a transudate (edema fluid) from an exudate (fluid resulting from

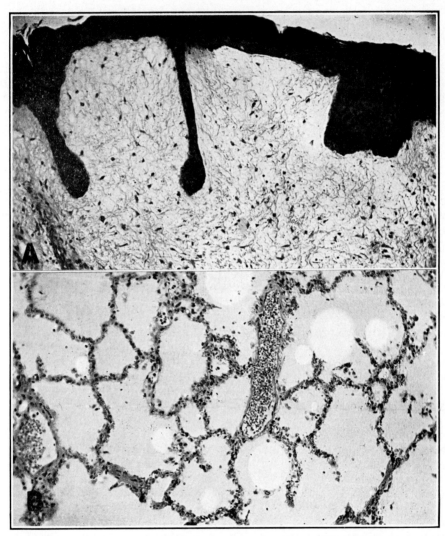

Fig. 71.—Edema showing *A*, elongation of the connective tissue cells of the dermis and their separation by intercellular fluid, and *B*, fluid filling the alveolar spaces. × 100.

inflammation) are unsatisfactory. The sediment from edema fluid is always scanty. Histologically it abounds in mesothelial cells but discloses few leukocytes.

Shock.—The term *shock* (Middle Eng. and Fr. = to shake or jolt) may be defined simply as acute peripheral circulatory failure. It may be divided into two varieties—primary and secondary.

Primary shock, also known as *neurogenic shock*, is a neurovascular reaction which, in its fully developed form is identical with *fainting* or *syncope* (Moon). It is attended by an acute reversible loss of voluntary control and consciousness due to dysfunction of the vital centers of the brain (Schroeder). This, in turn, results from inadequate oxygenation (Ostfeld). The two chief *causes* of inadequate oxygenation of the brain are vasodepression and sudden decrease in cardiac output. Of these *vasodepression* is the etiologic agent in about 95 per cent of cases. Since vasodepression eventuates in a fall in blood pressure when a person is in an upright position, such fainting is often referred to as *orthostatic syncope*. The causes of vasodepression are many. Emotions such as pain, fright, grief, anticipation, and horrifying visual experience are the most frequent precipitators. Other causes are stimulation of the carotid sinus, use of vasodilator drugs (nitrates and nitrites), and stimulation of vasosensory nerves as seen in connection with a blow to the solar plexus or testis, trauma to blood vessels or peritoneum, acute dilatation of a viscus, needle puncture of a pleura, etc. Of more permanent action are ganglion-blocking agents such as hexamethionium and sympathectomy. Sudden *decrease* in *cardiac output* accounts for only about 5 per cent of cases of syncope but is extremely important for it may be caused by serious underlying heart disease such as myocardial infarction or fibrosis. The physiologic basis for decrease in output of blood by the heart may be ventricular asystole or slowing brought about by carotid sinus stimulation or auricular tachycardia, arrhythmia, and fibrillation. Even these attacks, however, may be precipitated by fear, anger, or anxiety. Aside from vasodepression and decreased cardiac output as causes of syncope attacks may sometimes be precipitated by severe anemia, severe hemorrhage, and acute loss of water by perspiration. Syncope may also be faked by persons with hysteria or schizophrenia. The only *pathophysiologic* change in syncope is an acute loss of arteriolar tone in peripheral vessels, especially those of the muscles, with pooling of the blood in these areas. This results in decrease of available blood volume, drop in blood pressure, and the inevitable cerebral anoxia. The capillary walls and the blood itself show no qualitative alterations. While primary shock is usually transitory and reversible it may on occasion lead to secondary shock and sometimes, in the cases caused by decrease in cardiac output, it may even be *complicated* by sudden death. The *clinical manifestations* consist of pallor, retching, vomiting, sweating, giddiness, nausea, weakness, and collapse. The body slumps to the floor and becomes motionless and limp. Examination of the cardiovascular system discloses bradycardia and hypotension. The *diagnosis* of the syncope itself is readily made from the history and appearance of the patient. A further diagnosis as to the cause of the attack can be made only upon more careful complete physical, roentgenographic, and other examinations. This is especially important in patients with recurring attacks where organic cardiac lesions may exist. *Treatment* of the syncope itself consists of putting the patient in a recumbent position preferably with the legs elevated. When the patient assumes an erect posture he should move about in order to prevent pooling of blood in the vessels. Aside from these immediate measures, treatment should be directed toward removing or treating the underlying cause. The *prognosis* is generally good, for as indicated in the definition, the process is usually transitory and reversible.

Secondary shock, also known as *incipient* or *delayed shock*, is that form of circulatory failure characterized by capillary atony, abnormal capillary permeability, and changes in electrolytes of the blood. Although it may appear rapidly, it frequently develops slowly and insidiously. Some of the many *causes* of secondary shock together with its *vicious cycle* are exceptionally well illustrated in the accompanying chart constructed by Moon (Fig. 72). The key points in this cycle are (1) injury to capillary endothelium, (2) reduction in effective blood volume, and (3) anoxia. *Injury to capillary endothelium* may be brought about by trauma (accidental or surgical), burns, metabolic disturbances (especially those associated with adrenal glands such as Addison's disease, bilateral adrenalectomy, and previous cortisone therapy), infections (pneumonia, septicemia, peritonitis, empyema, pancreatitis, etc.), drugs (hexamethonium, dibenamine, chlorpromazine, nitrates, histamine, etc.), poisons (snake venoms, insect stings, etc.), pyrogens, prolonged labor, toxemia of pregnancy, obstruction gastrointestinal tract, perforation of a viscus, mesenteric artery thrombosis, serum sickness, transfusion reactions, irradiation sickness, and neurogenic stimuli as outlined in the preceding section on neurogenic shock (Breed). *Reduction* in *effective blood volume* is due in part to vasodilatation with increase in the vascular bed and in part to loss of blood or of its components either into the tissues and body cavities or outside of the body. Loss into the tissues and body cavities and spaces results from injury to capillary endothelium. Because of this, the endothelium becomes more permeable to fluids bringing about their escape into extravascular spaces. This results in hemoconcentration within the vascular tree, edema in the tissues, and effusions into mesothelial lined cavities. Such fluid (plasma) loss, which of course includes electrolytes, occurs chiefly in burns and peritonitis. Loss of blood (and electrolytes) outside of the body occurs in any acute or chronic hemorrhage be it traumatic, surgical, medical (bleeding peptic ulcer), or obstetrical. Loss of fluids other than plasma (and electrolytes) outside of the body may be seen in diarrhea, diabetic acidosis, low salt syndrome, Addison's disease, pyloric obstruction, intestinal obstruction, and fistulas (duodenum, biliary, pancreatic, and ileal). Reduction in effective blood volume produces a reduced volume flow of blood. This, in turn, may be aggravated by (1) cardiac insufficiency due to coronary artery occlusion and myocardial infarction, myocarditis, stab wound, cardiac tamponade, acute pericarditis, diphtheria, tachycardia, heart block, and valvular disease, (2) obstruction to the arterial or venous circulation as by embolism or thrombosis, and (3) sympatho-adrenal hyperactivity or administration of adrenalin. *Anoxia* is due to reduced delivery of oxygen and is brought about by anything which reduces the blood volume and volume flow. It is aggravated by asphyxia that results from any cause whatsoever. Its net effect is the production of tissue anoxia which further injures the capillary endothelium either directly or by increasing noxious catabolic products of tissues in general. *Experimentally* Moon has produced shock by a variety of methods outlined in Figure 72. Some of these are, while others are not, analogous to the causative factors in man.

Pathologically secondary shock is characterized by generalized hyperemia, capillary stasis, petechiæ, edema, and effusions. *Grossly* the superficial veins are collapsed and devoid of blood; the blood in the heart and larger intimal vessels is dark red and fails to clot readily; the mesothelial surfaces disclose numerous petechiæ, and the body cavities contain varying amounts of blood-tinged fluid. The lungs are enlarged, deep red, heavy, subcrepitant, and edematous (Fig. 73). Sectioning discloses an abundance of frothy fluid that drips freely from the cut surface. The gastrointestinal tract is relaxed; its mucosa discloses redness, swelling, numerous petechial erosions, and

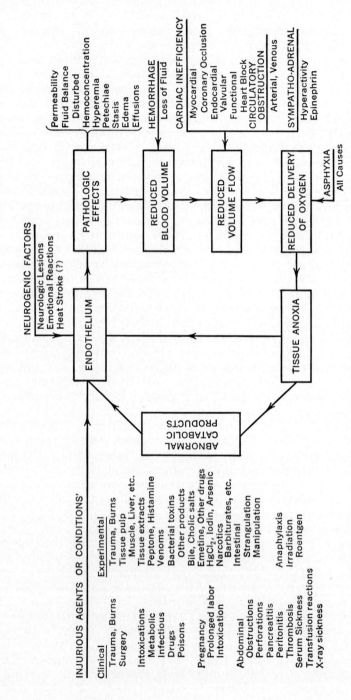

FIG. 72.—The vicious cycle of shock as illustrated by Moon. (Moon, *Shock*, Lea & Febiger.)

occasionally frank ulcerations, and its lumen contains recently extravasated or partly digested ("coffee ground") blood mixed with gastrointestinal juices. The other organs, especially the liver, kidneys, and brain reveal enlargement, hyperemia, and edema. The spleen, however, is contracted, firm, dry, and relatively bloodless. When death is delayed, the extravasated erythrocytes disintegrate and bring about diffuse pigmentation. The *histologic* changes consist of generalized capillary dilatation and engorgement, extravasation of erythrocytes, and escape of edema fluid into the tissue spaces. These changes are particularly marked in the lungs and gastro-

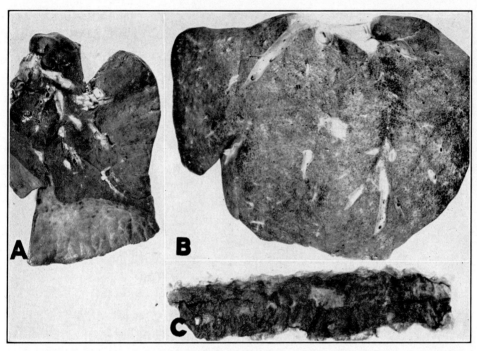

Fig. 73.—Secondary shock showing severe hyperemia of *A*, a lung, *B*, the liver, and *C*, a portion of the small bowel. The mucosa of the intestine discloses, in addition, frank ulcerations.

intestinal tract (Fig. 74). Parenchymatous degeneration is present in most of the organs, especially the kidneys, liver, heart, and adrenals. In addition, the kidneys show the changes of acute toxic nephrosis (p. 1064) and the liver, lymph nodes, spleen, pancreas, and adrenals may reveal focal areas of necrosis.

Physiologically, as a result of capillary atony and abnormal capillary permeability, secondary shock is attended by decreased blood volume, reduced volume flow, hemoconcentration, decrease of sodium and chlorides in the blood, increase of potassium in the blood, and renal functional deficiency. The electrolytic changes have already been considered in greater detail in the section on Disturbances of Fluid Balance (p. 199). In brief, the *physiologic sequence* of *events* in secondary shock may be listed as follows (Livermore): (1) fall in blood pressure due to loss of effective blood volume which results in (2) stimulation of the pressor receptors of the aortic arch and carotid sinus which produce (3) reflex sympathetic stimulation resulting in (4) increased heart rate and (5) selective vasoconstriction affecting principally the vessels of the skin, kidneys, muscle, and splanchnic areas and due to a *V.E.M.* (vasoexcitator material) released by the hypoxic kidneys. Initially, the vasoconstriction is beneficial for it reduces the vascular bed capacity thereby increasing the effective blood volume and thus compensating for the preceding chain of events. If, however, the patient continues to lose blood, the blood lost is not replaced, or the trauma or other causes of the shock continue, the vasoconstriction, if prolonged, is injurious for it aggravates the anoxic changes in the tissues and thus perpetuates the vicious cycle. A continuation of the factors producing shock

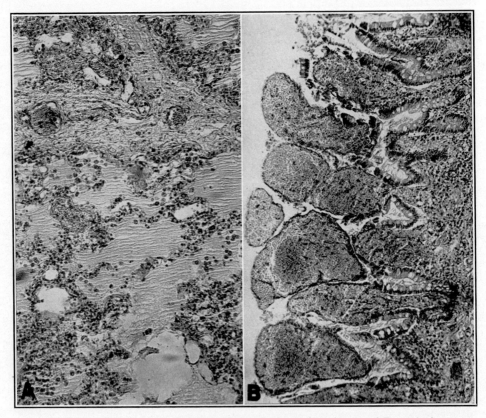

Fig. 74.—Shock showing *A*, severe congestion and edema of the lung, and *B*, marked engorgement of the capillaries of the submucosa of the jejunum with extravasation of erythrocytes. × 100.

leads to (6) a second fall in blood pressure which produces (7) a decrease in coronary and cerebral blood flow resulting in (8) myocardial failure with further depression of the circulation, (9) impairment of consciousness, and (10) depression of the vasomotor and respiratory centers. All of this results in a total collapse of the compensatory mechanism and the patient reaches the irreversible stage. Aside from the conditions already mentioned, two other factors that appear to play an important role in perpetuating and aggravating the cycle are *V.D.M.* and products of bacterial activity. *V.D.M.* (vasodepressor material) is an iron protein compound, ferritin, produced by the liver, spleen, and muscles which, as the name suggests, causes dilatation of the vascular bed and thus reduces the effective blood volume. When hypoxia is mild, the liver inactivates *V.D.M.* but when it becomes advanced, inactivation ceases and *V.D.M.* accumulates in the circulation, resulting in the pooling of large volumes of blood in the capillaries and venules. *Products* of *bacterial activity* are generally absorbed from the intestinal tract and are stored in the liver. They may, in addition, come from other areas, such as for example a gangrenous extremity. In either case, they are detoxified by a normal liver but not by a liver in the state of shock. The products thus accumulate and produce irreversible vasodepression.

The *clinical manifestations* in secondary shock vary with the severity of the condition. They may consist of any combination of the following: cold perspiration, tachycardia, feeble irregular pulse, low or unobtainable blood pressure, subnormal temperature, pallor, thirst, dehydration, hemoconcentration, nausea, vomiting, rapid and shallow respiration, suppression of urine, prostration, apathy, stupor, and electrolytic changes in the blood (p. 209). The *diagnosis* is made from a consideration of the history and the clinical manifestations listed and is readily checked by ascertaining the blood pressure and demonstrating hemoconcentration (erythrocytic count over 5,000,000 and hemoglobin over 15 gm./100 cc.) of the peripheral blood. *Treatment* is directed toward rectifying the fundamental causative factors. The aim should be to keep the systolic blood pressure over 70 mm. of mercury and to administer fluids in proportion to balance the urinary output (Livermore). More specifically, the following steps should be taken: elevate the legs, administer oxygen, control pain, apply heat in moderation, replace blood volume with blood, plasma, or plasma volume expanders, administer antibiotics to prevent infection, and judicially utilize vasoconstrictors and cortisone (which potentiates action of vasoconstrictors) when the patient does not respond. The *course* depends upon the severity of the process and the promptness and efficiency of treatment. Under appropriate conditions the cycle may be interrupted at any time and physiologic functions restored to normal. If interruption of the cycle is impossible the pathologic changes progress and culminate in death of the patient.

Thrombosis. — The term *thrombosis* (Gr. = coagulation) connotes *clotting* of blood within the cardiovascular system and the product of thrombosis is known as a *thrombus* (Gr. = plug) or *clot*. The mechanism of clotting of blood is a complicated chain reaction that, in part, is not yet well understood (Fig. 75). The process is initiated by contact of blood with a rough surface (usually in the form of injured endothelium) and is aided by decreased rate of flow or stagnation of blood. The actual clotting occurs in three phases (Wintrobe). The *first phase* consists of the formation of active thromboplastin as a result of the interaction of thromboplastinogenase (derived from ruptured platelets) and thromboplastinogen (present normally in plasma). Thromboplastin may also be derived from injured tissue cells, especially brain, lung, thymus, and testis. The *second phase* embraces the formation of thrombin (an albumin-like protein) as a result of the interaction of thromboplastin with calcium (normally present in the blood), prothrombin (inactive precursor of thrombin having properties of globulin), and the "labile factor" or "factor 5" (a catalytic plasma constituent the nature of which is not yet agreed upon). Prothrombin is formed in the liver and its formation depends upon the presence of vitamin K. It really consists of two components — a labile substance and the classical prothrombin. The *third phase* consists of the formation of fibrin as a result of the interaction of thrombin with fibrinogen. Fibrinogen is a labile plasma protein that is probably formed in the liver. Fibrin consists of a fine thread-like network that entangles the cellular elements of the blood (thus forming the clot) and, once formed, also possesses the power to contract.

Since all the elements necessary for clotting are always present in the blood there must be *factors normally* operating to *prevent thrombosis* of circulating blood. Some of these are (1) unbroken continuity of vascular endothelium, (2) anticoagulants consisting of (*a*) heparin (a mucopolysaccharide initially extracted from the liver but probably produced by mast cells), (*b*) fibrin regarded as an important antithrombin, and (*c*) anticephalin, and (3) fibrinolysin (Wintrobe). While fibrin is, of course, not normally present in the blood it does exist once clot formation gets under way. Its action as an antithrombin in preventing further coagulation is mediated through the absorption of thrombin. This interrupts the lysis of platelets which, in turn, diminishes the formation of thromboplastinogenase. The action of fibrinolysin is to dissolve fibrin once it is formed and

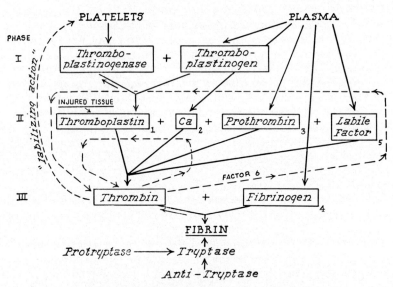

FIG. 75.—Diagram illustrating the mechanism of clotting of blood. (Wintrobe, *Clinical Hematology*, Lea & Febiger.)

thus not only prevent thrombosis by destroying the fibrin immediately upon its appearance but also dissolving the thrombus and accelerating its absorption. Such dissolution is sometimes seen after accidental death and, in living patients, after stimuli such as fear or severe exercise or following injection of adrenalin. Fibrinolysin (also known as plasmin and tryptase) is a proteolytic enzyme in normal blood formed from a precursor that has been called protryptase (by those calling the enzyme tryptase). Under normal circumstances, this enzyme is held in check by antitryptase. It is readily activated *in vitro* by bacteria and chemicals and *in vivo* by trauma, shock, and surgical procedures. Under *abnormal* circumstances *thrombosis is prevented* or *impaired* by (1) removal of fibrin and addition of oxalates or citrates (*in vitro*), (2) diminished formation of fibrinogen (diseases of the liver), (3) excessive formation of antithrombin (substances slowing rate of action of thrombin on fibrinogen) or antiprothrombin (substances slowing the formation of thrombin from prothrombin) consisting of such substances as herudin, heparin, cysteine, glutathione, taurine, and taurocholic acid, (4) deficient formation of prothrombin resulting from vitamin K deficiency or liver damage, (5) administration of Dicumarol, (6) abnormality of blood platelets, either quantitative or qualitative, as for example, that seen in thrombocytopenia, and (7) increase in antithromboplastin as occurs in hemophilia. Also, under *abnormal* circumstances thrombosis may be accelerated by (1) exposure to rough surfaces (*in vivo* or *in vitro*), (2) injection of substances like tissue extracts, trypsin, some snake venoms, *Staphylococcus aureus* toxins and (as in hemophilia) whole blood, fresh plasma, or globulin substance, and (3) application of thrombin or fibrin locally.

As already stated, the process of thrombosis is initiated by contact of the blood with injured endothelium and is aided by a decreased rate of flow or stagnation of blood. Some of the *causes* of *injury* to *vascular* (including endocardial) *endothelium* are (1) *degenerative processes* notably arteriosclerosis and phlebosclerosis, (2) a variety of acute and chronic *inflammations*, especially acute arteritis, periarteritis nodosa, thromboangiitis obliterans, and phlebitis, (3) *physical disturbances* in the form of blunt trauma (blow, crushing injury, surgical clamping, surgical ligation, etc.), penetrating trauma, severe spasm, (frostbite and ergot poisoning), irradiation, injection of irritating chemicals (arsenic, mercury, etc.), and (in the case of the heart) myocardial infarction, and (4) *tumors* by way of compression from outside or penetration of the wall and invasion of the lumen. Some of the *causes* of *slowing* of the blood stream are (1) severe cardiac damage or decompensation (affecting both the arterial and venous sides), (2) muscular inactivity (veins of the extremities as when a patient is confined to bed), (3) valvular stenosis (especially mitral and aortic), and (4) localized vascular dilatation with pooling of the blood (as in aneurysm or varices).

Changes in *constituents* of the *blood* as a cause of thrombosis are less well understood. They have already been mentioned above in connection with the mechanism of clotting but, from a more practical standpoint, may be considered somewhat more fully under the following five headings: thromboplastin deficiency, prothrombin and prothrombin conversion factor deficiencies, fibrinogen deficiency, fibrinolysin increase, and anticoagulants. *Thromboplastin deficiency* is best exemplified in *hemophilia*. This is a classical illustration of a hemorrhagic disorder due to failure of shed blood to clot properly (p. 944). The disease is characterized by severe and excessive bleeding from various parts of the body, often after the slightest trauma. It is inherited as a sex-linked mendelian recessive characteristic, is transmitted by females, but generally appears only in males. The results of the hemorrhage depend upon the location of, and the ability to stop, the bleeding. Examination of the blood discloses prolongation of the clotting time to several hours. The bleeding time is unaffected because platelets clump readily and occlude the induced pin-prick opening. Quantitatively prothrombin, calcium, and fibrinogen in the plasma are normal. There is, however, a lack of plasma thromboplastinogen which is responsible for the delayed conversion of prothrombin to thrombin. The active principle involved in this mechanism has actually been found to be a euglobulin. *Prothrombin* and *prothrombin conversion factor deficiencies* occur as congenital and acquired hemorrhagic disorders manifested clinically as bleeding due to defects in coagulation. Prothrombin is a sulphur-containing glycoprotein formed almost exclusively in the liver and requiring the presence of vitamin K for its production. Therefore, any disease that injures the liver, which incidentally is often manifested by *jaundice*, interferes with prothrombin formation and coagulation of blood and thus brings about bleeding. Evaluation of such circumstances is, of course, important where surgery is contemplated. Rarely prothrombin may be deficient in the presence of extreme inadequacy of food intake, biliary fistula, or fatty diarrhea. In *hemorrhagic disease* of the *newborn*, which occurs shortly after birth and is manifested by spontaneous external and internal hemorrhages, there is a low prothrombin concentration in the blood. The deficiency, however, appears to be only an exaggeration of the normally low prothrombin values found in the first few days of life. It is probably due to a lack of reserve vitamin K along with failure to produce vitamin K in the child's own intestinal tract until a bacterial flora is established. Administration of vitamin K corrects the defect. *Fibrinogen deficiency* is a rare cause of a defect in coagulation of the blood. In such instances the clots are thin, friable, and mechanically ineffective. The deficiency may be seen in *pernicious anemia, scurvy, pellagra, leukemia, metastatic carcinoma* of the *bone marrow*, and severe *liver damage*. Despite the fact that fibrinogen is formed chiefly in the liver and that hepatic injury may bring about its deficiency in the blood, bleeding in hepatic disorders usually results from prothrombin deficiency for the fibrinogen content of the blood is rarely depressed low enough to be responsible for hemorrhage. *Fibrinolysin increase* promotes absorption of clots and thus induces hemorrhage. It has been recorded in *toxemia* of *pregnancy*, after injection of *typhoid vaccine*, following *mercurial diuretics*, after *trauma* and *surgery*, and in *shock* from transfusion, hemorrhage, or burns. *Anticoagulants* are substances that slow down or prevent coagulation of blood. Clinically, they are used in conditions such as thrombosis of the coronary artery to prevent new thrombi or growth of thrombi that have already formed. Three anticoagulants that may be mentioned are heparin, hirudin, and dicumarol. *Heparin* is a mixture of compounds having a mucotin polysulfuric acid structure. It prevents coagulation by retarding the formation of thrombin and by acting as antithrombin. *Hirudin* is an extract of leeches. It renders blood incoagulable by preventing the action of thrombin on fibrinogen. *Dicumarol* is antagonistic to the function of vitamin K. It prevents coagulation of blood by inhibiting formation of prothrombin.

Pathologically thrombi may be divided into two varieties—postmortem and antemortem. *Postmortem thrombi* are generally referred to simply as postmortem clots. They develop terminally or shortly after death and are found in the heart, arteries, and veins. They are soft, jelly-like, moist, homogeneous, and unlaminated (Fig. 76). They are not closely adherent to the intima, and are easily detachable, leaving a smooth endothelial surface. They are of two types. The more common is called the *red*, *cruor*, or "*currant jelly*" *clot* and, as the name suggests, is red in appearance. It consists of an entanglement of all the elements of the blood and forms when the blood is coagulated rapidly (Fig. 76*A*). A less common type is called the "*chicken fat*" or *agonal clot* and, as the former name suggests, is yellowish gray in appearance (Fig. 76*B*). It consists of an entanglement of fibrin, leukocytes, and platelets and forms when the blood is coagulated more slowly, allowing the heavier erythrocytes to settle to the bottom.

Antemortem thrombi are generally referred to as true thrombi. They develop during life and are found in all portions of the cardiovascular tree including capillaries. They are composed of varying proportions of platelets, fibrin, leukocytes, and erythrocytes. They form slowly, are built up layer upon layer, and thus present a distinct laminated pattern (Fig.

76C). Grossly they are varicolored (mixtures of gray and red), firm, and friable. They are closely adherent to the intima and are detached with difficulty leaving a rough endothelial surface. *Histologically* they show the same laminated appearance seen grossly (Fig. 77A). The lamina are composed of layers of platelets and fibrin, intermingled with layers of leukocytes and erythrocytes. At first the outlines of the structures are distinct but later, as disintegration sets in, they become blurred and obscured.

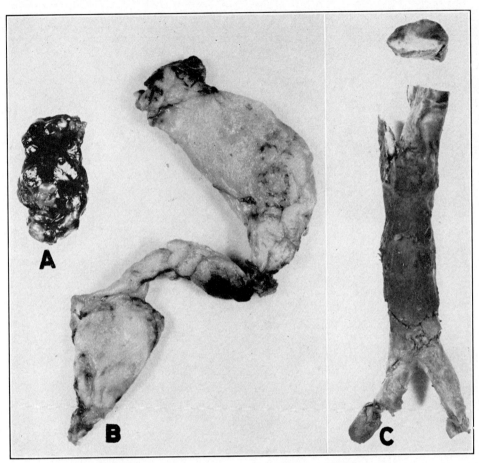

FIG. 76.—Thrombi showing *A*, red postmortem clot, *B*, "chicken fat" postmortem or agonal clot, and *C*, laminated, varicolored, antemortem thrombus.

Ultimately an *antemortem thrombus* may undergo any one of the following changes: (1) *Infection.* This occurs when the original cause of the thrombus is a pyogenic infection. An infected thrombus (also called a septic thrombus) becomes softened, often liquefied, and more friable. The increased friability, in turn, predisposes to embolism and pyemia. (2) *Softening.* Aside from infection, softening may occur as a result of action of enzymes such as fibrinolysin (tryptase). (3) *Complete absorption.* (4) *Contraction.* At first, shrinkage of a thrombus is due to contraction of fibrin while later it is due to contraction of fibrous tissue. In either case the final diminution in size may cause it to retract enough to re-open the lumen of the vessel. (5) *Organization.* At the point of attachment of the thrombus with the vessel the fibroblasts and capillaries of the vessel almost immediately begin to proliferate and invade the coagulum. Ultimately they completely replace the thrombus and then the latter is said to be organized. During the process of organizing the tissue shrinks, spaces are formed, and later the spaces become lined with endothelial cells. Both these endothelial-lined spaces and the anastomosing capillaries form direct communications with the lumen of the vessel thus re-establishing a certain degree of circulation (Fig. 77B). Such a thrombus is then said to be *canalized*. (6) *Calcification*.

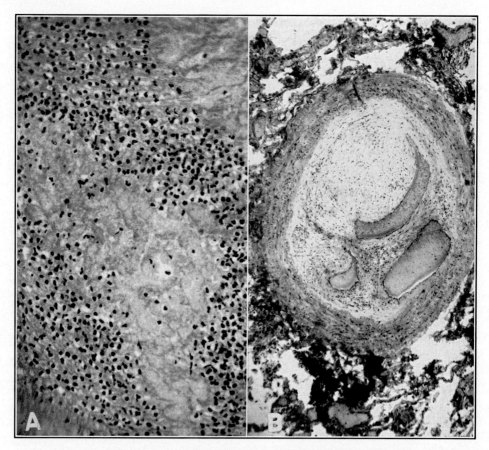

FIG. 77.—Antemortem thrombi showing *A*, early stage with distinct lamination. × 200, and *B*, late stage with organization and canalization. × 50.

Some of the thrombi ultimately become permeated with lime salts and are transformed into hard, round, radiopaque bodies. Such bodies in the veins are referred to as *pheboliths* (especially common in the pelvic veins) while those in arteries are called *arterioliths*.

The *clinical manifestations* of thrombosis depend upon the type of vessel affected (artery or vein), the completeness of the occlusion, the degree of collateral circulation, and the organ involved. In general, *arterial* involvement may result in ischemic atrophy, infarction, or gangrene, while *venous* involvement may result in edema, effusions into mesothelial-lined cavities, gangrene (as in the small bowel), embolism, or pyemia. In general

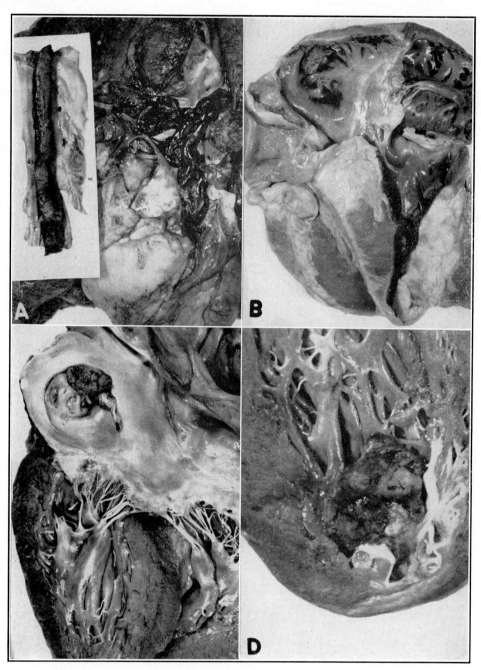

Fig 78.—Sources of emboli showing A, a thrombus in the inferior vena cava and an embolus in the pulmonary artery, B, a thrombus in the right auricle, C, a thrombus in the left auricle, and D, a thrombus opposite an infarct of the left ventricle.

also, involvement of the heart and brain is more serious than involvement of other organs.

Embolism.—The term *embolism* (L. and Gr. = in + to throw) means the transportation of any material not normally present in the bloodstream from one part of the cardiovascular system to an artery, vein, or capillary which it obstructs. The material transported is referred to as an *embolus* (Gr. = plug). A *saddle embolus* is one that straddles the bifurcation of a vessel. A *paradoxical embolus* is one that arises on the venous side of the circulation but gains entrance to the arterial side. This may occur in connection with (1) an interauricular or interventricular septal defect, (2) a

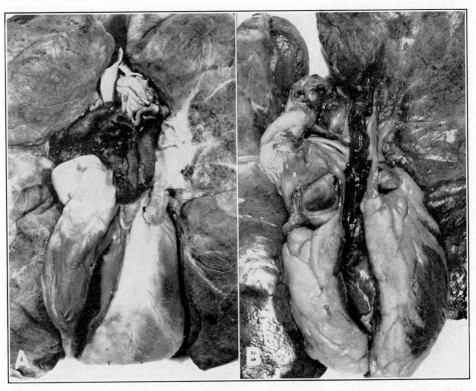

Fig. 79.—Pulmonary embolism showing *A*, the pulmonary artery filled with a coiled embolus that originated in a femoral vein. (Specimen submitted by Dr. H. T. Tamaki), and *B*, an embolus of the left pulmonary artery masked by a superimposed thrombus which has propagated proximally into the right ventricle.

direct communication between the pulmonary artery and aorta, or (3) material small enough to pass through the pulmonary capillaries. Emboli may conveniently be divided into solid, fluid, and gaseous.

Solid emboli generally consist of thrombi, tumor cells (a common method of spread), bacteria (responsible for bacteremia, septicemia, and pyemia), and some parasites. Of these, *thrombi* are the most important from the point of view of the topic at hand. As stated in the preceding section, thrombi may form in any part of the cardiovascular tree. From the points of origin, they may become dislodged either in part or *in toto* and thus produce *emboli*. The *sources* of such emboli are thus varied (Fig. 78). On the *venous side* of the circulation they most commonly originate in the veins of the lower extremities, veins of the pelvis, cavernous sinuses, right atrium, and right ventricle. The target organs are the lungs. On the *arterial side* of the circulation they usually originate in the left atrium, left ventricle, nitral and aortic valves (in the form of vegetations), and the aorta. The target organs are any of the organs located distal to the point of origin of the thrombus. The most common are the spleen, kidneys, lower extremities, and

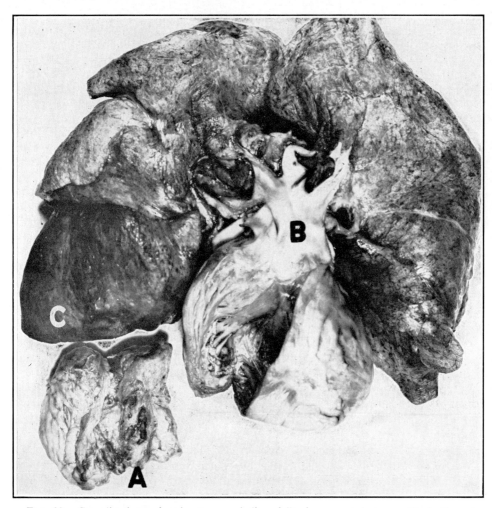

FIG. 80.—Complications of pulmonary embolism following prostatectomy illustrating *A*, thrombosis of periprostatic veins which gave rise to several emboli, *B*, pulmonary artery and its branches containing thrombi that have been superimposed upon the emboli, and *C*, infarct of the lower lobe of the right lung resulting from one of the emboli.

brain. *Pathologically* an embolus originating in a thrombus is, of course, identical with an antemortem thrombus. If the patient dies or is operated upon soon after embolism occurs, the embolus can be recognized as being foreign to the vessel in which it is impacted because it is often coiled upon itself in a serpiginous fashion, is not adherent to the adjacent endothelium, is removed with ease, and may be replaced to fit the vessel or structure where it first developed (Fig. 79*A*). If some time has elapsed between the time of embolism and the time of examination, the embolus may no longer be recognized as such for the coiled surfaces become adherent to each other and to the adjacent endothelium and a secondary thrombus completely covers and fuses with the original transported thrombus. In addition, the secondary thrombus has a tendency to propagate proximally (against the bloodstream) and fill the larger vascular tributaries (Figs. 79B and 80). In cases of embolism of the pulmonary arteries the proximal extension of a secondary thrombus may involve the main pulmonary artery, the right atrium, the right ventricle, and even the venæ cavæ. The *complications* following thrombotic emboli depend upon (1) the size of the recipient vessel (when it is small there may be no effect but when it is large there may be sudden death), (2) degree of collateral circulation (when insufficient the embolus may produce ischemia, infarction, or gangrene), (3) organ affected (involvement of the lungs, heart, or brain is more serious than involvement of other organs), and (4) presence or absence of infection (infected emboli produce embolic abscesses). Of all organs of the body the lungs are most commonly affected. The *frequency* of pulmonary emboli resulting from thrombi varies according to whether studies are made on necropsy material or on clinical material only, on whether they are reported as the cause of death or simply as an associated finding, and on the thoroughness of the examination (Israel). In a general hospital, however, massive embolism is observed in about 4 per cent of all necropsies while contributory embolism is seen in about 3 per cent of cases. In the over all, repeated studies have shown that about 10 per cent of all patients dying in hospitals have pulmonary embolism. In relation to all admissions to a medical or surgical service, the incidence is in the neighborhood of 0.5 per cent but regarding pulmonary disorders it almost equals the incidence of pneumonias and carcinoma combined. In the over all, approximately two thirds of the cases occur in "surgical" patients and one third in "medical" patients. The most common age period is between 30 and 80 years. The *clinical symptoms* in decreasing order of frequency are chest pain, dyspnea, abdominal pain, and syncope without pain. The signs are fever, rales, tachycardia, tachypnea, hemoptysis, hypotension, congestive failure, friction rub, rib tenderness, cyanosis, and jaundice. Varicosities and phlebitis of the lower extremities are detected in about two thirds of all cases. Electrocardiographic changes indicating acute cor pulmonale or coronary insufficiency are frequently observed. The *clinical diagnosis* is generally made from the symptoms and signs in conjunction with (1) evidence of thrombophlebitis in the deep veins of the legs, (2) characteristic roentgenographic changes in the lungs, and (3) characteristic electrocardiographic changes. The condition may be confused with myocardial infarction. Serum glutamic oxalacetic transaminase studies are significant in this respect for they are normal in pulmonary embolism and elevated in myocardial infarction. *Treatment* may be (1) medical—consisting of administration of anticoagulants to postoperative patients (heparin or dicumerol) or (2) surgical—ligation of the vena cava or both femoral veins. Early ambulation to prevent thrombosis is of distinct value. None of these measures, however, is entirely satisfactory. Once embolism has occurred, treatment consists of supportive measures only. In some patients, massive embolism is preceded by forewarning minor emboli or signs of phlebitis but in others the first and only indication of trouble is a massive fatal occlusion of the pulmonary circulation.

Fluid emboli are usually of two varieties—fat and amniotic fluid and rarely of oil (as following hysterosalpingography). Of these, *fat embolism* is by far the most frequent. Its precise incidence, however, is most difficult to determine for the frequency with which it is diagnosed is in direct proportion to the philosophy and keenness of the observer. Thus Peltier quotes figures that vary from less than 1 to over 80 per cent of traumatized patients. That fat embolism can and does occur is not questioned by most observers but the mechanism of its formation is not agreed upon. Since the condition is most frequently seen following fractures of long bones that contain an abundance of fatty marrow and following blunt or operative trauma on fat people and less often in connection with cutaneous burns, panniculitis (inflammation of fat tissue), acute pancreatic necrosis, and severe fatty change in the liver, most observers believe that the presence of intravascular fat droplets represents true embolism of fat from the fat depots of the body (Love). In order for the condition to develop, they further hold (1) that the envelope of the fat cell must be torn and liquid fat freed, (2) that veins in the vicinity must be torn, and (3) that increased pressure must be present to force the fat into the torn veins. All of these conditions are presumably met by trauma to fat depots. Other observers, however, maintain that the condition is not a true embolization of fat from fatty area but a local intracapillary precipitation of fat carried in the plasma (Johnson). They hold that the formation of the fatty droplets represents a change in a complex of symptoms encompassing shock, tissue injuries, and a change in emulsification of serum lipids. These conclusions are based on the following: (1) fat emboli are recorded in a large number of cases in the absence of trauma to long bones or fatty tissues, (2) there is no direct correlation between the severity or extent of the trauma and the frequency of fat embolism, (3) there is often a lag of a week or more between the trauma and onset of embolism, (4) fatty emboli are not limited to the lungs but are present in distant organs thus necessitating passage of the droplets through the pulmonary circulation, (5) ordinary necropsy material contains a high incidence of intracapillary fat droplets similar to those seen in fat embolism, and (6) in experiments on rabbits, fat droplets in tissue capillaries are as frequent in injuries to soft tissues as they are in fractures of bones. Regardless of the view held, it is certain that in a certain proportion of the types of cases listed *fat positive* droplets are readily visible in the capillaries of the lungs, brain, kidneys, heart, skin, and other organs. In most of the organs they do not produce any grossly visible alterations but in the skin they may be associated with tiny petechiæ, having a predilection for the upper torso. *Clinically* there is generally a history of severe injury (Love). Usually, after an interval of from 4 to 11 days, there develop cyanosis of the nail beds and lips, slow and stertorous breathing, restlessness, anxiety, delerium, coma, and death. The *diagnosis* may be made from a consideration of the history and clinical manifestations as outlined. In addition, fat droplets can be readily identified in the serum by using a water souble fluorochrome and fluorescence microscopy (Peltier). *Treatment*, by those who consider the condition as true embolism of fat, is directed toward prevention by proper immobilization of parts before transportation is attempted. Once the condition has developed symptomatic treatment, such as oxygen for cyanosis, etc. is instituted. Because fat is soluble in alcohol, intravenous administration of a 5 per cent glucose—5 per cent alcohol mixture has also been advocated. The *prognosis* depends upon the frequency of clinical diagnosis. When the condition is recognized in less severely affected patients, the recovery rate is high but when it is recognized only in the gravely ill patients, the recovery rate is low. Death is usually attributed to pulmonary, cerebral, cardiac, or renal failure.

Amniotic fluid embolism was first described by Steiner and Lushbaugh in 1941. It occurs, of course, only in connection with pregnancy. Although the pathogenesis of the condition is as yet poorly understood, it is thought that strong uterine contractions force the amniotic fluid (only after the membranes have ruptured) into myometrial veins at the placental site and thence into the general venous circulation. Grossly the lungs appear normal. Histologically the arterioles and capillaries contain squamæ, amorphous debris, mucus (derived from meconium), and rarely lanugo hairs. The hairs are readily identified microscopically using polarized light (Scofield). The same material may be found in the uterine and pelvic veins. Amniotic fluid embolism may account for some of the cases of otherwise unexplained sudden death during delivery.

Gaseous emboli may be separated into two groups—air emboli and caisson disease. *Air emboli* may be venous or arterial. *Venous air emboli* may occur in connection with (1) purposeful introduction of air into the pleural cavity (artificial pneumothorax), (2) operations on the neck when negative venous pressure during inspiration sucks air into partially severed veins, (3) transurethral resection of the prostate when air may enter transected and gaping prostatic veins, (4) intravenous therapy, and (5) uterine veins at the placental site. The last mentioned may result from a self-administered douche, from vaginal insufflation, or from an attempt to induce abortion by means of a syringe. At the time of delivery it may occur from simple entrance of air by way of the vagina, and in the postpartum period it may result from knee-chest exercises. The amount of air necessary to produce death by venous air embolism in man has not been accurately determined, although it is probably over 100 cc. Regardless of the site of the recipient veins the air ultimately collects in the form of frothy bubbles in the pulmonary arteries and the right side of the heart. As such it directly obstructs the pulmonary arteries and prevents the heart from contracting properly. The clinical manifestations, as would be expected, are entirely pulmonary. *Arterial air emboli* usually occur in connection with artificial pneumothorax in which case the air enters the pulmonary veins. Rarely they may be of a paradoxical nature. Air bubbles block the systemic arteries and are, therefore, responsible for a variety of clinical manifestations, the most serious of which pertain to the central nervous system and the heart.

Caisson disease, also known as compressed air illness and diver's paralysis, consists of a rapid liberation of air (mostly nitrogen) from the blood in people making a sudden transition from high to low atmospheric pressure. The condition thus occurs in caisson workers, deep sea divers, and aviators. The disorder is, in effect, arterial air embolism on a grand scale. Involvement of muscular and osseous arteries produces disseminated pains (bends); of cerebral and cerebellar arteries, vertigo and staggering gait (staggers); of pulmonary vessels, asphyxia (chokes); of coronary arteries, pain in the precordium; and of cutaneous vessels, pruritus (itch).

TRAUMA

Trauma (Gr. = wound) may be defined simply as an injury or a wound and a *wound* (L.) connotes an interruption by violence of the continuity of any tissue. Minor degrees of trauma are extremely common in everyday life but usually go unnoticed or are quickly forgotten. Major degrees of trauma sufficient to produce (1) a visible effect upon the body, (2) pain, or (3) loss of function and thus be indelibly recorded in the mind and remembered are, in comparison, infrequent. In this section only a few remarks will be made regarding trauma in general. Discussions of more specific effects of trauma to the individual organs will be considered in appropriate places in the text.

Abrasions (L. = a rubbing or scratching off) represent a superficial destruction of the epidermis by friction (Moritz). The corium may or may not be affected. The lesions may be produced by almost any suitably directed injury of not too great an intensity. From a medicolegal point of view, fingernail scratches or imprints of such objects as automobile grills and tires may be of extreme importance.

Contusions (L. = bruise) represent microscopic disruptions of tissues and smaller blood vessels together with extravasation of blood but with the surface (skin or organ) of the area remaining uninterrupted. Because of the bleeding, the affected area becomes discolored. The discoloration appears early in cases of superficial bruises but may not appear for several days in cases of deep bruises. While the initial color depends on the erythrocytes as such and is deep red to blue, subsequent discolorations depend upon erythrocytic degeneration products (hemosiderin and hematoidin) and range from brown to yellow and yellowishgreen.

Concussion (L.) is a clinical term connoting a sudden jarring resulting in functional disturbance. The term is usually applied to the brain but is not necessarily limited to this organ. Grossly, there are no detectable alterations. Microscopically, some cases reveal minute hemorrhages while others disclose no histopathologic changes.

Lacerations (L. = to tear) are wounds caused by crushing or stretching forces. They may involve the skin, subcutaneous tissue, or internal organs. Of these, the former is much more frequent. The disturbance is particularly apt to occur over bony prominences and usually results from a blunt impact. The defect may be linear, curved, flap-like, stellate, or otherwise irregular; the edges are usually ragged but, on occasion, are sharp and the defect is filled with blood and disrupted tissue often mixed with extraneous debris.

Incisions (L. = to cut) are wounds produced by objects with sharp edges and are formed as a result of both pressure and friction. Incisions may be classified as accidental, surgical, nonaccidental, self-inflicted, and those obtained as a result of assault. They may be single or multiple and superficial or deep. Unlike most of the other wounds already referred to, incisions are usually clean-cut, sharp, and associated with little damage to adjacent tissues.

Stab and *puncture wounds* are deep defects with relatively small diameters produced by rigid slender objects. They are incurred accidentally (falls, automobile accidents, etc.) or purposefully (homocide, suicide, or perversion). The external opening may be small and readily overlooked, especially if the object is in the nature of a hat pin, knitting needle, stilleto, or ice pick. The wound may be single or multiple; the tract may be straight or (due to shifting of organs) sinuous; the depth of the wound (due to indentation caused by the force) is frequently greater than the length of the object used, and injury to internal structures is much more serious than injury to the integument.

Bullet wounds are injuries sustained by rifled (revolvers, pistols, rifles, and machine guns) or smooth bore (shotguns and some smaller caliber revolvers and rifles) firearms. Of these, the former are by far the more frequent. In addition to the bullet, trauma is also incurred by burning gases, burning powder, substances from the detonator or powder charge, substances broken from the bullet, and debris left in the barrel by previous discharges. If the muzzle is three inches or less from the target, the clothes and skin will reveal powder deposits and burns. The entrance wound most frequently consists of a radial or cruciate laceration. Due to stretching of the structures before actual penetration, the opening hole is smaller than the bullet and the immediately adjacent skin discloses marks of the bullet known as the contact ring. In addition, if the muzzle of the gun is against the skin it will produce a contact wound that is readily identified by infra-red photography. Exit wounds are generally larger and more irregular than entrance wounds. This is due to flattening of the bullet, tumbling or wobbling of the bullet resulting from decreased velocity, and the penetration of shattered bony fragments. Internal injuries depend, among other things, upon the organs and structures involved.

Blast injuries are those sustained upon detonation of high explosives. If the victim is in the immediate vicinity of the explosive he may be blown to bits. If he is not in the immediate path of the explosive he may be severely burned by the combustion of gases and chemicals or by corrosive chemicals. Of equal or even greater importance are internal injuries that may be out of all proportion to the external wounds. They are due to (1) rapid atmos-pheric or, in the case of immersion, water movements with a swift change from normal to greatly increased and then greatly reduced pressures, (2) throwing the body against a resistant object, and (3) flying missiles. Briefly, the actual injury may consist of primary or secondary shock, cerebral concussion or hemorrhage, pulmonary damage (ranging from scattered foci of bleeding to extensive lacerations), hemorrhages or actual rupture of the gastrointestinal tract, rupture of eardrums and deafness, and psycho-logical trauma. Finally, detonation of high explosives may be accompanied by liberation of dangerous (chiefly carbon monoxide) gases.

The *complications* of *trauma* are numerous and varied. Some of the more important may be listed as follows: (1) *hemorrhage*—primary or secondary, (2) *inflammation*—aseptic, caused by tissue disintegration products, or septic, due to transfer of organisms from one part of the body to another (as from skin and mucous membranes to tissue spaces and body cavities) or to contamination from without (especially soil organisms such as *Clos-tridium welchii* and *Clostridium tetani*), (3) *loss* of *function*—particularly true when continuity of structures has been interrupted, (4) *necrosis* and *gangrene*—due to interruption of the blood supply (severance of vessels, thrombosis, or embolism) with or without the presence of contaminating organisms, and (5) *primary* or *secondary* shock. The latter may be moti-vated by any of the factors already considered in a preceding section. Of particular importance is the absorption of myohemoglobin (and other catabolites) in connection with persons sustaining extensive crushing injury to muscles. This has been referred to as the *crush syndrome*. It is charac-terized by the usual manifestations of secondary shock with emphasis on increasing oliguria culminating in death from anuria. The renal lesions are those of acute toxic nephrosis.

OBSTRUCTION OF HOLLOW ORGANS

The *hollow organs* of the body are those that are composed of a series of tubes. They consist of the following systems: respiratory, gastrointestinal, biliary, pancreatic, genital, urinary, cardiovascular, and central nervous. The *causes* of obstruction are numerous, are varied, and, to a great extent, are peculiar to the system or part of the system in question. They may be classified according to whether they affect primarily the lumen, the wall, or the adjacent tissues or they may be classified on the basis of congenital anomalies, degenerations, inflammations, physical disturbances, and tumors. The obstruction may be partial or complete. *Physiologically*, it is attended not only by impairment or complete cessation of normal function of the organ affected, but also by a consequent derangement of function of other organs. To give but one example, obstruction of the large bowel is attended by cessation of normal gastrointestinal function and by absorption of toxic products which causes a disturbance of the functions of both the circulatory and urinary systems. *Pathologically* the changes in the affected organ proximal to the obstruction consist of (1) accumulation of the contents normally carried by the tubes, (2) dilatation, thinning, and even rupture of the tubes, (3) atrophy, degeneration, and necrosis of the adjoining parenchymatous cells, and (4) secondary inflammation. Changes in distant organs are quite varied, are due to absorption of toxic products of metabolism, and consist essentially of retrogressive alterations of varying degrees. *Clinically* the manifestations depend upon the system affected and the degree and duration of the obstruction. The conditions as they pertain to each system are described in appropriate places in the text.

FOREIGN BODIES

Foreign bodies are concrete objects that are not native to the part. They may be *endogenous* (Gr. = in + to form), that is, formed within the body, or *exogenous* (Gr. = outside + to form), that is, formed outside of the body and brought to it secondarily. *Endogenous* foreign bodies usually consist of concretions initiated as a result of permeation of necrotic material with calcium and other salts. They are most common in the urinary, biliary, pancreatic, and respiratory tracts.

Exogenous foreign bodies are extremely varied in type. They usually gain entrance into the body through the opening of natural passages such as respiratory, gastrointestinal, urinary, and genital tracts. Sometimes, though, they gain entrance by way of abnormal openings such as stab or gunshot wounds, surgical incisions, etc. As a rule, foreign bodies produce ill effects because of their bulk, in which case they cause obstruction and secondary infection of hollow organs. Occasionally, however, as in the case of a peanut in the respiratory tract or talcum powder in the peritoneal cavity, they produce irritation and inflammation as a result of inherent chemical properties. Specific lesions as they pertain to specific organs are described in appropriate places in the text.

HERNIAS

A *hernia* (L. = rupture) may be defined as a protrusion of an organ, part of an organ, or tissue through an enlarged normal or an abnormal opening in the wall containing it. It is *named* according to (1) the protruding tissue, as omental, vesical, etc., (2) the cavity normally housing the part, as thoracic, abdominal, etc., (3) the anatomic part through which the tissue passes, as inguinal, umbilical, diaphragmatic, etc., (4) the cavity receiving the tissue, as scrotal, labial, etc., and (5) the name of the person first de-

15

scribing it, as Barth's, Richter's, etc. A hernia is of no *clinical significance* until it interferes with the physiologic function of the part or produces an anatomic change in the tissues affected. *Interference* in *function* is usually brought about by obstruction of the lumen of an organ (as for example, the lumen of the small bowel protruding through the inguinal ring). Some of the *anatomic changes* produced in herniated tissues or organs are (1) ulceration at the point of contact of the ring, (2) secondary infection, (3) gangrene, and (4) perforation with inflammation of the cavity normally housing the part (as for example, peritonitis). A hernia is said to be (1) *reducible* when the protruding tissue is replacable into its normal position, (2) *irreducible* when it cannot be replaced into its normal position, (3) *incarcerated* when the lumen of the organ is occluded but the blood supply to the wall is maintained, and (4) *strangulated* when it is irreducible, incarcerated, and the blood supply to the wall is occluded. Hernias of specific organs or systems are described in various portions of the text in connection with diseases of these organs or systems.

THERMAL DISTURBANCES

Thermal disturbances may be defined as local or systemic reactions of the body to excessive or subnormal temperatures. They may be considered under the following headings: burns, heat cramps, heat exhaustion, heat stroke, chilblains, trench foot, immersion foot, frostbite, and generalized hypothermia.

Burns.—A burn may be *defined* as a lesion sustained when tissue is exposed to a temperature greater than that consistent with normal metabolism. Burns are generally accidental injuries most commonly *acquired* at home and less commonly at places of employment. They are more frequent in children than in adults. The *cause* is excessive heat of any type (hot air, steam, hot water, fire, or light). *Pathologically* burns may conveniently be divided into three degrees—first, second, and third. A *first degree* burn grossly discloses erythema. The microscopic changes are confined to the superficial portion of the dermis and to the epidermis. The former discloses all the alterations seen in any early and slight inflammation. Epidermal changes consist of fleeting impairment of its anchorage to the dermis and nonspecific degenerative changes in the nuclei and cytoplasm of the outer and intermediate cell layers. The retrogressive alterations seen in this stage are reversible and the tissue is readily restorable to normal. A *second degree* burn is characterized by the formation of blisters, necrosis of the epithelium, and sloughing of varying amounts of the epidermis (Fig. 81). Blisters are formed within the epidermis and between the epidermis and dermis. They result mostly from an accumulation of extravascular edema fluid but also from liquefaction necrosis of epithelial cells. Second degree burns are generally followed by regeneration of epithelium and complete restoration of tissue to normal. A *third degree* burn is characterized by necrosis not only of the epidermis but also of the dermis and any of the underlying tissues (over bone). Grossly the affected area appears gray, red, brown, or black (charred) depending upon the amount of blood in the capillaries before coagulation occurs (Fig. 82). Histologically the dead tissue shows complete necrosis, while the adjacent viable tissue reveals varying degrees of degeneration. Healing occurs by the formation of granulation tissue and ultimately by extensive scarring. The most serious *complication* of burns is shock. When it occurs soon after the episode it is

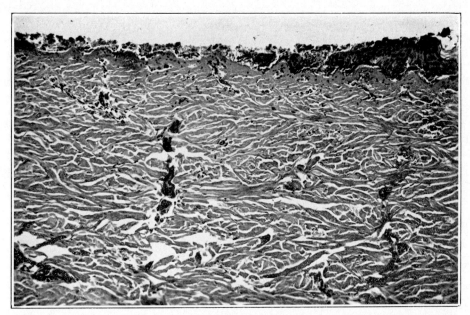

FIG. 81.—Second degree burn of the skin showing almost complete destruction of the epidermis. × 100.

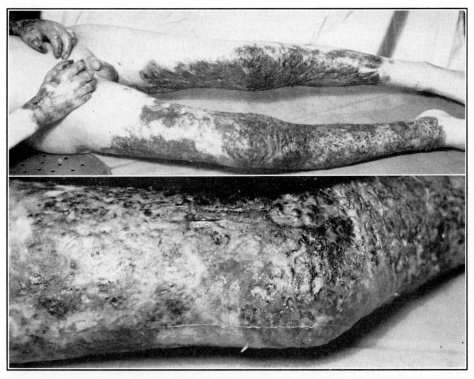

FIG. 82.—Third degree cutaneous burns. The close-up (lower picture) discloses extensive ulceration extending to the subcutaneous tissues.

of the primary variety but when it occurs after twenty-four hours it is of the secondary type. The latter is due both to loss of fluid into and from the burned area and to absorption of toxic products of the burned tissues. Morphologically fatal cases reveal all the changes already described in connection with Shock (p. 207). Of special importance perhaps is ulceration (Curling's ulcer) in the first portion of the duodenum. It occurs in about 4 per cent of all cases coming to necropsy. *Clinically* local symptoms in burns consist of severe pain, while general symptoms are those of shock. *Treatment* consists of restoration of plasma volume, prevention of local infection, and maintenance of a high protein and vitamin diet. The *prognosis* depends more on the extent of the burn than upon its depth. It is good when less than one-third of the body surface is affected and poor when more than one-half is involved. Annually about 4,600 people die in the United States from burns and scalds (Davis).

Heat Cramps.—Heat cramps are pains due to spasms of voluntary muscles. They frequently occur in freely perspiring laborers working in an intensely heated environment. The cause of the spasm and cramps is excessive loss of electrolytes, especially sodium chloride, in the perspiration. The temperature is normal or slightly subnormal (Malamud). The condition can be prevented by the ingestion of salt in amounts sufficient to compensate for that lost.

Heat Exhaustion.—Heat exhaustion results from prolonged exposure of the body to excessive heat. Some of the cases represent a progression of heat cramps and are due primarily to excessive salt depletion (Malamud). They exhibit muscle cramps, giddiness, anorexia, headache, vomiting, sweating, syncope on standing, dehydration, and oliguria. Other cases resemble those of heat stroke in that they are due to mild impairment of the heat regulating mechanism of the body. They are attended by dizziness, exhaustion, anorexia, insomnia, dyspnea, decreased sweating, polyuria, and "prickly heat" eruption. The condition is thus intermediate in position between heat cramps and heat stroke.

Heat Stroke.—Heat stroke (which includes sunstroke) results from paralysis of the heat-regulating *mechanism* of the hypothalamus. Normally this center causes dilatation or contraction of the peripheral capillaries and this brings about excessive loss or conservation of heat respectively. The temperature of the returning blood in turn stimulates or depresses the heat-regulating center. Normally, also, the mechanism of dissipation of heat from the body is by sweating and radiation. The former ceases when the medium surrounding the body is saturated with water vapor and the latter ceases when the temperature of surrounding medium is equal to or exceeds that of the body. Thus, when the atmospheric humidity and/or temperature reach a certain point, heat is no longer lost from the body, the temperature of the circulating blood rises, the heat-regulating mechanism becomes paralyzed, and heat stroke develops. The condition is particularly prone to occur in military personnel subjected to prolonged exercise under trying atmospheric conditions, in work shops where the humidity and temperature are high, and in older people whose heat-regulating mechanism is less adaptive. In general, it is most common in people over the age of 60 years and affects males more often than females (Austin). Alcoholism and cardiovascular disease are predisposing factors. The *pathologic changes* in various organs of the body are not specific and, in general, are those of Shock (p. 207). The alterations in the brain consist of degeneration, congestion, edema, and focal hemorrhages. *Prodromal manifestations* are similar to those in heat cramps and heat exhaustion. The important *clinical manifestations* of heat stroke as such are (1) fever, usually over 106°F, (2) a hot dry skin completely devoid of perspiration, (3) systolic blood pressure below 100 mm. of Hg., (4) central nervous system manifestations ranging from lethargy to coma, and (5) laboratory findings exhibiting hemoconcentration (erythrocytic count over 5,000,000 and hemoglobin over 15 gm. per 100 cc.), nitrogen retention in the blood, and increase of potassium and decrease of sodium and chlorides of the blood. The *diagnosis* is made from a history of exposure to excessive environmental temperatures coupled with the clinical manifestations listed. *Treatment* is directed toward rapid reduction of body temperature, restoring the electrolyte and fluid balance, prevention of bacterial invasion, and amelioration of associated diseases. The *prognosis* is guarded for the mortality is as high as 20 per cent.

Chilblains.—*Chilblains* (AS = cold + blister or sore) may be defined as degenerative, painful, cutaneous lesions affecting the heels, other parts of the feet, hands, ears, nose, legs, breasts, and buttocks (Williams). A common synonym for chilblain is *pernio* (Gr. = heel) signifying the common site of affection, namely, the heel. The *cause* of the condition is partly constitutional in that the arterioles of the skin react too spastically to cold and dilate too slowly to heat. The precipitating cause is exposure to damp, cold weather. The disorder *occurs* at all ages but is most common between 5 to 15 years and predominates in females. *Clinically* it is characterized by dusky red cutaneous patches that are attended by tenderness, burning, and intolerable itching, especially upon exposure to heat. In some, secondary infection is superimposed sooner or later, in which case the lesions crack and ulcerate. *Pathologically* the only noteworthy changes consist of edema and nonspecific inflammation of the corium. Some of the vessels show endothelial proliferation and thrombosis. Others reveal dilatation and engorgement with erythrocytes. Around the vessels are scattered lymphocytes and between the vessels is a proliferation of connective tissue. The *diagnosis* is made from the history and the appearance of the lesions. *Treatment* is symptomatic (for the lesions disappear with improvement of weather conditions) together with protection from the cold. Ointments are used for the chapping. The *prognosis* is good.

Trench Foot, Immersion Foot, and Frostbite.—These conditions may be collectively referred to as representing *local hypothermia* and may be conveniently considered together for they are similar, both physiologically and pathologically. *Trench foot* signifies injury to the feet (and occasionally to the hands) as a result of prolonged exposure to damp atmosphere (as soldiers in trenches) with the temperature in the neighborhood of 32° F. *Immersion foot* is a similar condition brought about by prolonged immersion of the extremities in water with the temperature around the freezing point. *Frostbite* constitutes injury to the peripheral portions of the body (feet, hands, ears, nose, and cheeks) consequent to exposure to atmosphere (high altitude to sea level) at a temperature below freezing. Regardless of the surrounding medium, the fundamental *cause* of the changes in local hypothermia is vascular occlusion. An added, but less important, factor is the action of the cold directly upon the cells. *Pathologically* the vessels first undergo constriction, then dilatation, and later thrombosis. The thrombi are rich in erythrocytes and platelets but are poor in fibrin (Friedman). Initially they are composed simply of agglutinations but in time they undergo complete organization. Changes affecting other tissues such as skin, fat, muscle, and nerves consist of degenerations, necrosis, nonspecific inflammations, and (later) fibrosis. In severe cases there is massive necrosis resulting in typical gangrene. *Clinically* slight to moderately severe cases may be divided into three stages—stage of exposure, hyperemic stage, and posthyperemic stage (Ungley). During the stage of *exposure* the blood supply becomes arrested because of vasoconstriction and the part affected becomes cold, numb, pale, swollen, and pulseless. The next stage is that of intense *hyperemia*. It occurs upon rewarming the area and is brought about by release of tissue metabolites. In addition to dilatation of the vessels (which is responsible for the hyperemia) there is escape of fluid into the tissues with marked swelling and severe pain. Within a week or ten days the final or *posthyperemic* stage appears. It consists of a gradual subsidence of the hyperemia and swelling and, as a result of degenerative changes, is accompanied by disturbances in sensation, disturbances in sweating, muscular atrophy, and paralysis. Within several weeks the affected part becomes sensitive to cold and is subjected to excessive sweating. In severe cases the stages of exposure and hyperemia are followed directly by blistering and gangrene.

Local Hypothermia.—*Local hypothermia*, as the name indicates, is a reduction of temperature locally below normal levels. Actually chilblains, trench foot, immersion foot, and frostbite are *naturally occurring* forms of local *hypothermia*. Purposeful local reduction of temperature may be referred to as *induced hypothermia*. This is usually performed in connection with exposed and peripheral portions of the body. One method in common use is *ethyl chloride spray*. Ethyl chloride is an inflammable, colorless liquid which, when expelled from its container in the form of a spray, acts as a local anesthetic and antispasmodic by rapidly reducing the temperature of the exposed tissues. It is used to allay pain in sprains and bursitis and to interrupt muscle spasm in stiff neck, trismus (spasm of jaw), lumbago (pain in the loin), sciatica (pain along the sciatic nerve), etc. Another form of locally induced hypothermia is that obtained by packing an *extremity in ice*. This has been advocated in preparation for amputation under the premise that it (1) avoids surgical shock, (2) prevents spread of infection and intoxication from a gangrenous limb, and (3) eliminates postoperative pain and edema.

General Hypothermia.—General hypothermia signifies a decrease in internal body temperature. The condition is analogous to hibernation in certain animals and has, therefore, also been referred to as induced hibernation. In man, general hypothermia has been *used* in the treatment of intractable pain, cancer, morphine addiction, and schizophrenia, as well as in surgery (Bierman). Originally, its surgical application was confined to correction of cardiac anomalies but more recently it has been used in operations on the aorta, general and abdominal surgical operations where prolonged interruption of critical blood supply to an organ or area of the body is required, in cirrhotic patients to minimize administration of hepatotoxic anesthetic agents, and as a hypotensive agent to minimize blood loss (Grosskrentz and Eiseman). The *objective* is to reduce tissue metabolism and oxygen requirements to a degree sufficient to allow susceptible tissues to survive prolonged partial or total ischemia without irreversible damage by interrupting their blood supply (Barnard). It has, for example, been determined that at normal body temperature clamping the venæ cavæ and azygos vein can be tolerated safely for one and one half minutes and that extension of the time to 3 to 4 minutes is attended by some risk (Bigelow). At a body temperature of 83° F there is 50 per cent reduction in oxygen demand and the circulation can be safely interrupted for 6 to 8 minutes. At a body temperature of 68° F the oxygen demand is reduced to 15 per cent and interruption of the circulation for as long as 20 minutes can be safely tolerated by the heart and brain. The *methods* of *induction* consist of cold bath, exposure to a draught of cold air, cooling room or chamber, cooling blanket or ice bags, connecting an artery to a vein by a polythene tube and cooling the blood as it passes through the tube, inserting a cooling coil into the thoracic or some other body cavity, and inserting a balloon into the stomach and then circulating cold water through the balloon (Ross and Barnard). Whatever method is used, induction must be gradual and in all instances must exceed an hour. Conversely, the warming process must also take place over a long period. *Physiologically*, the following are noted as the body cools: metabolic activity decreases, heart rate slows, cardiac output diminishes, circulating blood volume decreases, electrocardiogram shows elevation of the ST segment and inversion of the T wave in addition to a slow rate, steady decrease in oxygen consumption provided there is no shivering, hemoconcentration probably due to extravascular chloride concentration and withdrawal of fluid from the blood, prolongation of clotting time, tendency for the plasma potassium to drop, fall of pH of the blood to 7 due to retention of carbon dioxide, diminution to cessation of secretion of urine, and uniform drop in temperature of all tissues of the body (Ross). At 75 to 70° F the patient reveals drowsiness, stupor but no coma, unobtainable pulse and blood pressure, disappearance of pupillary reflexes, and slow respirations (Talbott). If the temperature does not drop below 68° F all of the above mentioned changes revert to normal, provided that the rewarming process is gradual. If the temperature goes below 68° F death ensues from cardiac standstill as the end point in asphyxia. Even at temperatures above 68° F an occasional untoward complication is ventricular fibrillation (Swan). The cause of this is unknown but is thought to stem from a disturbance in potassium of the blood or upset of the cholinesterase system. In some patients, pneumonia is a late complication.

LIGHT

Light consists of electromagnetic waves that travel at the rate of 186,300 miles a second. The *perceptible* waves have lengths varying from about 3.85 to 7.60 ten-thousandths of a millimeter. Waves beyond these lengths are known as *infrared* when they are longer than 7.60 ten-thousandths of a millimeter and as *ultraviolet* when they range from 3.85 to 1.0 ten-thousandths of a millimeter. As far as the body is concerned, *infrared* rays are poorly absorbed by the skin, penetrate deeply, and are responsible for the sensation of heat and immediate redness. *Ultraviolet* rays are filtered out by the superficial layers of the epidermis, are more irritating to the skin, and account for the latent (three to ten hours) redness that appears upon overexposure. If the exposure is of sufficient degree it will not only produce burns that are identical with those produced by heat, but will also be accompanied by similar systemic complications. As the acute reaction in the skin fades, melanin is deposited in the deeper portions of the epidermis. It accounts for the tanning that follows and then protects (as it does in dark complected people) against further exposure. *Chronic repeated* exposure of the skin (as in farmers and sailors) often results in hyperkeratosis of the epidermis and this in time may be transformed into cancer. An accelerated reaction of this type, known as *xeroderma pigmentosum*, is sometimes seen in children who are sensitive to light. Another reaction in hypersensitive people is *porphyria* (p. 76). Far from being entirely harmful, ultraviolet rays are also *beneficial*. In the plant world they are necessary for photosynthesis. In man they (1) kill bacteria, (2) transform harmful, ultraviolet rays are also *beneficial*. In the plant world they are necessary for photosynthesis. In man they (1) kill bacteria, (2) transform ergosterol in the skin to vitamin D, (3) have a tendency to elevate serum calcium, thus promoting bone growth in children and overcoming rachitic tetany, and (4) exert a salutary effect upon healing of wounds.

ELECTRICITY

Electricity is one of the fundamental forms of energy. While the tension varies, the following are generally the voltages in use: (1) for houses and workshops 100 to 250 V., (2) for driving streetcars and trains 400 to 600 V., and (3) for transmitting electric energy over long distances 100,000 V. The effect a given current has upon the body depends upon (1) tension or voltage, (2) intensity or amperage, (3) type of current, (4) resistance at points of contact, (5) path or current, and (6) individual susceptibility (McLaughlin). *Tension* is referred to as low tension when the current is below 1000 volts and high tension when it is over 1000 volts. Usually low tension currents are more effective than high tension ones but a current of even 65 volts may cause death if the person is well grounded. *Intensity* or *amperage* is determined by the tension divided by the conductor. In electrical shock the conductor is the body and, since the tissues and the circumstances dictate the intensity or amperage cannot be accurately calculated. The *type* of *current* is quite important for direct currents are less hazardous then alternating currents. Regarding cycles per second, those ranging between 30 and 150 are most dangerous whereas those with higher cycles are less dangerous. Frequencies of 400,000 or over are completely innocuous. *Resistance* at points of *contact* varies greatly in different areas and under different circumstances. Most important are duration of application of current and the thickness, cleanliness and dryness of the skin. The resistance of dry skin for example is 5,000 ohms whereas that at points of contact of moist saline electrodes is only 300 ohms. The *path* of the *current* through the body follows that of least resistance but converges and is of greatest intensity at the points of entrance and exit. Blood vessels and spinal fluid are good conductors whereas flat bones of the skull are poor conductors. In general, a current passing through the left side of the body and the heart or through the vital centers of the brain is more dangerous than that passing through other areas. A current entering one foot and emerging through another foot, for example, is rarely if ever fatal. *Individual susceptibility*, for some unexplained reason, is important for a current causing great damage to or death of one person may have little or no effect upon another.

Clinically, *death* from electric shock (artificial or lightning) may be (1) instantaneous—as soon as the current enters, (2) delayed—occurring during the passing of the current, (3) interrupted—recovery from a short unconsciousness, enabling the victim to free himself and perhaps wander off before he dies, (4) late—after a lapse of hours or days, and (5) the result of complications—burns, hemorrhages, infection, and embolism (Jaffe). Usually, however, death is instantaneous or delayed. The *mechanism* of instantaneous or early death is probably paralysis of the heart and/or the respiratory center.

The general *pathologic findings* are those of shock. Specific pathologic changes in tissues through which the *current* passes are characteristic but are not always found. Since the *skin* offers high resistance it discloses markings (due to heat and electric sparks) at the points of entrance and exit (contact) of the current in two-thirds of the cases. The markings are (1) round, oblong, linear, or rosette-like, (2) pale and elevated, (3) a few millimeters to several centimeters in diameter, and (4) depressed centrally, in which area the normal epidermal characteristics become erased. Histologically the changes consist of varying degrees of degeneration to complete necrosis and, if the survival of the patient extends beyond minutes, varying degrees of inflammatory reaction. The *voluntary muscles* undergo spasm which may be severe enough to produce rupture of its fibers, luxation of joints, or fracture of bones. Histologically the fine cross striations are replaced with coarse hyaline transverse bands. The *bones* may be exposed by destruction of overlying soft tissues or, in some cases, may actually be grossly perforated by the current. The *blood vessels* become brittle; the endothelium is damaged; thrombi are formed, and the nuclei of the media are destroyed. Coagulation of the blood is hastened by alternating current but delayed by direct current. The *heart* reveals fibrillations or twitchings but morphologically discloses no changes. The *nerves* show myelin degeneration and fragmentation of axis cylinders. The *brain* reveals congestion, edema, focal hemorrhages, ganglion cell degeneration, and demyelinization.

IRRADIATION

Irradiation—In medicine, *irradiation* (L. = into + to shine) or *radiation* connotes treatment with or exposure to roentgen or other forms (radium, radon, or radioactive isotopes) of radioactivity. In general, there are three important *types* of *rays*—alpha, beta, and electromagnetic (gamma and roentgen). Alpha rays are readily filtered out by the superficial layers of the skin where they cause the greatest damage; beta rays are intermediate in penetrating power; gamma rays are deeply penetrating and least damaging to the skin, and roentgen rays—having various wave lengths—vary in penetrability. From a practical irradiation point of view, alpha rays are of little or no significance. Beta and gamma rays are emitted directly by many radioactive isotopes and secondarily during roentgen therapy; beta rays are emitted by radioactive phosphorus and other isotopes; gamma rays account for most of the irradiation from radium and radon, and roentgen rays are, of course, emitted during roentgen therapy.

Over the years, the *sources* of material for pathologic study of the effects produced in man have been many. Some of them may be listed as follows: (1) excessive exposure of roentgen rays and radium during the early days after discovery, (2) moderate exposure in cyclotron workers, (3) introduction of naturally occurring radioelements into the body, especially radium preparations and thorotrast, (4) exposure of the population at Hiroshima and Nagasaki at the time of explosion of atomic bombs during World War II, (5) exposure of the population to fallout resulting from atomic bomb explosions, and (6) clinical exposure during the course of radiotherapy and the use of artificial radioactive isotopes (Warren). In *experimental animals*, the whole field has been covered even more intensely and completely than in man, for reasons that are quite obvious. The effects, whether local or general, are, for comparative purposes, fortunately quite similar to those in man (Schlumberger).

The *pathologic* effects of radioactive substances on tissues depend upon the amount absorbed rather than delivered, upon the rate of irradiation, and upon the sensitivity of the tissue itself. According to Warren and Bowers, the tissues of the body in order of decreasing sensitivity may be listed as follows: lymphocytes, erythroblasts, germinal epithelium of testis, myeloblasts, epithelium of intestinal crypts, germinal cells of the ovary, basal layer of the skin, connective tissue, bone, liver, pancreas, kidney, nerve, brain, and muscle. Depending upon the amount of irradiation absorbed and the rate of irradiation each of these tissues will show, in turn, no effect whatsoever, irritation, stimulation, degeneration, or necrosis. Fundamentally also, the changes are similar regardless of the tissue in question.

Since the *skin* is readily observable, the alterations in this structure may be taken as the prototype. The *first* change after adequate exposure is a transient erythema occurring in twenty-four hours and lasting one to two days (Teloh). The *next* change is a secondary erythema occurring ten to twenty-eight days later. Depending upon the severity of injury, this may be accompanied by vesication, edema, exudation of serum and fibrin, desquamation of the superficial layers of the epidermis, and epilation. The *third* stage consists of a variety of alterations and may appear as a continuation of the second stage or may not become manifested until a year or more after exposure. It consists of a combination of the following: (1) brown pigmentation, (2) atrophy and drying, (3) hyperkeratosis, (4) telangiectasis, (5) indolent and often painful ulceration, (6) secondary infection, and (7) spotting, brittleness, and furrowing of the nails (Fig. 83). While hyperkeratosis of the epidermis and changes in the nails are peculiar to the integument, the other changes listed may be found in any mucosal surface.

Histologically certain basic changes occur regardless of the tissue involved. The alterations affect both the cytoplasm and the nucleus of the cell. The *cytoplasmic* changes are not specific. They consist of parenchymatous, hydropic, hyaline droplet, and hyaline degenerations. Alterations in the mitochondria and Golgi apparatus are more subtle but have also been described (Warren). The changes in *nuclei* are more important than those in the cytoplasm. They are of two types—nonspecific and chromosomal (Hempelman). The nonspecific changes consist of the usual karyorrhexis, karyolysis, and pycnosis. The chromosomal changes are especially prone to occur in tissue that is actively proliferating. They consist of fragmentation of chromosomes, bridging between chromosomal fragments, swelling of nuclear material and chromosomal remnants, and multipolar mitotic figures. In some cells the daughters of damaged parents appear to be nonviable. In others, nuclear division continues but cytoplasmic division fails, leading to the formation of bizarre multinucleated giant cells. The ultimate result of the changes in the cytoplasm and nucleus just listed is complete dissolution of the cell.

While the alterations described above occur in all cells of the body they are particularly prominent in the *parenchymatous cells* of an organ. In addition, however, changes in the vessels and stroma of an organ have also a profound effect upon the ultimate fate of the area irradiated. The *vessels* reveal (1) swelling, vacuolization, endothelial proliferation, and foam cell replacement of the intima, (2) swelling, vacuolization, degeneration, fibrosis, and hyalinization of the media, (3) lymphocytic infiltration and fibrosis of the adventitia, and (4) thrombosis and later canalization in the lumen (Fig. 84, *A* and *B*). All these alterations produce narrowing or ob-

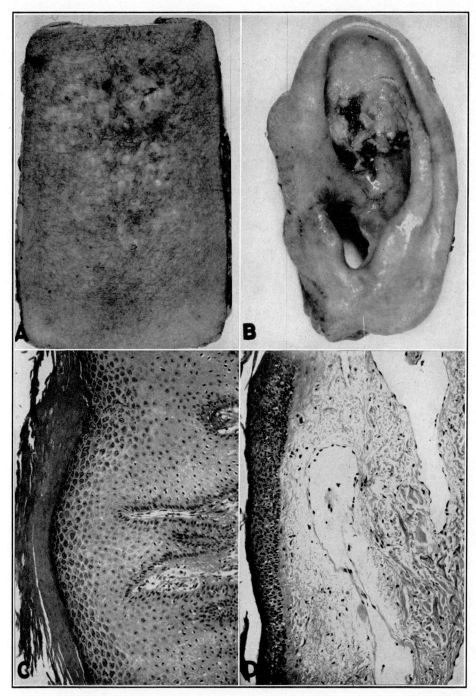

FIG. 83.—Irradiation effects showing *A* and *B*, atrophy, ulceration, and scarring of the skin of the back and left ear, *C*, hyperkeratosis of the skin. × 100, and *D*, atrophy of the epidermis and telangiectasia of the dermal capillaries. × 100.

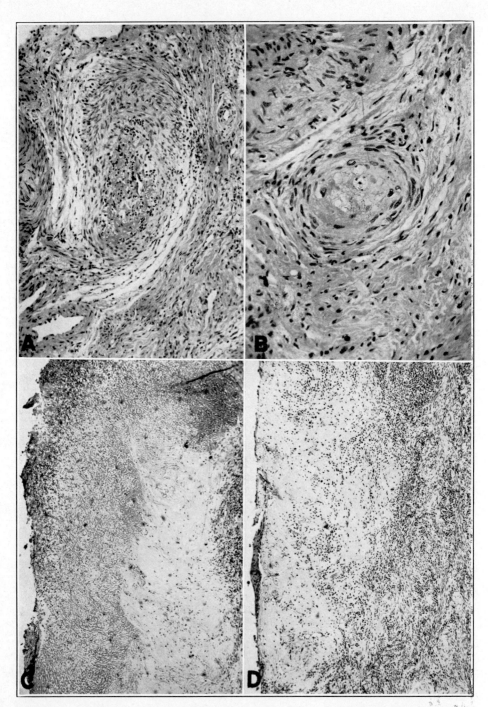

FIG. 84.—Irradiation effects showing *A*, an acute occlusion of a medium vessel by fibrinoid swelling of the intima. × 100, *B*, complete occlusion of a smaller vessel by proliferated and vacuolated endothelial cells. × 200, *C*, fibrinoid necrosis of the uterine cervix with underlying hyalinization in a "recent" response to radium. × 50, and *D*, complete fibrosis and hyalinization of the uterine cervix in an "old" response to radium. × 50.

literation of the bascular lumen. This results in ischemia and the ischemia, in turn, contributes to the necrosis. Early irradiation changes in the *stroma* are similar to those in any inflammation. They consist of capillary dilatation and exudation of serum, fibrin, and a variety of leukocytes. Later changes consist of fibrinoid degeneration, fibroblastic proliferation, and ultimately severe hyalinization (Fig. 84, *C* and *D*). These stromal alterations also contribute to ischemic degeneration and necrosis of the area as a whole.

While the basic pathologic changes in any organ or tissue exposed to sufficient irradiation are similar to those just described, some of the alterations peculiar to a few of the systems may be mentioned briefly. As already stated, the *hematopoietic* system is the most vulnerable. The first change is a depression of formation and release of white blood cells from the normal depots resulting in leukopenia. This is followed by disorders of the clotting mechanism and eventuates in a tendency to bleed from mucosal surfaces and into the tissues. The process is, of course, the same as that seen in acute radiation syndrome (see succeeding paragraph) and usually results only from total-body irradiation. Of the various theories advanced for the bleeding (see below), thrombocytopenia appears to be the most logical for hemorrhage is prevented or arrested by transfusion of intact platelets (Upton). Aside from leukopenia and bleeding, depression of the hematopoietic system is also attended by impairment of antibody (including properdin) formation, resulting in an acute illness during the second week. During the next few weeks there is, in addition, a deficiency in formation of erythrocytes with development of varying degrees of anemia. Just as it is vulnerable, the hematopoietic system has a remarkable capacity for regeneration and this occurs if the patient survives the first month. The *intestinal tract* is likewise quite vulnerable and may be disturbed as a result of local irradiation to the abdomen, irradiation of intra-abdominal organs such as the uterus, or total-body irradiation. The changes are also identical with those found in the acute radiation syndrome (see below). The early effects consist of degeneration, necrosis, and ulceration while the late effects consist of fibrosis and depletion of mucosal cells (Fig. 85). While the irradiation has a definite destructive effect upon the mucosal cells of the intestines, the extensive ulceration that occurs is probably due to the presence of bacteria and the passage of fecal material (Friedman). This is borne out in experiments on rabbits, where ulcers fail to develop when the fecal stream is deflected by colostomy. The complications of irradiation enteritis, colitis, or proctitis are perforation and adhesion formation. The earliest change in the *osseous* system is seen in growing children in the form of retardation of epiphyseal growth. In adults, the most obvious changes are noted around tooth sockets and at the ends of long bones (Marshak). They are especially prone to occur when radium is administered internally, for by such a route it has a propensity to lodge in bone. The changes noted are coarsing of the trabeculæ followed in time by areas of rarefaction, cyst formation, and sclerosis. The changes are due in part to the direct action of the rays on the bone and in part to vascular occlusion of the vessels supplying the bone. The ultimate result is softening, collapse, and destruction of weight-bearing bones. In the *lungs* the early changes consist of congestion, edema, some leukocytic infiltration, and increased secretion. The late changes are indicated by extensive fibrosis (Fig. 86). The *thyroid* responds by depression of secretory activity and later by destruction of the epithelial cells and diffuse fibrosis. The *gonads*, both male and female, react by degeneration and destruction of the sperm producing cells and ova. If the irradition is great enough permanent sterility results. The *uterus*, frequently irradiated for carcinoma of the cervix or endometrium, responds grossly by acute, necrotizing, ulceration followed later by fibrosis (Fig. 87, *A*). The microscopic changes consist of destruction of the epithelium, fibrinoid degeneration

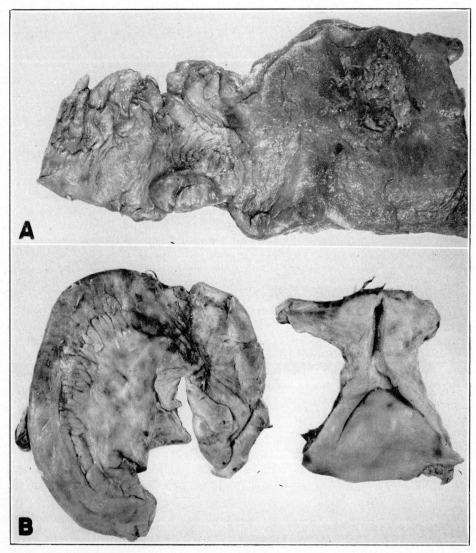

FIG. 85.—Irradiation effects showing *A*, acute inflammation and ulceration of the rectum caused by irradiation of the cervix for carcinoma and *B*, fibrosis and perforation of a loop of small intestine also resulting from irradiation of carcinoma of the cervix.

and necrosis of connective tissue followed later by extensive fibrosis, and vascular occlusion by endothelial proliferation and swelling (Fig. 84). The most common acute complications are irradiation cystitis, proctitis, and enteritis while the most common chronic complication is perforation of the ulcers with fistulas developing between the uterus and vagina on the one hand and the urinary bladder, rectum, and pouch of Douglas on the other (Fig. 87). The chief change in the *eyes* is the formation of cataracts. This is more prevalent with neutron (cyclotron workers) than with roentgen ray exposure. Irradiation of *embryos* results in the formation of a variety of congenital malformations—depending upon the stage of embryonic development. Such changes, however, are not transmittable to the off-spring and have therefore nothing to do with *genetic mutations*. The latter, while they definitely do occur, are more difficult to evaluate in man. They have, however, been specifically determined and established in plants,

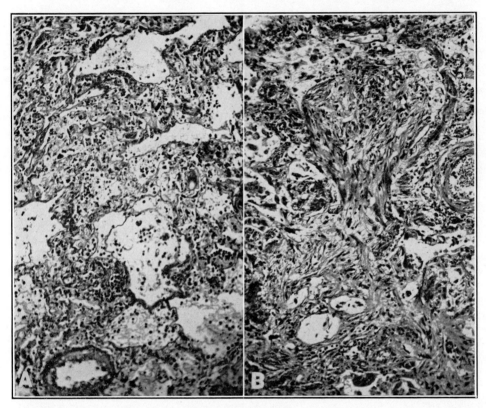

FIG. 86.—Irradiation effect Illustrating *A*, congestion, edema, and leukocytic infiltration of the lung and *B*, extensive diffuse fibrosis of the entire pulmonary parenchyma. × 100.

insects, and experimental animals (Glass). As a result of such work, there is not doubt that permanent hereditary alterations transmitted to progeny do develop in the genes of the chromosomes from exposure to irradiation. These alterations may or may not be visible microscopically. Finally, while all tissues respond to irradiation, the degree of pathologic change varies somewhat with *sensitivity* of the individual. This is greater in the young and in the old than in the age period between these extremes. Growing tissues are more susceptible than adult tissues and severe stresses, as for example burns and exhaustion, augment tissue reactions.

Aside from the untoward effects of irradiation described above two other serious *complications* that may arise are acute radiation syndrome and cancer. *Acute radiation syndrome* constitutes a symptom complex follow-

240 Physical Disturbances

ing total body exposure to damaging amounts of penetrating irradiation (Bowers and Lyon). While parts of the syndrome may occur in connection with (1) excessive roentgen treatment of generalized disorders such as leukemias, (2) over-administration of radioactive isotopes, or (3) heavy irradiation of the abdomen, the complete syndrome is seen only in connection with

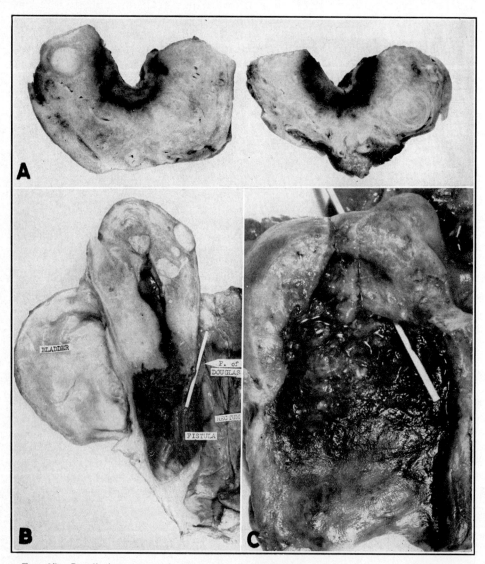

Fig. 87.—Irradiation changes in the uterus showing *A*, superficial ulceration and necrosis of the endometrium and adjacent myometrium, *B*, fistulas between the cervical portion of the vagina and pouch of Douglas and between the vagina and rectum, and *C*, a fistula between the uterine cavity and the pouch of Douglas and rectum.

over-exposure in the handling of atomic energy materials or explosion of an atomic bomb. The *pathologic* changes in the various tissues are similar to those already described with destruction of the cells of the hematopoietic system, skin, and mucosa of the gastrointestinal tract dominating the scene. As would be expected, therefore, the *symptoms* and *signs* are referable to the three systems most severely affected. Disturbances of the *hematopoietic system* result in hemorrhagic diathesis. This occurs in from four days to four weeks after exposure and is due to thrombocytopenia, increased permeability of blood vessels, and the appearance in the circulating blood of an anticoagulant resembling heparin. The bleeding consists of petechiæ, purpuras, melena, epistaxis, and metrorrhagia. If the patient survives he is apt to develop severe hypoplastic anemia. Disturbances of the *skin* are identical with those already described. Included in the untoward effects on the integument is epilation (loss of hair). This occurs only in areas of the skin exposed to the irradiation and, although all the hair may be lost, its regrowth in patients that survive is ultimately complete. Disturbances of the *gastrointestinal tract* consist of degeneration, necrosis, and extensive sloughing of the mucosa and are attended by nausea, vomiting, severe diarrhea with blood and mucus in the stools, and extreme dehydration. The *course* in acute radiation syndrome may be rapid with death from the acute destructive processes (including hemorrhage and infection) occurring in from one to six weeks or it may be more protracted with death from severe hypoplastic anemia occurring after six weeks. Patients with less exposure frequently recover.

The development of *cancer* is a late sequel of over-exposure to irradiation, usually occuring after lapse of several years. While the irradiation may act directly on the cells with resulting changes which progress to cancer in subsequent daughter cells, it is more likely that the effect is indirect and represents a sequence to chronic damage of tissue with resultant irregular repair (Brues). The latent period between irradiation and the development of cancer supports this contention. Without going into details there is ample evidence indicating the development of the following cancers as a sequel to irradiation: (1) carcinoma of the skin in areas irradiated for such benign conditions as acne vulgaris and in hands of physicians using roentgen rays in the early post-discovery days, (2) leukemia, especially in radiologists and in survivors of atomic bomb explosions in Japan (Lewis and Warren), (3) carcinoma of the thyroid in adults after irradiation of the thymus in infancy and in children after administration of radioactive iodine, (4) hemangio-endothelioma after parenteral administration of thorotrast, (5) carcinoma of the lung in Schneeberg miners after prolonged inhalation of radon dust, (6) osteosarcoma of bone after systemic absorption of strontium and radium as well as after irradiation of bones for benign conditions (Cruz), and (7) fibrosarcoma of soft parts after external irradiation (Pettit). Aside from retrogressive processes and repair producing cancer, direct hormonal stimulation may also be an important mechanism (Warren). In mice, for example, destruction of the thyroid by radioactive iodine results in the production of tumors of the pituitary gland by way of continued stimulation by thyrotropes. Similarly, irradiation of the ovaries depresses ovarian tissue. What is left is then stimulated to tumor formation by the continued action of gonadotropes.

Atomic Explosion.—Injury incurred as a result of an atomic explosion is essentially of three types—trauma, burns, and irradiation. The *trauma* sustained may be (1) a direct hit in which case, of course, the body just disintegrates, (2) air blast (p. 224), (3) indirect from flying objects (especially glass) and consisting of contusions, concussions, lacerations, fractures, etc., and (4) general resulting from the last two categories mentioned and consisting essentially of shock and crush syndrome. The *burns* sustained are of two types—flash and flame. Flash burns are the result of the direct action of radiant energy. The latter covers the entire width of the spectrum, resembles the sun, and consists essentially of ultraviolet rays, visible light, and infrared rays. The effects of these rays have already been considered in the earlier part of this chapter in the section on Light (p. 231). In an atomic explosion, the exposure is brief but intense and only parts of the body exposed directly to the rays are affected. Flame burns occur as a result of ignition of inflammable materials. They are not a serious problem because fires start in the area of explosion—an area where the victims are killed outright. The *irradiation* sustained is identical with irradiation from other sources. This has been discussed in the preceding section.

CHEMICALS

Chemicals causing retrogressive changes in tissues are too numerous to discuss here in any detail. The topic naturally falls in the realm of toxicology. In general, chemicals *gain entrance* into the body by ingestion, inhalation, parental administration, or absorption through the skin. Regardless of the portal of entry, many of the compounds are detoxified in the liver and, in an altered or unaltered form, are excreted by the kidneys or large bowel. Most chemicals are *poisonous* when received in appropriate amounts. Many produce damage to the tissues they first contact, while others affect distant organs more profoundly. In any given case, poisoning may be suicidal, homicidal, or accidental (including therapeutic and industrial). The *symptoms* and *signs* are protean and, of course, are referable to the tissues and organs sustaining the injury. While the *pathologic changes* may be characteristic of poisoning by a certain chemical they are not necessarily pathognomonic and the surest method of identifying the compound, therefore, is by *chemical analysis*. The materials to be saved at necropsy for analysis vary with the chemical compound in question. In a cursory fashion they have already been listed in connection with The Autopsy (p. 21). Because of the vastness of the topic, only a few of the more common poisons will be referred to and since there is no good method of classification, the chemicals will be listed alphabetically.

Acids causing bodily injury are usually taken by mouth for suicidal purposes. The immediate effects are burns involving the skin and the high spots of the upper gastrointestinal tract, namely, lips, mouth, pharynx, esophagus, and stomach. The discoloration of the burn varies with the acid. That produced by *sulphuric acid* is brown to black, by *nitric acid* yellow, by *hydrochloric acid* white, by *oxalic acid* brown, and by *carbolic acid* (phenol) white to pale brown or yellowish. If the patient survives, the affected area undergoes sloughing, ulceration, intense inflammation, and (later) fibrosis. *Cresols* (homologues of carbolic acid) and *lysol* (50% solution of cresol) have effects similar to those of carbolic acid.

Alcohol, as a cause of poisoning in man, usually exists in two forms—ethyl and methyl. *Ethyl* alcohol is that present in ordinary liquor. Concentrations in the blood up to 0.1 per cent result in some intoxication, from 0.1 to 0.2 per cent in severe intoxication, from 0.4 to 0.5 per cent in stupor or coma, and from 0.7 to 1.0 per cent in death. Acute poisoning results in severe gastritis, odor of alcohol in the stomach and lungs, and edema of the brain. Chronic poisoning is accompanied by lowering of resistance to infection, vitamin deficiency, and fatty change and cirrhosis of the liver. There is also injury to brain cells, for upon withdrawal of alcohol the patient often develops delerium tremens and acute insanity. *Methyl* alcohol is obtainable commercially as such and is often a component of "bootleg" liquor. Acute poisoning is accompanied by changes similar to those caused by ethyl alcohol. Recovery from a bout is followed by optic atrophy and blindness.

Alkalies are often ingested with suicidal intent by adults and accidentally by children. The common alkalies are caustic soda (sodium hydroxide), caustic potash (potassium hydroxide), quicklime (calcium oxide), ammonia water (ammonium hydroxide) and lye (sodium hydroxide with some sodium carbonate added). Except for the discolorations, the tissue changes are similar to those produced by acids.

Alkaloids as a cause of poisoning in man usually comprise opium, morphine, strychnine, cocaine, and atropine. A correct diagnosis is made from a consideration of the history, clinical findings before death, and chemical analysis. There are no characteristic pathologic changes.

Antibiotics (penicillin), when first introduced in 1943, were relatively safe, for their administration was not attended by any untoward reactions (Kern). With their continued use, however, sensitivity manifestations began to crop up until at present they cover almost the whole gamut of allergic reactions. While the sensitivities may occur in any person, they are most common and most severe in those with a history of allergy. The reactions (1) develop during the course of the second or subsequent doses of the drugs, (2) appear after topical, parenteral, or gastrointestinal routes of administration, and (3) develop in from a few minutes to 10 days after receiving the antibiotic. They consist of (1) a variety of skin eruptions including dermatitis medicamentosa, urticaria, erythema nodosa, erythema multiforme, contact dermatitis, exfoliative dermatitis, bullous dermatitis, and purpura, (2) serum sickness type of reaction manifested by pruritus, urticaria, joint pains, irregular fever, and eosinophilia, (3) agranulocytosis, (4) photosensitivity, (5) periarteritis nodosa, and (6) anaphylaxis. To prevent or minimize such reactions antibiotics (1) should not be given for minor ailments, (2) should not be applied locally, (3) should be given orally whenever possible, and (3) should not be combined parenterally with other possible antigens. Sensitivity can be readily identified by skin testing.

Antimony poisoning usually occurs as a result of ingestion of tartar emetic. It is generally accidental but may be suicidal or homicidal. Its action and the changes produced are similar to those caused by arsenic.

Arsenic is present in Paris green, rat poisons, Fowler's solution, fly paper, tree sprays, paper glazes, wall paper, etc. Poisoning may be suicidal, homicidal, or accidental (including therapeutic and industrial) and the chemical may gain entrance into the body by ingestion, absorption through the skin or vagina, or parenteral administration. In acute poisoning with death occurring up to twenty-four hours, the only pathologic change is hyperemia of the viscera. When death is delayed for several days there are severe inflammations of the entire gastrointestinal tract and necrosis of the liver. In either case, crystals of arsenic may be found between the folds of the gastric mucosa. In chronic poisoning, there are pigmentation and keratinization of the skin, loss of hair and nails, fatty change in the liver, heart, and kidneys, degenerative changes in the brain, optic atrophy, and neuritis.

Aspirin (acetylsalicylic acid) is the most commonly used medicinal agent in the world. While the vast majority of patients do not show any untoward reactions upon repeated use, a few, especially those with an allergic history, do develop sensitivity. This is manifested chiefly in the form of asthma, allergic rhinitis, and urticaria (Walton). Such allergic manifestations are usually seen in adults, are more common in males than females, and are attended by a mortality that is about four times as high as it is in other allergies. Aside from hypersensitivity, acetyl salicylic cid may produce poisoning, especially in children, as a result of overdosage (Harvie). Taken by ingestion the drug is promptly absorbed into the blood stream, reaching a peak level in about one and one half hours. Most of it is excreted by the kidneys in from 15 to 30 hours. Overdosage (poisoning) is attended by (1) hyperventilation (as a result of stimulation of the respiratory center) with resultant fall in plasma CO_2 and rise in plasma pH, (2) renal manifestations of diuresis followed by oliguria, (3) sweating and antipyresis, (4) hemorrhages from vasodilation and reduction in prothrombin, (5) ketosis, and (6) stimulation and then depression of the central nervous system encompassing excitement, disorientation, convulsions, stupor, and respiratory failure. Other manifestations include headache, tinnitus, deafness, vertigo, and hyperpnea. Death, when it occurs, is due to depression of the respiratory center.

Barbiturates comprise, among others, phenobarbital, veronal, and nembutal. They are used therapeutically as sedatives, are habit-forming, and are usually taken as an overdose. In acute poisoning there are no characteristic pathologic changes. In chronic poisoning the following may be present: mental confusion, ataxia, nausea, cutaneous rashes and ulcers, and rarely necrosis of the globus pallidus.

Benzene (benzol) is used in industry as a solvent. Poisoning may be accidental or suicidal. The chemical enters the body by ingestion or inhalation. Acute poisoning may result in death from respiratory failure and pathologically is not accompanied by any specific changes. Chronic poisoning is attended by destruction of the bone marrow and hypoplastic anemia.

Bismuth is usually administered orally in the form of bismuth subnitrate and bismuth subcarbonate, cutaneously in the form of salves, and intramuscularly in the form of a variety of preparations. Poisoning is generally accidental. Postmortem examination reveals (1) bluish-black spongy gums with loosened teeth, (2) ulcerative, pseudomembranous (grayish-black) enteritis and colitis which may lead to perforation, (3) parenchymatous degeneration of the liver, and (4) acute toxic nephrosis.

Boric acid (white powder) and *borax* (crystals) may cause accidental death in infants when used (mistakenly) subcutaneously instead of saline. The lesions consist of an acute dermatitis and acute toxic nephrosis.

Carbon dioxide is a gas that may cause death by asphyxiation. Such accidents may occur when an individual descends into a manhole or a well where the air has not been disturbed for a long time, or when he is imprisoned in a small room or safe where there is insufficient or no ventilation. The pathologic changes are those of asphyxia (p. 246). The gas is detected by analyzing a sample of the air.

Carbon monoxide is available in illuminating gas, mine explosions, and exhausts from automobiles. When it is present in concentrations up to 0.1 per cent it is responsible for headache, nausea, vertigo, and muscular weakness. When it is present in greater concentrations it produces unconsciousness and death. Pathologically the gas unites with hemoglobin to produce carboxyhemoglobin which is demonstrable both spectroscopically and chemically. The patient actually dies from asphyxia. At postmortem the tissues and blood are bright cherry red in color and the blood remains completely fluid. When death is delayed there are, in addition, bilateral necrosis of the globus pallidus and necrosis of the papillary muscles of the left ventricle of the heart.

Carbon tetrachloride is used as a solvent in industry and as a liquid cleaning agent for furniture and machines. Poisoning may occur by inhalation and, less commonly, by ingestion. Pathologically there are acute central necrosis of the liver and acute toxic nephrosis.

Chloral hydrate, also known as "knock-out" drops, is a favorite means of inducing submission when felony (especially rape or robbing) is contemplated. Occasionally an overdose is accidental. Death is usually rapid. At autopsy, crystals of the chemical may be found between the folds of the gastric mucosa. There are no other specific findings.

Chloroform used to be an important chemical when its use as an anesthetic was in vogue. Poisoning has also occurred as a result of its ingestion. When death is acute there is an odor of chloroform to the lungs, brain, and other tissues. When it is delayed there are frequently degenerations and necrosis of the liver and fatty changes in the heart and kidneys.

Copper is poisonous when in salt form. It is usually taken by mouth and death has been suicidal, homicidal, or accidental. At postmortem the following may be encountered: (1) green discoloration and ulceration of the upper gastrointestinal tract and colon, (2) fatty and parenchymatous change in the liver, and (3) acute toxic nephrosis.

Cyanides are used commercially in the form of salts in photography and silverplating and in the form of hydrocyanic acid in the disinfection of houses and ships. Poisoning may be suicidal, homicidal, or accidental and death is rapid. Pathologically, an odor of bitter almonds emits from various organs (especially the brain) and the blood is bright red and remains fluid for a prolonged period. If the chemical is taken by mouth the mucosa of the stomach is at first discolored crimson red and then rusty brown.

Gold salts have been used from time to time in the treatment of such chronic disorders as tuberculosis and arthritis. The compounds are administered by injection and poisoning is usually accidental. Locally there is yellow to violet necrosis of the tissues at the site of injection. Systemically, the skin shows dermatitis, keratosis, macules and papules; the hair and fingernails fall out; gold is deposited within the cells of the reticulo-endothelial system; there is a moderate to severe gastroenteritis, and there are hemorrhages of the gums.

Halogens consist of chlorine (yellowish-green gas or liquid), bromine (liquid or vapor), iodine (solid, liquid, or vapor) and fluorine (powder or liquid). They are strong corrosives. When inhaled they cause suffocation and irritation of the respiratory tract and when ingested they produce a gastroenteritis.

Lead poisoning, known also as plumbism, has already been considered in connection with Pigmentations (p. 83).

Mercury, often but not always, in the form of bichloride (corrosive sublimate) may be taken orally, cutaneously, parenterally, and by inhalation, and poisoning may be suicidal, accidental, or homicidal. When taken by mouth in the form of a strong solution it produces grayish-white coagulation necrosis of the high spots of the upper gastrointestinal tract similar to that produced by carbolic acid. When taken in tablet form it causes local necrosis and ulceration of the gastric mucosa. Regardless of the route of entrance, mercury is excreted by the large bowel where it produces a membranous colitis with extensive ulcerations and by the kidneys where it produces acute toxic nephrosis with early tubular calcification. Occasionally the gums become hemorrhagic and spongy and the teeth become loosened.

Paraldehyde is used as a quieting agent and is administered by mouth or rectum. Overdosage may cause death. The autopsy findings are not characteristic. The lungs and urine emit a distinct odor, but the other changes consist of inflammation of the stomach and generalized hyperemia of the viscera.

Phosphorus (yellow or white) was formerly used in the manufacture of matches and is still used in the manufacture of rat poison and fireworks. Poisoning may be homicidal, suicidal, or accidental (in children or when used as an abortifacient). Sudden death is due to central nervous system paralysis. It is accompanied by a garlic-like odor to the tissues and hyperemia of the viscera. Acute but delayed (several days) death is accompanied by hemorrhagic inflammation of the stomach, acute necrosis of the liver, and fatty changes in the kidneys, heart, and voluntary muscles. Chronic poisoning usually occurs in industry and is brought about by inhalation of phosphorous vapor. In addition to the fatty changes already referred to there is necrosis of the jaw ("phossy jaw") with loss of teeth.

Nitrous oxide is a colorless gas with a sweetish taste and smell and, in a mixture of 20 per cent oxygen, is used as an anesthetic. Death is usually due to an abnormally high concentration of nitrous oxide in the inhalant. The pathologic changes are those of *asphyxia* (cyanosis of the face, injection of conjunctiva, cyanotic hyperemia of all the organs, dark fluid blood, and petechiæ of the lungs, pericardium, pleura, and mucosal surfaces).

Silver poisoning, known also as argyria, has already been discussed in connection with Pigmentations (p. 84).

Smoke, as in burning buildings, produces death by way of carbon dioxide and carbon monoxide. If the patient survives he is likely to develop bronchitis and bronchopneumonia.

Sulfonamides are therapeutic agents used in the treatment of a variety of infections. They are administered by mouth and parenterally. Overdosages or sensitivity may cause death. The essential pathologic changes may consist of agranulocytosis, hepatic necrosis, dermatitis, and acute toxic nephrosis.

War gases actually consist of gases, smokes, volatilized liquids, and fine powders. Four general types of compounds are (1) *tear gas* (brombenzyl cyanide)—causing severe lacrimation and temporary blindness, (2) *lung irritants*—consisting of chlorine, phosgene, chlorpicrin, and chlormethyl chloroformate and producing severe inflammatory edema of the lungs with death from asphyxia, (3) *vesicant gases*—consisting of (*a*) mustard gas (dichlorethyl sulphide) which produces vesication of the skin, conjunctivitis, and inflammation of the respiratory tract and (*b*) lewisite (chlorvinyl dichlorarsin) which produces blisters of the skin and hemolysis of erythrocytes, and (4) *arsenic compounds*—consisting of fine powders that are irritating to the respiratory tract but are usually not lethal.

REFERENCES

Circulatory Disturbances

ALTSCHULE, M. D.: Medicine, *17*, 75, 1938 (Cardiac Decompensation).
BARTTER, F. C.: Metabolism, *5*, 369, 1956 (Aldosterone, Homeostasis, and Disease).
BLACK, D. A. K.: *Essentials of Fluid Balance*, Springfield, Ill., Charles C Thomas Co., 1957.

BRAHAM, J., and HOWELLS, G.: Brit. M. J., *1*, 830, 1948 (Milroy's Edema).

BREED, E. S.: Med. Cl. N. Amer., *41*, 669, 1957 (Shock).

CODY, M. L., and WINDROW, P. B.: J. A. M. A., *147*, 1760, 1951 (Air Embolism in Pregnancy).

DARROW, D. C., and YANNET, H.: J. Clin. Invest., *14*, 266, 1935 (Body Water and Extra-Extracellular Electrolytes).

DURANT, T. M., *et al.:* Am. Heart J., *38*, 481, 1949 (Arteriolar Air Embolism).

ELKINTON, J. R., and DANOWSKI, I. S.: *The Body Fluids. Basic Physiology and Practical Therapeutics*, Baltimore, Williams & Wilkins Co., 1955.

FADELL, E. J., and SULLIVAN, B. H.: Armed Forces M. J., *8*, 114, 1957 (Fat Embolism from Liver).

FAHR, G., and ERSHLER, I.: Ann. Int. Med., *15*, 798, 1941 (Capillary Pressure in Edema).

GAMBLE, J. L.: *Chemical Anatomy, Physiology, and Pathology of Extracellular Fluid*, Cambridge, Mass., Harvard University Press, 1950.

GARVIN, C. F.: Am. J. M. Sci., *205*, 515, 1943 (Cardiac Cirrhosis).

HARRISON, T. R.: *Failure of the Circulation*, 2nd Ed., Baltimore, The Williams & Wilkins Co., 1939.

ISRAEL, H. L., and GOLDSTEIN, F.: Ann. Int. Med., *47*, 202, 1957 (Pulmonary Embolism Clinically).

JOHNSON, S. R., and SVANBORG, A.: Ann. Surg., *144*, 145, 1956 (Fat Embolism).

KARSNER, H. P., *et al.:* J. A. M. A., *57*, 951, 1911, J. Med. Res., *27*, 205, 1912, and J. Exper. Med., *18*, 507, 1913 (Infarction).

LEVY, L. J.: Am. Surg., *18*, 637, 1952 (Fat Embolism).

LEWIS, H. B.: J. A. M. A., *138*, 207, 1948 (Proteins in Nutrition).

LIVERMORE, G. R.: Am. Practitioner, *7*, 20, 1956 (Shock).

LOVE, J. L., and STRYKER, W. S.: Ann. Int. Med., *46*, 342, 1957 (Fat Embolism).

MOON, V. H.: Am. J. Path., *24*, 235, 1948 (Pathology of Shock).

————: *Shock. Its Dynamics, Occurrence, and Management*, Philadelphia, Lea & Febiger, 1942.

MOON, V. H., *et al.:* J. A. M. A., *117*, 2024, 1941 (Shock and Hemorrhage).

OSTFELD, A.: Conn. State M. J., *19*, 159, 1955 (Syncope).

PARKER, F., JR., and WEISS, S.: Am. J. Path., *12*, 573, 1936 (Lungs in Mitral Stenosis).

PASS, I. J.: Am. J. Path., *11*, 503, 1935 (Hepatic Infarction).

PELTIER, L. F.: Internat. Abst. Surg., *104*, 313, 1957 (Fat Embolism).

RELMAN, A. S., and SCHWARTZ, W. B.: J. Clin. Invest., *34*, 959, 1955 (Nephropathy of Potassium Depletion).

SCHREADER, C. J.: A.M.A. Arch. Int. Med., *98*, 142, 1956 (Syncope).

SCHOFIELD, G. F., and BEAIRD, J. B.: Am. J. Clin. Path., *28*, 400, 1957 (Amniotic Fluid Embolism).

SHAPIRO, J. H., *et al.:* Am. J. Roent., *77*, 1055, 1957 (Oil Embolism).

SHARPEY-SCHAFER, E. P., *et al.:* Brit. M. J., *2*, 304, 1942 (Rapid Intravenous Injections).

SILVERBERG, M.: Physiol. Rev., *18*, 197, 1938 (Mechanism of Thrombosis).

SLUDER, H. M., *et al.:* Am. J. Obst. & Gynec., *64*, 118, 1952 (Amniotic Fluid Embolism).

SUNDERMAN, F. W.: Am. J. Clin. Path., *16*, 353, 1946 (Edema and Dehydration).

WARREN, S.: Am. J. Path., *22*, 69, 1946 (Fat Embolism).

WEECH, A. A., and LING, S. N.: J. Clin. Invest., *10*, 869, 1931 (Nutritional Edema).

WINTROBE, M. M.: *Clinical Hematology*, 3rd Ed., Philadelphia, Lea & Febiger, p. 244, 1951, (Coagulation of Blood).

WOOTTON, I. D. P., and KING, E. J.: Lancet, *1*, 470, 1953 (Normal Values Blood Electrolytes).

YOUNG, RAYMOND L., *et al.:* A. M. A. Arch. Path., *46*, 43, 1948 (Paradoxical Embolism).

Trauma

BYWATERS, E. G. L.: J. A. M. A., *124*, 1103, 1944 (Crush Syndrome).

COHEN, H., and BISKIND, G. R.: A. M. A. Arch. Path., *42*, 12, 1946 (Blast Injuries).

MORITZ, A. R.: *The Pathology of Trauma*, 2nd Ed., Philadelphia, Lea & Febiger, 1954.

Thermal Disturbances

AUSTIN, M. G., and BERRY, J. W.: J.A.M.A., *161*, 1525, 1956 (Heat Stroke).

BAKER, R. D.: Am. J. Path., *21*, 717, 1945 (Burns).

BARNARD, C. N.: Br. J. Surg., *44*, 296, 1956 (Methods Hypothermia).

BIERMAN, W.: J.A.M.A., *157*, 1189, 1955 (General Hypothermia).

BIGELOW, W. G.: J. Thor. Surg., *28*, 463, 1954 (Physiology Hypothermia).

BROWN, K. L., and GLOVER, D. M.: J.A.M.A., *165*, 643, 1957 (Burns, Mass Casualties).

COLEBROOK, L., and COLEBROOK, V.: Lancet, *2*, 181, 1949 (Burns).

DAVIS, J. H., and ABBOTT, W. E.: Surgery, *40*, 788, 1956 (Pathology Burns).

EDWARDS, E. A.: J. A. M. A., *149*, 1199, 1952 (Frostbite).

EISEMAN, B., *et al.*: New Engl. J. Med., *255*, 750, 1956 (Hypothermia General Surgery).
FRIEDMAN, N. B.: Am. J. Clin. Path., *16*, 634, 1946 (Frostbite, etc.).
————: Am. J. Path., *21*, 387, 1945 (Trench Foot).
FRIEDMAN, N. B., and KRITZLER, R. A.: Am. J. Path., *23*, 173, 1947 (High-altitude Frostbite).
GRISWOLD, M. L.: J.A.M.A., *164*, 861, 1957 (Treatment Burns).
GROSSKRENTZ, D. C., *et al.*: J.A.M.A., *165*, 949, 1957 (Hypothermia Aortic Operations).
LEWIS, R. B.: Military Surg., *110*, 25, 1952 (Frostbite).
MALAMUD, N., *et al.*: Military Surg., *99*, 397, 1946 (Heat Stroke).
MORITZ, A. R.: Am. J. Path., *23*, 915, 1947 (Burns).
ROSS, D. N.: Guy's Hosp. Rep., *103*, 97 and 116, 1954 (Physiology and Methods Hypothermia).
SMITH, R. S.: J.A.M.A., *164*, 511, 1957 (Treatment Burns Children).
SWAN, H.: Arch. Surg., *69*, 597, 1954 (Editorial, Hypothermia).
TALBOTT, J. H.: New England J. Med., *224*, 281, 1941 (General Hypothermia).
UNGLEY, C. C., *et al.*: Brit. J. Surg., *33*, 17, 1945 (Immersion Foot).
WILLIAMS, D. I.: Practitioner, *171*, 619, 1953 (Chilblains).

Light

BLUM, H. F.: Physiol. Rev., *25*, 483, 1945 (Review).
LAURENS, H.: Physiol. Rev., *8*, 1, 1928 (Review).

Electricity

ALEXANDER, L.: J. Indust. Hyg. & Toxicol., *20*, 191, 1938 (Neuropathology).
HELPERN, M., and STRASSMANN, G.: Am. J. Path., *17*, 592, 1941 (Electrocution).
JAFFE, R. H.: A. M. A. Arch. Path., *5*, 837, 1928 (Review).
McLAUGHLIN, C. W., and COE, J. D.: A.M.A. Arch. Surg., *68*, 531, 1954 (Variables Burns).

Irradiation

Atomic Bomb: A Message from the Surgeon General and Medical Department, 1948.
AUERBACH, O., *et al.*: Cancer, 1095, 1951 (Sarcoma after Irradiation).
BOWERS, J. Z.: J. A. M. A., *145*, 63, 1951 (Irradiation Syndrome).
BRUES, A. M.: Radiation Res., *3*, 272, 1955 (Carcinogenic Action).
CRUZ, M., *et al.*, Cancer, *10*, 72, 1957 (Osteosarcoma).
FRIEDMAN, N. B.: A.M.A. Arch. Path., *59*, 2, 1955 (Intestinal Ulcers).
GLASS, B.: Science, *126*, 241, 1957 (Genetics).
HEMPELMANN, L. H., *et al.*: Ann. Int. Med., *36*, 279, 1952 (Radiation Syndrome).
LEWIS, E. B.: Science, *125*, 965, 1957 (Leukemia).
LIEBOW, A. A.: Am. J. Path., *25*, 853, 1949 (Atomic Bomb).
LYON, G. M.: Mil. Med., *118*, 279, 1956 (Radiation Syndrome).
MARSHAK, R. H., *et al.*: J.A.M.A., *160*, 41, 1956 (Osseous Changes).
PETTIT, V. D., *et al.*: Cancer, *7*, 149, 1954 (Fibrosarcoma).
SCHLUMBERGER, H. G., and VAZQUEZ, J. J.: Am. J. Path., *30*, 1013, 1954 (Experimental Total-Body).
SPITZ, S., and HIGGINBOTHAM, N. L.: Cancer, *4*, 1107, 1951 (Sarcoma after Irradiation).
TELOH, H. A., *et al.*: Surg., Gynec. & Obst., *90*, 335, 1950 (Radiation Injuries Skin).
UPTON, A. C.: Blood, *10*, 1156, 1955 (Cause Bleeding).
WARREN, S.: Arch. Path., *34*, 443, 1942 (Radiation of Normal Tissues).
————: Cancer Res., *17*, 1, 1957 (Carcinogenesis and Experimental).
————: J.A.M.A., *162*, 464, 1956 (Leukemia).
WARREN, S., and BOWERS, J. Z.: Ann. Int. Med., *32*, 207, 1950 (Radiation Syndrome).
WARREN, S., *et al.*: Science, *124*, 60, 1956 (Pathology).

Chemicals

FAIRHILL, L. T.: *Industrial Toxicology*, Baltimore, The Williams & Wilkins Co., 1949.
GLAISTER, J.: *Medical Jurisprudence and Toxicology*, 9th Ed., Baltimore, The Williams & Wilkins Co., 1950.
GONZALES, T. A., *et al.*: *Legal Medicine and Toxicology*, New York, Appleton-Century-Crofts, 1937.
HARVIE, F. H., and SINGER, R. B.: A.M.A. Am. J. Dis. Child., *89*, 149, 1955 (Salicylates in Children).
KERN, R. A., and WIMBERELY, N. A.: Am. J. Med. Sc., *226*, 357, 1953 (Penicillin Reactions).
THIENES, C. H., and HALEY, T. J.: *Clinical Toxicology*, Philadelphia, Lea & Febiger, 1948.
VON OETTINGEN, W. F.: *Poisoning*, New York, Paul B. Hoeber, Inc., 1952.
WALTON, C. H., and RANDLE, D. L.: Canad. Med. Ass. J., *76*, 1016, 1957 (Aspirin Allergy).

Chapter

7

Tumors

GENERAL CONSIDERATIONS

THE fifth broad category of general disease processes may be grouped under the heading of *Tumors.* Contrary to common belief, the group doubtlessly represents a heterologous collection of disorders comparable to *Congenital Anomalies, Degenerations, Inflammations,* or *Physical Disturbances* rather than a distinct single entity. Although true tumors have been recognized as such for centuries, their importance has recently catapulted (1) as a result of more effective control of infectious diseases by the use of antibiotics and chemotherapeutic agents in the last two decades, and (2) as a result of the greatly increased longevity since the turn of the last century. Because the topic is vast, with the lesions affecting all organs and tissues of the body, it obviously cannot be covered in any detail in a single chapter. The aim of the present dissertation, therefore, is to present some general facts for purposes of orientation. Specific lesions affecting specific organs are considered in subsequent sections of the book. The ensuing discussion may be conveniently divided into the following: definition, classification, pathologic appearance, spread, incidence, cause in laboratory animals, cause in man, diagnosis, treatment, and prognosis.

DEFINITIONS

The word *tumor* (L. = to swell) means a swelling or a morbid enlargement. While it is still used in connection with inflammation and other swellings, more and more it is reserved to indicate a new growth — a mass of new tissue. A more elaborate definition would perhaps be phrased thus — a mass of new tissue which persists and grows independently of its surrounding structures and which has no physiologic function. This, however, says both too much and too little, for some tumors are independent only until they reach certain dimensions beyond which they cease to grow, while a few tumors (islet cell, ovarian, and thyroid) have definite physiologic functions. The word *neoplasm* (Gr. = new formation) connotes any new and abnormal growth and is thus synonymous with tumor. *Neoplasia* denotes the formation of a neoplasm.

Tumors are generally divided into two main groups — *benign* and *malignant.* The term *benign* (L.) is an adjective, is used in conjunction with tumor, neoplasm or growth, and signifies of mild character or innocent. The term *malignant* (L.) is either a noun or an adjective although usually it is employed as the latter and, as such, is also used in conjunction with tumor, neoplasm, or growth. It signifies virulence or a tendency to progress from bad to worse. The word *malignancy* is a noun that denotes the state or quality of being malignant. Its use in conjunction with the grading of

(249)

tumors (see a succeeding section) is proper but its use as a substitute for the phrase malignant tumor is still considered to be improper. A *benign tumor* grows slowly, is often limited in size, is encapsulated, does not infiltrate adjacent tissues, remains localized, does not kill the patient except when strategically located, reproduces its parent tissue well, discloses few and regular mitoses, and does not recur after removal. In contrast, a *malignant tumor* grows rapidly, is usually unlimited in size, is not encapsulated, infiltrates adjacent tissues, spreads to distant areas, kills the patient by sapping his strength, does not reproduce its parent tissue well, discloses many and often irregular mitoses, and has a tendency to recur after removal.

A *carcinoma* (Gr. = crab) is a malignant tumor arising from and composed of epithelium. Embryologically, epithelium usually arises from ectoderm and entoderm but occasionally, as in the case of the urinary and genital tracts, it also arises from mesoderm. A *sarcoma* (Gr. = fleshy tumor) is a malignant tumor arising from and composed of tissues of mesodermal origin excluding that which gives rise to the urinary and genital tract epithelium. The term *cancer* (Gr. or L. = crab) is a malignant tumor composed of epithelial cells and is, therefore, synonymous with carcinoma. Currently, however, its use has been broadened to indicate any malignant tumor and it thus encompasses both a carcinoma and a sarcoma. The word *precancerous* is an adjective used in conjunction with lesion and generally signifies a process that is not at present cancer but will, if given time, develop into cancer. The term is valid if used discreetly, although it is not acceptable by all workers in the field. *Hyperplasia* (Gr. = over + formation) signifies an abnormal multiplication of cells or an increase in number of normal cells in normal arrangement. *Hypertrophy* (Gr. = over + nutrition) indicates an enlargement of an organ or a tissue due principally to an increase in size of the cells but also to an increase in their number. *Anaplasia* (Gr. = backward + formation) denotes a reversion of the cells to a more primitive form. *Differentiation* signifies the degree to which a cell has matured. *Undifferentiation* connotes a lack of complete differentiation or maturity. *Dedifferentiation* implies that a cell has reached maturity and has then reverted to an immature state. A *carcinogen* is a substance that brings about or produces cancer. A *cocarcinogen* is a substance that augments the action of a carcinogen; an *anticarcinogen* is a substance that inhibits the action of a carcinogen, while a *tumor inhibitor* is a substance that delays or stops the growth of a tumor or destroys the cells once they have proliferated.

CLASSIFICATION

Although the divisions and subdivisions of tumors are many and varied, a classification based on histogenesis (the cells giving rise to the growth) is generally conceded to be the most acceptable. Since similar tissues are present in many widely separated portions of the body, it is at once apparent that a certain type of tumor may be found in more than one organ or site. Conversely, because certain tissues are highly specialized or, at the other end of the scale, are extremely primitive, some neoplasms are unique and are confined entirely to specific areas of the body. In addition, to further complicate the picture, almost every tissue is capable of giving rise to both a benign and a malignant growth.

As for nomenclature, a benign tumor is usually designated by the addition of the suffix -oma to the root of the word indicating the tissue of origin (*e.g.*, fat tissue = lipoma) while a malignant tumor is usually designated by the addition of the terms carcinoma when the tumor is of epithelial origin (*e.g.*, squamous cells = squamous cell carcinoma) and sarcoma when it is other than epithelial in origin (*e.g.*, fat tissue = liposarcoma). Less commonly, a malignant tumor like a benign tumor is also designated by the addition of the suffix -oma to the root of a word indicating a primitive cell (*e.g.*, neuroblast = neuroblastoma). If more than one type of mesodermal cell comprises the tumor the roots of the nouns indicating the component cells may be strung together (*e.g.*, myxomatous tissue, connective tissue, and fat tissue = myxofibrolipoma). Finally, and fortunately rarely, some tumors are named after the authors who first described them (*e.g.*, tumor of primitive renal cells = Wilms' tumor).

Some examples of the more common tumors are listed in the accompanying table. The classification is purposely incomplete for the objective here, as already stated, is simply orientation. More detailed listings are presented in connection with the different systems and organs in appropriate places in the text.

Tissue of Origin	*Benign Tumor*	*Malignant Tumor*
Squamous epithelium	Papilloma	Squamous cell carcinoma
	———————	Basal cell carcinoma
Glandular epithelium	Adenoma	Adenocarcinoma
Transitional epithelium	Papilloma	Transitional cell carcinoma
Connective tissue	Fibroma	Fibrosarcoma
Myxomatous tissue	Myxoma	Myxosarcoma
Fat tissue	Lipoma	Liposarcoma
Smooth muscle	Leiomyoma	Leiomyosarcoma
Striated muscle	Rhabdomyoma	Rhabdomyosarcoma
	Myoblastoma	Malignant myoblastoma
Blood vessels	Hemangioma	Hemangioendothelioma
Lymphatic vessels	Lymphangioma	Lymphangiosarcoma
Nerves	Neurofibroma	Neurofibrosarcoma
	Neuroma	———————
Nerve ganglia	Ganglioneuroma	Neuroblastoma
	Pheochromocytoma	Pheochromoblastoma
Nerve endings	Nevus	Melanoblastoma
Reticulum cells	Benign lymphoma	Lymphoblastoma
Cartilage	Chondroma	Chondrosarcoma
Bone	Osteoma	Osteosarcoma
Bone marrow	Dystrophies	Multiple myeloma
		Ewing's tumor
	———————	Lymphoblastoma
Placental trophoblast	Hydatidiform mole	Chorionepithelioma
Mixed tissues	Dermoid cyst	Teratoma

PATHOLOGIC APPEARANCE

As would be expected, the pathologic appearances of the various tumors vary to such an extent that any over-all description must serve only as an approximation. In addition, it should be pointed out from the onset that frequently gross appearances are not distinctive enough to permit a definitive diagnosis and that in order to accomplish this a microscopic examination is essential. For purposes of discussion, neoplasms may be conveniently divided into two broad groups—epithelial and nonepithelial mesodermal.

Epithelial tumors may be divided into those arising from a surface such as the skin and mucous membranes and those arising within an organ such as the liver, pancreas, kidney, gonad, etc. Each, in turn, may be divided into benign and malignant. *Benign surface epithelial growths* exfoliate out-

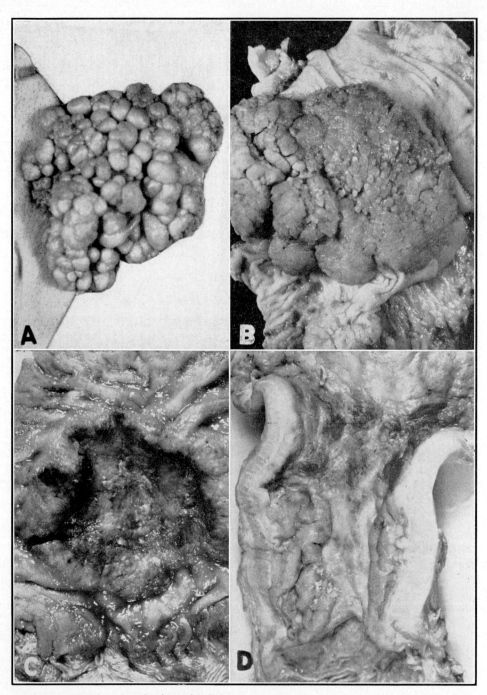

Fig. 88.—Showing *A*, a benign epithelial tumor (papilloma) of the nipple of a female breast, *B*, a protruding or papillary malignant epithelial tumor (carcinoma) of the mucosa of the colon, *C*, an ulcerating malignant epithelial tumor (carcinoma) of the mucosa of the rectum, and *D*, an infiltrating malignant epithelial tumor (carcinoma) of the mucosa of the stomach.

ward and are thus usually elevated, nodular, and pedunculated (Fig. 88*A*). Although they are firmly united with the subjacent tissues, they are not infiltrative and are, therefore, freely movable. The surface of the neoplasms located in the skin is usually rough, firm, and dry. That of tumors located in the mucous membranes is irregular, soft, and moist. In either case the surface is often serrated and the prongs are not adherent. Ulceration may or may not be present. Histologically the epithelial cells closely resemble the parent cells. They remain on the surface and do not penetrate the underlying structures. *Benign epithelial growths* arising *within organs* are grossly similar to benign nonepithelial mesodermal tumors (Fig. 89*A* and *C*). Histologically the cells reproduce the parent cells both in arrangement and appearance. *Malignant epithelial surface growths* are generally dividable into three groups—protruding or papillary, ulcerating, and infiltrating (Fig. 88*B*, *C*, and *D*). Protruding or papillary tumors resemble somewhat their benign counterpart with two exceptions—the prongs (when present) are often adherent to each other and, since the tumor always infiltrates the underlying tissue, it is not freely movable at its base. Ulcerating surface neoplasms are generally elevated above the adjacent tissues. The edges of the ulcer are somewhat undermined; the floor is covered with debris, and the base and sides are composed of firm white or gray tissue that is ill defined from its surroundings. Infiltrating surface growths differ from ulcerating neoplasms in that necrosis and sloughing of the tissue is minimal and permeation of adjacent structures is maximal. Histologically the neoplastic cells vary greatly from tumor to tumor and from area to area. At one extreme they still resemble closely, both in structure and arrangement, the cells whence they sprung. At the other extreme, they bear little or no similarity to the parent cells. In all instances the cells vary in shape, in size, and in staining qualities (usually being hyperchromatic) as compared with normal—characteristics which always differentiate a malignant growth from its benign counterpart. *Malignant epithelial tumors* arising *within organs* are small or bulky masses that are generally of a lighter (tan to white) color than the surrounding structures (Fig. 89*B*). They may merge imperceptibly with the adjacent tissues or they may be sharply defined but they are not encapsulated. They are usually quite firm and may even be hard. When they reach the surface of an organ they have a tendency to umbilicate centrally. This characteristic and the firmness are both due to the usual abundance of fibrous tissue that composes the stroma of the tumor. As a rule, larger tumors have a tendency to outgrow their blood supply and to undergo central necrosis and hemorrhage. Histologically the neoplasms in this group present essentially the same features as do the malignant surface epithelial growths.

Nonepithelial mesodermal growths always arise within, or at least beneath the covering of, an organ. They may be benign or malignant. Each of these, as in epithelial tumors, possesses the characteristics already outlined under Definitions above. *Benign nonepithelial mesodermal growths* measure from a few millimeters to many centimeters in diameter, are well encapsulated, are soft to hard depending upon the tissue comprising the tumor, are usually homogenous, and generally resemble the tissues whence they arose (Fig. 89*C*). As they increase in size they gradually protrude above the surface of the tissue that harbors them and when they become bulky enough the covering, whether skin or mucosa, gradually becomes attenuated and often ulcerated. Histologically, benign nonepithelial mesodermal

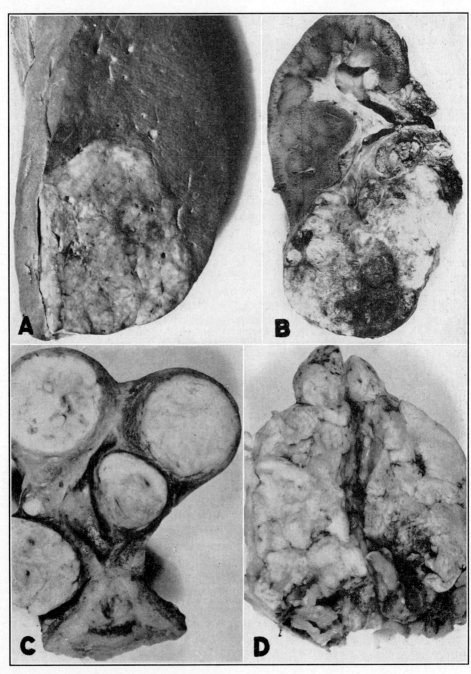

Fig. 89.—Showing *A*, a benign epithelial tumor (adenoma) arising within the liver, *B*, a malignant epithelial tumor (carcinoma) arising within a kidney, *C*, benign nonepithelial mesodermal tumors (leiomyomas or fibromyomas) arising within the uterus, and *D*, a malignant nonepithelial mesodermal tumor (liposarcoma) arising within the subcutaneous tissues.

growths resemble closely the parent tissues, be they fat, muscle, connective tissue, blood vessel, cartilage, or bone. *Malignant nonepithelial mesodermal growths* likewise measure from a few millimeters to many centimeters in diameter, appear sharply circumscribed but are not truly encapsulated, are generally quite soft and brainlike (except bony tumors), are fundamentally gray but because of necrosis and hemorrhage frequently present a mottled appearance, and, unlike malignant epithelial growths, do not present central umbilication upon reaching the surface (Fig. 89D). Histologically the tumors vary greatly in the degree of differentiation, although in all instances they too present variations in shape, size, and staining qualities of the cells. At one end of the scale they mimic the tissues whence they arose, while at the other end they bear little or no resemblance to the parent cells. As a rule, malignant nonepithelial mesodermal growths are more vascular and have a less abundant stroma than do comparable epithelial neoplasms.

In recent years considerable stress has been laid upon the relationship of the histologic appearance of a neoplasm to longevity. This is determined by what is known as *grading of tumors*. It is an attempt to predict the final outcome in the patient by noting the degree of departure (differentiation, undifferentiation, dedifferentiation, or anaplasia) of the neoplastic cells from normal. The basis underlying grading of tumors is the premise that the more primitive the cells the more rapidly do they spread and, conversely, the more mature the cells the more do they tend to remain localized. While this premise is generally true it does not always hold. One notable example is in cancer of the skin. A tumor reproducing basal cells is morphologically and chronologically more primitive than a tumor reproducing prickle or squamous cells, yet the latter is far more malignant than the former. Another exception to histologic grading of tumors (usually more apparent to pathologists than to clinicians) is the inescapable fact that a tumor frequently shows different degrees of maturity in different areas of the same mass and that microscopic examination confined, of necessity, to a minute area may thus be misleading. Then finally, it is also well known that a tumor composed of mature-appearing cells may have spread to distant portions of the body by the time the patient is first seen, while a neoplasm composed of immature cells may yet be entirely confined to a localized area. With these facts in mind it is apparent that grading of tumors has certain limitations but that it is of value provided it is considered in conjunction with the clinical picture. As to *nomenclature*, there are two classifications in vogue. The more commonly used classification divides the tumors into three groups—low grade, intermediate grade, and high grade. A tumor of low grade malignancy is one that histologically is quite mature—one that morphologically tends to mimic its parent cells (Fig. 90A and C and Fig. 91A). A tumor of high grade malignancy is one that histologically is quite immature—one that morphologically has no tendency to mimic its parent cells (Fig. 90B and D and Fig. 91B). A tumor of intermediate grade malignancy is one that morphologically is between these two extremes. Another classification that is used extensively, but that by many workers is considered to be too minute, is that of Broders. According to this classification, neoplasms are divided into Grades I, II, III, and IV. A comparison of the two classifications is as follows: Grade I corresponds to low grade, Grades II and III to intermediate grade, and Grade IV to high grade.

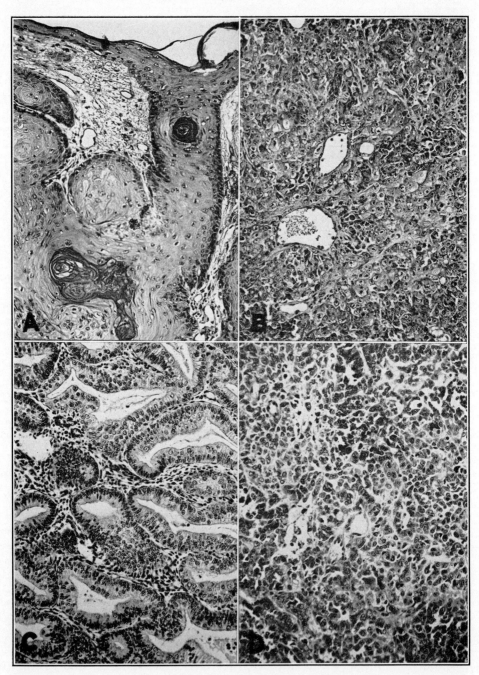

Fig. 90.—Histologic grading of tumors showing *A*, a squamous cell carcinoma of low grade malignancy, *B*, a squamous cell carcinoma of high grade malignancy, *C*, an adenocarcinoma of low grade malignancy, and *D*, an adenocarcinoma of high grade malignancy. × 100.

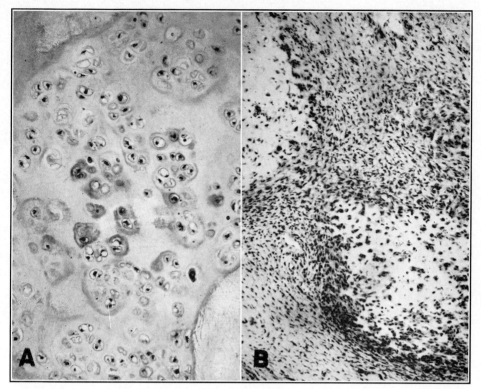

FIG. 91.—Histologic grading of tumors showing *A*, a chondrosarcoma of low grade malignancy, and *B*, a chondrosarcoma of high grade malignancy. × 100.

SPREAD

Benign tumors remain localized to the area of origin. As they enlarge they compress and distort the adjacent tissues. Frequently they become adherent to surrounding structures but this adherence is not due to infiltration by tumor cells but to adhesions which result from mechanical or chemical irritation. Sometimes the adhesions carry enough blood to secondarily revascularize the tumor. If, then, the original attachment of the growth becomes severed, the neoplasm loses its connection with the organ whence it arose and becomes parasitic on the tissue to which it has become adherent (common example is a pedunculated fibromyoma of the uterus becoming parasitic to another pelvic structure). Benign tumors do not spread to distant portions of the body. Although medical literature contains reports of "metastasizing adenomas of the thyroid" or "metastasizing leiomyomas of the uterus," such designations are incorrect for tumors behaving thus are really malignant despite their benign morphologic appearance.

Malignant tumors spread by three routes—infiltration, implantation, and metastasis.

Spread by *infiltration* occurs early in all malignant neoplasms. One of the characteristics of cancer cells is to insinuate themselves between adjacent normal cells and along tissue planes, set up secondary foci, and repeat the process. Although all tissues (including epithelium and bone) act as hosts,

17

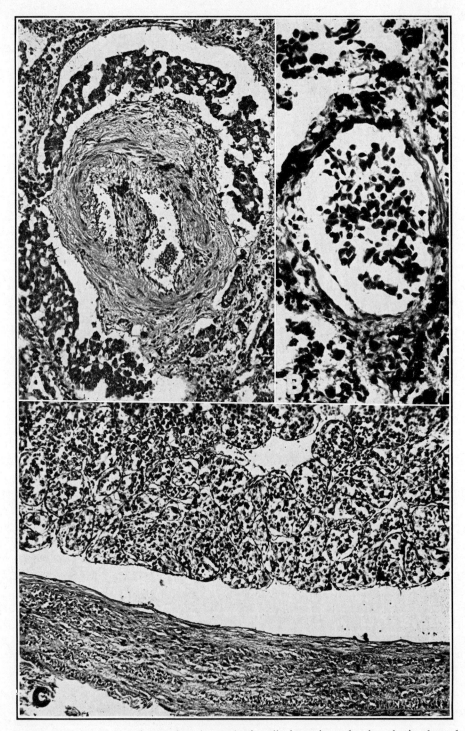

FIG. 92.—Tumor metastasis showing *A*, neoplastic cells in perivascular lymphatic channels, *B*, neoplastic cells in a pulmonary vein, and *C*, a mass of tumor tissue in a pulmonary artery. × 100.

spread by this route is especially easy in loose areolar or connective tissue (Fig. 90*A*).

Spread by *implantation* connotes the transfer of neoplastic cells from one organ or tissue through a space or potential space to another organ or tissue. Examples of such a method of spread are: cancer of the ovary seeding throughout the peritoneal cavity, cancer of the lung implanting on both pleural surfaces once the visceral pleura is reached, cancer of the larynx spreading to the lung by way of the tracheo-bronchial tree, and papillary carcinoma of the renal pelvis implanting on the vesical mucosa.

Spread by *metastasis* is perhaps the most important method of dissemination of the malignant tumor for it is by this means that the neoplasm often kills the patient. The word metastasis (Gr. = after + stand) literally means the transfer of any disease from one organ or part of the body to another not directly connected with it. With regards to malignant tumors, the term usually implies spread by way of vascular channels—both lymphatics and blood vessels. Metastasis by way of *lymphatic channels* occurs more frequently in carcinoma than in sarcoma. The tumor cells creep along the outside or inside of the lymphatic wall and are also carried with the lymphatic current as emboli (Fig. 92*A*). The direction of the latter is usually the same as the direction of the normal current but when a particular lymph channel is blocked, the direction of lymph flow and metastasis may be reversed. The first site of deposition of cancer spreading by lymphatic channels is the lymph nodes but beyond these cancer cells also reach the venous and (by way of the pulmonary capillaries) the arterial circulation and are then deposited throughout the body. Metastasis by way of *blood vessels* occurs both in carcinoma and sarcoma, but in the latter it is the chief method of dissemination. Both veins and arteries act as conveyors (Fig. 92*B* and *C*). The *veins* may be grouped into caval, portal, and prevertebral. The caval veins and their tributaries are responsible for metastasis to the lungs; the portal vein and its tributaries are responsible for metastasis to the liver, and the prevertebral veins are responsible for metastasis to the vertebræ. The *arteries* account for metastasis from one part of an organ to another but, if the tumor cells enter at the source of the systemic circulation, they also account for metastasis to several or many organs.

INCIDENCE

According to the United States Public Health Service, cancer as a cause of death in the United States ranked ninth in 1900 and second in 1940. It is now exceeded in frequency only by diseases of the circulatory system. This increase is due, in part, to a decrease in other diseases such as enteritis, pneumonia, and tuberculosis and, in part, to true increase in cancer itself. Actually, about 430 out of every 100,000 white persons living in cities in the United States are under treatment or observation for cancer and about 380 of these 430 persons have cancer. There are approximately 230 new cases per 100,000 white persons in cities that are diagnosed each year. The incidence in colored people is less than that in white people. In colored males, for example, the incidence is little more than 50 per cent as compared with white males, and in colored females it is about 80 per cent of that in white females. While some of this disparity may be due to a racial predisposition, a great portion of it may be accounted for on the basis of cancer going unrecognized in the colored population. *Sex* differences are quite definite, there being an excess of cancer in white females of about 12 per cent over white males, and in colored females of about 70 per cent over colored males. Here, as in the case of race differences, some of the disparity in figures may be due to lack of correct diagnoses. The actual incidence in the *sites* of *involvement* of various portions of the body also differ somewhat with the sex. Roughly the percentages in the male are as follows: respiratory system—8 per cent, urinary system—7 per cent, buccal cavity—10 per cent, skin—17 per cent, digestive tract—36 per cent, genital system—12 per cent, and other sites—10 per cent. The corresponding incidence in the female is as follows: respiratory system—2 per cent, urinary tract—3 per cent, buccal cavity—2 per cent, skin—11 per cent, digestive tract—23 per cent, genital system—51 per cent, and other sites—8 per cent. From these figures it is apparent that the digestive system is most commonly affected in males and the genital system is most commonly involved in females. *Age*, too, is a definite factor in the incidence of cancer. In general, there is a rapid increase during the latter half of life. White males over seventy-five years of age show an incidence of 100 times greater than that for the age group twenty to twenty-four years and 200 times that for the age group from birth to five years. In white females the figures are 76 and 191 respectively. The incidence in the colored population is about one-third that in the white population. The *mortality* rate per 100,000 population is 136 in white males, 136 in white females, 94 in colored males, and 134 in colored females. In 1940 there were 158,335 deaths from cancer in the United States while in 1946 there were 184,000 deaths.

CAUSES

The causes of cancer are not yet known. Over the years, however, there has accumulated through animal experimentation and clinical observation a massive amount of data. In fact, some investigators maintain that the discovery has, in all probability, already been made but that it is lost in the maze of accumulated knowledge. An attempt to summarize this phase of the work can best be done by attacking each of two natural lines of cleavage —knowledge gleaned from animal experimentation and that gathered from experience with the disease in man.

ANIMAL EXPERIMENTATION

Animal experimentation in the elucidation of the causes of cancer has been most fruitful not only because experiments can be better controlled and more precise, but because the life span of animals is short enough to enable one to work with many generations. Obviously, too, procedures can be carried out in animals that are taboo in man. By far the greatest amount of effort has been spent on the experimental production of cancer and only recently have reputable laboratories undertaken the experimental study of chemotherapy of tumors. Each of these two large divisions may be briefly considered separately.

EXPERIMENTAL PRODUCTION OF CANCER

Taking a broad view of the problem, there are two major factors concerned in the experimental production of cancer, namely, (1) the intracellular, inherent, or intrinsic, and (2) the extracellular, inciting, or extrinsic. With regard to the former, very little is known but, with regard to the latter, the data are massive. The first can, therefore, be dispensed with readily.

Intracellular Factors.—Intracellular factors concerned in experimental cancer may be considered under three headings—(1) heredity, (2) enzymes, and (3) chemical changes.

1. *Heredity.*—There is no question that heredity plays a factor in carcinogenesis in animals. By inbreeding, strains of animals can be produced which are either cancer resistant or cancer susceptible. The latter will, after a certain age, develop cancer of a certain organ such as the breast in a high per cent of animals. The development of these tumors can be appreciably hastened by the application of a carcinogen. The factors which determine the susceptibility or resistance of an animal to tumor formation must, therefore, be carried by the chromosomes (rod-shaped bodies seen in mitoses and made up of genes linearly arranged) and are currently located in genes. Some indication that chromosomes are at fault is seen in the atypical mitoses which are often encountered in cancers and in chromosomal aberrations studied under high magnification in specially prepared smears or imprints of tumors (Dillar). The mechanism in the initiation of cancer may be as follows: a normal gene acted upon by an endogenous or exogenous carcinogen is transformed into a tumor gene which produces the tumor, or the body may receive an already altered tumor gene (virus) which produces the tumor. Thus, the gene which is altered by the action of a carcinogen is equivalent to an already altered exogenous gene—the tumor virus. In this manner may be reconciled the viral and nonviral theories regarding the origin of cancer. Although heredity may produce cancer resistant and cancer susceptible strains of animals, the cancer resistant strains can be broken down if the carcinogen is powerful enough. This is seen, for example, in carcinoma developing after exposure to roentgen rays. Another example has been afforded by the work of Strong. He injected methylcholanthrene into cancer resistant NH mice and by inbreeding produced, by the twenty-fifth generation, cancers of the lungs and stomach and leiomyosarcoma of the uterus. Susceptibility and resistance, therefore, depend upon an interplay between heredity and environment, that is, chromosomal and extra-chromosomal factors (Morton). The carcinogenic process once started is irreversible for even if the inciting agent is withdrawn, cancer results. There is set off, therefore, an intracellular mechanism which is self-perpetuating. This change may be accomplished by one stroke or by a sequence of specific biologic changes similar to a chain reaction (Berenblum).

2. *Enzymes.*—In general, the range of enzymatic activity is less in tumors than it is in normal tissues. Many enzymes such as cathepsin, polypeptidase, and nuclease are normal in each. Others such as catalase and oxidase are decreased not only in the tumors but also in remote organs such as the liver and kidneys in mice and rats bearing tumors, and the liver in man with cancer. In the serum there is a decrease in fibrinogen, esterase, lipase, and, in carcinoma of the prostate, an elevation in acid phosphatase.

3. *Chemical.*—In tumor cells there is an increase of nucleic acids, pentoses, phosphates, and diamino acids. There is a decrease of coagulable protein factor and, in carcinoma of the skin, of calcium. The latter, according to Cowdry, may be responsible for the lack of cohesiveness of the epithelial cells and for their invasiveness and cancerous properties. In the blood there is a decrease of albumin and gamma globulin. Hemolysins for erythrocytes have been produced by extracting mouse tumors.

Extracellular Factors.—Extracellular factors may be conveniently considered under three headings—(1) physical agents, (2) biologic agents, and (3) chemical agents. Before discussing these it may not be amiss to say a word or two about the commonly used term—irritant. An *irritant* may be defined as any substance or agent injurious to living tissue and hence includes physical, biologic, and chemical agents. When used, therefore, it should be more precisely tagged. Its effects are partly passive in the form of actual physical damage to the cell and partly active in the form of tissue response such as inflammation and repair. Berenblum states that irritation is an "unphysiologic stimulation which, being potentially destructive, elicits a continued state of reparative hyperplasia."

1. *Physical Agents.*—These may be divided into mechanical irritants, thermal agents, and rays. *Mechanical irritants* consist of a few single blows sufficient to elicit demonstrable evidence of tissue damage or a frequent succession of mild injuries, each of which in itself is insufficient to produce damage but the cumulative effect of which is great enough to cause injury. Mechanical irritants loom forth as important items in human cancer (see succeeding section) but are of little significance in experimental cancer. Application, for example, of coal tar to the skin of a mouse produces irritation and carcinoma but its deleterious effect is not by way of a simple destruction of the cells followed by reparative hyperplasia but rather by its chemical effect upon the genes of the chromosomes. If trauma or mechanical irritation as such has anything to do with the initiation of cancer it must, according to present concepts, act similarly, that is, not through a simple destruction of cells but by an alteration of genes. *Thermal agents* include heat (burns) in the form of flame, solids, fluids, vapors, gases, and electricity, and cold in the form of frost. The latter is important from an experimental point of view because repeated freezing in mice may produce carcinoma of the skin. The other agents just mentioned are complicated for they are effective not only by imparting heat but also because of their chemical composition. Actinic *rays*, ultraviolet rays, or sunlight produce carcinoma of the hairless areas (ears, eyes, nose, and proximal portion of the tail) in albino or dark haired mice and rats and enhance the formation of cancer of the breast in cancer susceptible (C3H) mice. Roentgen rays, after prolonged exposure, will create carcinoma in a rabbit's ear. Roentgen rays and radium will produce various sarcomas in experimental animals. Dunlap, for example, fed 3 drops of radium chloride solution daily to 13 rats for twenty days. In an average of three hundred and sixty-five days, 9 rats developed osteosarcoma of the vertebræ and pelvic bones.

2. *Biologic Agents.*—Two important agents in the production of cancer belonging to this group are worms and viruses. With regard to *worms*, Fibiger, in 1913, fed cockroaches infested with eggs of spiroptera neoplastica to rats and produced cancer of the stomach. Bullock and Curtis, in 1920, fed ova of the cat tapeworm to rats. The usual cysts appeared in the liver and within the walls of the cysts sarcomas subsequently developed.

That *viruses* produce some tumors in animals there is no doubt, but that they are the cause of any cancer in man has not yet been proved. As already stated, the viral and nonviral theories of origin of cancer can be reconciled if the virus is considered to be an altered gene. Tumor viruses have all the properties of other viruses. They have a similar molecular weight; they pass through bacteria tight filters; they resist drying, and they are labile. Tumor viruses have a limited pathogenecity, that is, each produces a single type of tumor. Those who maintain that viruses cause all tumors postulate that there is one virus for each tumor and that this virus, present in many tissues, remains dormant until stimulated by some inciting agent or until the soil is prepared by such an agent. They further maintain that the virus has been neutralized by its own antibody in cases in which it cannot be isolated and that its presence is indicated by an antigen antibody reaction. Experience with Shope's papilloma virus in rabbits supports this contention. In the papilloma stage the virus is demonstrable but when the lesion becomes a carcinoma it can no longer be isolated. Unlike other carcinogens, the virus persists and multiplies and accompanies the changed cells as they multiply. In other words, it changes the cell directly.

The following *tumor viruses* are well established: (a) *Chicken Sarcoma of Rous.* This is found in domestic fowls and produces a variety of sarcomas together with fibroma, myxoma, osteoma, chondroma, endothelioma, and leukemia. Many sites of the body are affected. Each tumor has its specific virus. (b) *Lucke's Renal Carcinoma of the Frog (Rana pipiens).* These tumors arise in tubular epithelium, may be benign (adenoma) or malignant (adenocarcinoma), are transplantable, and if they are cancerous, metastasize. The nuclei of the tumor cells contain inclusion bodies. (c) *Shope's Papilloma Virus of Rabbits.* Cottontail rabbits are prone to develop epidermoid papillomas which, after a time, become cancerous and metastasize to lymph nodes and lungs. If the virus is rubbed into the scarified skin of a domestic rabbit there develops a rapidly growing papilloma which becomes cancerous at several points within a few months. (d) *Bittner's Milk Factor.* For the production of spontaneous mammary tumors in mice, three factors are necessary—a cancer susceptible strain, milk factor, and estrogens. The process can be enhanced by certain chemicals such as methylcholanthrene. If the young of a highly susceptible strain suckle a female of low susceptibility, they show a low incidence of carcinoma and vice versa. The tumors do not appear until estrus is established.

3. *Chemical Agents.*—In 1945 Hartwell, according to Spencer, compiled from the literature a list of 1,028 *chemical compounds* that were tested for carcinogenesis and found that 284 of these were active. Since then many others have been discovered. As would be expected, this list includes a wide variety of chemical classes although most of them contain the benzene ring. A review of these compounds also reveals that widely different chemical structures elicit similar carcinogenic responses and that some substances that are closely related to carcinogens have no carcinogenic activity. There is, thus, no invariable correlation between molecular structure and carcinogenic activity. Chemical carcinogens, therefore, act on more than one type of cell, and—if our previous definition is correct—they change a normal gene to a neoplastic gene. They first elicit a preneoplastic hyperplasia which is an unlimited or progressive proliferation of cells and this, in turn, goes on to cancer formation. *Carcinogenicity* is *influenced by* species, strains of animals, age, sex, diet, physical condition, chemical purity, dose, physical state of compound, solvent, vehicle, and route of administration. *Solvents* which are associated with a high incidence of tumor formation are chloroform, mineral oil, oleic acid, sesame oil, arachis oil, paraffin, synthetic glycerides, benzene, some lards, and probably cholesterol. The *diet* of animals appears to be quite important. Caloric restriction and diet deficient in carbohydrates inhibit genesis or decrease the incidence of all types of tumors in mice. Inadequate amounts of essential amino acids,

cystine, and lysine suppress ovarian function and prevent proliferation and cancer of mammary tissue. The incidence of hepatomas caused by azo compounds is lowered when the animals are fed a diet of rice, wheat, rye, yeast, liver, casein, and vitamin D. Pyridoxine and biotin enhance tumor growth and the effects of biotin are annulled by the use of avidin and egg white. Liver extracts and yeast supplements protect the liver against certain chemicals such as the azo dyes. Finally, choline deficiency alone produces tumors in livers of rats. Four of the most important classes of chemical carcinogens are hydrocarbons, azo compounds, hormones, and aniline dyes.

Carcinogenic hydrocarbons are available naturally and synthetically. Naturally occurring hydrocarbons are found in soot, tar, pitch, mineral oil, and creosote. The actual carcinogenic agents in tar are present in the higher boiling point fractions. Powerful carcinogenic tars can be made artificially by heating the following to temperatures of 700–920° C.: acetylene, isoproprene, turpentine, human skin, yeast, and cholesterol. Carcinogenic hydrocarbons can also be synthesized in pure form. Of these, benzanthracene, methylcholanthrene, cholanthrene, and benzpyrene or their derivatives are the most common and the most powerful. Structurally these compounds are related to bile acids and estrogens. Although the target organs vary, the skin of experimental animals has been the most widely used structure for the induction of carcinoma because it is easily accessible and because it can be observed accurately. For purposes of discussion, the action of carcinogenic hydrocarbons may be divided into the effects produced in (1) the skin, and (2) other organs and tissues.

Painting the *skin* of animals with soot, tar, pitch, oil, etc., was the first step in the production of cancer and followed the clinical observations that cutaneous cancer was higher in people working in such industries than it was in the general population. In 1889, Hanan painted the ears of rabbits with tar but obtained negative results. In 1894, Cazin painted the ears of dogs with tar and also obtained negative results. In 1914, Yamagiwa and Ichetawa painted rabbit's ears over a prolonged period with tar and produced both papilloma and carcinoma. Subsequently these experiments were not only confirmed many times but were extended using carcinogenic fractions and pure hydrocarbons. As a result of many investigations, it became apparent that the skin of the mouse and the rabbit was highly susceptible to hydrocarbons whereas that of the dog, guinea pig, and rat was resistant. The formation of carcinoma is hastened by the following: wounding the tarred area (Deelman phenomenon), injury to the wart, and addition of oleic acid. Lactic acid and lanolin delay or diminish the carcinogenic potency. More recently *Berenblum*, in working with mice, discovered that croton oil or a weak solution of turpentine produces only epithelial hyperplasia of the skin. If the application of these substances is preceded with but one painting with methylcholanthrene, carcinoma develops. His interpretation is that methylcholanthrene produces an irreversible change in the cells (latent cancer cells) and these, when subsequently irritated, develop into carcinoma. In this respect, croton oil is a cocarcinogen. The *stages* in the development of carcinoma of the skin in experimental animals are (1) induction or hyperplasia stage, (2) wart stage, and (3) cancer stage. Application of a carcinogen produces a latent preneoplastic stage which is indistinguishable histologically from reparative hyperplasia. In the rabbit, continued application of a carcinogen is necessary to produce carcinoma but in the mouse, removal of the carcinogen once the wart stage develops will, nevertheless, result in cancer. *Histologically* the initial changes are identical with a low grade inflammation. Then the epidermis increases in thickness, the cells and the nuclei increase in size, and the nucleoli become conspicuous. The basal layer proliferates to produce papillary outgrowths. Finally, after a certain period, carcinoma develops. Both the papillomatous and neoplastic changes are spotty. Local application of carcinogens to the skin gives not only carcinoma but also sarcoma of the underlying tissues and sometimes even tumors in susceptible remote organs or tissues.

Carcinogenic hydrocarbons will cause tumors in *other sites* than the skin of experimental animals, but specific cancers arise only in those organs and tissues that harbor spontaneous tumors, that is, the susceptible areas. The route of administration may be topical, parenteral, or oral and the tumors arise both locally and remotely. An example is the formation of tumors in the lungs, liver, and mammary glands of mice after intranasal administration of a carcinogen. The ultimate effect of the carcinogen varies with the drug used, its amount and concentration, the route of administration, and, as already stated, the genetic susceptibility of the host. Briefly, the following is a list of some of the cancers that have been produced by carcinogenic hydrocarbons: (1) breast—by injection into the breast, near the breast, or in the flank and by intratracheal administration, (2) lung—by intratracheal instillation and feeding, (3) liver— by local implantation, (4) thymus—lymphosarcoma and leukemia, (5) bone—sarcoma, (6) uterus—adenocarcinoma by local implantation, (7) salivary glands— squamous cell carcinoma after injection, (8) spleen—occasionally sarcoma, (9) stomach—carcinoma if injected directly into the stomach, and (10) brain—a variety of tumors. The following organs give rise to no tumors or to nonspecific growths: (1) testis—sarcoma at the site of injection, (2) prostate—squamous cell carcinoma and sarcoma but not adenocarcinoma, (3) vagina—none, (4) kidney—epidermoid carcinoma after direct introduction but not adenocarcinoma, and (5) lymph nodes—none.

Some of the carcinogenic *azo compounds* are: orthoaminoazotoluene, paradimethylaminoazobenzene, 2-aminofluorene, and 2-acetoaminofluorene. In 1932, Yoshida injected and fed orthoaminoazotoluene to mice and rats and noted the development of adenomas and carcinomas of the liver and papillomas and carcinomas of the urinary bladder. Kinosita, in 1937, readily produced hepatic tumors in similar animals by feeding butter yellow (dimethylaminoazobenzene). Subsequently, Groshowski produced hyperplasia of the thyroid by thiouracil and then by administering 2-acetoaminofluorene evoked carcinoma. For the azo compound the rat is the favored animal and by feeding 2-acetoaminofluorene, cancers have been produced in the following organs: breast, thyroid, lung, gastrointestinal tract, liver, pancreas, kidney, urinary bladder, uterus, lymph nodes, and bone marrow. It is thought that the azo compounds are converted into carcinogens by certain tissues in the body and that the resultant products initiate cancer of the tissue that does the converting. In the liver, for example, there is first destruction and then secondarily proliferation.

The most powerful carcinogenic *hormones* are estrogens. An estrogen is any chemical compound that produces cornification of the vagina of the adult mouse like that which occurs in estrus (L. = orgasm). Structurally, estrogens are related to methylcholanthrene. Evidence that estrogens are concerned with growth is seen in the development of the genital and extragenital organs at the time of puberty and the changes that occur during the menstrual cycles. Further, endometrium implanted into the peritoneal cavity of a rabbit grows better in the presence of ovaries and its atrophy is prevented by injection of estrogens. Also, castration in cancer susceptible strains of mice lowers the incidence of carcinoma and delays the time at which tumors will appear. The carcinogenic effects of estrogens are best outlined by considering, in turn, each target organ. In the *breast* the following have been recorded: (1) Mice of a cancer susceptible strain show an inhibition or delay in formation of cancer of the breast if the ovaries are removed before six months of age but reveal no inhibition or delay if they are removed after six months of age (Lathrop and Loeb, 1916 and Cori, 1927). (2) Ligation of mammary ducts or prevention of sucking (that is, stagnation of milk) and rapid breeding in mice and rats increases the incidence of carcinoma of the breast (Badd, 1925 and 1936). (3) Injection of estrogens into susceptible or nonsusceptible male or female mice results in the production of cystic changes, hyperplasia, and carcinoma of the breast (Bonser, and Lacassagne, 1932). (4) Transplantation of ovarian tissue (into organs other than the testis) in male mice results in the development of carcinoma of the breast. (5) Mice from a highly susceptible strain suckled on a female of low susceptible strain show a low incidence of carcinoma, while mice from a low susceptible strain suckled on a female of high susceptible strain show a high incidence of carcinoma (Bittner). Here, three factors are necessary — heredity, estrogens, and the milk factor. In the *endometrium* the following have been recorded: (1) Hyperplasia in mice, rats, guinea pigs, monkeys, and rabbits receiving estrogens. This effect is nullified if progesterone (C.L.) is added. (2) Carcinoma without metastasis in rabbits receiving corpus luteum extract and folliculin. (3) Squamous metaplasia of the uterine horn in rats, mice, and rabbits receiving estrogens. In the *myometrium* the following have been produced: (1) Hyperplasia in rats receiving large amounts of estrogens. (2) Fibromyomas in guinea pigs receiving large doses of estrogens. Here the process is enhanced by spaying the animals first and is prevented by the addition of progesterone or testosterone. In the *cervix* the following have been recorded: (1) Metaplasia of the columnar epithelium to a stratified squamous cell type in monkeys and guinea pigs receiving estrogens. (2) Squamous cell carcinoma in mice receiving estrogens. In mice the simultaneous injection of androgens or progesterone does not alter the final result. In the *testes*, administration of estrogens produces hypertrophy of the interstitial cells and atrophy of the tubules. In the *prostate*, estrogens produce hypertrophy of the smooth muscle in rats, ground squirrels, and dogs and metaplasia of the glands of the prostatic utricle and peri-urethra in dogs, rats, and monkeys. These changes are prevented by the administration of testosterone.

With regards to *aniline dyes* the subcutaneous and oral administration of beta naphthylamine to female dogs results in the formation of papillomas and carcinomas of the urinary bladder.

EXPERIMENTAL CHEMOTHERAPY

In connection with tumors, chemotherapy may be defined as the introduction of exogenous chemicals into an animal for the sole purpose of destroying the neoplastic cells and eradicating the cancerous process. Currently, a great deal of effort is being expended to discover chemicals with tumor-inhibitory properties. The animals generally used are mice and rats and the target tissues are usually transplantable and, to a lesser extent, spontaneously appearing tumors. Less frequently employed are (1) tissue cultures of both animal and human tumors and (2) human tumors grown in the anterior chamber of the eye of a rabbit, mouse, or guinea pig. In evaluating the tumor-inhibitory property of any chemical, such factors as species, strain of animal, age, sex, diet, and physical condition of the animal must be taken into consideration for, as already seen, these are often vitally concerned with retardation of tumor growth. Although literally thousands of chemicals have been tested, only a few have shown salutary effects. Some of these are acid chlorides, acriflavine, aldehydes, bromobenzene, cantharidin, carbon dioxide snow, colchicine, chloro compounds, folic acid antagonists, halogen compounds, nitrogen mustards, organic peroxides, phenolic fractions of tar, polysaccharides, sodium caccodylate, and urethane.

OBSERVATIONS IN MAN

Although less adaptable for experimental purposes than laboratory animals, man has served as a source from which much data on cancer have been derived. Furthermore, clinical observations are extremely important for the prime purpose in all experimental work is to benefit man and it is well known that many of the observations made in animals cannot be transferred to humans.

Intracellular Factors.—Intracellular factors in man are essentially the same as those already outlined in connection with animals. The role of heredity in cancer, however, is much more difficult to establish in man than it is in laboratory animals. Some of the reasons for this are as follows: man is too much of a mixture and not a pure strain; breeding cannot be controlled; the members in a family are not large enough to be of statistical significance; the life span is too long, and statistics are not reliable (Morton). Aside from these objections, there is a widespread feeling that heredity does play a part. This is proved beyond a shadow of a doubt in lower animals and so, presumably, should be a factor in man. Furthermore there are records of so-called cancer families where many members in successive generations developed cancer of even the same organ. In support of heredity playing a role are the facts that Europeans are more prone to cancer of the breast than are Japanese, polyposis of the colon and neuroblastoma of the eye are familial, and homologous twins sometimes develop symmetrical, similar, and simultaneous tumors.

Extracellular Factors.—Extracellular factors in man as a cause of cancer may be considered under the same headings as extracellular factors in experimental animals. Because of experimental limitations, however, the relative importance of the various factors concerned is altered. In general, exogenous factors fall in the category of occupational or environmental influence and account for a minority of cancers while endogenous factors consist chiefly of hormonal influence and probably account for most of the tumors.

1. *Physical Agents.*—Numerous examples of cancer occurring at the site of *mechanical irritation* or *trauma* can be quoted but it cannot be proved whether the irritation as such or some other concomitant factors are at fault. Some examples are as follows: (1) Carcinoma of the gallbladder may be caused not by the mechanical irritation of the almost invariably present gallstones but by the conversion of cholesterol in the stones into a carcinogen. (2) Carcinoma of the glans penis covered by a long prepuce may

be caused not by the irritation of nonspecific inflammation but by the conversion of smegma into a carcinogen. (3) Carcinoma in the sebaceous cyst may be caused not by mechanical irritation of sebum but by its conversion into a carcinogen. (4) Carcinoma of the tongue at the site of a jagged tooth may be caused not by simple irritation of the tooth but by irritants in the smoke of a heavy smoker. (5) Carcinoma of the bridge of the nose may be due not so much to the rubbing of glasses as it is to actinic rays. (6) Carcinoma of the cervix in multiparous women may be caused not by trauma and inflammation but rather by estrogenic stimulation. The question of trauma as a cause of cancer is most important from a medicolegal point of view. In this respect, the following criteria (Berenblum) must be met to establish an etiologic relationship: evidence of injury, identity of injured area with tumor site, histologic proof of cancer, type of cancer consistent with tissues injured, previous integrity of parts, reasonable time relationship between trauma and the apparent tumor, and absence of a known carcinogenic environment. *Thermal agents* appear to be important. It is well known that cancer is prone to develop in old cutaneous burns, usually many years after injury was sustained. As in the case of mechanical irritation, however, in some instances (as in railroad engineers) it may not be the heat as such that acts as the carcinogen but it may be rather the accompanying tarry combustion products. Ultraviolet *rays* from the sun acting upon exposed parts of the body result in chronic dermatoses, keratoses, and carcinoma. Radioactive substances (alpha, beta, gamma, and roentgen rays) produce radiodermatitis and in 25 per cent of cases are followed by carcinoma (Hueper). Bone sarcomas (as reported by Hatcher) follow irradiation of joints for tuberculosis. The incidence of leukemia in radiologists is eight times as frequent as leukemia in the average physician. Miners in cobalt mines in Schneeberg, uranium mines in Joachimsthal, and other pitchblende-containing mines in Canada and the Congo show an increased rate of carcinoma of the lung. In these cases it is not settled, however, whether the cause is radioactive material or other substances in the ores such as arsenic, nickel, chromium, or silica (Hueper).

2. *Biologic Agents.*—The role of biologic agents is not as definite in man as it is in animals. The only parasite of importance is a fluke—the *Schistosoma hematobium*—which is accompanied by a high incidence of carcinoma of the bladder and the liver. The only virus that is known to produce a tumor is that concerned with papilloma of the skin—verruca vulgaris.

3. *Chemicals.*—Chemical compounds as a cause of cancer in man may be divided into endogenous and exogenous. The most important endogenous chemicals are doubtlessly hormones. Although much is known about hormones, the mode of their action in carcinogenesis is still a complete enigma. Exogenous chemicals are many and varied. From a pathogenetic point of view, they may be divided into three groups (Hueper). Some, such as aromatic amines and those contained in tar, act directly upon cells, either in their original form or in the form of metabolites. The action may be catalytic or through interference with enzymes. Another group (certain metals) changes the normal constituents of cells or tissue fluids and transforms these into carcinogens. A third group (perhaps dietary) causes alterations of some endocrine glands or the liver and these, in turn, act upon the various tissues of the body. Aside from these generalities, the following compounds and conditions may be considered more specifically: hydrocarbons, aromatic amines, carbon tetrachloride, inorganic chemicals, dietary disturbances, and hormones.

Hydrocarbons are important carcinogenic agents in man. Contact with tar, soot (chimney sweeps), pitch, asphalt, crude petroleum, shale oil, creosote oil, paraffin oil, lubricating and fuel oils, greases, anthracene, and other distillates produces cancer of the skin. Inhalation of tar dust and fumes is said (without definite proof) to produce carcinoma of the lung in man. Contact with tar and inhalation of tarry fumes may be the cause of, or at least have some effect on, cancer of the lip, tongue, oral cavity, and pharynx. Tarry combustion plays a role in cancer of the abdominal skin in Kangri users in Kashmir, in Kairo users in Japan, in Change users in China, and in Chutta users in India (last mentioned producing cancer of the hard palate from smoking cigars with lighted ends in the mouth). Dhoti cancer of the loin and groin results from friction of soot that accumulates in a loin cloth. Betel nut cancer of the oral cavity in India and the Philippines is due to the tobacco present, and Khaini cancer (of the lower lip) in northern India also occurs from tobacco mixed with lime that is placed between the lip and gum. Finally, contact with mineral oils produces "mule-spinners'" cancer.

Aromatic amines consist of azo compounds and aniline dyes. While the former have not yet proved to be carcinogenic in man, the latter are definitely known to produce cancer of the urinary system.

Carbon tetrachloride is a cause of cirrhosis and indirectly a cause of cancer in workers exposed to the chemical over prolonged periods.

Inorganic chemicals are less important as carcinogenic agents in man than are the organic compounds referred to above. *Arsenic* is in a doubtful category. Some workers maintain that topical contact with arsenic produces cancer of the skin while others maintain that such a causative relationship has not been proved. Used medicinally, however, there appears to be no doubt that it can cause both squamous and basal cell carcinoma of the skin. By some authors it is also said to cause cancer of the lung. *Chromium* may be a factor in the production of some cancers of the lung for statistics show that pulmonary carcinoma is at least four times as frequent among chromate workers as it is among the general population. Cancers of the nasal sinuses and lungs in workers in copper and nickel refineries in South Wales and in nickel mines in Sudbury (Canada) are more prevalent than they are in the general population. The *asbestos* (polymerized SiO_4) industry also is said to be attended by an increase of pulmonary carcinoma.

Dietary disturbances are unequivocal factors in the production of carcinoma in animals. They have as yet, however, to be proved of definite etiologic significance in man although certain deficiencies do appear to play a contributory role. An imbalanced diet in Sweden and Finland (short in green vegetables) predisposes to the Plummer-Vinson syndrome. This is attended by a hyperkeratosis of the mouth and pharynx and later carcinoma of the nasopharynx. Dietary deficiencies in the Bantus (an African Negro tribe) are attended by cirrhosis and high incidence of carcinoma of the liver. In this connection, Gillman fed rats the diet consumed by the Bantus and produced both cirrhosis and carcinoma. Cancer of the thyroid gland is more prevalent in districts with endemic goiter (due to iodine deficiency) than it is in nongoiterous districts.

The role of *hormones* in the etiology of cancer is difficult to evaluate precisely but it is probable that hormones represent the most important single factor. It is certain that most deaths are due to cancer of endogenous origin. According to Spencer, "hormonal deficiency may set up internal environmental conditions which are unfavorable to proper functioning of normal cells." Of the many hormones present in the body, estrogens lead the list as possible carcinogenic agents. Clinical observations of value are confined almost entirely to the female genital organs and breast. Some information, however, has been obtained from study of carcinoma of the prostate. The effects of estrogens can be best considered by discussing briefly each of the target organs.

Fibroadenoma of the *breast* does not develop before puberty or after the menopause. It arises at the time of greatest hormonal imbalance, that is, in adolescence in both sexes and in senility in males. Normally estrogens produce a hyperplasia of the ducts and progesterone brings about differentiation into acini. Following menstruation there is involution. If there is an excess of estrogens or if the receptor is too sensitive, the hyperplasia may exceed the involution and the tumor (fibroadenoma) results. In *hyperplasia* of the *breast* progesterone levels in the blood are below normal. This allows the unopposed action of estrogens resulting in an excessive proliferation of the ducts, their failure to differentiate into acini, stagnation of secretion, dilatation of the lumens, and early cystic hyperplasia. That estrogens are concerned with *carcinoma* of the *breast* is evidenced by the fact that (1) carcinoma does not arise before puberty, (2) only 1 per cent of all mammary carcinomas are found in males, (3) hyperplasia predisposes to cancer, and (4) carcinoma grows faster during pregnancy. Hormonal influences on the growth of mammary tissue are also evidenced by their relative or absolute effects as therapeutic agents. *Androgens* (especially testosterone proprionate) in cases of cancer of the breast with metastasis to bones regardless of the age of the patient result in relief of pain, increase in appetite, gain in weight, ability to sleep, and an increased density in the bones by roentgen examination. They do not, however, produce any demonstrable effect on the cancer in soft tissues. *Castration* (chemical or medical) in premenopausal women results in changes in the tumors in both soft tissues and in bones. *Estrogens* given to older women (those passing the menopause at least five years previously) have a salutary effect on cancer of the breast in soft tissues in both the primary and metastatic sites. If given to younger women they tend to increase the rate of growth of the tumor. In cancer of the *prostate* castration and estrogens result in relief of pain, gain in appetite and weight, renewed vigor of the patient, and some disappearance of the lesions in bones roentgenographically. The effect is exerted by direct action on prostatic epithelium, inactivation of androgens, depression of gonadotropins, and depression of activity of the interstitial cells of the testes.

Estrogens have some effect on tissue growth in the *cervix* as evidenced by squamous metaplasia of the endocervical glands seen in women receiving estrogens and disappearance of these changes upon withdrawal of the therapy. Granulosa cell tumor of the ovary (which produces excessive amounts of estrogens) is rarely accompanied by carcinoma of the cervix. On a purely theoretical basis, Hoffbauer suggested that the increase in incidence of carcinoma of the cervix in multiparous females is due not to chronic irritation from inflammation but to the intensive stimulation by estrogens during pregnancy.

Hyperplasia of the *endometrium* is probably due to a long continued action of estrogens in the absence of a balancing effect of the corpus luteum. The estrogens from unruptured graafian follicles (during the reproductive period), adrenal cortex (postmenopausally), and granulosa cell tumor of the ovary (at any age). Hyperplasia occurs usually beyond the age of thirty-five years and infrequently after the menopause. Endocrine imbalance in cases of hyperplasia is indicated by (1) the frequent presence of a bloody menopause, (2) delayed menopause, and (3) increased incidence of sterility. Further, islands of squamous cell metaplasia often encountered in cystic hyperplasia of the endometrium are similar to metaplasia produced experimentally by the administration of estrogens. *Carcinoma* of the *endometrium* is a frequent accompaniment of hyperplasia and is also found to accompany granulosa cell tumor and theca cell tumor (each producing excess estrogens) of the ovaries with greater frequency than in normal women. *Fibromyomas* of the *myometrium* have long been regarded as reflectors of hyperestrogenism. Whether endometrial hyperplasia and follicular cysts are more frequent in these than in normal women is not agreed upon. It is agreed, however, that the tumors regress after the menopause and rapidly enlarge during estrogenic therapy.

The administration of gonadotropic hormones to females is reported to produce cystic degenerative changes in the *ovaries* and even follicular and corpus luteum cysts. Granulosa cell tumor and theca cell tumor, together with certain "luteomas" produce increased amounts of estrogens and feminizing syndromes while arrhenoblastoma and adrenocorticoid tumors produce increased amounts of androgens and masculinizing effects. In none of these, however, is there an endocrine factor known to cause the tumor itself.

TUMOR THERAPY IN MAN

The effects of estrogens and androgens on the generative system in man have been referred to in the preceding paragraphs. With regard to other chemicals, although many compounds have been tested, there is not one that has yet been proved to cure cancer. *Radioactive phosphorus* is almost specific for polycythemia vera but the effect is due to the irradiation and not to the phosphorus. *Hepbisul* is accompanied by symptomatic relief but has brought about no regression in the tumors themselves. *Nitrogen mustards* have a salutary effect on Hodgkin's disease, bringing about regression or complete disappearance of the lymph node enlargements. The effects, however, are only temporary. The response in lymphoblastomas other than Hodgkin's disease is less dramatic. *Urethane* (ethyl carbamate) brings about satisfactory remissions in chronic myeloid leukemia but has less influence on chronic lymphoid leukemia. *Myelokentric acid* (Miller) has prolonged life and brought about temporary remissions in acute lymphatic leukemia. Finally, *folic acid antagonists* have been tried in lymphoblastomas and have been shown to have some salutary albeit fleeting effect on the tumors.

DIAGNOSIS

A diagnosis of cancer in man encompasses most of the *procedures* used in the diagnosis of any disease process. The customary methods of approaching the problem may be briefly outlined under the following eight headings: (1) *History*. As in every disease the eliciting of a careful history is extremely important. Among others, the following should be noted: age, race, sex, occupation, precise symptoms, duration of symptoms, and any recent change in the symptoms. (2) *Physical Examination*. This encompasses the usual inspection, palpation, and percussion. The precise location, size (in centimeters or inches), and character of the tumor should be noted.

This is particularly true if, for some reason or other, the growth is not going to be removed immediately or if the effects of chemotherapy or radiotherapy are to be observed. (3) *Visual Aids.* In areas of the body that are not externally visible a great deal of information (both visual and securing material) can be obtained by pharyngoscopy, laryngoscopy, bronchoscopy, esophagoscopy, gastroscopy, proctoscopy, sigmoidoscopy, cystoscopy, thoracoscopy, and peritoneoscopy. (4) *Roentgenologic Examination.* This is accomplished by fluoroscopy or by roentgenography. The latter includes (*a*) ordinary roentgenograms, (*b*) planograms (tomograms), and (*c*) roentgenograms after using contrast media such as barium in lesions of the gastrointestinal tract and radiopaque oils in lesions of the lungs, gallbladder, urinary tract, female generative tract, and vessels. (5) *Biopsy.* The term biopsy (Gr. = life + vision) means the gross and microscopic examination of a piece of tissue removed from the body during life. Despite the innovation of newer techniques in the diagnosis of cancer, biopsy still remains the best single procedure at hand. Tissue is usually obtained by incision into the tumor and, less commonly, by needle aspiration. Once it is secured it may, if necessary, be sectioned and stained within a few minutes (frozen section method) or, if time is not of the essence and better preparations are desired, it may be processed by a more lengthy method. (6) *Cytology.* Although cytology (Gr. = cells + treatise) literally means the study of cells, as applied to tumors it connotes the microscopic study of neoplastic cells in smears prepared from any of the body fluids and secretions. This procedure is of special value in cancers of the lung, female generative system, and mesothelial-lined cavities. (7) *Clinical Laboratory Procedures.* These include a great variety of biochemical, immunological, and enzymological tests on the blood, urine, and other tissue fluids. Although many tests have, from time to time, been devised none has yet been developed that meets the necessary criteria to serve as a good general cancer detection or cancer exclusion procedure. The elevation of serum acid phosphatase in metastatic prostatic carcinoma of bone and the elevation of gonadotropic hormones in chorionepithelioma are not exceptions to this statement for they are applicable only to the two types of growth mentioned. (8) *Biologic Procedures.* Two methods applicable to the biologic study of tumors are transplantation of tumor tissue into the anterior chamber of the eye of the guinea pig, rabbit, or other animal and tissue culture. To date, each of these methods is of limited value as far as routine diagnosis of cancer is concerned.

TREATMENT

The best treatment of *benign tumors* is complete surgical excision performed in the operating room under aseptic precautions. While electric excision and electric or chemical destruction of the tumor is still practiced by some physicians, such procedures have generally been replaced by scalpel removal. The treatment of *malignant tumors* is less uniform. As in the case of benign growths, the procedure of choice is *complete removal* of the neoplasm and this is generally accomplished by surgical excision. When surgical excision is not feasible, either because of an inaccessible location or because of surrounding permeation of the tumor, the procedure of choice is *irradiation.* This may be accomplished by the use of roentgen rays, radon, radium, or radioactive isotopes. The response of the tumor to irradiation depends primarily on its histogenetic composition. In general (granting exceptions in each group) the radiosensitivity of neoplasms in decreasing order of susceptibility is as follows: (1) tumors of the hematopoietic and reticulo-endothelial systems, (2) carcinomas, (3) sarcomas of soft tissues, (4) sarcomas of bone, and (5) tumors of nerve tissue. The third method of attacking tumors is *chemotherapeutic*. Although this approach to the eradication of neoplasms is still in its infancy it appears to hold promise for the future. As indicated in preceding sections the currently acceptable procedures may be listed as follows: (1) hormones for carcinoma of the prostate and carcinoma of the breast, (2) nitrogen mustards for Hodgkin's disease and other lymphoblastomas, (3) urethane for myeloid leukemia, (4) myelokentric acid for acute lymphoid leukemia, and (5) folic acid antagonists for acute lymphoid leukemia and, to a lesser extent, for other lymphoblastomas.

PROGNOSIS

The prognosis in most *benign tumors* is good, for a cure can be expected in every case in which the lesion is completely excised. Even if no treatment is instituted, the outlook is good. Such an attitude, however, is not advocated because (1) one can never be sure that a given lesion is entirely benign until it is excised and examined microscopically, (2) if left within the body a benign tumor may, at any time, become malignant, and (3) if strategically located a benign tumor may produce profound physiologic disturbances by obstructing a hollow organ, by pressing upon vital structures, etc. Thus, the dictum that "no tumor is a good tumor" is a good principle to abide by and it follows, therefore, that all growths should be removed.

The prognosis in *malignant tumors* depends upon so many variables that generalization can scarcely be permitted. Some of the more important concerned are: (1) *Type of Lesion.* While most tumors are of unicentric origin some, lesions such as lymphoblastomas are usually of multicentric origin. Obviously, the prognosis in the former is better than it is in the latter. The outcome, even in malignant tumors of unicentric origin, varies with the histogenetic type of growth. For example, a basal cell carcinoma of the skin remains localized during its entire course while a melanoblastoma (malignant melanoma) disseminates early and widely. (2) *Duration.* In general, the longer the delay between discovery of the growth and the time of effective treatment, the poorer the prognosis. (3) *Localization.* Obviously the outlook is much better in cases in which the tumor remains localized to an accessible area than in cases in which it has spread to vital structures or distant tissues. (4) *Age of Patient.* As a rule, the younger the patient the more unfavorable is the outlook. (5) *Treatment.* The selection of the proper type of treatment and the thoroughness of its execution are of paramount importance in effecting a cure. More often than not, the statement that "the patient has but one chance" holds true. This chance usually rests with the first attempt at eradication.

REFERENCES

ANDRUS, S. B., *et al.*: Cancer, *4*, 1015, 1951 (Tumor Transplants in Eyes).
BERENBLUM, I.: A. M. A. Arch. Path., *38*, 233, 1944 (Irritation and Carcinogenesis).
————: Brit. M. Bull., *4*, 343, 1947 (Carcinogenesis).
BITTNER, J. J.: Cancer Research, *12*, 387, 1952 (Mammary Cancer in Mice).
BLACK, M. M., and SPEER, F. D.: Am. J. Clin. Path., *20*, 446, 1950 (Chemical Tests for Cancer).

BONSER, G. M.: Brit. M. Bull., *4*, 379, 1947 (Experimental Cancer of Bladder).

BOYLAND, E.: Cancer Research, *12*, 77, 1952 (Review of Carcinogens).

BURROWS, H., and HORNING, E. S.: Brit. M. Bull., *4*, 367, 1947 (Estrogens and Tumors).

Cancer Hemolysins: Editorial, J. A. M. A., *137*, 647, 1948.

CLARK, J. H., *et al.*: Cancer Research, *12*, 451, 1952 (Ultraviolet Radiation in C3H Mice).

CORSCADEN, J. A., and GUSBERG, S. B.: Am. J. Obst. & Gynec., *53*, 419, 1947 (Causes of Cancer of the Uterus).

COWDRY, E. V.: J. A. M. A., *135*, 408, 1947 (Epidermal Carcinogenesis).

CRABTREE, H. G.: Brit. M. Bull., *4*, 345, 1947 (Anti-carcinogenesis).

DICKENS, F.: Brit. M. Bull., *4*, 348, 1947 (Solvent in Carcinogenesis).

DORN, H. F.: U. S. Pub. Health Service, Reprint 2537, 1, 1944 (Statistics).

DYER, H. M.: *An Index of Tumor Chemotherapy*, Federal Security Agency, U. S. Pub. Health Service, 1949.

Environmental Cancer: Editorial, J. A. M. A., *126*, 836, 1944.

GARDNER, W. U.: A. M. A. Arch. Path., *27*, 138, 1939 (Estrogens in Carcinogenesis).

GREENE, H. S. N.: Cancer Research, *7*, 491, 1947 (Mouse Eye for Tumor Transplants).

GREENSTEIN, J. P.: J. A. M. A., *148*, 697, 1952 (Cancer and Liver Enzymes).

HADDOW, A.: Brit. M. Bull., *4*, 331, 1947 (Action of Carcinogens).

———————: Brit. M. Bull., *4*, 417, 1947 (Chemotherapy of Cancer).

HADDOW, A., and KON, G. A. R.: Brit. M. Bull., *4*, 314, 1947 (Carcinogenic Compounds).

HARRIS, R. S., *et al.*: Am. J. Path., *20*, 1, 1944 (Radium Osteosarcoma in Rats).

HARTWELL, J. L.: *Survey of Compounds Which Have Been Tested for Carcinogenic Activity*, Federal Security Agency, U. S. Pub. Health Service, 1941.

HATCHER, C. H.: J. Bone & Joint Surg., *27*, 179, 1945 (Osteosarcoma from Irradiation).

HENRY, S. A.: Brit. M. Bull., *4*, 389, 1947 (Occupational Skin Cancers).

HIRSCHBOECK, J. S., *et al.*: J. A. M. A., *136*, 90, 1948 (Urethane in Leukemia and Tumors).

HOMBURGER, F.: Cancer, *3*, 143, 1950 (Diagnostic Tests for Cancer).

HUEPER, W. C.: International Congress on Cancer Research, St. Louis, September, 1947 (Environmental and Occupational Causes of Cancer).

MENDELSON, R. W.: U. S. Armed Forces M. J., *2*, 1371, 1951 (Betel Nut Chewer's Cancer).

MORTON, J. J.: J. A. M. A., *135*, 957, 1947 (Cancer Problem).

MOULTON, F. R.: Approaches to Tumor Chemotherapy, Gibson Island Conference, 1945–46, American Association of Advancement of Science, 1947.

NATHANSON, I. T., and KELLEY, R. M.: New England J. Med., *246*, 135 and 180, 1952 (Hormonal Treatment of Cancer).

Nutrition in Relation to Cancer: Editorial, J. A. M. A., *135*, 644, 1947.

ORR, J. W.: Brit. M. Bull., *4*, 385, 1947 (Liver Tumors by Azo Compounds).

PAGE, R. C., *et al.*: Arch. Indus. Hyg. & Occupat. Med., *4*, 297–345, 1951 (High Boiling Oils and Cancer).

PETERMANN, M. L., and HOGNESS, K. R.: Cancer, *1*, 100, 1948 (Plasma Proteins in Cancer).

RAKOFF, A. E.: Radiology, *50*, 190, 1948 (Endocrine Factors in Pelvic Tumors).

RASK-NIELSEN, R.: Acta Pathol. et Microbiol. Scandinav., Supplementum 78, 1948 (Tumors in Various Tissues in Mice).

ROUS, P.: J. A. M. A., *122*, 573, 1943 (Causes of Cancer).

RUNDLES, R. W., and BARTON, W. B.: Blood, *7*, 483, 1952 (Triethylene Melamine in Tumors).

RUSSELL, W. O., *et al.*: Am. J. Clin. Path., *21*, 764, 1951 (Laboratory Tests for Cancer).

RUSSELL, W. O., and WYNNE, E. S.: Am. J. M. Sci., *222*, 485, 1951 (Viral Theory of Cancer).

SMITH, W. E.: Arch. Indust. Hyg. & Occupat. Med., *5*, 242, 1952 (Occupational Tumors).

SNEGIREFF, L. S., and LOMBARD, O. M.: Arch. Indus. Hyg. & Occupat. Med., *4*, 199, 1951 (Arsenic and Cancer).

SPENCER, R. R.: J. A. M. A., *127*, 509, 1945 (Cancer Biology).

STRONG, L. C.: Cancer, *1*, 120, 1948 (Methylcholanthrene and Cancer Resistance in Mice).

TAYLOR, H. C.: Am. J. Obst. & Gynec., *36*, 332, 1938 (Ovarian Hormone and Tumor Development).

TOWBIN, A.: A. M. A. Arch. Path., *52*, 199, 1951 (Tumor Transplant in Eye).

TRUHAUT, R.: Arch. Indust. Hyg. & Occupat. Med., *5*, 264, 1952 (Occupational Cancer).

Tumor Enzymology: Editorial, J. A. M. A., *122*, 509, 1943.

WILLIS, R. A.: *Pathology of Tumors*, St. Louis, C. V. Mosby Co., 1948.

WRIGHT, J. C., *et al.*: Arch. Int. Med., *89*, 387, 1952 (Triethylene Melamine in Tumors).

WYNNE, E. S., *et al.*: Am. J. Clin. Path., *22*, 28, 1952 (Serologic Reaction in Tumors).

Chapter

8

Heart

PATHOLOGIC PHYSIOLOGY

William A. Sodeman

The *heart* is one of the *vital* organs of the body for, upon its proper performance and co-ordination, depend the nutrition and physiologic functions of every other portion of the body. In this respect, the organ acts as a pump that forces the nutrition laden blood through the arteries, arterioles, and capillaries to supply the needs of all cells. The accomplishment of its task depends upon (1) an intactness of its partitions which prevents the blood from escaping into chambers not designated to receive it at the moment, (2) properly functioning valves which direct the flow of blood in the intended direction, and (3) an intact musculature which provides the force wherewith the blood is moved. Obviously, defects in any of these three structures prevent the designated propulsion of blood and bring about certain pathophysiologic alterations with consequences of varying degrees of gravity. In the following paragraphs, only the more important disturbances will be considered.

Uncomplicated *atrial septal defects* are characterized by left to right shunting of blood. Prevented in simple patency of the foramen ovale by an overlapping of the edges of the foramen, the flow of blood is from left to right because of the slightly higher atrioventricular resistance in the left side. Added flow into the right atrium increases the amount entering the right ventricle. Accordingly, the output of the right ventricle is increased and the systolic pulmonary pressure is increased along with pulmonary arterial pulsations. While the filling and output of the left ventricle remains unchanged, the increased output of the right ventricle produces dilatation and increased pulsations of the pulmonary artery, a systolic murmur, a thrill in the second left interspace, and accentuation of the second pulmonic sound (P_2). The changes may be seen fluoroscopically and electrocardiographically where there is evidence of right ventricular hypertrophy. If mitral stenosis also occurs with atrial septal defect, the combination is known as *Lutembacher's complex*. Mitral obstruction increases the blood shunted and the output of the left ventricle is reduced. Less blood returns to the right atrium by way of the general circulation and, with the increased shunt, the end output of the right ventricle is unchanged. There is less tendency for the left atrium to enlarge than in mitral stenosis without a shunt. Flow from right to left of sufficient degree to produce *cyanosis* appears when right atrial pressure is elevated. Heart failure may effect this change. In *congenital pulmonary stenosis* with incompletely closed foramen ovale, heart failure may produce this circumstance and simulate the tetralogy of Fallot.

In *ventricular septal defects*, disturbances in circulation vary according to the size of the defect.   Large defects cause sufficient embarrassment to produce death in infancy while *small* defects produce little physiologic disturbance.   *Medium sized defects* may not produce hemodynamic disturbances until early adult life.   Flow from left to right occurs in ventricular systole because of the higher left ventricular pressure.   In diastole, with equalization of the pressures, flow stops.   Hence, the murmur and thrill are systolic.   Since the blood returned to the right ventricle must recirculate through the lungs to the left ventricle, both ventricles have an increased load.   Therefore, electrocardiographic imbalance is not frequent.   If the *defect* is *large*, or if the aorta tends to be displaced to the right (dextroposition), fetal pulmonary resistance, in some unexplained fashion, persists, supposedly to prevent increased pulmonary blood flow.   Pulmonary hypertension results in pulmonary artery dilatation and right ventricular hypertrophy (which with ventricular septal defect and dextroposition of the aorta make up the Eisenmenger complex).   Left to right shunting may eventually give place to right to left shunting when pressure on the right side exceeds that on the left as pulmonary resistance becomes sufficiently high.   When ventricular septal defect and dextroposition of the aorta are *accompanied* by *pulmonary stenosis* and *right ventricular hypertrophy* circumstances change. Pulmonary stenosis produces increased resistance to flow and raises right ventricular pressure so that venous blood enters the aorta.   Lessened blood flow through the pulmonary circuit gives reduced blood in the lungs.   Still a jet effect through the stenotic valve may cause a dilatation of that artery. Polycythemia accompanies the cyanosis; clubbing of the fingers and toes appears, and growth and development may be retarded.

Valvular defects produce (1) insufficiency of valves from scarring, vegetations, and perforation, and (2) stenosis from adhesions or vegetations.   They bring about physiologic disturbances in circulation dependent upon the degree of the defect.   Mitral *insufficiency*, for example, permits a leak of blood into the left atrium causing, together with blood flowing into the atrium from the lung, dilatation and eventually hypertrophy of the chamber. Increased left ventricular filling is necessary to make up for the regurgitated blood.   This produces dilatation of the ventricle, increased ventricular output, and eventually hypertrophy.   Mitral *stenosis* interferes with flow of blood from the left atrium to left ventricle and increases the strain on the left atrium.   If the atrium dilates and finally becomes inadequate, pulmonary vein pressure increases, the veins become distended, and pulmonary hypertension ensues.   This results in right ventricular hypertrophy in order to maintain flow through the lungs. P_2 becomes accentuated and a pulmonic systolic murmur may appear.   Dyspnea, hemoptysis, and cough develop.   Due to the mitral stenosis, left ventricular filling may be reduced even with elevated left atrial pressure.   Left ventricular output is reduced and return flow to the right ventricle likewise is reduced.   Right ventricular output is then reduced, lessening strain on the pulmonary circuit.   Similar changes in the *aortic* and *other valves* produce like changes adapted to the valve and chambers involved.   *Aortic stenosis*, for example, produces increased resistance to outflow of blood and eventuates in left ventricular hypertrophy.   Aortic insufficiency through the need for increased output to compensate for the regurgitated blood, also results in dilatation and hypertrophy.   In aortic stenosis the murmur and thrill are systolic and, because of impaired action of the valve cusps, the second heart tone may be diminished. Slowed and prolonged ejection into the aorta produces a slowly developing prolonged pulse wave—the plateau pulse—of small amplitude. *Aortic insufficiency* permits backflow producing the characteristic diastolic murmurs. The sudden drop in pressure with regurgitation follows the increased pressure of a systolic contraction requiring increased output to compensate for the reflux. These changes create a wide pulse pressure, the Corrigan pulse, capillary pulse, and other peripheral signs of aortic regurgitation.

Dilatation and *hypertrophy* result from an increased demand on the myocardium. Exercise and fever increase the minute output of the heart by increasing the frequency of contractions as well as the output per stroke. Ventricular filling is augmented as is fiber length. These changes result in greater release of energy with resultant increased stroke output. Thus, compensation is maintained. In valvular defects, the dilatation produced effects a similar change in one or more chambers. Tissue demands in anemia and hyperthyroidism cause similar effects. Impaired circulation to heart muscle, as in coronary sclerosis, may reduce the limits to which the heart muscle may respond in this way and may reduce the ability of heart muscle to meet demands of exercise, fever, and even usual metabolic processes. The output of the heart becomes inadequate; a diastolic residue of blood remains in the ventricle, and dilatation ensues. If the process continues, hypertrophy of muscle develops to compensate. Similarly, hypertrophy ensues in the left ventricle in diastolic hypertension to meet the increased resistance.

The rise in ventricular filling, as described above, is normally accompanied by adequate rise in stroke output. When the response is not adequate, *congestive heart failure* (cardiac insufficiency with failure) occurs. A residue of blood, with increase in pressure, remains in, for example, the *left ventricle*, in diastole. Subsequent left atrial volume and pressure increase, leading to pulmonary hypertension. If the right ventricle ejects its load satisfactorily, blood accumulates in the pulmonary circuit with subsequent pulmonary congestion. As left ventricular output eventually reduces return to the right ventricle, the right ventricular output tends to be reduced to that of the left ventricle, with the increased accumulation of blood maintained in the pulmonary circuit. Since the reduced output of the left ventricle may occur in response to stress (such as exercise, fever, and anemia), producing increased cardiac output, the failure may appear with cardiac output above usual figures but still not adequate for the increased demand. Failure of the *right ventricle* may result (1) from failure of the left ventricle through its effects in producing pulmonary congestion and hypertension, (2) through the pulmonary hypertension of mitral stenosis, or (3) as the result of pulmonary disease which increases pulmonary resistance or increases blood flow because of anoxia. If and when the right ventricle cannot cope with the load or demands, it fails to empty adequately; diastolic volume and pressure rise, and this pressure represents the central venous pressure. Subsequent effects of disturbed renal clearance of sodium, with salt and water retention, along with elevation of venous pressure result in hepatic congestion and peripheral edema.

Pericardial disease, both pericardial effusion and fibrous constriction, compress the heart and restrict diastolic volume. Ventricular filling is impaired; cardiac output is diminished, and elevation of venous pressure ensues. The heart muscle may not be impaired at all. In trauma to or rupture of the heart, sudden hemopericardium may produce fatal tamponade from small amounts of extravasated blood, such as 300 cc. Rapid reduction in cardiac output, reduction in pulse volume and blood pressure, and elevation of venous pressure with distention of neck veins characterize the clinical picture. More slowly developing effusions (from tuberculous disease, pyogenic infections, or cancers) permit distention of the pericardium so that extensive effusion may occur before cardiac compression is serious. In constrictive pericarditis (due to an adhesive, thick, contracting pericardium) gradual constriction may lead to extreme elevations of venous pressure resulting in a large distended liver, ascites, and peripheral edema. The heart is not remarkably enlarged if at all.

Atherosclerosis involves the *coronary* system as well as the aorta and other arteries. The subintimal proliferation reduces the lumens of the coronary vessels with the severity of the process varying greatly from vessel to vessel. The left ventricle is especially vulnerable and the disorder occurs more frequently in men than in women. Concomitant diastolic hypertension, producing hypertrophy of heart muscle, increases the frequency of symptoms, for the increased size of muscle fiber increases the distance from capillary vessel to the muscle itself and adds to the difficulty of transfer of metabolites and nutritional factors. Impaired circulation of blood to the heart muscle fibers may lead to (1) inadequate contractions, eventuating in failure, (2) to disturbed irritability of muscle in certain foci, causing irregularities, or (3) to painful syndromes. Exercise increases demands on the heart muscle and if some areas are so deprived of circulation that metabolites cannot be removed in adequate amounts, they build up to the point of stimulating nerve fibers. Hence, pain occurs on exercise. With rest and reduced demands, circulation in the area again is adequate, metabolites are removed and the pain disappears. Thus, the *angina of effort* develops. If and when the atherosclerotic process leads to deposits of lipid and calcified materials, open ulcers and a heaping up of subintimal tissue develop to the point of slowing of the circulation and eventual clot may form. In addition, subintimal hemorrhage may cause sudden obliteration of the lumen. As a result, the circulation to a segment of heart muscle stops and acute *necrosis* of *heart muscle* in the area appears. Shock may develop. Resorption of cellular products from the infarcted area, such as the transaminase, may be measured in the blood. By indirect measurements, such as the white blood count elevation, increased sedimentation rate, or the appearance of C-reactive protein, similar changes may be detected. Electrical effects from the dead muscle disappear and, in the immediately surrounding partially injured area, currents of injury develop. These changes produce distinctive electrocardiographic abnormalities which are most helpful in diagnosis. Irritable areas in adjacent muscle at times act as foci for the development of premature beats or of ventricular fibrillation. If the circulation to the conducting system is involved, as frequently happens in the His system when posterior occlusion occurs, varying degrees of heart block may appear. Inflammation of the pericardium over the area of dead muscle may result in localized pericarditis often sufficient to produce an audible friction rub.

CONGENITAL ANOMALIES

Orientation.—The *incidence* of developmental abnormalities of the heart is difficult to determine with any degree of accuracy. They have been recorded as constituting from 0.27 to 0.9 per cent of all deaths, 1.33 per cent of deaths in patients under one year of age, 0.5 per cent of deaths in patients over one year of age, and 6 per cent of all cardiac patients under twenty years of age (White). Since the lesions are congenital they usually become manifest in *infants* and *young children* but, in some instances, they do not become apparent until later in life. The disorders occur in all *races* and in all strata of life. There is no particular preponderance in either *sex* when the anomalies are considered as a whole but in any single abnormality one sex is often favored over the other. While congenital anomalies arise as a result of an arrest of development, the *causes* for the arrest are not known. Most derangements are probably on the basis of hereditary defects in the germ plasm, but a few may be due to a viral (rubella) or some other infection incurred by the mother during the early weeks of pregnancy.

Embryology.—Before the developmental defects are classified and discussed, a brief review of the normal embryology of the heart appears to be in order. The heart arises from bilateral primordia which soon unite to form a primitive tubular structure. Due to a disparity in growth between the heart and the adjacent structures, the organ bends on itself in an S-shaped fashion as it elongates with the anterior part shifting to the right and the posterior part shifting to the left. Because of constrictions, the tube is divided into five parts—sinus venosus, primitive atrium, primitive ventricle, bulbus cordis, and truncus arteriosus. The *sinus venosus* receives the blood from the primitive veins. It first communicates with, and then forms part of, what is ultimately the right atrium. The connection between the primitive atrium and the primitive ventricle is known as the *atrial canal*. It grows less rapidly than the rest of the heart and thus remains as a narrowing. Its lumen is further reduced by a dorsal and a ventral thickening known as endocardial cushions. A meeting of these cushions in the midline forms the septum intermedium which divides the canal into right and left ventricular orifices. The *primitive atrium* grows rapidly and is divided into a right and left chamber by the septum primum which grows from above down. At first there is an opening between the septum intermedium and septum primum but later this closes and an opening called the foramen ovale occurs in the upper part of the septum primum. Another partition—the septum secundum—grows downward from the upper part of the atrium just to the right of the septum primum and foramen ovale. After birth it fuses with the primary septum to close the foramen ovale. The left atrium establishes communication with the lungs by uniting with the pulmonary veins which grow out from the lungs. The *primitive ventricle* becomes divided into a left and a right chamber by the ventral septum which grows upward from its lower part. The dorsal part of the ventricular septum unites with the dorsal part of the septum intermedium, leaving a patent interventricular foramen. This is ultimately closed by a merging of the ventral portion of the ventricular septum with the aortic septum. Most of the *bulbus cordis* becomes incorporated with the right ventricle. The distal portion of the bulbus cordis and the *truncus arteriosus* are then divided longitudinally by the aortic septum (which appears in three parts) into the aorta and pulmonary artery. The final oblique union of the aortic septum with the ventricular septum aligns the pulmonary artery with the right ventricle and the aorta with the left ventricle. The *valves* of the heart are formed from endocardial thickenings.

Classification.—In general, there are two types of classification of congenital diseases of the heart—clinical and pathologic. The *clinical* classification divides the disturbances into two groups—those attended by cyanosis and those unattended by cyanosis. The *pathologic* classification divides the conditions according to anatomical defects and since it is more precise it will be followed here. As seen from the above brief embryological considerations, the heart develops in many stages and since arrests of development may be multiple, the numerous combinations of the defects are still more complex. The more common abnormalities may be classified as follows: (1) heart as a whole—failure of development, ectopia, dextrocardia, idiopathic hypertrophy, rhabdomyoma (see tumors), cysts (see tumors), and diverticulum, (2) pericardium—defects and cysts (see tumors), (3) septal defects—atrial, ventricular, and aortic, (4) endocardium—fibroelastosis and bands, (5) valves—atresia, number of cusps, fenestrations, blood cysts, displacement, and aneurysm of sinus of Valsalva, (6) veins— pulmonary and venæ cavæ, and (7) coronary arteries.

Failure of Development.—Complete failure of development of the heart is known as *acardia* while failure of development of one-half of the heart is called *hemicardia*. The conditions are incompatible with life and, fortunately, constitute less than 1 per cent of all cardiac anomalies (White).

Ectopia.—Ectopia of the heart connotes its vertical displacement into the abdomen, into the neck, or (through a fissured sternum) outside of the thoracic cage. Although most of the patients die early in life, a few may live to adulthood.

Dextrocardia.—This anomaly consists of a misplacement of the heart into the right thoracic cage. It may be due to (1) a mirror image transposition of the cardiac chambers brought about by a reverse rotation of the primitive cardiac tube and usually seen in conjunction with a mirror image transposition of other organs (situs inversus), (2) lack of axial rotation of a normally formed heart resulting in the cardiac apex being formed by the right ventricle, or (3) simple shifting of the heart to the right as a result of absence of the right lung (Goldberger). Dextrocardia, unless complicated by other cardiac abnormalities, is of no clinical significance.

Idiopathic Hypertrophy.—This condition signifies simple congenital hypertrophy of the heart in the absence of any developmental defects. If the cases are carefully studied, anomalies of the coronary arteries, anemia, glycogen deposition, inflammation, etc., are found, so that there is doubt whether idiopathic hypertrophy is an entity (Levine).

Diverticulum.—A diverticulum of the heart is usually confined to the left ventricle. It consists of a sac-like protrusion of the entire thickness of the myocardium that may measure as much as 7 cm. in length and 3 cm. in diameter. As a rule, the defect herniates through the diaphragm into the abdomen but occasionally it is present entirely within the pericardial cavity. If the lesion is not resected surgically, death usually occurs from rupture.

Pericardial Defects.—These consist of an absence of the entire pericardium or a defect on the left side large enough to consider the left pleural cavity and the pericardial cavity as a single space.

Atrial Septal Defects.—Rarely the interatrial septa *fail* to *form* entirely leaving a single chambered atrium. Next in frequency (but still uncommon) are single or multiple *defects* in the *septum* other than the foramen ovale (Fig. 93). These defects may occur in any part of the septum but are commonly found in the lower portion (failure of union of the septum intermedium and septum primum). The size varies from a few millimeters to several centimeters. The most common and least important atrial defect is a *patent foramen ovale*. The size of the patency varies from barely visible to about 2 cm. in diameter and the opening may be uncovered or curtained by two overlapping (but not fused) membranes (Fig. 93). Some degree of patency of the foramen ovale occurs in about 10 per cent of the population.

Any *atrial septal defect* may occur in conjunction with other cardiac anomalies or it may be found by itself. The latter is of significance only when the defect is large. The direction of blood flow through the defect depends upon the relative pressures in the atrium. At birth and in infancy, pressure on the right side may be greater than that on the left, the flow of blood may thus be from right to left, and the baby may be cyanotic. As the child ages, the reverse is true and cyanosis disappears. In time, the volume of blood and pressure on the right side may increase to a degree sufficient to cause right-sided cardiac failure and this, in turn, may again produce a reversal of the blood flow from right to left. *Clinically*, in addition to the cyanosis, large defects may be attended by hoarseness, cough, hemoptysis, low blood pressure, small pulse pressure, right-sided cardiac enlargement, and variable

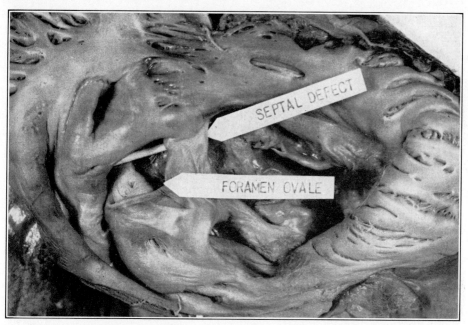

Fig. 93.—Interatrial septal defects showing a foramen ovale and failure of union of the septum intermedium and septum primum.

thrills and murmurs. *Roentgenographically* there is enlargement of the hilar vessels and right side of the heart together with diminution in size of the left atrium, left ventricle, and aortic knob.

Ventricular Septal Defects.—Defects in the interventricular septum, like those in the interatrial septum, represent arrests of development. *Complete failure* of septal formation results in a single common ventricle (Fig. 94*A*). If the interatrial septum develops normally there is a three-chambered heart—*cor biatrium triloculare*—but if, in addition, the interatrial septum fails to develop there is a two-chambered heart—*cor biloculare*. The latter is incompatible with life beyond a few months. The former is usually associated with a persistent bulbus cordis bearing the exit of the aorta. *Clinically* cor biatrium triloculare is not attended by cyanosis until heart failure develops and is accompanied by cardiac enlargement, prominent hilar markings, variable murmurs, and usually death in childhood. Partial failure of development of the interventricular septum results in an

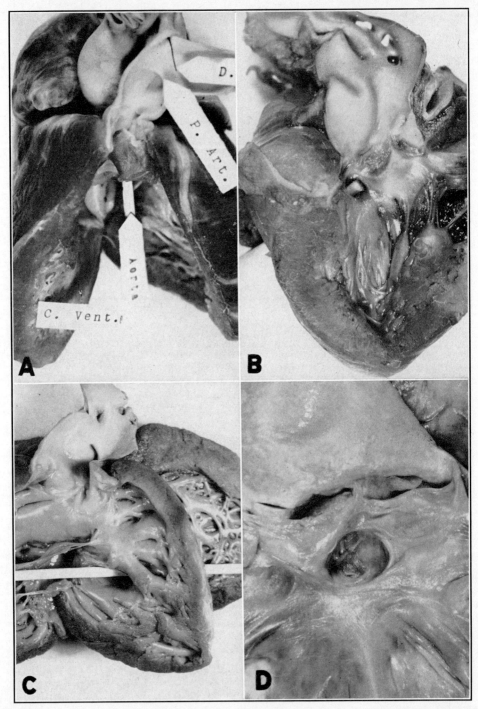

Fig. 94.—Interventricular septal abnormalities showing *A*, complete failure of formation of the septum resulting in a single common ventricle, *B*, patency of the upper and anterior (membranous) portion, *C*, patency of the muscular portion, and *D*, aneurysm of the upper and anterior (membranous) portion.

isolated septal defect often known as *Roger's disease* (Fig. 94*B* and *C*). The patency usually, but not always, occurs in the part of the septum that is last to close, namely, at the junction of the ventral portion of the ventricular septum with the aortic septum and is thus located superiorly and anteriorly. The size of the opening varies from a few millimeters to 2 cm. in diameter. *Clinically* cyanosis is absent (because the blood flow is from left to right), the heart may be enlarged to the right, a loud systolic murmur is present, and death (often from bacterial endocarditis) usually occurs before the age of forty years. Rarely, the ostium closes but the membranous covering undergoes *aneurysmal dilatation* with the protrusion encroaching upon the right ventricle (Fig. 94*D*). This abnormality is of no known clinical significance. Although the simple septal defects referred to above may exist alone, they are generally associated with other cardiac anomalies thus constituting definite syndromes. These are considered following a brief discussion of aortic and septal defects.

Aortic Septal Defects.—A defective development of the aortic septum affects both the pulmonary artery and the aorta and is generally associated with ventricular or atrial septal defects. Complete failure of development of the septum results in a common aorta and pulmonary artery—a *persistent truncus arteriosus*—while partial failure of development results in simply a communication between the aorta and the pulmonary artery (Fig. 95*A* and *B*). *Clinically* the former (and also the latter when the defect is large) is accompanied by varying degrees of cyanosis, right ventricular hypertrophy, systolic murmur and thrill, prominent aortic knob radiographically, and frequently death in several weeks. *Failure of the bulbus cordis* to *rotate* results in a *transposition* of the *great vessels* so that the pulmonary artery arises from the left ventricle and the aorta from the right ventricle (Fig. 95*C*). The anomaly is usually associated with other cardiac (septal) defects. *Clinically* there are cyanosis, clubbing of the digits, cardiac enlargement, variable murmurs, and usually death from cardiac failure within a few days or weeks. *Shifting* of the *septum* to the *right* results in *pulmonary artery hypoplasia, stenosis*, or *atresia* and concomitant *dilatation* of the *aorta* (Fig. 96) while *shifting* of the *septum* to the *left* results in *aortic hypoplasia, stenosis*, or *atresia* and *concomitant dilatation* of the *pulmonary artery*. In either case, the hypoplasia or dilatation affects the vessel as a whole, the atresia involves either the vessel as a whole or simply its valvular orifice, and the stenosis involves the orifice only. The *clinical* manifestations are variable. Narrowing of the pulmonary artery may be attended by cyanosis, right-sided cardiac enlargement, and ultimately cardiac failure and bacterial endocarditis. The patients generally live to adulthood. Congenital narrowing of the aorta is attended by manifestations similar to acquired aortic stenosis while aortic atresia is attended by marked cyanosis and death in a few days. *Subaortic stenosis* consists of a narrowing located about 1 cm. proximal to the aortic valve (Fig. 95*D*). It is due to a failure of complete absorption of the bulbus cordis by the left ventricle.

Tetralogy of Fallot.—This condition consists of (1) hypoplasia, stenosis, or atresia of the pulmonary artery, (2) interventricular septal defect, (3) dextroposition of the aorta so that its origin overrides the septal defect, and (4) hypertrophy of the right ventricle (Fig. 96). The pulmonic circulation may be maintained through the patent ductus arteriosus and/or hypertrophied bronchial arteries. *Clinically* there are cyanosis, intolerance to exertion, clubbing of the digits, a systolic murmur and thrill, right-sided

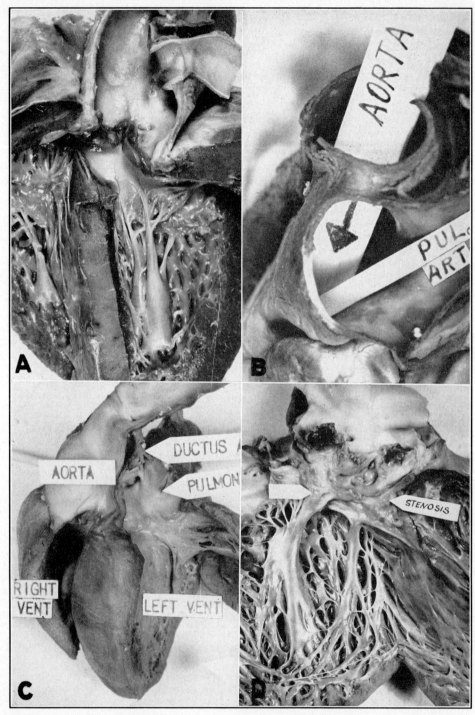

Fig. 95.—Aortic septal defects showing *A*, persistent truncus arteriosus with interventricular septal defect, *B*, aortic pulmonary communication, *C*, transposition of the great vessels with the aorta arising from the right ventricle and the pulmonary artery from the left ventricle, and *D*, subaortic stenosis with superimposed subacute bacterial endocarditis of the aortic valve proper.

cardiac enlargement, small pulmonary conus radiologically, and polycythemia. Formerly, death usually occurred in childhood or early adulthood. The condition can be corrected and the prognosis thus immeasurably improved by surgical anastomosis of the innominate or less often subclavian artery to a pulmonary artery (creation of an artificial ductus arteriosus).

Eisenmenger Complex.—This condition consists of a patency of the superior and anterior part of the interventricular septum with dextroposition of the aorta. The pulmonary artery is normal or dilated and the right ventricle is not hypertrophied unless heart failure supervenes. *Clinically* the anomaly is similar to that of a simple interventricular defect.

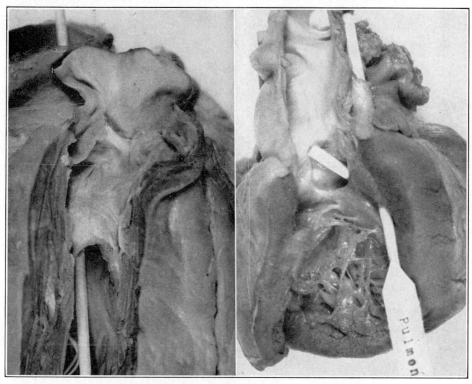

Fig. 96.—Tetralogy of Fallot (two specimens) showing (1) stenosis (to the left) and hypoplasia (to the right) of the pulmonary artery, (2) interventricular septal defect, (3) dextroposition of the aorta, and (4) hypertrophy of the right ventricle.

Fibro-elastosis.—Fibro-elastosis (endocardial sclerosis) of the heart represents a diffuse fibrous and elastic thickening of the endocardium of the left ventricle and less commonly of other chambers (Fig. 97). The lesion may also affect the valves and produce corresponding valvular stenosis. Rarely, endocardial thrombosis occurs. While there has been much speculation as to the *cause* of the condition, it is probable that anoxia is responsible for the changes (Johnson). The lack of oxygenation is based on a deficient circulation which, in turn, may be caused by anomalies of the coronary arteries, premature closure of the foramen ovale, or valvular atresia. While the disorder is generally seen in infancy it may make its appearance beyond 16 years of age, as indicated by the 25 cases recorded in adults by 1956 (Guraieb). *Clinically* the disorder usually starts with a sudden or more gradual onset of severe dyspnea, cough, vomiting and tachycardia. There are, in addition, cyanosis, cardiac enlargement, mitral murmurs, and hepato-megaly. *Death* usually occurs within six months from cardiac failure.

Endocardial Bands.—Endocardial bands containing muscle fibers or composed entirely of fibro-elastic tissue may be found stretching from one portion of the endocardium to another (Fig. 98). A network of such bands in the right atrium is referred to as a *Chiari network*. The significance of the bands is that they may produce adventitious sounds or may serve as a point of thrombus formation.

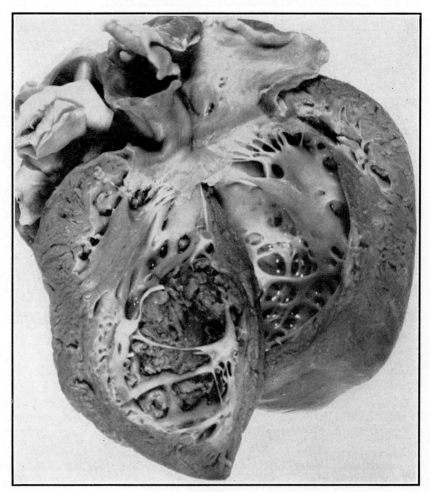

FIG. 97.—Fibro-elastosis of the heart illustrating marked thickening and fibrosis of the inner portion of the left ventricle with a superimposed mural thrombus.

Atresia of Valves.—Congenital stenosis and atresia of the aortic and pulmonic orifices and valves have already been mentioned. Similar changes may occur in the tricuspid and mitral valves. On the right side, such lesions are usually associated with a rudimentary or absent right-ventricle, an atretic pulmonary artery, and interauricular and interventricular septal defects. On the left side they are associated with hypoplasia of the chambers of the heart, aortic atresia, transposition of the great vessels, and atrial and ventricular septal defects. The *clinical* manifestations are obviously variable. The *prognosis* generally is poor.

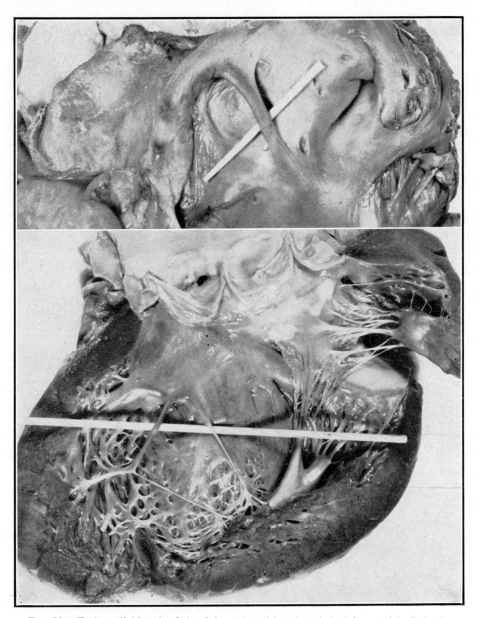

FIG. 98.—Endocardial bands of the right atrium (above) and the left ventricle (below).

Number of Cusps.—The aortic and pulmonic valves may disclose a fewer or greater *number* of cusps than normal with the usual digression in each being two or four (Fig. 99). Other things being normal, the number of cusps is of no clinical significance with the exception that a bicuspid aortic valve is more prone to bacterial invasion than a normal valve. Extremely rarely, the mitral or tricuspid valve may be completely *duplicated*.

Valvular Fenestrations.—Single or multiple congenital openings are not uncommon in the aortic or pulmonic cusps (Fig. 99). When small they are generally of no clinical significance although your author has seen subacute bacterial endocarditis developing along their margins. When large, they may be accompanied by sufficient regurgitation of blood to cause ventricular hypertrophy and even failure.

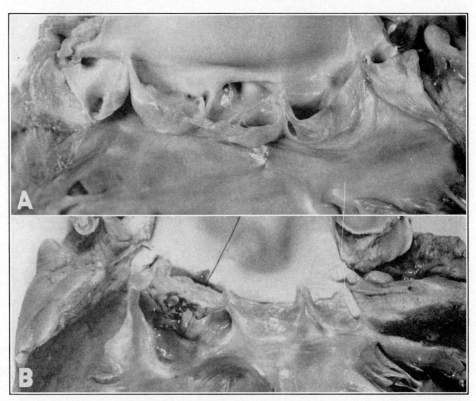

Fig. 99.—Fenestrations of aortic cusps showing *A*, simple defects in two of four cusps and *B*, a large defect (containing horse hair) surrounded by vegetations. Below the defect the endocardium is semilunarly thickened (pseudovalve). The patient died of cardiac failure and cerebral embolism.

Valvular Blood Cysts.—Small, 1 to 2 mm. sized, dark red, elevated, circumscribed, cystic spaces lined by endothelium and filled with blood may be found on the mitral and tricuspid (less often on the aortic and pulmonic) valves in as high as 75 per cent of infants that come to necropsy (Fig. 100). Although they have been considered to represent (1) hematomas, (2) vascular ectasias, and (3) angiomas, they probably represent endothelial-lined clefts into which blood is pressed (Levinson). They are of no known clinical significance.

Valvular Displacement.—Rarely, a portion of a tricuspid valve is attached to the wall of the right ventricle inferior to the atrioventricular junction (Ebstein's disease). Although the valve itself is usually normal and competent it may be deformed, resulting in hypertrophy and dilatation of the right atrium, increased blood pressure on the right side, shunting of blood from right to left through a patent foramen ovale, and chronic cyanosis.

Aneurysm of Sinus of Valsalva.—This consists simply of a congenital dilatation of a sinus of Valsalva. The condition is usually symptomless although a large dilatation may compress the superior vena cava and thinning may be of sufficient degree to produce rupture and hemorrhage.

Anomalies of the Pulmonary Veins.—One or all of the pulmonary veins may empty into the right atrium instead of the left atrium. When all veins are affected blood reaches the systemic circulation by way of a patent foramen ovale and, because the right atrium is overburdened, cardiac failure and severe passive hyperemia ultimately develop. Under these circumstances, the prognosis is poor but if only some of the veins empty into the right atrium, longevity need not be affected.

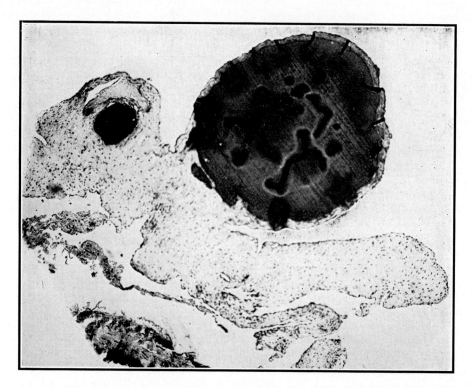

Fig. 100.—Blood cysts of the mitral valve. (Photomicrograph courtesy Dr. J. Stasney.)

Anomalies of the Venæ Cavæ.—Either vena cava or both venæ cavæ may open into the left atrium instead of the right atrium. The condition is accompanied by marked cyanosis, digital clubbing, and death within a few months after birth.

Anomalies of the Coronary Arteries.—Anomalies of the coronary arteries consist of (1) origin from other than the usual aortic sinuses, (2) presence of more than two (usually three and rarely four) coronary ostia and arteries, (3) absence of the right or left coronary artery, (4) origin of one or both coronary arteries from the pulmonary artery, and (5) origin of an anomalous vessel from the right ventricle. The abnormalities are significant when they convey a deficient supply of oxygenated blood to the myocardium, thus resulting in ischemia and infarction.

19

Clinicopathologic Correlation in Congenital Heart Disesae.—Although certain symptoms and signs are often peculiar to groups of congenital cardiac anomalies, most maldevelopments (if they are initially severe enough or if they are ultimately attended by cardiac decompensation) sooner or later disclose common clinical manifestations. These may consist of combinations of (1) dyspnea due to pulmonary hyperemia or tissue anoxia, (2) hemoptysis resulting from pulmonary hyperemia, (3) cerebral manifestations (headache, dizziness, syncope, and convulsions) caused by cerebral anoxia, thrombosis, or embolism, (4) polycythemia due to insufficient pulmonary ventilation, (5) hoarseness due to pressure of a dilated atrium on a recurrent laryngeal nerve, (6) cough resulting from similar pressure on a bronchus, (7) low blood pressure and small pulse pressure consequent to decreased amount of blood in the systemic circulation, (8) cyanosis caused by a deficient oxygenation of blood, (9) clubbing of the digits occurring in conjunction with cyanosis but not explained satisfactorily, and (10) cardiac murmurs and thrills due to blood rushing through small, incompetent, or abnormal openings (Goldberger).

DEGENERATIONS

Orientation.—Degenerations of the heart are of many varieties. They may predominate in the pericardium, the coronary arteries, the myocardium, or the endocardium. Most lesions of the pericardium and endocardium are preceded by inflammation and are considered in the succeeding section. Congenital lesions of the endocardium attended by degenerations have already been referred to in the first part of this section. Degenerations of the coronary arteries are followed by myocardial ischemia and infarction. They are discussed under Physical Disturbances. Degenerations of the myocardium are brought about by two divergent routes—by a direct attack upon the muscle fibers or by an indirect involvement (compression or lack of nutrition) by way of the stroma. Each may be acute or chronic in its course and each ultimately (if extreme enough and severe enough) may lead to myocardial failure and death of the patient. Some of the pathologic changes—*brown atrophy, amyloidosis, fatty infiltration* and *metamorphosis, calcification* and *ossification*, and *beriberi* have already been discussed under the general heading of Degenerations in Chapter 4, page 29. *Glycogen disease* is considered in Chapter 21, page 797, on the Liver. A few of the remaining disorders may be dwelt upon forthwith.

Parenchymatous Degeneration.—What has been said for parenchymatous degeneration in general in Chapter 4 holds for parenchymatous degeneration of the heart in particular. The condition is a common finding at postmortem in patients dying of any lingering or acute infectious process. It is not seen in a previously healthy person who meets with sudden death. In any case, it should be differentiated from postmortem autolysis. This may be achieved by considering the time elapsed between death and the necropsy, the temperature of the medium in which the body lay, and the comparative state of preservation of the rest of the tissues. Parenchymatous degeneration of the heart is manifested grossly by a soft, flabby, collapsible, cloudy myocardium and microscopically by swelling, granularity, and loss of striations of the muscle fibers. The condition includes such commonly used terms as "flabby heart" and "dishcloth heart."

Hypopotassemia.—While disturbances in potassium balance have already been considered in connection with Disturbance of Fluid Balance

(p. 199), the question of hypopotassemia in general and especially as it pertains to the heart, may be briefly mentioned at this point. The *normal* mean serum potassium concenration is 4.2 ± 0.25 mEq./L. While the figures vary, anything below 3.5 m.Eq./. may be considered as hypopotassemia (Surawicz). Normally, potassium balance is maintained as a result of an intake of potassium that averages about 1.0 m.Eq./Kg. of body weight and a proper excretion by way of the kidneys (at least 0.1 m.Eq./Kg./day) and gastrointestinal tract. A *depletion* of serum potassium concentration (hypopotassemia) *occurs* as a result of (1) when potassium intake is less than potassium output, (2) when there is excessive loss of potassium by the kidneys as in nephritis, (3) when there is a loss of potassium by the gastrointestinal tract as in diarrhea and vomiting, or (4) when steroids, such as aldosterone are administered (loss via the kidneys). More specifically, in a study of 557 patients with hypopotassemia, Surawicz recorded the following associated clinical conditions in decreasing order of frequency: inadequate diet, infusions of potassium-free solutions, vomiting, suction and gastrointestinal fistulas, diarrhea, renal disease, administration of steroids, prolonged diuresis, and insulin therapy in diabetic acidosis. In general, the *clinical manifestations* result from (1) disturbance of conduction of nerve impulses and (2) disturbance of cardiac function. More specifically, they may consist of anorexia, nausea, vomiting, abdominal distention, decreased motility and distention of the bowel, disturbances of respiration, decrease in blood pressure, cardiac dilatation, cardiac murmurs, loss of muscle strength, decrease in tendon reflexes, and mental disturbances that include increased irritability, stupor, listlessness, confusion, delerium, and coma. The general *pathologic* changes in hypopotassemia are those of the related or associated conditions rather than specific for, or even characteristic of, the chemical deficiency. This is particularly applicable to the heart. One reason for this is that the heart is often previously damaged so that the alterations are difficult to evaluate. When, however, overdoses of adrenal cortical hormones are given in Addison's disease, acute myocardial changes similar to those seen in *experimental animals* fed a potassium-deficient diet have been described. These consist of (1) focal degeneration, necrosis, and disintegration of fibers, (2) secondary infiltration with phagocytes, (3) edema, and (4) proliferation of connective tissue and blood vessels. Healing occurs by hypertrophy of the surviving muscle fibers and condensation of connective tissue. There is no evidence of regeneration of muscle fibers (French).

Anemia.—*Chronic anemia*, through deficiency in oxygenation, may result in (1) fatty metamorphosis (p. 54) and other degenerative changes in the myocardial fibers, (2) actual focal myocardial necrosis, (3) myocardial hypertrophy, and (4) dilatation of the cardiac chambers. Accordingly, the following may be noted *clinically*: dyspnea, cardiac enlargement, cardiac murmurs, dependent edema, and hepatomegaly. *Acute anemia*, as from any massive hemorrhage, is accompanied by a rapid depletion of erythrocytes in the peripheral blood, a corresponding anoxia of tissues, a decrease in blood volume and thus a drop in blood pressure, and shock. As far as the heart is concerned there is an increased work demand and an absolute and relative decreased oxygenation. This is particularly true when the coronary arteries are narrowed or occluded by a sclerotic process. Thus, the net result may be myocardial ischemia and infarction.

Digitalis Poisoning.—Large doses of digitalis produce the following changes in the heart of the cat and the dog: swelling and loss of striation of muscle fibers, pyknosis and branching of the nuclei, infiltrations with mono-nuclear cells and neutrophils, frank necrosis and infarction, and healing by fibrosis. Corresponding changes have not been recorded in man due, in part, to the relatively small doses of the drug employed and, in part, to the impossibility of distinguishing similar alterations caused by other processes which call for the use of digitalis in the first place.

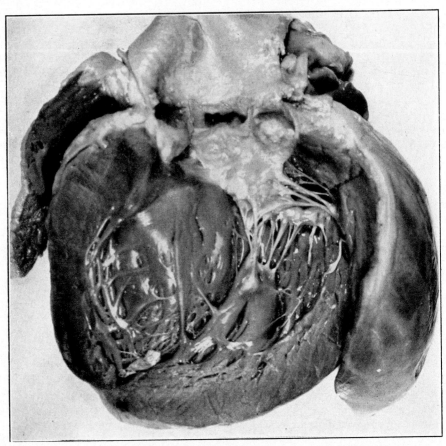

Fig. 101.—Myxedema heart showing thickening of the myocardium of the left ventricle, dilation of the corresponding chamber, and sclerosis of the aorta, aortic cusps, and mitral leaflet.

Myxedema Heart. —Myxedema heart simply indicates the cardiac changes in patients with hypothyroidism and myxedema. *Pathologically*, the alterations described consist of (1) general cardiac enlargement due to thickening of the myocardium of all chambers as well as dilatation of the chambers themselves (Fig. 101), (2) pseudohypertrophy or swelling, hydropic degeneration, loss of striations, and fragmentation of the myocardial fibers, (3) edema and leukocytic infiltration of the interstitial tissue, and (4) arteriosclerosis of the coronary arteries and aorta (Ibrahim). *Clinically* there are (1) cardiac enlargement, (2) feeble heart sounds, (3) diminished amplitude of pulsation, (4) slow heart rate, (5) normal blood pressure, (6) reduced voltage of the electrocardiogram, and (7) other manifestations of myxedema (p. 571). All the cardiac symptoms and signs are reversible upon treatment with thyroid extract.

INFLAMMATIONS

Orientation.—The three important anatomic subdivisions of the heart are endocardium, myocardium, and pericardium. Inflammation of the endocardium is known as *endocarditis*, of the myocardium as *myocarditis*, and of the pericardium as *pericarditis*. Although a lesion in any one portion of the heart may extend to or be concomitantly accompanied by inflammation of one or both of the remaining portions, the localization is generally of sufficient degree to render a classification into the three categories just mentioned of definite practical value.

ENDOCARDITIS

Orientation.—For practical purposes, endocarditis virtually resolves itself into inflammation of the valves (valvulitis) for, in the vast majority of cases, it is the valve cusps and leaflets that are involved and cause most of the untoward results. Further, the most frequently affected, and therefore the most important, valves are the mitral and aortic. The more common lesions may be considered under the following headings: rheumatic fever, bacterial endocarditis, atypical verrucal endocarditis, terminal endocarditis, spirochetal endocarditis, tuberculous endocarditis, and fungous endocarditis.

Rheumatic Fever.—Rheumatic fever may be defined as an acute to chronic degenerative and inflammatory disorder of the connective tissue of the body with the most profound changes occurring in the heart. It is a member of a group of "*collagen diseases*" that includes rheumatoid arthritis, disseminated lupus erythematosus, diffuse glomerulonephritis, and periarteritis nodosa. Rheumatic fever is responsible for about 90 per cent of heart disease in children and 35 per cent of heart disease in adults, has its greatest *incidence* between the ages of five and twenty years, has no predilection for any race or either sex, occurs with greater frequency in colder than in warmer (tropical) climates, is more prevalent in winter and early spring than in other seasons of the year, and is more common among the poor than the rich.

Although numerous theories have been propounded to explain the *cause* of rheumatic fever, it is now generally accepted that the disease results from a hypersensitivity to *Streptococcus hemolyticus*, *Streptococcus nonhemolyticus*, or *Streptococcus viridans* (Lancefield Group A)—a hypersensitivity to the whole organisms or their products. Such an explanation is favored by the fact that attacks of rheumatic fever are preceded by upper respiratory tract infections in about two-thirds of the cases, and that prophylactic antibiotic and chemotherapy in army camps has been attended by a low incidence of both upper respiratory tract infection and rheumatic fever. Since rheumatic fever does not follow every streptococcic infection in man there must be other added factors. Some of these appear to be heredity, hormonal imbalances (hyperinsulinism and hyperthyroidism), dietary (vitamin, fat, and protein) deficiency, exposure to cold and damp atmosphere, fatigue, overcrowding, and trauma. Although streptococci are now definitely incriminated as etiologic agents, the *mechanism* involved is not known. The theory that it works through a hyaluronic acid—hyaluronidase system has been more or less exploded. The explanation, according to this theory, was quite simple. Hyaluronic acid is present in the ground substance of connective tissue and protects against bacterial invasion. Hyaluronidase (an enzyme) polymerizes hyaluronic acid and thus enhances the spread of bacteria. Since some members of Group A streptococci produce hyaluronidase, it was thought that the excessive formation of this enzyme neutralized hyaluronic acid and thus brought about the lesions. The only difficulty with this explanation is that the strains of Group A streptococci that precede an attack of rheumatic fever elaborate hyaluronic acid but not hyaluronidase.

Experimentally, lesions (in the heart and other organs) similar to those found in rheumatic fever have been produced in sensitized laboratory animals (rabbits) by single or repeated intravenous injections of egg albumin and foreign (horse, duck, or bovine) serum. Intravenous injections of living or dead streptococci produce lesions more like those of subacute bacterial endocarditis rather than of rheumatic fever. A somewhat different experimental approach was used by Selye. He produced lesions resembling those found in rheumatic fever by first sensitizing animals by means of a high salt intake and unilateral nephrectomy, and then either administering large doses of adrenal cortical hormone or pituitary corticotrophin, or exposing them to cold or some other damaging agents (Waksman).

Pathologically the pathognomonic unit of rheumatic fever is the *rheumatic granuloma* or the *Aschoff nodule*. It is submiliary in size and is thus difficult to see with the naked eye. While the nodule is present in most organs of the body (albeit often in a modified form) it is seen in its complete and classical form in the myocardium. Characteristically it is paravascular (to one side of and not surrounding the vessel) in location (Fig. 102). Its development may be generally divided into four phases: (1) *Degenerative Phase*. The first noticeable change is a focal fibrinoid degeneration of connective tissue wherein the collagen swells, fragments, and stains deeply eosinophilic. (2) *Exudative Phase*. This stage consists of a permeation of the degenerated and adjacent tissues by monocytes, few neutrophils, and varying numbers of eosinophils. The degenerative and exudative alterations occur within the first two to four weeks of the illness. (3) *Granulomatous Phase*. This stage occurs in the fifth week of the disease and consists of the appearance of Aschoff giant cells in the peripheral portions of the original foci and beyond this of the appearance of epithelioid cells and fibroblasts. Aschoff cells are derived from mononuclear (reticulum) cells. They are large, rounded, or somewhat irregular, are sharply defined, have a moderate amount of lightly basophilic cytoplasm, and possess single or multiple, round, vesicular nuclei. (4) *Healing Phase*. This is the final stage and consists of an increase of connective tissue, a gradual accumulation of collagen, and scar formation. It occurs in from three to four months after the onset of the illness. Since the appearance and distribution of the lesions vary somewhat with the organ affected, a brief consideration of the changes in different sites of the body appears to be in order.

Involvement of the *endocardium* (endocarditis) is most profound in the valvular areas. The incidence of affliction of the valves in decreasing order of frequency is mitral, aortic, tricuspid, and pulmonary and the precise site of initial localization of the lesion is along the line of closure of the valves and the connective tissue of the cusps and leaflets. It consists of fibrinoid degeneration and exudation (Fig. 103). When the process reaches the surface the endothelium is damaged and the denuded area becomes covered with verrucæ. Grossly the latter consist of a row of small, pink to yellow, rough, closely adherent, wart-like vegetations located linearly along the line of closure of the leaflets and cusps (Fig. 104). Microscopically they are composed first of

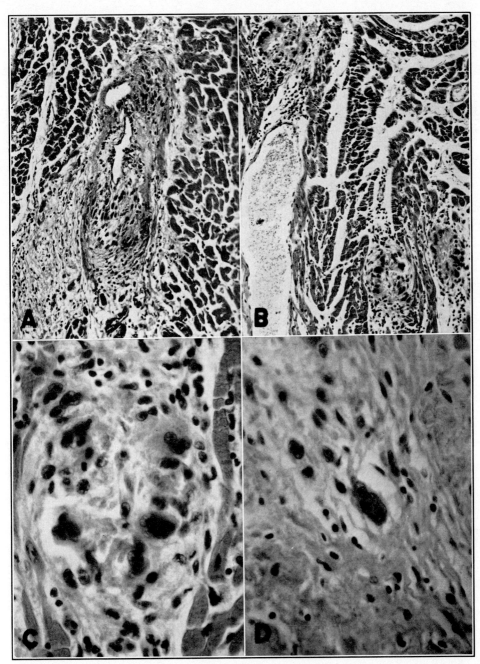

Fig. 102.—Rheumatic granulomas (Aschoff nodules) showing *A*, paravascular distribution of the lesions.   × 100, *B*, three acute nodules with central areas of fibrinoid degeneration and peripheral leukocytes and Aschoff cells.   × 100, *C*, high power view of a nodule with central fibrinoid degeneration and permeating Aschoff cells and leukocytes.   × 400, and *D*, healing nodule with a diffuse fibroblastic proliferation and an active multinucleated Aschoff cell.   × 400.

thread-like and then more conglomerate masses of fibrin surrounded, at their junction with the valve proper, by Aschoff cells and fibroblasts arranged at right angles to the surface. Ultimately, healing occurs by the usual invasion of connective tissue and deposition of collagen. Similar degenerative, exudative, granulomatous, and healing changes occur in the chordæ tendinæ and the endocardium of the left atrium, especially above the posterior leaflet of the mitral valve. As a result of these alterations, the affected areas ultimately become thickened, yellowish to brownish or grayish, firm, and rigid; the adjacent edges of the valve cusps and leaflets fuse and the cusps and leaflets contract, and the chordæ tendinæ also fuse, broaden, and become so short that the papillary muscles appear to arise

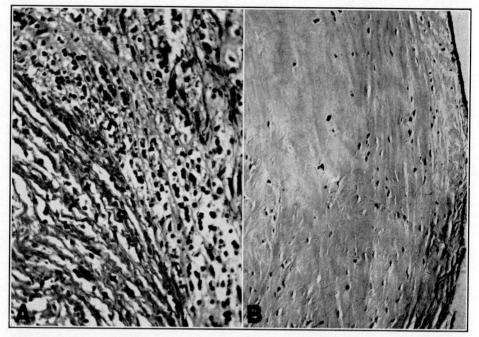

FIG. 103.—Rheumatic endocarditis showing *A*, an active lesion with fibrinoid degeneration and leukocytic permeation, × 200 and *B*, healed lesion with extensive fibrosis and collagen deposition. × 100.

directly from the leaflets themselves (Fig. 105.) In the end the newly formed collagenous tissue may undergo irregular calcification. The net result is valvular deformity, usually of sufficient degree to produce stenosis and/or insufficiency. Typical Aschoff nodules may affect any portion of the *myocardium* (myocarditis) but they prevail in the posterior part of the left ventricle, the base of the interventricular septum, and the left atrium. As already stated, they are submiliary in size and are scarcely visible grossly. The changes in the *mesothelial surfaces* (pericarditis, pleuritis, or peritonitis) may be focal or more general (Fig. 106). Grossly, they consist primarily of a fibrinous exudate with varying, but usually slight, amounts of straw-colored fluid. Histologically the tissue is permeated with fibrin, serum, and varying numbers of leukocytes (monocytes, neutrophils, and eosinophils). Sometimes the leukocytes are collected into clusters and when mononucleated or multinucleated giant cells are also present they form spurious

Aschoff nodules (Fig. 106). In mesothelial surfaces the process resolves or heals by fibrosis. In the latter instance, adhesions frequently form.

Vascular lesions in rheumatic fever may be widespread. Larger vessels such as the *aorta* and *pulmonary artery* may show Aschoff nodules or more diffuse inflammations distributed along the vasa vasorum. These changes may be of sufficient intensity to cause focal fraying of the elastic fibers of

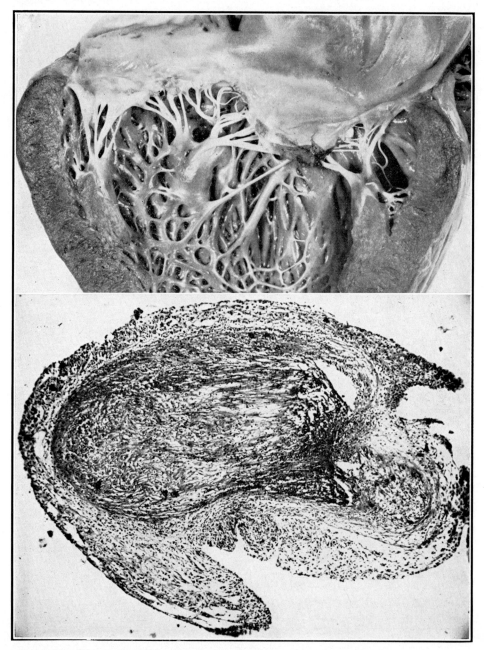

Fig. 104.—Rheumatic endocarditis showing (above) a row of fine bead-like verrucæ along the line of closure of the mitral valve and (below) profound fibrinoid degeneration and leukocytic infiltration of a mitral leaflet. × 50.

the media, but only rarely do they bring about enough weakening of the wall to cause appreciable dilatation (aneurysm) of the vessels. Sometimes the *ascending aorta* shows intimal involvement similar to that in the endocardium of the left atrium. Grossly it discloses yellowish to brownish transparent plaques or ridges while histologically it reveals fibrinoid degeneration and exudation. The process heals by fibrosis. The *smaller vessels* such as the pulmonary, coronary, renal, pancreatic, cerebral, celiac, hepatic, etc., show (1) fibrinoid degeneration of the intima and other portions of the wall, (2) fraying of the elastic fibers, (3) diffuse permeation with

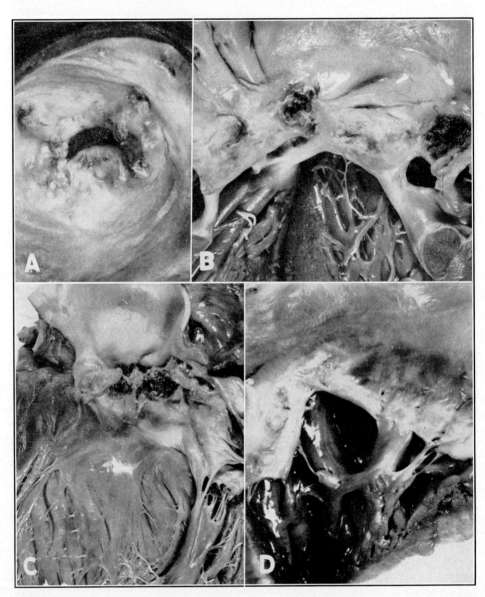

Fig. 105.—Healed rheumatic endocarditis showing fusion, fibrosis, and distortion of *A*, mitral leaflets (fish-mouth-like deformity of the valve), *B*, mitral leaflets (note also the fused thickened and shortened chordæ tendinæ), *C*, aortic cusps, and *D*, tricuspid leaflets. The mitral and aortic valves show, in addition, foci of calcification.

monocytes, neutrophils, and eosinophils, and (4) occasionally frank thrombosis (Fig. 107). The vascular lesions also heal by fibrosis.

Pulmonary involvement (rheumatic pneumonia) is said to occur in from
2 to 14 per cent of cases during the height of an attack of the disease. As
demonstrated roentgenographically the lesions are migratory in type.

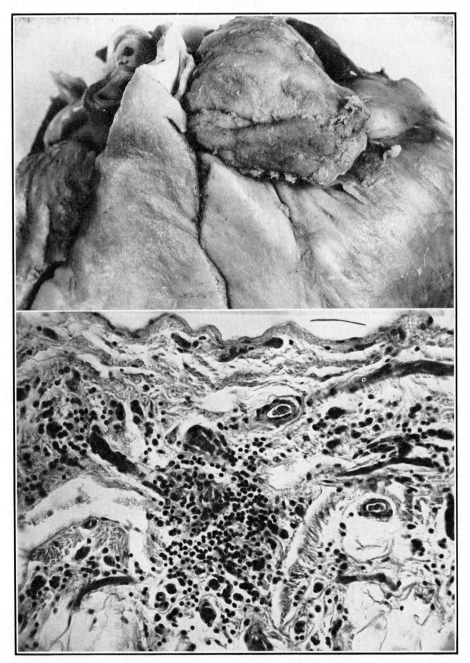

FIG. 106.—Rheumatic pericarditis illustrating (above) a fibrinous exudate on the surface of the
visceral pericardium and (below) an accumulation of leukocytes and Aschoff cells which, along
with some fibrinoid degeneration, produces a spurious Aschoff nodule. × 200.

Grossly the affected areas are firm, somewhat rubbery, and deep red. Histologically the alveoli contain edema fluid, scattered leukocytes, and a hyaline
membrane peripherally. The septa reveal fibrinoid necrosis and a permeation with monocytes, neutrophils, and Aschoff cells (Fig. 108A). Later the
exudate in the alveoli may organize to form globular masses called *Masson
bodies* and the alveolar septa become permanently thickened by a deposition
of fibrous tissue.

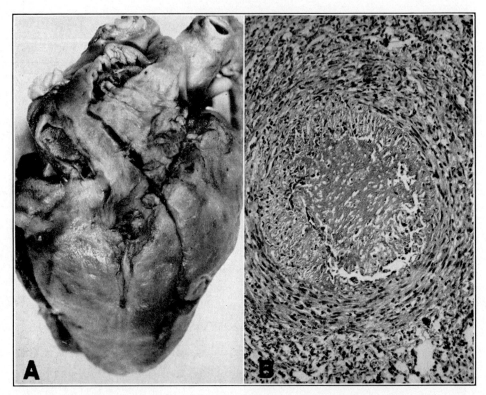

FIG. 107.—Rheumatic arteritis showing (to the left) thrombosis of a coronary artery in a two-
month-old child and (to the right) a histologic section of one of the branches of the same coronary
artery. The latter discloses fibrinoid degeneration of the intima, thrombosis of the lumen, and a
leukocytic infiltration of the media and adventitia. × 100.

In the *subcutaneous* tissues, small, ill-defined, moderately firm *nodules* measuring a few millimeters in diameter are frequently found overriding the bony
prominences of the elbow, wrist, knee, and ankle. Histologically they consist of a center of fibrinoid degeneration and a periphery of fibroblasts
containing varying numbers of monocytes, neutrophils, and eosinophils
(Fig. 108B).

The *joints* (rheumatic arthritis) may become swollen, reddened, tender,
and extremely painful. The joint spaces exhibit moderate amounts of
fluid containing fibrin and a few neutrophils. The lining membrane and
adjacent tissues reveal hyperemia, edema, fibrinoid necrosis, and a cellular
infiltration similar to that seen in other tissues. Classical Aschoff nodules
are not seen.

The *brain* is often affected in young patients. Grossly it discloses only
hyperemia. Histologically the gray matter, basal ganglia, brain stem, and

the tissue around the aqueduct reveal (1) engorgement, thrombosis, proliferative endarteritis, and perivascular mononuclear cell permeation of the terminal ramifications of the smaller vessels and (2) degeneration of the nerve cells. In addition, the larger vessels may show the changes already referred to above.

Renal involvement has been recorded in from 0 to 17 per cent of cases. The lesions have been described as consisting of focal interstitial nephritis, embolic nephritis, and acute diffuse glomerulonephritis.

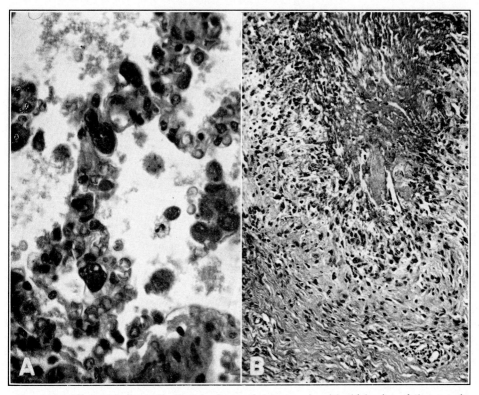

Fig. 108.—Rheumatic fever showing *A*, rheumatic pneumonia with thickening of the septa by fibrinoid degeneration, erythrocytic extravasation, and leukocytic (including Aschoff cell) infiltration. The alveoli contain similar cells. × 400, and *B*, subcutaneous nodule with central fibrinoid degeneration and peripheral fibroblastic proliferation and leukocytic infiltration. × 100.

Although the *complications* of rheumatic fever are referable to each of the many organs affected the most important sequel is cardiac failure. It may be acute—occurring at the height of the rheumatic infection, or it may be chronic—occurring weeks, months, or years after the acute infection has subsided. The *clinical manifestations* are quite varied. Jones (and later Bland and Jones) divided the symptoms and signs into two groups—major and minor. *Major manifestations* consist of (1) carditis—enlargement (due to involvement of the myocardium and dilatation of the chambers), murmurs (due to valvular stenosis and insufficiency), friction rub (due to pericarditis), congestive failure (due principally to endocardial and myocardial involvement), and electrocardiographic (prolongation of the auric, uloventricular conduction time) changes (due to myocardial involvement)- (2) arthralgia—migratory polyarthritis attended by swelling, redness, and tenderness of the joints (due to involvement of the synovial membranes and periarticular tissues), (3) chorea—consisting of involuntary jerky movements and found in approximately one-half of all children with rheumatic fever (due to involvement of the brain), (4) subcutaneous nodules—located over bony prominences (due to involvement of connective tissue), and (5) recurrences found in 70 per cent of young rheumatic fever patients. *Minor manifestations* are local (due to rheumatic involvement of the various organs) or general (due to absorption of toxic metabolites). They may be listed as follows: (1) fever, (2) abdominal pain (especially children), (3) precordial pain, (4) rashes (purpuric eruptions or rheumatic erythema consisting of reddish or bluish-red semicircular eruptions of the skin of the trunk), (5) epistaxis, (6) pulmonary signs (especially consolidation), and (7) miscellaneous, consisting of fatigue, pallor, sweating, loss of weight, headache, vomiting, hematuria, bursitis, and pleuritis. The *laboratory findings* include increase in size of the cardiac silhouette in roentgenograms, microcytic anemia, leukocytosis, and increased sedimentation rate. In addition, electrophoretic patterns on serum or plasma have shown a consistent decrease in albumin, a consistent increase in alpha globulin and fibrogen, and an inconsistent increase in gamma globulin (Robinson and Reid). Each of these reverts to normal with clinical improvement in the disease. Finally, from the laboratory standpoint, there is an appearance of, or a rise in, antistreptolysin O titer of the blood during the first 3 to 4 weeks of an attack of acute rheumatic fever (McCarty). Antistreptolysin O, incidentally, is an antibody directed against one of the extracellular hemolysins produced by Group A *Streptococcus*.

A *diagnosis* of rheumatic fever is based upon a correct interpretation of the various clinical manifestations listed above. Of added significance are geographic location, age of the patient (most prevalent between five and twenty years), and a salutary response to salicylates. A *differential diagnosis* includes many diseases. Some of the disorders listed by Hansen are appendicitis, poliomyelitis, osteomyelitis, emotional disorders, fulminating infection, rheumatoid arthritis, meningococcemia, sickle cell disease, bacterial endocarditis, pneumonia, brucellosis, and nephritis. One of the essentials of proper *treatment* is prolonged bed rest. In addition to other measures, salicylates, ACTH, and cortisone are administered during the acute phase, while antibiotics and sulfonamides are used to prevent recurrences. When valvular stenosis becomes marked, valvulotomy and commissurotomy are indicated. The *prognosis* varies somewhat with the locale, being worse in the colder than in the warmer climates. In a study of 588 children, Ash noted the following: two-thirds of the children developed heart disease, 10 per cent were dead at the end of the first year, one-quarter were dead at the end of ten years, one-third were dead at the end of fifteen years, and one-half were dead at the end of twenty years. When the initial attack occurs in adults, the prognosis is immeasurably better. In a study of 10,000 army personnel in World War II, the incidence of cardiac involvement was only 10 per cent.

Bacterial Endocarditis.—As the caption suggests, bacterial endocarditis is bacterial inflammation of the endocardium, especially the valve cusps and leaflets. In the past, bacterial endocarditis has been divided into two groups—*acute* and *subacute*. The main difference between the two groups was one of time—the acute being more fulminating while the subacute being more protracted. With the advent of antibiotic and chemotherapy, however, the courses of the conditions have been greatly altered. Thus, they may be discussed under the one heading and considered simply as a single disease with variations in intensity and quantity. Bacterial endocarditis is relatively common. The *incidence* at the Cook County Hospital is approximately 1.6 per cent of all autopsies with acute bacterial endocarditis being half as common as subacute. At the Philadelphia General Hospital, acute bacterial endocarditis constitutes approximately 2.5 per cent of all autopsies. There is no predilection for any race; the condition is as common in males as it is in females, and the usual age incidence is between twenty and sixty years with a preponderance in the fourth decade. Early spring appears to be the favored season. The ultimate *causes* are bacteria. While the organisms are interchangeable and sometimes mixed, *subacute bacterial endocarditis* is most commonly caused by *Streptococcus viridans*, any of the enterococcus group, and *Streptococcus nonhemolyticus* and *acute bacterial endocarditis* is generally caused by *Streptococcus hemolyticus*, *Staphylococcus aureus*, pneumococcus, gonococcus, and *Staphylococcus albus*. Some unusual causes of either form of the disease are *Streptobacillus moniliformis*, *Neisseria meningitidis*, *Brucella abortus*, *Clostridium welchii*, *Salmonella*, *Hemophilus influenzæ*, *Escherichia-Aerobacter*, and *Corynebacterium diphtheriæ*. In approximately two-thirds of the cases, the *source* of the organisms is not determinable. In the remaining third it may be ascribed to respiratory tract infection, dental caries (extraction of a tooth), cutaneous or other abscess, puerperal sepsis, osteomyelitis, genitourinary tract infection, or postoperative infection. The *route* of invasion is direct implantation on the endocardium from the bloodstream. In the acute form of the disease the valve cusps and leaflets are often previously normal although the disorder may also be superimposed upon previously damaged valves. In the subacute form of the disease the valve cusps and leaflets are almost always previously damaged. The most common *preexisting condition* is rheumatic fever. Other predisposing factors are arteriosclerosis (older age group) and congenital cardiac anomalies (including bicuspid aortic valve, patent ductus arteriosus both naturally occurring and the Taussig-Blalock types, coarctation of the aorta, tetralogy of Fallot, pulmonary stenosis, patent interventricular septum, and atrial septal defects). *Experimentally* bacterial endocarditis is readily produced in rabbits and dogs by repeated intravenous injections of streptococci obtained from a variety of lesions in man.

Pathologically both the subacute and acute forms of the disease attack the following valves in decreasing order of frequency: mitral, aortic, tricuspid, and pulmonary. In addition, subacute bacterial endocarditis may be found affecting a naturally occurring or artificially produced patent ductus arteriosus. As already stated, the valve cusps and leaflets are usually previously damaged in cases of subacute bacterial endocarditis but are frequently normal in cases of acute bacterial endocarditis. In either case, the *endocardial lesions* start along the line of closure of the cusps or leaflets as small pink to deep red vegetations. As they enlarge they spread laterally to involve adjacent leaflets or cusps and proximally on to the ventricular or auricular endocardium, as the case may be. In the fully developed form the vegetations are large, fungating, superficially irregular, pink or brown or intensely hemorrhagic, and quite friable (Figs. 109 and 111). In the subacute form of the disease, the underlying endocardium is usually only superficially eroded, while in the acute form of the disease it is usually extensively ulcerated to a degree that may cause complete perforation of the cusp or leaflet. In some instances the process extends along the

chordæ tendinæ which may also be ulcerated and ruptured. In cases of
patent ductus arteriosus, the vegetations occur in the ductus itself, at the
opening of the ductus into the pulmonary artery, and in the intima of the
pulmonary artery (Fig. 109). As the lesions become older they have a
tendency to heal by fibrosis and later by calcification. *Histologically* the
vegetations in the *subacute* form of the disease consist of masses of fused
fibrin and platelets intermingled with large colonies of bacteria. There are
present scattered mononuclear cells but there is a conspicuous paucity of
neutrophils (Fig. 110*A*). The lesions ultimately heal by replacement with
granulation and then fibrous tissue, both of which originate from the under-

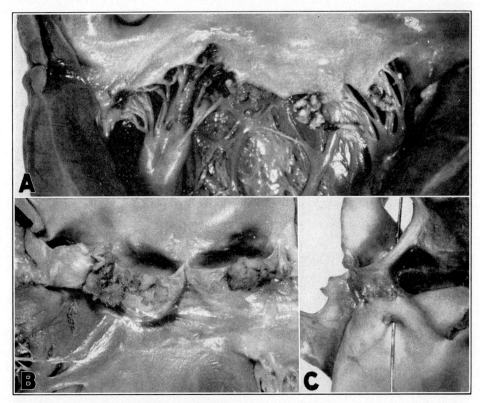

FIG. 109.—Subacute bacterial endocarditis showing *A*, healing vegetations on a mitral valve
that was previously damaged by rheumatic fever, *B*, exuberant friable vegetation covering two
aortic cusps that were previously damaged slightly by rheumatic fever, and *C*, several vegetations
surrounding the opening of the ductus arteriosus into the pulmonary artery.

lying endocardium. In the *acute* form of the disease the vegetations consist
essentially of a mixture of platelets, fibrin, and colonies of bacteria permeated and surrounded by great numbers of neutrophils (Fig. 112*A*). The
intense inflammatory reaction penetrates, ulcerates, and weakens any of
the underlying structures found in the path of its advancement. Here, as
in the subacute form, the lesion ultimately also heals by granulation and
fibrous tissue replacement. In time, the surface of the previous vegetation
becomes recovered with endothelium. Although the changes in the *myocardium* are perhaps ordinarily not as important in bacterial endocarditis
as they are in rheumatic fever, they are nevertheless quite frequent. They

may be due to (1) direct extension of the lesion from the endocardium. (2) coronary artery emboli from the vegetations, (3) toxins emanating from the growing and disintegrating bacteria, and (4) direct hematogenous bacterial seeding (Saphir). In *subacute bacterial endocarditis* the lesions in the myocardium are focal or diffuse. They generally consist of edema of the

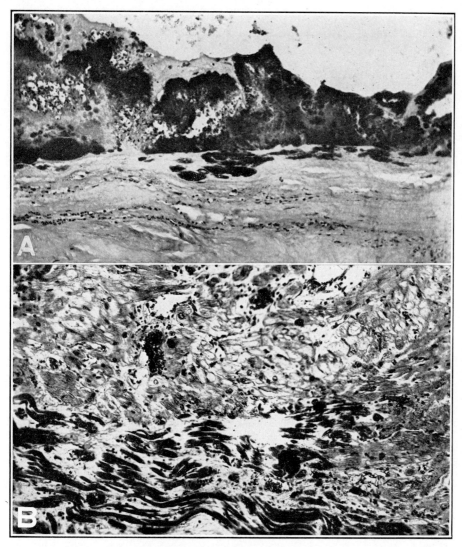

Fig. 110.—Subacute bacterial endocarditis showing *A*, masses of bacteria embedded in fibrinous and platelet thrombi. The vegetations are superimposed upon a sclerotic valve leaflet. Note the paucity of leukocytes, and *B*, myocardial edema, degeneration, and leukocytic permeation. × 100.

interstitial tissue, varying degrees of leukocytic infiltration, vascular engorgement, and slight to moderate degeneration of the myocardial fibers (Fig. 110*B*). Occasionally microscopic abscesses may be found in relation to the vessels and rarely a foreign body reaction to calcific emboli from the valvular vegetations may be recognized. In *acute bacterial endocarditis* the only difference is that the myocardial lesions tend to be more suppurative.

20

The involvement of the musculature may occur as a result of direct extension from the lesions in the endocardium or as a result of coronary artery embolism of the vegetation (Fig. 112B). In the latter instance, the lumen of the vessel is filled with colonies of bacteria and fused fibrin and platelet thrombi and the wall of the vessel together with the surrounding myocardium is densely permeated with neutrophils. Thus, frank abscess formation is the commonly encountered lesion. *Pericarditis*, usually as a direct

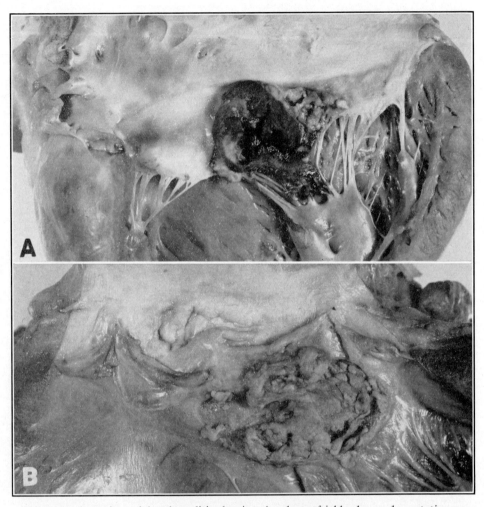

Fig. 111.—Acute bacterial endocarditis showing *A*, a large, friable, deep red vegetation on a previously normal mitral leaflet, and *B*, a similar but grayer vegetation covering an aortic cusp that was previously affected by rheumatic fever.

extension of the process from the myocardium, occurs in from 10 to 20 per cent of cases. Depending upon the type and virulence of the organism, the lesions vary from a fibrinous to a suppurative type.

The *complications* of bacterial endocarditis are (1) local valvular (insufficiency, stenosis, or rupture) and myocardial (weakness due to inflammation), (2) general toxemic, and (3) embolic. Embolism occurs in the systemic circulation when the lesions affect the left side of the heart or

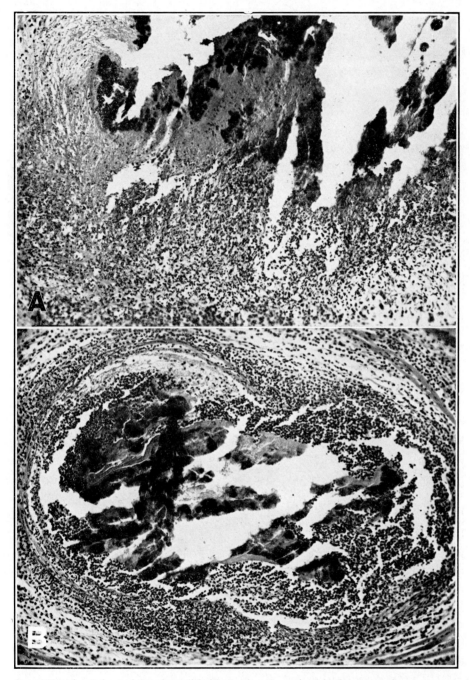

FIG. 112.—Acute bacterial endocarditis illustrating *A*, a mitral leaflet vegetation composed of masses of bacteria that are surrounded by numerous neutrophils and *B*, an embolic vegetation in a coronary artery. The central bacterial clumps are surrounded by an intense leukocytic infiltration of the wall of the vessel and adjacent myocardium. × 100.

when they affect the right side of the heart and there are septal defects. It involves the pulmonary circulation when the right side of the heart is involved. Small or microscopic emboli result in petechiæ while larger emboli produce infarcts. Embolic lesions in the subacute form of the disease are nonsuppurative (Fig. 113A and B) while in the acute form of the disease

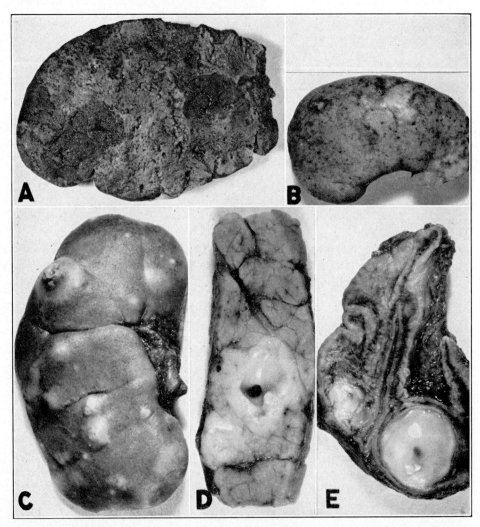

Fig. 113.—Complications of bacterial endocarditis showing A, massive bland infarction of the spleen, B, multiple bland infarcts of the kidney, and embolic abscesses of the C, kidney, D, pancreas, and E, adrenal.

they are suppurative with abscess formation (Fig. 113C, D, and E). Although any vessel, tissue, or organ may be affected the most commonly involved are the skin, brain, spleen, kidneys, eyes, myocardium, mesentery, lungs, and vasa vasorum. The last mentioned results in the formation of embolic (mycotic) aneurysms of the vessel and these may ultimately terminate in rupture and fatal hemorrhage. Aside from infarcts and abscesses the renal changes may consist of embolic glomerulonephritis and acute diffuse glomerulonephritis (see Chapter 31 on the Kidney, p. 1078).

Clinically (Loewe, Cates and Christie, and Dowling *et al.*) various combinations of the following manifestations may be encountered: (1) As a result of the general toxemia there may be fever, anemia, loss of weight, weakness, anorexia, sweating, chills, rigors, leukocytosis, and increased sedimentation rate. (2) Emboli affecting the following organs may be accompanied by the following respective manifestations: spleen—pain and enlargement, kidney—hematuria, albuminuria, casts in the urine, and elevated nonprotein nitrogen of the blood, central nervous system—a variety of paralytic manifestations, vessels—occlusions with corresponding symptoms and signs or mycotic aneurysms with rupture, lungs—cough, hemoptysis, pain, fever, dyspnea, and cyanosis, coronary arteries—symptoms and signs of coronary occlusion, and skin—petechiæ, *Osler's nodes* (tender, raised, purplish areas in the finger tips, pads of the toes, soles, and palms), and subungual splinter hemorrhages. (3) As a result of endocardial, myocardial, and pericardial involvement there may be a variety of murmurs, cardiac enlargement (clinically and roentgenologically), pericardial pain and friction rub, manifestations of cardiac failure, and a variety of electrocardiographic changes particularly alterations in the T waves. (4) Because the bacteria are exposed to and carried in the blood stream, positive blood cultures should be obtained in from 85 to 95 per cent of cases. (5) As a result of direct involvement of the synovia there may be inflammation (occasionally of a fleeting variety) of one or more of the larger joints. The *diagnosis* of bacterial endocarditis is made from a consideration of the clinical manifestations enumerated above and, more precisely, upon obtaining a positive blood culture. *Treatment* is divided into two phases—*prophylaxis* in the form of elimination of possible foci of infection and *active* consisting of antibiotics together with other supportive measures. The *prognosis* in untreated patients is poor for the mortality is 100 per cent. In antibiotic treated patients, the immediate mortality is about 15 per cent while the ultimate mortality should be less than 30 per cent. The secret of success lies in the early recognition of the disorder. Some of the more important *causes* of *death* are cardiac failure, cerebral and other embolisms, and pneumonia.

Atypical Verrucal Endocarditis.—Atypical verrucal endocarditis, also known as *Libman-Sack's disease* (1924), represents the endocardial lesions of a systemic disorder known as *disseminated lupus erythematosus*. The last mentioned is in essence an acute, subacute, or chronic degenerative, and to a lesser extent inflammatory disorder of the collagen tissue throughout the body. In this section the systemic disease, as a whole, may be conveniently considered. The condition *occurs* two to seven times as frequently in females as in males, is of greatest incidence between the ages of ten and forty years, and is as common in negroes as in the white population (Jessar). The *cause* is undetermined although many authors consider the disorder to be the result of an allergic hypersensitivity.

Pathologically, as indicated by the definition, the connective tissue throughout the body is affected and, therefore, every organ may be involved. The basic alteration consists of a granular, eosinophilic change in the *collagen* (Fig. 114*A*). As the lesion progresses there is ultimately complete disruption of the connective tissue cells but there is always only a slight leukocytic (mononuclear, lymphocytic, eosinophilic, and plasma cell) infiltration. In addition to the connective tissue change there is a similar alteration in the *vessels* (arterioles and venules) of the body. This consists essentially of a fibrinoid change affecting principally the media and the

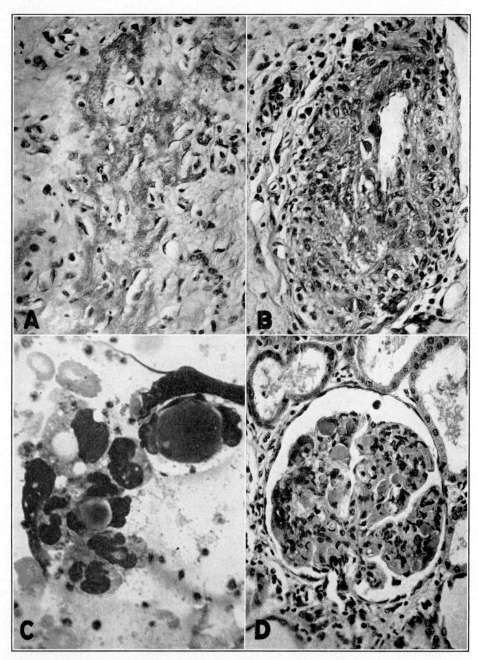

FIG. 114.—Disseminated lupus erythematosus showing *A*, fibrinoid change in the dermis. × 200, *B*, fibrinoid change and leukocytic reaction of an arteriole. × 200, *C*, L. E. cells in a bone marrow aspiration. × 1370, and *D*, wire-looping and intracapillary hyaline thrombi in a renal glomerulus. × 200.

intima but also extending for various distances out into the adventitia
(Fig. 114B). Here, also, the leukocytic infiltration is always sparse. Aside
from the connective tissue and vascular lesions, a word or two about each
of the organs appears to be in order. The *endocardial* lesions consist of
small, discrete or more conglomerate, gray to brown verrucal elevations

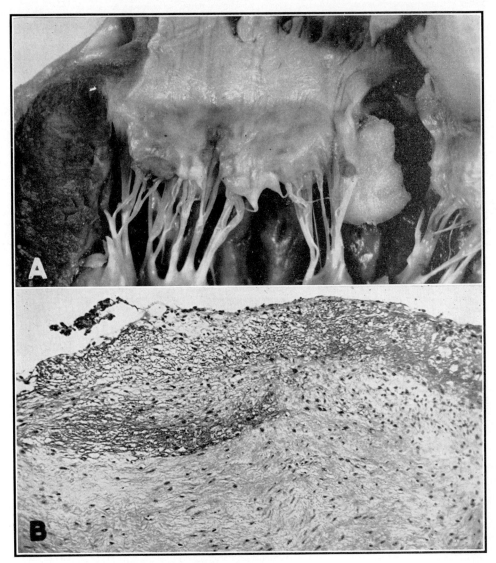

Fig. 115.—Disseminated lupus erythematosus illustrating *A*, three rather large, light brown
verrucæ on a mitral valve and *B*, fibrinoid change in the superficial portion of a mitral leaflet.
× 100.

located along the line of closure of the valve cusps and leaflets or spreading
over either surface of the valves and endocardium (Fig. 115A). Although
each of the valves may be affected, the lesion is most common in the mitral
and tricuspid valves. Histologically the verrucæ consist principally of
fibrinoid degeneration of the superficial portions of the endocardium with

frequently a superimposed precipitate of fibrin and platelets (Fig. 115*B*). The *myocardium* often reveals focal areas of collagen degeneration with slight leukocytic infiltration that may readily be mistaken for rheumatic nodules (Fig. 116*A*). The *mesothelial surfaces* (pericardium, pleura, and

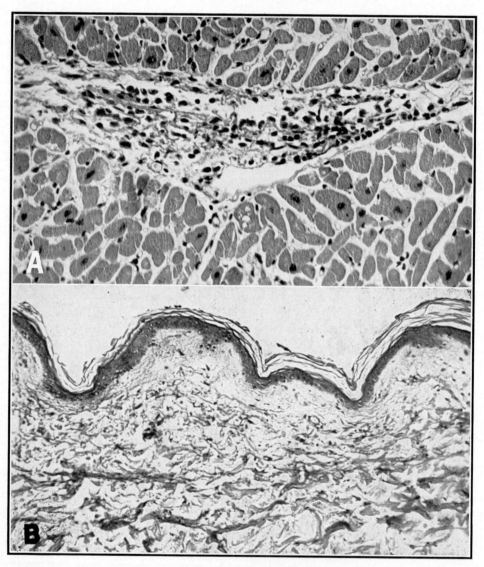

Fig. 116.—Disseminated lupus erythematosus showing *A*, focal myocarditis that superficially resembles an Aschoff nodule. × 200 and *B*, characteristic fibrinoid change in the dermis at its junction with the epidermis. × 50.

peritoneum) and *synovial membranes* (lining joints) usually disclose fibrinous or serofibrinous exudation. Histologically the surface is covered with an abundant amount of fibrin while the deeper tissue discloses the usual fibrinoid degeneration. In a typical case, the *skin* reveals erythematous macules and papules that charactistically cover the bridge of the nose and adjacent portions of the cheeks in a butterfly-like fashion and that are generally also present on the fingertips. In addition, of course, any portion of the body may be affected. Frank purpura or more hemorrhagic lesions are likewise sometimes noted. The cutaneous lesions usually heal, leaving a superficial roughening or scaling. Histologically the outer portion of the dermis, at its junction with the epidermis, discloses the usual fibrinoid degeneration and the adjacent epidermal cells reveal vacuolic and other degenerative changes (Fig. 116*B*). The deeper portions of the dermis show vascular alterations and fibrinoid degeneration. The *kidneys* disclose a

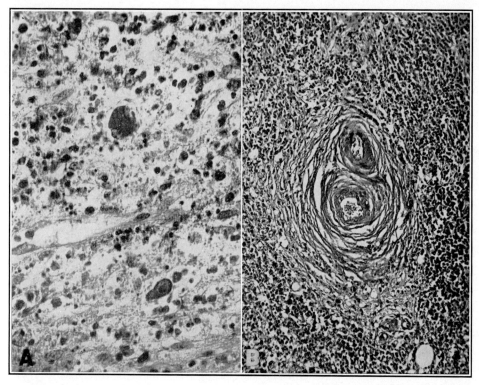

Fig. 117.—Disseminated lupus erythematosus illustrating *A*, two hematoxylin staining bodies in a lymph node. × 400, and *B*, an onion-skin lesion of the spleen consisting of peri-arterial bands of collagenous tissue. × 100.

hyaline thickening of the basement membranes of the glomerular capillaries, thus presenting what has been called wire looping (Fig. 114*D*). In addition, some of the capillaries contain solid hyaline bodies which Klemperer maintains are closely related to *L. E.* (lupus erythematosus) *cells*. In their typical form the latter are present both in the bone marrow and in the peripheral blood of patients with the acute type of the disorder. They consist of neutrophils containing large, round, homogeneous bodies that stain with basic dyes (Fig. 114*C*). The bodies probably represent nuclear material and contain depolymerized desoxyribonucleic acid. Klemperer has noted similar bodies which he termed "hemotoxylin staining bodies" in most tissues of the body prepared by the usual histologic technique. Teilum, in a study of 15 cases, noted them mostly in the endocardial vegetations and in lymph nodes and, to a lesser extent, in the spleen, pancreas, and kidneys. Histologically they resemble the structures seen in *L. E. cells* (Fig. 117, *A*).

The *spleen* characteristically reveals what are referred to as *onion-skin lesions*. They consist essentially of a concentric layering of collagenous connective tissue about the periphery of arterioles (Fig. 117, *B*). While such lesions are highly characteristic of disseminated lupus erythematosus, they are not pathognomonic of this condition, for similar changes have been noted in connection with sarcoidosis, thrombocytopenic purpura, and conditions associated with plasmocytosis and hyperglobulinemia (Teilum). In any of the organs of the body the lesions heal by resolution and/or fibrous tissue replacement.

The most serious *complications* attending disseminated lupus erythematosus are cardiac failure, renal insufficiency, and pneumonia. *Clinically* the symptoms and signs may all be explainable on the involvement of the various organs by the alterations in the connective tissue and the blood vessels. Soffer and Bader listed the following in decreasing order of frequency: fever, arthritis, L. E. cells, renal damage (hematuria, casts in the urine, and azotemia), increased sedimentation rate, anemia, loss of weight, leukopenia, lymphadenopathy, cutaneous rash, thrombocytopenia, focal ulcerations of the mucous membrane, pericarditis, pleuritis, organic mental syndrome (depression, euphoria, or psychosis), retinal changes, electroencephalographic abnormalities, petechiæ and purpura, cacchexia, palpable spleen, abdominal pain, Raynaud's phenomenon, and nephrotic syndrome. The cardiac manifestations are more frequently those of pericarditis than of endocarditis although a careful examination often discloses murmurs. The *diagnosis* of disseminated lupus erythematosus is made from a careful consideration of the clinical symptoms and signs listed above and is definitely determined by the finding of L. E. cells in the peripheral blood stream or the bone marrow. A *differential diagnosis* should include dermatomyositis, scleroderma, rheumatic fever, and rheumatoid arthritis. *Treatment* has been most varied and generally unsuccessful. Currently, ACTH and cortisone appear to be favored. They do not *cure* the condition but they do produce prompt and sometimes prolonged remissions. *Death* is usually due to renal failure, cardiac insufficiency, or pneumonia.

Terminal Endocarditis.—Terminal endocarditis has *also* been *called* degenerative verrucal endocardiosis, marantic thrombosis, nonbacterial thrombotic endocarditis, endocarditis simplex, and thromboendocarditis cachectica (Allen and Sirota). The condition is a *common* finding at autopsy. It occurs at any age and has no predilection for either sex. The *cause* of the disorder is not known although toxins, allergy, vitamin C deficiency, hemodynamic stresses, and valvular sclerosis have, from time to time, been incriminated. The condition may be an accompaniment of any acute or lingering illness and is commonly seen in conjunction with malignant tumors, cardiac failure, major operations, pneumonia, and nephritis. *Grossly* the lesion is found superimposed upon previously damaged valves (usually rheumatic) in about two-thirds of cases and upon previously normal valves in about one-third of cases. It may affect one or more valves and one or more cusps or leaflets in any individual case. The mitral valve is affected two times as frequently as the aortic and the right side of the heart is less often involved than the left. The lesion consists of small to large, single or multiple, gray, brown, or red verrucæ located along the line of closure of the valve cusps or leaflets (Fig. 118). It heals by resorption or fibrosis and nodulation. *Histologically* the condition consists primarily of fibrinoid degeneration of the superficial valvular collagen. When the endocardium is destroyed, there is a secondary deposition of blood elements, especially fibrin and platelets. Leukocytic infiltration (neutrophilic and lymphocytic) at the junction of the thrombus with the valve is either minimal or entirely absent. As the lesion ages it becomes replaced with the fibrous tissue. There are no known *complications* although Allen and Sirota suggest that the disorder may be a precursor of bacterial endocarditis. Clinically the condition is usually not recognized, and the *diagnosis* is made at autopsy. In some instances the lesions may be difficult to differentiate from those of rheumatic fever and bacterial endocarditis.

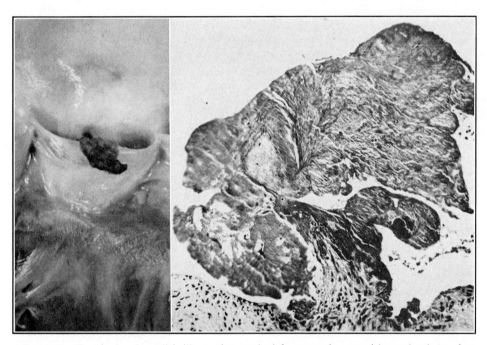

FIG. 118.—Terminal endocarditis illustrating, to the left, an aortic cusp with a rather large, deep red, pedunculated verruca and, to the right, fibrinoid degeneration of a cusp capped with a platelet and fibrin thrombus. × 50.

Spirochetal Endocarditis.—Most cases of spirochetal endocarditis are *syphilitic* in nature and affect the aortic valve. Since the disorder represents an extension of syphilitic aortitis it is considered in connection with other lesions of the aorta (Chapter 9, p. 375). Rarely, spirochetal endocarditis may be caused by the *Spirillum minus*. The lesion in this condition is similar to that in subacute bacterial endocarditis.

Tuberculous Endocarditis.—Tuberculous endocarditis is rare. Unlike other forms of endocarditis the process may involve any portion of the endocardium of either the right or the left side of the heart including the valve cusps and leaflets. *Mycobacterium tuberculosis* usually reaches the endocardium either by way of the coronary arteries or by way of direct implantation from the bloodstream. In either case, the endocardial lesion is generally part of a miliary process. Less commonly, the endocardium may be affected by direct extension of a tuberculous process from the pericardium or the myocardium. In miliary tuberculosis the endocardial lesions are usually small, measuring not more than 2 to 4 mm. in diameter, grayish-white, and sharply circumscribed. As a rule, they are not covered with thrombi. Lesions that extend from other portions of the heart are usually larger, more caseating, and covered with secondary thrombi that originate in the bloodstream.

Fungous Endocarditis.—Vegetative endocarditis caused by higher bacteria, yeast, or fungi is *rare*. The condition is much more common in males than it is in females and usually occurs beyond thirty-five years of age. Some of the more common *causative organisms* belong to the following genera: *Actinomyces, Histoplasma, Candida (Monilia), Erysipelothrix, Leptothrix,* and *Aspergillus.* A predisposing factor in allowing these organisms to gain a foothold and multiply is the widespread use of antibiotic therapy. Antibiotics accomplish this not only by suppressing bacterial growth but also by a direct enhancing effect upon the yeasts and fungi themselves. *Pathologically* the lesions are grossly identical with those in bacterial endocarditis. The valves are usually previously damaged (by sclerosis or endocarditis) although occasionally they may show no evidence of antecedent disease. The aortic, mitral, and pulmonic valves are affected in decreasing order of frequency. *Histologically* the vegetations are composed of the usual conglomeration of platelets, fibrin, and leukocytes. They contain, in addition, either free or engulfed causative organisms. The process heals by fibrosis and calcification. The *complications* and *clinical manifestations* are similar to those of bacterial endocarditis. The final *diagnosis* is made upon isolating the organisms from the blood or, of course, at postmortem. *Treatment* is not specific and has thus far been ineffective. The *prognosis* is poor, the average duration of life being six to eight months after the onset of the disease.

MYOCARDITIS

Orientation.—In former years the caption "myocarditis" was a catch-all for any degenerative, inflammatory, or obscure cardiac disorder that did not affect principally the endocardium or the epicardium. Now the term indicates, as it should, primary inflammation of the musculature itself and constitutes a distinct entity. The incidence of true myocarditis is low. It occurs at all ages and affects both sexes. The *causes* (see classification below) are protean. *Grossly* the myocardium may (1) appear normal, (2) be thin and soft, or (3) disclose irregular foci, depending upon the type and extent of the inflammation. *Histologically* the changes vary with the etiologic factors. The *clinical manifestations* are not prominent and are generally obscured by the primary disease process (Goldberger). There may be (1) a disproportionate increase in the pulse rate as compared with the increase in temperature (usually the pulse rises eight to ten points for every degree rise in temperature), (2) a feeble pulse, (3) low blood pressure, (4) substernal heaviness, (5) dyspnea and orthopnea, (6) cyanosis, (7) cardiac failure, (8) varying degrees of cardiac enlargement roentgenographically, and (9) a variety of nonspecific electrocardiographic changes. The *prognosis* depends upon the severity, extent, and type of inflammation. The condition may result in sudden death. Based upon the excellent review by Saphir, myocarditis may be *classified as* (1) fetal myocarditis, (2) myocarditis in infectious diseases, (3) isolated myocarditis, (4) myocarditis associated with bacterial endocarditis (p. 304), (5) metastatic pyemic abscess, (6) rheumatic myocarditis (p. 296), (7) myocarditis associated with infectious granuloma, (8) myocarditis in rickettsial diseases, (9) myocarditis in viral diseases, and (10) myocarditis in parasitic diseases.

Fetal Myocarditis.—Nonspecific inflammations of the myocardium often accompany congenital defects of the heart. They are infrequent in normal fetal hearts but undoubtedly account for some of the cases of idiopathic cardiac hypertrophy.

Myocarditis in Infectious Diseases.—Under this heading are included a wide variety of disorders. In *diphtheria* the myocardial fibers undergo severe degeneration and then necrosis. The interstitial tissue discloses edema and a diffuse perivascular infiltration with lymphocytes, neutrophils, and eosinophils. Healing occurs by resolution or scarring. In *enteric fever* (typhoid and paratyphoid) true myocarditis is rare but there have been recorded fatty change, multiplication of the nuclei of the muscle fibers, fragmentation of the myocardial fibers, foci of lymphocytes and neutrophils, and nuclear fragmentation of neutrophils. In *whooping cough*, myocardial alterations are rarely found and, even when present, are insignificant. They consist mostly of a fatty change and a few foci of lymphocytes. In *influenza*, inflammation of the myocardium has been infrequently recorded. It consists of degeneration to necrosis of the myocardial fibers and edema and focal lymphocytic infiltration of the connective tissue. In *pneumonia*, the myocardium may show parenchymatous degeneration, fatty change, hyaline degeneration, and interstitial infiltration with neutrophils and lymphocytes. In *scarlet fever*, the inflammation is primarily interstitial and the cells (principally lymphocytic) have a tendency to be grouped around vessels and thus produce a nodular arrangement. Secondarily, the adjacent myocardial fibers undergo degeneration and necrosis. In *meningococcic* and *gonococcic* infections, the myocardial lesions consist of foci of congestion, edema, and neutrophilic infiltration. Adjacent myocardial fibers show degeneration and necrosis. In addition, actual abscesses may be encountered in meningococcic infection. In *leptospirosis* the myocardium reveals focal hemorrhages, interstitial infiltration with lymphocytes and plasma cells and hyaline or granular degeneration of the myocardial fibers together with distinct feci of necrosis (Areán).

Isolated Myocarditis.—Isolated myocarditis, also known as Fiedler's, idiopathic, interstitial, acute, subacute, fibrinous, and productive myocarditis, was first described as an entity by Fiedler in 1899 (Gholmy). While its *cause* remains unknown, allergy (especially to drugs), viruses, and nutritional inadequacy have all been thought to be of etiologic significance. The condition is rather uncommon. It *occurs* most often in young adults but has also been described in infants and in the aged and it has no predilection for either sex. *Pathologically* the heart is diffusely enlarged; the myocardium is thickened and flabby; the chambers are dilated; the endocardium may contain mural thrombi, and the valve cusps and leaflets as well as the coronary arteries are devoid of pathologic changes (Fig. 119). Histologically there is a patchy but, in the areas affected, diffuse or granulomatous inflammation. The latter is uncommon and exists in the form of nodules (with foci of necrosis) that resemble tubercles or gummas. The diffuse inflammation is common and consists of a diffuse interstitial infiltration with lymphocytes and plasma cells with fewer neutrophils, monocytes, and eosinophils (Fig. 120). Giant cells may or may not be present and fibroblasts appear later. In addition, the myocardial fibers disclose parenchymatous and vacuolic degeneration, fragmentation and even necrosis. *Clinically* the patient presents himself with an abrupt onset of congestive heart failure that progresses rapidly and terminates fatally in a few weeks. The clinical *diagnosis* is generally established by a process of exclusion.

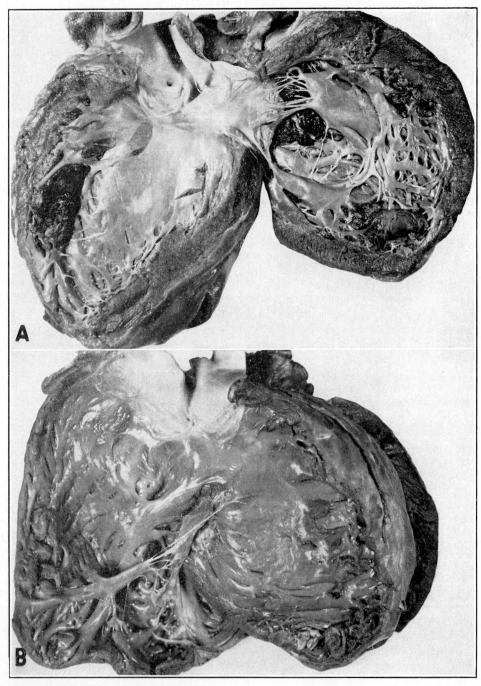

FIG. 119.—Isolated myocarditis showing *A*, a flabby myocardium of the left ventricle, dilatation of the chamber, and several endocardial thrombi and *B*, similar changes in the right ventricle.

Abscesses in the Myocardium.—Abscesses in the myocardium probably occur in all cases of pyemia. They are usually caused by staphylococci, streptococci, and pneumococci. They may be microscopic or macroscopic in size and when large, may bring about rupture of the heart.

Myocarditis Associated with Infectious Granuloma.—*Tularemia* may be accompanied by fatty change, parenchymatous degeneration, and fragmentation of the myocardium and, rarely, by diffuse interstitial lymphocytic infiltration. Typical granulomas have not been recorded. *Tuberculous* myocarditis is uncommon and is virtually always secondary to

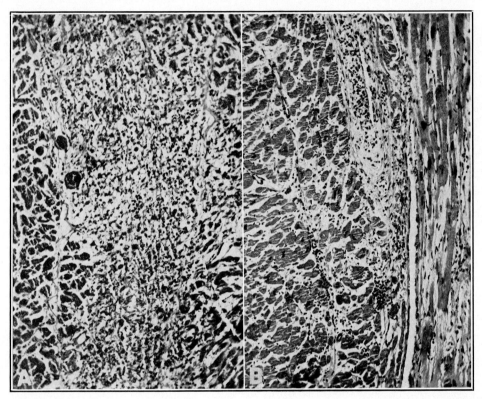

Fig. 120.—Isolated myocarditis illustrating *A*, degeneration and vacuolization of the myocardium and *B*, edema of the interstitial tissue with infiltration with plasma cells, lymphocytes, and neutrophils. × 100.

tuberculosis of the lungs and mediastinal lymph nodes. It may be nodular, miliary, or diffuse infiltrative and may affect any portion of the myocardium. The nodular and miliary forms are readily recognizable for they disclose typical tubercles. The diffuse form histologically presents tuberculous granulation tissue, although the specific nature of the lesion is not always characteristic. When it is not characteristic the diagnosis can be made with assurance only if *Mycobacterium tuberculosis* is isolated. *Boeck's sarcoid* may rarely affect any portion of the myocardium and sometimes the epicardium. Histologically the lesions disclose solid tubercles that are typical of the condition in other tissues of the body. *Syphilis* of the myocardium is rare and is almost always of the gummatous variety. It may involve any portion of the myocardium and when the gumma breaks down it may be accompanied by cardiac rupture. Diffuse syphilitic myocarditis is said to exist by some authors but not by others. The condition probably represents ischemic changes resulting from syphilitic occlusion of the coronary ostia. *Yeast* and *fungous* myocarditis may occur in generalized blastomycosis, torulosis, actinomycosis, moniliasis, sarcosporidiosis, and histoplasmosis. Any portion of the myocardium may be involved. The diagnosis is readily made histologically by finding the causative organisms within or without phagocytes and giant cells.

Myocarditis in Rickettsial Disease. —In *typhus* fever, the myocardium may be pale, soft, and present yellowish streaks. Histologically there are edema, vacuolization of the muscle fibers, and focal collections of monocytes, lymphocytes, plasma cells, neutrophils, and eosinophils around (often thrombotic and obliterated) vessels. In *Rocky Mountain spotted fever*, the following have been described: (1) fatty and other degenerations, fragmentation, and focal necrosis of muscle fibers, (2) vascular endothelial proliferation with necrosis and occlusion of lumens with necrotic material, and (3) perivascular accumulations of lymphocytes, plasma cells, basophils, and eosinophils.

Myocarditis in Viral Diseases. —In *measles* and *mumps*, myocardial changes are rare and consist principally of fatty changes and focal lymphocytic infiltrations. In *psittacosis*, there may be (1) edema and lymphocytic and neutrophilic infiltration of interstitial tissue and (2) parenchymatous and hydropic degeneration of the muscle bundles. In *yellow fever*, parenchymatous and fatty change of the myocardial fibers have been recorded but primary inflammation has not been noted. In fatal cases, *poliomyelitis* is accompanied by myocarditis rather constantly. The changes consist of (1) degeneration and necrosis of myocardial fibers, (2) separation of the fibers by edema fluid, (3) perivascular collection of neutrophils, lymphocytes, plasma cells, and monocytes, (4) congestion and hemorrhages, (5) edema, fibrosis, and cellular infiltration of nerves, and (6) later a diffuse or focal fibroblastic proliferation (Spain).

Myocarditis in Parasitic Diseases. —*Toxoplasma* may produce a myocarditis characterized by foci of coagulation necrosis with a heavy infiltration with neutrophils and eosinophils. In some instances the myocardial fibers show less damage and instead contain innumerable causative parasites. *Trypanosomiasis* may be accompanied by interstitial infiltration with monocytes, plasma cells, lymphocytes, and eosinophils and later by extensive fibrosis. *Trichinosis* affects the myocardium most severely between the fourth and sixth weeks of the disease. Histologically there are focal areas of myocardial necrosis permeated with lymphocytes, plasma cells, and eosinophils. Larvæ are rarely identifiable.

PERICARDITIS

Orientation. —Pericarditis *means* inflammation of the pericardium. The condition is seen in from 4 to 5 per cent of all autopsies. It *occurs* at all ages, affects all races, and has no predilection for either sex. The *causes* are quite varied (see classification below). The *pathologic changes* vary with the etiologic agent. Acute pericarditis may be "dry" consisting essentially of dulling and roughening of the surface by a precipitation of fibrin or it may be "wet" consisting, in addition, of an exudate of clear, hemorrhagic, or purulent fluid into the pericardial space. Chronic pericarditis discloses fibrosis, pericardial adhesions, and sometimes calcification. The *clinical* *manifestations* (excluding constrictive pericarditis) are quite similar regardless of the causative agent. They may be listed as follows: (1) a variety of noncardiac symptoms and signs due to the primary disease, (2) precordial pain occurring only when the parietal pericardium is affected and being localized or transmitted to the epigastrium, left shoulder and arm, or neck, (3) dry cough, dyspnea, and dysphagia caused by pressure of a distended pericardium on the tracheobronchial tree and the esophagus respectively, (4) pericardial friction rub due to rubbing of the visceral and parietal pericardium, (5) restlessness, paleness or cyanosis, distention of the veins of the neck, low blood pressure, small pulse pressure, enlargement of the heart, distant heart sounds, and disappearance of the apical impulse all due to pressure upon the heart and obstruction of the venous return by fluid accumulated in the pericardial cavity, (6) replacement of the normal contour of the heart by a bottle-shaped shadow fluoroscopically, and (7) normal or abnormal electrocardiograms (Goldberger). The chief *complication* is cardiac embarassment. The *diagnosis* is made from a consideration of the clinical manifestations listed above and examination of fluid received upon aspirating the pericardium. The *treatment* and *prognosis* depend upon the etiologic agent. For practical purposes, pericarditis may be *classified* as follows: rheumatic (page 296), acute idiopathic, pyogenic, uremic, granulomatous, constrictive, and miscellaneous.

Acute Idiopathic Pericarditis.—This condition, also known as acute primary, acute nonspecific benign, acute nonspecific, and acute relapsing pericarditis, is a clinical entity characterized by a sudden appearance of symptoms and signs of pericarditis following a respiratory tract infection by days or several weeks. The clinical manifestations are usually severe and often simulate myocardial infarction. The condition predominates in males and is most common between the ages of nineteen and forty-five years. The cause is unknown but a virus has been suspected since the disorder often follows primary atypical pneumonia. The condition responds quickly to antibiotics. The course is benign with the patients generally recovering readily although recurrences are common. Because of the unusually good outcome, the pathologic changes in the pericardium have not been described.

Pyogenic Pericarditis.—Pyogenic pericarditis includes all inflammations of the pericardium caused by the usual pyogenic organisms. The more common of these are pneumococci, streptococci, and staphylococci but other organisms such as gonococci, members of the Friedländer's group, influenza bacilli, etc., are also occasionally isolated. Although the inflammation of the pericardium may be the only site of involvement in the body, the caridac lesion is generally secondary to septicemia or a primary infection elsewhere in the thorax. Pathologically the exudation consists of varying amounts of fibrin, fluid, and leukocytes and is thus termed fibrinous, serous, purulent, or various combinations of these (Fig, 121*A* and *B* and Fig. 122*A*). The lesion may resolve completely or it may heal by organization and "milk spot" or adhesion formation (Fig. 121*C*). With the more effective antibiotic control of infectious diseases the incidence of pyogenic pericarditis has decreased and the prognosis has been immeasurably improved.

Uremic Pericarditis.—Uremic pericarditis usually develops in the end stages of uremia. Its cause is unknown. Pathologically the exudate is usually fibrinous with varying numbers of neutrophils, lymphocytes, plasma cells, and monocytes added. It usually makes its initial appearance at the base of the heart and then gradually extends to the apex. Grossly the

21

Heart

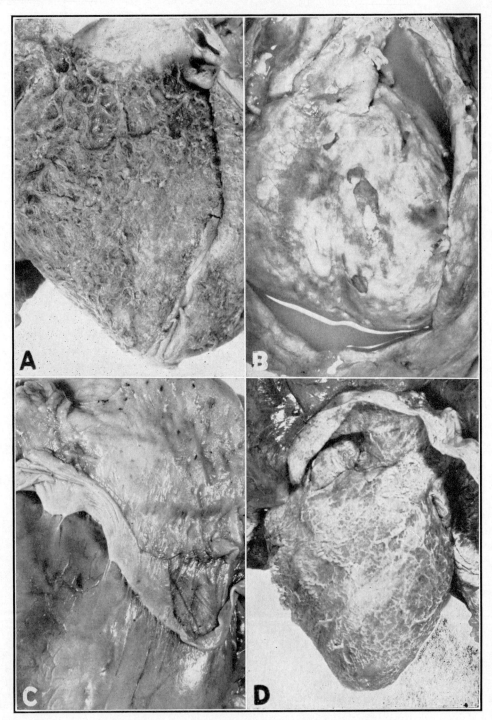

Fig. 121.—Pericarditis showing *A*, fibrinous, *B*, purulent, *C*, fibrous (healed), and *D*, uremic varieties of inflammation.

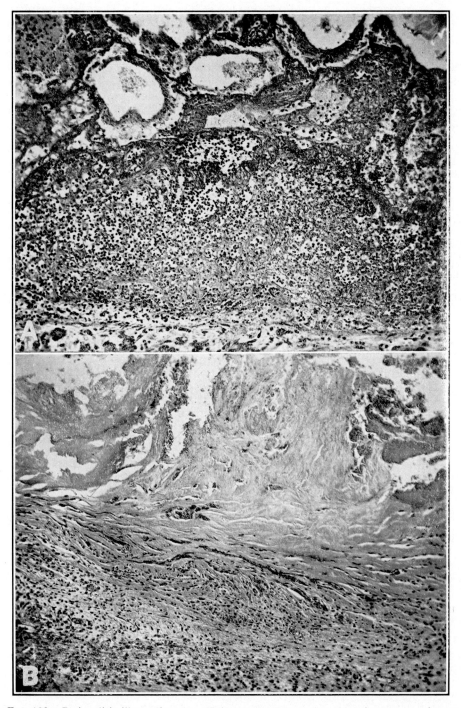

FIG. 122.—Pericarditis illustrating *A*, a fibrinopurulent type of exudate from a case of acute pericarditis and *B*, dense hyalinized fibrous tissue and bone from a case of constrictive pericarditis. × 100.

pericardium loses its smoothness and luster or becomes covered with fibrinous material (Fig. 121D). The condition is of little clinical significance since the patient generally dies within a few days of the more serious renal lesion.

Granulomatous Pericarditis.—Although many granulomatous diseases such as tuberculosis, actinomycosis, blastomycosis, histoplasmosis, coccidioidomycosis, tularemia, Boeck's sarcoid, etc., may affect the pericardium, all but tuberculosis are too rare to merit separate consideration. Even *tuberculous pericarditis* is uncommon. The condition is always secondary to tuberculosis elsewhere in the body and arises either as a hematogenous spread or as a direct extension. The primary lesions are usually in the lungs or mediastinal lymph nodes. The initial infection of the pericardium is generally accompanied by a serofibrinous, hemorrhagic, or somewhat greenish effusion. Later the lesion becomes granulomatous and finally, if healing occurs, it becomes replaced with fibrous tissue which may ultimately undergo focal calcification. Histologically the active process discloses typical tubercles or tuberculous granulation tissue. Although the outlook is better in cases treated with streptomycin, the prognosis is still not good. Death may occur as a result of tuberculosis of other tissues or of cardiac failure.

Constrictive Pericarditis.—Constrictive pericarditis, *also known* as chronic cardiac compression and chronic adhesive pericarditis, constitutes more or less a clinical syndrome. It affects males much more frequently than females and occurs at an average age of approximately thirty years. In most instances, the *cause* remains undetermined. Of the remaining cases, old tuberculous involvement appears to be definitely established while pyogenic pericarditis, rheumatic pericarditis, and hemopericardium may account for a minority of the cases. *Pathologically* the condition is characterized by extensive fibrous tissue replacement of both the visceral and parietal pericardium with widespread fusion of the two layers and corresponding obliteration of the pericardial cavity (Fig. 122B). The fused pericardial covering varies in thickness from 2 to 6 mm. Ultimately it undergoes diffuse, plaque-like or granular calcification and sometimes even ossification. Occasionally distinct fibrous bands are found to encircle and constrict the entrances of both the superior and inferior vena cava into the right side of the heart. The myocardium is usually thin, atrophic, soft, and inseparably fused with the pericardium. The cardiac chambers may be dilated. The heart, as a whole, is usually slightly enlarged although it may be normal or even subnormal in size. Simultaneous fibrous thickening of the pleuræ, diaphragm, and peritoneal surfaces may occur, constituting what is generally referred to as *polyserositis* or *Pick's disease* (Fig. 123). The important *complication* of constrictive pericarditis is cardiac failure. This is due to inability of the cardiac chambers to expand as they should and to fill properly during diastole. For similar reasons the important *clinical manifestations* are dyspnea, orthopnea, enlargement of the liver, ascites, swelling of the legs, distention of the veins of the neck, and elevation of the venous pressure. The heart is not appreciably enlarged and cardiac murmurs are generally not heard. Radiographically, calcification is readily apparent and, electrocardiographically, there are characteristic changes. The *diagnosis* is made from a consideration of the clinical manifestations as listed above. A differential diagnosis should include cirrhosis of the liver and cardiac failure due to other causes. *Treatment* is both medical and surgical. The latter consists of pericardiolysis or partial pericardiectomy. The *prognosis* varies from case to case. Without treatment the condition may be fulminating (death occurring in a few months) or protracted (death occurring in ten to twenty years). Definite improvement is said to occur in approximately two-thirds of the cases treated surgically.

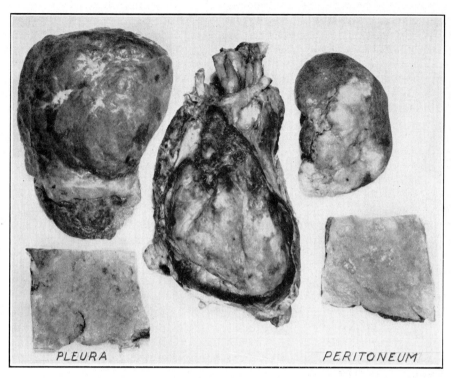

FIG. 123.—Polyserositis showing extensive fibrous thickening of the pericardium (subjected to pericardiectomy), liver, spleen, pleura, and peritoneum.

Miscellaneous.—There are still other types of pericarditis that have not been included in the above description. One of these is pericarditis following *trauma*. It is rare, results from penetrating or blunt injury, and may be aseptic or bacterial. Another is pericarditis consequent to a *myocardial infarction*. This is common, occurring in every case in which the infarct extends to the pericardium. The inflammation is aseptic. The exudate is localized to the area of infarction or covers most of the pericardium. It is usually fibrinous but it may also be serofibrinous or even hemorrhagic. The fate of the patient depends upon the myocardial lesion.

PHYSICAL DISTURBANCES

Orientation.—Under this heading may be included the following heterogeneous disorders of the heart: angina pectoris, myocardial infarction, myocardial hypertrophy, trauma, foreign bodies, myocardial rupture, hernia, hydropericardium, hemopericardium, pneumopericardium, cardiac tamponade, heart failure, and sudden death.

Angina Pectoris.—Angina pectoris (L. = pain + chest) is a *clinical syndrome* rather than a pathologic entity *caused* by fleeting relative anoxia of the myocardium. It is *characterized* by short episodes of localized or radiating precordial pain usually brought about by exertion and relieved by nitroglycerin or momentary rest (Goldberger). *Pathologically* the myocardium discloses only focal areas of degeneration and fibrosis. *Clinically* the syndrome may be differentiated from myocardial infarction in that the latter is usually accompanied by (1) pain while the patient is resting, (2) fever, (3) leukocytosis, (4) increased sedimentation rate, and (5) more profound electrocardiographic changes (Stein). The average age of patients with angina pectoris is about fifty-eight years; males are affected four times as frequently as females, and the ten-year survival is about one-half that of the normal population in the same age group (Block).

Myocardial Infarction.—Included under the heading of myocardial infarction are coronary occlusion, coronary artery disease, and coronary insufficiency. The combination of occlusion of the coronary arteries together with consequent myocardial damage accounts for the most *common* disturbance of the heart. The condition *occurs* at all ages from infancy on but, in three-quarters of the cases, is found in the fourth, fifth, and sixth decades of life. Negroes are affected much less frequently than white people and the incidence in males is three times that in females. The disorder has no specific relationship to occupation or social status (Master)' The *cause* of myocardial infarction is prolonged (at least of twenty minutes. duration) disproportion between the nutritional requirements of the heart and the actual amount or quality of coronary blood flow (Paterson). More specifically, the causes may be listed as follows: (1) *Congenital*—increased thickness of the intima of the coronary arteries as compared with other arteries of a similar caliber, and absence of one coronary ostia. (2) *Degenerations*—arteriosclerosis of the coronary arteries (accounting for about 90 per cent of all cases of myocardial infarction), and medionecrosis of the coronary arteries with subsequent dissecting aneurysm. (3) *Inflammations*—syphilitic aortitis (affecting the coronary ostia), rheumatic arteritis, nonspecific arteritis, periarteritis nodosa, thromboangiitis obliterans, and marked inflammatory deformity of the aortic valve. (4) *Physical Disturbances*—sudden fall in blood pressure consequent to shock, lowering of oxygen capacity of the blood from anemia, undue effort or excitement calling for increased cardiac output, direct trauma to the chest in the precordial area, coronary artery embolism, coronary artery thrombosis, intramural hematoma of the coronary arteries, and spasm of the coronary arteries. (5) *Tumors*—direct pressure upon, or invasion of, the wall of the coronary arteries by primary or secondary neoplasm of the heart, or tumor embolism of the coronary arteries. In addition to the above, two predisposing factors are diabetes mellitus (due to the increased incidence of arteriosclerosis) and hypertension (due to excessive demands in proportion to the arterial blood supply). Of all the factors listed, the most important, by far, is *arteriosclerosis*. Superimposed upon the arteriosclerotic lesion there may be (1) a sudden enlargement of the plaque from hematoma, (2) thrombosis, or (3) simply a sudden excessive demand on the heart (less than 5 per cent of cases). Thus, the relationship between the blood flow and the consequent myocardial damage is partly anatomic and partly physiologic. For this reason, all cases of coronary artery occlusion are not followed by myocardial infarction and, conversely, all cases of myocardial infarction do not disclose coronary artery occlusion. The relationship, however, is sufficiently constant to permit the use (among clinicians at least) of the two captions synonymously.

In most instances the primary *pathologic changes* are found in the *coronary arteries*. Although the lesions in the vessels vary with the precise etiologic factor, the most common change is arteriosclerosis (Fig. 124). While arterio-

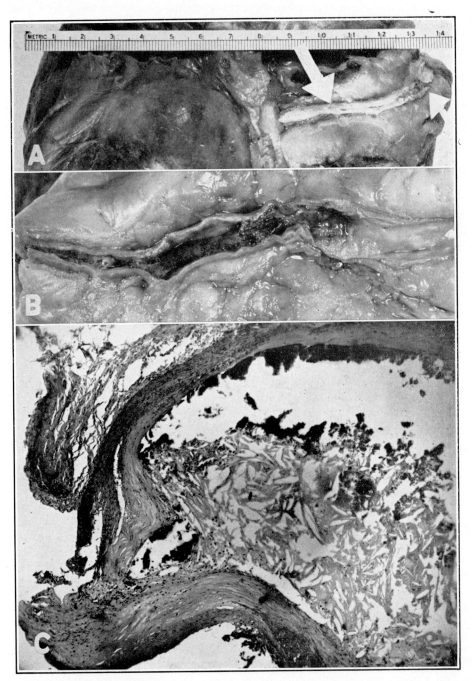

FIG. 124.—Coronary artery occlusion showing *A*, severe arteriosclerosis with complete obstruction of the lumen, *B*, thrombus superimposed upon an arteriosclerotic plaque, and *C*, great thickening of the intima by fibrous tissue with cholesterol deposition and calcification. × 50.

sclerosis is discussed in the section on the Arteries (p. 359), it may be stated here that the process starts in the intima and initially consists of foam cell formation together with connective tissue proliferation. The former consists of deposits of cholesterol and cholesterol esters within phagocytic cells. As the lesion progresses, the lumen is gradually encroached upon and the foam cells undergo complete degeneration followed by cholesterol crystal deposition and later even calcification. Although all portions of the coronary arteries may be affected, the proximal portion of the anterior descending

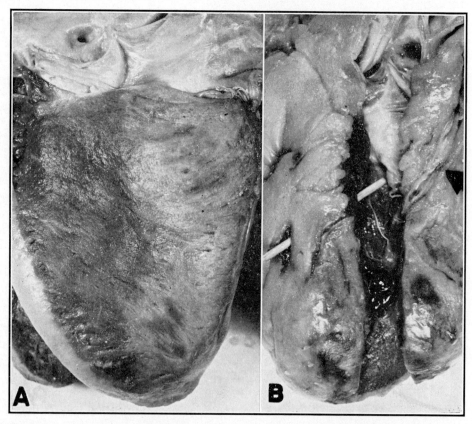

Fig. 125.—Myocardial infarction showing *A*, a mottled, light gray, ill-defined appearance of the myocardium and *B*, pericarditis opposite the infarcted area and perforation of the wall.

branch of the left coronary artery is most commonly involved, while next in frequency is the circumflex branch of the left coronary artery. Grossly, early lesions disclose simply a yellowish, plaque-like thickening of the intima. As the process ages the plaques become larger and larger, fuse with adjacent plaques, encircle the circumference, and encroach upon the lumen. Softening and calcification occur as the lesion ages. Ultimately (1) the intima disintegrates and the inner surface of the vessel is lined with gray, mushy material, and (2) small or large segments of the vessels may be converted into rigid, pipe-like structures. At any time, hemorrhage may occur within, or thrombi may be superimposed upon, the arteriosclerotic plaques, thus completing the occlusion of the lumen.

As far as the *myocardium* is concerned, the part most frequently affected is, of course, that supplied by the occluded vessel. Accordingly, the apex of the left ventricle or the apex and the adjacent anterior portion of the interventricular septum are most commonly involved. The earliest change consists of a focal, pale, blotchy red, or purplish discoloration of the myocardium (Fig. 125). The demarcation between the infarcted area and the normal tissue is ill defined. Later, as the lesion ages, the affected tissue becomes yellowish brown and dryer than normal. In time, as a result of healing by fibrosis, it becomes rather sharply demarcated from the adjacent myocardium, paler, and decreased in thickness. *Histologically* the changes

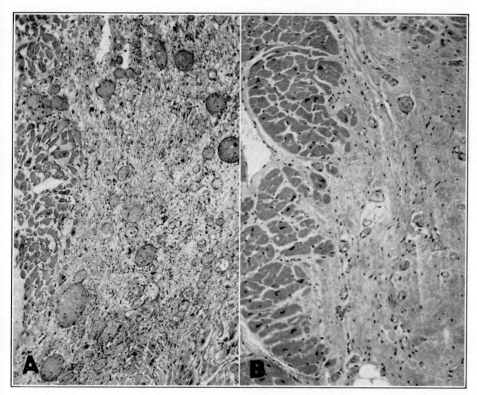

FIG. 126.—Myocardial infarction showing *A*, relatively early infarct with replacement of the muscle by recent granulation tissue and *B*, old infarct with extensive collagen deposition. × 100.

are those of ischemic atrophy, necrosis, granulation tissue replacement, and ultimately fibrosis (Fig. 126). When sections of the affected areas are carefully selected and properly studied microscopically, it is possible to *date* fairly accurately the time of the infarction (Mallory). Necrosis of the muscle as evidenced by hyalinization of the fibers, deeper staining, swelling of the fibers, disappearance of the normal striations, and appearance of eosinophilic granules begins within about five to six hours. Neutrophils appear as soon as the fibers become necrotic and reach their maximum concentration in approximately three days. Removal of the muscle and granulation tissue formation is initiated on the fourth or fifth day. Phagocytic activity of mononuclear cells in removal of the dead tissue becomes marked at approximately ten days. At this time the granulation tissue is

quite abundant, the fibroblasts are fairly numerous and somewhat basophilic, and eosinophils, plasma cells, and lymphocytes are quite prominent
(Fig. 126). By the end of the second week the necrotic muscle in small
infarcts is entirely removed and neutrophils have disappeared. By the
third week collagen makes its appearance, while by the fourth to sixth weeks
collagen becomes abundant and the vascularity and leukocytic infiltration
proportionately decrease. Subsequent changes consist of condensation
of the collagen and, in some instances, deposition of calcium. Regeneration
of muscle fibers is minimal if it exists at all.

The *complications* of myocardial infarction are many (Yater and Smith).
Pericarditis is seen in all instances in which the infarction reaches the
pericardium (Fig. 125B). It is usually of a fibrinous or serofibrinous variety
and when the lesion heals it either resolves or becomes replaced with fibrous
tissue bands. *Mural thrombi* are said to occur in about one-half of the cases
(Fig. 127A). They are found, of course, in areas in which the endocardium
is affected. *Rupture* of the heart is said to be present in about 9 per cent
of cases and usually occurs within the first ten days of the infarction (Fig.
125B). The usual site of rupture is the anterior wall of the left ventricle
midway between the apex and the base and near the interventricular
septum. Rarely the septum itself or the papillary muscles may be perforated. *Ventricular aneurysm* is said to occur in from 8 to 10 per cent of
cases. It forms as a result of fibrosis and weakening of the myocardium and
is most common in the anterolateral wall of the left ventricle followed by
the anterior wall and interventricular septum (Fig. 127B). *Emboli* from the
mural thrombi usually occur within the first two weeks of the infarction and
most commonly affect the lungs, brain, mesentery, extremities, spleen, and
kidneys. *Congestive heart failure* may occur in the early acute phase of the
infarction or it may occur later as a result of weakening and fibrosis of the
myocardium. *Secondary infection* of the infarct with abscess formation has
been recorded although it is extremely rare. *Acute pancreatitis*, generally
of a focal variety, is a fairly common concomitant finding. The reason for
its occurrence is not known.

Clinically the majority of cases of coronary artery occlusion and myocardial infarction occur during the routine living from day to day. Only a
few of the cases (less than 5 per cent) occur after unusually vigorous physical
activity. Briefly the clinical manifestations may be listed as follows
(Yater): (1) pain—anterior thoracic (with or without radiation down the
left arm or both arms), posterior thoracic, or abdominal (due to myocardial
ischemia and referred along the nerve pathways), (2) shock—varying degrees (due to acute myocardial insufficiency and absorption of tissue
metabolites), (3) respiratory embarrassment—consisting of dyspnea,
orthopnea, and a sense of suffocation (due to inadequate pulmonary ventilation), (4) gastrointestinal symptoms—nausea and vomiting (due to
anoxia of the gastrointestinal tract and the gastrointestinal centers in the
brain), (5) central nervous system manifestations—convulsions, syncope,
restlessness, and mental dullness (due to anoxia of the brain), (6) congestive
heart failure—low blood pressure, pulmonary edema, enlargement of the
liver, etc. (due to acute weakness of the myocardium), (7) abnormal cardiac
findings—tachycardia, enlargement, friction rub, murmurs, alterations in
rhythm, and electrocardiographic changes (due to myocardial necrosis,
pericarditis, and cardiac dilatation), (8) emboli—various organs (due to
breaking off of mural thrombi), and (9) leukocytosis, increased sedimentation rate, and fever—(due to absorption of metabolites from the infarcted

area).   Aside from *laboratory tests* already mentioned, a few additional words should be said concerning C-reactive protein and serum transaminase determinations as they pertain to myocardial infarction.   *C-reactive protein* is a highly sensitive test for acute inflammation (Kozonis).   It was originally applied to pneumococcal inflammations where it was demonstrated that the capsule of the *Pneumococcus* contains a C-polysaccharide which behaves

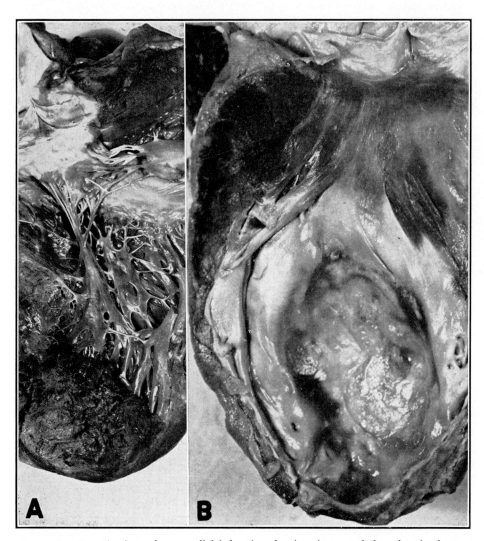

Fig. 127.—Complications of myocardial infarction showing *A*, a mural thrombus in the apex of the left ventricle and *B*, fibrotic and calcified aneurysm of the anterior wall of the left ventricle and the adjacent interventricular septum.

as an antigen and elicits the formation of a specific antibody.   The test now is known to be nonspecific.   In myocardial infarction the liberated proteins bring about an increase in serum beta globulin which contains C-reactive protein.   This, in turn, elicits antibody formation and a positive reaction. Such a reaction is strongly positive in acute infarction, persists in progressive infarction, and becomes negative as the infarction heals.   *Gutamic oxaloacetic transaminase* is an enzyme that is normally present in high concentration in heart, liver, kidney, muscle, and brain (Chinsky). It is also present in concentrations of 22 ± 7 units/milliliter in normal human serum. In acute myocardial infarction the level in serum becomes significantly elevated 6 hours after the onset of pain, reaches a peak in 24 hours, and then gradually subsides to normal over the next 1 to 4 days. A persistent elevation after 24 hours indicates progression of infarction and an ominous outlook. Since,

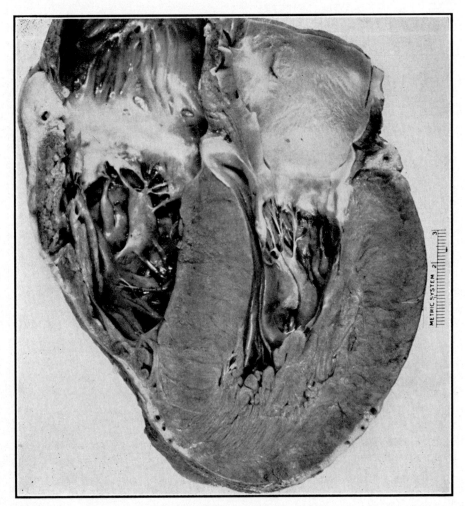

FIG. 128.—Marked myocardial hypertrophy of the left ventricle in longitudinal section.

however, serum transaminase is also elevated in various diseases of the liver, traumatic injuries (especially of muscles), and prolonged shock, the test must be evaluated in conjunction with other clinical manifestations.

The *diagnosis* of myocardial infarction is made from a consisdration of the clinical manifestations listed above. Clinically, the condition should be differentiated from angina pectoris, a variet yof other acute cardiac disorders, acute pancreatitis, perforated peptic ulcer, acute cholecystitis, and gallstone colic. *Treatment* consists of (1) physical rest, (2) control of pain by opiates, (3) attention to pulmonary edema by way of narcotics, administration of oxygen, and venesection, (4) combating shock by way of sedatives, vasospastic drugs, and intravenous fluids, (5) cardiac stimulants properly administered, (6) anticoagulant therapy, and (7) soft, easily digested diet (Sampson). The *prognosis* depends upon many factors. In general, the younger the person the poorer is the prognosis. The reason for this is that the collateral circulation is less well established in the younger age group than it is in the older age group. In a long-term follow-up of 100 cases, C. Smith listed the following mortalities: within twenty-eight days—15 per cent, within one year—25 per cent, within six years—34 per cent, within nine years, 55 per cent, and within the first two decades—80 per cent. The two chief *causes* of *death* are recurrent infarctions and congestive heart failure.

Myocardial Hypertrophy.—Anything that *causes* a prolonged extra demand on the heart results in hypertrophy of the myocardium. Most commonly, the extra demand is in the form of increased peripheral vascular resistance—benign or malignant hypertension when the systemic circulation is affected and pulmonic hypertension when the pulmonary arteries are involved. Some of the many other causes are congenital or acquired valvular defects, extracardiac vascular or intracardiac shunts, primary myocardial degenerative or inflammatory disorders, mild but prolonged coronary artery insufficiency, and endocrine (thyrotoxicosis) imbalances.

Normally the heart weighs between 275 and 325 grams, the left ventricle measures 8 to 10 mm. across, and the right ventricle measures 2 to 3 mm. in thickness. In *hypertrophy* these figures are slightly or greatly exceeded. The portion of the heart affected most severely is that which is immediately behind the disrupting factor. Thus, the musculature surrounding any chamber may be involved but, since hypertension is the most common cause of hypertrophy, the left ventricle is most commonly and most severely affected (Figs. 128 and 129). The heart, as a whole, may weigh 800 grams or more. The myocardium is generally concentrically thickened to two or more times normal. The consistency is firm; the color is light brown; the trabeculæ and papillary muscles appear of "good quality" and are several times the normal thickness, and the lumen of the ventricle is greatly reduced. In time, however, the myocardium becomes exhausted and since demands upon it continue, its fibers stretch and the cavity dilates. A large heart due predominantly to left ventricular hypertrophy is often called *cor bovinum*. A similar enlargement due to right ventricular hypertrophy is referred to as *cor pulmonale*.

Histologically, regardless of the site of hypertrophy, the myocardial fibers may, at first glance, appear normal although, if a direct comparison is made with a normal heart, they usually reveal enlargement, deeper eosinophilic staining of the cytoplasm, and hyperchromatism and irregularity of the nuclei. Gradually, as the hypertrophy outgrows its blood supply, focal areas of ischemic degeneration and necrosis of the myocardial fibers and residual replacement with connective tissue make their appearance (Fig. 129). Such foci have been referred to as *pseudoscars*.

Trauma.—Trauma to the heart may result from penetrating or nonpenetrating injury. *Penetrating* injury is generally due to knife or ice pick stabs and less commonly to gunshot wounds. Any part of the heart may be affected and the myocardium may be superficially or completely penetrated by defects of varying sizes and appearances. *Nonpenetrating* injury generally occurs as a result of trauma to the chest but on rare occasions may follow trauma to the abdomen or even the lower extremities. The injury may consist of a blow, fall, crush (as in a steering wheel accident), intense jarring, and blast (Bowman). The myocardium may or may not be previously diseased. The myocardial lesion may consist of a contusion, partial laceration, or complete rupture. Any part of the heart may be affected but the right ventricle and right atrium are most commonly involved. The

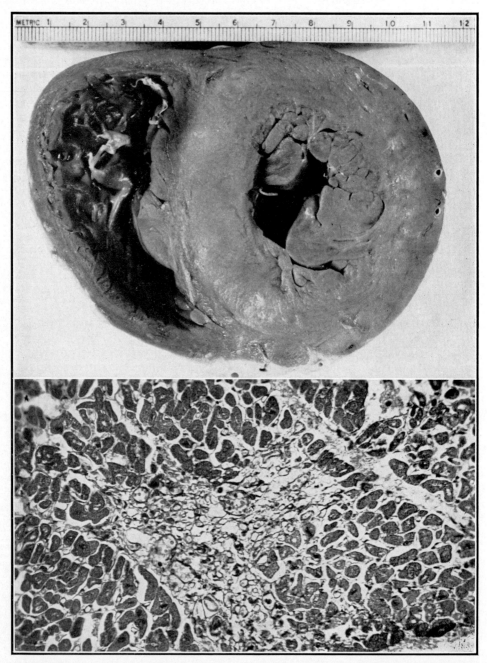

FIG. 129.—At the top, marked myocardial hypertrophy of the left ventricle in cross section. At the bottom, pseudoscarring of the myocardium showing degeneration and disappearance of the myocardial fibers and replacement with connective tissue. × 200.

mechanism of injury appears to be simple compression of the heart filled with blood between the sternum and vertebra together with increased intrathoracic pressure (Crane). Some of the *complications* are cardiac tamponade, hemothorax, accompanying injury to other organs, and, in penetrating wounds, subcutaneous emphysema. The chief *clinical manifestations* are those of shock and cardiac tamponade. *Treatment* of choice is pericardiotomy and primary cardiorrhaphy (Maynard). The *prognosis* is variable. About 50 per cent of the patients recover.

Foreign Bodies. — Foreign bodies of the heart are rare in civilian life but are fairly common in military service. In the latter, most consist of shell fragments and the usual portal of entry is directly from outside. The extraneous material may lodge within the pericardium, myocardium, endocardium, cardiac cavity, or combinations of these. Some of the *complications* are hemorrhage, embolism of the foreign body, thrombosis and embolism of the thrombus, pericarditis, myocarditis, endocarditis, myocardial fibrosis with subsequent aneurysm and rupture, injury to the coronary arteries, and cardiac neurosis (Swan). *Treatment* depends upon many factors. Removal is generally advocated in (1) symptomatic cases, (2) when the foreign body is large, and (3) when its location is such that complications may arise.

Myocardial Rupture. — Aside from direct trauma, cardiac rupture is generally secondary to myocardial infarction. Uncommonly it may follow bacterial endocarditis, syphilitic myocarditis, periarteritis nodosa, abscess of the myocardium, tuberculosis of the myocardium, and tumor. When the myocardium as a whole is affected the usual location of the perforation is the anterior wall of the left ventricle near the apex. Uncommonly the lower portion of the interventricular septum may be perforated and, rarely, the papillary muscles of the left ventricle may be ruptured.

Hernia. — Ectopia and diverticulum of the heart (p. 280) constitute the best examples of cardiac hernia. Of rare occurrence is herniation of the stomach, transverse colon, and part of the jejunum through the diaphragm and into the pericardial cavity. The latter lesions are acquired and follow industrial injuries or stab wounds (Crawshaw).

Hydropericardium. — Hydropericardium is a greater than normal accumulation of clear serous fluid in the pericardial cavity. It occurs in connection with cardiac edema, certain types of nephritis, nutritional edema, and chronic obstruction of the venous return to the heart.

Hemopericardium. — Hemopericardium is an accumulation of blood in the pericardial cavity (Fig. 130). It may occur in connection with rupture of the myocardium, rupture of the first part of the aorta, trauma to the heart, or rupture of a coronary artery. An accumulation of *hemorrhagic fluid* (but not frank blood) in the pericardial cavity is also sometimes referred to as hemopericardium but should be more accurately called hemorrhagic pericardial effusion, hemohydropericardium, or hemorrhagic pericarditis with effusion. It may occur in conjunction with tumors, tuberculosis, hemorrhagic diseases, and, occasionally, nephritis.

Pneumopericardium. — Pneumopericardium is the accumulation of air in the pericardial cavity. It may occur in conjunction with (1) introduction of air during pericardial aspiration of fluid, (2) perforation of the tracheobronchial tree, esophagus, or other hollow viscus, (3) penetrating external trauma, or (4) inflammation of the pericardium by gas-producing organisms.

Cardiac Tamponade. — Cardiac tamponade (heart + Fr. = plug or tampon) may be defined as a rapid accumulation of fluid, blood, or air in the pericardial cavity. It is accompanied by an elevation of intrapericardial pressure, compression of the heart, a fall in peripheral arterial pressure, and an elevation of the peripheral venous pressure. Such a sequence of events generally does not occur when the pericardial accumulation is slow because the pericardium has time to stretch and the physiologic action of the heart has time to readjust.

Heart Failure. — Virtually any lesion of the pericardium, myocardium, or endocardium may be associated with cardiac failure. The most common causes, however, are occlusion of the coronary artery, hypertension, and valvular disease. *Occlusion* of the *coronary artery* is generally due to arteriosclerosis and the sequel is *myocardial infarction* (p. 326). Heart failure con-

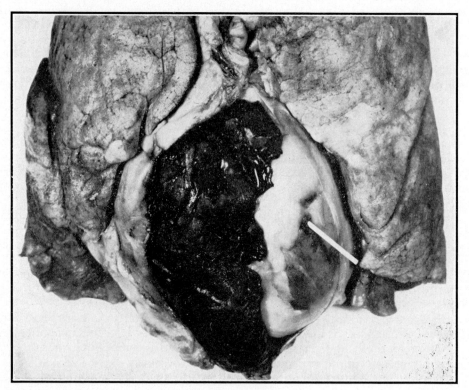

Fig. 130.—Rupture of a myocardial infarct with hemopericardium and cardiac tamponade.

sequent to this lesion may be acute if it occurs during the stage of the infarction or it may be chronic if it occurs sometimes after the infarct has healed. In either case, the pathologic changes are those of *passive hyperemia* or *congestion* (p. 193). The reason for the cardiac failure in myocardial infarction or subsequent fibrosis is simply interruption and weakening of the myocardial fibers leading to a decrease in myocardial force. For a time this may be compensated for by increased effort of remaining myocardial fibers but sooner or later these fibers become exhausted, the chambers dilate, and failure develops. With dilatation of the affected chamber or chambers the valvular rings also dilate and this, in turn, leads to incompetency of the valves which further aggravates the work load on the heart and embarrasses its output. The mechanism of heart failure in *hypertension* is somewhat similar, with the exception of course that the myocardial fibers are normal to begin with (p. 1057).   In hypertension there is increased peripheral vascular resistance consequent to arterial and arteriolar constriction and sclerosis.   Because of this increased resistance, the left ventricle must exert an extra force to raise the pressure sufficiently to force the blood through the vessels to the various organs and tissues of the body.   This extra force is attained by extra work on the part of the myocardium and this, in turn, is accomplished, over a long stretch, by hypertrophy of the fibers.   The continued extra demand, however, sooner or later is too much even for the

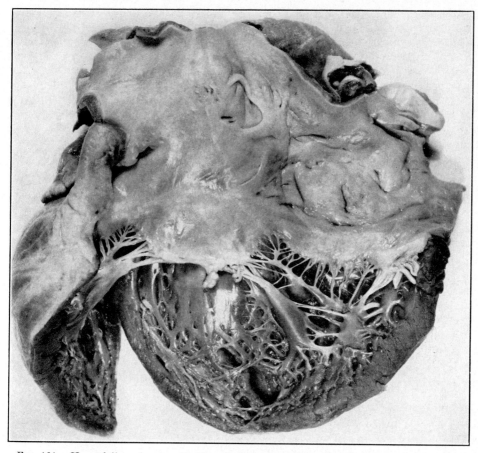

FIG. 131.—Heart failure due to mitral insufficiency consequent to dilatation of the mitral ring from rheumatic myocarditis. Note the rheumatic verrucæ along the line of closure of the mitral leaflets, dilatation of the mitral valve, and dilatation of the left atrium.

enlarged myocardial fibers.   As a consequence, they become exhausted and, contracting with decreased force, fail to pump all the blood out of the chambers.   Both the exhaustion and the incomplete emptying ultimately cause dilatation of the chambers.   This, in turn, is accompanied by stretching of the vascular rings, valvular incompetency, and further cardiac embarrassment.   Thus, a vicious cycle is established which ultimately leads to complete cardiac failure.

Heart failure from *valvular disease* may be acute, as in cases of bacterial endocarditis and less commonly acute rheumatic fever, but is more often

22

chronic as in cases of healed endocarditis consequent to either of these diseases. Of the two processes, rheumatic fever is the more frequent and of the valves involved the mitral is the most commonly affected. Normally, the area of the mitral orifice is 4 to 6 sq. cm. In acute rheumatic fever, both as a result of acute inflammation of the mitral leaflets and as a result of dilatation of the mitral ring due to the accompanying rheumatic myocarditis, the area of the mitral orifice enlarges and *mitral insufficiency* develops (Fig. 131). The latter mechanism is actually identical with that seen as an aggravating factor in myocardial infarction and hypertension. In any event, the blood from the left ventricle will thus be pumped both into the left atrium (through the insufficient mitral valve) and into the aorta. The relative amount going in each direction will depend upon the degree of mitral insufficiency as well as the relative differences in pressures exerted. In the latter instances, for example, even a minor degree of insufficiency may result in a large amount of regurgitation of blood into the left atrium if the pressure difference between the left ventricle and the left atrium is large. With escape of blood into the left atrium, this chamber first dilates temporarily and then hypertrophies. As the regurgitation is sustained, however, a second and permanent dilatation of the atrium ensues. At the same time, the ventricular intake of blood during diastole is increased. This, as in the atrium, leads to temporary dilatation followed by hypertrophy. If the defect, however, is not corrected the hypertrophy is followed by permanent dilatation and cardiac failure.

In old or healed rheumatic fever the leaflets of the mitral valve become fused, fibrotic, and calcified and as a consequence they become permanently fixed in a semi-closed position (Fig. 132). This, of course, leads to *mitral stenosis* and, to a lesser degree, to mitral insufficiency as well. As a result of encroachment upon the size of the mitral opening (to as little as 0.5 sq. cm. or even less) the left atrium must work harder to force the blood into the left ventricle. This results in hypertrophy of the muscle fibers. Since the increased work load continues, the myocardial muscle ultimately decompensates and the chamber dilates. This increases the blood volume in the pulmonary veins (which may even rupture and produce hemoptysis) and this, in turn, is transmitted to the right ventricle (Fig. 132, *B*). The same sequence of events takes place in the right ventricle leading to hypertrophy, dilatation, and decompensation. With dilatation and insufficiency of the tricuspid ring, the process is repeated in the right atrium and from here the venous congestion is passed onto all the organs draining into the right side of the heart.

Affliction of the *aortic valve* is next in frequency only to the mitral valve. Aortic *insufficiency* alone results from dilatation of the aortic ring and is due to such acute processes as acute rheumatic myocarditis or to such chronic processes as syphilitic aortitis or atherosclerosis. In any case, regurgitation of blood from the aorta into the left ventricle is greatest during each systole. This leads to an increase in diastolic volume of blood in the left ventricle and a decrease in diastolic pressure in the aorta and, of course, results in an increase in force of ejection of blood from the ventricle during systole. The extra work causes hypertrophy of the musculature of the left ventricle. This compensates for a while but ultimately the musculature fails, the ventricle dilates, and the mitral valve becomes insufficient. The consequent changes in the left atrium, pulmonary venous circulation, right ventricle, and right atrium are similar to those already described. Since the coronary arteries fill with blood during diastole, the decreased diastolic pressure in

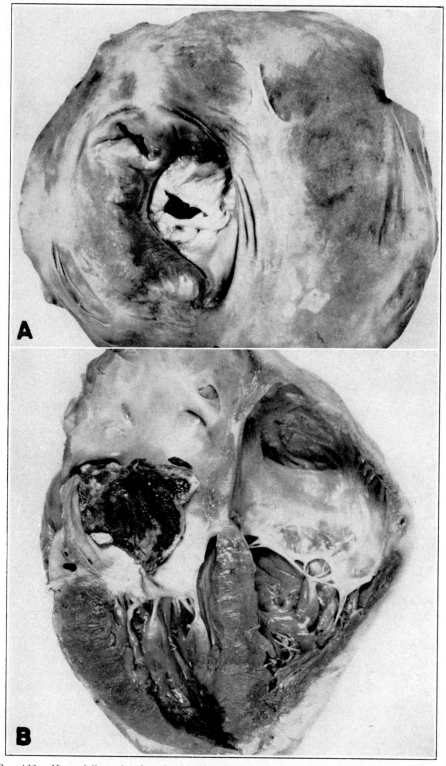

FIG. 132.—Heart failure showing *A*, old, fibrotic mitral stenosis and marked dilatation of the left atrium, and *B*, the same in longitudinal section with, in addition, a mural thrombus in the left atrium and hypertrophy and dilatation of the right side of the heart.

the aorta in aortic insufficiency may result in diminished blood flow in the coronary arteries and this, in turn, may bring about coronary artery insufficiency.

Aortic stenosis (decrease in area below the normal 3 sq. cm.) usually occurs as a result of healed rheumatic valvulitis or bacterial endocarditis. As in the case of the mitral leaflets, so the aortic cusps become fibrotic, thickened, fused, and permanently fixed in a semi-closed position (Fig. 133). This, of course, results in increased resistance to ejection of blood into the aorta, incomplete emptying of the blood from the ventricle during systole, increased volume of blood in the left ventricle, hypertrophy and then dilatation of the left ventricle, dilatation and insufficiency of the mitral ring, and a repeat of the processes already described in the left atrium, the pulmonary veins, and the right side of the heart. Because the valve cusps do not close completely there is also regurgitation of the blood into the left ventricle during diastole and this, of course, adds to the burden put upon the myometrium of the left ventricle. In aortic stenosis there is also diminutio in the coronary blood flow due to a decrease in pulse pressure and to encroachment on the coronary ostia by the same process that affects the aortic cusps.

Aside from changes in the myocardium, the accompaning *pathologic alterations* in heart failure are many. The left atrium, and to a lesser extent the right atrium, is frequently the seat of a mural *thrombus* due mainly to stagnation or pooling of blood in these areas (Fig. 132, *B*). The mesothelial-lined cavities (pericardial, pleural, and peritoneal) contain varied amounts of straw-colored fluid or *effusions* (Paul). The *lungs* are increased in weight and reveal congestion, hemorrhages, edema, infarction, fibrosis of alveolar walls, hemosiderosis, heart failure cells, and mild emphysema (Fig. 134). The liver discloses an increase in weight, central lobular congestion with or without hepatic cell degeneration, central lobular necrosis with or without inflammation, and varying degrees of cardiac cirrhosis. The *spleen* shows an increase in weight, dilatation of the sinusoids, engorgement and fibrosis of the red pulp, and atrophy of the white pulp. The *kidneys* are enlarged and congested and histologically reveal dilated glomerular spaces filled with protein precipitate, hypertrophy of the epithelium of the convoluted tubules, acute necrosis of the tubular epithelium, and edema of the interstitial tissue. The *remaining organs* and tissues disclose varying degrees of congestion, edema, and parenchymatous degeneration. The *net result* of all of these changes is impairment of physiologic functions of each of the organs affected.

Sudden Death.—Aside from physical trauma or certain poisonings (chloral hydrate and cyanide) the only conditions that will produce *instantaneous* death are coronary artery occlusion and acute anesthetic cardiac arrest. Some of the many other natural causes of sudden (but not instantaneous) death are rupture of the heart with cardiac tamponade, rupture of the aorta, cerebral apoplexy, severe hemorrhage in any area and from whatever cause, pulmonary embolism, fulminating respiratory or general infection, rupture of a viscus such as the liver or spleen, and shock from whatever cause.

Acute anesthetic cardiac arrest, as the caption implies, is arrest of contraction of the heart during the course of anesthesia (Ellis). Historically, the first anesthetic death was *recorded* in 1848; the first attempt at cardiac restoration by manual message was recorded in 1874, and the first successful cardiac restoration was recorded in 1901. The present incidence is given as varying between 1 in 1000 and 1 in 2000 consecutive operations. The

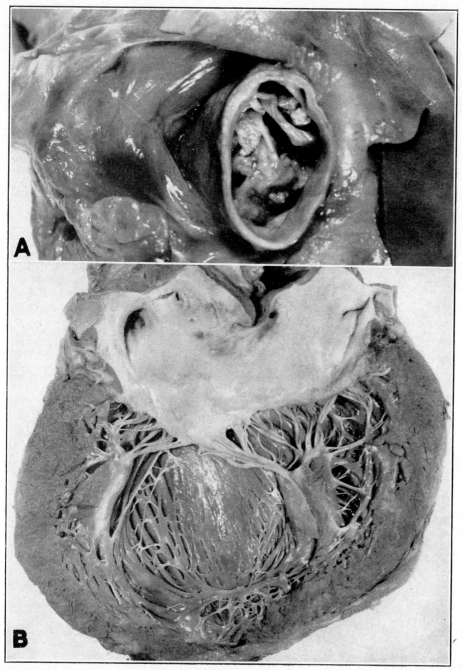

FIG. 133.—Heart failure illustrating *A*, healed aortic valvulitis with the fibrotic valves in a semi-closed position, and *B*, consequent hypertrophy and dilatation of the left ventricle, dilatation of the mitral ring, and dilatation of the left atrium.

absolute incidence is high between the ages of 1 to 5 years but reaches a peak between the ages of 30 to 50 years—probably due to the large number of operations performed during these periods of life. The relative incidence is about 20 times more common in people of 70 years of age and about 30 times more common in poor-risk patients. A recent upsurg in the number of recorded cases may be explained on (1) the greater awareness of the condition with more accurate diagnosis and (2) the increase in the number of

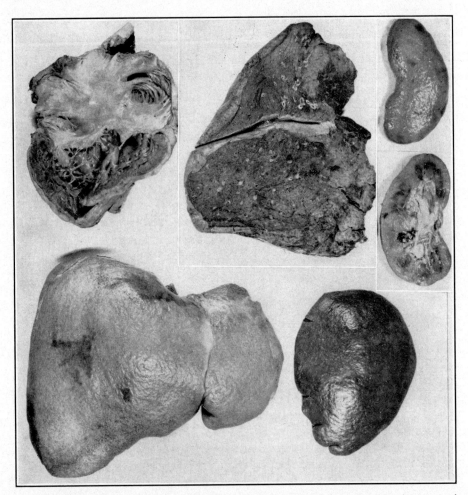

FIG. 134.—Heart failure showing a dilated right ventricle and atrium together with congestion and enlargement of the four organs most severely affected, namely, the lungs, kidneys, liver, and spleen.

surgical procedures on elderly and poor-risk patients. The most important *factor* responsible for cardiac arrest is cerebral anoxia. This is supplemented by the formation of small thrombi in the circulatory system of the entire body including the brain. The pre-existing *causes* eventuating in the stoppage of heart beat during anesthesia are (1) any pre-existing disease of the heart such as pericardial effusion, myocarditis, coronary artery disease, and valvular disorders or physiologic disturbances manifested as heart block or arrhythmias, (2) diseases of the respiratory tract attended by poor oxygen exchange, including hydrothorax, emphysema, and sudden pneumothorax, and (3) miscellaneous disturbances such as electrolytic upset and malnutrition. The precipitating causes are (1) hypoxia such as produced by shock, hypotension, anemia, excessive narcosis, and over curarization, (2) hypercarbia resulting from poor or exhausted soda lime in the anesthetic machine or mechanical defect of the machine, (3) vagal stimulation under any of the abnormal conditions already listed, (4) acute myocardial failure, (5) mechanical factors as, for example, tension, traction, or torsion applied to the heart or great vessels, and (6) combinations of anesthetic agents as, for example, administration of adrenalin in the presence of clyclopropane or chloroform anesthesia which results in increased myocardial irritability. The *diagnosis* of cardiac arrest is made by (1) absence of pulse or heart beat, (2) unobtainable blood pressure, and (3) cessation of bleeding into the wound. *Treatment* must be started within 3 minutes of the arrest and, for this reason, the physician must be forever on the alert. It should consist of (1) discontinuance of all anesthesia, (2) guarantee of continued delivery of oxygen by artificial respiration by way of endobronchial tube at a rate of flow of 10 to 20 liters per minute, and (3) guarantee of the transporting system by way of manual cardiac massage at the rate of 70 compressions per minute. Access to the heart should be by way of an emergency incision between the left fourth and fifth ribs, extending from the sternum to the left anterior axillary line. In the event of failure of immediate response, massage should be continued for at least 45 minutes.

TUMORS

Orientation. —Tumors of the heart are uncommon. They may be primary or secondary. Although the nomenclature regarding secondary growths is straightforward, that regarding primary growths is quite confused. At one time or another, virtually every tissue normally found in the heart has been described as giving rise to a primary benign and malignant tumor. Without attempting to list all of the tumors or combinations of terms that have been used, the following may be recorded as some of the more common and more important growths: (1) benign tumors—cysts, myxoma, fibroma, congenital glycogenic tumor, lipoma, angioma, and hamartoma, and (2) malignant tumors—mesothelioma, lymphoblastoma, and simply sarcoma. The categories listed may now be discussed briefly.

Cysts. —Cysts of the heart may be pericardial or myocardial. *Pericardial cysts* are sometimes referred to as pericardial celomic cysts. They may be located anywhere in the vicinity of the pericardium but are usually found in the anterior mediastinum at its angle with the diaphragm. They frequently reach a size of 15 cm. in diameter. Grossly they are composed of a thin, transparent wall, are usually unilocular, and are filled with clear, colorless, or straw-colored fluid. Histologically they consist of a layer of mesothelial cells covering a connective tissue wall. Their origin is not clear. They have been considered to arise as (1) failure of proper fusion of mesenchymal lacunæ that normally form the pericardium, (2) persistence of a ventral parietal recess, and (3) pulsion diverticulum of the parietal pericardium (Lillie). Clinically they are symptomless or, at most, produce epigastric and precordial pain. *Myocardial cysts* are generally incidental findings at autopsy. They may be located at any part of the heart but are most frequent in the left ventricle. They usually measure less than 2 cm. in diameter, are generally unilocular, contain gelatinous or rarely "sebaceous" material, and are lined by ciliated or nonciliated columnar or, less commonly, squamous epithelium. They have been considered to arise from entodermal inclusions and from multipotent mesodermal cells.

Myxoma.—Although there has been considerable discussion as to whether the so-called myxoma of the heart constitutes a true neoplasm or merely represents an organized thrombus, it appears that the former opinion prevails. If so, the lesion is the most common tumor of the heart, constituting approximately one-half of all primary cardiac neoplasms. Although it can occur in any part of the heart, the most common location (three-quarters of the cases) is the left atrium. The size varies from a few millimeters to 10 cm. in diameter. Most of the growths are polypoid with narrow or sessile pedicles. The external surface is smooth and glistening. The consistency is firm. Cut surfaces present soft, gelatinous or rubbery, white to light brown tissue. Histologically the growths consist of elongated, often stellate cells with round or oval nuclei, scanty cytoplasm, and varying amounts of intercellular mucoid material. The growths have occurred at all ages and, because they project into the lumen of the left atrium, they may give signs of mitral stenosis.

Fibroma.—Fibromas of the heart are closely related to myxomas. Most of the tumors are located in the left side and may be intramyocardial or subendothelial. The latter are often papillary or pedunculated and may be found in the vicinity of the valves. The tumors usually measure less than 5 cm. in diameter. Grossly they are sharply encapsulated and grayish-white. Histologically they are composed of whorls of connective tissue with varying amounts of intercellular collagen.

Congenital Glycogenic Tumor.—This tumor has also been referred to as *rhabdomyoma*. It is congenital in origin and is usually seen in infants or young children. The growth arises within the myocardium but may project beneath the pericardium or beneath the endocardium (Fig. 135*A*). It may consist of a single, fairly sharply circumscribed but not encapsulated nodule, of multiple nodules, or of innumerable nodules scattered throughout the myocardium. Histologically it is characteristically composed of so-called "spider cells," that is, cells disclosing a relatively large nucleus that appears to be enmeshed in threads of cytoplasm which, in turn, course between vacuoles that may contain glycogen. Some of the cells, in addition, contain cross striations. The tumor is frequently asymptomatic. It may be associated with tuberous sclerosis.

Lipoma.—Lipoma of the heart is relatively uncommon. It may arise within the pericardium, myocardium, or endocardium. The pericardial and endocardial growths are frequently pedunculated although the base in the latter is broader than the base in the former (Fig. 135*B*). The growths are generally sharply circumscribed, appear encapsulated, and are composed of light yellowish tissue. Histologically they disclose adult fat cells.

Angioma.—Angioma of the heart may be composed of blood or lymphatic vessels. In the recorded cases the tumors have been located within the myocardium, generally near the conducting system. Many of them have thus been associated with complete heart block. Grossly the growths are ill defined and generally somewhat spongy. Histologically they are composed of capillaries or cavernous spaces filled with blood or lymph.

Hamartoma.—The term hamartoma (Gr. = error + tumor) signifies a congenital, tumor-like nodule composed of tissue normally present in the area but bearing an abnormal arrangement. As far as the heart is concerned, the caption may be used to encompass benign tumor-like masses composed of mixtures of the following tissues: muscle, fibrous tissue, endothelial cells, blood vessels, fat, and nerves.

Mesothelioma.—A mesothelioma is generally considered to be a malignant tumor composed of cells lining the pericardial, pleural, peritoneal, or similar cavities. The lesion has also been called *endothelioma* (Reals). In general, the literature regarding mesothelioma as a group is so confused that many pathologists look upon any diagnosis of mesothelioma with some skepticism. Grossly the growths in the pericardium have been composed

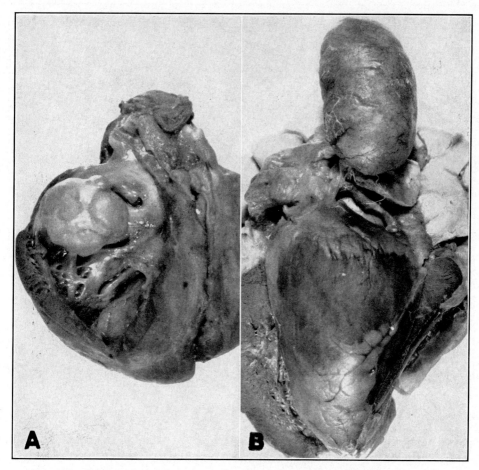

Fig. 135.—Benign tumors of the heart showing *A*, a congenital glycogen tumor of the left atrium (posterior view) and *B*, a lipoma of the pericardium.

more or less of closely packed nodules or sheets of grayish-white tumor tissue covering the heart in a plaque-like fashion. Histologically the tumors are composed of elongated cells with a tendency to whorl formation, of oval cells indiscriminantely arranged, or of cuboidal cells in definite glandular formation. The stroma varies from scanty and loose to abundant and collagenous. The greatest problem in making a diagnosis of mesothelioma is to make certain that the tumor is not metastatic.

Lymphoblastoma.—Any members of the lymphoblastoma group of diseases (see Lymph Nodes, p. 984) may affect the pericardium, myocardium, or endocardium. The lesions in the endocardium are usually extensions of tumors from the myocardium and not implants upon the surface. In any case, lymphoblastoma may affect the heart diffusely or may be localized in the form of small tumor nodules. Pericardial effusion, often of a hemorrhagic type, is frequent, especially in cases of leukemia. While in the majority of instances the effusion is due to direct involvement of the heart by the lymphoblastoma, occasionally the accumulation of fluid is entirely nonspecific (acute idiopathic pericarditis).

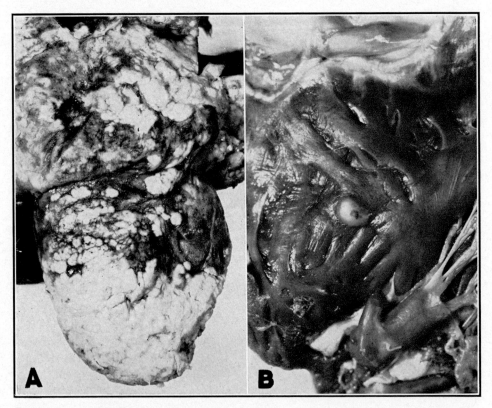

Fig. 136.—Secondary tumors of the heart showing *A*, a metastatic bronchogenic carcinoma of the visceral and parietal pericardium and *B*, a metastatic retroperitoneal sarcoma of the myocardium and endocardium.

Sarcoma.—Most malignant tumors of the heart have been recorded under the heading of sarcoma without any attempt at further differentiation. The tumors have been described at all ages without predilection for either sex. Primary sarcomas of the heart, unlike primary benign tumors, have a predilection for the right side, especially the right ventricle. Although the growths usually arise in the myocardium they may, as they enlarge, project either toward the pericardium or toward the endocardium. In general, the neoplasms are infiltrative but as they reach the surface they become sessile and even polypoid. Histologically they are extremely varied. Prichard, in summarizing the literature, listed the following tumors in decreasing order of frequency: fibrosarcoma, fibromyxosarcoma, myxosarcoma, leiomyosarcoma, rhabdomyosarcoma, and a variety of angiosarcoma.

Secondary Tumors.—Secondary tumors of the heart are from twenty to forty times as frequent as primary tumors (Prichard). The incidence has been given as varying from 0.03 to 1.4 per cent of all autopsies and from 1.0 to 7.5 per cent of all cases of cancer. The neoplasms reach the heart by direct extension or by metastasis by way of the blood vessels and lymphatic channels. The primary site of the tumor may be in any organ of the body with the stomach, lungs, breasts, esophagus, rectum, and the pancreas heading the list. Pathologically any portion of the heart may be affected although most of the tumors are deposited within the pericardium and myocardium (Fig. 136). Rarely, the tumor cells may be implanted upon (probably previously damaged) valves in a manner similar to vegetations in bacterial endocarditis. The metastasis may be single but more commonly it is multiple and frequently the nodules coalesce to form sheet-like plaques of tumor. Many of the pericardial lesions are accompanied by a hemorrhagic effusion. Histologically the tumors mimic the primary growths.

REFERENCES

Pathologic Physiology

BLOUNT, S. G., *et al.*: Circulation, *9*, 801, 1954 (Atrial Septal Defects).
FRIEDBERG, C. K.: *Diseases of the Heart*, Philadelphia, W. B. Saunders Co., 1949.
GOLDBERGER, E.: *Heart Disease*, Philadelphia, Lea & Febiger, 1951.
GOLDBERG, H., *et al.*: Am. Heart J., *47*, 527, 1954 (Dynamics Aortic Valvular Disease).
HARVEY, R. M., *et al.*: Circulation, *8*, 695, 1953 (Constrictive Pericarditis).
HULL, E.: Sodeman's *Pathologic Physiology*, Philadelphia, W. B. Saunders Co., 1956, p. 396.
LEVINE, S. A.: *Clinical Heart Disease*, 4th Ed., Philadelphia, W. B. Saunders Co., 1951.
WHITE, P. D.: *Heart Disease*, 4th Ed., New York, The Macmillan Co., 1951.

Congenital Anomalies

ADAMS, F. H., and KATZ, B.: J. Pediat., *41*, 141, 1952 (Endocardial Fibroelastosis).
ALEXANDER, W. S., and GREEN, H. C.: A. M. A. Arch. Path., *53*, 187, 1952 (Anomalous Coronary Artery).
BLUMBERG, R. W., and LYON, R. A.: A. M. A. Am. J. Dis. Child., *84*, 291, 1952 (Endocardial Fibroelastosis).
BOND, V. F., JR.: Am. Heart J., *42*, 424, 1951 (Eisenmenger's Complex).
EMERY, J. L., and ILLINGSWORTH, R. S.: Arch. Dis. Child., *26*, 304, 1951 (Congenital Mitral Stenosis).
FOWLER, R. E. L., and BEVIL, H. H.: Pediatrics, *8*, 340, 1951 (Aneurysm Sinus Valsalva).
GURAIEB, S. R., and RIGDON, R. H.: Am. Heart J., *52*, 138, 1956 (Fibroelastosis Adults).
JOHNSON, F. R.: A. M. A. Arch. Path., *54*, 237, 1952 (Endocardial Fibroelastosis).
LARGE, H. L., JR.: Am. J. M. Sci., *219*, 268, 1950 (Congenital Mitral Atresia).
LEVINSON, S. A., and LEARNER, A.: A. M. A. Arch. Path., *14*, 810, 1932 (Valvular Blood Cysts).
MAZAR, S. A., and BROWN, N.: New York State J. Med., *52*, 1295, 1952 (Bicuspid Aortic Valves).
McKINLEY, H. I., *et al.*: Pediatrics, *8*, 828, 1951 (Anomalous Coronary Artery).
PERKINS, G. B., *et al.*: J. Pediat., *35*, 401, 1949 (Tetralogy of Fallot).
ROGERS, H. M., and EDWARDS, J. E.: Am. Heart J., *41*, 299, 1951 (Cor Triloculare Biatrium)
RUBSAMEN, D., and KELLOGG, F.: Arch. Path., *51*, 658, 1951 (Duplication Mitral Valve).
SHAFIROFF, G. P.: J. Thoracic Surg., *21*, 30, 1951 (Absence Pericardium).
SKAPINKER, S.: A. M. A. Arch. Surg., *63*, 629, 1951 (Diverticulum Left Ventricle).
SOMMERS, S. C., and JOHNSON, J. M.: Am. Heart J., *41*, 130, 1951 (Congenital Tricuspid Atresia).
SPENCER, H., and DWORKEN, H. J.: Circulation, *2*, 880, 1950 (Communication Aorta and Pulmonary Artery).
TAUSSIG, H. B.: *Congenital Malformations of the Heart*, New York, The Commonwealth Fund, 1947.
WHITE, N. K., and EDWARDS, J. E.: A. M. A. Arch. Path., *45*, 766, 1948 (Anomalies of Coronary Arteries).

Degenerations

FINESTONE, A. J., and GESCHICKTER, C. F.: Am. J. Clin. Path., *19*, 974, 1949, (Ossification in Heart).
FRENCH, J. E.: A. M. A. Arch. Path., *53*, 485, 1952 (Hypoptassemia in Rats)
GASS, H., *et al.:* Medicine, *27*, 105, 1948 (Potassium and Periodic Paralysis).
GORE, I., and ARONS, W.: A. M. A. Arch. Path., *48*, 1, 1949 (Myocardial Calcification).
GRIFFITH, R. L.: A. M. A. Arch. Int. Med., *89*, 743, 1952 (Beriberi Heart).
GUTENKAUF, C. H.: Circulation, *3*, 352, 1951 (Beriberi Heart).
HELLERSTEIN, H. K., and SANDIAGO-STEVENSON, E.: Circulation, *1*, 93, 1950, (Atrophy of Heart).
HUNTER, A.: Quart. J. Med., *15*, 107, 1946 (Heart in Anemia).
IBRAHIM, M.: J. Lancet, *77*, 114, 1957 (Myxedema Heart).
JONES, R. S., and FRAZIER, D. B.: A. M. A. Arch. Path., *50*, 366, 1950 (Primary Amyloidosis).
KINNEY, T. D., and MALLORY, G. K.: New England J. Med., *232*, 215, 1945 (Heart in Acute Anemia).
LADUE, J. S.: J. Pharmacol. & Exper. Therap., *76*, 1, 1942 (Digitalis).
PERELSON, H. N., and COSBY, R. S.: Am. Heart J., *37*, 1126, 1949 (Periodic Paralysis).
SURAWICZ, B., *et al.*: Am. J. Med. Sc., *233*, 603, 1957 (Hypopotassemia).

Rheumatic Fever

ALTSCHULE, M. D., and BUDNITZ, E.: A. M. A. Arch. Path., *30*, 7, 1940 (Rheumatic Disease Tricuspid Valve).
ASH, R.: Am. J. Dis. Child., *76*, 46, 1948 (Rheumatic Infection in Childhood).
BENNETT, G. A.: Ann. Int. Med., *19*, 111, 1943 (Rheumatic Arthritis).
BENNETT, G. A., *et al.:* A. M. A. Arch. Path., *30*, 70, 1940 (Subcutaneous Nodules).
BLAND, E. F., and JONES, T. D.: Ann. Int. Med., *37*, 1006, 1952 (Natural History Rheumatic Fever).
CROSS, R. J.: Am. J. Med., *22*, 422, 1957 (Pathogenesis).
EPSTEIN, E. Z., and GREENSTAN, E. B.: A. M. A. Arch. Int. Med., *68*, 1074, 1941 (Rheumatic Pneumonia).
HANSEN, A. E.: J. A. M. A., *148*, 1481, 1952 (Early Diagnosis Rheumatic Fever).
HARTMAN, S. A., and BLAND, E. F.: Am. J. Med., *10*, 47, 1951 (Rheumatic Fever and Glomerulonephritis).
HOUSER, H. B., and ECKHARDT, G. C.: Ann. Int. Med., *37*, 1035, 1952 (Prevention Rheumatic Fever).
JOHNSON, A. L., *et al.:* Canad. M. A. J., *66*, 225, 1952 (Cortisone and ACTH).
JONES, T. D.: J. A. M. A., *126*, 481, 1944 (Diagnosis Rheumatic Fever).
KAGAN, B. M., *et al.:* A. M. A. Am. J. Dis. Child., *78*, 306, 1949 (Chorea).
KAUFMAN, P., and POLIAKOFF, H.: Ann. Int. Med., *32*, 889, 1950 (Rheumatic Heart Disease in Old Age).
KOBERNICK, S. D.: Am. J. M. Sci., *224*, 329, 1952 (Experimental Rheumatic Carditis).
KUTTNER, A. G., *et al.:* J. A. M. A., *148*, 628, 1952 (ACTH and Cortisone).
LAPIN, L., and STARKEY, H.: Canad. M. A. J., *60*, 371, 1949 (Pathology and Etiology Rheumatic Diseases).
LEARY, T.: A. M. A. Arch. Path., *13*, 1, 1932 (Rheumatic Endocarditis).
MASSELL, B. F., *et al.: Rheumatic Diseases*, Philadelphia, W. B. Saunders Co., p. 27, 1952 (Subcutaneous Nodules).
McCARTY, M.: Ann. Int. Med., *37*, 1027, 1952 (Diagnostic Tests Rheumatic Fever).
————: Bull. Rheumat. Dis., *7*, 23, 1957 (Antistreptolysin O).
RAICH, N. E.: Am. Pract. & Digest of Treatment, *2*, 328, 1951 (Uncommon Sites Rheumatic Fever).
REID, J., and SPROULL, D. H.: Br. Med. J., No. 5027, 1089, 1957 (Fibrinogen).
REITMAN, N.: Ann. Int. Med., *22*, 671, 1945 (Abdominal Manifestations Rheumatic Fever).
ROBINSON, J. J.: A. M. A. Arch. Path., *51*, 602, 1951 (Streptococcic Rheumatic Carditis in Animals).
ROBINSON, W. D., and ROSEMAN, S.: Bull. Rheumat. Dis., *7*, 31, 1957 (Serum Proteins).
SAPHIR, O.: A. M. A. Arch. Path., *32*, 1042, 1941 (Rheumatic Myocarditis).
SWIFT, H. F.: Ann. Int. Med., *31*, 715, 1949 (Etiology Rheumatic Fever).
VON GLAHN, W. C.: Am. J. Med., *2*, 76, 1947 (Pathology of Rheumatism).
WAKSMAN, B. H.: Medicine, *28*, 143, 1949 (Etiology Rheumatic Fever).
YOUNG, D., and SCHWEDEL, J. B.: Am. Heart J., *40*, 771, 1950 (Calcification Left Atrium Rheumatic Disease).

Bacterial Endocarditis

ABRAHAM, E., and JACKSON, M.: Am. Pract., *3*, 781, 1952 (Rupture Aortic Valve).
BARKER, P. S.: Am. Heart J., *37*, 1054, 1949 (Right-sided and Pulmonic).
CALL, J. D., *et al.*: Am. J. Clin. Path., *14*, 508, 1944 (Brucella).
CATES, J. E., and CHRISTIE, R. V.: Quart. J. Med., *20*, 93, 1951 (442 Cases of Subacute).
CORRELL, H. L., *et al.*: Ann. Int. Med., *35*, 45, 1951 (Clinico-pathologic Studies).
DICK, G. F., and SCHWARTZ, W. B.: A. M. A. Arch. Path., *42*, 159, 1946 (Experimental).
DORSET, V. J., *et al.*: Am. Heart J., *38*, 610, 1949 (Penicillin in Gonococcic).
DOWLING, H. F., *et al.*: Medicine, *31*, 155, 1952 (Staphylococcic).
FITZGERALD, W. M.: Wisconsin M. J., *49*, 131, 1950 (Seventy Cases).
FRIEDBERG, C. K.: J. A. M. A., *148*, 98, 1952 (Aureomycin in Subacute).
HAMBURGER, M., and STEIN, L.: J. A. M. A., *149*, 542, 1952 (Penicillin in Subacute).
JONES, H. E., and DALTON, E. G.: Arch. Dis. Child., *27*, 157, 1952 (After Taussig-Blalock Operation).
KAPLAN, S. R., *et al.*: J. A. M. A., *141*, 114, 1949 (Healed Subacute).
KURZ, E. R. H., *et al.*: Ann. Int. Med., *31*, 497, 1949 (Salmonella).
LOEWE, L.: Am. Pract., *1*, 349, 1950 (Subacute).
LOEWE, L., *et al.*: Ann. Int. Med., *34*, 717, 1951 (Enterococcal).
MACNEAL, W. J., *et al.*: Am. J. Path., *21*, 255, 1945 (Experimental).
MIDDLETON, W. S.: Ann. Int. Med., *31*, 511, 1949 (Hemophilus Influenzæ).
MORE, R. H.: Am. J. Path., *19*, 413, 1943 (Clostridium Welchii).
PETERSEN, E. S., *et al.*: J. A. M. A., *144*, 621, 1950 (Streptobacillus Moniliformis).
PIKE, C.: J. Path. & Bact., *63*, 577, 1951 (Corynebacterial).
PIRANI, C. L.: A. M. A. Arch. Path., *36*, 579, 1943 (Rupture Heart).
SAPHIR, O., *et al.*: Circulation, *1*, 1155, 1950 (Myocardium in Subacute).
TRAUT, E. F., *et al.*: Geriatrics, *4*, 205, 1949 (Ninety-four Autopsies in Elderly Patients).
WALLACE, C. S.: Ann. Int. Med., *34*, 1463, 1951 (Escherichia and Aerobacter).

Disseminated Lupus Erythematosus

ALLGOOD, J. W.: N. Carolina Med. J., *18*, 141, 1957 (General).
BENNETT, G. A., and DALENBACH, F. D.: Military Surg., *109*, 531, 1951 (Synovial Membrane Changes).
HUMPHREYS, E. M.: Ann. Int. Med., *28*, 12, 1948 (Cardiac Lesions).
JESSAR, R. A., *et al.*: Ann. Int. Med., *38*, 717, 1953 (Natural History).
KLEMPERER, P.: McManus—*Progress in Fundamental Medicine*, Philadelphia, Lea & Febiger, p. 51, 1952 (Pathology).
LEE, S. L., *et al.*: Am. J. Med., *10*, 446, 1951 (L. E. Cell).
LOWMAN, E. W., and SLOCUMB, C. H.: Ann. Int. Med., *36*, 1206, 1952 (Vascular Lesions).
MONTGOMERY, H., and McCREIGHT, W. G.: A. M. A. Arch. Dermat. & Syph., *60*, 356, 1949 (General Discussion).
SOFFER, L. J., and BADER, R.: J. A. M. A., *149*, 1002, 1952 (ACTH and Cortisone).
TEILUM, G., and POULSEN, H. E.: A.M.A. Arch. Path., *64*, 414, 1957 (Histopathology).

Other Endocarditis

ALLEN, A. C., and SIROTA, J. H.: Am. J. Path., *20*, 1025, 1944 (Terminal).
BAKER, R. D.: A. M. A. Arch. Path., *19*, 611, 1935 (Tuberculous).
BARON, E., and RITTER, D. W.: Ann. Int. Med., *33*, 1023, 1950 (Tuberculous).
BEAMER, T. R., *et al.*: Am. Heart J., *29*, 99, 1945 (Higher Bacteria and Fungi).
KUNSTADTER, R. H., *et al.*: J. A. M. A., *149*, 829, 1952 (Mycotic).
LOMBARDO, T. A., *et al.*: Am. J. Med., *22*, 664, 1957 (Mycotic).
ZIMMERMAN, L. E.: A. M. A. Arch. Path., *50*, 591, 1950 (Fungous).

Spirochetal Endocarditis

HITZIG, W. N., and LIEBESMAN, A.: A. M. A. Arch. Int. Med., *73*, 415, 1944 (Spirillum Minus).

Myocarditis

AREÁN, V. M.: Lab. Investig., *6*, 462, 1957 (Leptospiral Myocarditis).
GHOLMY, A. E.: Arch. Pediat., *71*, 203, 1954 (Isolated Myocarditis).
GOLDBERGER, E.: *Heart Disease*, Philadelphia, Lea & Febiger, p. 399, 1951.

Saphir, O.: A. M. A. Arch. Path., *32*, 1000, 1941; *Ibid*, *33*, 88, 1942 (General Review).
Scotti, T. M., and McKeown, C. E.: A. M. A. Arch. Path., *46*, 289, 1948 (Boeck's Sarcoid).
Spain, D. M., *et al.:* Am. Heart J., *40*, 336, 1950 (Poliomyelitis).

Pericarditis

Andrews, G. W. S., *et al.:* Quart. J. Med., *17*, 291, 1948 (Constrictive).
Chambliss, J. R., *et al.:* Circulation, *4*, 816, 1951 (Constrictive).
Freilich, J. K.: Ann. Int. Med., *37*, 388, 1952 (Acute Nonspecific).
Goldberger, E.: *Heart Disease*, Philadelphia, Lea & Febiger, p. 532, 1951.
Herrmann, G. R., *et al.:* Am. Heart J., *43*, 641, 1952 (130 Cases).
Myers, T. M., and Hamburger, M.: Am. J. Med., *12*, 302, 1952 (Tuberculous).
Nelson, A. A.: A. M. A. Arch. Path., *29*, 256, 1940 (Milk Spots).
Parker, R. C., Jr., and Cooper, H. R.: J. A. M. A., *147*, 835, 1951 (Acute Idiopathic).
Rosenow, O. F., and Cross, C. J.: A. M. A. Arch. Int. Med., *87*, 795, 1951 (Acute Benign).
Semple, E.: Edinburgh M. J., *55*, 731, 1948 (Tuberculous).
White, P. D.: Circulation, *4*, 288, 1951 (Constrictive).
Wood, J. A.: Am. Heart J., *42*, 737, 1951 (Tuberculous).

Myocardial Infarction

Blache, J. O., and Handler, F. E.: A. M. A. Arch. Path., *50*, 189, 1950 (Race Differences).
Block, W. J., Jr., *et al.:* J. A. M. A., *150*, 259, 1952 (6,882 Cases Angina Pectoris).
Blumgart, H. L.: Am. J. Med., *2*, 129, 1947 (Spasm of Coronary Arteries).
Brean, H. P., *et al.:* Radiology, *54*, 33, 1950 (Calcification).
Chinsky, M., and Sherry, S.: A.M.A. Arch. Int. Med., *99*, 556, 1957 (Transaminase).
Dack, S., *et al.:* Am. Heart J., *42*, 161, 1951 (Acute Hemorrhage).
Davis, H. A., *et al.:* A. M. A. Arch. Surg., *62*, 698, 1951 (Shock as Cause).
Ernstene, A. C.: J. A. M. A., *150*, 1069, 1952 (Complications).
Gans, R. H.: Am. Heart J., *41*, 332, 1951 (Rupture of Ventricle).
Geckler, G. E., *et al.:* J. A. M. A., *148*, 1413, 1952 (Perforation Interventricular Septum).
Goldberger, E.: *Heart Disease*, Philadelphia, Lea & Febiger, p. 243, 1951 (Angina Pectoris).
Horn, H., *et al.:* Am. Heart J., *40*, 63, 1950 (Pathology and Physiology).
Kozonis, M. C., and Gurevin, J.: Ann. Int. Med., *46*, 79, 1957 (C-Reactive Protein).
Lovitt, W. V., Jr., and Corzine, W. J., Jr.: A. M. A. Arch. Path., *54*, 458, 1952 (Medionecrosis and Hemorrhage).
Mallory, G. K., *et al.:* Am. Heart J., *18*, 647, 1939 (Histologic Study).
Master, A. M., and Jaffe, H. L.: J. A. M. A., *148*, 794, 1952 (Factors in Onset).
Moon, H. D., and Rinehart, J. F.: Circulation, *6*, 481, 1952 (Histogenesis of Coronary Arteriosclerosis).
Moyer, J. B., and Hiller, G. I.: Am. Heart J., *41*, 340, 1951 (Cardiac Aneurysm).
Oblath, R. W., *et al.:* J. A. M. A., *149*, 1276, 1952 (Cardiac Rupture).
Paterson, J. C.: McManus—*Progress in Fundamental Medicine*, Philadelphia, Lea & Febiger, p. 177, 1952 (Coronary Artery Disease).
Sampson, J. J.: Am. Pract. & Digest Treat., *2*, 1031, 1951 (Treatment).
Scharfman, W. B., *et al.:* Am. Heart J., *40*, 603, 1950 (Syphilitic Coronary Ostia).
Smith, C.: J. A. M. A., *151*, 167, 1953 (Length of Survival).
Smith, F. J., *et al.:* Am. J. M. Sci., *221*, 508, 1951 (920 Patients).
Stein, I.: Am. Heart J., *40*, 325, 1950 (Angina Pectoris).
Syner, J. C.: Armed Forces M. J., *3*, 699, 1952 (Myocardial Infarction).
Tedeschi, C. G., *et al.:* New England J. Med., *243*, 1024, 1950 (Abscess).
Thaler, R. W., and Wornas, C. G.: Am. J. Digest. Dis., *19*, 33, 1952 (Diabetes).
Yater, W. M., *et al.:* Ann. Int. Med., *34*, 352, 1951 (950 Autopsied Cases).

Other Physical Disturbances

Askey, J. M.: Am. J. Med., *9*, 528, 1950 (Rupture Papillary Muscle).
Bowman, H. S.: Am. J. Clin. Path., *23*, 33, 1953 (Trauma Heart).
Clagett, A. H., Jr., *et al.:* Am. J. M. Sci., *219*, 513, 1950 (Rupture Myocardium).
Connolly, E. P., and Littmann, D.: New England J. Med., *245*, 753, 1951 (Coronary Arteriosclerosis and Myocardial Hypertrophy).
Crane, A. P.: Military Surg., *110*, 346, 1952 (Trauma Heart).
Crawshaw, G. R.: Brit. J. Surg., *39*, 364, 1952 (Hernia into Pericardium).
Dale, W. A.: Ann. Surg., *135*, 376, 1952 (Cardiac Arrest).
Ellis, J. W.: Med. Times, *85*, 503, 1957 (Cardiac Arrest).

ELKIN, D. C., and CAMPBELL, R. E.: Ann. Surg., *133*, 623, 1951 (Cardiac Tamponade).

EVANS, L. R., and WHITE, P. E.: Am. J. M. Sci., *216*, 485, 1948 (Myocardial Hypertrophy).

HARRISON, C. V., and WOOD, P.: Brit. Heart J., *11*, 205, 1949 (Ischemic Heart Disease).

HUNT, W. E.: Arch. Dis. Child., *27*, 291, 1952 (Rupture in Infant).

KOEPSELL, J. E., *et al.*: A. M. A. Arch. Int. Med., *85*, 432, 1950 (Hypertension and Myocardial Hypertrophy).

LEVY, R. L., and VON GLAHN, W. C.: Am. Heart J., *28*, 714, 1944 (Cardiac Hypertrophy).

LIKOFF, W. B., and LEVINE, S. A.: Am. J. M. Sci., *206*, 425, 1943 (Thyrotoxicosis and Myocardial Hypertrophy).

MAYNARD, A. D. L., *et al.*: Surg., Gynec. & Obst., *94*, 605, 1952 (Penetrating Wounds of Heart).

METCALF, J., *et al.*: Circulation, *5*, 518, 1952 (Experimental Cardiac Tamponade).

PAUL, O., *et al.*: A.M.A. Arch. Path., *64*, 363, 1957 (Heart Failure).

ROSEMAN, M. D., and WASSERMAN, E.: New England J. Med., *245*, 450, 1951 (Hypertension and Mitral Stenosis).

SWAN, H., *et al.*: Ann. Surg., *135*, 314, 1952 (Foreign Bodies).

ZUCKER, R., *et al.*: A. M. A. Arch. Int. Med., *89*, 899, 1952 (Perforation Interventricular Septum).

Tumors

BIERMAN, H. R., *et al.*: Am. Heart J., *43*, 413, 1952 (Pericarditis in Leukemia).

BLANCHARD, A. J., and HETHRINGTON, H.: Canad. M. A. J., *66*, 147, 1952 (Malignant Hemangioendothelioma).

COLLER, F. C., *et al.*: Am. J. Clin. Path., *20*, 159, 1950 (Secondary Endocardial).

COULTER, W. W., JR.: A. M. A. Arch. Path., *49*, 612, 1950 (Myxoma).

FRIEDMAN, N. H., and SILVERMAN, J. J.: Blood, *5*, 916, 1950 (Benign Pericardial Effusion in Leukemia).

GREENBERG, M., and ANGRIST, A.: Am. Heart J., *35*, 623, 1948 (Primary Vascular Pericardial).

HERBUT, P. A., and MAISEL, A. L.: A. M. A. Arch. Path., *34*, 358, 1942 (Secondary).

KIDDER, L. A.: A. M. A. Arch. Path., *49*, 55, 1950 (Congenital Glycogenic Tumors).

KULKA, W.: Am. J. Path., *25*, 549, 1949 (Fibroma).

LAMBERTA, F., *et al.*: Dis. Chest, *19*, 528, 1951 (Secondary Pericardial).

LEACH, W. B.: A. M. A. Arch. Path., *44*, 198, 1947 (Primary).

LEIGHTON, J., *et al.*: A. M. A. Arch. Path., *50*, 632, 1950 (Myocardial Cysts).

LILLIE, W. I., *et al.*: J. Thoracic Surg., *20*, 494, 1950 (Pericardial Cysts and Diverticula).

LOEHR, W. M.: Am. J. Roentgenol., *68*, 584, 1952 (Pericardial Cysts).

MAINWARING, R. L., and AYRES, W. W.: Am. J. Path., *28*, 823, 1952 (Anitschkow Cell Sarcoma).

PRICHARD, R. W.: A. M. A. Arch. Path., *51*, 98, 1951 (Primary and Secondary).

REALS, W. J., *et al.*: A. M. A. Arch. Path., *44*, 380, 1947 (Mesothelioma).

SACHS, L. J., and ANGRIST, A.: Am. J. Path., *21*, 187, 1945 (Myocardial Cyst).

SHEA, J. P., and MUEHSAM, G. E.: Am. J. Clin. Path., *22*, 1081, 1952 (Lipoma).

SOLOMON, R. D.: A. M. A. Arch. Path., *52*, 561, 1951 (Malignant Teratoma).

STRAUS, R., and MERLISS, R.: A. M. A. Arch. Path., *39*, 74, 1945 (Primary).

SUSSMAN, W., and STASNEY, J.: Am. Heart J., *40*, 312, 1950 (Congenital Glycogenic Tumor)

Chapter

9

Vessels

PATHOLOGIC PHYSIOLOGY

William A. Sodeman

THE *vessels* form the second portion of the *cardiovascular system* and serve as the conduits for blood leaving and entering the heart. They consist of arteries, capillaries, veins. and lymphatics. Because the pressure of oxygenated blood leaving the heart is considerably greater than the pressure of carbon dioxide laden blood returning to the heart and lungs, the former vessels, that is arteries, have much thicker walls than do the latter, that is veins, and in the case of lymph, lymphatics. The larger arteries, such as the aorta and pulmonary are composed largely of elastic fibers with lesser amounts of smooth muscle; the medium sized arteries contain more smooth muscle than elastic fibers; the veins and larger lymphatics have lesser amounts of each, while the minute lymphatics and capillaries are composed mainly of endothelial lined tubules. As blood is forced into the greater vessels it is propelled with varying pressures and velocity. These depend upon the nature of the vessels, the amount of blood present, and the resistance to the outflow. Probably the most important single factor is *elasticity* of the vessel. Because of this property, the wall is first distended and, as a result of this distention, the vessel is then capable of exerting a continued force on the column of blood within its lumen and thus maintaining the blood pressure between systolic contractions of the heart. Were it not for this elasticity the blood pressure, in the interim, would drop to zero. Pathologically, thus, anything that interferes with this elasticity (arteriosclerosis) also interferes with the propulsion and distribution of the blood through the body. In the following paragraphs only a few of the more important pathophysiologic disturbances, as exemplified by selected disease processes, will be considered.

In *constriction* of the main *aortic trunk*, as in *coarctation* of the *aorta*, collateral channels develop connecting branches of the aortic arch with those of the descending aorta. Pulsations may be felt in these channels, especially the intercostals which also erode the ribs. Murmurs, either continuous or systolic, may be heard, especially in the interscapular area. The ventricular ejections enter the proximal aorta, an elastic reservoir of reduced capacity, and systolic pressure rises remarkably. The run off from this reservoir of small capacity in diastole accelerates fall in the pulse wave. Transmission of the waves through the collateral circulation with reflection of waves eventuates in a wave of greatly reduced amplitude in the lower aorta. In the lower extremities, therefore, the pulses are small and delayed or even absent.

In *shunting* of the *blood* between the greater and lesser circulations, as in *patent ductus arteriosus*, there occurs a continuous flow of blood from the aorta (high pressure) to the pulmonary artery (low pressure). This, along with acceleration in systole, produces a continuous murmur accentuated in systole. At times, up to one half the output of the left ventricle may be shunted through the ducts and returned to the left ventricle. Hence, the left atrium and ventricle are dilated and become hypertrophied. The increased output of the left ventricle maintains adequate flow to the periphery. The run off into the pulmonary artery, as with any arteriovenous fistula, produces lowered diastolic pressure. In some instances, developing pulmonary hypertension results in right ventricular hypertrophy. If pulmonary pressure becomes sufficiently high, reversed flow through the shunt occurs and cyanosis appears. Since the ductus enters the aorta distal to the left subclavian artery, a greater part of this flow is directed downward producing a deeper cyanosis in the lower rather than the upper extremities.

In *hardening* of the *arterial* walls, as in *arteriosclerosis*, the dynamics pertaining to *elasticity* are interfered with. Normally, the ejected blood enters the large, elastic arteries which act as a compression chamber to buffer the more peripheral arteries from too sudden an increase in pressure and flow. In systole, only a portion of the blood is moved along and a portion is stored by expansion of the vessels to allow a "run off" into the capillaries during diastole. Changes in the vessel walls affect not only the diameter of the vessels but also hemodynamic factors based upon the characteristics of the blood vessel wall. Thus, with reduction in the elasticity of the vessels, other things being constant, a higher pressure is found at the height of injection and a lower pressure in the interval. In man, the increased size of the aorta may partially compensate for such changes. Comparable change may occur in pressure relations if the vessel is distended beyond its usual limits, as in hypertensive disease, for the vessel is then more rigid. Aortic arteriosclerosis is one of the most common of all conditions affecting arterial elasticity. Atheromatosis (p. 359) may result in two changes responsible for inadequacy of the arteries; rupture of the vessel and obstruction. Both these changes produce serious results and, if they occur in a vital organ (heart, brain), may lead to death. General narrowing of vessels from arteriosclerosis must be greatly advanced to reduce blood supplies to a point at which symptoms appear, unless an accident of the type mentioned occurs. When occlusion does occur, the *symptoms* depend upon the location, the degree of involvement of branches, and the rapidity of development. They vary from those of acute occlusion to chronic insufficiency with claudication, muscle weakness, atrophy of skin and deeper structures, stiffness of joints, and finally gangrene. Infection may be a serious problem by aggravation, through pressure, of impaired circulation and by increased metabolic need which the vessels cannot supply.

Peripheral vascular disease implies disturbances in blood flow through the periphery, especially the extremities, whether due to structural disturbances, either remote or in the area, or not. The terms "functional" and "organic" are in common use. *Functional disturbances* imply the absence of structural changes in the vessels as a cause of the disorder as, for example, Raynaud's disease. Organic changes may result from such functional disorders. *Organic disturbances* imply disturbed circulation as the result of structural damage to vessels, for example, thromboangiitis obliterans involving the vessels of the area, or cervical rib involving the vessels beyond the structural defect. If such disturbances prevent an adequate circulation through the arteries, *arterial insufficiency* develops and may result in a train of *symptoms* including reduced or absent pulsations, pain, color change with change in position, coldness, pallor, ulceration, and gangrene.

23

Pain is an outstanding symptom in many peripheral vascular disorders. It may be of several types and varies in mechanism. Pain at rest, in sudden arterial occlusion, may be sudden and severe. At times, it may come on gradually over several hours. Usually pain due to embolism or thrombosis is associated with coldness, loss of or diminished pulsations and sensation, and some paresis—all resulting from ischemia and all being manifestations of *acute arterial insufficiency*. The cause for such pain is not entirely clear. Slowly developing complete occlusions often occur without any pain at all. However, in acute occlusion there is spasm of associated collateral vessels, a factor which some believe important in the causation of the pain, for sympathetic block relieves it. Spasm is partially responsible, also, for pallor and the other ischemic symptoms mentioned. In *ulceration* and *gangrene*, as seen for example in thromboangiitis obliterans and before ulceration in so-called pretrophic pain of ischemia, pain is common. It is, however, different in type and may be constant and severe, interfering with sleep so that the patient sits up, with the feet dependent, for relief. Heat may give partial relief, as may the dependent position. *Elevation* and *cold* accentuate the pain. The fact that cold and elevation do this suggests that the cause is related to ischemia of the part. Necrosis from impaired circulation is responsible for gangrene and, when severe, ulceration is a common part of the picture. Less marked changes result in a number of disturbances, such as thickened nails, large corns, and callus formation on the parts exposed to friction or weight bearing.

Skin color is an important sign of changes in the peripheral circulation, for a portion of the color of the skin is attributable to the vessels down to and including those of the subpapillary plexus. Changes in color may result from changes in the color of the blood itself or in the amount of blood contained in the vessels. Constriction or spasm of the vessels, as in *Raynaud's disease*, exemplify such changes. In the early stages of an attack, exposure to cold causes arteriolar spasm leading to pallor. Later, with dilatation of the arterioles and capillaries, redness, dusky cyanosis, or cyanosis may develop. Thus, pallor, redness and cyanoisis are produced by Raynaud's disease, the color varying with the state of the small vessels. Venous obstructon may lead to stasis and cyanosis also. In Raynaud's disease, color changes are produced by cold or, at times, by emotion. Attacks may be artificially produced by immersion of the hand in iced water. In general, in Raynaud's disease no cause can be assigned, such as cervical rib, arterial obstruction, or the like, and spontaneous attacks are bilateral. Obstruction to arteries may be secondary and, if present, involves only minute peripheral arteries, so that gangrene, if produced, is superficial and usually only on the finger tips or acral parts.

CONGENITAL ANOMALIES

Orientation.—In the course of normal development the vascular patterns throughout the body follow certain fixed lines of evolution resulting ultimately in a network which is called normal. The major channels of each of the three systems are rather constant while the minor channels are most constant in the arterial system, less constant in the venous system, and least constant in the lymphatic system. Deviation from the usual courses of the vessels are referred to as Congenital Anomalies. They are most important in connection with arteries, less important in connection with veins, and least important in connection with lymphatics. Also, in the arterial circulation, the greater the size of the vessel the more disturbing is its abnormality. For this reason anomalies of the *Aortic Arch* overshadow all others in importance. They alone will thus be considered in this section under the following headings: coarctation of the aorta, patent ductus arteriosus, posterior right subclavian artery, right-sided aortic arch, and double aortic arch. First, however, a brief discussion of the embryology appears to be in order.

Embryology of the Aortic Arches.—Early in embryonic life there are two primitive aortas which fuse anteriorly to form the aortic sac and posteriorly to form the descending aorta (Fig. 137). On each side, six sprouts

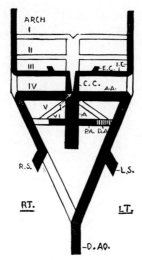

Fig. 137.—Larger vessels as shown in a diagrammatic sketch of the aortic arches. Blocked areas represent the definitive arteries, unblocked areas those that disappear. *I, II, III, IV, V* and *VI* are the arches. *E.C.*, external carotid. *C.C.*, common carotid. *I*, innominate. *A.A.*, aortic arch. *A.*, aortic sac. *P.A.*, pulmonary artery. *D.A.*, ductus arteriosus. *R.S.*, right subclavian. *L.S.*, left subclavian. *D.Ao.*, descending aorta. (Herbut, *Surgical Pathology*, 2nd Ed., Lea & Febiger.)

from the aortic sac unite with six sprouts from the dorsal aorta to form a series of six aortic arches. Ultimately, only portions of these arches persist while the remaining portions disappear resulting in a system of channels that is called normal. The following arches contribute to, or form, the following arteries: first arch—mandibular artery, second arch—hyoid and stapedial arteries, third arch—carotid arteries, fourth arch—aortic arch (left arch) and right subclavian and innominate arteries (ventral portion right arch), fifth arch—no permanent arteries, and sixth arch—pulmonary artery (proximal portion) and ductus arteriosus (distal portion left arch).

Coarctation of the Aorta.—Coarctation (L. = together + to make tight) connotes a partial or complete constriction of the aorta in the vicinity of the entrance of the ductus arteriosusor ligamentum arteriosum (Fig. 138). The condition is found in less than 2 per cent of all autopsies. The blood supply to the lower part of the body is maintained by the establishment of a collateral circulation between the segmental vessels above the constriction and the segmental vessels below the constriction. *Clinical manifestations* may consist of the following: precordial pain, headache, dizziness, epistaxis, vomiting, enlargement of the heart to the left, cardiac murmurs, hypertension in the upper extremities, hypotension in the lower extremities, pulsation of the vessels proximal to the constriction, erosion of the inferior margins and posterior portions of the ribs roentgenographically, radiologic demonstration of the constriction after intra-arterial injection of diodrast, and evidences of cardiac failure. *Treatment* consists of surgical reestablishment of the lumen in the constricted portion. The *prognosis* is good. The *causes* of death in untreated cases are myocardial failure, rupture of the ascending aorta, endocarditis, and cerebral hemorrhage.

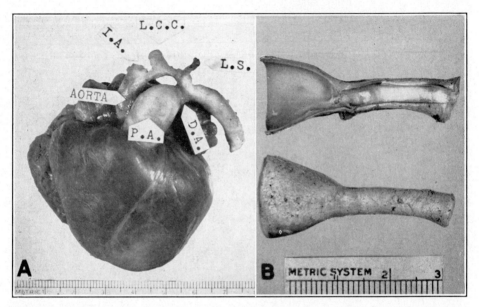

Fig. 138.—Coarctation of the aorta showing *A*, an infant's heart with the constriction near the entrance of the ductus arteriosus and *B*, a resected surgical specimen with a funnel-shaped dilatation of the aorta proximal to the constriction.

Patent Ductus Arteriosus.—In intra-uterine life the ductus arteriosus shunts the blood from the pulmonic to the systemic circulation. Under normal circumstances such a shunt is not necessary in postnatal life and, accordingly, the ductus arteriosus obliterates within the first eight weeks in almost 90 per cent of cases. In most of the remaining cases, obliteration occurs within the first year. Occasionally, however, the shunt persists and the condition is referred to as a patent ductus arteriosus (Fig. 139). The length of the ductus varies from a few millimeters to 3 or 4 cm. while the width varies from barely patent to 1 cm. Initially the ductus arteriosus appears as any other artery but, as the patient ages, it has a propensity to become arteriosclerotic and calcified. The pulmonary artery may undergo the following changes: diffuse or focal (aneurysmal)dilatation, arteriosclerosis and calcification, rupture, or infection with *Streptococcus viridans*. The *clinical manifestations* may consist of the following: retardation of growth, enlargement of the heart, precordial thrill, cardiac murmurs, prominent pulmonary conus and pulmonary congestion roentgenographically, and evidences of cardiac failure. *Treatment* consists of surgical ligation or severance of the ductus arteriosus. The *prognosis* in surgically treated patients is good while in medically treated cases the ultimate outcome is poor. In the latter group, two-thirds of the patients die by the age of forty from *Streptococcus viridans* infection, congestive heart failure, or rupture of the pulmonary artery.

Posterior Right Subclavian Artery.—Normally the right subclavian artery arises in part as a persistence of the anterior portion of the right fourth aortic arch. Abnormally, when this portion of the arch disappears and the dorsal portion persists, the right subclavian artery arises from the last portion of the aortic arch distal to the left subclavian artery and courses to the right between the esophagus and the vertebral bodies (Fig. 139). The incidence of the anomaly is recorded as varying from 0.4 to 2.4 per cent of all autopsies. The condition, as a rule, is *symptomless* although the following

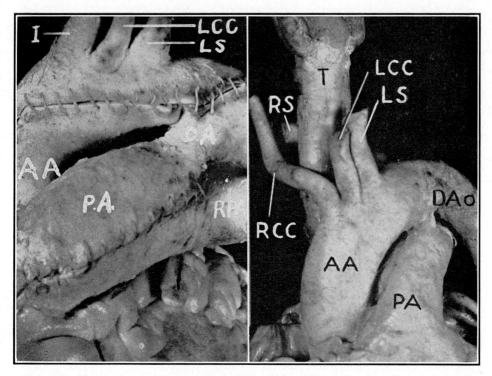

Fig. 139.—Patent ductus arteriosus (on the left) and posterior right subclavian artery (on the right) showing *A.A.*, ascending aorta, *P.A.*, dilated pulmonary artery, *R.P.A.*, right pulmonary artery, *D.A.*, ductus arteriosus, *I*, innominate artery, *L.C.C.*, left common carotid artery, *L.S.*, left subclavian artery, *R.C.C.*, right common carotid artery, *R.S.*, right subclavian artery, *D.Ao.*, descending aorta, and *T*, trachea.

have been recorded: dysphagia, inequality in radial pulses, pressure on the thoracic duct, and atrophic changes in the upper extremity. *Treatment* is generally unnecessary. The *prognosis* is good.

Right-sided Aortic Arch.—This abnormality arises as a result of a persistence of the right fourth aortic arch and partial disappearance of the left fourth aortic arch—a reversal of the normal events. The incidence is recorded as varying from 0.07 to 0.6 per cent of all autopsies. The definitive arch passes to the right of the trachea and esophagus, and the descending aorta usually crosses posteriorly to the esophagus at some point before it traverses the diaphragm. In approximately one-third of the cases the left subclavian artery arises from a left innominate artery. In the remaining two-thirds it arises as the last branch of the aortic arch and traverses to the left between the esophagus and vertebra or it arises from a persistent left aortic root.   The right common carotid artery and the right subclavian artery arise directly from the right arch.   In the presence of a left innominate artery and an anterior left subclavian artery, the ligamentum arteriosum is found on the right side whereas in the presence of a posterior left subclavian artery it is located on the left side, connecting the left aortic root or the left subclavian artery with the pulmonary artery.   At times the entire left aortic arch persists as a fibrous cord.   *Clinically* the anomaly is usually asymptomatic although pressure upon the esophagus, trachea, or recurrent

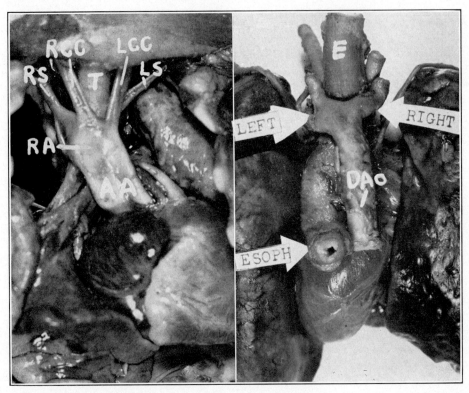

Fig. 140.—Right-sided aortic arch (on the left) and posterior view of a double aortic arch (on the right) showing *A.A.*, ascending aorta, *R.A.*, right-sided aortic arch, *R.S.*, right subclavian artery, *R.C.C.*, right common carotid artery, *L.C.C.*, left common carotid artery, *L.S.*, posterior left subclavian artery, *T*, trachea, *E*, esophagus, and *D.Ao.*, descending aorta.

laryngeal nerves has produced dysphagia, stridor, hoarseness, cough, pain in the chest, and a tingling sensation in the left arm.   During life, the arch may be demonstrated on the right side of the trachea and esophagus by means of bronchoscopy, esophagoscopy, fluoroscopy, and roentgenography.   *Treatment* is generally unnecessary unless a persistence of a fibrous left aortic arch produces tracheal or esophageal obstruction.   In such instances, surgical severance is indicated.   The *prognosis* is good.

   Double Aortic Arch.—A double aortic arch is the least common of all vascular anomalies in this area.   It comes about as a persistence of both the right and left fourth aortic arches and thus forms a complete arterial collar about the trachea and esophagus (Fig. 140).   Both the right and left common carotid and subclavian arteries arise independently from their respective arches. As a rule, the right arch is somewhat smaller than the left and, in all cases, the vagus and recurrent laryngeal nerves are symmetrically distributed about the corresponding arches. *Clinically* some patients go through adult life without any pertinent manifestations. Others, however, disclose dyspnea, stridor, cyanosis, cough, dysphagia, and loss of weight (due to compression of the trachea and esophagus). The anomaly may be demonstrated roentgenographically and bronchoscopically. In symptomatic patients, *treatment* consists of severance of one of the aortic arches. In such cases and in asymptomatic cases the *prognosis* is good.

DEGENERATIONS

Orientation.—While virtually all of the degenerative processes that affect other organs of the body (Chapter 4, p. 29) may also affect the various layers of the vessels, it is more important, at this point, to discuss degenerative vascular disease processes as a whole. Accordingly, the following conditions may be considered: arteriosclerosis, Mönckeberg's sclerosis, Ayerza's disease, medionecrosis, and phlebosclerosis.

Arteriosclerosis.—The term *arteriosclerosis* (Gr. = artery + hardness) signifies hardening of the arteries and may be defined as a thickening of the vascular wall with loss of elasticity. When other conditions such as Mönckeberg's sclerosis are removed from the group, the caption connotes a degenerative change of the intima characterized by focal yellowish thickenings which contain stainable lipids. *Arteriolar sclerosis* is a similar condition that affects arterioles. *Atheroma* (Gr. = porridge or mush), as it pertains to an artery, signifies a swelling of the intima composed of porridge-like or pultaceous material. *Atheromatosis* simply signifies an atheromatous condition. *Atherosclerosis* (Gr. = porridge + hardness) is a form of arteriosclerosis characterized by porridge-like or pultaceous softening of the intimal plaques. In this section, as throughout the book, arteriosclerosis is used as defined above and atherosclerosis is employed to designate an advanced stage of arteriosclerosis in which the plaques undergo necrosis and pultaceous softening. Arteriosclerosis is *widespread* affecting most races (notable exceptions being the Chinese and Eskimos). The condition is seen in all ages from infancy to senility but does have a definite sex and age distribution within these extremes. The incidence of arteriosclerosis with its complications (coronary disease) is low in females before the menopause. In comparison, the incidence in males between the ages of 20 to 40 years is much higher. After the age of 60 years the incidence in females equals that in males (Rosenfeld).

Although numerous theories have been proposed in the past to explain the genesis of arteriosclerosis, its precise *causes* are not yet known. As a result of a tremendous amount of work carried out in the last two decades, however, it appears that the development of the disorder is definitely related to disturbances of lipid metabolism and local factors in the arterial wall (Duff and McMillan).

Actually, the process may be summed up by the statement that it represents a *metabolic disturbance* in which plasma lipids accumulate in the arterial wall (Rosenfeld). In general, it may be stated that the disorder starts in childhood and progresses with increasing age and that it is due, in part at least, to a hereditary fault transmitted as a mendelian dominant. The *deposits* in the arterial wall have been *ascribed to* (1) imbibition of lipid from the blood stream, (2) extravasation of serum or blood from the vasa vasorum, (3) reaction of the intima to injury, (4) necrotic debris of degenerated subintimal tissue, and (5) local production of lipid consequent to some disorganization of the intima such as mechanical strain or abnormal action of lipolytic enzymes. Morphologically, the lesions disclose a great local accumulation of cholesterol and cholesterol esters together with neutral fat, lecithin, and sphingomyelin. In other words, the lipid content of the arteriosclerotic lesions is similar to the lipid content of blood serum or plasma. In fact, the local quantity of these material is so great that it could not possibly come from degeneration of tissue locally. It follows, therefore, that the alternate *source* is the *plasma* that bathes the intima. Normally, the intima is nourished by plasma in the vascular lumen. Abnormally, a disturbance of this nourishment probably accounts for the mechanism in the development of arteriosclerosis. Physiologically, the intima acts as a semipermeable molecular filter for constituents of the plasma, and the passage of materials from the plasma into and through the wall is aided by the normal arterial pressure. Pathologically, increase in arterial pressure, change in molecular size of the active constituents of the plasma, and changes in permeability of the intima affect the rate and amount of filtration. Thus an *increase* in *arterial pressure* as occurs in hypertension causes an increase in amounts of plasma constituents penetrating the intima. This would apply especially at the points of greatest pressure and hence would explain the greater distribution of the arteriosclerotic plaques (1) in the aorta and its larger branches rather than in the smaller arteries and (2) around the orifices of the emerging vessels rather than between the points of exit of the branches. The *molecular size* of the *plasma constituents* has a significant bearing on their penetration of the intima. The smallest lipoproteins pass through the vascular wall into the perivascular lymphatic channels; the intermediate sized (macromolecular) particles (those from 12 to 100 Svedberg units) are caught intramurally, while the largest cannot enter the wall at all and remain in the plasma. Actually, it is the medium sized (macromolecular) lipoproteins that are chiefly responsible for the arteriosclerotic lesions. The only cholesterol that is deposited in the plaques initially is that carried with the medium sized lipoprotein molecules. An increase in *permeability* of the *intima* is important in the genesis and localization of arteriosclerosis. It may result from (1) lack of oxygen, (2) local increase in acidity, (3) effect of noxious substances such as histamine, and (4) thyroid deficiency. Conversely, a decrease in permeability of the intima results from (1) thyroid hormone, (2) calcium, (3) ascorbic acid, and (4) iodides. Once the tissue is injured locally, cholesterol is deposited in greater amounts and at this stage hypercholesterolemia enhances the formation of the lesion.

As already noted, the intermediate sized (macromolecular) plasma *lipoproteins* are all important in the genesis of arteriosclerosis. Lipoproteins represent large complex molecules of serum lipids of different sizes and densities that contain varying amounts of free cholesterol, cholesterol esters, phospholipid, neutral fat, and protein. They are classified according to their rate of flotation during ultracentrifugalization in a medium of higher specific gravity and their concentration or amount present is expressed in Svedberg units of flotation. Using this as a basis, it has been determined that molecules of small size are increased in fasting blood, that molecules of large size (macromolecular) are increased in nonfasting blood, that molecules of larger size (macromolecular) are involved in the early steps of metabolism of exogenous food especially rich in fatty materials, and that the concentration of molecules of larger size (macromolecular) is reduced by dietary restrictions of fats and cholesterol. It has further been determined that hypercholesterolemia correlates with arteriosclerosis only when it is associated with elevation of macromolecular lipoproteins of the size of 12 to 100 Svedberg units. Corroborative evidence in support of the latter statement consists in the finding of macromolecular lipoproteins in (1) high concentration in patients with coronary artery disease and arteriosclerosis, (2) low concentration in children and young women, and (3) low concentration in animals not addicted to spontaneous arteriosclerosis. If hypercholesterolemic rabbit serum or plasma is injected intravenously into control rabbits, arterial lesions like those seen in arteriosclerosis develop within 2 days. Ultracentrifugalization of the same serum separates it into an upper and a lower fraction. The upper fraction, composed of lipoproteins of largest molecular size, produces no arterial lesions when injected intravenously into rabbits while the lower fraction, composed of lipoproteins of smaller size, produces typical arteriosclerotic lesions. Once again, it thus appears that lipoproteins of particular size are much concerned in the genesis of arteriosclerosis. That size of the molecules is important is further borne out by the fact that macromolecular polysaccharide substance when injected intravenously into rabbits produces vascular lesions resembling those in arteriosclerosis. Turning again to man, it has been shown that the particle size of lipoprotein increases in normal people after a fatty meal and that there is a sustained level of lipoproteins of similar size in people with conditions (diabetes mellitus, nephrosis, and xanthomatosis) predisposing to arteriosclerosis. It has further been shown that a fatty meal in a young person produces a sustained increase of particle size of lipoproteins for only a short period, whereas in older people the concentration is maintained at a high level for as long as 24 hours. In the latter, as in those with conditions predisposing to arteriosclerosis, there is thus a permanent increase in "atherogenic" lipoprotein particles in the circulating blood. The reason for this sustained increase is not entirely clear. It may, perhaps, be concerned with changes in fat metabolism such as, for example, a decrease of secretion in pancreatic lipase with a lower concentration of this enzyme in the blood. It may also have something to do with a deficiency in heparin for this may eventuate in a blockage of utilization of fat molecules. Rabbits receiving cholesterol develop arteriosclerosis with ease but when given heparin in addition they disclose retardation of formation of the arterial lesions. Heparin probably acts by reversing conditions that predispose to arteriosclerosis in that it (1) breaks down larger lipoprotein molecules of low density into smaller lipoprotein molecules of high density and (2) increases alpha and decreases beta lipoproteins (for importance of this see succeeding paragraph).

Variation in the *chemical constituents* of the *lipoproteins* is likewise extremely important in the genesis of arteriosclerosis. In normal and atherosclerotic sera all of the cholesterol and phospholipid are combined with either alpha or beta globulins. Normally the ratio of cholesterol to phospholipid is less in the alpha than in the beta globulins. Abnormally, as in cases of myocardial infarction and in diseases predisposing to arteriosclerosis such as diabetes mellitus, nephrosis, and xanthomatosis there is (1) an increase in cholesterol, (2) an increase in the ratio of cholesterol to phospholipid, (3) an increase of cholesterol in the beta globulin, (4) a decrease of cholesterol in the alpha globulin, (5) a decrease in alpha lipoproteins, and (6) an increase in beta lipoproteins. Further determinations have shown that the amount of cholesterol in the alpha fraction decreases in people in the following groups in the order listed: infants, young women, young men, older adults, survivors of myocardial infarction, and those with diseases predisposing to arteriosclerosis.

The influence of *hormones* on the development of arteriosclerosis is quite substantial. The role of sex and age has already been mentioned in the first paragraph of this section. A more detailed analysis of the level of macromolecular lipoproteins of the order of 12 to 100 Svedberg units ("atherogenic" lipoproteins) in the different age groups of the two sexes discloses the following: (1) between 1 to 20 years equal levels in males and females, (2) between 25 to 30 years a striking elevation in males, (3) over 30 years a steady increase in males until the age of 60 years, (4) between 60 to 70 years a decrease in males, and (5) over 30 years a steady increase in females. The level in males at 30 years equals the level in females between 50 to 60 years. The level of "atherogenic" lipoproteins thus appears to be related to *sex hormones*. This is supported by the fact that administration of *estrogens* to survivors of myocardial infarcts reverses the conditions predisposing to arteriosclerosis in that it (1) increases the cholesterol in the alpha fraction, (2) decreases the cholesterol in the beta fraction, (3) produces a fall in the serum cholesterol, (4) drops lipid levels to those in healthy normal people, and (5) proportionately increases those lipoproteins that are composed of smaller relatively stable molecules. Stoppage of estrogenic therapy or the addition of *testosterone* to the estrogens reverses the blood picture to the pre-estrogenic treatment spectrum.

The effect of *diet* on the development of arteriosclerosis has already been referred to. It has been stated, for example, that (1) fasting increases plasma lipoproteins of small molecular size, (2) eating fatty foods increases plasma lipoproteins of larger (macromolecular) size, and (3) a diet low in fats and cholesterol decreases the concentration of plasma macromolecular lipoproteins. Repeated clinical observations in *man* have also shown (1) that a low fat and cholesterol diet is attended by a decrease in serum cholesterol, (2) that there is a higher incidence of arteriosclerosis in groups where the diet is rich in fats and cholesterol, (3) that unsaturated vegetable oils in the diet are attended by decreased cholesterol levels and are less "atherogenic" than saturated vegetable or animal fats which increase cholesterol levels, (4) that starvation (as in wartime) decreases the concentration of serum cholesterol esters and this, in turn, decreases the incidence of general arteriosclerosis and myocardial infarction, and (5) over eating and obesity are attended by a high concentration of serum cholesterol and macromolecular lipoproteins whereas restricted diets and normal weights are attended by lower concentrations of these substances in the serum. *Experimentally*, the administration of cholesterol (in a naturally occurring form as egg yolk and cream or in purified form) to rabbits, chickens, dogs, hamsters, and guinea pigs results in the formation of arteriosclerosis. The degree of development of the arterial change is directly proportionate to the amount of cholesterol administered and to the duration of the experiment. Also experimentally, thyroidectomy and the administration of thiouracil results in hypothyroidism and arteriosclerosis. Experimental arteriosclerosis, however, is inhibited in cholesterol-fed animals that are first rendered diabetic by alloxan or that simultaneously receive Tween 80 or Triton A 20 intravenously. In such animals there is also a marked elevation of serum phospholipid and neutral fat. When the latter two are not elevated, arteriosclerosis develops in the presence of hypercholesterolemia despite the alloxan

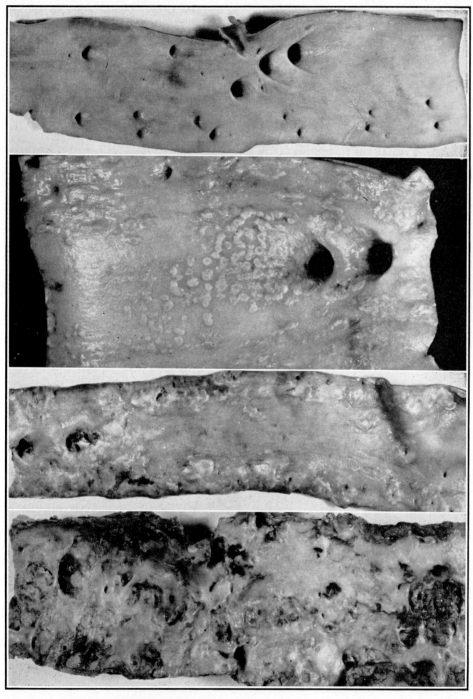

FIG. 141.—Arteriosclerosis of the aorta illustrating increasing involvement of the intima from above down. The lowest photograph shows numerous atheromatous ulcers.

diabetes or the administration of Tween 80 or Triton A 20. Several investigations in severe coronary arteriosclerosis developing in man at an early age and in patients with hypercholesterolemia and severe arteriosclerosis have shown similar findings, that is, a decrease of serum phospholipid. Thus, it appears that the stability of cholesterol in the serum depends upon the proportion of other blood lipids, especially phospholipid. These act as emulsifying agents and thus keep the molecules of lipoproteins in relatively small size. Finally, it has been demonstrated that certain lipotropic agents, such as choline, inositol, and methionine have a salutary effect in arteriosclerosis. This is probably accomplished not by a direct action on the arteriosclerotic plaques but rather by increasing the phospholipid content of the serum and thus returning the cholesterol-phospholipid ratio to normal.

Pathologically all vessels of all organs of the body may be affected. While the localization or severity of involvement in any given case is unpredictable, in general the arteries most commonly involved in decreasing order of frequency are aorta, coronary arteries, larger branches of the aorta, cerebral arteries, arteries of the abdominal organs, arteries of the extremities, and pulmonary arteries. Arteriolar changes are more variable. Although they too occur in all organs they are probably most conspicuous in the adrenals, spleen, and kidneys. For descriptive purposes the lesions may be divided into three groups—aorta, medium-sized arteries, and arterioles.

The *aortic* lesions may be taken as the prototype for other large vessels. Most of the changes occur in the intima. The earliest alterations occur in the ascending aorta and then gradually progress inferiorly. In time, however, the changes in the abdominal aorta overtake those in other portions so that ultimately the part below the diaphragm is most severely affected. The earliest changes consist of round, oval, or irregular yellow flecks projecting above the intimal surface and located around the exit of intercostal and other arteries (Fig. 141). Gradually the flecks become larger and coalesce to give distinct plaques. As they enlarge, they become paler, more protruding, firmer, and even calcified. In time, the central portions of the larger deposits become necrotic, softened, and filled with soft, mush-like material (atheroma). In these lesions the intimal covering becomes thinner and thinner until ultimately it breaks through, producing irregular ulcers (atheromatous ulcers) that discharge their contents into the bloodstream. At the same time, the necrotic lesions also extend outwardly causing erosion, thinning, and weakening of the muscular coat. *Histologically* the earliest change consists of an increase of intimal ground substance containing fat positive droplets. Simultaneously the fatty material is engulfed by macrophages which are thus transformed into foam cells. These cells are large and rounded, disclose an abundant amount of reticulated or even vacuolated cytoplasm and reveal central or slightly eccentric, round, relatively small nuclei (Fig. 19, p. 60 and Fig. 142). As the lesion progresses, connective tissue deposition becomes greater and greater, collagen makes its appearance, the foam cells and adjacent tissues disintegrate, cholesterol crystals and other fatty substances are liberated, and calcification supervenes. Extension of the lesion into the media causes fraying, fragmentation, and rupture of the internal elastic lamina and destruction of the muscle fibers. Here, as in the intima, there is a fibroblastic reaction and there may be necrosis and calcification.

Alterations in the *medium-sized arteries* are essentially similar to those in the aorta. The initial lesion consists of fatty flecks and streaks while later lesions are characterized by extensive fibrosis, necrosis, ulceration, and calcification. The changes in the *coronary arteries* have been described in Chapter 8 (p. 327). They occur at a relatively early age and, as already stated, may be seen even in infancy. Involvement of the *cerebral arteries*, as a rule, occurs much later than that of the coronary vessels. The arteries at the base of the brain are practically never affected before the age of thirty years and those of the basal ganglia are usually involved after the age of fifty years. Lesions in the *arteries* of the *abdominal organs* are most severe at the origins of these vessels from the aorta. The changes in the *arteries* of the *extremities* are predominantly of a fibrous tissue nature with only small deposits of fat but with frequent vacuolization and calcification

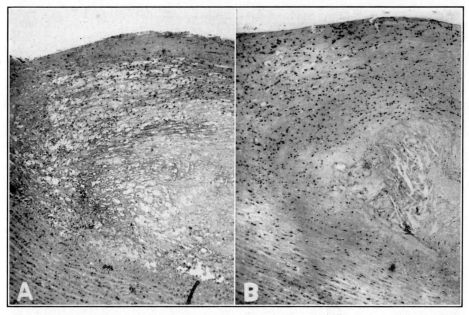

FIG. 142.—Arteriosclerosis showing *A*, marked thickening of the intima with foam cells intermingled with connective tissue and *B*, an older lesion with formation of cholesterol crystals within necrotic material covered by a broad band of dense fibrous tissue. × 50.

(arteriosclerosis obliterans). Atherosclerosis of the arteries of the extremities is infrequent except in conjunction with diabetes mellitus. The recorded incidence of involvement of the *pulmonary arteries* varies from 6 to 70 per cent (Duff and McMillan). The sites of predilection are the larger intrapulmonary branches, with the main extrapulmonary portions and the smaller intrapulmonary portions usually remaining relatively free.

The lesions in the *arterioles* are generally of three types—necrotic, proliferative, and hyaline (Fig. 143). The type of change depends essentially upon the rapidity of the development. *Necrotic* arteriolar changes are generally seen in severe, rapidly progressing hypertension. They are probably caused by a sudden increase in intravascular tension with sudden overstretching of the muscle fibers. The most outstanding morphologic characteristic is smudging of the entire wall of the arteriole with special emphasis on the muscle coat. The individual fibers are no longer apparent but are replaced with granular, eosinophilic material within which are

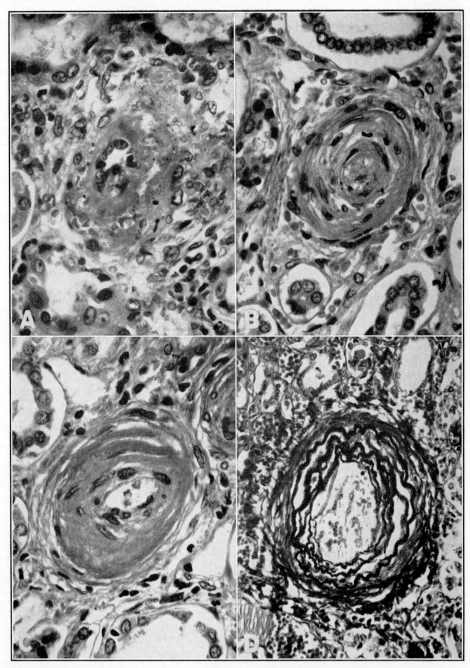

FIG. 143.—Arteriolar sclerosis illustrating *A*, necrosis of the wall, erythrocytic extravasation, and smudging of the entire arteriole. × 400, *B*, endarteritis obliterans with marked "onion-skin" proliferation of the intima. × 400, *C*, replacement of the intima with hyalin. × 400, and *D*, reduplication and splitting of the internal elastic lamina. × 200.

frequently seen intact erythrocytes. Because of the swelling of the wall the lumen is encroached upon and may even be obliterated. *Proliferative* lesions consist of an increase in number and concentric lamellation of the cells of the intima producing what has been referred to as an "onion skin-like" effect. The changes are frequently of sufficient degree to produce complete obliteration of the vascular lumen. *Hyaline* alterations occur when the arteriolar lesions develop slowly. They consist of a great thickening of the intima by homogeneous, eosinophilic material. When the deposition is severe enough, the lumen of the vessel may be entirely obliterated. In both the proliferative and the hyaline types of arteriolarsclerosis the internal elastic lamina undergoes splitting, reduplication, and fragmentation.

The *complications* of arteriosclerosis are (1) obliteration of the lumen of the vessel by thickening of the intima, (2) ulceration of the intimal plaque with superimposed thrombosis, (3) arterial embolism from the contents of the atheroma or from the superimposed thrombus, and (4) aneurysmal dilatations due to weakening of the media. In medium-sized and smaller vessels the consequences of obliteration of the lumen are, of course, atrophy, infarction, and gangrene. The *clinical manifestations* are extremely varied and depend primarily upon the vessel affected and the degree of its occlusion. A *diagnosis* of arteriosclerosis may be arrived at by direct palpation of the vessels if they are peripherally located, by direct visualization as in the case of fundal arteries, by roentgen demonstration of calcification, and by an analysis of the symptoms and signs which the vascular occlusions may produce. *Treatment* is both surgical and medical. Surgical treatment is limited to some of the complications which arterial occlusion produces. Medical treatment is symptomatic and, in addition, consists of (1) a low cholesterol-fat diet to reduce the serum cholesterol levels, (2) use of lipotropic agents (choline and inositol) to increase serum phospholipid levels, and (3) use of endocrine preparations when they are indicated (Morrison). The *prognosis* depends, of course, upon the vessels affected and the degree of their involvement.

Mönckeberg's Sclerosis.—This condition, also known as calcinosis of the media, is a degenerative disturbance of the larger and medium-sized arteries of the extremities and of some of the internal organs (such as the ovaries and uterus) characterized by calcification and sometimes ossification of the media (Fig. 144). The deposits are usually segmental and ring-like but they may also be more diffuse. They are readily visualized roentgenographically. The cause of the medial changes is not definitely known although it is thought that prolonged vasospasm plays a role. The disorder is of little practical significance until intimal changes (atheromatous) are superimposed upon the medial alterations. Such a sequence of events occurs in about 12 per cent of cases and the condition then behaves like the usual arteriosclerosis (Silbert).

Ayerza's Disease.—Although opinions vary as to exactly what constitutes Ayerza's disease, it appears to be the consensus that the condition consists of primary pulmonary vascular sclerosis with subsequent right-sided cardiac hypertrophy and dilatation. The syndrome has no predilection for either sex and although it may occur at all ages it is more common before the age of fifty years. Clinically there are dyspnea, orthopnea, cyanosis, and evidences of right-sided cardiac failure. Radiologically there is prominence of the pulmonary conus and the heart is enlarged to the right. Death may occur suddenly.

Medionecrosis.—This condition, known also as idiopathic cystic medionecrosis, consists of mucoid degeneration of the media of the aorta and,

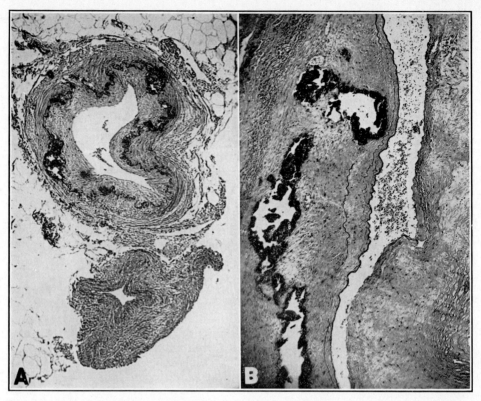

FIG. 144.—Mönckeberg's sclerosis showing calcification of the media of *A*, a medium sized artery in a thyroid gland and *B*, a larger artery in a uterus. × 50.

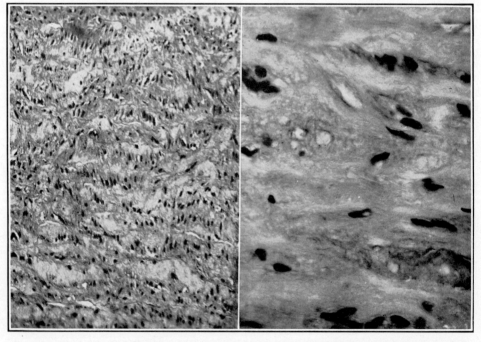

FIG. 145.— Medionecrosis of the aorta showing the muscle fibers separated by masses of mucoid material. × 100 and 400.

less often, of the larger arteries.   Grossly, the vascular wall may be thickened but shows no other abnormalities.   Histologically the media reveals slit-like or more rounded and cystic defects filled with mucoid material (Fig. 145).   The cause of the retrograde process is probably arterial ischemia resulting from hypertrophy of the media and proliferation of the intima of the vasa vasorum.   The lesion is important because it predisposes to the formation of a dissecting aneurysm.

Phlebosclerosis. — *Phlebosclerosis* (Gr. = vein + hardness) connotes hardening and thickening of veins.   The vessels affected are generally the inferior vena cava, the iliac veins, the popliteal veins, and the portal vein. Most commonly the thickening consists of endophlebohypertrophy and endophlebosclerosis (Lev and Saphir).   *Endophlebohypertrophy* starts at birth, occurs at the mouths of the tributary veins, and consists of long streaks or plaques composed of proliferated elastic, muscle, and connective tissue cells of the intima and adjacent media.   *Endophlebosclerosis* is superimposed upon phlebohypertrophy with advancing age.   The changes are retrogressive and consist of (1) mucoid degeneration of the ground substance, (2) loss of elastic fibers and muscle cells, (3) fragmentation of the intimal elastic lamina, and (4) replacement by collagenous connective tissue.   Deposits of lipids and calcium are not found.   *True phlebosclerosis* (venous atheroma or senile sclerosis of veins) is infrequent.   It occurs most commonly in the lower portion of the inferior vena cava and the proximal portions of the common iliac veins, that is, at points of maximal mechanical stress.   Grossly the lesion consists of white to yellow, raised, irregular plaques measuring as much as 2.5 cm. in greatest diameter.   Histologically the plaques are composed essentially of proliferations of subendothelial connective tissue of the intima with subsequent hyalinization.   Deposition of lipids in small droplets and calcification are present in the more advanced lesions (Geiringer).

INFLAMMATIONS

Orientation. — Inflammation of vessels is known as *angiitis* or *vasculitis*, of arteries as *arteritis*, of veins as *phlebitis*, and of lymphatic channels as *lymphangiitis*.   These designations are generally further qualified according to (1) the *time element* as acute, subacute, or chronic, (2) the *anatomic site* as temporal, pulmonary, radial, etc., (3) their *behavior* as localized or migrating, (4) their *relation* to *other diseases* as primary or secondary, (5) the presence of *thrombus* formations as thrombophlebitis, etc., (6) the *etiologic agent* as syphilitic, tuberculous, etc., and (7) the *pathologic appearance* as nonspecific, granulomatous, necrotizing, etc.   Since none of these classifications is entirely satisfactory it is necessary to use a combination of terms.   The more important lesions may thus be listed under the following headings: nonspecific arteritis, rheumatic arteritis (Chapter 8, p. 176), periarteritis nodosa, granulomatous giant cell arteritis, thromboangiitis obliterans, syphilitic vasculitis, tuberculous vasculitis, migrating phlebitis, thrombophlebitis and phlebothrombosis, pylephlebitis, lymphangiitis, and filariasis.

Nonspecific Arteritis. — Nonspecific inflammation of arteries may be primary or secondary.   *Primary nonspecific arteritis* is rare.   The cause is unknown, although *Streptococcus hemolyticus* has been suspected.   Both large and small arteries are affected but the latter bear the brunt of the infection.   Histologically all the coats are permeated with a variety of leukocytes, the intima is swollen and may show proliferation, and the lumen

24

is occluded by a thrombus. The lesion heals by organization and fibrosis. In the acute stage the skin and subcutaneous tissues disclose hemorrhages, necrosis, ulcerations, and focal gangrene (Kramer). Death may occur as a result of the overwhelming toxemia from absorption of tissue metabolites. *Secondary nonspecific arteritis* may occur as a result of (1) direct extension of a local inflammatory process and (2) hematogenous spread of organisms during the course of infectious diseases such as pneumonia, enteric fever, septicemia, pyemia, bacterial endocarditis, etc. The organisms may attack the vessel from the luminal side or, by way of the vasa vasorum, from the adventitial side. The pathologic changes are nonspecific, consisting of edema, degeneration, leukocytic infiltration, necrosis, thrombosis, and healing by resolution and organization.

Periarteritis Nodosa.—Periarteritis nodosa is an acute inflammatory and necrotizing disorder of the medium-sized and smaller arteries throughout the body. The condition has *also* been *referred* to as polyvasculitis, necrotizing angiitis, polyarteritis nodosa, and panarteritis. The disorder was first described in 1866 by Kussmaul and Maier (Zeek). At first it was thought to be rare but with freer application of biopsies it has been shown to be quite common. By December, 1952, about 500 cases were recorded in the literature (McNeil). The disorder is about three times as common in males as it is in females and, while it occurs at any age from infancy to senility, it is most prevalent in the third and fourth decades of life. The *cause* of the disease is not definitely known. In the past, specific toxins, bacteria, spirochetes, rickettsia, viruses, and parasites have been incriminated as direct etiologic agents but now it is generally conceded that if any of these cause the disorder, they do so through the medium of hypersensitivity. Other agents considered to be of significance in man are sulfonamides, antibiotics, thiouracil, allergens, and anything that produces the alarm reaction (McNeil and Simon). Some indication that the disorder is a result of hypersensitivity lies in the fact that similar vascular lesions are found in other allergic disorders such as rheumatic fever, glomerulonephritis, severe asthma, and serum sickness. Experimentally, the condition may be produced in rabbits by repeated injections of foreign serum and in rats by the administration of desoxycorticosterone acetate and by wrapping the kidneys in silk or cotton (Kobernick).

Pathologically the disorder affects the medium and smaller arteries although, on occasion, it may also be seen in the larger arteries and sometimes the veins. The lesions are irregularly distributed. Any vessel in any part of the body may be affected. In fatal cases the distribution, in approximate order of decreasing frequency, is as follows: heart, liver, gastrointestinal tract, kidney, pancreas, mesentery, muscles, skin, peripheral nerves, central nervous system, and other organs. *Grossly* there is little to be seen in early lesions. The skin may disclose purpura, petechiæ, erythema, vesicles, or a scarlatiniform eruption. The remaining organs may reveal infarctions, hemorrhages, or no changes whatsoever. Occasionally the gastrointestinal tract may disclose extensive ulcerations of the mucosa. The vessels may appear entirely normal or they may show thickening of the walls, thrombosis of the lumens, irregularly scattered aneurysmal dilatations, or rupture with frank hemorrhage. *Histologically* the lesions are segmental in distribution, often being more pronounced at the bifurcations of the vessels. Sometimes only part of the circumference may be affected while at other times all of it may be involved (Fig. 146). The earliest lesion starts in the media and consists of edema and fibrinoid necrosis. From this

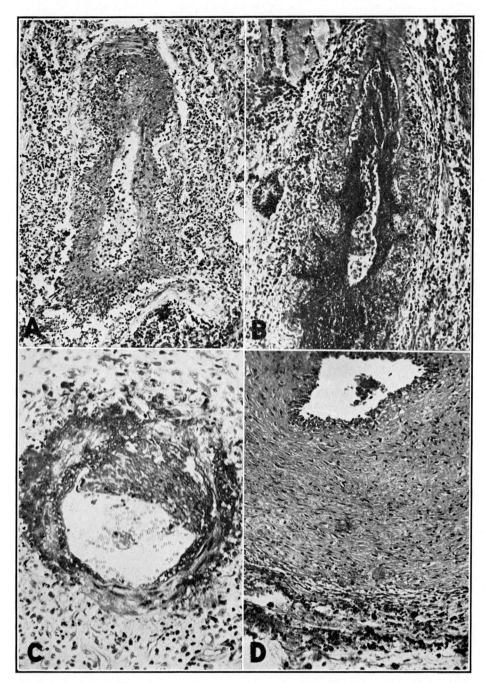

Fig. 146.—Periarteritis nodosa showing A, a vessel with severe fibrinoid necrosis of the media, beginning thrombosis, and a diffuse infiltration with mostly neutrophils and eosinophils. $\times$ 100, B, a similar vessel (stained for elastic tissue) with necrosis and fraying of the elastic tissue. $\times$ 100, C, segmental (lunar) involvement by a similar process. $\times$ 200, and D, a healed stage characterized by extensive fibrosis and perivascular hemosiderin deposition. $\times$ 100.

location it extends both toward the lumen and toward the adventitia. As a result, the internal elastic lamina becomes frayed, fragmented, and replaced with intensely eosinophilic amorphous material. The second stage is one of exudation. It is characterized by edema and an intense infiltration with neutrophils and eosinophils with lesser numbers of plasma cells, lymphocytes, mononuclear cells, and occasional giant cells. When the intima is reached thrombosis generally supervenes. Also, because of the intensity and nature of the reaction, the wall is weakened and aneurysmal formation or complete rupture occurs. The final stage is replacement with granulation tissue and healing by fibrosis. This fibrosing process affects not only the media and intima but also the thrombus and adventitia. In healed lesions, aside from the fibrosis, telltale evidence of the inflammation exists in the adventitia in the form of hemosiderin granules both free and within phagocytic cells.

The *complications* are thrombosis, ischemic atrophy, infarction, aneurysmal formations, vascular rupture, and hemorrhage. *Clinically* the manifestations are extremely varied. They depend upon the degree of vascular occlusion and the organ affected. Thus, in some instances, there may be no symptoms or signs while in others some combination of the following may exist: fever, leukocytosis, albuminuria, abdominal pain, hypertension, edema, neuritis, hematuria, anemia, tachycardia, rapid onset, weakness, loss of weight, dyspnea, cough, emaciation, sensory involvement, muscle soreness, visual disturbances, nodules, nausea, history of allergy, coma, atrophy, cyanosis, hematemesis, pain in the chest, uremia, icterus, convulsions, adenopathy, positive serologic reaction, chills, diarrhea, vertigo, and hemoptysis (King). The *diagnosis* should be suspected in the presence of fever, leukocytosis, albuminuria, and abdominal pain. It can be proved without doubt only by biopsy. In this connection, it should be stated that since the lesions are segmental, a single negative biopsy does not necessarily rule out the condition. *Treatment* has been quite unsatisfactory with general reliance being placed upon spontaneous remissions. Cortisone seems to enhance the healing of arterial lesions but apparently does not cure the condition. In fact, malignant hypertension has been recorded following its use. The *prognosis* varies with the extent and severity of the lesions. In some cases prolonged remissions are noted; in others the course terminates in death within four years, and in others still, especially in cases of renal involvement, death may occur within a few months. The *causes* of *death* are "debility," infarction of vital organs, hemorrhage, cardiac failure, and renal insufficiency.

Granulomatous Giant Cell Arteritis.—This condition has also been referred to as giant cell arteritis, temporal arteritis, and cranial arteritis. The last two terms are misnomers for, in fatal cases, lesions have been shown to be widespread. The condition is a nonsuppurative granulomatous inflammation of arteries in which there is a peculiar destruction of the elastic fibers of the internal elastic lamina with resulting giant cell formation (Kimmelstiel). The disorder was first described in 1932 and by 1948 there were at least 48 cases recorded in the English language (Crosby). The lesions occur chiefly in women beyond the age of fifty years. The *cause* of the disorder is not known although staphylococci, streptococci, gram-positive cocci, and allergy have been incriminated.

Pathologically, the lesions are characteristically found in the temporal arteries but, in cases coming to necropsy, most vessels of the body have been involved. Some of these are retinal, carotid, hypogastric, radial, subclavian, iliac, femoral, coronary, renal, celiac, mesenteric, and pulmonary arteries, and the aorta (Cardell and Heptinstall). *Histologically*, the initial lesion consists of intimal proliferation together with segmental swelling, fragmentation, and destruction of the internal elastic lamina (Fig. 147) The destroyed elastic fibers are then engulfed by multinucleated giant cells and this, according to Kimmelstiel, is the pathognomonic lesion. Subsequently, the process spreads into the media where large segments of muscle fibers are destroyed. Throughout these areas there is a diffuse permeation with

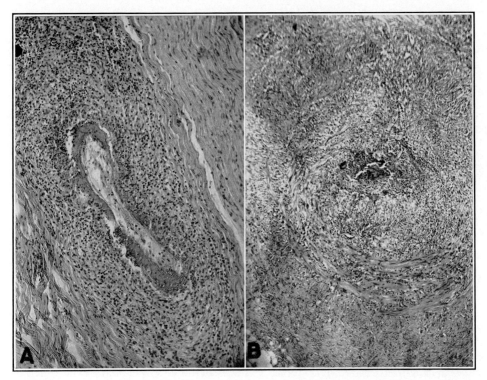

Fig. 147.—Granulomatous giant cell arteritis illustrating *A*, intimal proliferation to a degree that virtually obliterates the lumen, swelling and degeneration of the internal elastic lamina, and a diffuse permeation of the rest of the wall and surrounding tissue with leukocytes. ×100, and *B*, similar changes with, in addition, multinucleated giant cells engulfing fragment elastic fibers. ×50.

monocytes, lymphocytes, and fewer numbers of eosinophils and neutrophils. Simultaneously the intima may become necrotic and the lumen may be filled with a thrombus. Beyond the media, the inflammatory process may affect not only the adventitia but also the periarterial nerves. Ultimately the entire lesion heals by granulation tissue formation and fibrosis. Aside from death, the most serious *complication* is blindness (due to involvement of the retinal artery) which occurs in approximately one-third of the cases. *Clinically*, *systemic* manifestations (due to the widespread nature of the disorder) consist of fever, anorexia, malaise, loss of weight, and weakness. *Local* manifestations (due to inflammation and thrombosis) consist of tenderness, swelling, nodularity, redness, and thrombosis of the involved cranial vessels together with severe throbbing headache. In addition, there may be pain in the scalp, face, jaws, eyes, and the temporomandibular joints. The *diagnosis* is made by eliciting the typical local manifestations just described in a woman beyond fifty years of age. It is confirmed by biopsy. There is no satisfactory *treatment*. The *prognosis* is generally good, although the mortality rate is approximately 10 per cent. The *causes* of *death* are cardiac failure and cerebral hemorrhage or thrombosis.

Thromboangiitis Obliterans.—This condition, also known as Buerger's disease and spontaneous juvenile gangrene of extremities, is a segmental inflammatory and obliterative disease of the medium and small-sized arteries of extremities and less often of the viscera (Allen). The disorder affects males in approximately 98 per cent of cases and is most commonly seen between the third and the fifth decades of life. The *causes* of the condition are not known (Burt). A hereditary factor probably plays a significant role since the disorder has been found to be familial and has a predisposition for Jews. As to other more precise factors, bacteria, viruses, a variety of vaso-spastic drugs, hormones, trauma, and a hypersensitivity to nicotine have all, at one time or another, been incriminated. Personality wise hostility, aggressiveness, and negativism have been implicated (Baker).

Pathologically the lesions are most common in the lower extremities, are less common in the upper extremities, and are occasionally found in internal organs such as the brain, lungs, heart, liver, mesentery, intestine, and spermatic cord. *Grossly* the changes consist of segmental vascular occlusions. The vessels are indurated but are not brittle (Allen). The arteries are involved first, then the veins, and occasionally the nerves are incorporated in the inflammatory process. Early, the obliterating intra-luminal mass is red or brownish while later it becomes yellowish and then grayish. In old lesions the artery, veins, and nerves are frequently bound together in a fibrous mass. *Histologically* the condition is a panarteritis and panphlebitis with thrombosis and without suppuration. The initial lesion appears to be a proliferation of the endothelial cells with a moderate degree of lymphocytic infiltration. Superimposed upon the intimal changes there is a luminal thrombus which gradually undergoes organization (Fig. 148). The internal elastic lamina is well preserved. The media undergoes a gradual permeation with fibroblasts and capillaries, but the muscle fibers, for the most part, remain well preserved. The adventitia discloses fibrosis and perivascular lymphocytic infiltrations. As already stated, the fibroblastic proliferation sometimes extends to encircle the nerves.

The *complications* consist of (1) ischemic atrophy involving the muscles, bones, fat, skin, nails, and nerves, and (2) ulcers and gangrene of especially the digits of the lower and upper extremities. The *clinical manifestations* are due to vascular ischemia and perhaps to pressure upon the nerves. They consist of intermittent claudication, pain, decreased skin temperature of the involved extremity, cyanosis of the extremity when in a lowered position, pallor of the extremity when in an elevated position, loss of pulsation of the larger arteries, and migrating superficial phlebitis (Hueper). Chemical studies on the blood are normal. The *diagnosis* is readily made in the presence of an obliterative, often bilateral, vascular disease occurring in a young, especially Jewish, male, particularly in the presence of a familial history. *Treatment* has been most varied. Cessation of smoking has brought about an arrest of the disease. Some of the other therapeutic measures are bed rest, heat cradle, exercises, pain-relieving drugs, and, more recently, sympathectomy (Marshall and Messinger). The *prognosis* is variable. In some cases the disease undergoes spontaneous arrest; in others repeated attacks lead ultimately to the complications listed above, and in still others the disorder is rapidly progressive.

Syphilitic Vasculitis.—*Primary* syphilitic inflammation of the vessels is essentially arterial and may be divided into two groups—(1) aorta, its larger branches, and medium-sized arteries, and (2) smaller arteries such as those of the brain. *Secondary* syphilitic inflammation of vessels affects the arterioles, capillaries, smaller veins, venules, and lymphatic channels. In any case the causative organism is *Treponema pallidum*.

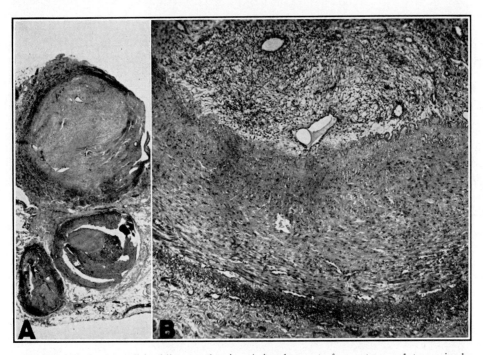

Fɪɢ. 148.—Thromboangiitis obliterans showing *A*, involvement of an artery and two veins by an organized thrombotic process. × semigross, and *B*, an artery with the intima and lumen replaced by granulation tissue, a media containing some fibrosis tissue and capillaries, and an adventitia disclosing considerably more fibrous tissue replacement. × 50.

Syphilitic aortitis is much more common than, but pathologically is similar to, syphilis of the larger branches of the aorta and the medium-sized arteries. The condition is six times as common in Negroes as it is in the white population, occurs between the ages of thirty and seventy years in over 80 per cent of cases, and is about four times as frequent in males as it is in females. *Pathologically* the process is most severe in the first part of the ascending aorta and becomes less prominent as the diaphragm is approached. For some unexplained reason the inflammation seldom extends below the level of the diaphragm. The route of infection is by way of the vasa vasorum. The initial lesions consist of a perivascular infiltration with lymphocytes and plasma cells and, to a lesser extent, of endothelial proliferation of the vasa vasorum. Sometimes the perivascular and paravascular infiltrates consist of minute gummas (Fig. 149). From the adventitia the lesion extends into the media and as it does so it destroys both the muscle bundles and the elastic fibers. Healing occurs by fibrous tissue replacement. Simultaneously, as the inflammation proceeds toward the lumen, the intima undergoes connective tissue replacement and later hyalinization. Grossly these changes are represented by the formation of pearly white, elevated, irregular, intimal plaques. As the lesion ages, the fibrous tissue within the wall of the aorta contracts, producing longitudinal, transverse, and radiating intimal scars. In time, atheromatous changes supervene in

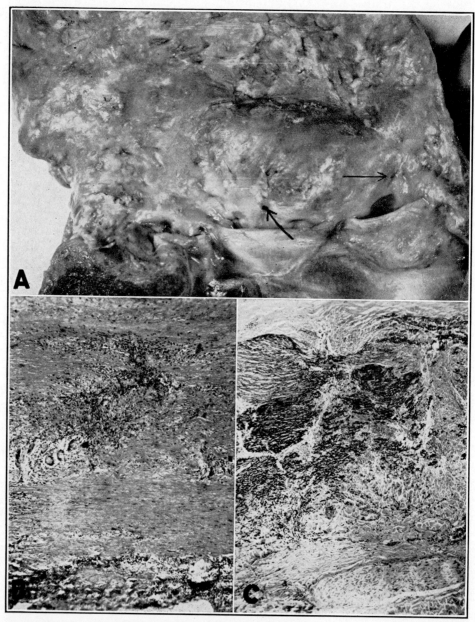

FIG. 149.—Syphilitic aortitis showing A, irregular plaque-like thickening and atherosclerosis of the intima, marked stenosis of the coronary ostia (arrows), fibrosis and widening of the commissures of the aortic cusps, and fibrosis of the free edges of the aortic cusps, B, lymphocytic, plasma cell, and gummatous infiltration of the vasa vasorum of the adventitia and media. × 50, and C, disruption of the elastic fibers of the media by the syphilitic process (elastic tissue stain). × 50.

the plaques causing considerable distortion of the original picture (Fig. 149). The *coronary ostia* are usually caught in the process. They become surrounded by the intimal plaques and undergo marked stenosis. Similarly the *aortic valve* is characteristically involved. The commissures become shortened, broadened, and separated and the free margins of the cusps become greatly thickened and rolled. The *complications* of syphilitic aortitis are as follows: (1) dilatation of the aorta with or without aneurysmal formation (due to destruction of elastic fibers and muscle tissue and replacement with fibrous tissue), (2) subsequent rupture of the aneurysm with fatal hemorrhage or pressure of the aneurysm upon vital structures, (3) aortic valvular insufficiency and myocardial failure (due to stretching of the aortic valvular ring and to scarring of the aortic cusps), (4) occlusion of the coronary ostia with myocardial infarction or sudden death (due to an insufficient coronary arterial supply), and (5) miscellaneous, consisting of bacterial endocarditis, mural cardiac thrombi, pulmonary thrombosis and infarcts, etc. (Montgomery). *Clinically* a latent period between contraction of the disease and the development of clinical manifestations varies from a few months to fifty years. Simple syphilitic aortitis is generally asymptomatic. When complications develop they are referable to the aneurysm, aortic insufficiency, or coronary artery occlusion. The *diagnosis* is made from a consideration of the symptoms and signs together with a history of syphilis and positive serologic tests for syphilis. *Treatment* is that of syphilis in general, together with symptomatic relief when complications develop. The *prognosis* varies from patient to patient. According to Rich and Webster, 15 per cent of cases of uncomplicated syphilitic aortitis develop aneurysm or aortic insufficiency after an average of three to five years. According to Montgomery, the average duration of life in patients with aortic insufficiency is one and one-half years.

Syphilis of the *smaller arteries* may affect the coronary arteries but is much more common in the vessels of the brain. Here the lesions are confined to the smaller meningeal arteries, the arteries at the base of the brain, and the larger tributaries of these vessels. The changes occur both in the adventitia and the intima. In the adventitia the characteristic alterations are perivascular infiltrations of the vasa vasorum of the larger arteries and of the entire vessel in the smaller ramifications. The intimal changes consist of concentric proliferations of connective tissue with marked encroachment upon the vascular lumen. The latter, in turn, produces cerebral ischemia, degeneration and disappearance of the ganglion cells, or frank liquefaction necrosis.

While the lesions described above are usually seen in connection with acquired tertiary syphilis, involvement of the *arterioles, small veins, capillaries*, and *lymphatic channels* does occur as a secondary phenomenon in any of the stages of syphilis. Such lesions consist essentially of an invasion of the vessels from the outside by syphilitic granulation tissue, be it of the diffuse or the gummatous variety. When the granulation tissue is relatively young, the outlines of the structures mentioned may be readily discerned in ordinary preparations. When, however, the granulation tissue is older the outlines of the vessels fuse with the inflammatory cells, the newly formed fibroblasts, the proliferating capillaries, and the necrotic material to such an extent that they can be identified only with the aid of elastic tissue stains. The changes in the smaller vessels account for local ischemia, necrosis, and ulcer formation but since they occur in a limited area they are not of as grave a consequence as those in the larger vessels.

Tuberculous Vasculitis.—*Secondary* involvement of arteries, veins, and lymphatic channels by extension of a tuberculous process from neighboring tissues is common. *Primary* tuberculous involvement of these structures is, in comparison, rare and, in recorded cases, has been confined to the larger arteries. Some of these are the aorta and the femoral, common iliac, and hepatic arteries. The organisms gain entrance with the bloodstream by way of vasa vasorum and are deposited in the adventitia, media, and intima. The characteristic lesion is the tubercle. Weakening of the wall of a larger vessel may be of sufficient degree to produce an aneurysm or rupture and fatal hemorrhage.

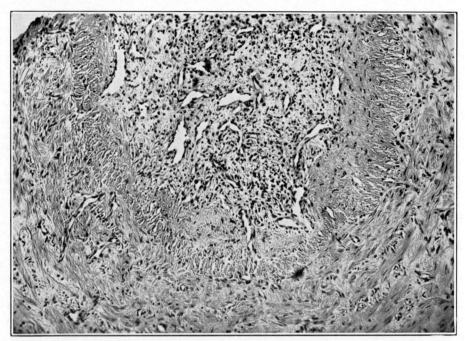

FIG. 150.—Migratory phlebitis disclosing a vein with a recanalized luminal thrombus. × 100

Migratory Phlebitis.—As the term suggests, migratory phlebitis is an inflammation of the veins that skips from one portion of the body to another (Vinther-Paulsen). The condition does not include multiple thrombophlebitis that accompanies various infectious diseases. The *cause* is unknown. *Pathologically* either the peripheral or the visceral veins may be affected. The lesion consists of a nonspecific inflammation of the entire wall of the vessel with a superimposed luminal thrombus (Fig. 150). *Clinically* peripheral lesions are characterized by the appearance of small, red, tender nodules in relation to the vein. Visceral lesions are accompanied by extremely varied symptoms and signs depending upon the site (coronary, cerebral, mesenteric, portal, hepatic, splenic, adrenal, or renal) and severity of involvement. The *diagnosis* is usually made by a process of exclusion. *Treatment* has been varied, with Dicoumarol appearing to have the best effect. The *mortality* is recorded at approximately 20 per cent. The *cause* of *death* is usually circulatory disturbance in a viscus.

Thrombophlebitis and Phlebothrombosis.—*Thrombophlebitis* (Gr. = clot + vein + inflammation) connotes inflammation of a vein associated with thrombosis. The inflammation is primary. The thrombus is secondary, and, because of the inflammatory reaction, is firmly attached to the intima. *Phlebothrombosis* (Gr. = vein + clot) means thrombosis of a vein of noninflammatory origin with the clot (at least initially) loosely adherent to the intima. *Clinically*, and even pathologically, it is sometimes difficult or even impossible to distinguish thrombophlebitis from phlebothrombosis and it has, therefore, become customary to combine the two conditions under the caption *venous thrombosis, thromboembolism,* or *thromboembolic disease.* In practice the disorder is seen most frequently postoperatively, during and after pregnancy, in connection with infectious diseases, and in any person confined to bed for whatever reason. The most important complications are embolism and (when the deep veins are affected) chronic venous insufficiency. The latter is attended by edema, ulceration, infection, and even gangrene. Since the topics of venous and arterial thrombosis and embolism have been discussed in some detail in Chapter 6 (pp. 211 and 218) there, is no need for further reiteration here.

Pylephlebitis.—*Pylephlebitis* (Gr. = gate + vein + inflammation) is inflammation of the portal vein and its tributaries. The condition *stems* from inflammation of intestines (especially appendicitis) and is usually *caused* by streptococci, staphylococci, or colon bacilli. *Pathologically* the inflammation and accompanying thrombosis start in the terminal mural radicals of the venous system. Proximal extension occurs by way of continuity or embolism. In either case the organisms ultimately lodge in the liver where they produce multiple acute abscesses. The *clinical manifestations* are those of the initial disease followed later (when the liver is affected) by chills, fever, profuse sweating, abdominal pain, malaise, anorexia, loss of weight, and (terminally) jaundice. Formerly the mortality rate was 100 per cent but with the advent of antibiotics and chemotherapy, cures are recorded with increasing numbers and the *prognosis* is thus immeasurably improved.

Lymphangiitis.—Inflammation of lymphatic channels may be acute or chronic. *Acute lymphangiitis* follows any infection with pyogenic (and even other) organisms, especially streptococci. The inflammatory process spreads along the draining lymphatic channels to the interrupting lymph nodes and sometimes beyond these to the second chain of nodes. *Grossly* the vessels are seen as fine, red, tender, elevated streaks while *histologically* they are perfused with neutrophils and may show thrombosis. The draining lymph nodes are enlarged and tender. Histologically they disclose nonspecific inflammation or, in some cases, abscess formation. *Clinically*, in addition to the local reaction, there may be chills and high fever (Allen). The condition may subside spontaneously but antibiotics and chemotherapeutic agents are generally indicated. *Chronic lymphangiitis* results from repeated attacks of acute lymphangiitis or from a smouldering, low-grade, initial infection. *Pathologically* the condition may be attended by endothelial proliferation, mural fibrosis, luminal occlusion, stasis of lymph, and lymphedema.

Filariasis.—Filariasis is a parasitic infection of the lymphatic channels caused by *Wuchereria bancrofti* and seen throughout the tropics (Sawitz). The adult worms live in the lymphatic channels where the microfilariæ are deposited by the female. Upon reaching the bloodstream, the microfilariæ linger in the visceral blood vessels during the day and the peripheral blood vessels during the night. From the latter they are picked up by mosquitoes where, in two weeks, they become infective. Infective larvæ then reach

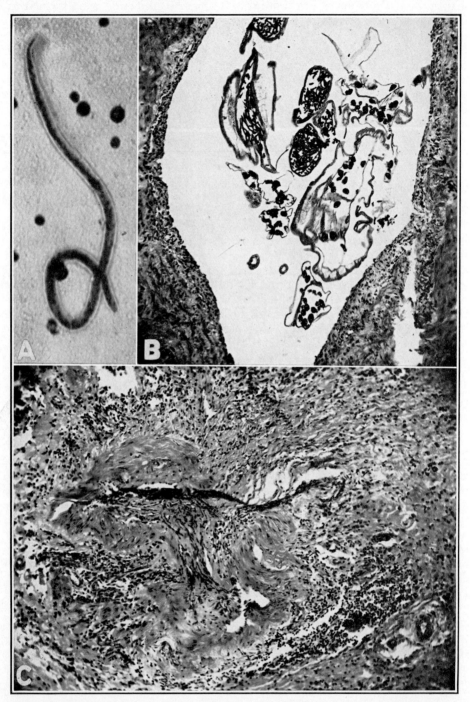

FIG. 151.—Filariasis showing *A*, a microfilaria.   × 400, *B*, sections of adult worms in the
lymphatic channels.   × 100, and *C*, extensive fibrosis in a lymph node.   × 100.

man through the bite of the mosquito and mature in the lymphatic channels. Adult worms are thread-like, the male measuring about 4 cm. and the female about 7.5 cm. in length. Microfilariæ have a rounded anterior and a tapered posterior end and measure approximately 300×7 microns (Fig. 151). *Pathologically* the adult worms may cause characteristic changes in the lymphatic channels and lymph nodes (Hartz). The lesion is a granuloma consisting of central epithelioid cells, occasional peripheral giant cells of the Langhans' type, and a surrounding mantle of lymphocytes and plasma cells. When the worms have died before biopsy there may be present, in addition, an eosinophilic infiltration. In time, some of the worms disintegrate, others calcify, and the lesion tends to heal by fibrosis. Both the inflammation and the presence of the worms within the lymphatic channels causes stasis and lymphedema of the extremities and external genitals. After repeated infections, this swelling becomes permanent—a condition known as *elephantiasis*. *Clinically*, aside from the local swelling, discharged metabolites of the worms may cause leukocytosis and eosinophilia. The *diagnosis* of filariasis is established by identifying microfilariæ in the peripheral (night) blood, by biopsy, and by immunologic and serologic tests. *Treatment* consists of (1) prevention by destroying the mosquitoes, (2) administration of hetrazen to kill the microfilariæ, and (3) surgical excision of enlarged parts. The *prognosis* is good in early cases and fair in others.

PHYSICAL DISTURBANCES

Orientation.—The more important physical disturbances of the vessels are aneurysms, thrombosis, embolism, vasospasm, varicose veins, phleboliths and arterioliths, superior vena cava syndrome, lymphedema, and trauma. Venous thrombosis and embolism have been considered in a preceding section and thrombosis and embolism in general have been discussed in Chapter 6 (pp. 211 and 218). The remaining conditions may now be expounded upon briefly.

Aneurysms.—An *anuerysm* (Gr. = a widening) may be defined as a localized dilatation of an artery or vein containing blood in a fluid or coagulated state. The *incidence* is difficult to determine but it can be said with assurance that the condition is common. Aortic aneurysms are recorded as constituting from 0.8 to 2.6 per cent of all autopsies (Maniglia and Gregory). Aneurysms may occur at all ages but are most common after the age of fifty years. They affect all races (syphilitic aneurysms predominate in Negroes while arteriosclerotic aneurysms predominate in the white population) and have a two or three to one predilection for males. The *cause* of aneurysmal formation is anything that weakens the vascular wall. Some of the more important etiologic factors are (1) *congenital*—malformations of the layers of the vascular walls, (2) *degenerations*—arteriosclerosis, medionecrosis, and pressure atrophy, (3) *inflammations*—syphilis, periarteritis nodosa, adjacent nonspecific inflammation, rheumatic fever, and septic emboli, (4) *physical disturbances*—trauma, hemorrhage into the wall, pressure from the outside and increased intraluminal pressure, and (5) *tumors*—erosion from the outside and, rarely, primary of the vessel wall itself.

The *classifications* of aneurysms are many, varied, and overlapping. Aneurysms may be captioned according to the (1) *anatomic structure involved*—arterial, venous, or arteriovenous, (2) *location*—external (not in the body cavity), internal (within the body cavity), abdominal, thoracic, intracranial, aortic, subclavian, popliteal, etc., (3) *etiologic agent*—arteriosclerotic, inflammatory, bacterial, syphilitic, embolic, traumatic, etc., (4) *source of etiologic agent*—endogenous or exogenous, (5) *size*—miliary or massive, (6) *gross appearance*—berry, fusiform, cylindroid, tubular, saccular, ampullary, circumscribed, dissecting, etc., (7) *composition of the wall*—true or ectatic (all layers present), false or spurious (some layers only present), or hernial (inner coat protruding through the outer layers), (8) *complications*—ruptured or eroding, and (9) *persons* who first described them—Rasmussen's (one associated with a tuberculous cavity), Richet's (fusiform), Shekelton's (dissecting), etc.

Pathologically (1) any vessel may be affected, (2) the size of the aneurysm varies from microscopic to many centimeters in diameter, (3) the shape of the aneurysm is likewise variable (see classification above), (4) the lumen of the aneurysm always communicates with the lumen of the vessel, (5) the ostia between the aneurysm and the vessel may measure only a millimeter across or may be as wide as the aneurysm itself, (6) the cavity of the aneurysm contains fluid, clotted, or organized blood, (7) the inner surface of the aneurysm is generally rough, (8) the wall of the aneurysm is composed either of all the layers of the wall of the vessel (albeit stretched) or one or more of the layers may be absent, and (9) the vessel wall adjacent to the ostium and the wall of the aneurysm often reveal evidences of the process that primarily weakens the wall.

The most important *complications* are (1) rupture with massive or fatal hemorrhage, (2) pressure upon or erosion of any adjacent structure, (3) occlusion of the vascular lumen at the point of origin of the aneurysm by a thrombus or by pressure of extravasated blood, and (4) thrombotic embolism distal to the origin of the aneurysm. The clinical manifestations vary with the vessel affected and the type of complication that arises. The *diagnosis* is arrived at from (1) a consideration of the history, (2) a careful physical examination, (3) establishment of etiologic factors such as syphilis, arteriosclerosis, periarteritis nodosa, etc., and (4) roentgen visualization of the defect. The *treatment* and *prognosis* depend, among other things, upon the vessel affected, the exact location of the aneurysm, the size of the aneurysm, the etiologic agent, and the complication that arises.

Aside from the general considerations outlined above a few specific words may be profitably devoted to the following more common and more important aneurysms: congenital, arteriosclerotic, dissecting, embolic, syphilitic, and arteriovenous.

Congenital Aneurysms.—Congenital aneurysms (also referred to as miliary, berry, bifurcation, or developmental aneurysms) result from a developmental failure of fusion of the media of an artery with the media of its branch. The internal elastic lamina is at first normal but, as a result of the weakened wall, it gradually degenerates, stretches, and ultimately bulges, forming the aneurysm. Congenital aneurysms are generally *small*, measuring not more than two to three centimeters in diameter. They are frequently *multiple* and are found at the bifurcations of medium-sized vessels (Fig. 152). While they have been described in the pulmonary, coronary, splenic, pancreaticoduodenal. and other arteries, they are most common in the *intracranial vessels* where the incidence is recorded as varying from 0.8 to 1.5 per cent of all autopsies.

Arteriosclerotic Aneurysms.—As longevity has increased, arteriosclerotic aneurysms have become more frequent and, at present, they lead the list in *incidence*. They are most numerous after the age of fifty years and preponderate in males. The *aorta* is their favorite vessel. While statistics vary, it may be stated that in the abdominal aorta, approximately nine-tenths of all aneurysms are arteriosclerotic and only one-tenth are syphilitic, while in the thoracic aorta the reverse is true. Also, as far as the abdominal aorta is concerned, syphilitic aneurysms are limited to the segment between the diaphragm and the origins of the renal arteries. Aside from the aorta, almost all *large* and *medium-sized arteries* of the body have been known to harbor arteriosclerotic aneurysms. Some of these are popliteal, iliac, femoral, uterine, colic, pancreaticoduodenal, gastric, mesenteric, celiac, renal, splenic, cystic, hepatic, pulmonary, subclavian, innominate, and carotid. *Grossly* the aneurysms are either fusiform or saccular; they vary in size from a few to many centimeters; their walls are sclerotic and of

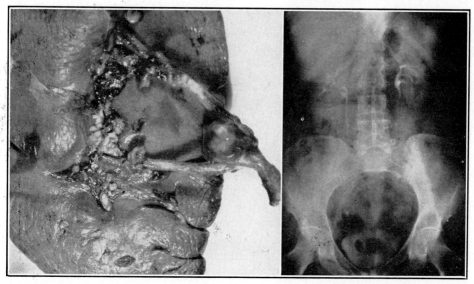

FIG. 152.—Congenital aneurysm at the bifurcation of the splenic artery with secondary calcification. The latter shows well in the roentgenogram.

varying thickness; the lumens contain fluid, clotted, or organized blood, and the vessel whence the aneurysm arose usually shows advanced arteriosclerosis (Fig. 153). The histologic changes are primarily those of the causative disease. Other pertinent aspects are similar to those outlined at the beginning of this section in connection with aneurysms in general.

Dissecting Aneurysms.—A dissecting aneurysm consists of a massive hemorrhage in the wall of an artery, spreading longitudinally along its course and ultimately rupturing through the intima or the adventitia or both. The predisposing *cause* is medionecrosis and the initial lesion is hemorrhage into such a media from the vasa vasorum. The condition is usually seen in the *aorta* (constituting about 0.36 per cent of all autopsies) but other vessels (such as the splenic artery) may, on rare occasions, be affected. In the aorta the process generally initiates in the ascending portion, descends inferiorly to involve even the femoral arteries, and also affects the other main branches (Fig. 110*B*). The intimal tear is usually located just above the aortic valve while the adventitial rupture may occur anywhere along the course. In decreasing order of frequency the latter results in hemorrhage into the pericardial, pleural, and peritoneal cavities. *Clinically* dissecting aneurysm of the aorta predominates in males with an average age of 40 to 70 years (Fisher). The important manifestations are (1) sudden onset of pain usually in the chest or epigastrium with radiation to the back, neck, flanks, or extremities, (2) syncope, and (3) secondary symptoms consisting of dyspnea, vomiting, nausea, orthopnea, etc. The physical signs include shock, hypertension, cardiac enlargement and murmurs, pericardial friction rub, diminished pulsations in the peripheral

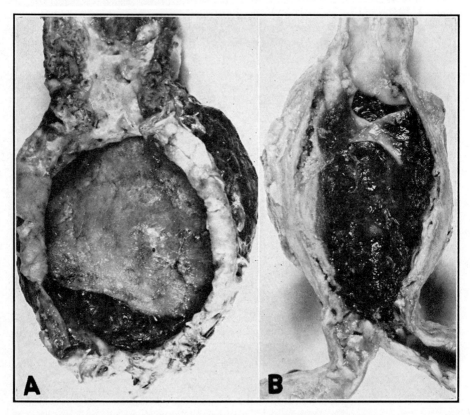

FIG. 153.—Arteriosclerotic aneurysms of the lower portion of the aorta showing *A*, a saccular and *B*, a fusiform type of dilatation. Each contains coagulated blood.

vessels, protean neurologic findings, a palpable abdominal mass, and variable EKG findings. *Treatment* is similar to that in myocardial infarction. The *prognosis* is poor. In 58 cases studied by Levinson, the immediate mortality was 36.2 per cent, the three- to six-day survival was 35 per cent, and the three-month to eight-year survival was 25.9 per cent.

Experimentally, dissecting aneurysms can be produced readily in the aorta of rats fed a diet of the sweet pea—*Lathyrus odoratus* (Bean and Walker). The active principle in the sweet pea has actually been determined as beta aminopropionitrile (Lalich). The aneurysms, with or without rupture, are generally limited to the arch of the aorta. In this area the elastic fibers of the media are normally irregularly aligned in relation to the lumen. Elsewhere in the aorta they are arranged parallel to the longitudinal axis. The spaces between the fibers are filled with collagen fibers, ground substance, and smooth muscle. In sweet-pea-fed rats the initial changes in the media of the arch consist of edema and swelling followed by fragmentation and dissolution of elastic fibers (Bachhuber). All of this produces weakening of the wall with resultant dilatation, aneurysm, or dissecting medial hemorrhage. The ultimate result is rupture or healing. The latter is accomplished by the appearance first of granulation and then of connective tissue in the intima, media, or adventitia. Inflammation is present only when the rupture is contained by fibrous tissue. Aside from the aortic lesions, the rats also develop osteoporosis, skeletal deformities, and hindlimb spasticity with or without paralysis. The experimental syndrome is comparable to *lathyrism* (poisoning by *Lathyrus cicera*) in man. This is attended by muscle weakness, paresthesias, and transient paralysis of the lower extremities.

Infective Aneurysms. —Infective aneurysms are more often called mycotic aneurysms, but since the term mycotic generally refers to fungous infections the latter caption is confusing and should be dropped. An infective aneurysm *results from* weakening of the wall caused by the lodgment of septic material or bacteria either within the lumen of the vessel or within the vasa vasorum (intravascular origin) or by extension of a neighboring inflammatory process in adjacent perivascular tissues (extravascular origin). Intravascular infective aneurysms may be further subdivided into (1) those caused by infected emboli lodging (as already stated) in the lumen or the vasa vasorum, (2) those due to deposition of microorganisms directly on the intima or in the vasa vasorum, and (3) those resulting from extension of infection from aortic or pulmonic valves (Hankins). Of all these causes, the most common are septic emboli arising in bacterial endocarditis. Aneurysms caused by intraluminal occlusion with septic emboli must occur in vessels small enough to stop such material while those occluding vasa vasorum may occur in arteries of any caliber. Most of the recorded cases in the latter category have occurred in the aorta and the coronary, cerebral, subclavian, gastroepiploic, celiac, superior mesenteric, axillary, ulnar, iliac, popliteal, tibial, and femoral arteries (Revell and Shnider). Depending upon the location of the vessel affected, the *cases* may be *grouped into* those (1) affecting the brain and producing what may be called the *intracranial syndromes* —attended by manifestations of intracranial hemorrhage or vascular occlusion, (2) affecting the abdominal vessels and producing what may be called the *abdominal syndromes* —attended by pain and other manifestations of an acute abdominal emergency, (3) affecting the intrathoracic arteries and producing what may be called the *thoracic syndromes* —attended by manifestations simulating coronary artery occlusion, and (4) affecting the arteries of the extremities and producing what may be called the *extremity syndromes* —attended chiefly by pain and local swelling (Shnider). *Pathologically*, the vessels affected (especially the aorta), frequently disclose some underlying disease such as arteriosclerosis, cystic medionecrosis, congenital hypoplasia, and even syphilis (Parkhurst). *Grossly* the aneurysms are saccular and may measure as much as 8 cm. in diameter. *Histologically* they reveal the underlying pathologic process (when such exists), destruction and disruption of the wall, and superimposed acute to chronic inflammation which may or may not abound in bacteria. The most noteworthy *complication* is rupture attended by hemorrhage and shock. The *clinical* manifestations, as already indicated, vary with the vessel and area of the body affected. The *diagnosis* can be readily established clinically when vessels of the extremities are affected but is usually made only at autopsy when internal arteries are involved. The *prognosis* is generally poor.

25

Syphilitic Aneurysms.—Syphilitic aneurysms are most common in Negro males before the age of fifty years. They *occur* in the aorta, in the larger branches of the aorta, and in larger vessels of the extremities. They are not seen in the small arteries because syphilitic lesions of such vessels are of a proliferative nature. In the aorta (as already stated above) the lesions affect the ascending aorta, the aortic arch, and the descending aorta to the level of the origins of the renal arteries with decreasing order of frequency. They are rare below this level. Syphilitic aneurysms comprise

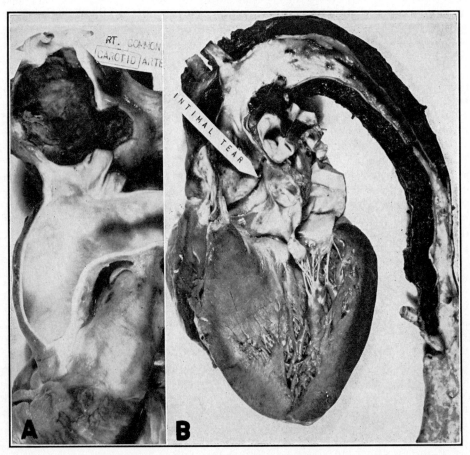

Fig. 154.—Aneurysms showing *A*, a syphilitic saccular dilatation of the innominate artery and *B*, a dissecting type of the aorta and its main branches.

about 90 per cent of all thoracic aneurysms. *Grossly* they are fusiform or saccular (Fig. 154*A*) and, both grossly and microscopically, they present the usual evidences of syphilitic aortitis or arteritis (p. 375). The *complications, clinical manifestations*, and *diagnosis* are covered in the general dissertation on the subject at the beginning of this section. *Treatment* has been both medical and surgical. The prognosis is poor, death usually being caused by rupture and fatal hemorrhage.

Arteriovenous Aneurysms.—Arteriovenous aneurysms, also known as arteriovenous fistulas, may be congenital or acquired. *Congenital arteriovenous aneurysms* are frequently called *cirsoid* or *racemose aneurysms*. It is thought that congenital telangiectasis or hemangioma may serve as a starting point for their development. There is usually no history of trauma. The *lesion* consists of a mass of dilated, tortuous, intercommunicating arteries and veins of over-all varying sizes (Fig. 155). It may affect the following areas of the body: scalp, other portions of the head, neck, upper extremities, lower extremities, lungs, pancreas, duodenum, stomach, kidneys, spleen, vertebræ, and uterus. The *complications* are erosions, hemorrhage, and, if located in an extremity, hypertrophy of the limb. *Clinically* the progression is slow and it may be years before manifestations develop

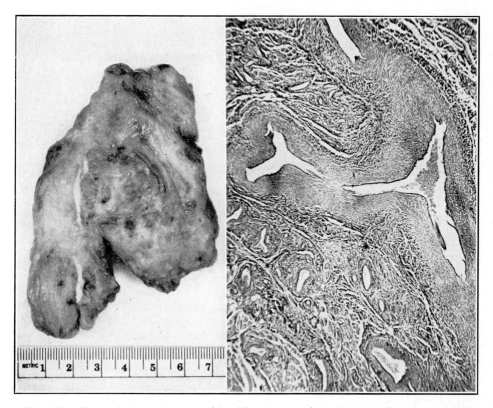

Fig. 155.—Congenital arteriovenous (cirsoid) aneurysm from the arm of a 12 year old boy showing an ill-defined mass of fibrous tissue and vascular channels grossly and intercommunicating arteries and veins microscopically. × 25.

(Adams). Locally, external lesions are usually attended by palpable and visible venous pulsations, thrill, and audible bruit continuous throughout the cardiac cycle. Internal lesions are usually detectable when hemorrhage occurs. Regardless of the location, when the aneurysms are large shunting of the blood results in elevated venous pressure, elevated oxygen content of the venous blood, and ultimately in cardiac hypertrophy and decompensation. Pulmonary shunts are also accompanied by polycythemia, cyanosis, dyspnea, and clubbing of the fingers. In obscure cases, angiography is a good diagnostic aid. *Treatment* consists of doing nothing, of ligation of the feeding arteries, or of surgical excision. The *prognosis* varies with the location and extent of the lesion.

Acquired arteriovenous aneurysms are also referred to as traumatic arterio-venous fistulas. As the latter caption indicates they are usually *caused* by penetrating injury and are, thus, more common in warfare than in civilian life. Rarely, they result from rupture of an arterial aneurysm into an adjacent vein. *Pathologically* the communication is generally small, of variable size, and may be direct or indirect (connected by an aneurysm or a channel composed of extravasated blood and connective tissue). In recorded cases most of the vessels of the body have been affected. Some of these are aortic arch and left innominate vein, aorta and superior inferior vena cava, common carotid artery and internal jugular vein, and the fol-lowing arteries and veins: brachial, external iliac, femoral, popliteal, axillary, tibial, and radial. The more common *complications* are (1) local vascular degenerative and calcific changes, (2) arterial aneurysm (which may rupture) proximal to the shunt, (3) cardiac hypertrophy and decom-pensation (when the shunt is large and affects the larger vessels), and (4) bacterial arteritis and endocarditis (usually streptococcic). The *clinical manifestations* are similar to those outlined in connection with the con-genital variety. *Treatment* consists of arterial reconstruction in lesions of short duration and quadruple ligation of the artery and vein in lesions of longer duration. The *prognosis* is generally good.

Vasospasm.—Contraction of vessels or vasospasm is a physiologic property whereby the flow of blood to a portion or portions of the body is regulated. Abnormally the contraction may be of sufficient severity to result in pathologic processes. Some of the more important vasospastic conditions may be listed under the headings of visceral, Raynaud's disease, acrocyanosis, livedo reticularis, ergotism, and local hypothermia. The last mentioned, consisting of chilblains, trench foot, immersion foot, and frostbite has been considered in Chapter 6 (p. 229). The others may be discussed briefly forthwith.

Visceral vasospasm of a sufficient degree to produce local ischemia and infarction undoubtedly does occur, although admittedly the phenomenon is difficult to prove. A few acceptable examples of such vasospasms are angina pectoris, some infarcts of the spleen and kidneys, bilateral diffuse cortical necrosis of the kidneys, and some infarcts of the central nervous system. In all fairness, however, it must be stated that some authors do not accept the contention that contraction of vessels can be severe enough to produce permanent tissue damage.

Raynaud's disease consists of paroxysmal spasm of the digital arteries occurring in response to cold and emotions and producing bilateral sym-metrical ischemia and cyanosis of the digits (Blain). Other protruding parts, such as the nose, cheek, and ears, may also be affected. The con-dition is generally seen in women between the ages of twenty and forty-five years in whom there is other evidence of vasomotor instability. The *cause* of the vascular susceptibility to spasm is unknown. During an *attack*, the skin becomes white and cold and the affected area becomes parasthetic. Upon exposure to warmth the area becomes blotchy, blue, swollen, and finally hyperemic (Hueper). Ultimately, as a result of re-peated attacks, the tips of the fingers and toes may disclose blisters, kera-toses, fissures, scars, atrophy, and, rarely, necrosis, and gangrene. Because of lack of examination the early *changes* in the vessels are unknown. In advanced cases, proliferative and sclerosing alterations are seen in the in-tima and inner portions of the media of the medium-sized and smaller arteries. Changes in sympathetic ganglia are considered to be nonspecific.

Treatment consists of an avoidance of cold and application of warmth. In severe cases, sympathectomy appears to offer permanent relief. *Raynaud's syndrome* or *phenomenon* is a condition similar to Raynaud's disease but having as a basis for the disorder some recognizable primary alteration in the affected arteries or definite causative agents that bring about the characteristic clinical manifestations (Duff).

Acrocyanosis (Gr. = extremity + cyanosis) is a condition characterized by painless persistent coldness and diffuse cyanosis of the distal parts of the extremities (Allen). The cause is unknown. Physiologically, the disorder is thought to be due to arteriolar constriction and distal capillary dilatation. Pathologically the capillaries are said to be dilated and elongated but other changes have not been noted. The condition is distinguished from Raynaud's disease in that the discoloration is persistent rather than intermittent.

Livedo reticularis is a condition characterized by a reddish-blue mottling of the skin of the greater portions of the extremities (Allen). The cause is doubtlessly some vascular instability. Physiologically the disorder results from arterial obstruction (spastic or organic) and distal capillary dilatation. The mottled appearance of the skin distinguishes the entity from acrocyanosis.

Ergotism is poisoning due to ergot. In man, ergotism usually results from medicinal use of various ergot preparations and is characterized by convulsions and gangrene (Allen). The latter is due primarily to vasospasm. Pathologically the severe spasm causes intimal proliferation, endothelial damage, and secondary thrombosis. The net result is ischemia and gangrene. The latter usually affects the distal portions of the extremities.

Varicose Veins. —Varicose veins, also referred to simply as varices, may be defined as dilatation of veins. Without further specification the caption refers to veins of the lower extremities. The *incidence* is generally recorded as varying between 10 and 17 per cent of the population (Allen). The condition occurs at all ages but is most common beyond the age of thirty years and affects females about two or three times as frequently as males. The *causes* are generally dividable into predisposing and precipitating. The *predisposing* cause is usually considered to be some hereditary weakness of the wall as evidenced by a high incidence of the disorder in families. As a rule, it is implied that the weakness is within the venous wall itself and in no particular location. Our own studies have indicated that there is normally an absence of smooth muscle and internal elastic lamina in the sinus wall of the great saphenous vein in the valve area at the saphenofemoral junction. Because of this finding, it has been postulated that similar defects may occur in other perforating veins and that such defects may cause dilatation of the veins, incompetency of the valves, flow of blood from the deep to the superficial veins, and varicosities of the latter. *Precipitating causes* are mechanical. They are due to increased intravascular pressure and this, in turn, may result from (1) erect posture over prolonged periods (best example being occupational, such as policemen), (2) increased intra-abdominal pressure as occurs in ascites, pregnancy, coughing, lifting, straining, etc., (3) organic obstruction of proximal veins such as seen in thrombophlebitis, tumors, etc., and (4) loss of tone of supporting tissues as seen with increasing age (bringing about relative increase of intraluminal pressure).

Pathologically the veins affected in decreasing order of frequency are long saphenous and its tributaries, short saphenous and its tributaries, communicating branches between the superficial and deep veins, collateral veins of the lower abdomen, and smaller cutaneous veins. The deep veins are rarely involved (Allen). The pathologic changes in the affected veins consist of dilatation, elongation, tortuosity, loss of elasticity, irregular thickening of the walls due to hypertrophy of the various layers and fibrosis, irregular thinning of the wall between the thickened areas due to dilatation, and disappearance or complete atrophy of the valves. Later, as a result of endothelial damage (due to infection, trauma, or degeneration from anoxia) and stasis of blood, secondary thrombosis may supervene.

Complications are due to venous stasis, trauma, and infection. They consist of eczematoid pigmentation, ulceration, hemorrhage, cellulitis, and thrombophlebitis. *Clinically* the condition is usually symptomless until the varicosities become large. At this stage, combinations of the following symptoms may be noticed: easy fatigability of the leg muscles, sensation

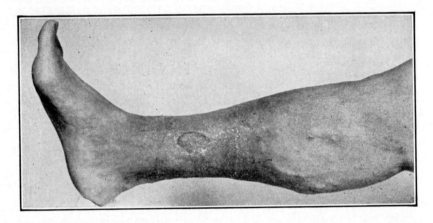

Fig. 156.—Varicose veins of a lower extremity. The channels are dilated, tortuous and knotty. The skin of the lower portion is pigmented and ulcerated. (Herbut, *Surgical Pathology*, 2nd Ed., Lea & Febiger.)

of fullness and congestion, soreness in the regions of the veins, muscle cramps, burning, pain, itching, and symptoms referable to the complications listed above (Allen). Examination reveals irregular dilatations, tortuosities, and knots of the venous channels together with edema of the extremity and, later, evidences of the complications already referred to (Fig. 156). The *diagnosis* is usually readily arrived at from the characteristic gross appearance of the extremity. *Treatment* has been varied. In general, it consists of (1) eliminating the cause, (2) palliative relief in the form of bandages, elevation of the extremity, change of occupation, etc., (3) injection of sclerosing solutions, (4) surgical, in the form of ligation of the great saphenous vein at its origin or excision of the larger trunks, and (5) attention to the complications. The *prognosis* is variable but, in general, adequate treatment in early or moderately advanced cases gives good results.

Phleboliths and Arterioliths.—*Phleboliths* (Gr. = vein + stone) are calculi or stones found within veins. Similar masses within arteries are known as *arterioliths* (Gr. = artery + stone). The former are common, the latter are rare. They occur as a result of organization and calcification of vascular thrombi. Although phleboliths may be found anywhere in the body, the most common locations are the veins of the pelvis and lower extremities. They are of various shapes and sizes, may partially or completely occlude the vein, are adherent at one or more points, are smooth externally, appear gray, and are extremely firm (Fig. 157). On rare occasions they may become detached and thus form emboli. They are usually readily demonstrable radiographically.

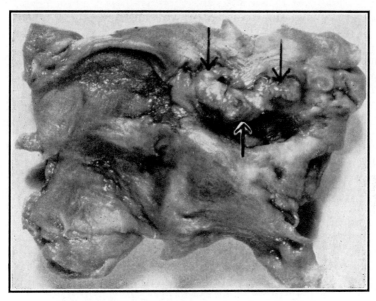

FIG. 157.—Phlebolith showing an irregular, elongated, calcified nodule within the lumen of a vein.

Superior Vena Cava Syndrome —This syndrome may be due to obstruction of the superior vena cava, bilateral obstruction of the innominate veins, or fistula between the ascending aorta and superior vena cava (McIntire and Sykes). Of these, *obstruction* of the *superior vena cava* is the most common and most important. The greatest *incidence* is between thirty and sixty years of age and the male-female ratio is approximately three to two. The *causes* of the obstruction are usually aneurysms of the aorta, primary or secondary mediastinal tumors, chronic fibrous mediastinitis (tuberculous, syphilitic, or idiopathic), and localized phlebitis with thrombosis. *Pathologically* the obstruction is brought about by compression of the vessel from without, invasion of the wall of the vena cava with superimposed secondary thrombosis or intraluminal occlusion by tumor, or a combination of these. Further, the obstruction may be partial or complete. Once the thrombus is formed or a tumor penetrates the intima, the intraluminal mass may propagate in either direction to involve other tributaries or even the heart itself. *Clinically* the manifestations (aside from the primary condition) are due to the venous obstruction. They consist of (1) dilatation of the veins and increased venous pressure proximal to the obstruction, (2) edema of the upper extremities, head, and neck, (3) cyanosis, (4) dyspnea, (5) pain in the head and neck, and (6) miscellaneous consisting of hoarseness, dysphagia, drowsiness, and convulsions. *Treat-*

ment consists of eradication of the primary disorder. The *prognosis* is poor since most of the cases are caused by a malignant tumor or aneurysm of the aorta.

Lymphedema.—Lymphedema is a swelling of the soft tissues (usually of an extremity) due to an abnormal accumulation of lymph. The *causes* are varied. In some cases, no etiologic agent is demonstrable; in a few instances the condition is congenital (simple or familial), while in the majority of cases it is due to obstruction of the lymphatic channels. The obstruction may occur locally or in the draining lymph nodes. The causes of the obstruction are malignant tumor, surgical interruption of the lymphatic channels (as in radical operations), fibrosis following irradiation, recurrent lymphangiitis, and filariasis (Lowenberg). *Pathologically* the disturbance is characterized by thickening of the skin and subcutaneous tissue, appearance of many enlarged, thin-walled lymphatic spaces, increase of connective tissue, accumulation of lymph between the tissue cells, atrophy of normal structures of the limb (epidermal appendages, nerves, and muscles), and varying degrees of leukocytic infiltration (Allen). *Clinically* the involved extremity undergoes progressive and uniform enlargement until it becomes several times the normal size. At first, the tissue is soft but later it becomes indurated. The skin is thick, often becomes rough, and, in advanced cases, may even become ulcerated. *Treatment* consists of elimination of the cause. If this is impossible (and if the lesion is not due to a malignant tumor in which case death is inevitable) surgical excision of the redundant tissues is indicated. The *prognosis* depends upon the cause. The lymphedema as such is not lethal.

Trauma.—Trauma to vessels is more important in warfare than in civilian life. Of the three vascular systems in the body, injury to arteries is generally more important than injuries to veins and lymphatic channels. The *incidence* of vascular injuries in the American Theaters of Operation in World War II was 0.96 per cent (DeBakey and Simeone). The *cause* of the injury is, of course, trauma. It may be direct as a result of stabbing, gunshot, or shell fragments or indirect by way of a blunt blow, dislocation, or fracture. The *injury* may thus be opened or closed and the arterial lesion may be one of spasm, contusion, or laceration (Gardner). *Spasm* occurs in conjunction with severance, laceration, or contusion and is seen not only in the injured segment but also reflexly in the arterial trunk, both proximal and distal to the injury. If prolonged, it results in ischemia and gangrene. *Contusion* of an artery may result in occlusion by thrombosis or spasm. *Laceration* of an artery is the most common injury. It, of course, results in loss of continuity of a vessel and complete impairment of the circulation. Although any vessels in the body may be affected, the *arterial trunks* most commonly involved are the brachial, tibial, femoral, and popliteal. As a rule, the larger the vessel the more serious the consequences. Some of the more common *complications* are primary or secondary hemorrhage, ischemia, gangrene, infection, traumatic aneurysm, arteriovenous fistula, Volkmann's contracture, and causalgia (intense local sensation of pain and burning). Other pertinent data in connection with vascular injuries are found in general discussions on Hemorrhage and Trauma in Chapter 6 (pp. 196 and 222).

A rare but important vascular injury is that sustained by the larger *lymphatic trunks*, especially those in the thorax. The consequence is escape of lymph or chyle and when this takes place into the thoracic cavity, the disorder is called *chylothorax*. In this condition, the thoracic duct harbors the *defect*. When the defect is located in the lower portion of the thoracic duct, the effusion is on the right. When it is located in the superior portion, the effusion is on the left. The defect results from (1) destructive damage (indirect trauma to the chest, perforating wound, accidental severance at operation, etc.), (2) obstruction (tumor, filaria, tuberculosis, thrombosis left subclavian vein, etc.), and (3) spontaneous (Jahsman). The *effused fluid* discloses the following: milky appearance, creamy layer on standing, emulsified fat globules, odor of food eaten, alkaline reaction, specific gravity over 1.012, constant degree of opalescence, absence of bacteria, fat content 0.4 to 4 per cent and similar to the fat in the food, total solids over 4 per cent, total proteins over 3 grams per hundred cc., and salts and organic substances like those in the chyle from the thoracic duct. *Clinically* the following may be noted: (1) a period of latency before onset of symptoms, (2) rapid reaccumulation of fluid after tapping, (3) progressive emaciation, (4) collapse or shock (due to change in intrathoracic pressure), and (5) inanition, oliguria, and thirst (probably from breakdown of lipid metabolism). The *prognosis* is poor, for in traumatic cases the mortality is over 50 per cent while in cases caused by a malignant tumor it is 100 per cent and these two etiologic factors account for the majority of cases of chylothorax.

TUMORS

Orientation.—Primary tumors of vessels follow the distribution of vessels in the body and are, therefore, located in virtually every organ and tissue. While some of the nomenclature is well standardized, much of it is not and, thus, there exists a profusion of terms which greatly complicates the study of the growths. At the risk of oversimplification, the following benign and malignant tumors may be considered: hereditary hemorrhagic telangiectasia, hemangioma, sclerosing hemangioma, glomus tumor, lymphangioma, hemangioendothelioma, Kaposi's sarcoma, hemangiopericytoma, and lymphangiosarcoma.

Hereditary Hemorrhagic Telangiectasia.—This condition, also known as Osler-Weber-Rendu disease, is not a true tumor but consists simply of groups of abnormally dilated capillaries and veins. The disorder is *inherited* as a dominant, affects both sexes with equal frequency, and may be transmitted by either the male or the female (Kushlan). Although hereditary, it does not appear until adult life. The *sites* of affliction are: skin, nail beds, conjunctivæ, nose, mouth, pharynx, larynx, trachea, esophagus, stomach, intestines, urethra, bladder, kidneys, brain, meninges, liver, and spleen. *Grossly* the lesions are small, measuring only millimeters in diameter, but are multiple and often coalescing. They may be pinpoint, spiderlike, or nodular; they are sharply circumscribed, bright, and slightly raised, and they blanch on pressure or after hemorrhage. *Histologically* they are composed of thin-walled dilated capillary channels composed of but a single layer of endothelium. *Clinically* the only symptom is hemorrhage (epistaxis, hemoptysis, hematemesis, melena, hematuria, etc.) which is usually recurrent and may be severe enough to cause death. The advocated *treatment* is cauterization of the bleeding area only, leaving the remaining lesions alone.

Hemangioma.—Hemangiomas are benign tumors composed of proliferating blood channels. They *originate* from clusters of unipotent angioblastic cells that have failed to form regular vascular connections (Pack and Miller). The lesions, therefore, arise from embryonic rests and are of congenital origin. They are thus usually *found* at birth although, on rare occasions, they may not be noticed until adulthood. As a rule, they grow with the growth of the child and stop increasing in size when general growth ceases. Sometimes, however, they fade with increasing age and entirely disappear within a year or two after birth. They affect both sexes and are rare in Negroes.

Although any *organ* may be involved, most of those that are recognized occur in the skin, subcutaneous tissues, and mouth. About one-half of the cutaneous lesions affect the head and neck. *Pathologically* hemangiomas of the skin are variously classified depending upon their appearance. The *capillary* type varies from a few millimeters to several centimeters in diameter and is bright red. It is flat or elevated and, when elevated, is sessile or pedunculated (Fig. 158). It is composed of thin-walled capillaries

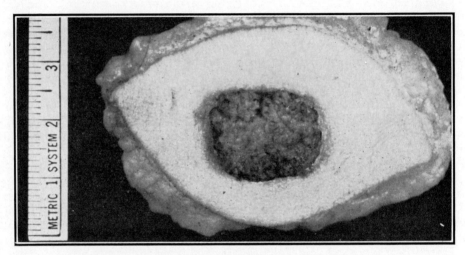

FIG. 158.—Hemangioma showing an elevated, pedunculated, rough, deep red, cutaneous mass measuring about 1.5 cm. in diameter.

that are empty or filled with blood (Fig. 159*A*). The stroma is usually loose and scanty. The *port wine* stain is pink to purplish, flat, and blotchy. It usually occurs on the face and is composed of thin-walled dilated capillaries located in the outer portion of the dermis. The *spider angioma* consists of a central solid hub measuring a few millimeters in diameter encircled by fine radiating strands for distances up to 1 cm. This lesion may be part of hereditary hemorrhagic telangiectasia. The *cavernous* hemangioma consists of a mass of intercommunicating cavernous spaces that are often directly connected with the systemic circulation. They usually affect the deeper portions of the skin and the subcutaneous tissues. Grossly they appear as ill-defined, boggy, compressible, colorless or bluish masses and, when located in an extremity, they may be associated with enlargement of the limb. Cavernous hemangioma is frequently found in internal organs, especially the liver. Histologically the spaces are lined with endothelial cells (Fig. 159*B*). The stroma may be loose and scanty or it may be abundant and collagenous.

The *complications* of hemangiomas are infection and hemorrhage. They are especially apt to occur when the lesions are so located that they are subjected to trauma. A malignant transformation does occur but is extremely rare. *Clinically* hemangiomas are usually symptomless until they bleed or produce pressure. The *diagnosis* is generally readily apparent from the gross appearance. *Treatment* has been quite varied. Some lesions disappear spontaneously while others can be successfully treated by irradiation, freezing, surgical excision, or injection of sclerosing solutions. The *prognosis* is good as far as preservation of life is concerned, but the cosmetic results are often disappointing.

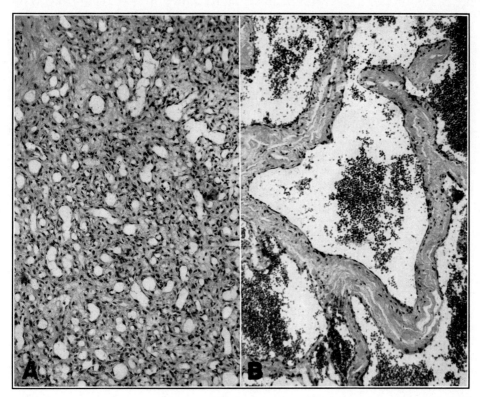

Fig. 159.—Hemangioma showing *A*, a capillary type composed of numerous thin-walled, small, endothelial-lined spaces supported by a connective tissue stroma and *B*, a cavernous type composed of large spaces lined by endothelium filled with blood and supported by a collagenous stroma. × 100.

Sclerosing Hemangioma.—Sclerosing hemangiomas are, in reality, capillary hemangiomas that have gone or are undergoing retrogressive changes. The lesions are of *congenital* origin but the patient usually seeks treatment when he is between the ages of thirty and fifty years. The *tumors* more commonly involve the extremities than they do the trunk. They are usually limited to the skin and subcutaneous tissue, may measure as much as 5 cm. in diameter, are raised but flat, are usually covered with smooth skin, and vary in color from gray to pink, yellow or tan-brown. Cut surfaces show a sharp demarcation but no encapsulation. *Histologically* the lesions are essentially capillary hemangiomas with varying degrees of overgrowth of connective tissue (Fig. 160). The capillaries may be clearly outlined and intact or they may be broken up and represented merely by endothelial cells. Connective tissue overgrowth may be cellular or collagenous and may be slight or so abundant as to overshadow all other elements. Other components that vary in amount from slight to severe are hemosiderin, foam cells, and giant cells. Sclerosing hemangioma is an *innocent lesion*, the chief significance of which is its recognition and differentiation from the pigmented nevus or the more ominous melanoblastoma.

Glomus Tumor.—A glomus tumor is a benign neoplasm of the neuromyoarterial glomus (a subcutaneous arteriovenous anastomosis that regulates the peripheral circulation of blood). A *normal glomus* consists of an afferent artery, an arteriovenous anastomosis proper, collecting veins,

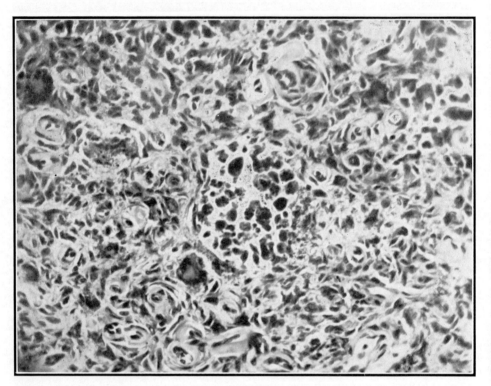

FIG. 160.—Sclerosing hemangioma showing a thin-walled space containing phagocytes with engulfed hemosiderin, capillaries surrounded by hyalinized bands, cellular connective tissue stroma, and giant cells. × 200.

neuroreticular tissue, and an encircling collagenous capsule (Riveros and Pack). Surrounding the arteriovenous anastomosis are elongated cells that resemble smooth muscle cells on the one hand and epithelioid cells on the other. They are the pericytes which give the glomus, and the tumor that develops from it, a characteristic appearance (Murray and Stout). The *growths* may be located anywhere in the skin (and even in the middle ear) but are most common on the distal portions of the extremities, especially the digits. They are rounded, elevated, firm, red to blue, extremely painful nodules that usually measure from 0.5 to 2 cm. in diameter. They may be single or multiple. *Histologically* the lesions present the organoid structure of a glomus with the most characteristic structure consisting of endothelial-lined spaces surrounded by pericytes (Fig. 161). Pericytes are elongated or more rounded, ill-defined cells containing a moderate amount of lightly eosinophilic cytoplasm and elongated oval or even rounded, evenly stained nuclei. The arrangement of the pericytes varies. In some instances they are closely packed around the endothelial cells; in others they may be separated from the endothelial cells and from each other by collagen fibers, and in others still they may be clumped together in large masses between the endothelial-lined spaces. *Treatment* consists of surgical excision. The *prognosis* is good. Malignant transformations do occur but are extremely rare.

Glomus Jugulare Tumors.—*Glomus jugulare tumors* arise from glomus bodies found in the adventitia of the dome of the jugular bulb, along the course of the tympanic branch of the glossopharyngeal nerve, along the

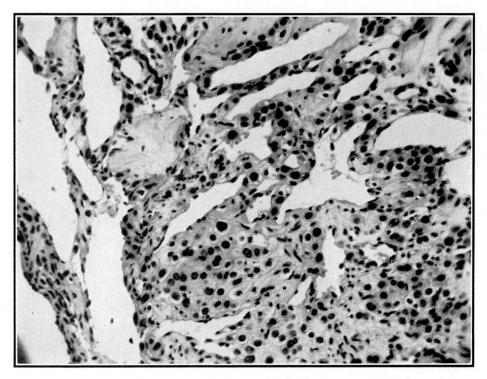

Fig. 161.—Glomus tumor showing endothelial-lined spaces separated
by a stroma containing pericytes. × 200.

course of the cochlear promontory, and along the course of the auricular branch of the vagus nerve (Aquino). Among others, they have also been called tympanic body tumors and nonchromaffin paraganglioma. While the tumors can occur elsewhere, they are most common in the *middle ear*, whence they project into the external auditory canal. They are found at all ages, predominate in females, and are attended by (1) the presence of an aural polyp that bleeds readily, (2) discharge from the ear, (3) tinnitus, (4) impairment in hearing, (5) pain in the ear, (6) facial paralysis, and (7) cloudiness of the mastoid cells (in more extensive lesions) radiologically. *Histologically* the tumors are composed of clumps or masses of closely packed cells encircled by fibrillar or more collagenous bands and bordered by numerous, engorged, thin-walled capillaries (Fig. 162). The cells are polyhedral, have a moderate amount of pink cytoplasm, and disclose round, rather uniform appearing nuclei. The *clinical diagnosis* is made from the appearance of a bleeding "polyp" in conjunction with the aural manifestations listed. It is confirmed by biopsy. The usual *treatment* is surgical excision with radical mastoidectomy. The *prognosis* is guarded for recurrences do occur.

Lymphangioma.—Lymphangiomas are benign tumors of lymphatic channels that originate in displaced fetal cells of the lymphatic system (Watson and McCarthy). The tumors are of *congenital* origin with most being noted at birth or within the first year of life. Both sexes are affected with equal frequency. Over one-half of the tumors affect the head and neck and most of the rest involve the extremities. Only a few are found on the

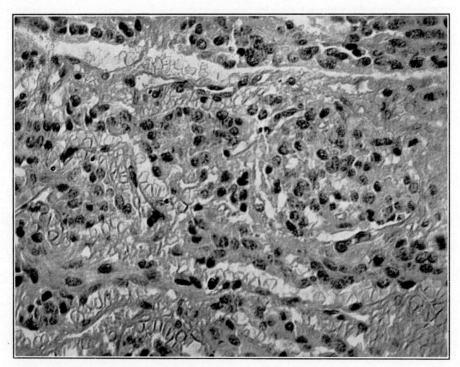

FIG. 162.—Glomus jugulare tumor illustrating clumps of rather uniform appearing polyhedral cells surrounded by numerous engorged capillaries. × 400.

trunk, in the mediastinum, and retroperitoneally. *Pathologically* the growths may be divided into three types—simple, cavernous, and cystic. *Simple lymphangiomas* consist of local dilatations of lymphatic channels rather than true tumors. They are small, sharply circumscribed, verrucal-like, superficial elevations composed of endothelial-lined capillaries or cavernous spaces filled with lymph. They show little or no propensity for growth. *Cavernous lymphangiomas* are the most common. They are composed of endothelial-lined dilated cavernous spaces that are empty and filled with lymph or occasionally with blood (Fig. 163). The stroma may consist of connective tissue, lymphoid cells, fat, or muscle. Grossly the tumor discloses an ill-defined mass of small, compressible, sponge-like spaces (Fig. 163). The lesion generally affects the skin and subcutaneous tissue and is also found between muscles, in the mouth, in the mesentery, and retroperitoneally. *Cystic lymphangiomas* or *cystic hygromas* are gener-

ally found in the neck and, less commonly, in the axilla and retroperitoneum. They are composed of multiloculated, ill-defined, endothelial-
lined, cystic spaces of varying sizes filled with serous fluid. The lesions
in the neck appear to grow rapidly, insinuating themselves along fascial
planes and encircling all structures they contact. They extend into the
mediastinum and the axilla. The *complications* of lymphangiomas are extension of the tumor with compression of vital structures and infection
(local and systemic). The latter has been minimized with the advent of
antibiotics and chemotherapeutic agents. The *clinical manifestations* vary
with the location of the growth and consist mainly of swelling and pressure.

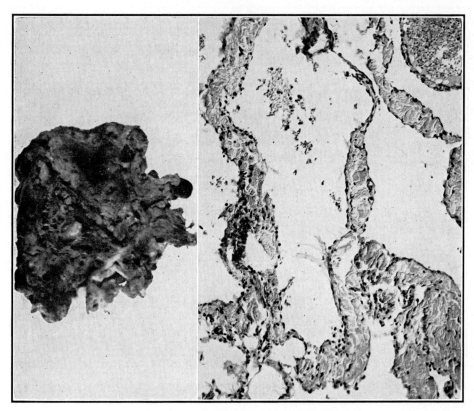

FIG. 163.—Lymphangioma showing (to the left) a spongy tumor and (to the right)
cavernous spaces lined by endothelial cells. × 100.

The *diagnosis* is established from the location and gross appearance of the
lesion. The *treatment* of choice is surgical excision. If this cannot be
accomplished, irradiation may be attempted although the response is
generally poor. The *prognosis* is guarded for recurrences are common.

Hemangioendothelioma.—This is a malignant tumor of blood vessel
that is commonly known as *hemangiosarcoma.* The growth is relatively
uncommon. It *occurs* at all ages, with a preponderance in childhood and
youth, and affects both sexes with approximately equal frequency (Stout).
It may *originate* in any organ or tissue of the body with the majority of
cases occurring in the spleen, liver, bones, skin, and subcutaneous tissues.
Grossly the tumors may reach large proportions, measuring as much as

20 cm. or more in diameter. They are ill-defined, usually quite hemorrhagic, and moderately firm and soft. Although the *histologic* picture may
vary, fundamentally there are two patterns that are constantly seen —
proliferation of atypical endothelial cells and formation of anastomosing
vascular tubes supported by a delicate reticulum (Fig. 164). The endothelial cells may be elongated, rounded, or polygonal with ill-defined cytoplasm and elongated or rounded, deeply stained, irregular nuclei. Characteristically they line the vascular spaces but they also exist as sheets
within the stroma. The vascular channels are of varying shapes and sizes.

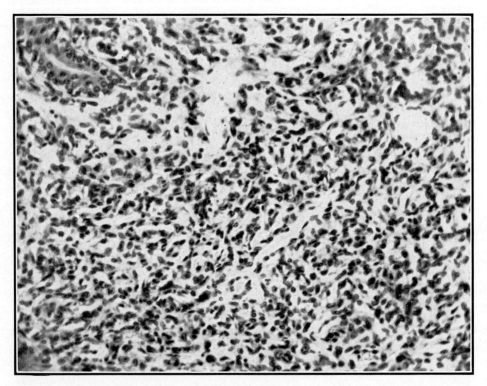

Fig. 164.—Hemangioendothelioma illustrating ill-defined vascular spaces lined by somewhat
irregular elongated endothelial cells and a stroma composed of similar cells. × 200.

Their inner surfaces may be smooth or they may be interrupted by heaps of
endothelial cells protruding into the lumens. The latter also contain
variable amounts of blood. The tumor *spreads* by local extension and by
lymphatic and, more commonly, bloodstream metastasis. Secondary
deposits may occur in any organ of the body. Aside from metastasis, a
common complication of superficial growths is hemorrhage. The *clinical
manifestations* are those of pressure or obstruction and vary with the location of the growth. The *diagnosis* can be made only upon histologic examination. The *course* may be fulminating with death occurring in a few weeks
or it may be protracted with survival as long as nineteen years. Of 18 cases
studied by Stout, 10 were dead of metastasis at the time of reporting. Some
of the remaining cases were lost to follow-up and others were treated too
recently for a definitive evaluation.

Kaposi's Sarcoma.—Kaposi's sarcoma is also referred to as multiple idiopathic hemorrhagic sarcoma. *Geographically* the condition is prevalent in Central and Southeastern Asia but also occurs elsewhere (Aegerter and Peale). It is most *common* in *patients* in the fifth to seventh decades of life, is rare in children, affects twenty males to every female, and prevails in laborers and outdoor workers. *Pathologically*, although the tumor is recorded as primary in almost all parts of the body, it most commonly

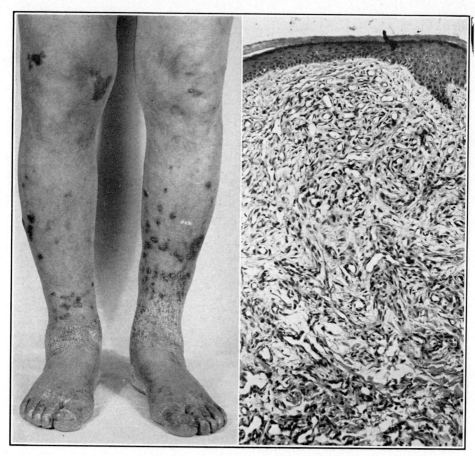

FIG. 165.—Kaposi's sarcoma showing (to the left) the typical distribution and appearance of the lesions and (to the right) actively proliferating capillaries in the dermis. × 100.

originates in the skin of one or both extremities (Fig. 165). The original lesions exist as sharply circumscribed, irregular, red, macular areas. As they age, the color deepens to reddish-blue and finally brown to black. Simultaneously, the areas become elevated and in time they lose some of the discoloration, become firmer, and show superficial scales. New lesions appear in the adjacent healthy skin, resulting eventually in involvement of a large segment of the integument. As a result of blockage of the lymphatic channels, the skin becomes indurated and the extremity becomes enlarged and edematous. *Histologically* the lesion starts in the corium and then infiltrates the underlying structures (Fig. 165). The first changes are those of a capillary or cavernous hemangioma. Later the lesion may develop

26

along one of two lines. Less commonly, there is a proliferation of the capillaries and a diffuse permeation with plasma cells, lymphocytes, neutrophils, and eosinophils giving the tumor a granulomatous appearance. More commonly, the endothelial-lined spaces become less distinct and the intersinusoidal tissue becomes replaced with elongated spindle cells that fuse with and resemble endothelial cells, thus giving a true sarcomatous appearance. *Complications*, aside from local infection and ulceration, consist of metastasis to lymph nodes, lungs, liver, spleen, heart, intestines, and almost any other viscus. Of the metastatic sites, the intestines are the most important for here the tumors have a tendency to (1) ulcerate, (2) cause fatal hemorrhage, (3) perforate and produce peritonitis, and (4) serve as

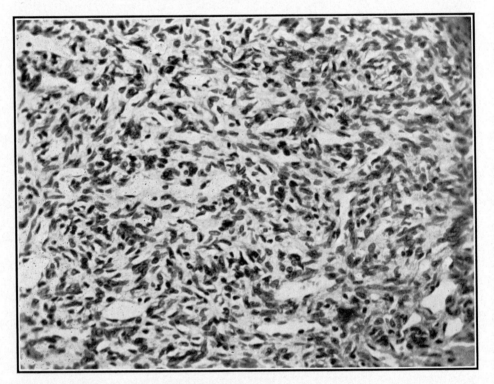

FIG. 166.—Hemangiopericytoma illustrating thin-walled capillary spaces supported by elongated, deeply staining pericytes. × 200. (Slide submitted by Dr. William C. Herrick.)

starting points for intussusception. *Clinically* the only manifestations (until metastasis occurs) are referable to the local lesion. The *diagnosis* is made from the characteristic distribution and appearance of the tumor. *Treatment* has been most varied with surgical excision and irradiation being favored. The ultimate *prognosis* is poor for the disease invariably terminates fatally in from eight months to twenty-five years.

Hemangiopericytoma.—This tumor is akin to the glomus tumor but differs from it in that (1) it does not present the organoid arrangement or encapsulation of the glomus tumor and (2) it has a tendency to become malignant more frequently (Stout). The lesion is seen at all ages and has no predilection for either sex. It may occur whenever capillaries are found but the *locations* in recorded cases have been the skin, subcutaneous tissues, muscles, retroperitoneum, omentum, orbit, tongue, pericardium, diaphragm, ileum, uterus, bone, and meninges. *Grossly* the growths usually measure as much as 3 or 4 cm. in diameter. They are sharply circumscribed, nodular, pinkish gray, and, occasionally, partially calcified. *Histologically* the basic lesion consists of a profuse proliferation of capillaries surrounded by a thin or thick connective tissue sheath and beyond this by collars, masses, or sheets of tumor cells (Fig. 166). The neoplastic cells are quite variable. They are of moderate sizes, ill defined, and elongated to rounded or polyhedral. The cytoplasm is lightly eosinophilic and the nuclei are round,

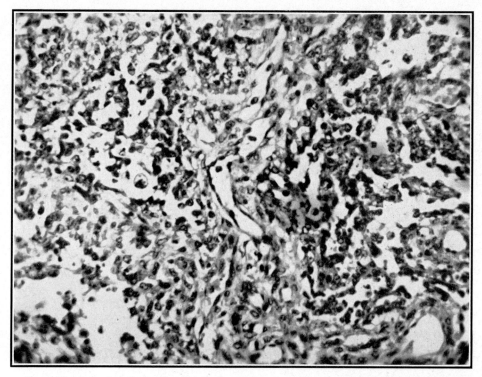

Fig. 167.—Lymphangiosarcoma in postmastectomy lymphedema showing well-formed and poorly formed capillary spaces lined by irregular endothelial cells. × 200.

oval, or irregular and uniform or deeply stained. The advocated *treatment* is surgical excision. The *course* is generally protracted for the tumors grow slowly and usually remain localized. Metastasis to lymph nodes, lungs, peritoneum, retroperitoneum, and subcutaneous tissue occurred in approximately 16 per cent of the recorded cases.

Lymphangiosarcoma.—Lymphangiosarcoma is a malignant tumor of lymphatic channels. The condition is extremely rare. Recently, Stewart and Treves have drawn attention to such tumors occurring in 6 cases of postmastectomy lymphedema. In these instances, the swelling of the extremity occurred immediately or within the first year and the duration of the edema until the appearance of the lymphangiosarcoma varied from six to twenty-four years. The *lesions* appear as purplish-red, subdermal, slightly raised, macular or polypoid areas that have a tendency to coalesce and enlarge. The surface epithelium stretches, ulcerates, discharges a serosanguinous fluid, crusts, heals, breaks down again, and repeats the process. Ultimately the lesion extends over most of the arm and even onto the chest and metastasizes to the lungs. *Histologically* the tumors are composed of proliferating, endothelial-lined, lymphatic channels supported by a stroma of small round cells or of elongated cells similar to the endothelial lining cells (Fig. 167).

REFERENCES

Pathologic Physiology

ALLEN, E. V., BARKER, N. W., and HINES, E. A.: *Peripheral Vascular Disease*, 2nd Ed., Philadelphia, W. B. Saunders Co., 1955.

SODEMAN, W. A.: *Pathologic Physiology*, 2nd Ed., Philadelphia, W. B. Saunders Co., 1956, p. 285.

Congenital Anomalies

BURTON, W. Y., *et al.*: Northwest Med., *44*, 118, 1945 (Right-sided Aortic Arch).

CLAGETT, O. T., and JAMPOLIS, R. W.: A. M. A. Arch. Surg., *63*, 337, 1951 (Coarctation Aorta).

DODRILL, F. D.: Surgery, *31*, 304, 1952 (Double Aortic Arch).

DOLTON, E. G., and JONES, H. E.: Lancet, *1*, 537, 1952 (Anomalies Aortic Arch.).

FELSON, B., *et al.*: Radiology, *54*, 340, 1950 (Posterior Right Subclavian Artery).

GAERTNER, R. A. and BLALOCK, A.: Surgery, *40*, 712, 1956 (Experimental Coarctation).

GROSS, R. E.: Circulation, *1*, 41, 1950 (Coarctation Aorta).

GROSS, R. E., and LONGINO, L. A.: Circulation, *3*, 125, 1951 (412 Cases Patent Ductus Arteriosus).

HERBUT, P. A.: A. M. A. Arch. Path., *35*, 719, 1943 (Anomalies Aortic Arch).

HERBUT, P. A., and FOX, J. R.: Am. Heart J., *31*, 490, 1946 (Right Aortic Arch).

HERBUT, P. A., and SMITH, T. T.: Arch. Otolaryng., *37*, 558, 1943 (Double Aortic Arch).

KEYS, A., and SHAPIRO, M. J.: Am. Heart J., *25*, 158, 1943 (Patent Ductus Arteriosus).

OLESEN, O. L.: Danish M. Bull., *4*, 33, 1957 (44 Cases Coarctation).

RUMEL, W. R., *et al.*, J.A.M.A., *164*, 5, 1957 (1601 Cases Coarctation).

TOUROFF, A. S. W.: Am. Heart J., *25*, 187, 1943 (Patent Ductus Arteriosus and Bacterial Endarteritis).

Degenerations

ALDERSBERG, D., *et al.*: J. A. M. A., *141*, 246, 1949 (Genetics of Atherosclerosis).

BRILL, I. C., and KRYGIER, J. J.: A. M. A. Arch. Int. Med., *68*, 560, 1941 (Pulmonary Vascular Sclerosis).

BURCHELL, H. B., *et al.*: J. A. M. A., *147*, 1511, 1951 (Clinical Manifestations of Arteriosclerosis).

DUFF, G. L., and McMILLAN, G. C.: Am. J. Med., *11*, 92, 1951 (Pathology of Atherosclerosis).

Editorial: J. A. M. A., *141*, 266, 1949 (Arteriolar Necrosis).

GEIRINGER, E.: A. M. A. Arch. Path., *48*, 410, 1949 (Venous Atheroma).

HEUPER, W. C.: A. M. A. Arch. Path., *38*, 162, 1944 (Arteriosclerosis—Review).

KRAMER, D. W.: Angiology, *1*, 53, 1950 (Obliterative Endarteritis).

LEV, M., and SAPHIR, O.: Am. J. Path., *28*, 401, 1952 (Endophlebohypertrophy and Endophlebosclerosis).

McCLOSKEY, J. F., and CHU, P. T.: A. M. A. Arch. Path., *52*, 132, 1951 (Medionecrosis and Dissecting Aneurysms of Aorta).

McCLUSKEY, R. T., and WILENS, S. L.: Am. J. Path., *29*, 71, 1953 (Sclerotic Veins).

McLRETCHIE, N. G. E.: Am. J. Path., *28*, 413, 1952 (Pathogenesis Atheroma).

MOSRISON, L. M.: Ann. Int. Med., *37*, 1172, 1952 (Diet and Atherosclerosis).

MOCHCOWITZ, E.: J. A. M. A., *143*, 861, 1950 (Arteriosclerosis and Atherosclerosis).

PRIOR, J. T., and JONES, D. D.: Am. J. Path., *28*, 937, 1952 (Arteriosclerosis in Infancy).

ROSENFELD, L.: Am. J. Clin. Met., *5*, 286, 1957 (Genesis Arteriosclerosis).

SILBERT, S., *et al.*: J.A.M.A., *151*, 1176, 1953 (Mönckeberg's Sclerosis).

Inflammations

ALLEN, E. V., BARKER, N. W., and HINES, E. A., JR.: *Peripheral Vascular Diseases*, Philadelphia, W. B. Saunders Co., p. 403, 1946 (Thromboangiitis Obliterans).

BAGGENSTOSS, A. H., *et al.:* Am. J. Path., *27*, 537, 1951 (Cortisone and Periarteris Nodosa).

BAKER, G., and MASSELL, T. B.: Angiology, *7*, 319, 1956 (Thromboangiitis Obliterans).

BURT, C. C.: Postgrad. M. J., *32*, 232, 1956 (Thromboangiitis Obliterans),

CARDELL, D. S., and HANLEY, T.: J. Path. & Bact., *63*, 587, 1951 (Autopsies in Temporal Arteritis).

CHURG, J., and STRAUSS, L.: Am. J. Path., *27*, 277, 1951 (Allergic Angiitis and Periarteritis Nodosa).

COHEN, M. B.: Am. J. Surg., *80*, 44, 1950 (Treatment Thrombophlebitis).

CROSBY, R. C., and WADSWORTH, R. C.: A. M. A. Arch. Int. Med., *81*, 431, 1948 (Review Temporal Arteritis).

DENHAM, S. W.: A. M. A. Arch. Path., *51*, 661, 1951 (Syphilis Coronary Artery).

EHRENREICH, T., and OLMSTEAD, E. V.: A. M. A. Arch. Path., *52*, 145, 1951 (Malignant Hypertension Following Cortisone in Periarteritis Nodosa).

FAGER, D. B., *et al.:* J. Pediat., *39*, 65, 1951 (Polyarteritis Nodosa in Infancy).

FARMER, D. A., and SMITHWICK, R. H.: Angiology, *1*, 291, 1950 (Thromboembolic Disease).

FISHER, R. L., *et al.:* Angiology, *2*, 132, 1951 (Thromboangiitis Obliterans in Women).

FOWLER, N. O., JR.: Angiology, *1*, 257, 1950 (Thromboembolism).

GRIFFITH, G. C., and VURAL, I. L.: Circulation, *3*, 481, 1951 (Polyarteritis Nodosa—17 Cases).

HARTZ, P. H.: Am. J. Clin. Path., *14*, 34, 1944 (Filariasis).

HEPTINSTALL, R. M., *et al.:* J. Path. and Bact., *67*, 507, 1954 (Giant Cell Arteritis).

HERBUT, P. A., and PRICE, A. H.: A. M. A. Arch. Path., *39*, 274, 1945 (Periarteritis Nodosa of Renal Arteries).

HUEPER, W. C.: A. M. A. Arch. Path., *38*, 278, 1944 (Thromboangiitis Obliterans).

JERNSTROM, P., and STASNEY, J.: J. A. M. A., *148*, 544, 1952 (Ulcerative Enteritis and Polyarteritis).

KIMMELSTIEL, P., *et al.:* A. M. A. Arch. Path., *54*, 157, 1952 (Granulomatous Giant Cell Arteritis).

KING, B. G.: Ann. Int. Med., *32*, 466, 1950 (Clinical Diagnosis Periarteritis Nodosa).

KOBERNICK, S. D.: Am. J. M. Sci., *224*, 329, 1952 (Experimental Periarteritis Nodosa).

KRAMER, D. W.: *Peripheral Vascular Diseases*, Philadelphia, F. A. Davis Co., p. 126, 1948 (Nonspecific Arteritis).

LOGAN, P. J., *et al.:* J. Obst. & Gynaec. Brit. Emp., *58*, 433, 1951 (Thrombophlebitis in Pregnancy).

MARSHALL, W.: Am. J. Surg., *82*, 448, 1951 (Thromboangiitis Obliterans).

MARTORELL, F.: Angiology, *3*, 271, 1952 (Thromboangiitis Obliterans in Brothers).

MCNEIL, N. F., *et al.:* Ann. Int. Med., *37*, 1253, 1952 (Polyarteritis Nodosa and Deafness).

MESSINGER, W. J., *et al.:* Am. J. Med., *6*, 168, 1949 (Thromboangiitis Obliterans).

MONTGOMERY, B. M., *et al.:* Ann. Int. Med., *37*, 689, 1952 (Syphilitic Heart Disease).

NEUMANN, M. A.: Am. J. Path., *28*, 919, 1952 (Tuberculous Vasculitis).

O'BRIEN, J. F., *et al.:* Br. J. Vener. Dis., *31*, 74, 1955 (578 Cases Syphilis).

OCHSNER, A., *et al.:* J. A. M. A., *144*, 831, 1950 (Venous Thrombosis).

OCHSNER, A., and DEBAKEY, M.: J. A. M. A., *139*, 423, 1949 (Postphlebitic Sequelæ).

REIMANN, H. A., PRICE, A. H., and HERBUT, P. A.: J. A. M. A., *122*, 274, 1943 (Trichinosis and Periarteritis Nodosa).

RICH, C., JR., and WEBSTER, B.: Am. Heart J., *43*, 321, 1952 (Uncomplicated Syphilitic Aortitis).

SAWITZ, W. G.: *Medical Parasitology*, New York, The Blakiston Co., p. 94, 1950 (Filariasis).

SIMON, R.: Med. Times, *85*, 275, 1957 (Periarteritis Nodosa).

VINTHER-PAULSEN, N.: Angiology, *3*, 194, 1952 (Migratory Phlebitis).

WAUGH, D.: Am. J. Path., *28*, 437, 1952 (Penicillin Arteritis).

WISHART, J. H., and PETERSON, L. J.: J. A. M. A., *133*, 539, 1947 (Pylephlebitis).

ZEEK, P. M.: Am. J. Clin. Path., *22*, 777, 1952 (Critical Review Periarteritis Nodosa).

Physical Disturbances

ADAMS, H. D.: Surg., Gynec. & Obst., *92*, 693, 1951 (Cirsoid Aneurysms).

ALLEN, E. V., BARKER, N. W., and HINES, E. A., JR.: *Peripheral Vascular Disease*, Philadelphia, W. B. Saunders Co., 1946.

BACHHUBER, T. E., and LALICH, J. J.: A.M.A. Arch. Path., *59*, 247, 1955 (Sweet Pea Meal, Rat Aortas).

BEAN, W. B., and PONSETI, I. V.: Circulation, *12*, 185, 1955 (Diet and Dissecting Aneurysm).

BLADES, B., *et al.:* Circulation, *2*, 565, 1950 (Pulmonary Artery Aneurysms).

BLAIN III, A., *et al.:* Surgery, *29*, 387, 1951 (Raynaud's Disease).

DeBakey, M. E., and Simeone, F. A.: Ann. Surg., *123*, 534, 1946 (Arterial Injuries).
de la Pena, A., and Reig, J.: J. Internat. Coll. Surg., *16*, 419, 1951 (Phleboliths).
Duff, R. S.: Br. J. Clin. Pract., *10*, 855, 1956 (Raynaud's Disease).
Elkin, D. C.: Ann. Surg., *123*, 591, 1946 (Cirsoid Aneurysm).
Fields, A.: Ann. Western Med. & Surg., *6*, 162 and 441, 1952 (Diagnosis Varicose Veins) and Am. Pract., *2*, 686, 1951 (Varicose Ulcer).
Fisher, H. W.: Med Times, *85*, 530, 1957 (Dissecting Aneurysm).
Gardner, C. E., Jr.: Am. J. Surg., *77*, 181, 1949 (Arterial Injuries).
Gerbode, F., et al.: Surgery, *32*, 259, 1952 (Arteriovenous Fistulas).
Gold, H.: Canad. M. A. J., *65*, 427, 1951 (Abdominal Aortic Aneurysm).
Gordon, B. S., et al.: Am. Heart J., *44*, 51, 1952 (Vertebro-arteriovenous Aneurysms).
Gore, I., and Seiwert, V. J.: A. M. A. Arch. Path., *53*, 121 and 142, 1952 (Dissecting Aortic Aneurysm).
Hammer, J. M., et al.: J. Internat. Coll. Surg., *16*, 289, 1951 (Fistula Carotid Artery and Internal Jugular Vein).
Hankins, J. R., and Yeager, G. H.: Surgery, *40*, 747, 1956 (Mycotic Aneurysm).
Heckler, G. B., and Tikellis, I. J.: J. A. M. A., *150*, 1301, 1952 (Acquired Arteriovenous Fistula and Endocarditis).
Heuper, W. C.: A. M. A. Arch. Path., *38*, 283, 1944 (Raynaud's Disease).
Hudson, C. L., and Murray, J. B.: J. A. M. A., *141*, 130, 1949 (Typhoid Infection Arteriovenous Aneurysm).
Jackson, A., et al.: J. A. M. A., *150*, 1106, 1952 (Aortic Aneurysm into Superior Vena Cava).
Jahsman, W. E.: Ann. Int. Med., *21*, 669, 1944 (Chylothorax).
Janes, J. M., and Ivins, J. C.: Surgery, *29*, 398, 1951 (Popliteal Aneurysms).
Javett, S. N., and Kahn, E.: A. M. A. Arch. Dis. Child., *27*, 294, 1952 (Mycotic Aortic Aneurysm).
Kirby, C. K., et al.: Ann. Surg., *130*, 913, 1949 (Aneurysm Common Carotid Artery).
Lalich, J. J.: A.M.A. Arch. Path., *61*, 520, 1956 (Beta Amino-propionitrile and Aortic Rupture).
Lazarus, J. A., and Marks, M. S.: J. Urol., *52*, 199, 1944 (Aneurysm Renal Artery).
Levinson, D. C., et al.: Circulation, *1*, 360, 1950 (Dissecting Aneurysm of the Aorta).
Lindskog, G. E., et al.: Ann. Surg., *132*, 591, 1950 (Pulmonary Arteriovenous Aneurysm).
Lowenberg, E. L.: Virginia Med. Monthly, *79*, 351, 1952 (Lymphedema).
Maniglia, R., and Gregory, J. E.: A. M. A. Arch. Path., *54*, 298, 1952 (Arteriosclerotic Aortic Aneurysm).
McCloskey, J. F., and Chu, P. T.: A. M. A. Arch. Path., *52*, 132, 1951 (Dissecting Aortic Aneurysm).
McCook, W. W.: J. Thoracic Surg., *23*, 299, 1952 (Arteriovenous Fistula Aortic Arch).
McIntire, F. T., and Sykes, E. M., Jr.: Ann. Int. Med., *30*, 925, 1949 (Superior Vena Cava Syndrome).
McSwain, B., and Diveley, W.: Southern Surg., *16*, 501, 1950 (Arterial Aneurysms).
Mitchell, R. G., and Claireaux, A. E.: A. M. A. Arch. Dis. Child., *27*, 147, 1952 (Aortic Aneurysm).
Palmer, T. H.: New England J. Med., *243*, 989, 1950 (Splenic Artery Aneurysms).
Parkhurst, G. F., and Decker, J. P.: Am. J. Path., *31*, 821, 1955 (Mycotic Aneurysm Aorta)
Pemberton, J. deJ., et al.: Ann. Surg., *123*, 580, 1946 (Fistula Aorta and Inferior Vena Cava).
Prioleau, W. H.: J. A. M. A., *149*, 922, 1952 (Treatment Varicose Veins).
Ravell, S. T. R., Jr.: Ann. Int. Med., *22*, 431, 1951 (Mycotic Aneurysms).
Reynolds, R. P., et al.: J. A. M. A., *141*, 841, 1949 (Uterine Arteriovenous Aneurysm).
Rukstinat, G. J.: J. A. M. A., *149*, 1129, 1952 (Coronary Artery Aneurysms).
Scott, V.: Am. J. Syph., *28*, 682, 1944 (Abdominal Aneurysms).
Shallow, T. A., Herbut, P. A., and Wagner, F. E., Jr.: Surgery, *19*, 177, 1946, (Aneurysm Pancreaticoduodenal Artery).
Silver, G. B., and Kahn, J. W.: Ann. Int. Med., *36*, 888, 1952 (Syphilitic Popliteal Aneurysm).
Shnider, B. I., and Cotsonas, N. J.: Am. J. Med., *16*, 246, 1954 (Mycotic Aneurysm).
Stalker, L. K.: Am. J. Surg., *84*, 195, 1952 (Treatment Varicose Veins).
Temple, L. J.: J. Thoracic Surg., *19*, 412, 1950 (Aneurysm Subclavian Artery).
Viar, W. N., and Lombardo, T. A.: Circulation, *5*, 287, 1952 (Aneurysm Aorta into Inferior Vena Cava).
Wagner, F. B., Jr., and Herbut, P. A.: Am. J. Surg., *78*, 876, 1949 (Etiology Varicose Veins).
Walker, D. G., and Wirtschafter, Z. T.: A.M.A. Arch. Path., *61*, 125, 1956 (Aorta in Lathyrism).

Tumors

AEGERTER, E. E., and PEALE, A. R.: A. M. A. Arch. Path., *34*, 413, 1942 (Kaposi's Sarcoma)

ANDREWS, G. C., *et al.*: Am. J. Roentgenol., *67*, 273, 1952 (Treatment Angiomas).

AQUINO, J. A.: A.M.A. Arch. Otolar., *65*, 263, 1957 (Glomus Jugulore Tumors).

BROWN, J. B., and FRYER, M. E.: A. M. A. Arch. Surg., *65*, 417, 1952 (Treatment Hemangiomas).

CAMPBELL, J. L., JR.: J. Urol., *62*, 80, 1949 (Hereditary Hemorrhagic Telangiectasia).

DAWSON, E. K.: Edinburgh M. J., *65*, 655, 1948 (Sclerosing Angioma).

FISHER, E. R., *et al.*: Am. J. Path., *28*, 653, 1952 (Hemangiopericytoma).

GROSS, R. E., and WOLBACH, S. B.: Am. J. Path., *19*, 533, 1943 (Sclerosing Hemangioma).

KINKADE, J. M.: Ann. Otol., Rhin. & Laryng., *58*, 159, 1949 (Angiosarcoma).

KUSHLAN, S. D.: Gastroenterology, *7*, 199, 1946 (Hereditary Hemorrhagic Telangiectasia).

LEMMER, K. E.: A. M. A. Arch. Surg., *57*, 531, 1948 (Glomus Tumors).

McCARTHY, W. D., and PACK, G. T.: Surg., Gynec. & Obst., *91*, 465, 1950 (Malignant Vascular Tumors).

MITCHEL, N., and FEDER, I. A.: Ann. Int. Med., *31*, 324, 1949 (Kaposi's Sarcoma).

MURRAY, M. R., and STOUT, A. P.: Am. J. Path., *18*, 183, 1942 (Glomus Tumor).

PACK, G. T., and MILLER, T. R.: Angiology, *1*, 405, 1950 (Hemangiomas).

RIVEROS, M., and PACK, G. T.: Ann. Surg., *133*, 394, 1951 (Glomus Tumor).

STADLER, H. E., and JOHNSON, T. W.: J. Pediat., *41*, 100, 1952 (Hydroma).

STEWART, F. W., and TREVES, N.: Cancer, *1*, 64, 1948 (Lymphangiosarcoma).

STOUT, A. P.: Ann. Surg., *118*, 445, 1943 (Hemangioendothelioma).

————————: Cancer, *2*, 1027, 1949 (Hemangiopericytoma).

TEDESCHI, C. G., *et al.*: A. M. A. Arch. Path., *43*, 335, 1947 (Kaposi's Visceral Disease).

WATSON, W. L., and McCARTHY, W. D.: Surg., Gynec. & Obst., *71*, 569, 1940 (Hemangioma and Lymphangioma).

Chapter

10

Upper Respiratory System

PATHOLOGIC PHYSIOLOGY

Fred Harbert

THE *function* of the *nose* is to warm, moisten, and filter inspired air at an approximate rate of 500 cubic feet in 24 hours (Fabricant). On inspiration, air courses high in the nasal vault where it is exposed to olfactory epithelium. This epithelium is unique in that its submucosal lymphatics communicate with the subarachnoid space (Walls). During respiration there is a negligible exchange of air between nose and sinuses. The mucosa is covered by a thin film of mucus which acts as a moveable blanket propelled by cilia. The rate of movement is about 5 mm. per minute and it takes from 5 to 10 minutes for a particle deposited on the mucus blanket to propelled to the nasopharynx. The cilia in *sinuses* beat toward the ostea. If the lining of a sinus is exenterated it regenerates, complete with cilia, in about 9 months. Ciliary activity is suspended by cold, heat, drying, and changes in pH or tonicity. The normal pH varies from 5.5 to 6.5 but shifts to the alkaline side in the presence of infection.

Cilia can only function efficiently when covered with a thin film of mucus. *Abnormally*, when a sinus becomes filled with fluid, they are ineffective. To restore function the fluid must be removed by irrigation in subacute cases or an artificial window in chronic cases. The vestibule is lined by squamous epithelium and protected by vibrissæ. The widespread habit of deep wiping with tissue on a finger tip often causes squamous metaplasia of the epithelium of the septum and inferior turbinate above the vestibule with resultant bleeding and crust formation. When an air passage is closed there is metaplasia to nonciliated epithelium and an increase in goblet cells. This also occurs when the nasal passages are not used for respiration as after laryngectomy.

The *defenses* of the upper respiratory tract may be listed as follows: (1) protective mucous barrier, (2) ciliary action, (3) phagocytosis, (4) lysozyme fermentation, (5) local inflammation, (6) natural immunity, and (7) acquired immunity. The *size* of *particles* in inspired air is important in determining site of deposition. Particles greater than 12 microns are deposited in the nose while those of 0.1 to 4 microns tend to lodge in the bronchioles and alveoli (Walls). Inhaled particles are usually in droplet form and considerably larger than the above, resulting in their deposition primarily in the nose. *Crystalloids* pass readily through the mucosa but colloids are only partially absorbed. *Bacteria* and *viruses* must establish themselves on the surface before they can penetrate.

Among *laboratory tests* usually employed, cytologic examination of stained smears is of value. A high percentage of eosinophils indicates

(408)

allergy while a preponderance of neutrophilis is characteristic of an acute infection. In the diagnosis of neoplasms, cytologic studies may be used but biopsy of suspicious areas is usually preferable. In the common cold there are mainly degenerative changes characterized by loss of cilia, desquamation of superficial cells, and pyknosis. Normally, the nose and sinuses are free of pathogenic organisms. In the presence of infection smear, culture, and sensitivity tests will reveal the offending organisms and indicate effective therapy.

CONGENITAL ANOMALIES

Orientation.—An understanding of the developmental malformations of the nose, paranasal sinuses, and nasopharynx can be acquired only if the intricate embryology is appreciated. It will thus behoove the reader to refresh his memory on this phase of the topic. Further, since the nose, mouth, and pharynx develop in part from common structures, abnormalities of one of these structures are often associated with abnormalities of the other.

Nose.—Congenital anomalies of the nose occur most commonly along the lines of fusion of the various tissues (Keogh). They may consist of the following: complete *absence* of the nose, *double* nose, *bifid tip*, *humped* nose, *depressed* nose, single or double *lateral cleft* between the nose and the mouth (harelip and cleft palate), single or double *cleft* between the *nose* and *cheek* (continuation of harelip and cleft palate), *median cleft* between the nose and mouth (median harelip and cleft palate), *flattened nostrils* (associated with harelip), exposure of *lower* edge of *septum* (in harelip), *perforations* in *septum*, *absence* of *septum*, *deflection* of *septum*, *atresia* of external or posterior nares, and *cysts*. Congenital cysts of the nose may consist of fissural cysts, dermoid cysts, and encephalomeningomyeloceles.

Fissural cysts are cysts developing along the lines of fusion of the various processes (Rosenberger). They occur principally in two locations—facial cleft and incisive canal. Cysts of the *facial cleft* are found in the lateral nasal cleft in the area of union of the premaxilla and maxilla. They enlarge superiorly and anteriorly, producing a fluctuant tumor that obliterates the nasofacial fold and fills the superior lateral tissues. Cysts of the *incisive canal* occur at the junction of the nasal septum and floor about 2 cm. posterior to the anterior nares and may protrude into the nose or the mouth. The *contents* of fissural cysts are mucoid and the *lining* consists of ciliated epithelial cells. *Treatment* of choice is surgical excision.

Dermoid cysts originate at the bridge of the nose as a result of epidermal inclusions between the fissural lines of closure. Most are apparent at or shortly after birth but a few may not be noted until later in life. They are usually *located* at the bridge of the nose but they may be found at any point between the bridge and the tip with the stalk, nevertheless, extending to the point of origin. They may measure as much as 2 or 3 cm. in diameter. They are *filled* with cheesy material, may harbor hair, and are lined with squamous epithelium containing the usual epidermal appendages. If left alone, they have a tendency to break down and produce draining sinuses. *Treatment* consists of surgical excision.

Encephalomeningomyeloceles, also known as encephaloceles, are herniations of the meninges or meninges and brain tissue through the skull. In the region of the nose the herniations occur as a result of faulty fusion of the cranial fissures. They may be *located* at the base of the nose and protrude beneath the skin, but, more commonly, they are found internally protruding into the nasal cavity in the sphenopharyngeal area. *Path-ologically* they are rounded or polypoid cystic swellings of varying sizes that have a tendency to ulcerate, discharge cerebrospinal fluid, and become infected. In addition, those protruding into the nasal cavity also produce obstruction of the respiratory tract. *Treatment* is surgical excision. Prior to the era of antibiotics, the *prognosis* was poor for the mortality from postoperative meningitis was high. Now the outlook is good.

Sinuses.—Congenital abnormalities of the paranasal sinuses are relatively unimportant. They may consist of complete absence of development, increase in size, decrease in size, variations from the normal shape, variations in number of air sacs (as in the ethmoid sinuses), and abnormalities in location and size of the ostia. The last-mentioned may be important in connection with the maxillary sinuses where abnormally located and small ostia may impede drainage and predispose to inflammation.

DEGENERATIONS

Degenerations of the epithelium, blood vessels, connective tissue, bone, and other tissues of the nose and sinuses are prevalent but they occur only in conjunction with other disease processes such as inflammations, physical disturbances, and tumors. They will not, therefore, be discussed separately.

INFLAMMATIONS

Orientation.—Inflammation of the nose is called *rhinitis* and inflammation of the paranasal sinuses is known as *sinusitis*. The infections are common, important, and quite varied. They may be considered under the following headings: acute nonspecific rhinitis and sinusitis, chronic nonspecific rhinitis and sinusitis, allergic rhinitis and sinusitis, atrophic rhinitis, rhinitis caseosa, syphilis, tuberculosis, Boeck's sarcoid, scleroma, leprosy, glanders, fungous rhinitis, and malignant granuloma.

Acute Nonspecific Rhinitis and Sinusitis.—Acute nonspecific rhinitis is also known as the common cold, acute coryza, and catarrh. It may start in the nose (and spread downward) or the pharynx or larynx (and spread in either direction) (Bloomfield). Acute nonspecific sinusitis is generally a complication of acute nonspecific rhinitis. The common cold outnumbers by far all other acute disease processes in man. The *causes* are predisposing and precipitating. The most important single *predisposing factor* is impairment of ciliary action. This occurs as a result of improper ventilation of the nasal passages, rapid alterations in temperature, changes in pH of the mucous membrane, and inadequate supply of moisture. The initial *precipitating factor* is a virus that may be grown on chorioallantoic membranes and may be transmitted to ferrets, monkeys, and man. The viral infection is short-lived, lasting not more than two or three days. Colds that continue beyond this period are due to superimposed bacterial invasion, especially streptococcic. The common cold is endemic, epidemic, and pandemic. In the northern hemisphere it is particularly prevalent in winter and early spring.

Pathologically the initial changes in the mucosa consist of redness, dullness, and dryness. Subsequently the mucosa becomes thickened and the surface becomes covered with watery or purulent secretion. *Histologically* the epithelial cells disclose hyperactivity in the form of excessive secretion of mucus which eventually leads to degeneration and destruction of the cells. When the latter is advanced, the epithelium may be completely denuded in focal areas. The basement membrane may be prominent while the underlying submucosa discloses congestion, edema, and varying degrees of neutrophilic, eosinophilic, plasma cell, and lymphocytic infiltration. The submucosal glands likewise disclose hyperactivity of the lining epithelial cells and the lumens of these glands may become distended with mucus. In a period of five to seven days, the congestion and edema decrease, the leukocytes either disintegrate or wander off, the epithelium regenerates, and the structures return to normal.

The *complications* of the common cold are bronchitis, sinusitis, and otitis media. Of these, the most common and most important is *acute sinusitis*. Although any and all of the sinuses may be affected, the most commonly involved are the maxillary sinuses. The pathologic changes are identical with those found in the nasal mucosa. When the draining ostium becomes occluded, mucus accumulates under pressure and forms what is known as a *mucocele*. Other complications of sinusitis are osteomyelitis, meningitis, intracranial abscess, and cavernous sinus thrombosis. The *clinical manifestations* may be (1) *general* consisting of malaise, chilliness, dullness, aching, fever, and leukopenia and (2) *local* consisting of sneezing, burning sensation, dryness, discomfort, and discharge. When the sinuses become involved there are, in addition, headache, nasal voice, local pain, and sometimes swelling of the skin covering the affected sinuses. The *diagnosis* is arrived at from the patient's symptoms and the local appearance of the mucosa. *Treatment* is unsatisfactory. Specific antiviral medicines are, at present, unknown, while antibiotics and chemotherapeutic agents, at most, only shorten the bacterial infection by a day or two. The *course* of the disease is usually limited to about a week unless complications arise.

Chronic Nonspecific Rhinitis and Sinusitis.—This condition represents a continuation of the acute infection just described. The *cause* is bacterial infection in which allergy may play a role. *Pathologically* the disturbance may be unilateral or bilateral. The mucosa is diffusely or irregularly thickened to a degree that it may actually form polypoid projections. It is gray, firm, and may or may not be covered with an exudate. *Histologically* the epithelium may be hyperplastic, ulcerated, or metaplastic (transformed to a stratified squamous cell type). The basement membrane is thick and the submucosa discloses congestion, edema, fibrosis, and a leukocytic infiltration predominating in plasma cells, lymphocytes, and monocytes. The submucosal glands may show changes similar to those seen in the mucosal epithelium. Frequently they become cystic as a result of accumulation of mucus. The chief *clinical manifestations* are those of obstruction to the airway, nasal voice, and pain over the sinuses. The *morbidity* is high for the infection persists and tends to recur.

Allergic Rhinitis and Sinusitis.—Although allergic reactions of mucosa of the nose are generally associated with similar reactions of the mucosa of the sinuses, it is the nasal lesions that usually draw attention and the condition is thus frequently referred to simply as allergic rhinitis. Some of the *synonyms* are vasomotor rhinitis, perennial hay fever, and atopic coryza (Stoesser). The condition *occurs* at all ages from infancy to old age. The ultimate *cause* is an allergen or a group of allergens consisting essentially of the following: (1) inhalants—pollens or spores of molds occurring seasonally (referred to as hay fever), animal danders, orris root, wool, insecticides, cotton linters, and house dust, (2) foods—milk, eggs, wheat, fish, nuts, vegetables, and some fruits, (3) drugs—coal tar derivatives, salicylates, iodides, bromides, argyrol, sulfonamide, etc., (4) physical agents—heat, sunlight, and cold, and (5) bacteria—especially protein disintegration products (Criep).

Pathologically the lesions are usually bilateral. The turbinates are swollen; the mucosa is bluish gray and boggy; the nasal cavities are reduced in size, and there may be few or many mucosal polyps filling the nasal cavities. In some cases the mucosal surfaces appear rather dry while in others they are covered with an abundant watery, mucoid, or even purulent secretion. The changes in the mucosa of the sinuses are similar to those in the nasal passages. *Histologically* the epithelium frequently discloses an agglutination or complete disappearance of the cilia. It may be hyperplastic, atrophic, ulcerated, or metaplastic. The basement membrane, as a rule, is greatly thickened, hyalinized, eosinophilic, and prominent. The submucosa reveals congestion, edema, fibrosis, and a diffuse permeation with leukocytes chief among which are eosinophils. Neutrophils, lymphocytes, plasma cells, and monocytes are likewise present but are generally evident in lesser numbers. The changes in the submucosal glandular epithelium are similar to those in the covering epithelium. The lumens of the glands may be filled and distended with mucus.

The *complications* of allergic rhinitis and sinusitis are (1) local obstruction of the air passages and sinus cavities and (2) other manifestations of allergy, chiefly in the form of asthma and eczema. In some cases there are also profound emotional disturbances culminating in loss of appetite, loss of sleep, interference in general efficiency, and a universal sense of ill-being. *Clinically* the most common symptom is recurrent perennial nasal obstruction. Associated with this are generally watery nasal secretions, postnasal discharge, sneezing, coughing, loss of sense of taste and smell, headache, fatigue, etc. (Criep). As corroborative evidence of the allergic nature of the condition, one may find eosinophilia of the peripheral blood and nasal secretions. Roentgenograms of the sinuses frequently disclose clouding. The *diagnosis* of allergic rhinitis and sinusitis is generally arrived at from a family history of allergy, other manifestations of allergy, skin tests with specific allergens, and response to antihistaminic drugs and epinephrine. *Treatment* consists of elimination of the cause (if this can be determined), local topical applications, surgical interference, and psychotherapy. The *prognosis* is guarded for regardless of what treatment is carried out the condition tends to recur.

Atrophic Rhinitis.—Atrophic rhinitis has also been called ozena, rhinitis sicca, atrophic catarrh, fetid coryza, sclerotic rhinitis, and "stink nose." The condition is *characterized by* atrophic changes in the nasal mucosa and turbinates, abnormal roominess of the nasal passages, and a mucopurulent discharge which drys, crusts, and produces a characteristic odor (Cullom). The disorder usually *starts* before twelve years of age and is five times as common in females as it is in males. The *cause* of atrophic rhinitis is still undetermined. Some of the many etiologic factors that have been suggested are heredity, anatomic variations in the nasal passages, rhinitis in childhood (with vascular occlusion), osteitis, disease of the paranasal sinuses, a deficiency state, infection with specific bacteria, endocrine disturbances, etc. *Histologically* the important changes consist of the following: (1) replacement of the ciliated epithelium with stratified squamous epithelium that occasionally shows cornification, (2) disappearance or thickening and collagenization of the basement membrane, (3) diffuse submucosal increase of fibrous tissue, (4) atrophy and disappearance of the submucosal glands, (5) intimal proliferation, hyalinization, and obliteration of the submucosal vessels, and (6) varying degrees of plasma cells and lymphocytic infiltration. The chief *clinical manifestations* consist of offensive odor, nasal obstruction (due to pus formation), and occasionally headache. The *diagnosis* is arrived at from the history and local appearance of the mucosa. *Treatment* consists of local cleanliness in the form of intranasal sprays with removal of the crusts. Other efforts to restore the mucosa to normal have been of little or no avail.

Rhinitis Caseosa.—Rhinitis caseosa is a rare type of unilateral nasal disorder *characterized by* (1) an accumulation of extremely offensive, soft, cheese-like material in the nose and sinuses, (2) presence of a seropurulent discharge from the sinuses, and (3) ultimate external and internal deformity of the nose (Myersburg). It occurs at all ages with a peak *incidence* in the third and fourth decades, has no predilection for either sex, and is most common in continental Europe. The *cause* is unknown. It has been considered to be (1) nasal erysipelas, (2) a form of scrofula (tuberculosis), (3) a specific bacterial infection, (4) a cholesteatoma, (5) the result of a foreign body, (6) necrosis of polyps, and (7) secondary infection and degeneration to anything that causes an interference with drainage of the sinuses and nose. *Pathologically* the cheesy material is composed of debris, cholesterol crystals, and necrotic bits of mucosa containing foreign body giant cells. The cavity is devoid of an epithelial surface (Eggston and Wolff). The lining is composed of dense fibrous tissue containing lymphocytes and plasma cells. *Treatment* consists of complete removal of the material followed by local cleanliness. The *prognosis* is excellent.

Syphilis.—While the topic of syphilis is discussed in the section on the Skin, Chapter 39 (p. 1331), its local manifestations in the nose may be mentioned here briefly. The condition may be acquired or congenital (Scott-Brown). *Acquired nasal syphilis* may exist in the primary, secondary, or tertiary stages of the disease. The *primary stage* consists of the chancre and constitutes less than 1 per cent of all extragenital sores. It is usually located just within the alae or on the lower part of the septum and exists as a round or oval, red, flattened ulcer with an over-all diameter of less than 2 cm. (Ballenger). The *second stage* is manifested as a rhinitis with superficial ulceration. The *tertiary stage* is the most common and usually consists of the gumma. The lesion affects the mucous membrane, periosteum, and bone. It is generally located on the nasal septum but may also affect other portions of the nasal cavity. Early, the area appears as a local swelling covered by a reddened mucosa. Later it breaks down, ulcerates, and even perforates the bones contacted. When the nasal support is lost, the nose collapses. *Congenital nasal syphilis* appears within the first two to six weeks after birth, consists of lesions similar to the second stage of acquired syphilis, and manifests itself mainly in the form of snuffles. Congenital lesions analogous to the tertiary stage of acquired syphilis usually become manifested about the time of puberty. Lesions corresponding to the chancre do not occur.

Tuberculosis.—Tuberculosis of the upper respiratory system is almost always *secondary* to pulmonary tuberculosis. Although it may affect the nose, sinuses, and nasopharynx, it has been determined from studies at autopsy that *nasopharyngeal* tuberculosis is the most common, being found in as high as 80 per cent of all patients dying of the pulmonary condition (Szanto and Hollander). In half of these the nasopharyngeal *lesions* exist in the form of irregular, ovoid, superficial ulcers with yellowish-gray bases and undermined edges, while in the remaining half they are discoverable only by microscopic examination. In most instances, the disease of the upper respiratory system produces no *symptoms* or at least is overshadowed by the disorder in the lungs. In others it may produce nasal discharge, nasal or sinus discomfort, and nasal obstruction.

Boeck's Sarcoid.—Boeck's sarcoid is usually a widespread systemic disorder that affects primarily the reticulo-endothelial system (p. 501). In the nose the lesions exist as nodules in the mucosa and vestibule (Scott-Brown). Histologically they are composed of small, hard tubercles.

Scleroma.—Scleroma is a specific, infectious, granulomatous disease affecting the nose, pharynx, larynx, trachea, and bronchi. Originally the disorder was called rhinoscleroma (Gr. = nose + hard swelling) but because the disorder is not limited to the nose the name has been recently changed to scleroma. When first described, scleroma was limited to Eastern Europe but now it is known to be worldwide in *distribution* (Kline and Brody). It is more common in females than in males and although it may occur at any age from the second decade on, it is most frequent in the third decade of life. Predisposing *causes* appear to be overcrowding, vitamin deficiency, and lack of local hygiene. Although the precipitating cause is still questioned by some observers, most authors agree that *Klebsiella rhinoscleromatis* (von Frisch bacillus) is probably the causative organism. This is a gram-negative encapsulated rod that belongs to the Friedländer's group of organisms. It is readily grown on artificial media but its experimental transfer to man and laboratory animals fails to produce the disease.

Pathologically the disorder usually begins in the nasal septum or alæ and progresses by extension to involve the nasopharynx, larynx, trachea, bronchi, and even the lip, tongue, uvula, soft palate, orbit, lacrimal passages, eustachian tubes, and tympanic cavity (Kline and Brody). Grossly *four stages* are identifiable—(1) catarrhal—consisting of mucosal atrophy and crusting and of diffuse submucosal thickening and induration, (2) localized nodular—developing as circumscribed nodules of varying sizes with a tendency to coalescence, (3) diffuse nodular—comprising a progression of the second stage, and (4) cicatricial—constituting a terminal replacement with fibrous tissue. *Histologically* the initial lesion consists of dilatation of the capillaries, edema of the stroma, and a diffuse infiltration with eosinophils, neutrophils, plasma cells, lymphocytes, and monocytes. Gradually the monocytes increase in size to form foam cells that are called Mikulicz cells (Fig. 168*A*). These are large, sharply circumscribed cells with small nuclei and reticulated or finely vacuolated cytoplasm that contains the causative organisms. Older lesions show (1) increasing numbers of Russell bodies (round hyaline structures that measure 20 to 40 microns in diameter and that probably develop from plasma cells) (Fig. 168*B*), (2) increasing collagen deposition, (3) decreasing leukocytic infiltration, and (4) thrombosis and hyalinization of the vessels.

The *complications* consist of secondary infection and asphyxia. The *clinical manifestations* are those of obstruction and impairment of function of the upper respiratory system. They may consist of epistaxis, nasal discharge, hoarseness, cough, dyspnea, and asphyxia. The *diagnosis* is made from the appearance of the lesions (location, gross appearance, and biopsy) together with isolation of the causative organism. *Treatment* has been most varied consisting of the use of a wide variety of medicines, surgical excision, electric destruction, irradiation, and more recently of the administration of antibiotics and chemotherapeutic agents. The *prognosis* is guarded for, despite treatment, the condition usually recurs and progresses.

Leprosy.—Leprosy is a specific granulomatous disease of an infectious nature affecting principally the skin, peripheral nerves, and mucous membranes and occurring endemically in most parts of the world but being especially prevalent in tropical and subtropical countries. Although the condition is usually diagnosed in adults, it has been clearly demonstrated that the *initial infection* occurs in children and is well established before the age of ten years (Elliott). The cause is *Mycobacterium lepræ*. This is

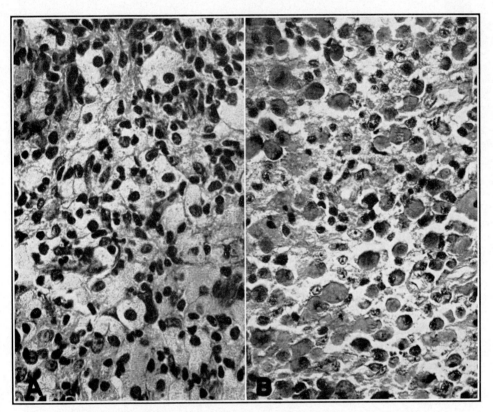

Fig. 168.—Scleroma showing *A*, many large rounded and polyhedral Mikulicz (foam) cells and *B*, numerous Russell bodies. × 400.

a gram-positive, slightly curved, often beaded, acid-fast organism that morphologically resembles *Mycobacterium tuberculosis*. It has not been successfully cultivated on artificial media and when injected into experimental animals has been incapable of reproducing the disease. Its route of entrance into the body has not been definitely determined although some authors believe that the mucosa of the upper respiratory system may serve as a portal of entry.

Pathologically the lesions are essentially of two types—lepromatous and tuberculoid (Zeluff and Hayes). *Lepromatous* leprosy (also referred to as nodular leprosy) initiates as macules and then indurated nodules and appears on the forehead, nose, face, ears, and limbs (especially digits). The *lesions* about the face result in furrowed thickenings with gross disfigurement, producing an appearance that has been likened to that of a lion. Nodular and ulcerating lesions appear early in the mucosa of the nose, pharynx, and larynx, and granulomatous lesions are also found in the spleen, bone marrow, liver, and adrenals. In the respiratory system the process has

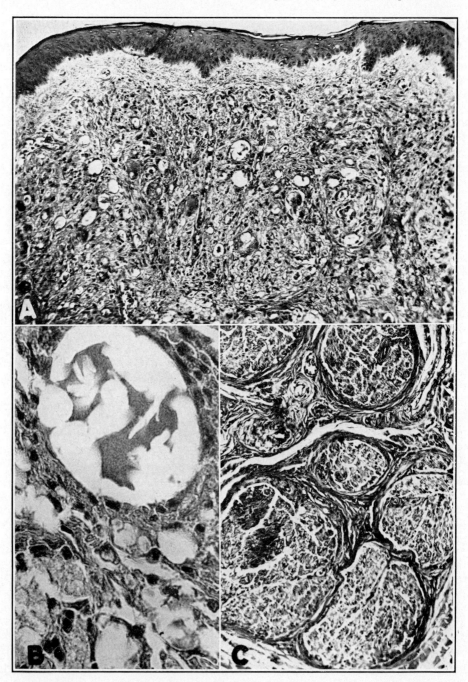

FIG. 169.—Leprosy showing *A*, fairly well-defined tubercles in the dermis.   × 100, *B*, leprosy (foam) cells and a globus.   × 400, and *C*, perineural and intraneural fibrosis.   × 100.

a tendency to coalesce, ulcerate, fibrose, and produce deformity of all structures affected. *Histologically* lepromatous lesions initially consist of perivascular infiltrations of plasma cells and lymphocytes. Later, they form irregular tubercles composed of central masses of epithelioid cells surrounded peripherally by plasma cells, lymphocytes, and occasional giant cells (Fig. 169). In both early and late lesions, leprosy cells and globi are generally prevalent. The former are large foam cells that frequently abound in *Mycobacterium lepræ*. The latter are clumps of *Mycobacterium lepræ* that are found (1) free between the tissue cells, (2) within vacuolated spaces that have been mistaken for lymphatic channels, and (3) within grotesque giant cells. *Tuberculoid* leprosy (also known as neural and maculoanesthetic leprosy) is generally confined to the skin and *initiates* as erythematous or hypopigmented macules. The central area of these macules is atrophic, depigmented, and anesthetic to heat and pinprick. Later, irregular swellings occur along the course of the nerves and when the nerve fibers are destroyed there is complete segmental loss of sensation. *Histologically* the dermis discloses a nonspecific infiltration with plasma cells and lymphocytes while the nerves reveal encasement and permeation with bundles of dense collagenous connective tissue.

The *complications* of cutaneous leprosy are those consequent to loss of sensation and anesthesia and consist essentially of traumatic ulcers and infections. The chief complications of lesions in the upper respiratory system are those consequent to obstruction and secondary infection. In childhood and adolescence the initial *course* is similar to that of measles. The manifestations may consist of fever, malaise, rash, and then nodules and indurations developing about the eyes, face, nose, and ears. The nodules and indurations gradually progress and ultimately (usually after many years) produce the typical lion-like facies. The most important nasal symptoms comprise discharge, epistaxis, and obstruction. When the process extends to the larynx there are, in addition, hoarseness and dyspnea. The *diagnosis* is made from the typical appearance of the lesions, from finding numerous *Mycobacterium lepræ* in smears of scrapings of the mucous membrane, and from biopsy. *Treatment* in the past has been quite varied. Currently segregation of infants and children from diseased persons and administration of antibiotics and sulfonamides appear to be generally practiced. The *prognosis* in early cases is better now than in the past for, with the advent of sulfonamides and antibiotics, the lesions of the mucous membranes tend to heal and the nodular masses tend to regress. In older fibrotic lesions the prognosis is poor.

Glanders.—Glanders (also known as farcy) is a contagious disease affecting horses and asses and transmitted to man by direct inoculation, usually through an abraded surface (Ballenger). It is *caused* by *Bacillus mallei*. *Pathologically* either the skin or the mucous membrane of the nose may be affected. The lesion starts as an abscess which then breaks down to produce an ulcer with undermined edges. It extends by continuity and coalescence and, in the respiratory tract, may ultimately affect the pharynx and even the larynx. The microscopic appearance is nonspecific, consisting of a mixture of bacteria and leukocytes supported by a stroma of capillaries and connective tissue. As the lesion ages, the connective tissue becomes more prominent. *Clinically* the disorder exists in an acute and a chronic form. The acute form simulates typhoid fever with the exception that within three or four days after the onset of symptoms, lesions appear in the skin and nasal mucosa. Death often results within two to three weeks. The

27

chronic form simulates tuberculosis and terminates fatally in about 50 per cent of cases in from a few months to two years. The *diagnosis* is arrived at from a consideration of the history, cutaneous sensitivity tests, serologic tests, and isolating the causative organisms. This is accomplished by inoculating material from the lesion into the peritoneal cavity of a male guinea pig, noting an inflammation of the spermatic cord and tunica vaginalis, and culturing the inflammatory material from the tunica vaginalis on a potato.

Fungous Rhinitis.—Inflammations of the nose and rest of the upper respiratory system with fungi and yeast-like organisms is uncommon. Some of the infections are rhinosporidiosis, aspergillosis, blastomycosis, actinomycosis, moniliasis, histoplasmosis, and sporotrichosis (Scott-Brown). What has been said in the general dissertation on fungous infections in Chapter 5 (p. 157) also applies to lesions in the upper respiratory system. Of all the infections listed above, *histoplasmosis* appears to be gaining in importance in the United States. In 1943, Moore and Jorstad assembled 22 recorded cases involving the ear, nose, and throat, and since then several others have been reported in the literature. The local lesions are chiefly ulcerative but are not characteristic. The diagnosis is established upon isolating the causative organism. The disorder is discussed in greater detail in Chapter 12 (p. 513).

Malignant Granuloma.—*Malignant granuloma* of the face has also been called midline lethal granuloma, nasal malignant granuloma, idiopathic granuloma of the face, gangrenous granuloma, facial mycosis fungoides, malignant reticulosis, etc. (Lopes de Faria). The disorder consists of a relentlessly progressing ulcerating and necrotic process of unknown etiology that starts in the nose and gradually destroys the nose as well as the infraorbital, buccal, zygomatic, and palatine regions. As it extends it spares the esophagus but may progress to involve the pharynx, hypopharynx, larynx, trachea, and main bronchi. *Grossly* the lesion usually appears as a nonspecific ulcer covered with watery, purulent, or hemorrhagic exudate. Less frequently the initial lesion exists as a reddish tumor mass. *Histologically* the basic cells are of moderate sizes and rounded or polyhedral. They possess a moderate to scanty amount of often vacuolated cytoplasm and deeply stained round nuclei. From the angulations of the cell borders, processes may stream out between the adjacent cell. Other cells are strictly inflammatory, consisting of plasma cells, monocytes, lymphocytes, and neutrophils. Thin-walled capillaries are generally numerous. Aside from local *manifestations* of discharge, bleeding, and pain, the patients usually disclose fever that does not respond to antibiotics. The *diagnosis* is made from the location and nature of the lesion, its lack of permanent response to therapy, and the nonspecific histologic alterations. *Treatment* consists of radiotherapy, hormonal (cortisone and ACTH) therapy, and surgical excision. The *prognosis* is poor for most of the patients ultimately die of the disorder. In this respect, it behaves like a malignant tumor.

PHYSICAL DISTURBANCES

Orientation.—Some of the more important physical disturbances of the upper respiratory system may be considered under the following headings: foreign bodies, rhinoliths, epistaxis, cerebrospinal rhinorrhea, trauma, aerosinusitis, and mucocele.

Foreign Bodies.—In the *nose* foreign bodies are usually of exogenous origin and are introduced through the anterior nares. Occasionally, they may be introduced by way of the posterior nares as a result of coughing or sneezing and, rarely, they may enter directly through the skin as a result of external force such as gunshot or trauma. A few of the extremely varied exogenous *foreign bodies* of the nose that have been recorded in the literature are beans, peas, straws, cherry stones, nuts, gauze sponge, marbles, shoe buttons, twine, cotton, paper, pencil erasers, beads, rubber bands, coal, and stones. In comparison, endogenous nasal foreign bodies are rare and consist essentially of bony fragments and, less often, teeth. The *symptoms* are those of the *complications* which consist of obstruction, infection, and bleeding. *Treatment*, of course, is removal.

Foreign bodies of the *paranasal sinuses* are, in comparison, much less common. While the maxillary sinuses are most frequently affected the ethmoid, frontal, and sphenoid sinuses may also occasionally be involved. The *foreign bodies* usually gain entrance as a result of injury (automobile, industrial, war, or surgical) and generally consist of fragments of bones, teeth, metals, sticks, pencils, and parts of operative instruments. The *symptoms* may be entirely absent or those of sinusitis. The *diagnosis* is made by eliciting a careful history, from a careful examination, and from the roentgen appearance. *Treatment* is removal. The *prognosis* is good.

Rhinoliths.—Rhinoliths (Gr. = nose + stones) are nasal stones or concretions. Although they are uncommon, there were over 350 cases recorded in the literature by 1952 (Van Alyea and Makart). They occur at all ages but are most common in the second and third decades and they prevail in females. The *cause* is generally a foreign body that stimulates secretion which, with removal of water, allows a precipitation of salts. *Pathologically* the condition is usually unilateral and the stone is generally single. The size varies from a few millimeters to as much as 5 cm. in greatest diameter and from a few milligrams to 110 grams in weight (Terrafranca and Zellis). The stone is usually located in the floor of the nose or at the inferior meatus and the enlargement is, as a rule, toward the septum. The calculus generally possesses a central nucleus which may be composed of an exogenous or an endogenous foreign body. The latter may consist of a fragment of a tooth, a fragment of a bone, blood clot, desquamated epithelium, leukocytes, or bacteria. *Chemically* the stones are composed chiefly of calcium phosphate with varying amounts of calcium carbonate, magnesium phosphate, organic matter, and water. The *complications* are (1) deviation, ulceration, or destruction of the septum, antral wall, or palate, (2) rhinitis caseosa, and (3) otitis media. *Clinically* the condition may be asymptomatic for years but in time there usually develop unilateral purulent and offensive nasal discharge, unilateral nasal obstruction, epistaxis, headache, swelling of the nose, and conjunctivitis. The *diagnosis* is arrived at by (1) eliciting a careful history, (2) a careful examination, and (3) the roentgenographic appearance. *Treatment* is removal. The *prognosis* is good.

Epistaxis.—Nosebleed is a symptom and not a disease. It may be slight or copious and single or recurrent. In children and young adults, its point of origin is usually in the anterior part of the nasal septum while in older adults it may also be in the posterior or superior part of the nose. According to Cody, the *causes* of epistaxis may be listed as follows: (1) trauma— fracture, postoperative injury, epistaxis digitorium, and foreign bodies, (2) cardiovascular disease—hypertension, arteriosclerosis, and hereditary hemorrhagic telangiectasia, (3) blood dyscrasias—leukemia, hemophilia, polycythemia vera, and purpura hemorrhagica, (4) inflammations—acute rhinitis, chronic rhinitis, atrophic rhinitis, acute xanthomas, and granulomas such as tuberculosis, syphilis, and scleroma, (5) neoplasms—benign and malignant, and (6) miscellaneous—vicarious menstruation, vitamin deficiency, chronic irritation (chemical irritant, irradiation, and excessive smoking), diseases of the liver and spleen, and spontaneous anterior septal hemorrhage (childhood). *Treatment* consists of eliminating the cause. Until this can be accomplished, local therapy in the form of tamponage and/or electrocoagulation are generally indicated. The *prognosis* depends entirely upon the causative factor. The nosebleed as such, while alarming, is rarely fatal.

Cerebrospinal Rhinorrhea.—Cerebrospinal rhinorrhea is the escape of spinal fluid from the nose. The condition is uncommon in civilian life but is not infrequent in warfare. The *causes* may be listed as follows: congenital defect in cribriform plate, nasal encephalomeningomyelocele, trauma to the head, operation on paranasal sinuses or cranium, tumor erosions (primary of the sinuses or within the cranium), infection, and spontaneous (MacDonald). *Pathologically* the communication between the cranial cavity and the nose is usually through the cribriform plate. The fluid discloses the following characteristics: watery, clear, faintly alkaline, tasteless or slightly salty, no precipitate with acetic acid, trace of coagulum on boiling, trace of sugar, precipitation on addition of cold nitric acid, cell count 0 to 20, and specific gravity 1.005 to 1.010. The most important *complication* is meningitis. *Clinically* the condition is characterized by a nasal discharge of copious amounts of clear watery fluid. Premonitory symptoms (due to the primary condition) may consist of headache, dizziness, eye symptoms, failing vision, optic neuritis, scotomas, bitemporal hemianopsia, etc. The *diagnosis* is made from a consideration of the history and the characteristics of the fluid. *Treatment* consists of correction of the etiologic factors. The *prognosis* depends upon the cause. With the advent of antibiotics and chemotherapeutic agents, deaths from infection are now rare.

Trauma.—Trauma to the nose and paranasal sinuses may consist of a blunt or a penetrating injury. In the *nose* it may result in epistaxis, hematoma (especially of the nasal septum), and simple or compound fractures of any of the nasal bones. In the *sinuses* it may result in hemorrhage, disarticulation of the malar bone, fracture of the wall of the sinus or base of the stall, fragmentation and dislodgment of bony fragments into the sinus cavity, dislodgment of a tooth into the antrum, and deposition of an extraneous foreign body within the sinus. In any case, the important *complications* that may arise are cerebrospinal rhinorrhea, infection, deformities, nasal obstruction, and nasal concretions.

Aerosinusitis.—Areosinusitis is an acute or chronic inflammation of the paranasal sinuses caused by a difference of barometric pressure within the sinuses as compared with that of the outside atmosphere (Campbell). The condition is seen in high-altitude flyers. It is characterized by congestion and inflammation of the mucosa and submucosa and, in some cases, by actual mucosal or submucosal hemorrhages. The latter is referred to as *aerohematoma* (Wright and Boyd).

Mucocele.—A *mucocele* (Gr. = mucus + tumor) of the paranasal sinuses represents a walled-off collection of mucus in usually the frontal, ethmoid, or sphenoid sinuses and less often in the maxillary sinus (Kaplan). It originates on the basis of mechanical obstruction to the drainage of the sinus or to the drainage of the submucosal glands.   Some of the many *causes* of *obstruction* are previous operations, tumors (polyps and osteomas), fractures of the sinuses, deviated nasal septum, and inflammation.   Once the drainage has been obstructed the *secretions* from either the lining cells or the submucosal glands or both *accumulate* within the cavity.   As they do so they produce pressure upon and erosion of the confining bony structures, ultimately perforating them and extending into the adjacent structures (Fig. 170).   The latter include the nose, orbit, other sinuses, or intracranial

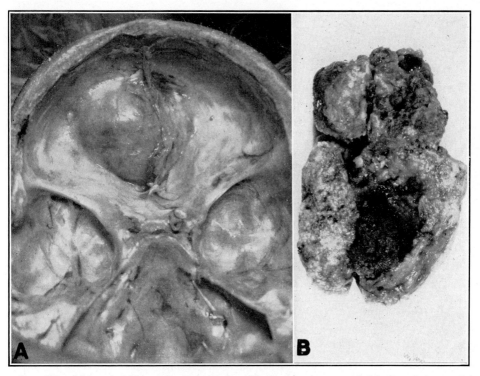

FIG. 170.—Mucocele of the left ethmoid sinus illustrating *A*, a rounded bulge of the cranial fossa due to erosion through the bone beneath the dura, and *B*, a greatly thickened sac subsequently removed from the cavity.

cavity.   The last mentioned is especially important for here the extension may result in meningitis, brain abscess, encephalitis, and death.   Thus, clinically, the condition may behave in a "malignant" fashion although *histologically* the lining cells show only hyperactivity and secretion and are entirely benign.   The *clinical manifestations* are those of pressure on surrounding structures.   The *diagnosis* is made from the history, careful examination, roentgenographic changes, and (often) exploratory procedures. *Treatment* consists of removing the cause of the obstruction and promoting adequate drainage.   The *prognosis* is good.

TUMORS

Orientation.—Tumors and tumor-like conditions of the upper respiratory system affect the nose proper, the nasopharynx, and the paranasal sinuses.

Some are common; others are rare. They occur at all ages, have no over-all predilection for either sex, and are found in all races.

Pathologically the growths are as varied as the protean tissues that anatomically compose this area of the body. Some of the diverse lesions that have been recorded may be listed as follows (Eggston and Wolff): dermoid cyst, encephalomeningomyelocele, rhinophyma, polyp, adenoma of submucosal glands, carcinoma, papilloma, myxoma, myxosarcoma,

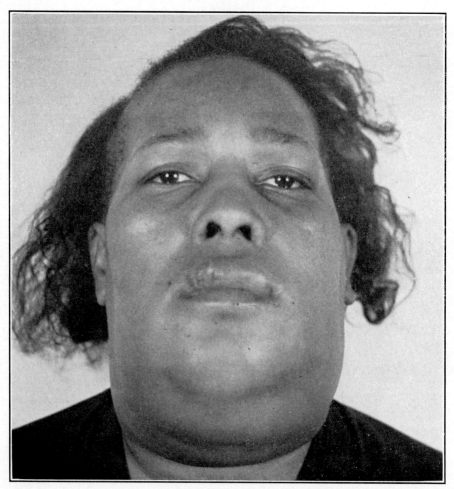

FIG. 171.—Carcinoma of the nasopharynx showing bilateral cervical lymph node metastases.

fibrosarcoma, ossifying fibroma, angioma, juvenile angiofibroma, osteoma, osteosarcoma, chondroma, chondrosarcoma, chordoma, rhabdomyoma, leiomyoma, myoblastoma, lipoma, neurofibroma (neurinoma or schwannoma), lymphoblastoma, plasmacytoma, melanoblastoma, nasopharyngioma (Rathke's pouch tumor), and secondary tumors consisting of extension from the mouth as odontoma or adamantinoma and metastasis from distant areas such as carcinoma of the kidney, osteosarcoma, etc. As seen from this listing, some of the lesions are benign while others are malignant.

The chief *complications* are (1) infection, (2) hemorrhage, (3) obstruction,

(4) pressure atrophy and erosion of adjacent structures, and (5) metastasis to distant areas (malignant tumors). The *clinical manifestations* are those of the complications enumerated. They vary somewhat with the location of the growth. In the *nose proper* they generally consist of nasal obstruction, increased nasal discharge, pain, and (especially in the case of malignant tumors) bleeding (Havens). The bleeding may be spontaneous or it may follow slight trauma. In the *nasopharynx* the symptoms may be the same as those in the nose proper with, in addition, pain in the temporoparietal region, ringing in the ears, and occasionally double vision. In cases of carcinoma, however, the first indication of the lesion is often unilateral or bilateral metastasis to cervical lymph nodes (Fig. 171). In the *paranasal*

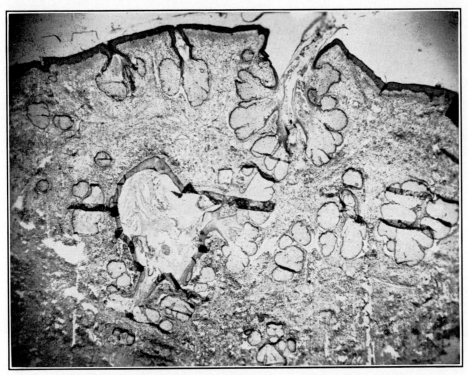

Fig. 172.—Rhinophyma disclosing greatly hypertrophied sebaceous glands with scattered dilatations. × 7.

sinuses they may consist of obstruction of the lacrimal duct, increased unilateral discharge, loosening of the upper teeth (tumors of the antrum), bulging of the cheek and floor of the orbit (tumors of the antrum), bulging of the forehead (tumors of the frontal sinuses), and pain. When the growths break into the nose the symptoms are similar to those in tumors of the nose proper. Direct and indirect visual *examination* discloses the presence of the tumors in the nose and nasopharynx. Advanced tumors of the paranasal sinuses may also be seen bulging or extending into the nasal passage. *Roentgenograms*, especially in neoplasms of the paranasal sinuses, disclose clouding of the air spaces and destruction of bones (Figs. 174 and 175). The *diagnosis* is made from (1) a consideration of the history, (2) the findings on physical and roentgenographic examination, and (3) biopsy. Depending upon the type of growth, its location, and its size, *treatment* consists of surgical excision, electrocoagulation, or irradiation. The *prognosis* depends upon the nature of the tumor. In benign growths it is good, while in malignant growths it is fair to poor.

Aside from the general dissertation just concluded, the following tumors and tumor-like conditions may be singled out for brief separate considerations: rhinophyma, polyp, ossifying fibroma, angiofibroma, papilloma, neurogenic tumors, carcinoma, and melanoblastoma.

Rhinophyma.—This condition is not a true tumor. It consists of a marked hypertrophy, hyperplasia, and cystic dilatation of the sebaceous glands of the tip of the nose together with an increase of supporting fibrous

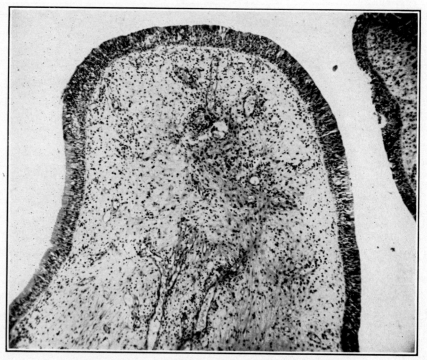

FIG. 173.—Nasal polyp disclosing a covering of hyperplastic but still ciliated epithelium and a core composed of edematous, well-vascularized, connective tissue permeated with leukocytes. × 50.

tissue, prominence of dilated capillaries, and a diffuse infiltration with lymphocytes and plasma cells (Fig. 172). Grossly it appears as an irregular bulbous protrusion of the skin of the anterior third of the nose. The disorder is practically confined to men in the sixth and seventh decades of life and appears to represent the end stage of *acne rosacea* (p. 1348).

Polyp.—Polyps of the upper respiratory system are not true tumors but represent rather a form of hyperplastic rhinitis and sinusitis. They are more common in males and usually become apparent in the third decade of life. The ordinary *causes* are bacterial infection and allergy. The masses *grow* from the middle turbinate, uncinate process of the ethmoid bone, maxillary sinus, frontal sinus, and sphenoid sinus (Ballenger). They *consist of* one or more, smooth, pink to cyanotic, usually soft and boggy, pedunculated masses that measure as much as 4 to 5 cm. in length. *Histologically* the epithelial covering may be pseudostratified ciliated, stratified squamous, attenuated, or ulcerated (Fig. 173). The basement membrane may be inconspicuous or thick, broadened, and hyalinized. The core is composed of varying proportions of the following: edematous connective tissue, collagenous connective tissue, engorged capillaries, dilated vascular

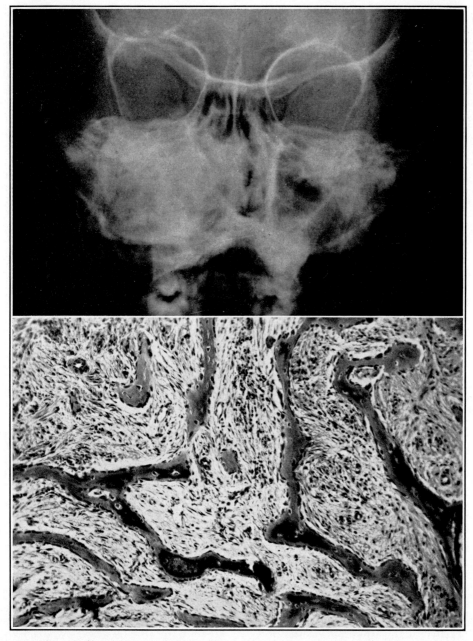

Fig. 174.—Ossifying fibroma of the maxilla showing, above, opacity of the right antrum and, below, a fibrous tissue stroma supporting trabeculæ of centrally calcified and peripherally osteoid bone. × 100.

channels, hyperplastic and/or cystic glands, and leukocytes (eosinophils, neutrophils, plasma cells, lymphocytes, and monocytes). Depending upon which of these elements predominates, the polyps are called myxomatous, fibromatous, angiomatous, adenomatous and granulomatous respectively.

Ossifying Fibroma.—As the name suggests, this is a tumor of the maxillary (and less commonly other) sinuses composed of fibrous tissue with osseous elements added. It is *also known* as osseous fibroma, fibro-osteoid osteoma, central osteoma, sclerosing fibroma, hyperplastic localized osteitis,

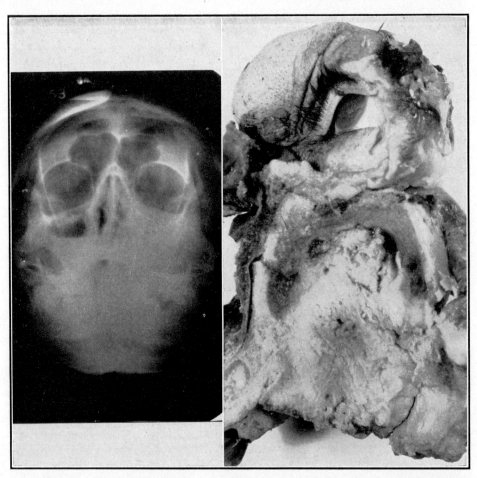

Fig. 175.—Carcinoma of the left maxillary sinus showing, to the left, opacity of the sinus and, to the right, a hemisection of the resected maxilla with the sinus filled with gray tumor tissue.

localized osteodystrophic fibroma, and localized osteitis fibrosa (Hara). It is probable that most, if not all, of the previously described benign giant cell tumors of the maxilla fall into this category. The growth *affects* females more frequently than males and prevails between the ages of ten and thirty years. *Pathologically* the neoplasm is generally unilateral. It grows slowly, filling, expanding, and ultimately eroding the antrum (Fig. 174). In time it may encroach upon the orbit, nose, or alveolar ridge. *Grossly* it is gray to creamy in color, moderately vascular, and gritty. *Histologically* it consists of a stroma of mostly compact collagenous connective tissue arranged in whorls and strands (Fig. 174). Embedded within the stroma are thin, irregular, osseous trabeculæ composed of central calcified bone and peripheral osteoid tissue or of osteoid tissue throughout. Immediately surrounding the trabeculæ, the connective tissue is generally loose. Giant cells of the foreign body type are scattered here and there but are not numerous.

Angiofibroma.—An *angiofibroma*, usually called a juvenile masopharyn-geal angiofibroma and less often simply a fibroma, is a benign fibrous and vascular tumor that arises from the periosteum of the nasopharynx, that grows into the adjacent cavities, and that infiltrates the adjacent soft and bony tissues. Described as a relatively rare tumor (Sternberg), the *incidence*

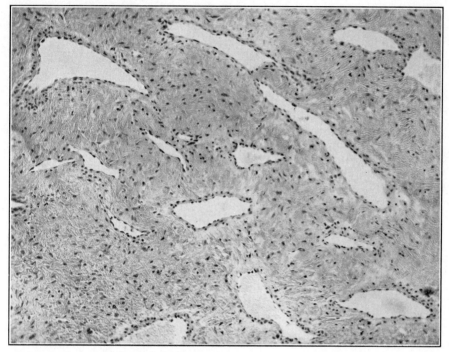

FIG. 176.—Angiofibroma illustrating a stroma of collagenous connective tissue containing varisized endothelial-lined spaces. × 100.

in Egypt is given as 1 in 50,000 ear, nose, and throat patients and in New York as 1 in 16,000 patients in the same category (Handousa). The tumor usually affects males in the second decade but has also been described in women as old as 50 years. The *cause* is unknown, although an association with hormones has been suggested because of the predilection for young males. *Grossly* the tumor is generally sessile, rounded, nodular, tan or gray and smooth or superficially ulcerated. As it fills the nasopharynx it pushes the palate down and forward and as it erodes the adjacent bones it fills the maxilla, the orbit, or even extends into the base of the brain. Cut surfaces reveal resistant gray tissue that appears spongy because it is permeated with vascular channels. Occasionally it undergoes myxomatous degenera-tion. *Histologically* the tumor is composed of two elements—connective tissue and vascular channels (Fig. 176). The connective tissue generally possesses a collagenous and rarely almost a cartilagenous matrix. The cells are elongated or stellate and, as a rule, are not too numerous. The nuclei are plump, oval, deeply stained, and sometimes irregular. While the tumor usually resembles fibrous tissue, sometimes clear spaces are present around the cells and the tissue then resembles embryonic cartilage or even fat. The vascular component of the older portions of the tumor consists of large endothelial-lined spaces that may be occluded by recent or organized thrombi. In the advancing edge of the tumor, however, the vessels consist of thick-walled capillaries similar to those seen in granulation tissue. The covering mucosa is atrophic, hyperplastic, ulcerated, or transformed into a squamous cell type. While conservative *treatment* and irradiation have been

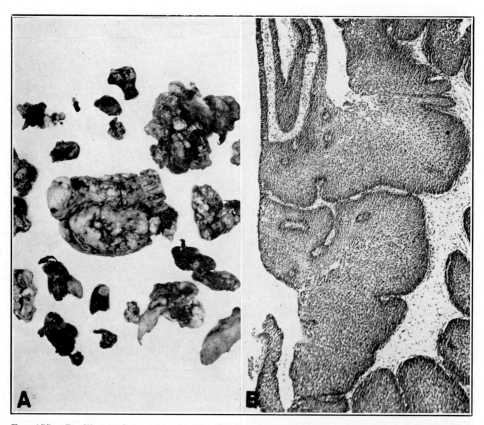

FIG. 177.—Papilloma of the nose showing *A*, the tumor removed in a piece-meal fashion and *B*, the typical histologic proliferation of regular transitional cell type of epithelium. × 50.

tried, the most acceptable therapy is surgical excision. The *prognosis* is good if treatment is radical enough and instituted in time. Deaths from intracranial infection and bronchopneumonia have, however, been recorded.

Papilloma.—A *papilloma* of the nasal cavity, as papilloma elsewhere, is a benign tumor arising from the epithelial lining (Som). It is a reddish gray, lobulated, indurated mass that bleeds readily upon manipulation and that may attain a size large enough to fill the nasal cavity and produce deformity of the nose, sinuses, and face. As it grows it destroys any bony structures that it may contact. *Histologically* it is composed of markedly hyperplastic epithelium that resembles a cross between transitional epithelium on the one hand and nonkeratinizing squamous epithelium on the other (Fig. 177).

While much of the overgrowth is above the surface epithelium some of it is into the submucosa. For this reason, some authors have referred to the lesion as a *schneiderian carcinoma*. Such a designation, however, is incorrect for the masses are surrounded by an intact basement membrane and the cells are regular. *Treatment* consists of generous surgical excision. Because of the peripheral spread of the tumor, this can generally be accomplished only by piece-meal dissection (Fig. 177). The *prognosis* is guarded for recurrences are common and a frankly carcinomatous transformation does occur.

Neurogenic Tumors.—*Neurogenic tumors* of the nose are found in the nasal fossa and are related in origin to the olfactory area (McCormack). They have been called *esthesioneuroepithelioma*, *neuroblastoma*, and *neurocytoma*. They are said to comprise about 3 per cent of all intranasal tumors (excluding polyps), usually occur in adults, and have no predilection for either sex. *Pathologically* some are benign while others are malignant but the delineation between the two is not definite. *Grossly* the tumors are composed of varisized masses of gray, moderately firm tissue with areas of necrosis and hemorrhage. As in most other tumors in this area, these growths produce erosion and destruction not only of the soft but also the the bony tissues, as they expand in neighboring directions. *Histologically* the more mature neoplasms resemble neuroblastoma of the adrenals and sympathetic ganglia. They are composed of small round cells with round evenly stained nuclei and scanty cytoplasm. The latter is drawn out into polar fibrils which can be discerned by special stains. While in most areas the cells are more or less diffusely arranged, occasionally true rosettes are readily visualized. The stroma is scanty and contains moderate numbers of thin-walled capillaries. The less mature tumors are composed of larger, somewhat more irregular cells with less tendency to rosette formation.

Carcinoma.—Carcinoma of the upper respiratory system usually occurs after the age of thirty years and is more common in males than in females. It may affect the nose proper, the nasopharynx, or the paranasal sinuses. In the *nose* the disease is unilateral and generally originates on the septum or high on the lateral wall. Grossly the tumor may be primarily ulcerating or fungating. The ulcerating lesion consists of an irregular defect in the mucosa with raised and firm edges, a gray floor, and a firm, grayish-white, ill-defined base. The fungating lesion consists of an irregular, pinkish-gray, polypoid mass or masses of varying dimensions. The tumor is friable and bleeds easily. In the *nasopharynx* the most common locations of the growths are the posterior part of the orifice of the eustachian tube, the vault, and the tonsillar areas. The tumor is generally flat or ulcerating, small, and easily overlooked. Rarely, it may be polypoid and bulky. In the *paranasal sinuses* the neoplasm is generally polypoid, bulky, and similar to the fungating lesion in the nose. In advanced cases the tumor fills the entire sinus cavity as a rather soft, friable, pinkish-gray mass (Fig. 175). Carcinoma of the sinuses is generally unilateral and is five times as common in the maxillary sinuses as in all other sinuses combined (Watson). *Histologically*, regardless of the point of origin, carcinoma of the upper respiratory tract may be of a squamous cell, transitional cell, or adenomatous variety (Fig. 178). *Squamous cell carcinoma* may be of low to high-grade malignancy. The former exists as strands, nests, or masses of sharply defined, polyhedral cells with abundant cytoplasm and round to irregular hyperchromatic nuclei. Some tumors disclose keratin and epithelial pearls while others do not. Squamous cell carcinoma of high-grade malignancy exists as diffuse sheets or single, relatively small, rounded or elongated cells with scanty

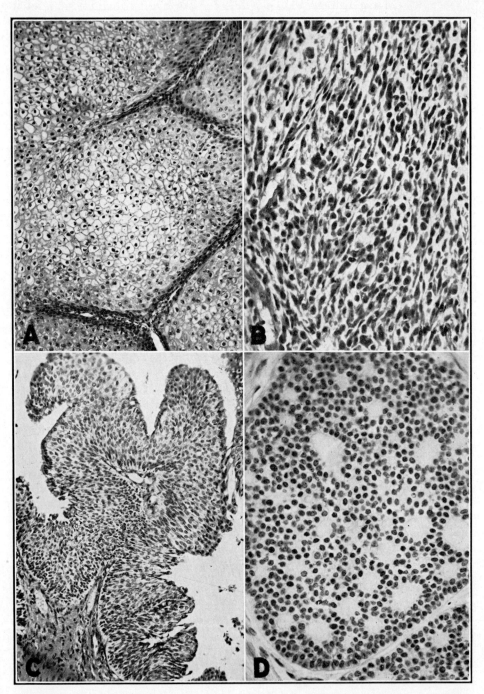

FIG. 178.—Carcinoma of the upper respiratory tract showing *A*, a squamous cell type of low-grade malignancy without pearl formation. × 100, *B*, a squamous cell type of high-grade malignancy with rounded and spindle-shaped cells. × 200, *C*, transitional papillary type. × 100, and *D*, adenocarcinoma (low-grade malignancy or adenoma, potentially malignant) with the lumens filled with mucoid material. × 200.

cytoplasm and round to oval hyperchromatic nuclei. Squamous cell carcinoma of intermediate grade malignancy is between these two extremes. *Transitional cell carcinoma* is composed of strands, nests, or irregular clumps of rather uniform-appearing polygonal cells with moderate amounts of cytoplasm and round, evenly stained nuclei. In infiltrating tumors of the nasopharynx the cells are often intermingled with existing lymphoid tissue and the tumor is then frequently referred to as *lymphoepithelioma*. *Adenocarcinoma* is the least common. It originates in the submucosal glands and is generally of low-grade malignancy (some authors referring to it as adenoma or cylindroma). It is usually composed of masses of ill-defined cuboidal cells in acinar formation. The lumens of the glands may be empty or filled with mucoid material. In any case the *stroma* may be scanty or abundant and may be composed of loose or collagenous connective tissue. In addition to the tumor cells, it always contains varying numbers of plasma cells, lymphocytes, and neutrophils. Regardless of its exact site of origin, carcinoma of the upper respiratory system *spreads* to adjacent structures by direct extension and erosion and metastasizes to cervical lymph nodes (Fig. 171) and distant areas. The latter consists of lymph nodes, lungs, pleura, heart, bones, liver, etc. In general, carcinoma of the nose proper and sinuses tends to remain more localized while carcinoma of the nasopharynx tends to metastasize early.

Melanoblastoma.—This neoplasm, known more often as malignant melanoma, is a rare, highly malignant tumor of the nose. It may be primary or metastatic. *Primary* melanoblastoma usually originates in the anterior part of the chamber at approximately the level of the mucocutaneous junction. *Secondary* melanoblastoma may be found anywhere within the nose, nasopharynx, or paranasal sinuses. Grossly the tumor is indistinguishable from carcinoma except when it contains melanin in amounts adequate enough to render a black or brown color. Aside from its location, the growth is similar to that seen in the skin (see Chapter 39, p. 1397).

REFERENCES

Pathologic Physiology

FABRICANT, N. D.: *Nasal Medication. A Practical Guide*, Baltimore, Willams & Wilkins Co., 1942

WALLS, E. W.: J. Laryng. & Otol., *71*, 519, 1957.

Congenital Anomalies

ANDERSON, F. M.: A. M. A. Arch. Otolaryng., *46*, 644, 1947 (Encephalomeningocele).

KEOGH, C. A.: Scott-Brown's *Diseases of the Ear, Nose, and Throat*, New York, Paul B. Hoeber, Inc., p. 74, 1952 (Congenital Anomalies).

RANDALL, R. G.: J. Iowa State M. Soc., *41*, 257, 1951 (Dermoid Cysts).

ROSENBERGER, H. C.: A. M. A. Arch. Otolaryng., *40*, 288, 1944 (Fissural Cyst).

Inflammations

BALLENGER, W. L., and BALLENGER, H. C.: *Diseases of the Nose, Throat, and Ear*, 10th Ed., Philadelphia, Lea & Febiger, 1957.

BAYON, P. J.: Southern M. J., *32*, 211, 1939 (Histopathology of Sinusitis).

BLOOMFIELD, A. L.: J. A. M. A., *144*, 287, 1950 (Common Cold).

CRADDOCK, W. H.: Ann. Otol., Rhin. & Laryngol., *58*, 671, 1949 (Nasal Allergy).

CRIEP, L. H.: J. A. M. A., *136*, 601, 1948 (Allergic Rhinitis).

CULLOM, M. M.: J. A. M. A., *117*, 987, 1941 (Ozena).

EAGLE, W. W., *et al.*: A. M. A. Arch. Otolaryng., *30*, 319, 1939 (Atrophic Rhinitis).

EGGSTONE, A. A., and WOLFF, D.: *Histopathology of the Ear, Nose, and Throat*, Baltimore, The Williams & Wilkins Co., 1947.

ELLIOTT, D. C.: J. Pediat., *35*, 189, 1949 (Leprosy).

FITE, G. L.: A. M. A. Arch. Path., *35*, 611, 1943 (Leprosy).

FOX, N., *et al.:* A. M. A. Arch. Otolaryng., *33*, 1033, 1941 (Atrophic Rhinitis).

HODGES, R. G.: J. A. M. A., *147*, 1335, 1951 (Epidemiology Upper Respiratory Tract Diseases).

JOHNSON, E. D.: A. M. A. Arch. Otolaryng., *47*, 165, 1948 (Acute Frontal Sinusitis).

KERN, R. A., and SCHENCK, H. B.: J. Allergy, *4*, 485, 1933 (Allergic Nasal Polyps).

KLINE, P. R., and BRODY, E. R.: A. M. A. Arch. Dermat. & Syph., *59*, 606, 1949 (Scleroma).

LEVINE, M. G.: Am. J. Clin. Path., *21*, 546, 1951 (Scleroma).

LOPES DE FARIA, J.: A.M.A. Arch. Otolar., *65*, 355, 1957 (Malignant Granuloma).

MEYERSBURG, H., *et al.:* A. M. A. Arch. Otolaryng., *23*, 449, 1936 (Rhinitis Caseosa).

MILLER, M. W.: Pennsylvania M. J., *53*, 1274, 1950 (Allergic Rhinitis).

MOORE, M., and JORSTAD, L. H.: Ann. Otol., Rhin. & Laryng., *62*, 779, 1943 (Histoplasmosis).

RADNER, D. B., and PINKERTON, F. J.: Am. Rev. Tuberc., *50*, 313, 1944 (Tuberculosis of Antrum).

REYES, E.: A. M. A. Arch. Dermat. & Syph., *54*, 531, 1946 (Scleroma).

RUSSELL, D. A., *et al.:* J. A. M. A., *148*, 642, 1952 (Scleroma).

SCOTT-BROWN, W. G.: *Diseases of the Ear, Nose, and Throat*, New York, Paul B. Hoeber, Inc., Volume I, 1952.

SEMENOV, H.: J. A. M. A., *111*, 2189, 1938 (Pathology of Sinusitis).

STOESSER, A. V.: J. Lancet, *69*, 198, 1949 (Allergic Rhinitis in Pediatrics).

SZANTO, P. B., and HOLLANDER, A. R.: Ann. Otol., Rhin. & Laryng., *53*, 508, 1944 (Tuberculosis of the Nasopharynx).

WIGH, R.: Radiology, *54*, 579, 1950 (Mucoceles of Sinuses).

ZELUFF, G. W., and HAYES, G. J.: J. A. M. A., *150*, 582, 1952 (Leprosy).

Physical Disturbances

CAMPBELL, P. A.: Ann. Otol., Rhin. & Laryng., *54*, 69, 1945 (Aerosinusitis).

CODY III, C. C.: Texas State J. Jed., *48*, 256, 1952 (Epistaxis).

DICKIE, J. K. M.: Canad. M. A. J., *58*, 121, 1948 (Nasal Hemorrhage).

HIRSCH, O.: A. M. A. Arch. Otolaryng., *56*, 1, 1952 (Cerebrospinal Rhinorrhea).

HOWARD, J. C., JR.: Ann. Otol., Rhin. & Laryng., *54*, 186, 1945 (Foreign Bodies of Maxillary Sinus).

KAPLAN, S., *et al.:* A.M.A. Arch. Otolar., *51*, 172, 1950 (Mucocele).

MACDONALD, R.: Laryngoscope, *55*, 552, 1945 (Cerebrospinal Rhinorrhea).

MEYERS, P. T.: Pennsylvania M. J., *51*, 540, 1948 (Foreign Bodies Maxillary Sinuses).

SHEA, J. J.: J. A. M. A., *120*, 745, 1942 (Fractures Paranasal Sinuses).

TERRAFRANCA, R. J., and ZELLIS, A.: Radiology, *58*, 405, 1952 (Rhinoliths).

VAN ALYEA, O. E., and MAKART, C. D.: Ann. Otol., Rhin. & Laryng., *61*, 490, 1952 (Rhinoliths).

WRIGHT, R. W., and BOYD, H. M. E.: A. M. A. Arch. Otolaryng., *43*, 357, 1946 (Aerohematoma).

Tumors

BALLENGER, W. L., and BALLENGER, H. C.: *Diseases of the Nose, Throat, and Ear*, 10th Ed., Philadelphia, Lea & Febiger, 1957.

DIEHL, K. L.: A. M. A. Arch. Otolaryng., *49*, 275, 1949 (Adenocarcinoma Nasopharynx).

EGGSTONE, A. A., and WOLFF, D.: *Histopathology of the Ear, Nose, and Throat*, Baltimore, The Williams & Wilkins Co., 1947.

FOX, C. C.: A. M. A. Arch. Otolaryng., *48*, 390, 1949 (Carcinoma Nasopharynx).

HARA, H. J.: A. M. A. Arch. Otolaryng., *40*, 180, 1944 (Ossifying Fibroma).

HAVENS, F. Z.: S. Clin. North America, *21*, 109, 1941 (Carcinoma Nose, Nasopharynx, and Sinuses).

HANDOUSA, F. H., and ELWI, A. M.: J. Lar. Otol., *69*, 647, 1954 (Angiofibroma).

McCORMACK, L. J., and HARRIS, H. E.: J.A.M.A., *158*, 318, 1955 (Neurogenic Tumors).

O'KEEFE, J. J., and CLERF, L. H.: Ann. Otol., Rhin. & Laryng., *55*, 312, 1946 (Malignant Tumors Maxillary Sinus).

SCHOLMAN, J. G., and ANDERSON, H. W.: Ann. Otol., Rhin. & Laryng., *59*, 124, 1950 (Melanoblastoma Nose and Sinuses).

SEELIG, C. A.: Ann. Otol., Rhin. & Laryng., *58*, 168, 1949 (Carcinoma Antrum).

SHALL, L. A.: J. A. M. A., *137*, 1273, 1948 (Malignant Tumors Nose and Sinuses).

SIMMONS, M. W., and ARIAL, I. M.: Surg., Gynec. & Obst., *88*, 763, 1949 (Carcinoma Naso-pharynx).

SOM, M. L., and WITCHELL, T. S.: N. York State M. J., *57*, 1634, 1957 (Papilloma).

STERNBERG, S. S.: Cancer, *7*, 15, 1954 (Angiofibroma).

STEWART, T. S.: J. Laryng. & Otol., *65*, 560, 1951 (Nasal Melanoblastoma).

THOMPSON, E. A.: A. M. A. Arch. Otolaryng., *54*, 390, 1951 (Lymphoepithelioma Naso-pharynx).

VAN METRE, T. E., JR.: Bull. Johns Hopkins Hosp., *82*, 42, 1948 (Malignant Tumors Naso-pharynx).

WATSON, W. L.: Laryngoscope, *52*, 22, 1942 (Carcinoma Sinuses).

Chapter

11

Larynx

PATHOLOGIC PHYSIOLOGY

FRED HARBERT

THE primary *function* of the larynx is protection of the airway from foreign bodies, especially during deglutition. This is accomplished by three sphincters. The first is incomplete and consists of the epiglottis, arytenoids, and aryepiglottic folds. The second is also incomplete, being deficient posteriorly, and consists of the ventricular bands. The third is complete and consists of the true cords which are also the organs of phonation. Complete sphincteric occlusion of the airway is necessary to efficiently clear the trachea and bronchi of accumulated secretions by coughing. An effective cough is produced when the glottis is closed and intrathoracic pressure is built up by contraction of abdominal muscles and diaphragm, followed by sudden opening of the glottis to produce a bechic blast. After tracheotomy, cough is very inefficient, particularly in the first postoperative days. Under such circumstances, deep as well as superficial aspiration of the tracheobronchial passages is necessary to maintain a satisfactory airway. This is particularly important when tracheotomy is done because of impaired cough reflex as, for example, in an unconscious neurosurgical patient or one with paralysis of the diaphragm.

The *blood supply* of the larynx is from branches of the superior thyroid artery. The *lymphatics* of the true cords are few in number. This has a distinct bearing on the lateness of spread to adjacent lymph nodes of neoplastic or inflammatory processes restricted to the cords proper. Contrarily, the lymphatics of the supraglottic and infraglottic tissues are numerous. The former pass by way of the thyrohyoid membrane and pharyngo-epiglottic folds to the deep cervical nodes while the latter pass through the cricothyroid membrane to the deep nodes. Lymph nodes in these areas are therefore often enlarged by infective or neoplastic processes.

The main *nerve supply* is by way of the superior laryngeal and the recurrent laryngeal nerves. The superior laryngeal nerve is sensory except for its external branch which supplies the cricothyroid muscle. When the cricothyroid muscle is paralyzed there is loss of tone in the cord. This results in the cord becoming bowed and the arytenoid being tilted forward. The recurrent laryngeal nerve supplies all the other intrinsic muscles of the larynx. When this nerve is affected, varying degrees of paresis may occur although, in general, the tone of the cords is preserved and the voice shows little or no impairment. The greatest effect of such an affliction is on the airway, which becomes impaired because of failure of abduction (Semon's Law). Contrarily, when failure of abduction occurs either a functional aphonia (hysteria) or bulbar involvement, as in poliomyelitis, should be considered. Breathing is controlled by the medulla while vocalization is controlled by the cortex. Asphyxia by volition is impossible because when anoxia causes loss of consciousness, the involuntary centers resume respiration.

Trauma due to faulty use of the voice, to excessive coughing, or to irritants (such as excessive smoking) may cause reversible changes in the true cords such as edema and submucosal hemorrhage. When the abuse continues, however, permanent changes may occur in the form of fibrosis, polyps, or nodules and these necessitate surgical removal to restore the voice. As opposed to chronic irritation, acute infections and allergic reactions (such as angioneurotic edema) may produce acute swelling of the mucosa thereby impairing the airway and requiring tracheotomy.

Laboratory procedures employed in establishing a diagnosis of laryngeal disease include smears and cultures taken preferably by direct laryngoscopy and biopsy. Smears and cultures (including animal inoculations) are used in the diagnosis of bacterial, spirochetal, and fungal disorders while biopsy, although important in similar lesions, is mandatory in the case of neoplasms.

GENERAL CONSIDERATIONS

Although diseases of the larynx may be grouped under those of either the upper respiratory system or the lower respiratory system, it is nevertheless convenient to consider them separately, for many of the disorders are peculiar to this organ. Conditions that usually represent extensions from the nose, pharynx, or trachea will be merely listed for the sake of completeness. As in other areas, the disorders may be conveniently divided into the five usual broad groups of disease processes.

CONGENITAL ANOMALIES

Orientation. —Developmental abnormalities of the larynx may be listed as follows: absence (rare and incompatible with life), hypoplasia (of the entire larynx or of the epiglottis), asymmetry (anomalies of development of a portion of the larynx), clefts in the interarytenoid space, web, cyst, laryngocele, and stridor.

Web. —Congenital webs of the larynx are also known as diaphragms, adhesions, or bands (McHugh and Loch). Although the condition is present at birth it may not be discovered until adulthood. It has a slight preponderance for the female. At an early age in embryonic development, an epithelial overgrowth normally occludes the larynx. The persistence of this occlusion results in web formation. The precise *cause* of the persistence is unknown but heredity appears to play a definite role. *Pathologically* three-quarters of the lesions occur at the level of the vocal cords while the rest affects the subglottis, supraglottis, posterior wall of the laryngeal cavity, and rarely the entire larynx. In any given case the web is located anteriorly and extends posteriorly for varied distances until, in an extreme instance, it forms a complete diaphragm. *Grossly* it is pink to gray and measures up to 1.5 cm. in thickness. *Histologically* it is covered on the superior surface with stratified squamous epithelium and on the inferior surface with respiratory epithelium. Between these two there is a core of vascularized connective tissue containing varying numbers of mucous glands and varying amounts of fat, striated muscle, and cartilage. The chief *complication* (when encroachment on the airway is marked) is laryngeal obstruction. *Clinically* there may be hoarseness (when the cords are affected), dyspnea, cyanosis, cough, and suffocation. The *diagnosis* is made by direct or indirect laryngoscopy. *Treatment* is indicated only when there is serious interference with respiration. It consists of incision or excision of the web with placing of a keel (tantalum) between the anterior margins. The *ultimate results* are often poor.

Cyst.—Cysts of the larynx are either congenital or acquired. *Congenital cysts* have been seen at all ages (Fox and Dinolt). They probably arise from embryonic cells displaced from the appendix of the ventricle. Other sources of origin are branchiogenic and thyroglossal. *Acquired cysts* result from traumatic or inflammatory occlusion of the excretory ducts of the lands or from traumatic transplantation of epithelium into the deeper

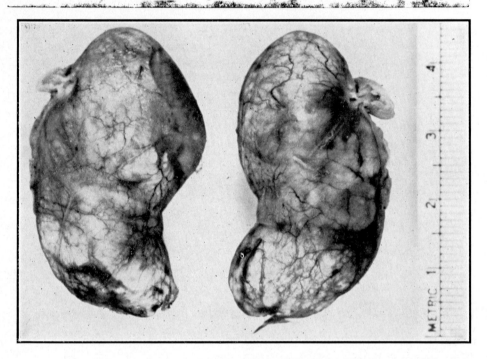

Fig. 179.—Laryngocele showing a hemisected, thin-walled, elongated sac.

tissue. *Pathologically*, regardless of origin, the cysts may be located on the epiglottis, vocal cords, lateral wall of the larynx, and the aryepiglottic folds. They vary in size from a few millimeters to several centimeters. The contents are serous, gelatinous, or hemorrhagic. The lining is composed of columnar, cuboidal, pseudostratified columnar, or squamous epithelium and may or may not be attenuated. The rest of the wall consists essentially of connective tissue. *Symptoms* are due to obstruction of the airway and may consist of hoarseness, dyspnea, fullness in the throat, and dysphagia. The *diagnosis* is made by direct or indirect laryngoscopy. *Treatment* consists of complete excision accomplished best by thyrotomy. The *prognosis* is excellent.

Laryngocele.—A laryngocele is an outpouching or cystic dilatation of the appendix of the ventricle (O'Keefe). The condition is found in both sexes and at all ages. The *cause* is a congenital weakness of the wall with a superimposed increase in intraglottic pressure. This may be enhanced by anything (tumors or inflammations) that encroaches upon the orifice of the ventricular appendage and thereby produces a check value effect. *Pathologically* the condition is generally dividable into three varieties—(1) internal—consisting of a swelling with in the larynx located above the false cords and extending superiorly to the aryepiglottic folds or base of the tongue, (2) superior external—consisting of a sac that has perforated the thyrohyoid membrane and that appears as a swelling in the neck, and (3) combined internal and external. *Grossly* the sac is usually elongated and may measure up to 5 or 6 cm. in greatest diameter (Fig. 179). The wall is thin and transparent. The inner surface is smooth. The lumen contains air. *Histologically* the lining consists of respiratory epithelium supported by a wall of connective tissue. *Complications* consist of asphyxia and infection. The *clinical manifestations* are due to encroachment upon the vocal cords and/or the airway. They may consist of alterations in voice, cough, dyspnea, and a collapsible cystic swelling in the neck. The *diagnosis* is made upon careful physical examination and roentgenography. *Treatment* is surgical excision. The *prognosis* is good.

Stridor.—Congenital laryngeal stridor is a symptom and not a disease. The condition results from abnormally short aryepiglottic folds and an associated omega-shaped epiglottis. The larynx is thus an exaggeration of the infantile type of organ (Trimby). Under such circumstances inspiration causes a trap-door-like closure of the aperture by sucking the epiglottis down in contact with the arytenoids and aryepiglottic folds. The diagnosis is made upon direct laryngoscopy. The disorder must be differentiated from any obstructive lesion of the larynx. It has nothing to do with enlargement of the thymus.

DEGENERATIONS

As elsewhere in the body, degenerative conditions of the larynx are common in conjunction with other disease processes. Aside from these, *calcification* of laryngeal cartilages is one of the more common retrogressive processes that is found in an otherwise normal larynx. The disorder occurs as early as the second decade, is hereditarily determined, and is not influenced by mineral or metabolic disturbances (Vastine). The condition is without clinical significance.

INFLAMMATIONS

Orientation.—Inflammation of the larynx is known as *laryngitis*. The condition is important because it is frequent and because it may produce encroachment upon the lumen of the airway sufficient to cause suffocation. While classifications are diverse the following listing is generally sufficient to include most of the common infections: acute nonspecific laryngitis, chronic nonspecific laryngitis, edema, diphtheria, syphilis, tuberculosis, Boeck's sarcoid, scleroma, leprosy, glanders, and fungous laryngitis. Of these, diphtheria is considered in connection with disorders of the Upper Digestive System (p. 605); scleroma, leprosy, and glanders have been discussed in the preceding Chapter; fungous infections are similar to those in the nose (p. 501), while Boeck's sarcoid generally forms part of a systemic infection (p. 418). The remaining conditions may now be considered briefly in the order mentioned.

Acute Nonspecific Laryngitis. —Acute nonspecific laryngitis is generally preceded by infection of the upper respiratory tract and accompanied by tracheitis and bronchitis. Because of the latter, the condition is often referred to as *acute laryngotracheobronchitis.* The disorder occurs at all ages but it is drawn to the physician's attention more often in infants and children because of the gravity of the disease at this age. In a large series of cases it predominates in males in the ratio of 2 to 1. It is most prevalent in the winter and early spring. In some cases, the *cause* is doubtlessly a virus with subsequent bacterial (influenzal, streptococcic, staphylococcic, pneumococcic, etc.) invasion. In others, it is bacterial (especially influenzal and streptococcic) from the start.

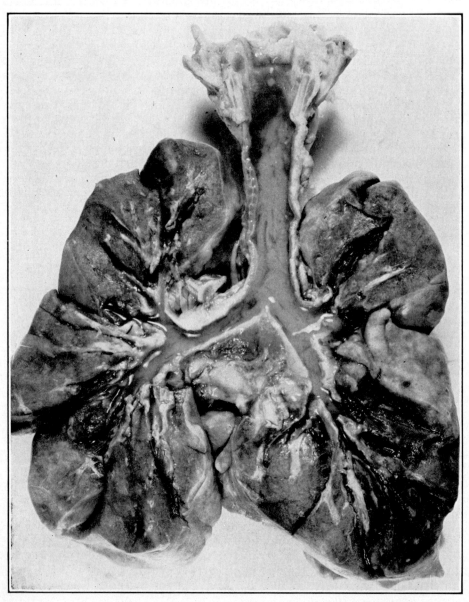

Fig. 180.—Acute laryngotracheobronchitis in a child showing swelling of the laryngeal mucosa and filling of the trachea and bronchi with thick purulent material.

Pathologically the process usually affects the larynx, trachea and bronchi, although the severity of involvement of each of these structures varies from case to case. As a rule, the initial lesion consists of severe hyperemia and this, in turn, is followed by exudation and edema. The type of exudate varies from serous to mucoid, purulent, or even somewhat hemorrhagic. The exudate fills the lumen of the larynx, trachea, and bronchi and is often closely adherent to the underlying mucosa (Fig. 180). Sometimes the exudate is less fluid and exists in the form of a pseudomembrane that covers and is densely adherent to the lining of the respiratory tract. Such cases may be difficult to differentiate from diphtheria. As a result of occlusion of the airway, the pulmonary parenchyma discloses alternating areas of atelectasis and emphysema and, in some instances, it may also reveal focal areas of bronchopneumonia. *Histologically* the epithelium generally shows varying degrees of hypersecretion, degeneration, and even complete necrosis with sloughing. The basement membrane may be prominent. The submucosa reveals varying degrees of congestion, edema, and leukocytic infiltration. The leukocytes consist primarily of neutrophils with varying numbers of plasma cells, lymphocytes, and monocytes added.

The *complications* of acute laryngotracheobronchitis consist of (1) obstruction of the larynx, trachea, and bronchi (as a result of exudation and edema), (2) atelectasis and emphysema of the pulmonary parenchyma with varying degrees of pneumonia, (3) septicemia, and (4) pneumothorax (after tracheotomy). The *clinical manifestations* may develop gradually (especially in cases that follow an upper respiratory tract infection) or they may develop with great rapidity (especially in cases that start as an acute laryngotracheobronchitis). They are explainable on the basis of mucosal irritation, obstruction to the airway, and absorption of local toxic products. They may consist of laryngeal discomfort, laryngeal pain, change in voice, obstruction (evidenced by respiratory stridor, cyanosis, and retraction of tissues about the thoracic cage), dysphagia, fever, rapid respirations, and increase in pulse. The *diagnosis* is generally made from the history, physical examination, indirect laryngoscopy, and, when necessary, direct laryngoscopy. Bacteriological studies usually reveal the type of organism involved but treatment should not be withheld until these results are known. A differential diagnosis includes diphtheria. *Treatment* is primarily prophylactic in the form of preventing an acute infection of the upper respiratory system spreading inferiorly. Once the condition has developed, treatment consists of steam inhalations, administration of oxygen, administration of antibiotics and chemotherapeutic agents, and, when necessary, intubation or tracheotomy. The *prognosis* is generally good. Without treatment, the course is unpredictable for many patients recover spontaneously in a few days, while others progress until they present an alarming picture of respiratory obstruction (Morgan and Wishart). The response to treatment that is initiated early in the disease is good. The mortality rate in 1,077 cases studied by Everett was 2.0 per cent. In general, the younger the patient the greater is the danger of death. The *causes* of *death* are anoxia, cardiac failure, and spread of the infection locally or systemically.

Chronic Nonspecific Laryngitis.—Although most authors divide chronic nonspecific infections of the larynx under headings such as diffuse or local hypertrophic laryngitis, vocal nodules, pachydermia laryngis, and atrophic laryngitis (Ballenger) the conditions may conveniently be considered under one heading. In general, the infections *occur* more frequently in males than in females and although they may be present at all ages they usually predominate in older people. The *causes* are many. In some instances no definite etiologic factor can be determined. In others the following play a definite role: continuation of an acute infection of the larynx, improper use of the voice, excessive use of tobacco or alcohol, inhalation of irritating chemicals or other substances, allergy, mouth breathing, local chronic passive hyperemia (such as occurs in connection with heart disease, pressure by tumors, etc.), and direct local trauma such as that following intubation.

Pathologically, as seen from the variety of terms employed to designate the different appearances, the gross and microscopic changes are quite variable. Although any portion or portions of the larynx may be involved, the condition especially affects the vocal cords. The lesion may be diffuse or local and single or multiple. The mucosa may be (1) reddened, gray, or grayish-white, (2) hyperplastic or atrophic, and (3) intact or ulcerated. Sometimes the affected area is locally elevated to produce a pedunculated mass. In such instances it is frequently reddened, soft, friable, and bleeds easily upon manipulation. *Histologically* the epithelium may be relatively normal, hyperplastic, hyperkeratotic, atrophic, or ulcerated. The submucosa discloses an increase in thick-walled capillaries and connective tissue and a diffuse infiltration with plasma cells, lymphocytes, monocytes, neutrophils, and eosinophils. The submucosal glands may be hyperplastic and hyperactive, atrophic, or cystically dilated.

The *complications* are generally referable only to the changes in the voice. Sometimes, however, as a result of fibrous tissue formation there may be encroachment upon the lumen of the larynx with obstruction of the airway. The *clinical manifestations* are usually those pertaining to alterations in the voice. These may consist of simply a change in the tone of the voice, hoarseness, huskiness, or aphonia. In addition, there are frequently local discomfort, dryness, occasionally pain, cough, and dyspnea. The *diagnosis* is made from obtaining a careful history, direct or indirect laryngoscopic examination, and biopsy. *Treatment* consists of eradication of the etiologic factor, rest of the vocal cords, and operative removal of the nodules or thickenings. The *prognosis* is generally good.

Edema.—Edema of the larynx is a state of the soft tissues characterized by swelling, bogginess, and an accumulation of fluid in the tissue spaces and between the cells. It is not a disease process. It may *occur* at all ages. The many *causes*, as outlined by Miller, may be local or general. *Local* factors may be (1) laryngeal and consist of bacterial infection, irritation by a foreign body, trauma, inhalations of steam or chemicals, and contracture of scar tissue after operation, or (2) extralaryngeal and consist of a wide variety of bacterial infections, wounds to the base of the tongue and pharynx, tumors or scars interfering with venous drainage, enlargement of the thyroid, and exposure to irradiation. *General* factors may consist of allergy, cardiac disease, renal disease, pulmonary disease, and medications. The *clinical manifestations* are those of encroachment upon the functions of the vocal cords and laryngeal obstruction. They may appear insidiously or abruptly. The *diagnosis* is made from the history and direct or indirect laryngoscopy. *Treatment* consists of eliminating the cause. Otherwise it is similar to that in acute laryngitis. The *prognosis* depends on the etiologic agent, age of the patient, and severity and duration of the edema.

Syphilis.—Syphilis of the larynx may be congenital or acquired (Ballenger). *Congenital syphilis* may consist of a diffuse thickening and superficial ulceration of the lining or of a gumma. The former appears at or soon after birth while the latter may become apparent at any time between birth and puberty. *Acquired syphilis* may occur in all three stages of the disease although the chancre is extremely rare. Secondary acquired syphilis, as elsewhere, exists as mucous patches. Gummas usually predominate in the anterior part of the larynx. They consist of local swellings which soften and then ulcerate producing deep craters that extend to and destroy the underlying cartilages. The *clinical manifestations* may consist of cough, hoarseness, and aphonia. The infection responds to antisyphilitic *treatment* and the *results* depend entirely upon the amount of tissue destroyed before treatment is instituted.

Tuberculosis.—Tuberculosis of the larynx is practically always secondary to tuberculosis of the lungs. In a study of 811 cases of pulmonary tuberculosis at postmortem, Auerbach discovered involvement of the larynx in 304 (37.5%). The condition occurs most frequently in the third and fourth decades of life and has no predilection for either sex. The *cause* is *Mycobacterium tuberculosis.* Usually the organisms are implanted upon the laryngeal mucosa by way of infected sputum and only rarely is the infection hematogenous. Local trauma in the form of coughing or bronchoscopy predisposes to the formation of the lesions.

Pathologically any and all portions of the larynx may be affected with the vocal cords, epiglottis, and ventricular bands being most commonly involved. Although there is some controversy as to what constitutes the initial lesion, it appears to be the concensus that the first change is indicated by a patchy, intense hyperemia of the mucosa (Cody). Following this, the lesion may become ulcerative or proliferative. The *ulcers* are usually multiple, irregular in outline, and at first superficial. As they increase they develop distinctly undermined edges and they penetrate to varying depths, affecting even the cartilages. The floor is covered by the usual gray, caseous, necrotic material. *Proliferative* lesions appear to be more diffuse, sometimes affecting the greater portion of the laryngeal mucosa (Fig. 181). They exist as a diffuse thickening and swelling of the tissues with the surface thrown into innumerable tubercles or larger projections. Such a mucosa is generally pale, gray, and glistening. In time, however, the surface breaks and typical tuberculous ulcers form. In either case, the lesions tend to heal by resolution and fibrosis and, when the original destruction is severe, the fibrosis produces marked distortion and obliteration of the usual anatomic demarcations. *Histologically* the characteristic lesions consist of the usual tubercles and tuberculous granulation tissue.

In early lesions, the most important *complication* is edema of the larynx while in old lesions it consists of laryngeal destruction. Local *clinical manifestations* consist of hoarseness, dysphagia, dryness, and burning pain. These manifestations, in the presence of active pulmonary tuberculosis, along with indirect laryngoscopy and, occasionally, biopsy enable a correct *diagnosis* to be made. Specific *treatment* consists of the administration of antibiotics and chemotherapeutic agents. Other treatments in the past have consisted of rest of vocal cords, local applications of a variety of medicines, inhalations of protean compounds, diathermy, irradiation, electrocoagulation, and surgical excisions (Cody). The *prognosis* as far as the laryngeal lesion is concerned is, as a rule, good for in the presence of antibiotics and chemotherapeutic agents, not only do the symptoms disappear but the lesions heal in the majority of patients.

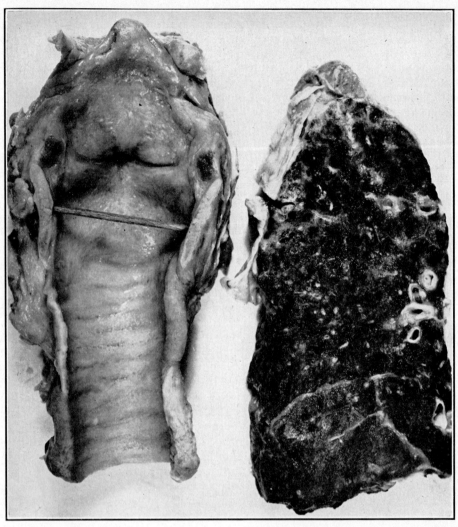

Fig. 181.—Laryngeal tuberculosis showing a proliferative lesion. The mucosa is diffusely swollen and roughened by innumerable coalescing tubercles. The specimen to the right is a lung disclosing tuberculosis in its superior half.

PHYSICAL DISTURBANCES

Orientation.—Under this heading the following disorders of the larynx may be briefly considered: paralysis, spasm, trauma, irradiation chondronecrosis, obstruction, and foreign bodies.

Paralysis.—Paralysis of the vocal cords of the larynx results from interruption of the motor nerve pathways to these structures. The interruption may occur centrally (cortical or bulbar) or peripherally. The latter may be found anywhere along the courses of the vagus nerves or their recurrent laryngeal branches (Ballenger). *Cortical* lesions are often traumatic (frequently occurring at birth) or are functional. *Bulbar* lesions occur as a result of injury, progressive bulbar paralysis, syphilis (tabes dorsalis), apoplexy, syringomyelia, and multiple sclerosis. *Peripheral* lesions may be due to enlarged cervical lymph nodes, trauma, thyroid enlargements, operations (especially on the thyroid), aneurysms, mediastinal tumors, pleurisy, scoliosis of cervical vertebra, tuberculosis, and toxins (bacteria, lead, arsenic, alcohol, etc.). The *paralysis* varies with the type of lesion. In cortical and bulbar lesions it is often unilateral (for the centers are separated) but it may be bilateral (birth trauma); in peripheral lesions of a nonoperative nature it is usually unilateral, while in peripheral lesions of an operative nature it may not only be bilateral but it may also affect only parts of a single vocal cord. The vagaries of the paralysis following surgery are explainable on the anatomic distributions of the recurrent laryngeal nerves. It has been shown by careful dissection that these nerves bifurcate two, three or more times before they enter the larynx (Morrison). Thus, it is apparent that the postoperative paralysis will involve those portions of the cord innervated by the branches of the destroyed nerves.

Spasm.—Spasm of the larynx may be tonic or clonic (Ballenger). *Tonic spasm* consists of rigidity of the muscles which persists for a considerable time. It may be caused by (1) irritation of the motor centers in the brain (as seen in tetanus and hydrophobia), (2) irritation of the trunks of the recurrent laryngeal nerve before destruction and paralysis occurs (as seen in pressure from aneurysm of the aorta, carcinoma of the esophagus, pleuritic adhesions of the apex of the right lung, and tumors pressing upon the nerves), and (3) reflex irritation (generally seen in sensitive children as a result of tapeworm, tight prepuce, constipation, etc.). *Clonic spasm* consists of rhythmic, involuntary, jerky, movements of the vocal cords, soft palate, or other laryngeal or pharyngeal muscles. It may be associated with similar contractions of voluntary muscles in other portions of the body. It is of central origin and is seen in connection with epidemic encephalitis, chorea, hemorrhage of the brain, multiple sclerosis, and tumors of frontal lobes. *Clinically* laryngeal spasm may be associated with crowing inspiration, cyanosis, aphonia, and coughing.

Trauma.—In *military life*, trauma to the larynx constitutes at least 1 per cent of all casualties (Lynch). In *civilian life* it is considerably less common and occurs in conjunction with industry, accidents, criminal attacks, and suicide attempts. In either case, the *injurious agent* may be applied from within in the form of inhalation of hot vapors, poisonous gases, chemicals, or foreign bodies or from without in the form of direct or indirect penetrating or nonpenetrating injury in the form of bullet, shrapnel, or blow (Ledderer and Howard). The *injury* may affect the larynx proper, the trachea, or the cervical tissues. It consists of lacerations, fractures, hematoma, hemorrhage, and laryngeal edema. Later it may be associated with infection (local, mediastinal, or pulmonic), laryngeal fibrosis and deformity, and obstruction to the airway. The immediate *treatment* is directed toward securing an adequate dry airway, controlling hemorrhage, and combating shock. If a tracheotomy is necessary it should be performed as low as possible. Subsequent treatment consists of determining the extent of the injury, attention to the wound, and, finally, reconstruction of the larynx and rehabilitation of the patient.

Irradiation Chondronecrosis.—Chondronecrosis of the larynx after therapeutic doses of irradiation occurs in cartilage that has a lowered radio-resistance (Goodrich and Lenz). The lowered resistance is *caused* by penetrating carcinomas and infections wherein the nutrition and circulation of the cartilage is interfered with. During irradiation therapy, laryngeal edema occurs early but subsides in four to six weeks after treatment has been concluded. In patients *developing chondronecrosis*, the edema not only persists or recurs but becomes more pronounced. The laryngeal structures become distorted; the airway becomes narrowed; the breath becomes foul; sequestrated cartilage is expectorated or aspirated; pneumonia or lung abscess may develop, and the patient may die of pulmonary complications, sepsis, or cachexia. *Microscopically* the early changes consist of disappearance of cartilage cells, while the later alterations encompass varying degrees of degeneration to complete disintegration of the tissue. The condition usually appears within six months after the conclusion of the irradiation therapy. The *epiglottis* is affected more often than other cartilages. Advocated *treatment* in impending or early cases of chondronecrosis is laryngectomy.

Obstruction.—Anything that encroaches upon the lumen of the larynx results in obstruction to the airway. Some of the more important conditions may be listed as follows: (1) congenital—hypoplasia, web, cyst, laryngocele, and stridor, (2) inflammations—acute nonspecific laryngitis, chronic nonspecific laryngitis, edema, diphtheria, syphilis, tuberculosis, Boeck's sarcoid, scleroma, leprosy, glanders, etc., (3) physical disturbances—paralysis, spasm, trauma, irradiation chondronecrosis, stenosis, and foreign bodies, and (4) tumors—benign or malignant and laryngeal or extralaryngeal.

Foreign Bodies.—Foreign bodies lodged in the larynx are quite *diverse*. They are usually located at or above the vocal cords but may also be found inferiorly. Generally, however, when they pass the vocal cord barrier they uninterruptingly proceed to the bronchi. *Clinically* there may be sudden death from asphyxia or there may be violent coughing, hoarseness, aphonia, and dyspnea (Scott-Brown). Later the foreign body may be (1) dislodged and coughed up or aspirated into the lungs, or (2) bring about local infection (especially if it is a penetrating object such as a fish bone). The *diagnosis* is generally made from the history and indirect laryngoscopy. *Treatment* is removal.

TUMORS

Orientation.—Some tumors and tumor-like conditions of the larynx are common while others are rare. They *affect* all races; some predominate in one sex, others in the other, and, depending upon the growth, they have certain predilections for various ages. The *cause* of the tumor-like conditions is irritation, generally consisting of infection, smoke, and trauma. The cause of true tumors is unknown.

Pathologically the tumors are quite diverse. Most of those that have been recorded in the literature may be listed as follows: polyps, keratosis, papilloma, adenoma, carcinoma, fibroma, amyloid tumor, fibrosarcoma, neurofibroma, lipoma, hereditary hemorrhagic telangiectasia, lymphangioma, hemangioma, hemangioendothelioma, chondroma, chondrosarcoma, chordoma, osteoma, osteosarcoma, plasmocytoma, lymphblastoma, leiomyoma, leiomyosarcoma, myoblastoma, rhabdomyosarcoma, and secondary tumors consisting of extension from adjacent structures such as thyroid, pharynx, and esophagus, and metastasis from distant areas.

The *complications* consist of obstruction, inflammation, hemorrhage, and (in malignant growths) extension into the neck and metastasis. The *clinical manifestations* depend upon the location of the growth and not upon the type of neoplasm (Scott-Brown). They generally produce symptoms by interfering with the function of the vocal cords or by obstructing the

airway. Growths situated on the outside of the aryepiglottic folds or on the
epiglottis may become quite large before they produce obstruction. Tumors
displacing muscle fibers may cause discomfort in the throat with perhaps
variable alterations in the tone of the voice. Neoplasms located on the
vocal cords usually prevent proper apposition of the cords and thus, even
when tiny, bring about hoarseness. Other manifestations may consist of
pain, paroxysmal cough, dyspnea, stridor, asphyxia, and dysphagia. The
diagnosis is made from a consideration of the history, direct and indirect
laryngoscopic examination, and biopsy. The usual *treatment* is surgical
excision (local or laryngectomy) although in certain tumors irradiation is
advocated by some authors. The *prognosis* varies with the neoplasm.

Of all the tumors or tumor-like conditions mentioned above, the following
are frequent enough to merit separate consideration: polyps, keratosis,
amyloid tumor, papilloma, and carcinoma.

Polyps.—Polyps of the larynx are not true tumors. They are found in
adults and predominate in males. They occur as a response to trauma and
inflammation. *Grossly* they occur on the anterior two-thirds of the vocal
cords as rounded, smooth, gray to red, pedunculated or sessile nodules that
usually measure as much as 8 mm. in greatest diameter. *Histologically* the
surface is covered with squamous epithelium which may be hypertrophic,
attenuated, or ulcerated. The core is composed of dense connective tissue,
of myxomatous connective tissue, of capillaries or dilated sinuses, or of
granulation tissue. Accordingly, the lesions have been called fibromatous,
myxomatous, angiomatous, or granulomatous polyps respectively. The
condition is cured by local excision.

Keratosis.—Keratosis of the larynx is not a true tumor. It represents a
localized benign hyperplasia of the epithelium with abundant keratinization. The *synonyms* that are usually used are hyperkeratosis and leukoplakia. The condition is found only in adults and is more common in males.
The *cause* is anything that irritates the mucosa over a prolonged period.
Some of the agents usually listed are tobacco, excessive use of alcohol,
vocal abuse, chronic postnasal discharge, syphilis, endocrine dyscrasias,
avitaminosis A and B, viral infection, and mycosis (Grossman and Matthews). *Pathologically* the lesions are located on the upper surface and edge
of one or both vocal cords (Clerf). They exist as single or multiple chalk-
white thickenings of the mucosa that may at times present a papillomatous
appearance (Fig. 182). *Histologically* the process consists of excessive deposition of keratin on the surface, slight hyperplasia of the prickle cells,
and often marked hyperplasia of the basal cells. The basement membrane
is intact. The submucosa is composed of collagenous or edematous connective tissue that contains varying degrees of leukocytic infiltration and varying numbers of dilated vascular channels filled with fluid or clotted blood.
The chief *complication* is a carcinomatous transformation. *Treatment*
consists of removal of the cause if this can be determined. Otherwise it
consists of stripping the vocal cord of its mucosa and submucosa or, if the
lesion suggests carcinoma, of laryngofissure and cordectomy. The *prognosis* is unpredictable and the patients should, therefore, be kept under close
observation.

Amyloid Tumor.—An amyloid tumor is probably a fibroma that has been
permeated with amyloid. It is not confined to the larynx for the mass has
also been *described* in the tongue (base), trachea, nose, pharynx, mouth,
lungs, skin, urinary bladder, etc. In the larynx the condition is most common in the sixth decade of life (Kreissl). *Pathologically* the lesion is rounded

or polypoid and grossly consists of a reddish mass that usually measures as much as 1 cm. in diameter. It may be found in the vocal cords, subglottis, or ventricular bands. *Histologically* the surface is covered with regular, hyperplastic, or atrophic epithelium and the mass is composed of homogeneous hyaline material that takes a positive amyloid stain.

Papilloma.—Papilloma is the most common benign laryngeal tumor (Holinger). It is equally divided between both sexes and it occurs at all ages. Single lesions, however, prevail in patients over sixteen years of age while multiple lesions prevail in those under sixteen years of age. The

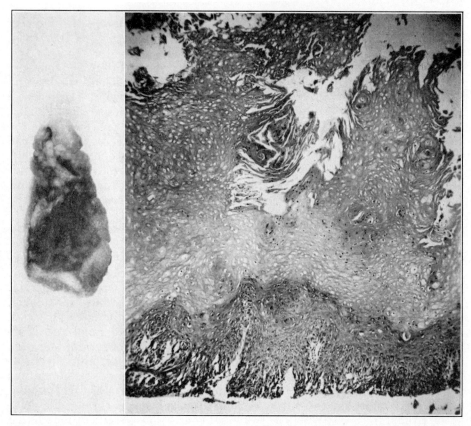

Fig. 182.—Keratosis of the larynx showing, to the left, a removed cord containing white papillary areas and, to the right, the surface covered with a thick layer of keratinized material.

cause of the growths in children is probably viral and possibly endocrine (for they frequently disappear spontaneously at puberty) while the cause in adults is unknown. *Pathologically* the growths may be located anywhere in the larynx but they predominate on the true and false vocal cords. They exist as glistening, elevated, mulberry-like, pink to red, friable excrescences or nodules that have a tendency to bleed upon manipulation. *Histologically* they consist of a core of well-vascularized connective tissue covered with hyperplastic but otherwise regular adult squamous epithelium (Fig. 183). Aside from encroachment upon the airway an important *complication* in adults is an occasional malignant transformation. *Treatment* has been diverse with surgical removal being favored. As already stated, the tumors that appear in childhood have a tendency to disappear spontaneously as puberty is approached.

Carcinoma.—It has been estimated that cancer of the larynx (which is composed mostly of carcinoma) comprises about 4 per cent of all cancers in the body (Clerf). It may *occur* at any age from the third decade on and is about fourteen times as frequent in males as it is in females. The *cause* is unknown. Heredity appears to play a role. In some instances benign lesions such as papilloma or keratosis precede the growth but in others there seems to be no antecedent pathologic change. Other etiologic factors that have been incriminated from time to time are abuse of the larynx and inhalation of irritating materials such as smoke, dust, etc.

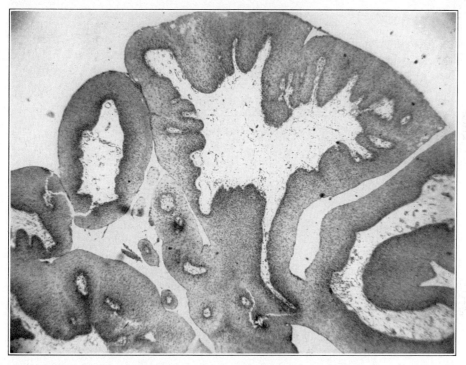

Fig. 183.—Papilloma of the larynx illustrating cores of connective tissue covered with hyperplastic but otherwise regular stratified squamous epithelium. × 7.

Pathologically carcinoma of the larynx is generally dividable into two broad groups—*intrinsic* occurring in or below the ventricles and *extrinsic* occurring on or above the ventricular bands. Approximately two-thirds of all cases originate on the vocal cords. Usually one cord is affected, the anterior third of the cord is more commonly involved, and the lesion is single. In the remaining one-third of cases, other portions of the laryngeal mucosa are affected with predominant involvement of the subglottic area. The *original lesion* appears as a circumscribed or more diffuse, gray to pink thickening with a smooth or granular surface (Altman). As it extends, the tissue becomes more fixed and rigid. When the vocal cord is involved, its motility becomes impaired. Later the lesion becomes papillary or infiltrating and, in either case, may become ulcerated (Fig. 184). Well-established growths measure from a few millimeters to 5 or 6 cm. in greatest

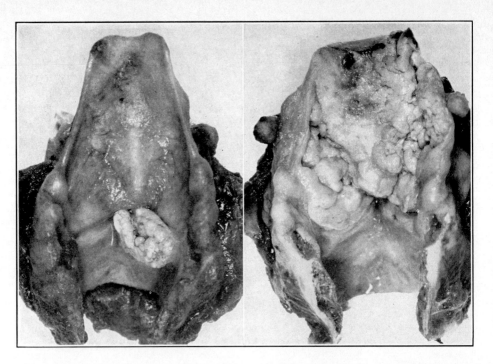

Fig. 184.—Carcinoma of the larynx showing, to the left, a fungating growth that has replaced most of the right vocal cord and, to the right, a fungating tumor that has covered the entire epiglottis.

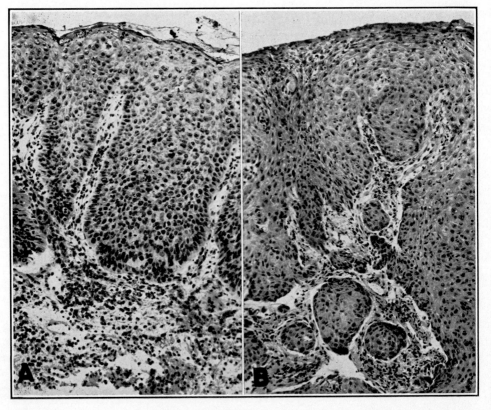

Fig. 185.—Carcinoma of the larynx showing A, a tumor that is still confined by the basement membrane (intraepithelial carcinoma) and B, a squamous cell carcinoma of intermediate grade malignancy permeating the submucosa. × 100.

diameter. They are usually gray, firm, friable, and bleed upon manipulation. *Histologically* the tumors are usually squamous cell carcinomas and only rarely are they adenocarcinomas. They start in the lining epithelium as an intraepithelial carcinoma (Fig. 185). Such a lesion is confined by the basement membrane. The cells are mostly of the prickle variety but vary considerably in shape, size, and staining qualities. The cytoplasm is usually abundant and the nuclei are round, oval, or irregular, and hyperchromatic. Mitoses may be numerous and the normal polarity of the cells is distorted. As the lesion advances it breaks through the basement membrane and infiltrates the submucosa in the form of strands, nests, and individual cells. The cells are similar morphologically to those found in the intraepithelial tumors, although they vary in their degree of malignancy. In decreasing order of frequency they are of an intermediate, low, and high grade malignancy. Most of the tumors, thus, show well-defined prickle cells and have a tendency to undergo keratinization and pearl formation. The supporting stroma is usually of a loose connective tissue variety and is permeated with leukocytes.

Carcinoma of the larynx *spreads* by (1) direct extension (intraepithelially and subepithelially) to involve other portions of the larynx, trachea, pre-epiglottic space, and perilaryngeal tissues and (2) by metastasis to affect, in decreasing order, the following organs: cervical lymph nodes, mediastinal lymph nodes, lungs, thyroid, liver, kidneys, heart, bones, spleen, adrenal, jejunum, mesenteric lymph nodes, and submaxillary gland (Latella). In general, both extension of the tumor to perilaryngeal tissues and metastasis of the tumor to extralaryngeal organs is about four times as common in extrinsic growths as it is in intrinsic tumors.

A definitive *diagnosis* of carcinoma of the larynx can be made only by biopsy. The condition should be differentiated clinically from syphilis and tuberculosis. Although both surgical excision (by way of laryngofissure or laryngectomy) and irradiation therapy have been recommended, it appears to be the concensus that the *treatment* of choice is surgical removal. The over-all five-year *survival* rate in large series of patients treated (1) by irradiation is approximately 35 per cent, (2) by laryngofissure about 80 per cent, and (3) by laryngectomy about 50 per cent. The survival rate of patients with intrinsic carcinoma is about four times that of patients with extrinsic carcinoma. The *causes* of *death* listed by Latella in a series of 117 cases were as follows: cachexia, bronchopneumonia, local hemorrhage, lung abscess, pulmonary tuberculosis, renal disease, hypoproteinemia, tracheo-esophageal fistula, pulmonary artery thrombosis, myocarditis, and brain damage from carotid artery ligation.

REFERENCES

Congenital Anomalies

Fox, N., and DINOLT, R.: A. M. A. Arch. Otolaryng., *37*, 552, 1943 (Cysts).
KEIM, W. F., and LIVINGSTONE, R. G.: Ann. Otol., Rhin. & Laryng., *60*, 39, 1951 (Laryngocele).
McHUGH, H. E., and LOCH, W. E.: Laryngoscope, *52*, 43, 1942 (Webs).
O'KEEFE, J. J.: A. M. A. Arch. Laryngol., *54*, 29, 1951 (Laryngocele).
TRIMBY, R. H.: J. A. M. A., *122*, 740, 1943 (Laryngeal Stridor).

Degenerations

VASTINE II, J. H., and VASTINE, M. F.: A. M. A. Arch. Otolaryng., *55*, 1, 1952, (Calcification Laryngeal Cartridges).

29

Inflammations

Auerbach, O.: A. M. A. Arch. Otolaryng., *44*, 191, 1946 (Tuberculosis).
Ballenger, W. L., and Ballenger, H. C.: *Diseases of the Ear, Nose, and Throat*, 10th Ed., Philadelphia, Lea & Febiger, 1957.
Brown, L. A.: A. M. A. Arch. Otolaryng., *56*, 521, 1952 (Granuloma Following Intubation).
Cody III, C. C.: A. M. A. Arch. Otolaryng., *53*, 1, 1951 (Tuberculosis).
Davison, F. W.: Pennsylvania M. J., *53*, 250, 1950 (Obstructive Laryngitis).
Everett, A. R.: Laryngoscope, *61*, 113, 1951 (Acute Laryngotracheobronchitis).
Miller, M. V.: A. M. A. Arch. Otolaryng., *31*, 256, 1940 (Edema).
Morgan, E. A., and Wishart, D. E. S.: Canad. M. A. J., *56*, 8, 1947 (Laryngotracheobronchitis).
Sinclair, S. E.: J. A. M. A., *117*, 170, 1941 (Influenzal Laryngitis).
Wallner, L. J., *et al.*: J. A. M. A., *145*, 1252, 1951 (Tuberculosis).

Physical Disturbances

Ballenger, W. L., and Ballenger, H. C.: *Diseases of the Ear, Nose, and Throat*, 10th Ed., Philadelphia, Lea & Febiger, 1957.
Fien, I., *et al.*: A. M. A. Arch. Otolaryng., *55*, 689, 1952 (Tabes Dorsalis).
Goodrich, W. A., and Lenz, M.: Am. J. Roentgenol., *60*, 22, 1948 (Irradiation Chondronecrosis).
Lederer, F. L., and Howard, J. C.: A. M. A. Arch. Otolaryng., *43*, 331, 1946 (Trauma).
Lynch, M. G.: A. M. A. Arch. Otolaryng., *47*, 413, 1948 (Trauma).
Morrison, L. F.: Ann. Otol., Rhin. & Laryngol., *61*, 567, 1952 (Recurrent Laryngeal Nerve Paralysis).
Scott-Brown, W. G.: *Diseases of the Ear, Nose, and Throat*, New York, Paul B. Hoeber, Inc., 1952.

Tumors

Altmann, F., *et al.*: A. M. A. Arch. Otolaryng., *56*, 121, 1952 (Intraepithelial Carcinoma).
Clerf, L. H.: A. M. A. Arch. Otolaryng., *32*, 484, 1940 (Carcinoma).
——————: A. M. A. Arch. Otolaryng., *40*, 177, 1944 (Preepiglottic Space and Carcinoma).
——————: A. M. A. Arch. Otolaryng., *44*, 517, 1946 (Sarcoma).
——————: J. A. M. A., *132*, 823, 1946 (Keratosis).
Cunning, E. S.: J. A. M. A., *142*, 73, 1950 (Diagnosis and Treatment of Tumors).
Cutler, M.: J. A. M. A., *142*, 957, 1950 (Carcinoma).
Friedberg, S. A., and Segall, W. H.: Ann. Otol., Rhin. & Laryngol., *50*, 783, 1941 (Polyps).
Garland, L. H., and Sisson, M. A.: Surg., Gynec. & Obst., *94*, 598, 1952 (Carcinoma).
Grossman, A. A., and Matthews, W. H.: Canad. M. A. J., *66*, 39, 1952 (Keratosis).
Harris, H. H., and Wattleworth, K. L.: A. M. A. Arch. Otolaryng., *53*, 640, 1951 (Tumors).
Holinger, P. H., *et al.*: Ann. Otol., Rhin. & Laryngol., *59*, 547, 1950 (Papilloma).
Kreissl, L. J., *et al.*: A. M. A. Arch. Otolaryng., *50*, 309, 1949 (Amyloid Tumors).
Lachmann, J.: A. M. A. Arch. Otolaryng., *53*, 299, 1951 (Sarcoma).
Latella, P. D.: Ann. Otol., Rhin. & Laryngol., *61*, 265, 1952 (Carcinoma).
McCall, J. W., and Fisher, W. R.: Laryngoscope, *62*, 475, 1952 (Carcinoma).
Scott-Brown, W. G.: *Diseases of the Ear, Nose, and Throat*, New York, Paul B. Hoeber, Inc., 1952.
Tucker, G.: J. A. M. A., *149*, 119, 1952 (Carcinoma).

Chapter

12

Lower Respiratory System

PATHOLOGIC PHYSIOLOGY

Richard T. Cathcart

The chief *normal function* of the lungs is to effect the transfer of oxygen and carbon dioxide between the ambient air and the circulating blood. This requires the integration of both the airway and the circulatory systems. There is a series of steps which is necessary in order for gas exchange to take place. First is the mass movement of air into and out of the lungs. This is the process of *ventilation* and is a function of the bellows action of the chest. It is essentially a mechanical process and demands the coordination of the musculo-skeletal apparatus of the thorax, the diaphragm, and the accessory respiratory muscles. An additional requirement for effective ventilation is the presence of a patent airway system as well as normal elastic pulmonary tissue. Once the air has been introduced into the lungs it must be distributed to the innumerable pulmonary alveoli which are surrounded by a vast capillary network and perfused by pulmonary arterial blood. This is a more subtle function and its clear understanding is essential for a knowledge of the manner in which pulmonary function is altered by disease.

In normal man the *inspired air* is distributed very evenly throughout the lungs. This means that the concentration of oxygen from alveolus to alveolus is very nearly identical. At the same time there is an even distribution of the blood perfusing the alveoli. The *normal volume* of the lungs is in the neighborhood of 5000 cc. Under resting conditions, only about one tenth of this volume, or 500 cc., would be utilized in any one breath. Much of the time, many of the alveolar sacs are at least partly collapsed and are not distended with inspired air. It is of great physiologic importance that the capillaries which supply such nonventilated alveoli are also collapsed, and consequently do not perfuse under such conditions. As the *tidal volume* becomes larger, more alveoli are ventilated and at the same time their attendant capillaries open up and are perfused with blood. There is then a perpetual readjustment of capillary perfusion to alveolar ventilation. This maintenance of a fairly constant *ventilation-perfusion* ratio is essential for normal function to continue.

In certain *diseased states* the stability of this *ratio* is upset and symptoms of pulmonary dysfunction appear. Such a situation might arise under a variety of circumstances. When there occurs an increase in ventilation without a proportionate increase in perfusion, there will of necessity be ventilation of alveoli which are not perfused. Such ventilation is of no value to the subject because it involves the delivery of air to portions of the lungs which are unable to participate in the gas exchange. Similarly, if there were an increase in perfusion without a proportionate increase in ventilation, blood would pass through nonaerated areas and full saturation could not be attained.

The third step in the process of gas transport is that of *diffusion*. This refers to the diffusion of oxygen across the alveolar membrane into the capillary blood. It involves also the simultaneous diffusion of carbon dioxide from the blood into the alveolar space from where it is breathed out in the expired air. The lungs are extremely efficient in this regard. At any one time at rest, only 60 cc. of blood are present in the pulmonary capillaries. The transit time through the capillary is only about three fourths of a second. Yet the lungs are capable of oxygenating some 5000 cc. per minute at rest and under conditions of physical stress as much as 25,000 cc. The amount of gas which can diffuse is indirectly proportional to the thickness of the membrane. For the rapid transfer of the gas which normally occurs, an easily permeable membrane is mandatory.

Pathologic conditions which interfere with pulmonary function may interfere with ventilation, with distribution, with diffusion, or with circulation. In the discussion which follows they have been separated only for purposes of analysis. In practice it is uncommon for one function to be affected to the exclusion of all others.

In order to *understand* the *dysfunction* which pathologic conditions might produce, it is first necessary to *know* where the pathologic lesion in the lung is, what structures are involved, and finally, how malfunction of these structures may affect each specific function of the lungs. It is further necessary to have a concept of the enormous *reserve* which the lungs possess. This is true not only of their capability to hold air, but of their circulatory capacity as well. Depending somewhat on size and age, a normal individual is capable of breathing somewhere between 100 to 200 liters per minute. Resting minute ventilation is in the neighborhood of 5 liters per minute and even following moderate degrees of exercise does not exceed 20 liters per minute. The brreathing reserve is thus extremely high and is of some significance. This means that for any disease to produce pulmonary insufficiency it must be either extensive or most fortuitously situated.

The *pulmonary capillary bed* has similar properties. Its total cross sectional area is about 60 square meters. Under extreme circumstances it can accomodate as much as 25 liters of blood per minute. At rest, the normal pulmonary blood flow is about 5 to 6 liters per minute. Here again, the reserve capacity is extremely large. This is related in part to the large volume of the capillary bed but also to its enormous distensibility. The vessels of the pulmonary circuit contain little muscle, have thin walls, and are highly distensible. Their capacity then is far above the usual demands which are placed upon them. Consequently, any pathologic lesion which affects the pulmonary vasculature must be so diffusely situated that the vascular bed is reduced by more than one half before there can result any increase in pulmonary artery pressure or right-sided heart failure.

Ventilatory dysfunction may be conveniently subdivided into restrictive and obstructive insufficiency. The phrase *restrictive ventilatory insufficiency* is used to indicate a decrease in ventilatory capacity which results from a limitation of the normal expansion and contraction of the lungs. To a very great extent this is mechanical and may be the result of both pulmonary and *extrapulmonary causes*. Among the latter, hydrothorax, arthritis of the spine, kyphoscoliosis, and pleural fibrosis are common. In this group, marked insufficiency is unusual and dyspnea perhaps the only symptom. Of more importance are the *intrapulmonary causes*. Prominent among them are the various pulmonary fibroses. These may be the result of irradiation, pneumoconioses, or infection such as might be a sequel to chronic bronchitis and bronchiectasis. In any case, there is replacement of normal pulmonary parenchyma by masses of fibrous tissue of varying sizes. These are inelastic and rigid and, when diffusely situated, may markedly limit the excursion of the lungs. The degree of insufficiency closely parallels the degree of fibrosis. The most prominent *symptoms* are dyspnea and hyperventilation. In advanced cases, arterial anoxia may result but it is rare for carbon dioxide retention to occur. It is characteristic of this type of disease that the *vital capacity* is *reduced* proportionately more than is maximum breathing capacity.

Obstructive ventilatory insufficiency implies narrowing or partial obstruction to the airway system of sufficient degree to impair ventilation. This is characteristically the result of obstruction in the smaller bronchi, particularly the terminal and respiratory bronchioles. The obstruction may be the result of spasm, edema, secretion, or fibrosis of the bronchial wall. Not infrequently several, or all, of these factors may be implicated at the same time. There may be numerous physiologic consequences to such a situation. Since obstruction is present it will require greater physical effort to blow air beyond it. The work of breathing increases and *dyspnea* becomes more marked as the obstruction becomes more severe. The diameter of the tracheobronchial tree is largest during inspiration and smallest during expiration. Hence, when any obstruction is present, it will be more critical during expiration. The *expiratory phase* will be *prolonged* and the timed *vital capacity diminished*. The presence of obstruction favors the distention and distortion of alveoli distal to it. They tend to become progressively larger and are emptied with great difficulty. The *residual volume increases*. These are progressive events which may *occur in* bronchial asthma, chronic bronchitis, and pulmonary emphysema. The degree to which they occur will depend upon the degree of obstruction, its duration, and the presence or absence of antecedent emphysema.

Uneven distribution of the inspired air is a common feature of many types of pulmonary diseases. As has been previously noted, the oxygen breathed in is normally distributed evenly throughout the lung. In diseased states where there exist irregular alterations in the consistency of the lung, this will not occur. Alveoli adjacent to fibrotic or consolidated areas tend to be restricted in their expansion and are ventilated less well than alveoli surrounded by normal lung. Similarly, air spaces which are distal to obstructed bronchi may receive little or no air at all. This is particularly true when the alveoli are dilated and distorted as in pulmonary emphysema. If perfusion of these alveoli continues, it is impossible for the blood passing through them to become fully saturated with oxygen. Such blood which perfuses non-ventilated alveoli is returned then to the left heart without having been oxygenated. This blood has all the characteristics of venous blood and is referred to as *"venous admixture."* It contaminates the fully aerated blood and *arterial unsaturation* occurs. In normal individuals there is always some perfusion of nonventilated alveoli and this is partially responsible for the fact that the normal oxygen saturation is only 96 per cent. As pulmonary disease advances, this tendency becomes more marked and is intensified by the irregular distribution of the pathologic lesion. It is the most common cause of *cyanosis* in lung disease. This combination of poor distribution of inspired air and uneven perfusion of alveolar capillaries reaches a zenith in *pulmonary emphysema*. In this condition, overbreathing is frequent but much of the air goes to alveoli which are not perfused. The patient becomes progressively *dyspneic*. At the same time, much of the pulmonary artery blood perfuses areas which are poorly ventilated or not ventilated at all. The amount of venous admixture increases and cyanosis becomes more marked. This is the most important factor associated with the cyanosis seen in *lobar pneumonia*. A region of consolidation is filled with exudate and leukocytes precluding the entrance of air. Although such areas are perfused and, in fact, may be even hyperemic because of the inflammation present, nonetheless the blood passing through such sections of the lung is not oxygenated and returns to the left heart unaltered.

Impairment of *diffusion* has been associated with a variety of diseases which have the following features in common: (1) a striking similarity in the clinical picture regardless of etiology, (2) fairly uniform physiologic findings, and (3) a predilection for the pathologic process to involve the alveolar septa. They are all associated then with a decrease in the permeability of the alveolar-capillary membrane. *Interstitial pulmonary fibrosis* is a classical example of this type of disease. The deposition of connective tissue, the growth of capillaries, and the round cell infiltrations cause marked thickening of the septa rendering the diffusion of gas more difficult. A similar disturbance of function is typically found in *berylliosis* where interstitial granulomas may cause a decrease in membrane permeability. Actually, any pathologic process which may cause thickening of the alveolar septa and is sufficiently diffuse may produce this same syndrome. The *basic lesion* may be fibrosis, edema, or tumor but the physiologic effect is the same. Other conditions in which this has been reported to date are *scleroderma*, *Boeck's sarcoid*, *hematogenous tuberculosis*, and *alveolar cell carcinoma*. The *symptoms* of this group of diseases are primarily dyspnea and cyanosis. *Physiologic studies* reveal a decrease in vital capacity and are relatively normal in maximum breathing capacity. Hyperventilation is characteristic and extreme on exercise. The arterial oxygen saturation is usually only slightly lower than normal but falls precipitously on exercise. The carbon dioxide level is low. It is important to note that as much as oxygen diffusion may be hindered, carbon dioxide diffusion is rarely affected. Carbon dioxide diffuses through the alveolar membrane some twenty times more readily than does oxygen.

In *general*, an attempt has been made to outline the normal function of the lungs and the manner in which this might be altered by pathologic changes. It should be pointed out that no absolutely rigid *classification* of disease according to *function* is possible. It is uncommon for any pulmonary lesion to affect one structure alone. Therefore, more than one function is usually altered. When many structures are involved, it is infrequent that they are affected to the same degree. One would expect that in almost any pathologic process of the lungs a combination of factors might be present, each of which might influence function in a different manner and to a different degree. And such is the case. It becomes necessary to *appraise* the *morphologic changes* in the lung, determine what *physiologic function* they might modify, and to estimate the extent to which this would occur. The latter consideration is fully as important as the first two in view of the enormous reserve of the lung. The alveoli are so numerous and the vascular bed so large and distensible that much adaptation is possible. It is not infrequent then that considerable disease may be present with little disturbance of function. By the same token, when symptoms of pulmonary insufficiency do appear they are usually indicative of the fact that the pathologic process is either diffusely situated or advanced in degree.

Physiologic *tests* of *pulmonary function* have proved to be most helpful in the evaluation of pulmonary disability. They have permitted not only the analysis of the functional derangement but have provided a means of quantitating it as well The more common tests are vital capacity, residual volume, minute ventilation, maximum breathing capacity, breathing reserve, index of mixing, and arterial blood analysis.

Vital capacity may be defined as the maximum volume of air which can be expired following a maximum inspiration. It is preferably recorded on a spirometer with a rotating drum. This permits the analysis of a curve from which more information is gained than from measurement of volume alone. The normal values vary greatly according to the age, sex, and height of the patient but range between 2500 and 5000 cc. A convenient method of reporting the vital capacity is by timing the expiratory phase. A subject should be able to expire 87 per cent of the volume in 1 second, 90 per cent in 2 seconds, and 95 per cent in 3 seconds. Diminution of the vital capacity is a measurement of the air space available. Prolongation of expiration as may be demonstrated in the timed curve is usually indicative of bronchial obstruction.

Residual volume is that volume of air which remains in the lungs following a maximum expiratory effort. Since this gas is not expired, it cannot be measured directly, but must be calculated by a gas dilution technique. Although more cumbersome to measure, it is an important determination and is an index of the ability of the lungs to empty. The normal residual volume measures 1000 to 1500 cc. and in no case should it exceed 30 per cent of the total capacity of the lungs. Elevation of the residual volume is strongly suggestive of the presence of pulmonary emphysema and the degree of elevation is closely related to the degree of emphysema which is present.

Minute ventilation is the volume of air breathed by the lung in one minute. It is expressed in liters per minute and, of course, varies with the state of activity of the subject. At rest, in a basal state, this should be no more than 3.5 to 4 liters per minute per square meter of body surface area. An excess is indicative of a state of hyperventilation.

Maximum breathing capacity is the maximum volume of air which the patient can breathe in and out of his lungs per unit of time. The patient is instructed to breathe into a spirometer as rapidly and as deeply as he can for a period of 12 seconds. The expired gas is collected and measured, and the breathing curve is recorded. The volume is expressed in liters per minute. The normal range is wide, 100 to 200 liters, but the normal value is closely related to the age, sex, and size of the patient. This is perhaps the best single test of ventilatory ability available. It provides a definite measure of breathing capacity. The study of the breathing record clearly separates restrictive from obstructive lung disease.

Breathing reserve represents the difference between the maximum breathing capacity and the actual minute ventilation at any one time. It is customarily expressed as a percentage of the maximum breathing capacity and is used as a convenient index of the degree of dyspnea present. A study of this relationship is important since it reveals that dyspnea is more closely related to a diminution of the maximum breathing capacity than to increased ventilatory requirement.

Index of *mixing* pertains to the dilution of nitrogen with oxygen. The subject inhales 100 per cent oxygen for a period of 7 minutes. At the end of this time, a maximum expiration is performed and a gas sample is obtained. This end expiratory sample is delivered from alveolar air and is analyzed for nitrogen. The percentage of nitrogen remaining in alveolar air following a 7 minute oxygen washout is termed the index of intrapulmonary mixing. The normal determination should be less than 2.5. A value above this figure is indicative of the poor distribution of inspired air and an excellent measurement of the degree that this function is impaired.

Arterial blood analysis for oxygen and carbon dioxide is the best overall test of pulmonary function. The arterial oxygen saturation should be 96 per cent or above. In the absence of a veno-arterial shunt, a reduction in the oxygen saturation indicates either that there is impaired diffusion across the alveolar capillary membrane or that a significant amount of blood is circulating through poorly ventilated areas of the lungs. The carbon dioxide level of the arterial blood reflects the result of the subject's ventilatory status. It tends to be low in conditions associated with hyperventilation. On the other hand, an elevated carbon dioxide content in the presence of a low or normal pH is indicative of ventilatory insufficiency. It is important that a sample of arterial blood should be analyzed both at rest and following standard exercise. There is ample evidence that arterial blood values may be normal when activity is minimal, only to become markedly altered following physical stress.

Other tests are available for the more detailed study of lung function and, of those described, there are numerous modifications (Comroe and Baldwin). Nonetheless, a knowledge of the few mentioned above allows for a comprehensive evaluation of pulmonary function as well as the manner and degree to which normal physiology may be modified by disease.

GENERAL CONSIDERATIONS

This Chapter on the Lower Respiratory System will include disorders of the trachea, bronchi, lungs proper, pleura, and mediastinum. The consideration of disturbances of the mediastinum is incomplete for a few of the conditions (as, for example, congenital vascular anomalies, aneurysms, and tumors of vessels) have already been discussed while others (thymic diseases and lymph node enlargements) will be included in subsequent chapters. As elsewhere, the disorders are conveniently dividable into the usual five broad categories of disease processes.

CONGENITAL ANOMALIES

Orientation.—Some congenital abnormalities of the respiratory system are common while others are rare. In either group some are important (to the point of being incompatible with life) while others are inconsequential. They may be listed as follows: tracheal obstruction, tracheo-esophageal fistula, tracheal diverticulum, mediastinal bronchogenic cysts, accessory and aberrant bronchi, bronchial obstruction, variations in pulmonary lobes, pulmonary maldevelopment, cystic disease of the lungs, Kartagener's triad, alveolar dysplasia, arteriovenous fistula, abnormalities of the larger vessels, defect in the anterior mediastinum, and thoracic meningocele. Tracheo-esophageal fistula is discussed in the Chapter on the Esophagus (p. 633) while arteriovenous fistula is discussed in the Chapter on the Vessels (p. 386). The other anomalies may now be briefly considered in the order listed.

Tracheal Obstruction.—Congenital obstruction of the trachea may be extrinsic or intrinsic. *Extrinsic* obstruction is due to compression of the lumen from without. It may be caused by any tumor mass in the mediastinum or by vascular anomalies (double aortic arch). Thymic enlargement (not tumor) is considered by some authors to be capable of producing external pressure but its capacity to do so is quite doubtful. *Intrinsic* factors may consist of atresia, complete absence of the lower portion, stenosis, and transient narrowing (Evans). The last mentioned is probably due to soft tracheal rings.

Tracheal Diverticulum.—Diverticula of the trachea may be congenital or acquired. They arise as an outpocketing between the muscle bands of the membranous part of the trachea. They are usually located 3 or 4 cm. distal to the larynx, generally protrude to the right, have a narrow ostium, may measure up to 5 cm. in diameter, and are lined with respiratory epithelium. They have been known to erode into the innominate artery, become infected, and, by pressure, cause recurrent laryngeal nerve paralysis (Drymalski).

Mediastinal Bronchogenic Cysts.—Mediastinal bronchogenic cysts arise as a pinching off of diverticula of the trachea. They are generally found on the right side of the trachea at any point between the larynx and the right main bronchus but are most commonly located opposite the sternoclavicular joint. They are round or oval, thin-walled, unilocular cysts that are filled with serous fluid or mucus and that may measure as much as 9 cm. in diameter (Healy and Heller). They may or may not be connected by fibrous tissue with the trachea. Histologically they are lined with respiratory epithelium and, within the wall proper, often disclose submucosal glands and smooth muscle bundles. They are usually asymptomatic but occasionally may produce pressure symptoms. Sometimes they become infected.

Accessory and Aberrant Bronchi.—The level of the tracheal bifurcation into the right and left main bronchi is fairly constant but the bifurcation of the main bronchi into various subdivisions is not. The latter dictates the length of the mainstem bronchi and these lengths, in turn, are important to the surgeon in performing a pneumonectomy. An accessory bronchus is rare. It usually stems from the right side of the trachea above the tracheal bifurcation, but it may also arise from the right main bronchus and occasionally it may be found on the left side.

Bronchial Obstruction.—Like tracheal obstruction, congenital bronchial obstruction may be extrinsic or intrinsic. *Extrinsic* obstruction is caused by external pressure and may be due to a tumor or an abnormally located pulmonary vein. *Intrinsic* obstruction may occur in the form of stenosis, atresia, or web. A web consists of a diaphragm spanning the bronchial lumen. It may be complete or incomplete.

Variations in Pulmonary Lobes.—This caption may embrace variations in *number* of lobes and accessory pulmonary tissue. The former generally consists of two lobes on the right side and/or three lobes on the left. *Accessory lung* tissue may consist of (1) a *tracheal accessory lung*—usually located superiorly on the right side and communicating with the right accessory bronchus, (2) *esophageal lobe*—a mass of lung tissue communicating by a "fistula" with the esophagus, (3) *azygos lobe*—located in the apex of the right lung and caused by pleural grooving by the azygos vein (Fig. 186), and (4) *intralobular sequestration*—consisting of aberrant, usually cystic, lung tissue that (*a*) is located within the medial portion of either lower lobe,

(b) has no communication with the main tracheobronchial tree, and (c) possesses a separate blood supply directly from the aorta (Fig. 187). Regardless of the location of the accessory lung tissue, the chief *complication* is pyogenic infection. *Roentgenographically* the extra density may be mistaken for a tumor or for tuberculosis.

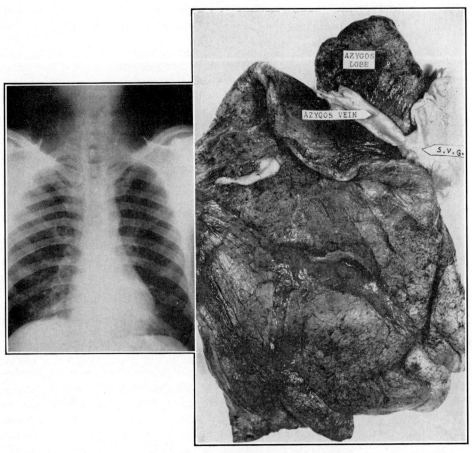

FIG. 186.—Azygos lobe of the right lung showing a roentgenographic shadow that could be mistaken for a tumor and the azygos vein segmenting the upper lobe.

Pulmonary Maldevelopment. — Improper development of the lungs occurs in various degrees. It may affect a portion of one lung, an entire lung, or both lungs. Simple underdevelopment is referred to as *hypoplasia;* complete absence of lung substance, bronchial tree, and vascular structures on the affected side is called *agenesis,* and the presence of small, rudimentary bronchi with absence of pulmonary and vascular structures is known as *aplasia* (Tuynman). The changes are slightly more *common* in males than they are in females and predominate on the right side. The *clinical manifestations* vary with the anomaly and consist of (1) none when the defect is slight, (2) dyspnea and cyanosis when the maldevelopment is greater, and (3) death when agenesis or aplasia is bilateral.

Cystic Disease of the Lungs. — Cystic disease of the lungs may be congenital or acquired. *Congenital cysts* are frequently referred to as broncho-

genic cysts, polycystic disease, honey-combed lung, congenital cystic malformations, congenital bronchiectasis, etc. Their *incidence* at the Walter
Reed Army Hospital was recorded as 42 cases in 100,000 hospital dispositions
with the estimated general incidence being 5 per 100,000 population (Cooke
and Blades). They *develop* as a result of separation of portions of the lung
buds or their derivatives. If this comes about early in the development of
the embryo a solitary large cyst is likely to develop proximally, while if it
comes about late multiple small cysts are more apt to develop peripherally.

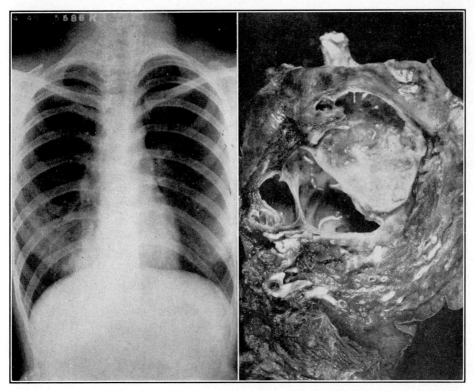

Fig. 187.—Intralobar sequestration of the lung showing a roentgen opacity in the medial portion
of the right lower lobe and the resected cystic lung tissue with its aberrant blood supply.

Once separation of pulmonary tissue occurs, the pull of the thoracic cage
and accumulation of fluid are responsible for the distention. Later the
fluid drains into a bronchus and is replaced with air. *Pathologically* the
cysts may be located in any portion of either lung. They may be single or
multiple and may measure from a few millimeters to twenty centimeters
or more in diameter. They are always connected with bronchi. In small
cysts the communications are direct, large, and easily demonstrable but in
large cysts they are oblique, small, and usually difficult to locate (Fig. 188).
The lumens are filled with fluid, air, or sometimes pus. The inner surfaces
are smooth, gray, and often trabeculated and the walls are generally thin.
Histologically the cysts are lined with respiratory epithelium which, on
occasion, may be attenuated, ulcerated, or metaplastic. The wall is composed of connective tissue and may contain submucous glands, fat, smooth
muscle, and cartilage. The chief *complications* are infection, hemorrhage,

and rupture with spontaneous pneumothorax. The *clinical manifestations* are those of (1) progressive enlargement with encroachment upon the respiratory capacity resulting in attacks of dyspnea and cyanosis, (2) infection resulting in fever, cough, expectoration, loss of weight, pain in the chest, etc., and (3) hemorrhage resulting in hemoptysis. Radiologically

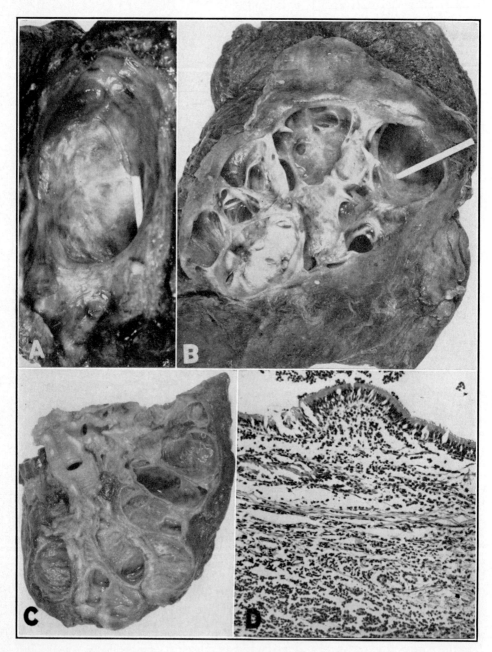

FIG. 188.—Congenital cysts of the lung showing *A*, a solitary, large, smooth-walled cyst with an applicator inserted through a bronchial opening, *B*, multiple large cysts, *C*, many small cysts communicating directly with bronchi, and *D*, cyst wall with a lining of pseudostratified columnar epithelium and a connective tissue wall permeated with leukocytes. × 100.

the pulmonary fields may show areas of decreased (when the cysts are filled with air) or areas of increased (when the cysts are filled with fluid) density and the cystic spaces may be outlined by instillation of radiopaque material into the tracheobronchial tree. The *diagnosis* is based upon the clinical manifestations and the radiologic appearance. *Treatment* is surgical excision. The *prognosis* is good.

Acquired cysts of the lungs are of two varieties—(1) healed, drained, pulmonary abscesses that have become epithelialized, and (2) emphysematous blebs or bullæ. Neither of these is a true cyst. The former represents an end stage of pulmonary infection while the latter represents a breakdown and coalescence of overdistended alveoli in pulmonary ephysema (p. 529).

Kartagener's Triad.—This syndrome consists of situs inversus (a mirror-imaged transposition of the thoracic and abdominal organs), bronchiectasis, and inflammation and/or abnormal development of the paranasal sinuses. Although the condition is congenital and hereditary it may not be recognized until adulthood. Clinical manifestations are generally referable to the sinuses and/or the lungs.

Alveolar Dysplasia.—This is a congenital malformation of the alveoli characterized by a reduction in their numbers, a connective tissue thickening of the walls, and a diminution in the size of their spaces (MacMahon). Grossly the lungs are well formed but are rubbery, reddish, and subcrepitant. The condition may be complicated by atelectasis, congestion, edema, hemorrhage, or inflammation. The disorder is found in either premature or full-term infants. It may be responsible for death within the first forty-eight hours after birth. If the infant survives this period the condition predisposes to pneumonia.

Abnormalities of Larger Vessels.—Abnormalities of the larger vessels concern both the veins and the arteries. *Venous abnormalities* may consist of (1) presence of a common right or left pulmonary vein, (2) increase in number consisting of three and rarely four veins (instead of two) entering either the right or the left atrium, and (3) drainage of a portion or the entire pulmonary circuit into the right side of the heart either directly (right atrium) or indirectly (by way of the superior vena cava, innominate vein, subclavian veins, etc.) (Healey). *Clinically* variations in number of pulmonary veins have little significance beyond mechanical difficulties encountered at operation. Drainage of the pulmonary veins into the pulmonic circulation is incompatible with life when such a connection is complete unless there are compensating cardiac anomalies or it may be accompanied by varying degrees of improper oxygenation when the connection is incomplete.

Arterial abnormalities may consist of (1) persistent truncus arteriosus (p. 283), (2) absence of pulmonary artery with persistent ductus arteriosus, (3) absence of pulmonary artery with hypertrophied bronchial arteries, (4) absence of pulmonary artery with anomalous pulmonary arteries arising from arteries such as the subclavian, intercostal, esophageal, phrenic, common carotid, inferior thyroid, lower thoracic aorta, upper abdominal aorta, celiac, or superior mesenteric, and (5) combinations of these (Manhoff and Howe). The *clinical manifestations* are like those in tetralogy of Fallot or other similar congenital anomalies of the heart (p. 283).

Defect of the Anterior Mediastinum.—This anomaly is extremely rare. It consists of a small or complete opening in the anterior mediastinum with a free communication between the two pleural cavities (Gross and Lewis). The condition is of significance only when air enters the anterior mediastinum or either pleural cavity, in which case it may be responsible for bilateral pneumothorax, atelectasis, and death.

Thoracic Meningocele.—This is a rare congenital malformation, there being only 14 cases recorded up to 1952 (Rubin and Stratemeier). It consists of a protrusion of the meninges of the spinal cord through an intervertebral foramen. The mass varies from a few to many centimeters in diameter and causes an enlargement of the foramen, erosion of adjacent portions of the ribs, and kyphoscoliosis. Ordinarily the condition produces few or no symptoms. Treatment consists of surgical excision with closure of the spinal meninges.

DEGENERATIONS

Orientation.—In the Lower Respiratory System, as in other areas of the body, degenerative processes are generally intimately bound with specific diseases. Despite this, however, the following conditions may be listed in this category: tracheopathia osteoplastica, Ayerza's disease (p. 367), pulmonary calcifications, pneumoconiosis, and lipid pneumonia.

Tracheopathia Osteoplastica.—This condition, known also as *osteoma* of the trachea, consists of the formation of innumerable nodules of bone in the lower portion of the trachea and the main bronchi. The excrescences originate in the perichondrium of the tracheobronchial cartilages and protrude inwardly, gradually but surely narrowing the lumen. They are composed of calcified cartilage, osseous tissue, and bone marrow. The covering epithelium usually undergoes metaplasia to a stratified squamous cell variety. The condition occurs in middle-aged adults. The *clinical manifestations* are due to stenosis and infection and consist of increasing dyspnea, cough, expectoration, and hemoptysis. The *diagnosis* is made from bronchoscopy and biopsy. There is no adequate *treatment*. The *prognosis* is poor.

Pulmonary Calcification.—Formerly it was thought that most if not all calcifications of the lungs were *due to* tuberculosis. Now it is known that a variety of chronic healed inflammatory processes such as histoplasmosis, coccidioidomycosis, aspergillosis, blastomycosis, etc., account for even a greater number of cases than does tuberculosis. The *incidence* of pulmonary calcifications in the general population varies with the locality from 1.5 per cent in Toronto to 20 per cent in the Mississippi Basin (Heaton). While the *deposits* vary in number, size, and location they are usually single, rounded, and located in the upper half of the lung fields. Sometimes, however, they may be diffuse and miliary (Doub). *Pathologically* the foci consist of a background of collagenous connective tissue permeated with calcium salts and occasionally containing true bone.

Pneumoconiosis.—Pneumoconiosis (Gr. = lung + dust) is a lung condition due to inhalation of dust particles. It is an all-inclusive term that encompasses a wide variety of both harmful and inert substances. Sometimes the dusts are relatively pure but more often two or more are inhaled simultaneously and the clinical and pathologic picture is thus complicated. A few of the more important conditions that may be mentioned are: anthracosis, silicosis, talc pneumoconiosis, asbestosis, siderosis, berylliosis, bauxite fume pneumoconiosis, and bagassosis.

Anthracosis.—Anthracosis connotes the deposition of carbon particles in the lungs. The condition is seen to some extent in all city dwellers and industrial workers but reaches its zenith in coal miners. In soft coal miners the disorder is often pure, but in hard coal miners it is complicated by the invariable presence of silica (*anthracosilicosis*). *Carbon particles* are relatively inert. They are inhaled with the air, ingested by phagocytes, and transported to the alveolar septa and to the peribronchial, perivascular, subpleural, and mediastinal lymph nodes (Fig. 189*A*). When the phagocytes die the particles are liberated and may accumulate locally in great numbers. They do not, however, elicit a fibrous tissue reaction. The carbon appears black. Depending upon the amount present, the lung discloses peppery deposits, nodular accumulations, or masses replacing virtually the entire parenchyma (Fig. 189*B*). The central areas of the large accumulations have a tendency to liquefy and form cavities. Pure anthracosis does

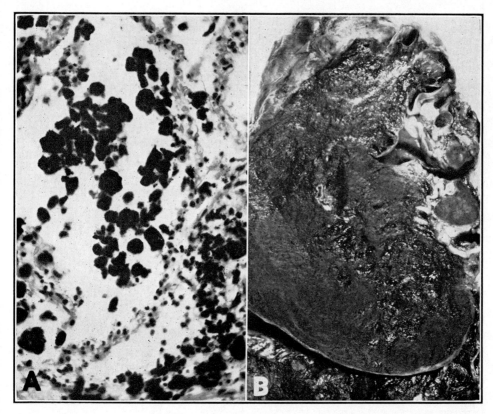

Fig. 189.—Anthracosis showing *A*, carbon pigment in alveolar spaces and septa within and without phagocytes, and *B*, replacement of most of the upper lobe and draining lymph nodes with carbon. The lung tissue shows several small irregular cavities.

not predispose to infection and generally does not produce cardiac embarassment. The fibrosis that accompanies *graphite pneumoconiosis* is thought to be due to the 30 per cent silica content of graphite (Wyatt).

Silicosis.—Silicosis is caused by the deposition of silica (SiO_2) which is also known as free silica or silicon dioxide. It exists in either crystalline (quartz) or amorphous form (Forbes). It is common in nature, constituting about 60 per cent of the earth's crust and is thus found in abundance in connection with the mining, sand blasting, metal grinding, and other *industries*. Silica exerts its *effect* on the lungs because of its inherent chemical, rather than its physical, properties. In the United States it has been generally adopted that a concentration of less than 5,000,000 silica particles per cubic foot does not constitute an industrial health hazard. It has also been shown that silica particles 10 microns or more in diameter are not dangerous because they are filtered out before they reach the alveoli, and that the most injurious particles are those that measure less than two microns across.

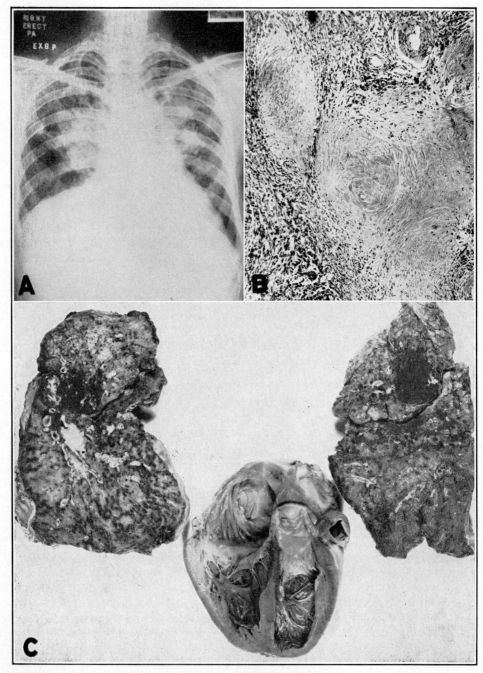

FIG. 190.—Anthracosilicosis showing *A*, multiple, bilateral opacities in a roentgenogram, *B*, coalescing, lamellated, fibrous tissue nodules.   × 50, and *C*, coalescing and single masses in each lung and right-sided cardiac hypertrophy and dilatation from the same case illustrated in *A*.

Pathologically once the particles reach the alveoli they are picked up by phagocytes and distributed in a manner similar to carbon particles. Upon liberation, however, they provoke a characteristic progressive tissue response. The initial reaction is one of tubercle formation. It consists of a central loose collection of epithelioid cells surrounded at the periphery by Langhans' giant cells and leukocytes (neutrophils, plasma cells, lymphocytes, and monocytes). Occasionally the center undergoes necrosis. As the lesion ages it becomes less cellular and more and more fibrous (Fig. 190*B*). The connective tissue is deposited in concentric lamellations and undergoes progressive collagenization. Individual nodules then coalesce

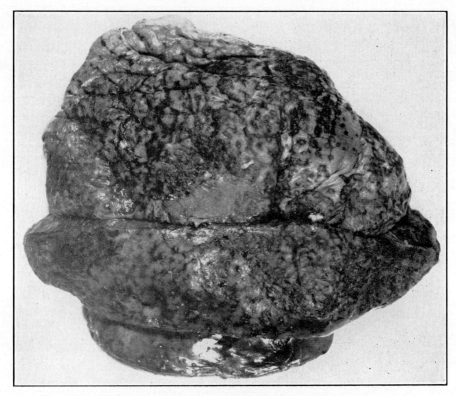

Fig. 191.—Silicosis illustrating innumerable small gray subpleural foci rimmed with carbon pigment.

to produce larger conglomerations. *Grossly* the initial lesion appears as grayish white to black (because carbon is almost always present) pinpoint firm nodules distributed for the most part along the course of the pulmonary lymphatic channels (Fig. 191). As they enlarge they coalesce until ultimately they form large conglomerate gray to black masses occupying most of the lung fields (Fig. 190*C*). Occasionally they may undergo spontaneous central necrosis and cavitation. As a rule, both lungs are affected symmetrically, the masses have no particular predilection for any portions of the lungs and, as the lesions age, they tend to migrate medially.

The *complications* are pulmonary emphysema, pneumothorax, pyopneumothorax, tuberculosis (silicotuberculosis), chronic bronchitis, and right-sided cardiac decompensation (cor pulmonale). The *clinical mani-*

festations depend upon the degree of pulmonary fibrosis and the complications that develop. Generally they consist of dyspnea, pain in the chest, cough, expectoration, hemoptysis, loss of weight, and gastrointestinal disturbances. The *diagnosis* is made from the history, the clinical picture, and the roentgenograms which disclose shadows that correspond to the pathologic deposits (Fig. 190*A*). *Treatment* is prophylactic (by way of proper industrial hygiene) and symptomatic. The *prognosis* is variable. Some people develop rapid progressive fibrosis upon short exposure to minimal amounts of the dust while others are highly resistant upon prolonged exposure to large amounts of the dust.

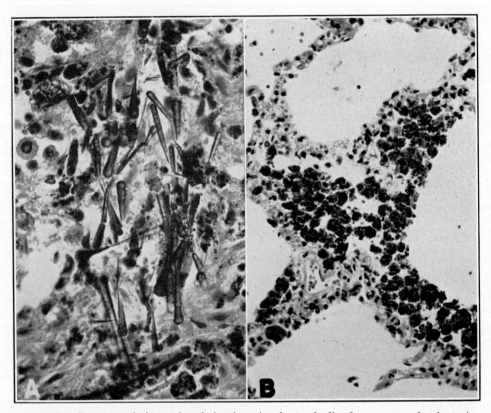

FIG. 192.—Pneumoconiosis continued showing *A*, asbestos bodies from a case of asbestosis. × 400, and *B*, intraseptal granules of iron free and within phagocytes without a fibrous tissue reaction. × 200.

Talc Pneumoconiosis.—Talc pneumoconiosis occurs in miners, millers, and occupations where talcum powder fills the atmosphere (Friedman). Since talcum powder is native hydrous magnesium silicate and contains about 0.5 per cent free silica it is probably the silica that produces the pulmonary changes. The pathologic and clinical characteristics are the same as those in silicosis.

Asbestosis.—Asbestos is a *mineralogical vegetable* known for its insulating and fire-resistant properties (Wyatt). It *contains* about 40 per cent silica, 40 per cent magnesium, and 3 per cent iron oxide. It is inhaled by *workers* in weaving, sorting, or carding rooms and in crushing houses in two forms — black granular pigment and *asbestos fibers*. In the lungs the latter appear as elongated structures measuring from 5 to 10 microns in diameter and as many as 300 microns in length. They consist of a central fiber covered by a corrugated, golden yellow, iron-positive crust (Fig. 192A). The asbestos bodies are incarcerated in the bronchiolar and alveolar walls where they evoke an exudation of protein fluid and cells. The *reaction* is, in part, of a simple foreign body type and, in part, may be due to the silica content. Early, it consists of an exudation of leukocytes and foreign body giant cells. Later, it is replaced with fibrous tissue. The fibrosis is more common in the lower lobes and is characteristically distributed about affected bronchioles, subpleural areas, and pleuras. The *complications*, less frequent than in silicosis, consist of tuberculosis, formation of carcinoma, and,

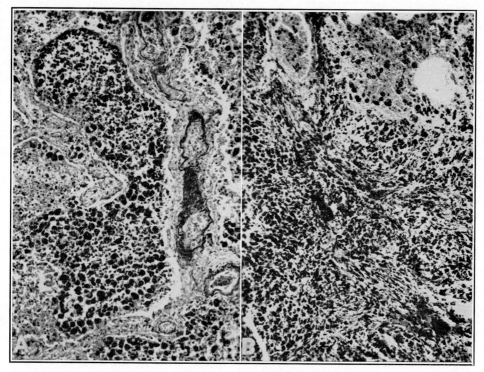

Fig. 193.—Idiopathic pulmonary hemosiderosis illustrating *A*, an abundance of hemosiderin granules, fibrosis of the alveolar septa, and disruption of elastic tissue in the septa and vessels and *B*, extensive fibrosis and many filaments covered with iron. × 100.

uncommonly, right-sided cardiac failure. *Clinically* there is a gradual onset of dyspnea, dry cough, and clubbing of the fingers. *Roentgenographically* the lung fields show a ground glass appearance. The *diagnosis* is made from the history, roentgenograms, and finding asbestos fibers in the sputum. *Treatment* is preventative and symptomatic. The *prognosis* is fair but the course is generally protracted.

Siderosis.—Siderosis connotes the deposition of *iron* in the lungs. The condition occurs *exogenously* in connection with oxyacetylene grinding of steel alloys and ocher mill turneries (Wyatt) but is also found *endogenously* in cases of long-standing cardiac failure (Lendrum) or idiopathically (Wyllie). The latter is called *idiopathic pulmonary hemosiderosis*. In either case, the iron particles (1) are phagocytosed by monocytic cells, (2) are deposited within the alveoli, alveolar septa, and peribronchial, perivascular, subpleural, and mediastinal lymphatics and lymph nodes (Fig. 192), and (3) evoke both a destructive and inflammatory response (Fig. 193). The retrogressive process consists of fragmentation, disruption, and disappearance of the elastic fibers of the alveolar septa and pulmonary vessels. Some of the fibers become impregnated with iron and then present as yellowish-green filamentous structures both within the alveolar septa and, less often, in the draining lymph nodes (Soergel). Some of them become surrounded by foreign body giant cells. The inflammatory response is insidious and mild. It is chiefly monocytic in type. Ultimately, however, there is a concomittant deposition of collagenous connective tissue, although this is never as extensive as that seen in silicosis. As would be expected, the iron content of the lungs is increased several thousand fold. *Grossly* the lungs are enlarged, heavy, irregularly firm, and more or less diffusely brown. Radiologically they disclose either multiple, blotchy, confluent shadows or smaller, almost miliary-like, tiny nodules spreading peripherally from the hilum.

Of special interest is the group of cases usually labeled *idiopathic pulmonary hemosiderosis* and also referred to as essential pulmonary hemosiderosis, allergically conditioned pulmonary purpura, and hemorrhagic asthma (Soergel, Browing, and Schaar). Although not too frequently recorded, it is the consensus that the condition is more common than supposed and that many cases go unrecognized. In the cases recorded, the disorder has been about 4 times as frequent in children as in adults, has predominated in males, and has been recognized in the age periods from 4 months to 40 years. As the name suggests, the *cause* of the condition remains unknown, although theoretically it has been thought to be due to (1) an abnormality of lung tissue in the form of an acquired or congenital low grade inflammation or of a defect in pulmonary elastic fibers, (2) formation of auto-antibodies against an unknown sensitizing agent with their localization in the alveolar walls and with subsequent antigen-antibody reaction in these areas, and (3) a defect in vasomotor contraction of pulmonary vessels resulting in an intermittent increase in pressure and hemorrhages. *Clinically* there are acute attacks of pulmonary hemorrhage attended by dyspnea, tachycardia, and hemoptysis. Actually, it is thought that the bleeding is more or less continuous with exacerbations resulting in the acute episodes. In time there are pallor, anemia, weakness, and loss of weight. The bone marrow is hyperplastic. The *diagnosis* is made from the history, roentgenograms, and needle aspiration biopsy. Treatment is symptomatic and supportive. Iron compounds, and even transfusions, are administered for the anemia. Splenectomy and adrenal hormones have been tried with equivocal success. The *prognosis* is guarded, for the immediate mortality is about 25 per cent and the average duration of life is about 3 years.

Berylliosis. — Beryllium is a *metal* that is used in the ceramic industry, lamp manufacturing, precision tooling, electric welding, radio and television industry, atomic projects, etc. (Wyatt). The metal gains entrance into the body by contact or inhalation and produces lesions in the skin and lungs. The *cutaneous* lesions are in the form of a contact dermatitis in susceptible people occurring about two weeks after exposure or of ulcers that fail to heal. The latter occur when the surface has been abraded. The *pulmonary* lesions may be acute or chronic. *Acute pneumonitis* is rapid in onset. It consists of severe congestion, outpouring of alveolar fluid rich in proteins, hyaline membranes lining the alveoli, occasionally scattered fibrinoid ma-

terial, cuboidal swelling of alveolar cells, and a permeation with mononuclear cells, plasma cells, and lymphocytes. *Chronic pneumonitis* is
insidious in onset with fatigue, loss of weight, cough, dyspnea, cyanosis,
and clubbing of the fingers as prominent *clinical* features. It consists of
diffuse nodulations measuring as much as 4 mm. in diameter, of scarring,
and of intervening emphysema. *Histologically* the chronic pulmonary
lesion is similar to the indolent ulcer of the skin (Fig. 194). It is a granuloma consisting of tubercles composed of epithelioid cells with surrounding
giant cells, mononuclear cells, lymphocytes, and plasma cells. Central

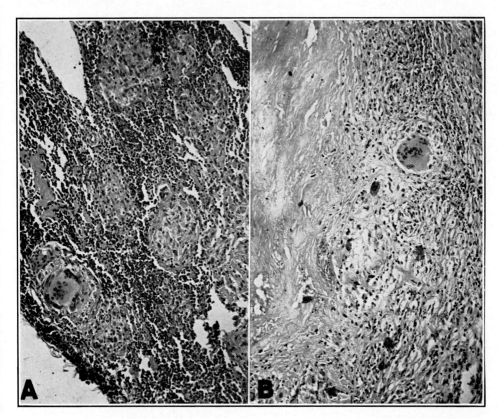

Fig. 194.—Berylliosis showing *A*, an early lesion with tubercles composed of epithelioid cells
and giant cells, and *B*, a late lesion consisting of necrosis surrounded by spurious tubercles and
collagenous fibrous tissue. × 100.

granular necrosis may be present and extensive, especially in coalescing
lesions. Ultimately, healing occurs by fibrosis and collagenization. The
mortality rate in cases with the pulmonary condition is recorded as varying
from 1 to 20 per cent.

Bauxite Fume Pneumoconiosis.—This disorder is caused by the inhalation of bauxite fumes in the manufacture of artificial corundum (Wyatt).
The *clinical* manifestations may consist of dyspnea, substernal pain, fatigue,
and (because of spontaneous pneumothorax) cyanosis. *Pathologically*
there is a diffuse interstitial fibrosis of the lungs, rather than nodulation,
with prominence of alveolar lining cells. The *mortality rate* is about 30
per cent.

Bagassosis.—Bagasse consists of the fibrous residue resulting from crushing of sugar cane and the expression of its juices (Koven). *Industrially* it is used (1) in the manufacture of boards for interior decorating, (2) for insulating purposes, and (3) in the manufacture of bricks. Inhalation of this material gives bagassosis. *Clinically* and *radiologically* the condition is similar to miliary tuberculosis. *Histologically* the lesion consists of a foreign body giant cell and foam cell reaction about the bagasse fibers (Wyatt). Since spores and fungi are found in association with the fibers and the lesions, it is not certain which of these evokes the reaction.

Lipid Pneumonia.—Lipid pneumonia is also known as lipoid pneumonia and, less commonly, as paraffinoma. The condition is relatively *common*, there having been over 300 cases recorded in the literature by 1951 (Volk). It occurs at all ages and affects both sexes with equal frequency. The *causes* are usually mineral, animal, or vegetable lipids of *exogenous* origin. In recorded cases they have consisted of mineral oil, chaulmoogra oil, cod liver oil, milk fat, petrolatum, lard, egg yolks, olive oil, sesame oil, poppy seed oil, and, rarely, iodized vegetable oils used in roentgenography (Hoffman and Bell). The materials enter the lungs by way of the tracheobronchial tree during the course of infant or tube feeding, vomiting, swallowing, or administration of nasal medication. Predisposing factors are infancy, old age, debilitating disorders, and paralysis of the pharynx. Occasionally the lipids are of *endogenous* origin occurring as a result of low-grade pulmonary infection in connection with bronchial obstruction (Morgan).

Pathologically the posterior portions of the lower lobes are more commonly affected than other areas of the lungs. The disorder is more common on the right side than on the left but occasionally it may be bilateral and symmetrical. The condition is generally divided into two types—infantile and adult. *Infantile* lipid pneumonia consists of irregular, diffuse, pneumonic consolidations that are indistinctly outlined, light yellowish in color, and rubbery in consistency. *Histologically* the predominating lesion consists of large foam cells filling alveolar spaces and infiltrating alveolar septa (Fig. 195D). Occasionally free oil droplets are present but there is little or no fibrous tissue formation or giant cell reaction. The changes in the draining lymph nodes are similar. *Adult* lipid pneumonia consists of coalescing masses that are more sharply defined. They are yellowish gray, are firm to hard, and present a spongy appearance (Fig. 195B). *Histologically* the phagocytic and foam cell reactions are similar to those in the infantile type. In addition, the alveolar spaces and alveolar walls contain droplets of oil that are often surrounded by foreign body gaint cells and reveal a diffuse increase in fibrous tissue (Fig. 195C). Sometimes the lesions reveal central necrosis and rarely they disclose calcification. The reaction in the draining lymph nodes is similar to that in the lung parenchyma.

The *complications* consist of emphysema, pulmonary abscess, nonspecific pneumonia, empyema, tracheobronchitis, and bronchiectasis. *Clinically* the condition is insidious and is asymptomatic until the lesion becomes extensive. In the latter the manifestations are due principally to depletion of functioning lung parenchyma. They may consist of rapid respirations, dyspnea, dry cough, cyanosis, dullness to percussion, and moist rales. *Roentgenograms* reveal opacities that correspond to the distribution of the pathologic lesions (Fig. 195A). Other symptoms and signs correspond to the complications that accompany some of the cases. The *diagnosis* is made from the history and roentgenographic appearance. The finding of foam cells and droplets of oil in the sputum may be of considerable aid in

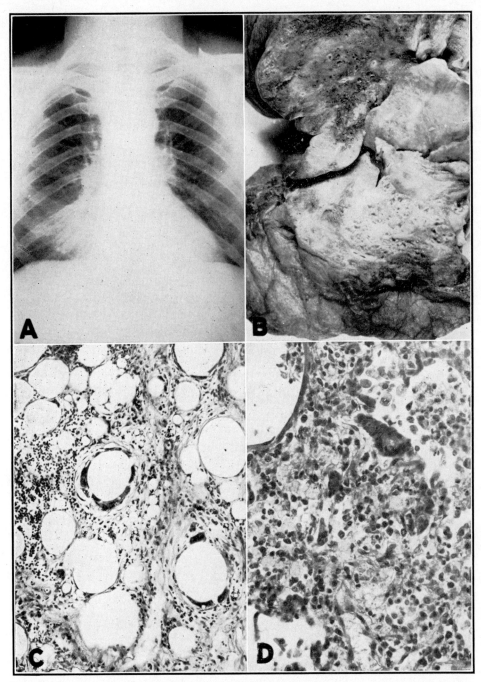

FIG. 195.—Lipid pneumonia showing *A*, a roentgenographic shadow in the medial portion of the right lung, *B*, a spongy gray appearance of the affected areas in the removed specimen, *C*, large fat vacuoles surrounded by foreign body giant cells and fibrous tissue in the adult type. × 100, and *D*, foam cells in the alveolar spaces and septa in the infantile type. × 200.

arriving at a proper evaluation. Among others, a differential diagnosis in the adult type of lipid pneumonia should include carcinoma. *Treatment* is not specific and consists mostly of prevention and removal of the causative agent. Sometimes complications (such as bronchiectasis) necessitate a lobectomy. The *prognosis* is good if the lesion is minimal and contact with the causative agent is severed early. It is only fair in advanced cases.

INFLAMMATIONS

Orientation.—Inflammation of the trachea is known as *tracheitis*, of bronchi as *bronchitis*, of trachea and bronchi as *tracheobronchitis*, of bronchioles as *bronchiolitis*, of the lung parenchyma as *pneumonitis* (Gr. = lung + inflammation) or *pneumonia*, of the pleura as *pleuritis* or *pleurisy*, and of the mediastinum as *mediastinitis*. While inflammations of the structures enumerated are many and varied, for purposes of discussion they may be listed under the following headings: tracheobronchitis, fibrinous bronchitis, bronchiectasis, pneumonia, pulmonary abscess, pleurisy, empyema, and mediastinitis.

Tracheobronchitis.—Unless otherwise specified, the caption tracheobronchitis refers to infection of the trachea and bronchi with ordinary pyogenic organisms. The condition may be acute or chronic. *Acute tracheobronchitis* is generally an extension of acute laryngitis (p. 438). *Chronic tracheobronchitis*, or *chronic bronchitis* as it is more commonly known, may result from a persistence of the acute process but more commonly it is secondary to tonsillitis, chronic rhinitis, chronic sinusitis, dental infection, etc. (Prior). It may also be secondary to heart disease, industrial fumes, or, most frequently, tobacco smoke. *Pathologically* the mucosa is reddened, thickened, and covered with mucus or pus. Histologically the epithelium is hyperplastic, attenuated, or metaplastic. The submucosal glands are hyperactive and the submucosa shows congestion, edema, and a diffuse infiltration with plasma cells, lymphocytes, and mononuclear cells. The important *complications* are pulmonary fibrosis and emphysema. The chief *clinical manifestations* are cough, expectoration, and later dyspnea. The *diagnosis* is made from the history and by a process of exclusion. A word of caution, however, should be raised in making a diagnosis of chronic tracheobronchitis for only too frequently such a diagnosis is a catchall, often for much more serious pulmonary disease (carcinoma). *Treatment* consists of elimination of the cause and administration of antibiotics. The *prognosis* is variable.

Fibrinous Bronchitis.—This is a special type of bronchitis, characterized chiefly by (1) cough, (2) dyspnea, and (3) expectoration of white casts of various shapes and sizes (Fig. 196). The casts are composed mainly of fibrin and mucin with varying amounts of cellular debris, bacteria, and Charcot-Leyden crystals added. The condition may be primary or it may be secondary to tuberculosis, asthma, fungous infection, etc. The prognosis in the primary type is good while that in the secondary type is dependent upon the underlying disease. Asphyxia has been recorded.

Bronchiectasis.—The term bronchiectasis (Gr. = bronchus + dilatation) means simply dilatation of bronchi. Actually, however, it connotes bronchial dilatation with superimposed infection. The condition *affects* all races, has no predilection for either sex, and occurs at all ages with a preponderance between twenty and sixty years and a mean age of thirty years. The *causes* are variable. A minority of cases is of congenital origin while the vast majority is acquired (Herbut and Everts-Suarez). The initial lesion in the latter is *bronchial obstruction*. In some cases the obstruction, in the form of congenital stenosis, inflammation, foreign body, or tumor, is apparent at the time the lesion is discovered while in others no obstruction is demonstrable. Even in these cases, bronchial occlusion in childhood, in the form of mucous plug, pus, blood, foreign body, etc., doubtlessly antedates the development of the condition. In any case, the occlusion is followed by atelectasis and by inflammation of the bronchial wall distally. The inflammation weakens the bronchial wall while the atelectasis increases the negative intrathoracic pressure and the two bring about bronchial dilatation. Infection, in turn, is perpetuated in the dilated

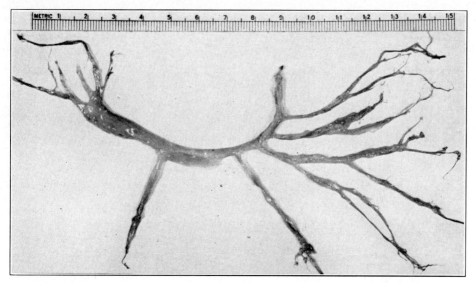

Fig. 196.—Bronchial cast expectorated by a patient with fibrinous bronchitis.

segments and the vicious cycle is maintained. In analyses of large series of cases the following conditions are frequently found to precede bronchiectasis: pneumonia, pleurisy, asthma, abscess, pertussis, influenza, measles, and tuberculosis (Ochsner and Souders). Cultures of the bronchial pus generally yield a variety of pathogenic (the usual pyogenic) and saprophytic organisms.

Pathologically the process is as common on the right side as on the left, is bilateral in slightly less than one-half the cases, may affect one or more lobes simultaneously or consecutively, is most common in the lower lobes, and decreases in frequency from below up. Proximally the bronchi are absolutely (due to inflammations, tumors, etc.) or relatively narrowed (Jones and Cole), while distally they are fusiformly or saccularly dilated (Fig. 197*B* and *C*). The lumens of the affected bronchi usually contain mucoid material or pus. The inner surfaces of the bronchi are smooth, gray or hemorrhagic, and intact or ulcerated. In long-standing cases they have a tendency to disclose transverse corrugations. The walls are thick, unyielding, gray, and fibrotic. The peribronchial tissue discloses varying degrees of fibrosis; the parenchyma reveals atelectasis, emphysema, fibrosis, and even abscesses, and the pleura usually discloses adhesions. *Histo-*

logically the changes in the bronchi in early cases are indistinguishable from severe, acute, necrotizing bronchitis (Fig. 198*A*). As such, the epithelium is ulcerated, the wall is permeated with neutrophils, and the muscle and elastic fibers are destroyed. In cases of less rapid onset or in those that are already well established, the epithelium may be hyperplastic, attenuated, focally ulcerated, or metaplastic (Fig. 198*B* and *C*). The submucosa is

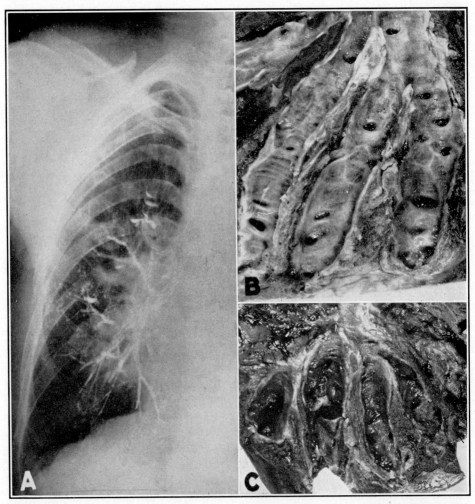

Fig. 197.—Bronchiectasis illustrating *A*, a bronchogram with pooling of the oil, *B*, cylindrical dilatation and cross striations of bronchi, and *C*, cylindrical and saccular dilatation of bronchi.

thickened and replaced with chronic inflammatory cells or distinct granulation tissue. In time, not only the muscle and elastic fibers tend to disappear but the glands become less numerous. Extension of the inflammatory process through the bronchial wall produces a similar reaction in the peribronchial tissues. The pulmonary parenchyma discloses alternating areas of emphysema and atelectasis. The latter reveals thickening and fibrosis of the alveolar septa, lining of the alveoli with cuboidal epithelial cells, the presence of Masson bodies (organized globs of exudate) within the alveoli, and a diffuse permeation with plasma cells, lymphocytes, monocytes, and foam cells (Fig. 198D).

The *complications* of bronchiectasis are pneumonia, pulmonary abscess, empyema, brain abscess, and, rarely, amyloidosis. Paranasal sinusitis is a concomitant infection in about one-third of the cases. Despite chronicity of the bronchial irritation, the development of bronchogenic carcinoma is a

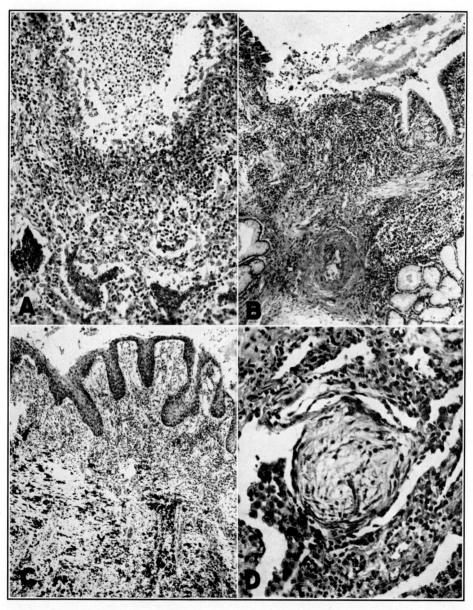

FIG. 198.—Bronchiectasis showing *A*, acute inflammation and destruction in an early phase of the disease (severe bronchitis). × 100, *B*, chronic inflammation of the wall and denudation of the lining epithelium in a fully-developed case. × 50, *C*, squamous metaplasia of the lining epithelium also in a well-established case. × 50, and *D*, Masson body (organized exudate) in an alveolus. × 200.

rare complication (Konwaler). The *clinical manifestations* are explainable on the basis of bronchial irritation, pulmonary suppuration, replacement of functioning by nonfunctioning pulmonary parenchyma, and absorption of toxic products from the lungs. They consist of cough, expectoration of sputum (from slight to copious), hemoptysis, pain in the chest, dyspnea, frequent colds, malaise, and weakness. Physical examination may be entirely negative or may reveal transient ronchi, suppressed breath sounds, and clubbing of the digits (in about one-fifth of cases). Plain roentgenograms show some abnormalities in most of the cases while *bronchograms* reveal pooling of iodized oil in the bronchi in virtually all instances (Fig. 197*A*). *Bronchoscopy* discloses mucosal changes and luminal pus and rules out other conditions. The *diagnosis* is made from the clinical manifestations, roentgenography (ordinary and following instillation of iodized oil), and bronchoscopy. *Treatment* is variable. Good palliation is obtainable by medical methods such as postural drainage and administration of antibiotics. A cure, however, can only be affected by surgical excision of the involved portions. Some of the postoperative complications (less formidable now with the advent of antibiotics and chemotherapeutic agents) are pneumonia, empyema, and bronchial fistula. The *prognosis* varies with the severity, extent, and duration of the condition and the age of the patient.

Pneumonia. — Pneumonia is not a single disease but is a protean collection of disease processes incited by a variety of agents. It has been *classified* according to the (1) *causative agent* as pneumococcic, staphylococcic, streptococcic, tuberculous, allergic, viral, etc., (2) *anatomic* distribution of the lesions as lobar, lobular, bronchial, double (both sides), interstitial, etc., (3) *gross appearance* as hemorrhagic, fibrinous, purulent, etc., (4) *clincial course* as typical or atypical, (5) *duration* of the process as acute or chronic, (6) *route* of *entrance* of the inciting agent as aspiration, hematogenous, or pleuritic, and (7) *relation* to *other disorders* as postoperative, postembolic, post-traumatic, terminal, etc. The ideal classification is one based on etiologic agents but because these are often multiple or cannot always be determined and because different organisms or unrelated agents may produce identical clinical pictures and pathologic changes, a combination of the above listings appears to be the most satisfactory. Accordingly, the following pneumonic conditions may be considered in the order mentioned: lobar pneumonia, bronchopneumonia, terminal pneumonia, aspiration pneumonia, allergic pneumonia, eosinophilic granuloma, tularemia, tuberculosis, Boeck's sarcoid, syphilis, plague, pertussis, interstitial pulmonary fibrosis, rickettsial pneumonia, viral pneumonia, fungous and yeast-like pneumonia, and parasitic infection.

Lobar Pneumonia. — Lobar pneumonia is an acute sporadic and endemic inflammation of a greater portion of a lobe, an entire lobe, or more than one lobe of the lungs. While it may occur at any *season* of the year it is more common in winter and early spring. Although the *incidence* of lobar pneumonia has probably not changed as a result of antibiotic and chemotherapeutic agents, the severity of the disease necessitating hospitalization has declined and the mortality rate has been greatly reduced (Reimann). The age incidence of the disorder has apparently shifted in recent years. Formerly lobar pneumonia was most common between the third and the fifth decades of life while at present it preponderates in the fifth and sixth decades. The disease is about four times as common in males as it is in females and it affects all races. In most instances, lobar pneumonia is *caused* by pneumococci and in only rare instances does it result from one

of the Friedländer's group of organisms. While it is no longer of any practical importance to type the pneumococci (because treatment is the same
regardless of the type of organism) the incidence of the various types at
the Jefferson Medical College Hospital has been approximately as follows:
I, III, VIII, VI, II, V, and others. In some instances, patients developing
lobar pneumonia may be in previously good health but in the majority,
careful questioning will uncover some previous *predisposing* disorder. Most
commonly, this exists in the form of an upper respiratory tract infection.
Less commonly, it may consist of the following: chilling of the body, acute
or chronic alcoholism, cardiac disease, pulmonary infections, and penetrating or nonpenetrating trauma to the chest. In any case, the pneumococci gain entrance by way of the tracheobronchial tree. Once they initiate
the infection they are dispersed through the lung by the flow of edema fluid
through the pores of Cohn and contiguous air passages (Gunn and Robertson). The organisms multiply rapidly in the edema fluid as long as it is
poor in leukocytes, that is, in the early part of the infection. *Experimentally*
lobar pneumonia has been produced in dogs by implanting pneumococci
suspended in starch paste into the terminal air sacs (Robertson) and in
rats by intratracheal insufflation of pneumococci suspended in mucin
(Gunn).

Pathologically the condition may be unilateral or bilateral and it may
affect the greater portion of a lobe, an entire lobe, or more than one lobe.
The inflammation is a dynamic process that differs in no way from any
other nonspecific inflammation (p. 106). Despite this, however, it has been
customary to divide the stages of lobar pneumonia into four categories —
congestion, red hepatization, gray hepatization, and resolution. The stage
of *congestion* occurs within the first few hours after entrance of the pneumococci. The affected portion of the lung becomes enlarged, red, firmer than
normal, and subcrepitant. When cut, hemorrhagic fluid drips freely from
the exposed surface. Histologically the following are noted: engorgement
of the alveolar capillaries with blood, thickening of the alveolar septa, and
a beginning outpouring of edema fluid and erythrocytes (Fig. 200*A*). The
stage of *red hepatization* is characterized by a further enlargement of the
lung, not only to the point where the entire pleural space may be occupied
with lung tissue, but to a degree sufficient to produce imprints of the bony
structures of the thoracic cage upon the pulmonary substance. Externally
the pleura covering the affected tissue shows beginning pleuritis exhibited
by a rough, dry, dull surface often covered with fibrinous material. Cut
surfaces disclose a diffuse uniform replacement of the involved parenchyma
by a solid mass of dark red, firm, friable tissue that resembles liver (hence
the name red hepatization). The histologic changes represent a progression
of the first stage with, in addition, the presence of increasing numbers of
neutrophils and increasing deposition of fibrin (Fig. 200*B*). In the stage of
gray hepatization the lungs remain voluminous and still bear the imprints
of the bony structures of the thoracic cage. The pleura covering the involved portion of the lung usually reveals a definite fibrinous exudate while
the affected parenchyma is solid, at first dry but later moist, diffusely gray,
and quite friable (Fig. 199). Histologically the alveolar septa become
thinner and less prominent (due mostly to the diffusion of the alveolar
exudate) to a point where in the late phases of this stage their delineations
are discernible only with difficulty. The exudate itself consists primarily
of neutrophils with varying amounts of fibrin added (Fig. 200*C*). The
erythrocytes have laked and disappeared and the edema fluid has been re-

placed by the cellular elements. The red and gray stages of hepatization occur consecutively and overlappingly and consume the interval from the second to the sixth or seventh days of the disease. The stage of *resolution* normally appears on about the sixth or seventh day. Grossly the lung diminishes in size, becomes softer, regains some of its crepitations, and assumes a gray, moist, somewhat gelatinous appearance. Histologically it is characterized by a fluidification of the leukocytes and fibrin, the appearance of large numbers of actively phagocytic monocytes, absorption of the fluid, reappearance of the alveolar septa, and gradually a restoration of the

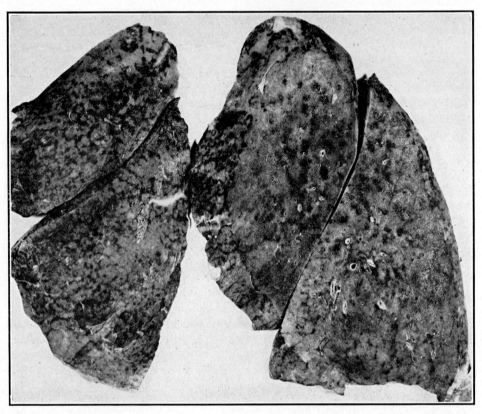

Fig. 199.—Lobar pneumonia, early gray hepatization, showing (to the right) complete consolidation of both lobes and (to the left) a fibrinous exudate covering the pleura.

lung parenchyma to normal (Fig. 200*D*). The histologic changes in the *pleura* are similar to those in the lung proper. Initially they consist of congestion and edema and, in turn, are followed by an exudation of leukocytes and fibrin, fluidification of the exudate, and ultimately resolution.

The *complications* of lobar pneumonia are much less frequent now (with the advent of antibiotics and chemotherapy) than formerly. They may consist of pericarditis, endocarditis, meningitis, arthritis, peritonitis, empyema, pulmonary atelectasis, pulmonary abscess, and failure of resolution with organization. Pulmonary abscesses secondary to lobar pneumonia are rare but are similar to other nonspecific abscesses. They are usually multiple and consist of focal areas of complete destruction of tissue surrounded by an acute inflammatory process in various stages of healing

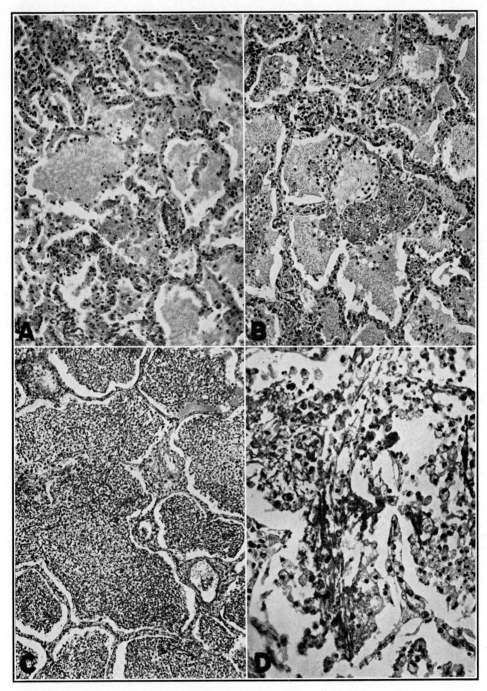

Fig. 200.—Lobar pneumonia showing A, stage of congestion with distended alveolar capillaries and escape of edema fluid and erythrocytes into the alveolar spaces. $\times$ 100, B, stage of red hepatization with exaggeration of changes shown in A along with beginning leukocytic exudation. $\times$ 100, C, stage of gray hepatization with diffuse extravasation of leukocytes and fibrin. $\times$ 100, and D, stage of resolution with fluidification of the exudate and presence of many phagocytes. $\times$ 200.

(Fig. 201*A*). Failure of resolution is followed in due course by an organization of the exudate resulting in a thickening of the alveolar septa and a filling of the alveolar spaces with plugs of granulation and fibrous tissue (Fig. 201*B*). Because of the early administration of antibiotics and chemotherapeutic agents the *clinical manifestations* and course of lobar pneumonia have been considerably modified in recent years. Characteristically, however, the disease is generally preceded by a mild upper respiratory tract infection and, in a few days, is ushered in abruptly with chills, fever, pain in the chest, cough, and expectoration of bloody or rusty sputum. The

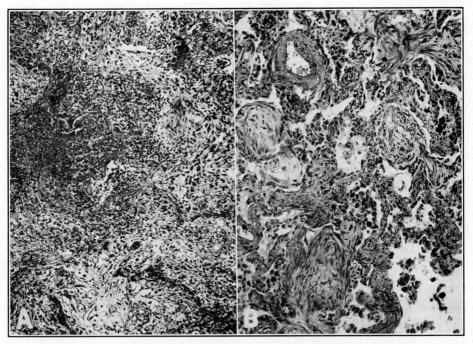

FIG. 201.—Complications of lobar pneumonia illustrating *A*, acute abscess formation and *B*, organization of the exudate. × 100.

chills correspond to the stage of bacterial invasion and usually occur when the fever is ascending; the fever is due to the absorption of toxic products from the lungs; pain in the chest results from inflammation of the parietal pleura; the cough is due to irritation of the bronchial mucosa, and the blood-tinged or rusty sputum is consequent to escape of the erythrocytes from the alveolar capillaries into the alveolar spaces. In addition to the above the following are also noted: prostration, delirium, dyspnea, cyanosis, sweating, signs of pulmonary consolidation (respiratory lag, dullness, blowing breath sounds, and increased vocal fremitus), rales in the chest, sweating, increased respiration, rapid pulse, increased sedimentation rate, leukocytosis, and, roentgenographically, pulmonary opacities. Of these, the local pulmonary manifestations are due to exudation and consolidation while the systemic manifestations result from absorption of toxic products, peripheral vascular collapse, physiologic weakness of myocardial fibers, and anoxia. The *diagnosis* of lobar pneumonia is made from (1) a characteristic history (as noted above), (2) physical findings, (3) massive pulmonary consolidation as demonstrated roentgenographically, and (4) isolation of the causative organisms (early in the course of the disease) from the sputum and the blood. *Treatment* consists mainly of the early administration of antibiotics and chemotherapeutic agents. The *prognosis* is good for the current mortality rates have varied between 5.7 and 9.3 per cent. Before the era of antibiotics and chemotherapeutic agents, the recorded mortality varied from 19 to 37 per cent (Reimann). In general, the mortality rate is higher in infants and in the aged than it is in patients of intervening ages.

Bronchopneumonia.—The term bronchopneumonia as used here encompasses all patchy primary bacterial pneumonias that originally affect the bronchi and bronchioles, and then spread to involve the rest of the pulmonary parenchyma. Bronchopneumonia is much commoner than lobar pneumonia. While it may occur at any age, it predominates at the two extremes of life, namely, infancy and old age. The *causes* are precipitating and predisposing. The usual *precipitating* causes are the ordinary pyogenic organisms occurring approximately in the following decreasing order of frequency: hemolytic streptococcus, staphylococcus of the aureus variety, member of the Friedländer's group of organisms, pneumococcus, influenza bacillus, colon bacillus, etc. The *route* of invasion of the organisms is the tracheobronchial tree. While occasionally bronchopneumonia may develop in a previously healthy individual, usually it is engraphed upon some other condition. Some of the *predisposing* factors are upper respiratory infection, viral infection (notably influenza and measles), and any debilitating condition.

Pathologically, while lobar pneumonia is characterized by a uniformity of pattern with one stage following the other, bronchopneumonia is characterized by an irregular response with new areas of inflammation beginning while others are already receding. The lesions are always multiple, involve more than one lobe, and are generally bilateral. The areas of consolidation are distributed along the course of the bronchial tree (Fig. 202*A* and *B*). They are large or small, usually appear ill defined, vary in color from deep red to gray, and are moist to dry and granular. As they increase in size, adjacent lesions coalesce to form solid masses of inflammation that sometimes are difficult to distinguish from lobar pneumonia. The areas of the pulmonary parenchyma between the lesions appear relatively normal, congested, atelectatic, or emphysematous. Since many of the infiltrations are situated peripherally the pleura is frequently involved and reacts with a fibrinous, purulent, or hemorrhagic type of exudation. *Histologically* the primary infection is in the bronchi and bronchioles (Fig. 202*C*). The changes in these areas are similar to those of acute bronchitis with the degree of inflammation varying from case to case. The lumens of the bronchi and bronchioles are usually filled with neutrophils, nuclear fragments, debris, mucus, and bacteria. The epithelial cells show varying degrees of hypersecretion, degeneration, or complete necrosis. The walls reveal congestion, edema, intense neutrophilic infiltration, and destruction of tissue. The peribronchial and peribronchiolar areas disclose an extension of the bronchial and bronchiolar inflammation. Ultimately the inflammation affects the alveolar spaces and septa (Fig. 202*D*). Here the stages of the inflammation are similar to those in lobar pneumonia with, as stated before, the age of the lesion varying from area to area. The response thus consists of congestion and edema, precipitation of fibrin, exudation of erythrocytes and leukocytes (chiefly neutrophils), and resolution by

31

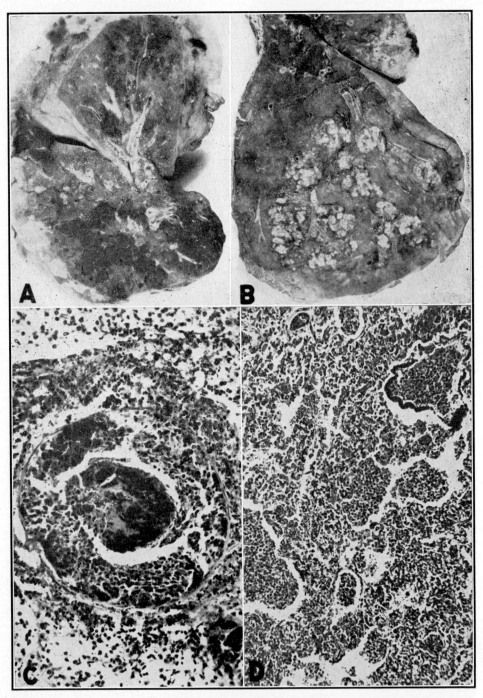

FIG. 202.—Bronchopneumonia showing *A*, a patchy hemorrhagic consolidation following the distribution of the bronchial tree, *B*, multiple early abscesses similarly distributed, *C*, a bronchiole filled with debris and colonies of bacteria (staphylococci) and the bronchial wall and peribronchial tissues permeated with neutrophils. × 200, and *D*, pulmonary parenchyma infiltrated with leukocytes and erythrocytes. × 100.

fluidification and mononuclear cell invasion. Unlike lobar pneumonia the proportion of each of these elements varies greatly from case to case, depending upon the type, numbers, and virulence of the invading organisms and upon the resistance of the individual. Thus, in some instances, it may be mostly hemorrhagic, in others fibrinous, and in others still purulent. Also, unlike in lobar pneumonia, the lesions in bronchopneumonia have a greater tendency to undergo suppuration with abscess formation, organization, and fibrosis. In any case the parenchyma between the areas of inflammation discloses collapse of the alveoli (atelectasis) in some areas and overdistention of the alveoli (emphysema) in other areas.

The *complications* of bronchopneumonia are similar to those of lobar pneumonia with the exception that local pulmonary complications outnumber others and that the complications as a whole are more numerous. The usual untoward effects are empyema, pulmonary abscess, organization of the pulmonary lesions, and bronchiectasis. The *clinical manifestations* are similar to those in lobar pneumonia with the exceptions that the onset is usually less dramatic and the course is more protracted. The *diagnosis* is made from the history, physical examination, roentgenographic presence of irregular areas of pulmonic consolidation, and culturing the causative organism from the sputum. *Treatment* consists primarily of the administration of antibiotics and chemotherapeutic agents and other supportive measures. When complications (empyema, pulmonary abscess, or bronchiectasis) arise, surgical intervention may be necessary. The *prognosis* with modern forms of therapy is generally good. Whereas previously the mortality was as high as 90 per cent it has now been reduced to less than 10 per cent.

Terminal Pneumonia.—Terminal pneumonia, also known as hypostatic pneumonia, is common, being found to a greater or lesser extent in everyone who does not die suddenly. It has as its basis a failing circulation, escape of edema fluid into the alveoli, and multiplication of bacteria (already present) in the excellent medium thus provided. *Pathologically* the process is bilateral and starts in the dependent portions of the lungs. Thus, it usually affects the lower lobes or the posterior portions of all lobes. Grossly the lungs are heavy and congested and, when cut, allow the escape of an abundant amount of frothy fluid. The areas of pneumonia are ill defined, usually occupy a good portion of each lung, appear red to gray, and are firm and noncrepitant. *Histologically* there are varying proportions of edema fluid, erythrocytes, and neutrophils filling the alveolar spaces and there is a conspicuous absence of fibrin (Fig. 203). Bronchi and bronchioles are involved in a similar process, but these structures are not primarily or as severely affected as they are in bronchopneumonia.

Aspiration Pneumonia.—Aspiration pneumonia may be divided into two groups—that resulting from aspiration of food and that found in the newborn. *Food aspiration pneumonia* is a relatively common finding at autopsy. Fetterman and Moran encountered the condition in 5.7 per cent of 469 consecutive autopsies. The disorder is not only noted in postoperative patients as a result of aspiration of vomitus, but is also seen in nonsurgical patients (whose swallowing mechanism is not functioning properly as in marasmus, stupor, or central nervous system disorders) as a result of aspiration of food that is being ingested. Aspiration pneumonia has been produced in healthy guinea pigs injected intratracheally with various types of foods (Moran). In man, the condition is generally accompanied by bronchopneumonia or terminal pneumonia. The lumen of the tracheobronchial tree may or may not contain *grossly* recognizable food particles; the mucosa is reddened, and the areas of consolidation grossly are nonspecific (Fig. 204). *Histologically* the parenchymal reactions vary, consisting of (1) congestion and edema, (2) neutrophilic infiltration, (3) acute abscess formation, or (4) granulomas composed of focal proliferations of fibroblasts and capillaries permeated with neutrophils, plasma cells, lymphocytes, mono-

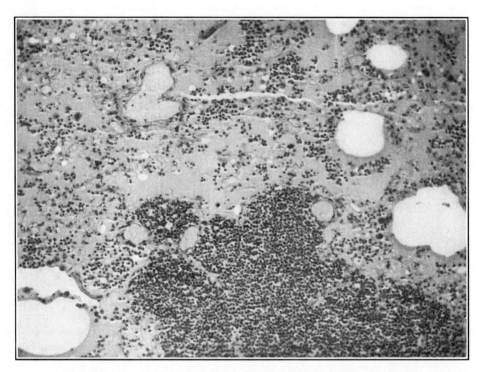

Fig. 203.—Terminal pneumonia showing severe edema, absence of fibrin, and an infiltration with neutrophils. × 100.

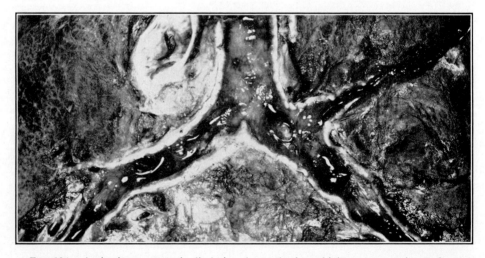

Fig. 204.—Aspiration pneumonia disclosing the tracheobronchial tree to contain vomitus.

cytes, and giant cells of the foreign body type (Fig. 205 *A*).   Food particles may be identified in the bronchioles and in the vicinity of the foreign body giant cells.

Aspiration pneumonia of the *newborn*, also called *hyaline membrane dssease*, is usually seen in immature infants who are limp, feeble, or cyanotic at birth and, in whom, respiration is initiated and maintained with difficulty (Tregillus and De).   Death occurs as a result of asphyxia.   *Pathologically*, the tracheobronchial tree contains frothy fluid, and aeration of the pulmon-

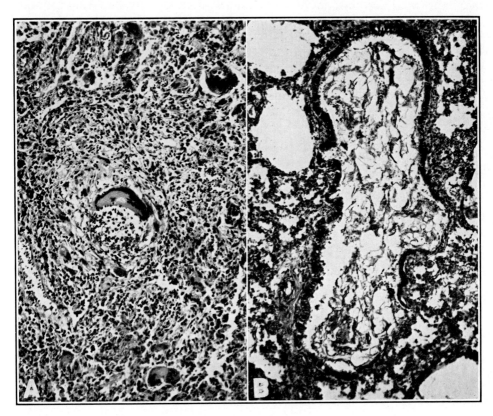

Fig. 205.—Aspiration pneumonia showing *A*, a granulomatous reaction to aspirated food, consisting of fibroblasts, leukocytes, and foreign body giant cells, and *B*, a bronchiole filled with meconium and vermix caseosa and the parenchyma atelectatic and emphysematous in a case of death shortly after birth.   × 100.

ary parenchyma is often limited to the anterior borders.   The rest of the lungs are nonaerated, bluish red, and heavy.   *Histologically* the bronchial and bronchiolar epithelium may be intact or degenerated and sloughed. The lumens of the bronchi, bronchioles, and even the air sacs contain meconium, vernix caseosa (sebum and desquamated twisted epithelial cells from the skin of the fetus), and pulmonary cellular debris (Fig. 205*B*). The alveoli are lined by a hyaline membrane and contain leukocytes, erythrocytes, and nuclear fragments (Fig. 206*A*). The nature of the hyaline membranes is not agreed upon, being considered to represent (1) concentrated protein of aspirated amniotic fluid (Blystad), (2) degeneration products of bronchial epithelium (Tregillus), (3) vernix caseosa, or (4) pushed aside and concentrated edema fluid arising in the lungs. Of these, the last named appears to be the most logical explanation. Histochemical studies disclose the membrane to be positive for fat and polysaccharide aldehyde (De). Electron microscopic studies reveal it to be composed of a finely fibrillar matrix similar to fibrin and containing enmeshed cell debris such as nuclei, mitochondria, endoplasmic reticulum, and vacuoles (van Breemen). In addition, the rest of the pulmonary parenchyma shows alveolar dysplasia and atelectasis. That the condition is entirely nonspecific and not limited to newborn infants is demonstrated by the fact that similar

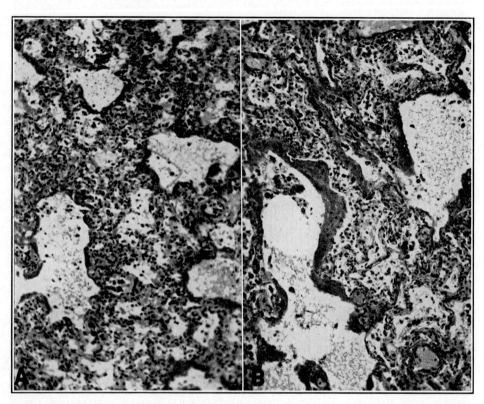

FIG. 206.—Hyaline membranes lining alveolar septa from a case of A, hyaline membrane disease in a newborn infant and B, a 39 year old woman who died of salicylate poisoning and in whom a terminal pneumonia was also present. × 100.

hyaline membranes are found in adults in conjunction with a variety of pulmonic inflammations including influenza, bronchopneumonia of any type, rheumatic fever, terminal pneumonia, septicemia, pneumonia associated with uremia, irradiation pneumonitis, etc. (Fig. 206, B).

Allergic Pneumonia.—The generally recognized allergic conditions of the lungs are rheumatic pneumonia (p. 299), asthma, and Loeffler's syndrome.

Asthma (Gr. = panting) is an allergic disorder of the lungs characterized by recurrent attacks of paroxysmal dyspnea, a wheezing cough, and a sense of constriction of the chest. It *occurs* at all ages, affects both sexes with equal frequency, and has no predilection for any race. The attacks are brought about by bronchial occlusion due to muscle spasms and presence of tenacious secretions in the bronchial lumens. The *cause* of the bronchial changes is hypersensitivity to a variety of agents including dusts, foods, drugs, and bacteria. *Pathologically* the lungs at autopsy are voluminous, not only filling the entire pleural space but bulging through the thoracic incision (Fig. 207). The pleural surfaces are smooth, moist, glistening, and free of adhesions (Fig. 208*A*). The lungs, externally, are irregular due mostly to large areas of emphysema intermingled with small, often deeply depressed areas of atelectasis. The weight is decreased and the consistency is soft. Cut surfaces are dry and disclose pinkish-gray parenchyma dotted with bronchi and bronchioles that are filled with thick tenacious secretions.

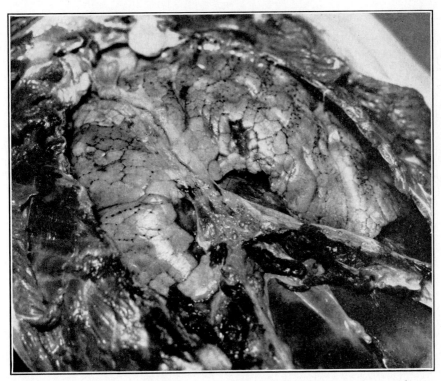

FIG. 207.—Asthma showing voluminous lungs that fill the pleural spaces and encroach upon the anterior mediastinum and heart.

Histologically the lumens of the bronchi and bronchioles are filled with mucus mixed with debris (Fig. 208*B* and *C*). The lining epithelium shows hypersecretion and degeneration; the basement membrane is prominent, and the submucosa contains a variety of leukocytes with eosinophils predominating. The distal pulmonary parenchyma shows emphysema alternating with areas of atelectasis. Both in the lungs and in other tissues of the body, the smaller arteries may show an acute arteritis. The *complications* are thoracic deformities (indrawn sternum or pigeon breast in children and barrel-shaped chest in adults), fracture of ribs (due to coughing), fibrous bronchial stenosis, bronchiectasis, tuberculosis, mediastinal emphysema, pneumothorax, right-sided cardiac failure, and prolongation of an attack known as status asthmaticus (Derbes). *Treatment* consists of (1) avoidance of allergens to which the individual is sensitive, (2) desensitization, (3) administration of antispasmatic drugs such as adrenalin, ephedrine, aminophylline, etc., (4) sedation, and (5) other measures (Unger). The *mortality rate* in hospitalized asthmatics has been recorded by Bullen as 9 per cent.   *Death* may result from the asthma itself (asphyxia), from pneumonia, or from cardiac failure.

Loeffler's syndrome, also known as transitory pulmonary infiltration with eosinophilia, tropical eosinophilia, etc., is a fleeting disorder of the lungs *characterized by* malaise, an irritating cough, mucoid sputum containing eosinophils, slight fever, scattered rales and perhaps a pleural friction

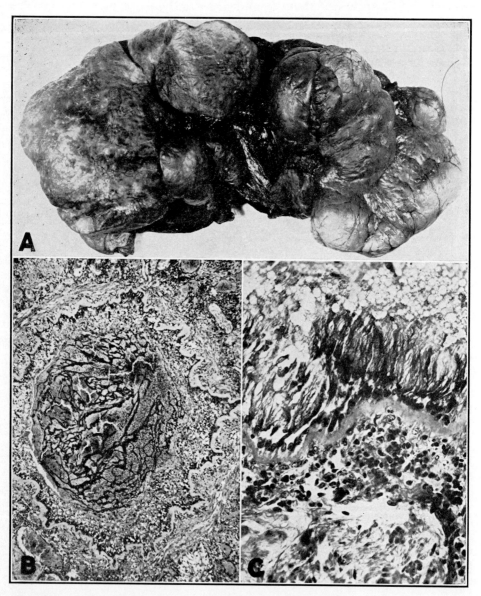

Fig. 208.—Asthma illustrating *A*, a lung with marked emphysema and depressed areas of atelectasis, *B*, a large bronchiole with the lumen filled with secretion and cellular debris and a conspicuous basement membrane.   × 50, and *C*, a portion of the wall of a bronchus with degenerating epithelial cells, a prominent hyalinized basement membrane and eosinophilic infiltration of the submucosa.   × 200.

rub, leukocytosis to 15,000, eosinophilia, increased sedimentation rate, irregular migratory shadows roentgenographically, and usually recovery in from one to two weeks but with a tendency to recurrence. The condition *occurs in both sexes* and at all ages. The causative *allergens* are many, consisting of animal parasites, bacteria, fungi, dusts, pollen, etc. The condition has been produced *experimentally* in sensitized rabbits by intra-tracheal injection of horse serum (Herbut and Kinsey). *Pathologically* the bronchial and bronchiolar changes are similar to those in asthma. The alveoli disclose a true eosinophilic pneumonia characterized by congestion, edema, and a leukocytic infiltration that predominates in eosinophils. In some of the cases, granulomatous lesions have been recorded. Generally, there are no *complications*. The *diagnosis* is made from the clinical mani-festations and roentgenograms. The condition should be differentiated, among others, from tuberculosis. *Treatment*, is, as a rule, unnecessary. The *prognosis* is good for most patients recover spontaneously.

Eosinophilic Granuloma. —This is a relatively new condition, being first described as a separate pulmonary lesion by Farinacci *et al.* in 1951 (Auld). As the name suggests, it is a granulomatous inflammation of the lungs characterized especially by the presence of eosinophils. It *occurs* more often in males than females and has been encountered mostly in the second decade of life. The *cause* is unknown. Such agents or conditions as bacteria, fungi, viruses, Hodgkin's disease, berylliosis, and sarcoidosis have been ruled out. Hypersensitivity is a definite possibility, since the lesion is characterized by an eosinophilic infiltration and a hypersensitivity-type of arteriolitis and since the condition is accompanied by eosinophilia. In your author's opinion, however, the disorder is more likely related to eosino-philic granuloma of bone (p. 919) since similar pulmonary lesions have been demonstrated in this condition and also in the allied Hand-Schüller-Christian and Letterer-Siew diseases.

Pathologically, pleural adhesions may or may not be present. The pleural surfaces may reveal cysts or blebs and, where they overly the granulomas, they do disclose puckering. The parenchymal lesions are diffusely scattered, appear grayish white or tan, and measure up to 1.5 cm. in diameter. *Histo-logically*, the granulomas are composed essentially of histiocytes and eosino-phils (Fig. 209, *A*). The former are large, pale, and either sharply defined or confluent. Their cytoplasm is abundant and usually granular. Occa-sionally it contains vacuoles. Their nuclei are round or oval, uniform, and vesicular. Sometimes giant cells are encountered. The eosinophils are mostly of the bilobed variety. In the granuloma these two types of cells are intermingled with generally the histiocytes predominating. Fibroblasts are also present in greater or lesser numbers. The granulomas are located in the interstitial and parabronchiolar tissues. In the latter position, they frequently communicate with the bronchiolar lumen. Aside from the gran-uloma, the interstitial tissue may show a more diffuse infiltration with eosinophils and histiocytes. In addition, the arterioles disclose fibrinoid degeneration of especially the aventitia, eosinophilic infiltration of the entire wall, endothelial proliferation, and lumenal thrombosis. Beyond the granulomas, the pulmonary parenchyma shows emphysema and air-filled blebs.

The only noteworthy *complication* is pneumothorax, which results from rupture of the subpleural blebs. *Clinically* the onset of the disorder is insidious and the symptoms are mild. The manifestations include cough, sputum, moderate dyspnea, chest pain, weight loss, and the presence of rales. The laboratory data discloses leukocytosis over 10,000, neutrophilia, eosinophilia (3 to 10%), elevated sedimentation rate, and diffuse bilateral linear or nodular infiltrations roentgenographically (Fig. 209,*B* and *C*). The *diagnosis* is made with certainty only by biopsy. *Treatment* is symptomatic. The *prognosis* is good. The condition has improved or become stabilized in from a few months to a year in all recorded cases.

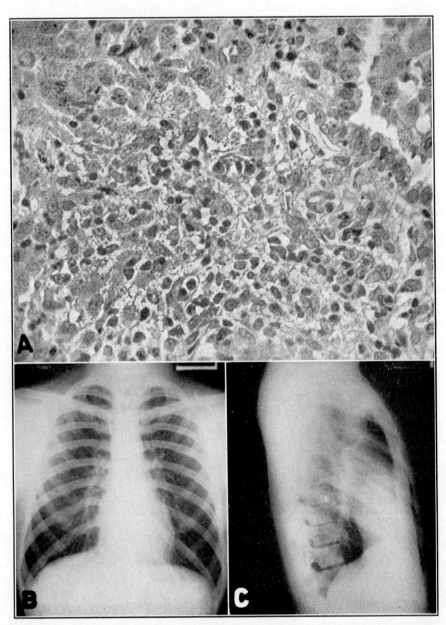

FIG. 209.—Eosinophilic granuloma of the lungs showing *A*, histiocytes and eosinophils permeating the tissue adjacent to a bronchiole and histiocytes within the bronchiolar lumen. × 400, and *B*, diffuse bilateral pulmonary shadows roentgenographically.

Tularemia.—Tularemia is an infectious disease named after Tulare County in California where the disorder was first recognized in man. Normally it is a disease of rodents and is transmitted to man by direct contact (butchers, hunters, etc.) or, less often, by bites of infected ticks, flies, fleas, or bedbugs. The condition is widespread in the United States, there being about 2000 new cases recorded annually (Pullen and Stuart). The *causative organism* is the *Pasturella tularensis*—a nonmotile, gram-negative, pleomorphic bacillus that grows well on cystine beef agar and, in the laboratory, is pathogenic for the mouse and guinea pig.

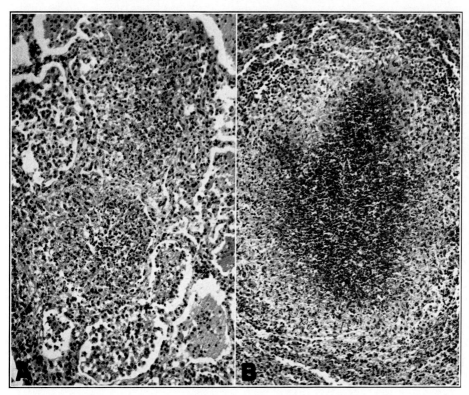

Fig. 210.—Tularemia showing *A*, an early lesion with mostly mononuclear and epithelioid cell reaction, and *B*, a more advanced lesion with extensive central necrosis and nuclear fragmentation and distinct peripheral epithelioid reaction. × 100.

Pathologically tularemia may affect the skin and lymph nodes (ulcero-glandular), the conjunctivæ and lymph nodes (oculoglandular), the lymph nodes primarily (glandular), or many tissues throughout the body (typhoid or febrile form). Usually the initial lesion is on the hand. It consists of a red papule which progresses to form an indolent ulcer with a necrotic floor, overhanging edges, and indurated base. Simultaneously, the draining lymph nodes become enlarged and tender and frequently break down to form draining sinuses. The disease may end here, may spread to other lymph nodes, or may then be distributed throughout the body. Regardless of the organ affected (lymph nodes, lungs, spleen, liver, etc.) the pathologic changes are similar. *Grossly* the lesions resemble tuberculosis. They may exist as tiny, discreet, yellowish tubercles, as coalescing nodules, or as ulcerating, caseating, and fibrosing masses. In the lungs they may, in addition, produce consolidations that resemble those of bronchopneumonia and lobar pneumonia. *Histologically* early lesions resemble soft tubercles. They are composed of mononuclear and epithelial cells or of foci of central necrosis surrounded by masses of mononuclear and epithelioid cells (Fig. 210). Older lesions reveal central caseation necrosis, scattered Langhans' giant cells in the cellular zone, and peripheral fibrosis.

The *complications* (aside from the septicemic or typhoid form of the disease) are generally limited to the lungs and consist of bronchiectasis, fibrosis, empyema, and abscess. Rarely, there may be pericarditis, peritonitis, meningitis, encephalitis, enteritis, venous thromboses, and thrombophlebitis. *Clinically* after an incubation period of from two to six days, there is a sudden onset of malaise, chills, fever, headache, nausea and vomiting, sweating, and prostration. Following this the manifestations depend upon the organ or organs affected. The *diagnosis* is made from the history, clinical findings, agglutination tests, skin tests, and isolation of the causative organism. *Treatment* is prevention, local applications, and administration of antibiotics. The *prognosis* is fair to good. Pullen and Stuart recorded a mortality of 7.55 per cent in 225 cases studied, while Corwin and Stubbs recorded a good response to streptomycin and dihydrostreptomycin.

Tuberculosis.—Tuberculosis, also known as phthisis (Gr. = consume), is an acute to chronic infectious disease that (1) is worldwide in distribution, (2) affects all races with particular preponderance in Negroes, (3) occurs at all ages from infancy on but predominates in children and young adults, (4) in the over-all has no predilection for either sex, (5) is more common in large cities than in rural areas, and (6) prevails among the poorer and overcrowded population. The *cause* is *Mycobacterium tuberculosis*—a grampositive, acid-fast, slender, slightly curved, beaded, aerobic bacillus that grows well on special artificial media and is particularly pathogenic for the guinea pig. Of the three common types of *Mycobacterium tuberculosis* (human, bovine, and avian), the human and bovine types cause most if not all of the infections in man. The three varieties of organisms can be differentiated culturally and by animal inoculation. *Chemically Mycobacterium tuberculosis* contains proteins, lipids, and carbohydrates. The protein fraction is responsible for the tissue damage and the constitutional symptoms in the hypersensitive patient. The lipid fraction accounts for the acid-fastness and the epithelioid cell, giant cell, and tubercle formation. The carbohydrate fraction is responsible for bacterial virulence and host immunity. The *sources* of the organisms are (1) *exogenous*—most commonly by way of droplet or dust infection from man, occasionally by way of infected milk, and rarely through the placenta from the mother, and (2) *endogenous*—breakdown of previous tuberculous foci in the body. The *route* of infection in man is usually by inhalation, less frequently by ingestion, uncommonly (and locally) by cutaneous inoculation, and rarely (as already stated) hematogenously by way of the placenta. Because of the preponderance of the respiratory and gastrointestinal routes, the most commonly affected tissues of the body are the lungs and mesenteric lymph nodes. Once the organisms gain a foothold they spread by direct extension, lymphatic channels, natural passages (pulmonary passages, pleural or peritoneal space, lumen of the urinary tract, etc.), or blood vessels.

Pathologically the location, spread, and appearance of the lesions depend upon the virulence of the organisms, the number of organisms, and the resistance of the host. They differ also according to whether the invasion represents a primary or a secondary infection. The former is referred to as primary tuberculosis while the latter is known as reinfection tuberculosis.

Primary tuberculosis represents the first infection with *Mycobacterium tuberculosis*. It generally occurs in infancy or childhood but it may also be found in adults. Usually the primary infection is in the lung but, on occasion, it may be found in the tonsil or the small intestine. The primary *pulmonary lesion* is usually single, affects any lobe of either lung, and is located just beneath the pleura in any part of the lobe (Fig. 211). The

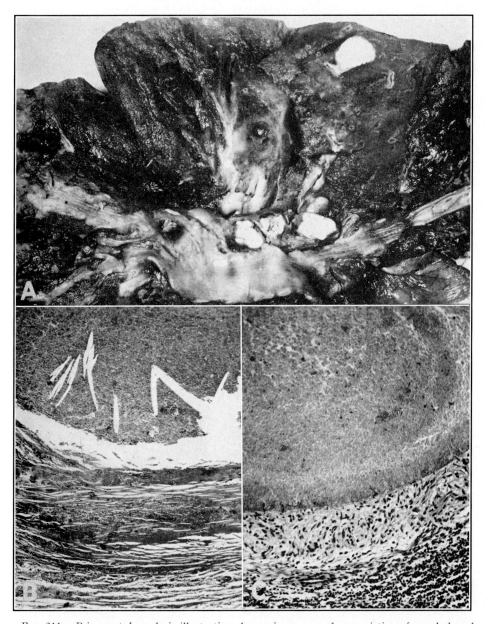

Fig. 211.—Primary tuberculosis illustrating *A*, a primary complex consisting of a subpleural caseous nodule and three similar hilar masses, *B*, primary pulmonary mass of caseation necrosis surrounded by a fibrous capsule.   × 50, and *C*, hilar lymph node with a caseous center and capsule of epithelioid cells.   × 100.

lesion is sharply circumscribed, often well encapsulated, grayish white, firm, and frequently calcified. As a rule, it measures less than 1.5 cm. in diameter. Careful inspection discloses multiple involvement of the draining lymph nodes along a peribronchial path extending from the primary subpleural focus to the hilar and mediastinal lymph nodes. These secondary deposits represent tuberculous involvement of lymphoid tissue. They vary in size but otherwise the hilar and mediastinal lesions are similar to the subpleural deposit. The original focus beneath the pleura is known as the *primary tuberculous lesion* or the *Ghon lesion*, while the original subpleural focus together with the lesions in the draining lymph nodes are referred to as the *primary tuberculous complex* or the *Ghon complex*. *Histologically* the original lesion consists of the tubercle. At first it is composed of a focal exudation of neutrophils. Within twenty-four hours mononuclear cells appear and within the first week, these are transformed into epithelioid cells. Within the second week, giant cells of the Langhans' type and lymphocytes become discernible about the periphery of the original focus. Caseation necrosis becomes apparent toward the end of the second week. Ultimately, the smaller foci coalesce to give a large central area of caseation necrosis. Originally the tissue about this area is composed of mononuclear cells, epithelioid cells, and lymphocytes in which there are distinct tubercles. As the lesion ages, the peripheral area is gradually replaced with collagenous connective tissue which ultimately forms a distinct limiting fibrous capsule (Fig. 211*B*). Calcium salts and cholesterol crystals may or may not appear within the central caseous area. The chain of events in the draining lymph nodes is similar (Fig. 211*C*). In addition to the primary lesion and the primary complex, some of the patients with primary tuberculosis disclose, roentgenographically, a triangular area of density with the base located peripherally and the apex at the hilum of the lung. This lesion is referred to as *epituberculosis*. Originally it was thought to be due to a pneumonia caused by dead organisms and their toxic products but, as a result of numerous bronchoscopic studies, it is now known that most cases represent bronchial compression or direct luminal breakthrough by tuberculous peribronchial lymph nodes causing atelectasis of the peripheral pulmonary segment. Most primary tuberculous lesions heal and remain arrested for varying periods of time or throughout life. A few, however, progress and *result in* tuberculous pneumonia with or without cavitation, miliary tuberculosis, tuberculous meningitis, or tuberculous osteoarthritis. A late sequel may be bronchiectasis.

Reinfection tuberculosis generally occurs in adults and, less frequently, in young children. Usually (but not always) the lesion is localized to one or both apices of the lungs within the first 2 centimeters of the surface. The reason for this localization is not known, although it is thought to have something to do with low arterial pressure and high oxygen tension in these areas of the lung as compared with other portions. In any case of reinfection tuberculosis there are two opposing factors at work—destructive processes and reparative processes. The former are characterized by necrosis, cavitation, and extension of the inflammation while the latter are characterized by resolution and healing by fibrosis. Depending upon which predominates, the pulmonary disease may assume one of several forms. The usual types of pulmonary and other lesions are apical scarring, fibrocaseous tuberculosis, tuberculous tracheobronchitis, tuberculous pneumonia, miliary tuberculosis, disseminated tuberculosis, organ tuberculosis, and tuberculoma.

Apical scarring occurs when resistance is good and represents the healed end stage of reinfection tuberculosis. It consists of an irregular, rounded or linear, ill-defined, depressed mass of fibrous tissue located just beneath the apical pleura and measuring up to 3 or 4 cm. in greatest diameter (Fig. 212*A*). It is composed of dense, sclerotic, fibrous tissue, is usually permeated with carbon pigment and calcium, may contain bone, and generally shows little evidence of residual tuberculous infection (Fig. 212*B*).

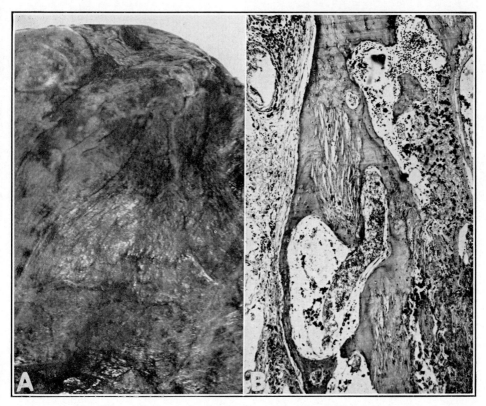

Fig. 212.—Apical scar showing *A*, depressed and wrinkled pleura and
B, connective tissue containing bone and carbon pigment. × 50.

Fibrocaseous tuberculosis occurs when the destructive process overshadows the reparative process. It is seen in the presence of heavy doses of virulent organisms with only fair resistance on the part of the body. The infection starts at original points of reinfection tuberculosis and spreads throughout the lung by contiguity and air passages. As the lesions progress they coalesce, forming small or large areas of caseation necrosis surrounded by active tuberculous tissue and varying degrees of fibrosis. When the caseous tissue reaches a bronchus it is discharged, leaving large, frequently intercommunicating, irregular cavities (Fig. 213*A*). Sometimes fibrous tissue forms in overabundance despite the spreading caseous nature of the infection, resulting in massive pulmonary fibrosis (Fig. 213*B*). Thus, ultimately, a part of a lobe, an entire lobe, an entire lung, or both lungs are composed of (1) masses of yellowish-gray caseous material, (2) varisized ragged cavities lined by gray necrotic tissue and traversed by bronchi and vessels, and

(3) varying degrees of peripheral fibrosis. *Histologically* fibrocaseous tuberculosis is represented by tubercle formation (Fig. 213C), caseation necrosis, tuberculous granulation tissue (Fig. 213D), and fibrosis (p. 167).

Tuberculous tracheobronchitis is usually seen in conjunction with fibrocaseous tuberculosis. It develops as a result of direct extension of the

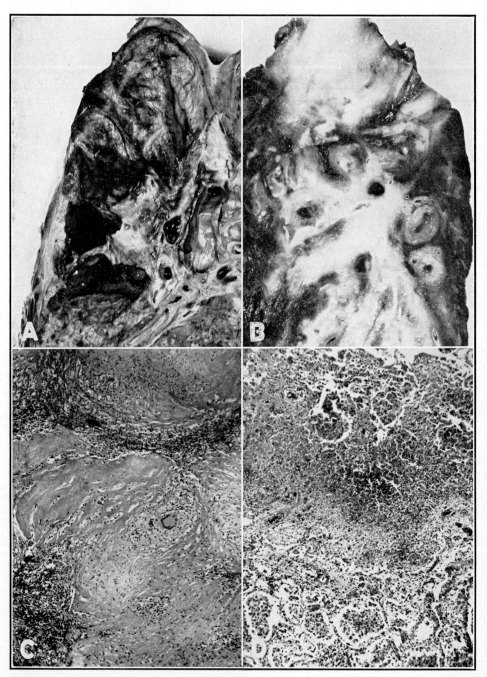

Fig. 213.—Fibrocaseous tuberculosis illustrating *A*, multiple cavities surrounded by active lesions and fibrous tissue, *B*, extensive fibrosis, *C*, solid tubercles with collagenization of the connective tissue. × 50, and *D*, tuberculous granulation tissue. × 50.

parenchymal lesion, submucosal lymphatic permeation, direct implantation on the mucosa, or breaking through of a peribronchial or peritracheal lymph node. The initial lesion consists of elevation and edema of the mucosa followed by breakdown, ulceration, and granulation tissue replacement. The ulcers are irregular and have overhanging edges and gray floors. Healing occurs by resolution or by fibrosis. The latter results in bronchial distortion and stenosis. *Histologically* the process consists of tubercles or tuberculous granulation tissue (Fig. 214*A*).

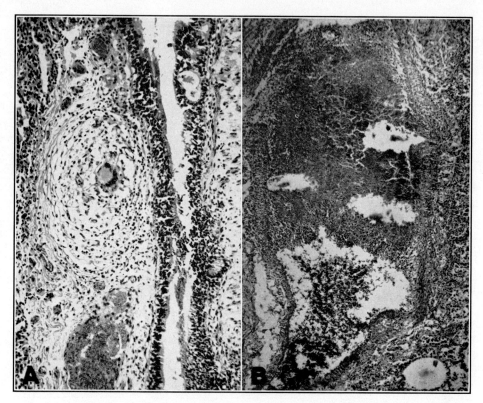

Fig. 214.—Tuberculosis showing *A*, a tubercle in the submucosa of a bronchus. × 100, and *B*, a pulmonary vessel filled with caseous tuberculous tissue. × 50.

Tuberculous pneumonia, also known as acute phthisis and "galloping consumption," occurs when the resistance on the part of the body is poor, the dose of tubercle bacilli is large, or the organisms are unusually virulent. Once the infection is established it sweeps through the entire lung or both lungs (by direct extension or aerogenously) with great rapidity. Grossly the involved portions of the lung are enlarged, diffusely gray, and firm. They possess a striking resemblance to gray hepatization of lobar pneumonia (Fig. 215*A*). Aside from the diffuse parenchymal lesion there may be present small, ragged cavities, bronchial ulceration, and pleural inflammation. *Histologically* the lesion is represented by a diffuse mononuclear cell infiltration with foci of early necrosis and liquefaction (Fig. 215*B*). Tubercles are not recognizable, or at least are poorly formed, and acid-fast bacilli are readily demonstrable in properly stained histologic sections.

32

Miliary tuberculosis occurs when a caseous focus breaks into an artery, vein, or lymphatic vessel and keeps discharging tubercle bacilli into the passing current (Fig. 214*B*). As a result, myriads of tubercle bacilli are sprayed throughout the tissues. Wherever they are deposited, tubercles develop. The distribution of the tubercles and bacilli will depend upon the vessel or vessels affected. Thus, the lungs are primarily involved when a larger lymphatic trunk or a pulmonary artery is eroded, while all tissues of the body are involved when a pulmonary vein is penetrated. Grossly the tubercles appear as uniformly distributed, gray foci less than a milli-

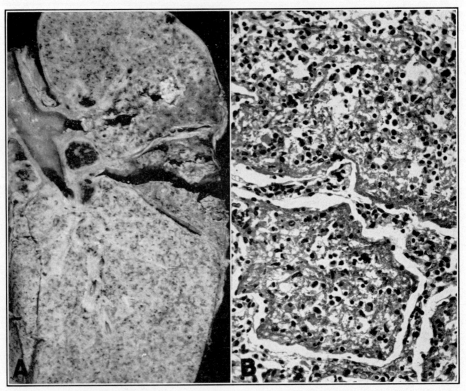

FIG. 215.—Tuberculous pneumonia illustrating *A*, a diffuse involvement that appears like gray hepatization in lobar pneumonia (note early, ragged cavities), and *B*, an exudate composed mostly of mononuclear cells. $\times$ 200.

meter in diameter, while microscopically they consist of small, soft or hard tubercles (Fig. 216). Healing occurs by resolution, fibrosis, or calcification.

Disseminated tuberculosis is a term applied to active or healed (fibrotic and calcified) tuberculous foci scattered throughout the organs (especially the spleen and liver) of the body. The lesions are sharply circumscribed, grayish white or caseous, firm, and measure 2 to 4 mm. in diameter. They represent residues of a hematogenous spread, wherein other tuberculous foci disappeared but scattered points of infection persisted.

Organ tuberculosis means simply tuberculosis of any organ of the body. With the exception of the lungs, the organisms usually reach the organ by the hematogenous or lymphatic route. The explanation for the infection is similar to that in disseminated tuberculosis, that is, the foci in other tissues disappear while those in the organs affected persist. The lesions are generally of a fibrocaseous type.

Tuberculoma is a term applied to a circumscribed mass of encapsulated tuberculous tissue that measures more than 2 cm. in diameter. It may represent (1) an encapsulation of a giant primary tuberculous focus, (2) an encapsulation of a restricted reinfection focus of tuberculous tissue that has a capacity for regression, and (3) a blocked tuberculous cavity with inspissation of necrotic material (Culver). The lesion is found most frequently in the lungs where it is asymptomatic and usually discovered roentgenographically (Fig. 217) but it may also occur in other organs.

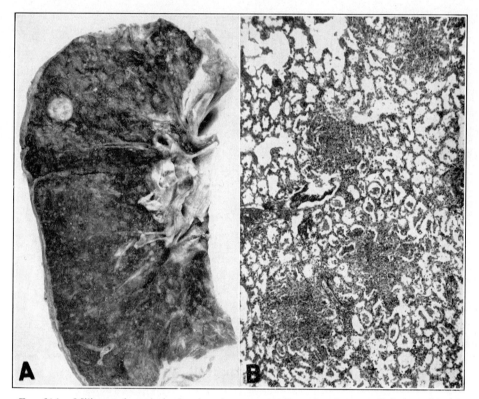

Fig. 216.—Miliary tuberculosis showing *A*, numerous tiny pinpoint gray foci throughout the lung (note also subpleural primary focus), and *B*, several soft tubercles in the pulmonary parenchyma. × 50.

The most favorable *result* of reinfection tuberculosis is healing by resolution or fibrosis. Unfavorable results consist of (1) extension of the process throughout the lungs (as already described) and throughout other tissues and organs of the body, (2) extensive pulmonary fibrosis, (3) pulmonary emphysema, (4) empyema, and (5) bronchopleural fistula (usually following operation or pneumothorax). In addition, it must not be forgotten that tuberculosis offers no immunity to other pulmonary diseases so that because a patient has tuberculosis there is no reason why he may not have, in addition, a pyogenic pneumonia, fungous infection, carcinoma, etc. *Clinically, primary tuberculosis* is frequently attended by few or no symptoms. In some instances, there may be low-grade fever (from absorption of toxic bacterial and tissue products) and (if the patient is a child) failure to gain weight. The lesions in primary tuberculosis are best demonstrated roentgenographically. *Reinfection tuberculosis* is likewise generally asymptomatic at the onset. Sooner or later, however, systemic and local manifestations develop. General *systemic* manifestations are due to the absorption of protein products from the destroyed bacteria and tissues. They consist of various combinations of weakness, fatigue, anorexia, loss of

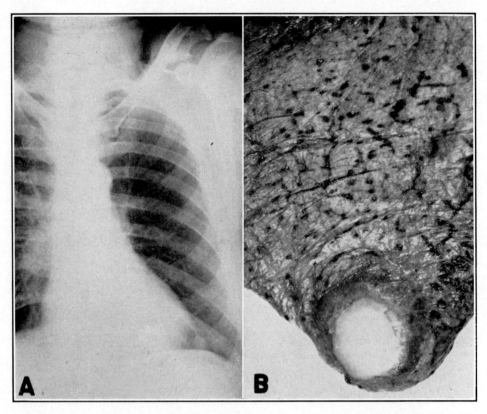

FIG. 217.—Tuberculoma illustrating *A*, a rounded opacity just lateral to the apex of the heart, and *B*, a circumscribed encapsulated mass of caseous material.

weight, fever, and night sweats. *Local* pulmonic manifestations consist of cough (due to irritation of the bronchial mucosa), expectoration (due to discharge of tuberculous material into the bronchial lumens and to secondary bronchial infection) hemoptysis (due to erosion of pulmonary vessels), and pain (due to involvement of the parietal pleura). *Physical examination* varies with the lesion. It depends upon the extent of the consolidation and cavitation and upon the pulmonic complications that arise. Manifestations pertaining to other organs and systems of the body are varied depending upon the dissemination of the tuberculous process. A *diagnosis* of pulmonary tuberculosis is made from (1) the clinical manifestations, (2) the roentgenographic appearance of the lungs, and (3) isolation of *Mycobacterium tuberculosis* from sputum by way of smears, culture, or animal inoculation. In this connection it is important to note that all acid-fast organisms do not represent *Mycobacterium tuberculosis* for butter, milk, hay, and smegma also contain acid-fast organisms which, however, are nonpathogenic. Also, in connection with diagnosis, a word or two should be said about *tuberculin reactions*. A positive tuberculin reaction means that the person has or has had tuberculosis. A negative reaction may be found in a healthy person who has never had tuberculosis or in a person acutely ill with overwhelming tuberculosis or some other disease. *Treatment* is varied and must be individualized for the patient at hand. In general, *medical* treatment consists of rest, diet, symptomatic relief, administration of antibiotics and chemotherapeutic agents, pneumothorax, and pneumoperitoneum. *Surgical* treatment consists of paralyzing the diaphragm, thoracoplasty, and pulmonary resection. The *prognosis* depends upon many factors. As already stated, most persons with primary infection recover, while the outcome in patients with reinfection tuberculosis depends upon the age of the patient, the extent of the lesion when the patient is first seen, the natural resistance of the patient, the type of treatment, etc. In general, the mortality rate in the United States and most other countries is steadily decreasing. It is about equal in males and females until the age of puberty, is greater in females from the age of puberty to the end of the third decade, and is greater in males from the fourth decade on. Tuberculosis is still a common cause of death in the age period between puberty and the beginning of the fifth decade.

Boeck's Sarcoid. —This condition was originally called sarcoid because the lesions resembled a sarcoma. The disorder is also referred to, among others, as sarcoidosis, lupus pernio, and Besnier-Boeck-Schaumann disease. It is virtually impossible to determine the exact *incidence* of the disorder except to say that it is common and worldwide in distribution. It occurs at all ages but is more frequent in young adults and it predominates in females and in Negroes. The *cause* remains undetermined. The disorder is thought by some to be related to tuberculosis and to be caused by the lipid fraction of *Mycobacterium tuberculosis*. In addition, other etiological agents such as other acid-fast organisms, spirochetes, protozoa, viruses, fungi, parasites, foreign bodies, chemicals, etc., have been incriminated but without proof.

Pathologically Boeck's sarcoid is primarily a disorder of the reticuloendothelial system but with all tissues and organs of the body affected. The major organs and systems involved in decreasing order of frequency are lungs, lymph nodes, spleen, skin, liver, bone marrow, and uveal tract (Jaques). The cutaneous lesions exist as papules, nodules, or diffuse infiltrations and they measure as much as 3 or 4 cm. in diameter. Initially the covering epidermis is red but later it becomes bluish and even brownish. Although it may be scaly it does not ulcerate. Otherwise, regardless of the location of the inflammation, the gross appearance is similar. The earliest lesion consists of gray or yellowish granules that resemble miliary tubercles in tuberculosis (Longcope and Freiman). As the lesions age they cluster and ultimately appear as sharply circumscribed, gray to yellow, noncaseating, non-necrotic masses that measure as much as 4 or 5 cm. in diameter. In the thorax the lesions are characteristically bilateral and symmetrical and may affect, primarily, the mediastinal and hilar lymph nodes, the pulmonary parenchyma, or both (Fig. 218*A*). In the marrow they affect principally the bones of the hands and feet. In other organs they are irregularly distributed. *Histologically*, too, the lesions are similar, regardless of location. The characteristic unit is the hard tubercle (Fig. 218 *B*). It is composed of a solid mass of epithelioid cells in whorl formation surrounded by a mantle of lymphocytes and fewer monocytes, plasma cells,

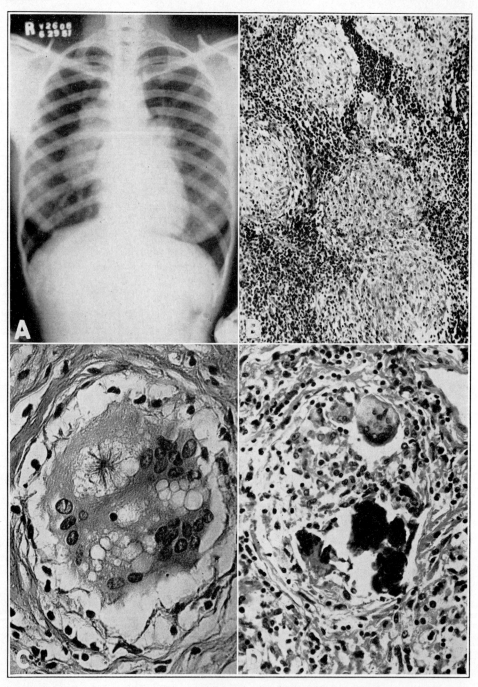

Fig. 218.—Boeck's sarcoid showing *A*, bilateral hilar infiltrations in a roentgenogram of the chest, *B*, hard tubercles composed of epithelioid cells. × 100, *C*, an asteroid body. × 400, and *D*, Schaumann bodies. × 200.

eosinophils, and giant cells of the Langhans' type. Slight central fibrinoid degeneration may occur, but caseation necrosis is not present. In addition, there are frequently present two types of inclusions—asteriod bodies and Schaumann bodies. Neither of these, however, is specific for sarcoidosis (Ricker and Clark). *Asteroid bodies* are usually seen in vacuoles of giant cells and consist of a central hub of eosinophilic material with radiating spoke-like processes (Fig. 218C). Although their nature is not known they may represent crystalline forms of fat. *Schaumann bodies* are deeply bluish staining, concentric, lamellated, multiple contoured, iron- and calcium-positive concretions of variable sizes (Fig. 218D). They are also usually found within giant cells but occasionally may be seen within the tubercles or within adjacent tissue spaces. The lesions in Boeck's sarcoid heal by resolution or fibrosis.

The *complications* may be listed as follows: (1) tuberculosis occurring in from 15 to 25 per cent of autopsied cases (Longcope and Freiman), (2) pulmonary fibrosis, (3) pulmonary emphysema, (4) right-sided cardiac failure occurring in as high as 8 per cent of cases (Jaques), and (5) others due to involvement of the different organs throughout the body. *Clinically* the disease is insidious in its onset and is often devoid of symptoms and signs, being discovered only incidentally during roentgenography. The most common manifestations are due to the lesions themselves and consist of ocular disturbances, enlargement of the peripheral lymph nodes, cough, and shortness of breath. Constitutional symptoms are probably due to absorption of toxic protein products and consist of anorexia, loss of weight, weakness, and, less frequently, fever. In addition, the following may be noted: increased sedimentation rate, eosinophilia, relative monocytosis, slight hypochromic microcytic anemia, hyperproteinemia, hyperglobulinemia, and reversal of the albumin-globulin ratio (Jaques). The *diagnosis* is made from the clinical manifestations, laboratory findings, radiological findings (increased densities in the chest and rarefactions of the terminal portions of the bones of the hands and feet), and biopsy. *Treatment* is unsatisfactory. The *prognosis* is variable. The disease is characterized by exacerbations and regressions and is completely unpredictable. Prolonged follow-ups indicate that the process remains inactive or clears in about one-third of the cases while it progresses or culminates in death in the remaining two-thirds. The *causes* of *death* are usually one of the complications listed above.

Syphilis.—Syphilis of the lung may be congenital or acquired. *Congenital syphilis* of the lungs, also known as *pneumonia alba*, is seen in infants that are dead upon delivery or die shortly thereafter. The condition represents more an arrest of development than actual inflammation. The lungs are small, nonaerated, noncrepitant or subcrepitant, firm, and gray. Histologically the alveolar septa are broad, cellular, and lined with prominent cells (Fig. 219). The alveolar spaces are poorly expanded or completely collapsed.

Acquired syphilis of the lungs is uncommon, usually occurs in adults, and is a manifestation of tertiary syphilis (Morgan). The lesion may be of four varieties—bronchial, fibrotic, gummatous, and vascular. *Bronchial* and *tracheal* syphilis consist of ulceration, scarring, deformity, and stenosis of the tracheobronchial tree. *Fibrotic* syphilis may appear rapidly or insidiously and consists of a diffuse interstitial type of infiltration that is indistinguishable from any interstitial pneumonia. *Gummatous* syphilis is more specific. The gummas are often multiple, occur in any part of the lung, and measure as much as 4 to 5 cm. in diameter. They consist of sharply circumscribed masses of grayish-white necrotic (but not caseous) tissue that may or may not cavitate. The surrounding parenchyma is fibrotic. Histologically the essential changes consist of central necrosis (with maintenance of the elastic tissue pattern) and surrounding epithelioid and fibroblastic cells and, beyond these, plasma cells and lymphocytes (p. 184). Spirochetes are difficult or impossible to demonstrate. *Vascular* syphilis of the lungs consists of a productive type of lesion like the usual syphilitic aortitis and of a gummatous variety (Segal). The former may cause aneurysmal formations, while the latter may result in arterial necrosis, rupture, and fatal hemorrhage. The *diagnosis* of syphilis of the lung

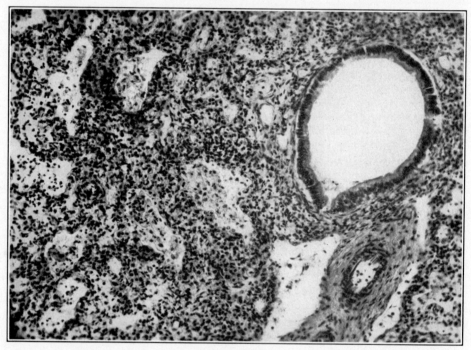

Fig. 219.—Congenital syphilis of the lung (pneumonia alba) illustrating broad alveolar septa and poorly expanded or completely unexpanded alveolar spaces. × 100.

is difficult to make, both clinically and pathologically. One is justified in arriving at such a diagnosis (1) in the presence of a history of syphilis, positive serologic tests, evidence of syphilis in other parts of the body, and typical pulmonary lesions, and (2) by ruling out other disease processes (Royce).

Plague.—Plague is a highly infectious disease that has ravaged the Old World for centuries and still occurs in endemic, epidemic, and pandemic forms in many parts of the world (especially Burma, China, and Africa). The causative organism is the *Pasteurella pestis*—a small, gram-negative, pleomorphic bacillus that can be identified in smears of infected material, cultured on blood agar media, and recovered from inoculated guinea pigs. The organism affects rodents (especially rats and squirrels) and is transmitted to man by bites of fleas (less often bedbugs and body lice) or by direct inoculation (Meyer and Hampton). After an incubation period of three to five days there may *develop* headache, malaise, chills, fever, and prostration. Following these, the disease may assume one of three forms — bubonic, septicemic, or pneumonic. In *bubonic* plague the lymph nodes (especially inguinal or axillary) become enlarged and painful, and rapidly break down and suppurate. In *septicemic* plague the organisms are distributed throughout the body and produce similar lesions wherever they lodge. In *pneumonic* plague the lesions affect principally the lungs where they produce patchy areas of intensely hemorrhagic consolidation with early breakdown of tissue. *Histologically*, regardless of their location, the lesions are characterized by intense hemorrhagic necrosis with little leukocytic infiltration. *Treatment* is prevention and administration of sulfonamides. The *prognosis* depends upon the severity, extent, and type of infection, and these very from epidemic to epidemic. The mortality rate may be extremely high.

Pertussis. — Pertussis (L. = intensive + cough), also known as whooping cough, is an acute infectious disease that occurs endemically and epidemically, is generally seen in late winter and early spring, and usually affects infants and children. It is probably *caused* by the *Hemophilus pertussis* — a small, gram-negative, nonmotile, pleomorphic bacillus that grows readily on blood agar.

Pathologically the lesion is essentially a bronchopneumonia that is associated with a mucopurulent exudate poor in fibrin (Smith). The tracheobronchial mucosa is swollen, shows patchy areas of degeneration to necrosis, and is covered with clumps of *Hemophilus pertussis;* the submucosa contains mononuclear cells and lymphocytes; the peribronchial tissues are permeated with a similar exudate; the alveoli contain a mononuclear exudate, and the tracheobronchial lymph nodes are hypertrophic and show infiltration with mononuclear cells and phagocytes. Focal hemorrhages may be found in the mesothelial-lined cavities, meninges, brain, muscle of the anterior abdominal wall, etc.

The *complications* of pertussis are hemorrhages (nasal, pulmonary, intracranial, etc.), fracture of the ribs (due to violent coughing), subcutaneous emphysema (resulting from rupture of pulmonary alveoli and escape of air), secondary pneumonia, atelectasis (due to plugging of the bronchi with tenacious mucus), and bronchiectasis (Lees). *Clinically* the disease is characterized by four stages — (1) an incubation period of seven to ten days, (2) catarrhal stage lasting one to two weeks and characterized by an upper respiratory infection with cough and fever, (3) paroxysmal stage lasting four to six weeks and characterized by attacks (10 to 40 in a twenty-four hour period) of the following: deep inspiration followed by several short coughs, cyanosis, congestion of the eyes, distention of the cervical veins, a long whooping inspiration (due to closure of the glottis), and frequently ending in vomiting, and (4) convalescent stage where the paroxysms become less severe and less frequent and gradually fade away. From the laboratory standpoint the most outstanding feature is leukocytosis (mostly lymphocytes) to 50,000 or more. The *diagnosis* is made from a history of exposure, lymphocytosis, typical clinical manifestations, and isolation of *Hemophilus pertussis* on a cough plate containing blood agar medium. *Treatment* is prevention by way of vaccination with killed *Hemophilus pertussis* and, during the disease, administration of chemotherapeutic agents and convalescent serum. The over-all *prognosis* is fair to good. The death rate in the United States in 1950 was about 0.1 to 0.2 per 100,000 population—approximately one-twelfth of that in 1900 (Gordon and Hood). The mortality is particularly high in infants.

Interstitial Pulmonary Fibrosis.—Interstitial pulmonary fibrosis, *known also* as diffuse fibrosing interstitial pneumonitis and interstitial fibrosis of the lung, is a progressive pulmonary disorder characterized by fibrosis of the alveolar septa. Although there are only a few autopsy cases recorded (about fifteen up to 1952), the condition does seem more common than these few reports would tend to indicate. It occurs in adults over twenty years of age and affects both sexes with approximately equal frequency. The *cause* of the condition is not known although a virus, chemical irritants, etc., have been mentioned as etiologic agents.

Pathologically both lungs are diffusely involved. The pleural surfaces are usually smooth and glistening although fibrous adhesions may occur. The lungs are rubbery, subcrepitant, diffusely gray, and, on cut surface, disclose irregular map-like patterns with ill-defined gray granularities (Fig. 220*B*). *Histologically* the alveolar septa are thickened by an increase of connective tissue, capillaries, and infiltrations with plasma cells, lymphocytes, and occasionally eosinophils and phagocytes (Fig. 220*C* and *D*). The inner surfaces of the septa are frequently lined by prominent cuboidal cells and may also be covered by thick, eosinophilic, hyaline membranes. The alveolar lumens contain an exudate primarily of mononuclear cells with varying degrees of organization and Masson body formation. In many areas, rounded or streak-like segments of the pulmonary parenchyma are completely replaced with scar tissue. The intervening portions of the lung substance may show varying degrees of emphysema. The bronchi reveal (1) sloughing or metaplasia of the epithelium, (2) plasma cell and mononuclear cell infiltration of the submucosa, and (3) fibrosis of the entire wall.

The *complications* generally consist of right-sided cardiac hypertrophy, dilatation, and ultimately failure. *Clinically* the condition is heralded by what appears to be an acute respiratory infection or early congestive cardiac failure. This is followed by progressive dyspnea and cyanosis. *Radiologically* increasing linear or finely nodular areas of increased density are scattered uniformly throughout both lung fields (Fig. 220*A*). The *diagnosis* is made from the history, from the radiologic appearance, and by a process of exclusion. A differential diagnosis should include pneumoconiosis, tuberculosis, fungous pneumonia, rickettsial pneumonia, primary atypical pneumonia, and other established viral pneumonias. There is no satisfactory *treatment*. The *prognosis* is poor. In the recorded cases death occurred as a result of asphyxia in from a few weeks to three years.

Rickettsial Pneumonias.—Some of the common features of rickettsial inflammations have already been mentioned in Chapter 5 (p. 153). Rickettsial pneumonia occurs almost invariably in Q fever, in one-half the cases of scrub typhus, and less often in typhus fever and Rocky Mountain spotted fever (Anderson). Grossly and histologically the lesions are similar to interstitial pulmonary fibrosis and atypical pneumonia (Allen and Spitz). The lungs are increased in weight; the pleural surfaces are usually smooth but may disclose fibrinous material or fibrous adhesions, and the cut surfaces reveal irregular areas of infiltration characterized by a gray appearance and rubbery consistency. *Microscopically* the bronchi and bronchioles disclose the following: (1) lumens filled with mucus, leukocytes, and sloughed epithelial cells, (2) degeneration of the mucosa, and (3) an infiltration of the walls with plasma cells and mononuclear cells. The alveolar septa are thickened by fibrous tissue deposition and are lined by cuboidal cells. Foci

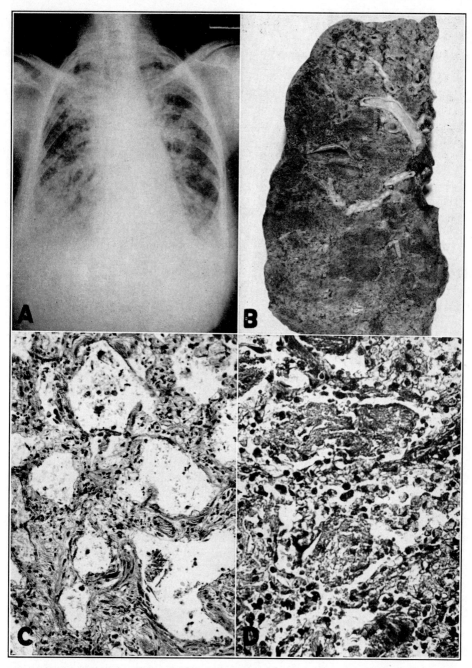

Fig. 220.—Interstitial pulmonary fibrosis showing *A*, diffuse opacities radiologically, *B*, diffuse, rubbery consolidation grossly, *C*, fibrosis of the alveolar septa. × 100, and *D*, organization of the pneumonic exudate. × 100. (Some photographs used by Cox and Kohl, Am. J. Clin. Path.)

of atelectasis alternate with foci of emphysema. Vascular changes are inconspicuous and consist of platelet thrombi with only occasional infiltrations of mononuclear cells about veins and arteries.

Viral Pneumonia.—Under this heading may be included a variety of lesions, some of which are thought to be caused by a virus, but from which a virus has never been isolated, and others of which are proved to be of viral origin. The former comprise primary atypical pneumonia, viral pneumonia of infancy, pneumonia of infectious mononucleosis, and pneumonia of erythema multiforme exudativum, while the latter include the pneumonias of rubeola, variola, vaccinia, varicella, lymphocytic choriomeningitis, influenza, and ornithosis (Reimann).

Primary Atypical Pneumonia.—This type of pneumonia is known by many other names, some of which are nonbacterial pneumonia, atypical pneumonia, and viroid, viral, or virus pneumonia. The *incidence* varies from year to year, but in general, the condition may be said to constitute about 15 to 20 per cent of all pneumonias in hospitalized patients, 25 per cent of all respiratory tract disease in the Army, and 2.78 per 1,000 enlisted men in the Navy. It occurs at all seasons with most of the epidemics being recorded in the cold months. The disorder affects both sexes with equal frequency and is found at all ages but with a preponderance in young adults. The *cause* is probably a virus although, as already stated, such an agent has never been isolated. The condition parallels closely upper respiratory tract infection.

Pathologically the lungs are enlarged and heavier than normal (Parker). The surface is covered with fibrinous material in about one-half of the cases. The general appearance of the lungs is that of congestion, especially in the posterior and inferior portions. In addition, there are present dark, purplish areas of atelectasis and scattered indefinite gray nodulations that measure as much as 3 mm. in diameter. The tracheobronchial mucosa is red and the smaller bronchial ramifications contain small amounts of mucopurulent material. *Histologically* the process is that of interstitial pneumonitis. The alveolar septa are (1) thickened by hyperemia, edema, increase of connective tissue, and infiltration with plasma cells, lymphocytes, and basophils, (2) lined by prominent cuboidal or oval alveolar cells, and (3) exhibit peripheral eosinophilic hyaline membranes in about one-half of the cases. The alveolar lumens are filled with an exudate composed mostly of the mononuculear cells with or without evidence of phagocytosis. As the process ages, the exudate tends to undergo organization. The bronchi and bronchioles disclose a nonspecific ordinary type of inflammation.

Complications are recorded as varying from 7 to 42 per cent of cases (Reimann). Some of the unfavorable results are pleural effusion, empyema, delayed resolution, bacterial pneumonia, atelectasis, bronchiectasis, abscess, otitis media, sinusitis, pericarditis, encephalitis, jaundice, and hemolytic anemia. *Clinically* the onset is usually gradual and is generally preceded by an upper respiratory tract infection (Billings). The usual manifestations are slight fever, chilliness, headache, nonproductive cough, slight respiratory distress, paucity (rales only) or absence of physical signs, normal leukocytic count, normal sputum, and varying pneumonic shadows radiographically. The *diagnosis* is made from the clinical manifestations, absence of any specific etiologic agent, roentgenograms, and serologic tests. The serologic demonstration of at least a fourfold increase of cold hemagglutinins and *Streptococcus MG* agglutinins in convalescent as compared with the acute phase serum favor the diagnosis of primary atypical pneumonia (James). A differential diagnosis includes virtually all other types of pneumonic infiltrations. *Treatment* is symptomatic and supportive. Antibiotics and chemotherapeutic agents have been used but it is still questionable whether they do or do not shorten the course of the disease. The *prognosis* is good for most patients recover on an average of from seven to eight days. The mortality rate is around 0.1 per cent but figures up to 3 per cent have been recorded. Most deaths occur in the aged or in patients with pre-existing respiratory or cardiac disorders.

Viral Pneumonia of Infancy.—This disorder, *also known* as interstitial giant cell pneumonia and inclusion disease, is seen at anytime during infancy and is characterized by fever, diarrhea, and a variety of respiratory

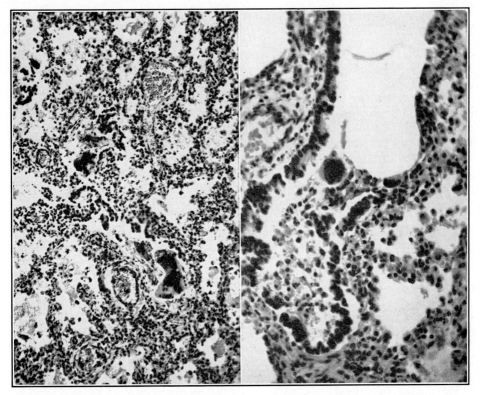

FIG. 221.—Viral pneumonia of infancy showing thickened alveolar septa and large multinucleated giant cells. The giant cell in the bronchiole discloses a cytoplasmic inclusion. × 100 and 200.

symptoms including cough, rapid respirations, dyspnea, and cyanosis (Wolman and Pinkerton). In epidemics the mortality may be as high as 20 per cent (Anderson). Death may occur suddenly. *Grossly* the lungs reveal a diffuse firmness or irregular areas of consolidation. *Histologically* the alveolar septa are thickened and the lining cells are prominent. Some of the alveoli are atelectatic while others are emphysematous. The pathognomonic change consists of the presence of multinucleated giant cells (derived from bronchial epithelial cells or alveolar septal cells) containing intracytoplasmic and, less often, intranuclear inclusions (Fig. 221).

Pneumonia of Infectious Mononucleosis.—There is no proof that infectious mononucleosis is caused by a virus but pneumonia may complicate the condition in as high as 14 per cent of cases and, clinically, the pneumonic process is similar to that of primary atypical pneumonia (Reimann). To further indicate the possible relationship of the two disorders a positive heterophile antibody reaction (which is diagnostic of infectious mononucleosis) has been recorded in as high as 36 per cent of cases of primary atypical pneumonia.

Pneumonia of Erythema Multiforme Exudativum. — In one series, pneumonia has been recorded in 14 of 17 cases of this disease (Reimann). Histologically the pneumonic process is characterized by a mononuclear exudate similar to that in primary atypical pneumonia.

Pneumonia of Rubeola. — Rubeola (measles) is accompanied by pneumonia clinically in as high as 25 per cent of cases (Weinstein and Franklin) but abnormal roentgenographic shadows may be seen in as high as 80 per cent of cases (Reimann). The pneumonia is usually encountered in children under five years of age and occurs at any time from the eruptive to the fading stages of the disease. *Grossly* the lungs show slight emphysema and basilar hyperemia. *Histologically* the following are noted: interstitial pneumonia, mononuclear cell infiltration of the bronchial walls and adjacent alveoli, acute emphysema, and giant cells similar to those in viral pneumonia of infancy but without inclusions (Corbett).

Pneumonia of Variola. — Variola (smallpox) may disclose vesicles, pustules, and hemorrhages in the mucosa of the entire respiratory tract and a pneumonia in the lung parenchyma characterized by hemorrhages, various types of exudates (predominating in monocytes, lymphocytes, or neutrophils), prominence of alveolar lining cells, and the presence of Guarnieri bodies within fixed or desquamated alveolar cells (Lillie). The neutrophilic infiltrations are thought to be due to secondary bacterial invasion.

Pneumonia of Vaccinia. — Vaccinia (cowpox) is capable of producing a penumonia similar to that in variola. The lesions have been produced many times in experimental animals (Reimann).

Pneumonia of Varicella. — The incidence of pneumonia in varicella (chickenpox) is less than 1 per cent (Frank). The changes are similar to those in other types of viral pneumonia including thickening of the alveolar septa, prominence of alveolar septal cells, occasional foci of necrosis, hemorrhage, and intranuclear inclusions in bronchial and septal cells.

Pneumonia of Lymphocytic Choriomeningitis. — This type of pneumonia is also of the interstitial variety with an alveolar exudate composed principally or entirely of mononuclear cells.

Influenzal Pneumonia. — Influenzal pneumonia is *caused* by the virus of influenza A and B (Reimann). The virus primarily attacks the *mucosa* of the respiratory tract causing degeneration, necrosis, and sloughing of the epithelial cells, and inflammation of the submucosa with mononuclear cells (Fig. 222) (Parker). The *parenchymal changes* are primarily those of interstitial pneumonitis with thickening of the alveolar septa and exudation of mononuclear cells. The capillaries show intense congestion and the alveoli are filled with edema fluid. As a consequence the lungs are voluminous, frothy pink, and heavy (Fig. 223). This picture, however, is almost invariably clouded by secondary infection with staphylococci and streptococci, bringing about severe congestion and edema, formation of an alveolar hyaline membrane, atelectasis alternating with areas of emphysema, and later suppuration in the bronchi, bronchioles, and alveoli (Fig. 223). The *complications* consist of chronic bronchitis, abscess, bronchiectasis, and pulmonary fibrosis. The *clinical manifestations* vary greatly from epidemic to epidemic and from case to case but, in typical instances, there is a sudden onset of chilliness, fever, malaise, preorbital pain, sore throat, cough, and fever (Thalmann).   *Treatment* is prophylactic (administration of vaccine) and symptomatic.   Antibiotics are of value in combating secondary bacterial infection.   The *prognosis* is generally good but in some epidemics the mortality may reach 50 per cent or higher.

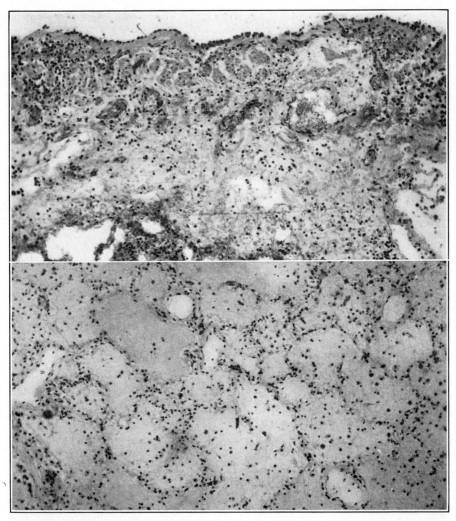

Fig. 222.—Influenzal pneumonia illustrating (above) almost complete denudation of the bronchial epithelium and a mononuclear cell infiltration of the wall and (below) intense congestion and edema of the parenchyma.   × 100.

Ornithosis.—*Ornithosis* (Gr. = bird) is an all-inclusive term connoting a viral infection of birds (Wolins).   It includes the viral infection of parrots known as *psittacosis* (Gr. = parrot).   The *causative agent* is usually referred to as one of the psittacosis group of viruses.   The viruses occur in a variety of domesticated and wild birds, are infective for white mice, and produce complement fixing antibodies.   Man is usually infected by inhaling contaminated dust and, less often, by a bite of an infected bird.   *Pathologically,*

the lungs show the usual type of viral response consisting of thickening of
the alveolar septa, prominence of alveolar lining cells, and a mononuclear
type of exudate. *Complications* are few, those recorded being myocarditis
and peripheral vascular thrombosis. *Clinically,* after an incubation period
of seven to fifteen days, there develop headache, photophobia, sweating,
malaise, anorexia, abdominal distention, slow pulse, continuous fever,

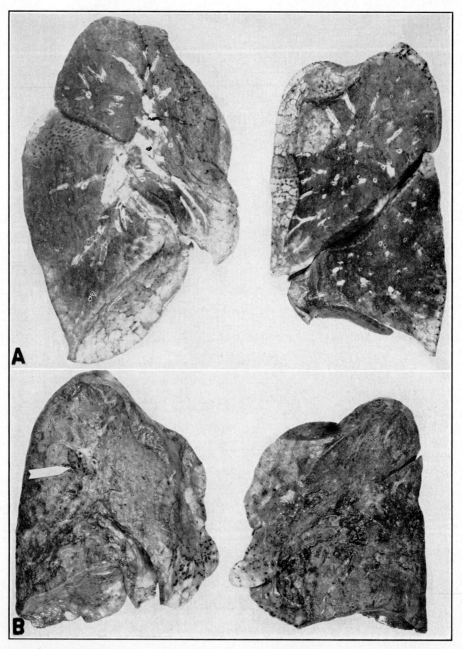

Fig. 223.—Influenzal pneumonia showing *A*, voluminous and edematous lungs from an uncomplicated case, and *B*, congested and edematous lungs with gray foci of suppuration and an abscess
cavity from a case complicated by staphylococcic inflammation.

cough, and (demonstrated roentgenographically) pulmonic shadows. A positive *diagnosis* is made from a history of contact with infected birds, the clinical manifestations, and isolation of the virus. *Treatment* is generally symptomatic. Chemotherapeutic agents and antibiotics are of doubtful value. The *prognosis* is good for the mortality is generally less than 10 per cent.

Fungous and Yeast-like Pneumonias. —Some of the common features of fungous and yeast-like infections have already been considered in Chapter 5 (p. 157). Involvement of the lungs by this group of organisms was once considered rare but, with increasing awareness on the part of the medical profession, such infections are now known to be rather common. The *sources* of the organisms are (1) endogenous (from the normal body flora) — such as those causing moniliasis and one type of actinomycosis, and (2) exogenous (from soil) — such as those causing histoplasmosis, coccidioido-mycosis, cryptococossis, etc. (Kligman). The *route* of infection is by inhala-tion or hematogenously (from other foci in the body such as the skin, gastrointestinal tract, etc.). *Clinically, roentgenographically,* and *grossly* early lesions closely resemble viral and various bacterial infections while older lesions are virtually indistinguishable from healed, calcified, fibro-caseous, miliary, or other types of tuberculosis (Kligman, Hobby, and Good). *Histologically* the infections are granulomas, many of which may also be readily mistaken for tuberculosis unless the causative organism is identified. Thus, aside from the clinical, roentgenographic, and pathologic findings, identification of the organism remains the only positive method of *diagnosis.* The sources of material for this purpose are sputum, broncho-scopically removed secretions, pus (from draining cutaneous sinuses, ulcers, or abscesses), and tissue (secured bronchoscopically or at thoracotomy). Whatever the source of material, the organisms can be identified in fresh or unstained smears, by culturing (on Sabouraud's or other media), by animal (mice, rabbit, guinea pig, etc.) inoculation, and in histologic sections (Conant). In addition, cutaneous sensitivity tests (with appropriate antigens) and serologic (complement fixation, agglutination, etc.) tests are of distinct value. The *complications* are (1) extension of the process to involve the pleura, thoracic wall, and mediastinal structures, (2) hema-togenous dissemination to involve virtually all tissues of the body, and (3) involvement of the pulmonary parenchyma to a degree producing pulmonary insufficiency and/or cardiac failure. *Treatment* (except for surgical excision) is unsatisfactory. There is as yet no effective antibiotic or chemothera-peutic agent available. Iodides are definitely of limited value only. The *prognosis* is variable. Most infections, however, are minimal and self-limited. Only a small minority progresses and results in death of the patient.

Aside from the general characteristics of the pulmonary manifestations outlined above, a few additional words may be said about the following more important diseases: histoplasmosis, coccidioidomycosis, blastomycosis, cryptococciosis, actinomycosis, nocardiosis, moniliasis, and aspergillosis.

Histoplasmosis. —Histoplasmosis is an acute to chronic disease that may affect primarily the skin, oropharynx, gastrointestinal tract, or the lungs or that may be systemic in distribution affecting especially the organs of the reticulo-endothelial system, that is, lymph nodes, spleen, liver, and bone marrow (Hodgson, Reid, and Bass). The disorder is common in the United States, particularly along the Mississippi Basin. It is caused by the *Histoplasma capsulatum* —a rounded, slightly oblong organism that measures 2 to 4 microns in diameter and discloses a doubly refractile rim and basophilic unipolarly, bipolarly, or irregularly clumped chromatin (Fig. 224*A*). In tissues, the organisms are generally located within phagocytic cells but they may also be found free between the cells. They are seen best in recent lesions and are found with increasing difficulty as the process ages.

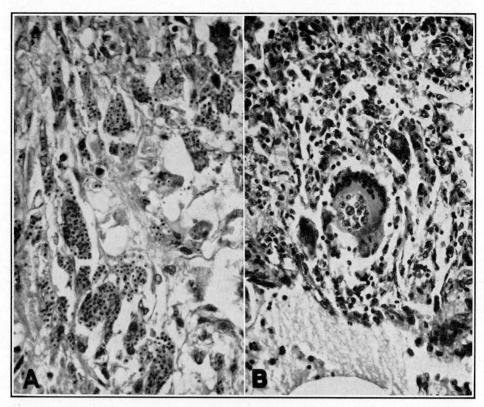

Fig. 224.—Fungous and yeast-like pneumonia showing *A*, *Histoplasma capsulatum* within and without phagocytic cells. × 400, and *B*, *Coccidioides immitis* within a giant cell. × 200.

Coccidioidomycosis.—Coccidioidomycosis is an infectious, primarily pulmonary disease that is generally benign and self-limited but that occasionally may progress, becoming widely disseminated throughout the body and causing death within a short period. The disease is endemic in San Joaquin Valley, California, but has also been recorded in other Southwestern States (Bass, Schwarz, and Forbus). The causative agent is the *Coccidioides immitis*. In tissues the organisms appear as spherules and endospores (Fig. 224*B*). The latter represent end stages of development of the former. The spherules attract, and are engulfed by, phagocytes and giant cells. They are round, doubly refractile structures that, in their free state, measure about 5 microns in diameter but, with maturity, measure 40 microns or more across. As the spherules age, they develop endospores which, with rupture of the capsule of the original spherule, are released to repeat the cycle.

Blastomycosis.—This disease, also known as *North American blastomycosis* and *Gilchrist disease*, is a chronic infection characterized by the formation of suppurative and granulomatous lesions affecting any organ of the body, especially the skin, lungs, and bones (Starrs and Bonoff). The disorder is limited more or less to North America, but sporadic cases have been recorded in foreign countries. The causative organism is the *Blastomyces dermatitidis* —a round or oval, sharply circumscribed, often budding organism with a doubly refractile rim and an over-all diameter of from 5 to 20 microns (Schwarz and Baum). The organisms are especially abundant in pus from the lesion and, in tissues, are seen both intracellularly and extracellularly (Fig. 225*A*).

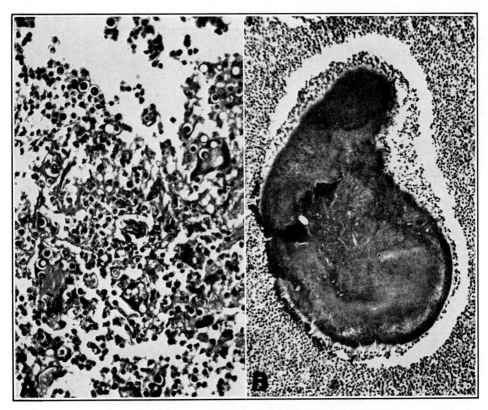

Fig. 225.—Fungous and yeast-like pneumonia showing *A*, *Blastomyces dermatitidis* both free and within giant cells. × 200, and *B*, a colony of *Actinomyces bovis*. × 100.

Cryptococcosis.—Cryptococcosis, also called *torulosis*, is a subacute to chronic disease that may affect all portions of the body (including the lungs) but that has a special predilection for the brain and meninges (Ratcliffe, Cohen, and Berk). In Europe the disorder is called blastomycosis and, of course, it should not be confused with North American blastomycosis. The causative organism is the *Cryptococcus neoformans* (*Torula histolytica*) —a rounded organism measuring about 8 to 20 microns in diameter, possessing (in tissues) a thick gelatinous capsule, and prone to budding.

Actinomycosis.—Actinomycosis is a chronic infectious disease that is worldwide in distribution and that produces lesions in all parts of the body with particular predilection for the cervicofacial area, iliocecal region, and lungs. It is caused by the *Actinomyces bovis* (*israeli*)—an anaerobic normal inhabitant of the mouth (especially teeth and tonsils). In tissue the organisms appear grossly in tiny varicolored (usually yellowish) granules often referred to as "sulphur granules." Histologically the granules consist of a central tangled mass of gram-positive mycelia surrounded at the periphery by gram-negative, club-shaped rods arranged at right angles to the main mass. Grossly the lesion consists of an ill-defined, firm mass of inflammatory and fibrous tissue perforated with abscesses and draining sinuses. Microscopically the most prominent features consist of colonies of organisms embedded in a sea of neutrophils (Fig. 225 *B*).

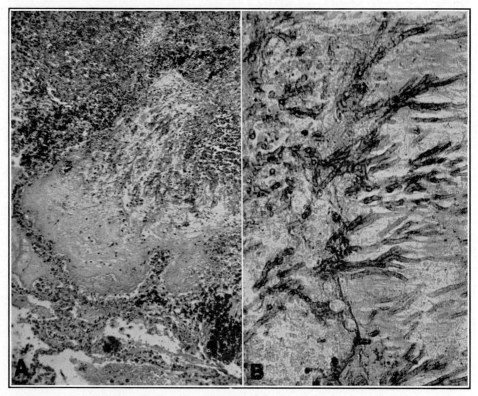

Fig. 226.—Moniliasis showing *A*, a tangled mass of organisms surrounded by a nonspecific inflammatory reaction. × 100, and *B*, a higher magnification of the organisms. × 400. The patient had been treated intensively with antibiotics.

Nocardiosis.—Nocardiosis is an acute to chronic infectious disease that usually affects the lungs, skin (often the lower extremities), and brain but may also be found in other tissues of the body. It is caused by an aerobic, gram-positive, inconstantly acid-fast species of the family *Actinomycetaceæ* called *Nocardia asteroides* (Bernstein). It grows well on the ordinary culture media under aerobic conditions. The lesions differ from those of actinomycosis in that there is no formation of "sulphur granules" or clubbed forms (Hager). The characteristic reaction consists of an abscess with branching organisms scattered throughout the tissue.

Moniliasis.—Monaliasis is generally a surface infection of mucous membranes especially the mouth (when it is known as *thrush*), esophagus, vulva, vagina, and urinary tract but that occasionally may affect other organs, particularly the lungs. It is caused by the *Candida (Monilia) albicans*. In surface lesions the organisms, existing as tangled masses of mycelia, form a superficial, loosely adherent, grayish-white membrane (Fig. 226). The underlying reaction is nonspecific. In the lungs, tubercles with giant cell formations have been described (Oblath). Moniliasis is more frequent now with the advent of antibiotics and chemotherapeutic agents. Apparently these compounds upset the bacterial-monilial relationship and permit the latter to flourish (Wolff).

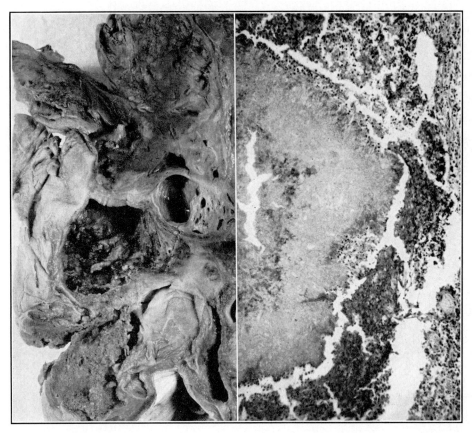

Fig. 227.—Aspergillosis illustrating cavities in the lung containing necrotic material and a microscopic section of a tangled mass of mycelia covering the wall of a small cavity. × 100.

Aspergillosis.—Aspergillosis, like moniliasis, is more common now with the widespread use of antibiotics and chemotherapeutic agents (Abbott). The condition is caused by the *Aspergillus fumigatus*—a fungus that often contaminates grain. The disease is thus seen in agricultural workers and pigeon feeders. Usually the infection is a contaminant of surface wounds but occasionally it may affect the lungs and other organs. In most pulmonary lesions the disorder is probably superimposed upon a previous cavitary disease. The cavities are lined by a layer of fungal mycelia and occasionally conidia (Fig. 227).

Parasitic Infections.—The chief parasitic infections that may affect the lungs are toxoplasmosis, amebiasis, ascariasis, hookworm disease, strongyloidiasis, echinococcosis (hydatid disease), and paragonimiasis. Of these, toxoplasmosis and paragonimiasis only may be considered here, echinococcosis is discussed in the Chapter on the Liver (p. 828), while the others are considered in the Chapters on the Small and Large Intestines (pp. 714 and 769).

Toxoplasmosis.—Toxoplasmosis (Gr. = bow or arc + plasm) is a protozoan disease found in animals such as mice, rats, rabbits, guinea pigs, dogs, and pigeons, and in man (Sawitz). It is caused by *Toxoplasma*—a rounded, elongated, or crescentic organism that measures 4 to 6 × 2 to 3 microns. It possesses basophilic cytoplasm and an acidophilic nucleus. In man, the disease is usually seen in newborn infants but may also be encountered in older children and even in adults (Frenkel and Sultin). While the infection may be found in any of the *tissues* of the body, it has a predilection for the central nervous system, eyes, heart, lungs, and the organs of the reticulo-endothelial system. The organisms are found phagocytosed within cells and are also present in cysts. They elicit a granulomatous reaction that may undergo calcification. In the lungs they are responsible for an interstitial pneumonitis similar to that found in viral pneumonia. The *diagnosis* is made by recovering the organisms from mice or other animals inoculated with spinal fluid, blood, or infected tissues. Cutaneous sensitivity tests and complement fixation are also of diagnostic value.

Paragonimiasis.—Paragonimiasis is an infection caused by *Paragonimus westermani* and limited to the Orient. The organism is a fluke that measures about 1 cm. in length (Sawitz). It usually lives in cavities in the lungs (but may be found in other organs) where it deposits ova (Craig and Faust). The latter are then coughed up or swallowed and passed in the stools. The intermediate stages are spent in snails and crayfish or crabs. *Pathologically* the cysts may measure 1 to 2 cm., are composed of a thick, fibrous wall, and contain the fluke surrounded by hemorrhagic pus. *Clinically* there are cough, expectoration of rusty sputum, and hemoptysis. The *diagnosis* is made by identifying the ova in the sputum or feces. *Treatment* of choice is administration of emetine hydrochloride. The *prognosis* is fair.

Pulmonary Abscess.—Pulmonary abscess is localized suppuration in the lung attended by cavitary destruction of tissue. Actually it is a clinico-pathologic condition and not a single entity (Brock). The process is usually spoken of as a *fetid* or *putrid* abscess when it is rapidly progressive and foul smelling (usually caused by anaerobic organisms), and as *nonfetid* or *non-putrid* when it is less rapidly progressive and not attended by a foul odor (usually in cases of aerobic infection). The exact *incidence* of pulmonary abscess is difficult to determine but it may be said with assurance that the condition is still common. While it may occur at any age, it is usually found in patients beyond the third decade of life. It has no predilection for either sex. The *causes* are predisposing and precipitating. *Predisposing* causes may be listed as follows: (1) tracheobronchial aspiration of septic material (saliva, oronasal pus, and blood or other material consequent to tonsillectomy, extraction of teeth, etc.), (2) bronchial obstruction (congenital, inflammatory, foreign body, or tumor), (3) unresolved pneumonia, (4) infarction, (5) septicemia or pyemia, (6) pre-existing congenital or acquired pulmonary cysts, and (7) fatigue, malnutrition, and exposure (such as seen in alcoholics). *Precipitating* causes consist of aerobic, micro-aerophilic, and anaerobic organisms among which may be listed the fol-

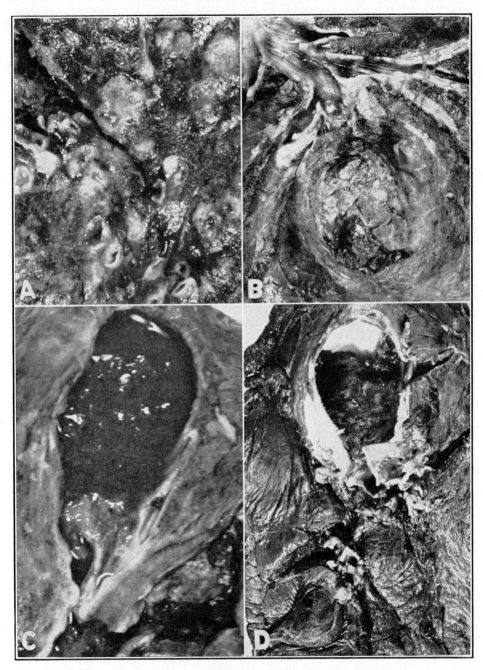

Fig. 228.—Pulmonary abscesses showing A, multiple acute abscesses following unresolved pneumonia, B, acute solitary abscess in a lower pulmonary segment with the contents evacuated, the inner surface lined with gray material, and the wall composed of nonfibrous tissue, C, chronic solitary abscess with the cavity filled with black granular material, and D, chronic solitary perforated abscess with a fibrotic wall.

lowing: staphylococci, streptococci, Friedländer's organisms, pneumococci, influenza bacilli, colon bacilli, spirochetes and fusiform bacilli, and *B. melaninogenicum.*

Pathologically the lesion may consist of a single abscess, two or three coalescing abscesses, or multiple abscesses (Fig. 228). Depending upon the cause, any portion of either lung may be involved but the most common location is the posterior and axillary portion of the subapical part of the upper lobe (Brock). The process usually follows and is limited to a bronchopulmonary segment and, only later, does it spread by direct extension or aerogenously to other portions of the lung. In most cases the lesion is peripheral in location and the pleura becomes affected and adherent early. An *acute fetid abscess* is, in reality, acute suppurative pneumonia with local gangrene added. The lesion is characterized by a rapidly spreading extensive destruction of tissue locally. There is little encapsulation, an incompletely separated, gray, soft slough and an ill-defined wall of varied thickness. The odor, as previously stated, is strong and highly offensive. Early in the process the bronchi are occluded due both to inflammation of the bronchial mucosa and to compression by the adjacent abscess. When the bronchial wall is finally penetrated the contents of the abscess are discharged and the cavity then contains both air and pus. Since the wall of the abscess is soft and composed mostly of necrotic tissue and leukocytes, it is collapsible. An *acute nonfetid abscess* differs from a fetid abscess in the following respects: absence of a slough, generally smaller cavity, usually less rapid spread, sharper delineation, and absence of a foul odor. In either case, when the abscess becomes *chronic* it is generally sharply defined; the wall is firm, fibrotic, and not collapsible; the lumen contains completely liquefied tissue and debris which, however, may undergo inspissation; the lumen may or may not communicate with a bronchus, and the tissue surrounding the abscess discloses an acute to chronic pneumonitis with or without the formation of new satellite abscesses. *Histologically* the process is entirely nonspecific consisting of varying degrees of tissue necrosis, leukocytic infiltration, granulation tissue formation, and fibrosis.

Some of the many *complications* that may arise are empyema, mediastinitis, bronchopleural fistula, pulmonary fibrosis, bronchiectasis, metastatic abscesses (especially to the brain), and even amyloid disease. The *clinical manifestations* are due to the local suppuration and the absorption of toxic products resulting from the inflammatory process. They may consist of any combination of the following: fever, chills, pleural pain, cough with or without expectoration of abundant sputum, choking sensation, hemoptysis, dyspnea, cyanosis, anorexia, loss of weight, weakness, and anemia (Levin and Weisel). *Roentgenograms* (showing pulmonary opacities and actual cavities with fluid levels) are indispensable in localizing and showing the extent of the lesions. *Bronchoscopy* is of distinct value not only in precisely localizing the pulmonary segment involved but also in eliciting some of the predisposing causes of the infection. The *diagnosis* is arrived at from a consideration of the clinical manifestations, roentgenography, and bronchoscopy. *Treatment* consists of (1) removal of the predisposing cause if possible, (applicable chiefly in cases of obstruction by a foreign body or inspissated secretion) (Samson), (2) bronchoscopic and postural drainage, (3) administration of antibiotics and chemotherapeutic agents, and (4) surgical drainage or pulmonary resection (Jewett, Drake, and Touroff). The *prognosis*, in cases not associated with carcinoma, is generally excellent for recovery should be close to 100 per cent.

Pleurisy.—Pleurisy (pleuritis), as already stated, is inflammation of the pleura. That the condition is common is attested by the frequency with which fibrous pleural adhesions (residues of pleurisy) are noted at autopsy. Smith, for example, found adhesions in 66 per cent of an unselected series of 400 autopsies and in 94 per cent of patients with a history of pneumonia and/or pleurisy. Inflammation of the pleura occurs in conjunction with any condition that *causes* irritation of the pleura. Usually the etiologic agents are bacteria and the underlying process is pneumonia, bronchiectasis, pulmonary abscess, and septicemia. Other causes, however, are pneumoconiosis, pulmonary infarcts, irradiation, trauma, foreign bodies, and even tumors. *Pathologically* the pleura initially becomes rough, dry, and dull. Beyond this, its appearance varies with the dominance of its component elements—fibrin (fibrinous), serum (serous), leukocytes (purulent), erythrocytes (hemorrhagic), etc. (p. 131). Further, the condition is referred to as dry pleurisy when there is little or no fluid present, and moist or wet pleurisy when fluid is present in sufficient proportion to cause a moist appearance. The disorder heals by resolution and/or fibrosis with adhesion formation. The chief *complication* of pleurisy is empyema. The *clinical manifestations* are primarily those of the underlying disease. The chief symptom of the pleurisy as such is pain (occurring only when the parietal pleura is affected) while the chief sign is friction rub (due to the rubbing of the two roughened pleural surfaces against each other). The *diagnosis* is made from the history, physical findings, and roentgenographic appearance. The *treatment* and *prognosis* are essentially those of the primary disorder.

Empyema.—Empyema (Gr. = within + pus) is an accumulation of pus in a body cavity and, unless otherwise specified, it usually connotes the pleural cavity. As stated above, the condition represents a complication of pleurisy. The *causes*, therefore, are the same as the causes of pleurisy with the precise etiologic agents always being bacteria (generally staphylococci, streptococci, pneumococci, Friedländer's organisms, and tubercle bacilli) and the usual underlying process being pneumonia. The condition (1) occurs at all ages but is more frequent in early adult and adult life, (2) has a predilection for males, and (3) is most common in the late winter and early spring (Sellors and Cruickshank).

Pathologically the process is usually unilateral and may affect an entire pleural cavity or may be loculated in any portion of the pleural cavity. The loculation is usually in the basal and posterior portion. In *nontuberculous* empyema the appearance of the exudate varies with the causative organism from thick and creamy (pneumococcic and staphylococcic infection) to mucoid (Friedländer's infection) and gray and watery (streptococcic infection). Variations, however, do occur and the gross characteristics thus may not be used to indicate the type of infection. The pleura varies in thickness with its inner (empyema) portion being composed of necrotic material and its outer portion consisting of fibrous tissue. The histologic changes indicate a nonspecific granulation tissue reaction in varying degrees of resolution or fibrosis. In *tuberculosis* the effusion is nonpurulent (serous, serofibrinous, or hemorrhagic) in about 60 per cent of cases and purulent (empyema) in the remaining 40 per cent (Gordon). Grossly tuberculous empyema is indistinguishable from nontuberculous empyema. Microscopically it discloses tubercles or tuberculous granulation tissue.

The *complications* of empyema are pulmonary abscess, bronchiectasis, metastatic infection (brain, etc.), bronchopleural fistula, pericarditis, fibrosis of the pleura, permanent pulmonary atelectasis, and hemorrhage.

Clinical manifestations (due to toxemia) consist of fever, lassitude, anorexia, loss of weight, anemia, and leukocytosis. Occasionally there are also clubbing of the digits, cardiac disturbance, cyanosis, dyspnea, and amyloidosis. Locally the following may be noted: restriction of movement, flattening of the chest, spinal deformity, dullness on percussion, and absence of vocal fremitus and breath sounds (Sellors and Cruickshank). The *diagnosis* is made from the clinical manifestations, roentgenograms, and aspiration of pleural fluid. A differential diagnosis should include hydrothorax, hemothorax, large pulmonary abscess or cyst, diaphragmatic hernia, and tumor. *Treatment* consists of administration of antibiotics and chemotherapeutic agents, needle aspiration of the fluid contents, and surgical drainage (Brown, Sellors, and Frazier). The *prognosis* varies with the age of the patient, the duration of the process, and the underlying condition. The mortality in nontuberculous empyema should be less than 10 per cent (Frazier and Shank).

Mediastinitis.—Inflammation of the mediastinum is relatively uncommon. It is *caused* by bacteria, chief among which are streptococci. The lesion is generally secondary to (1) infection of the larynx with or without retropharyngeal abscess, (2) perforation of the esophagus (traumatic as a result of instrumentation or foreign body, or spontaneous as a result of carcinoma), and (3) miscellaneous comprising an ascending infection from the retroperitoneal space, hematogenous infection, extension of an infection from the vertebræ or other adjacent structures, and perforation of the trachea or main bronchi (Neuhof and Rabin). *Pathologically* the process is entirely nonspecific. The infection may (1) spread throughout the tissues (cellulitis) and be characterized by diffuse induration, edema, and permeation with pus, (2) spread rapidly and be attended by massive necrosis (gangrene) of the tissues, or (3) become localized and form a distinct abscess. The location of the primary infection depends upon the predisposing causative factors. Generally, however, the posterior mediastinum is affected at any point between the level of the neck and the diaphragm. The chief *complications* are pulmonary abscess and pericarditis. The *clinical manifestations* consist of (1) pain in the throat aggravated by swallowing, fever, and increase in pulse rate, (2) remission of symptoms (within twenty-four to forty-eight hours), and (3) subsequent recovery or reappearance and progression of the manifestations just listed together with tissue emphysema, tenderness in the lower portion of the neck, leukocytosis, and irregular roentgenographic shadows (Korkis). The *diagnosis* is arrived at from a consideration of the clinical manifestations (especially history) and roentgenographic changes. *Treatment* consists of antibiotic and chemotherapy, early surgical drainage, and gastrostomy (Adams). With the advent of antibiotic and chemotherapy, the *prognosis* is immeasurably improved. If the diagnosis is made early, and treatment is instituted promptly, recovery (except in cases of carcinoma) should be close to 100 per cent.

PHYSICAL DISTURBANCES

Orientation.—Under the heading of Physical Disturbances may be included a variety of unrelated conditions of the lungs, pleural cavities, and mediastinum. Some of these (as indicated below) have already been discussed in preceding chapters while others may be considered briefly here. The more common disorders are hyperemia and edema (Chapter 6, pp. 191 and 203), thrombosis (Chapter 6, p. 211), embolism (Chapter 6, p.

218), infarction, gangrene (Chapter 4, p. 89), tracheal and bronchial obstruction, foreign bodies, microlithiasis, emphysema, atelectasis, irradiation
pneumonitis, fistulas, trauma, herniation of the lung, hydrothorax, hemothorax, chylothorax (Chapter 9, p. 392), pneumothorax, and hemoptysis.

Edema.—*Pulmonary edema* was defined by Laennec, in 1834, as "the
infiltration of serum into the substance of the organ, in such degree as
evidently to diminish its permeability to the air in respiration" (Luisada).
This definition is still acceptable. The condition is seen in a great variety
of disorders both clinically and at autopsy and, in the latter instance, is not
necessarily simply a "terminal" or "agonal" phenomenon. A few of the
many *causes* may be listed as (1) arterial hypertension associated with
uremia, (2) coronary artery occlusion with myocardial failure, (3) cerebral
disorders such as meningitis, encephalitis, brain tumor, subarachnoid hemorrhage, trauma to the skull, and cerebrovascular accidents such as hemorrhage, embolism, or thrombosis, (4) pulmonary artery embolism necessitating sudden diversion of the blood stream to the opposite lung,
(5) sudden strain in chronic cor pulmonale, (6) trauma to the chest, (7)
mitral stenosis, (8) pneumonias, and (9) shock from whatever cause.
Experimentally, pulmonary edema has been produced in a variety of animals
by diverse procedures. Some of these are (1) acute left ventricular strain
by ligation of the aortic arch, (2) acute right ventricular strain by inducing
pulmonary embolism, (3) damaging the right or left ventricular myocardium,
(4) obstruction of pulmonary veins, (5) intravenous injection of adrenalin,
methyl salicylate, muscarine, alloxan, thiourea derivatives, or ammonium
chloride, (6) production of hypoglycemia, (7) trauma to the chest, (8) rapid
intravenous infusions, (9) inhalation of toxic gases, and (10) production of
cerebral damage by way of occlusion of the carotid artery or by direct
trauma.

While many theories have been advanced to explain the *pathogenesis*
of pulmonary edema, it is apparent that three fundamental factors, acting
in varying combinations, are responsible. The first factor is an increase in
pulmonary capillary pressure in excess of 25 mm. of mercury. It is consequent to a sudden displacement of blood from the greater to the lesser
circulation. This in turn results from severe peripheral vasoconstriction
and may be due to (1) release of adrenalin as in anger, fright, or exposure
to cold, (2) release of angiotonin by way of renal ischemia, or (3) vasomotor
stimulation by way of lesions of the central nervous system or by reflex
action. Vasoconstriction brings about increased arterial resistance which,
in turn, produces an increased strain on the left ventricle. This is especially
significant if the left ventricle is already embarrassed by previous disease
of the myocardium (infarction) or valvular disorders. In addition, vasoconstriction is also accompanied by an increase in venous return to the
heart. This further elevates the pulmonary capillary pressure. The second
factor is increased permeability of pulmonary capillary endothelium. This
is favored by an increase in pulmonary blood flow (resulting in capillary
dilatation), allergy, poisons, anoxia, dyspnea from sudden effort, chronic
heart failure, and inhalation of toxic gases. The third factor is decrease
in osmotic pressure of the blood as seen in connection with prolonged saline
infusion, nephrosis, starvation, and liver disease. The net result of these
three factors is escape of the fluid portion of the blood through the capillary
walls into the pericapillary spaces and alveoli. This, of course, constitutes
pulmonary edema.

Pathologically, the lungs are enlarged, heavy, and subcrepitant. Frothy pink edema fluid bubbles from the trachea and bronchi spontaneously and upon compression of the pulmonary parenchyma. Cut surfaces reveal excessive amounts of pink fluid dripping freely from exposed alveoli. *Histologically*, the capillaries are congested, the alveoli are broadened, and the alveolar spaces are filled with finely granular eosinophilic fluid (Figs. 71*B* and 74*A*). When the latter contains an abundant amount of protein it takes a deep eosinophilic stain and appears more solid but when it contains lesser amounts of protein it takes a light eosinophilic stain and appears more watery.

Clinically, attacks of pulmonary edema may occur at any time. *Premonitory manifestations* consist of precordial oppression or pain, restlessness, weakness, and dry nonproductive cough. The *attack* is accompanied by (1) labored and accelerated respirations, (2) assumption of a characteristic sitting-up and forward-bent position, (3) the presence of gurgling sounds in the chest and appearance of pink frothy sputum in the passages of the upper respiratory tract, (4) cold, clammy extremities, (5) paroxysms of suffocation and vomiting, (6) the presence of a rapid and weak pulse, and (7) a drop in blood pressure to shock levels. Physical examination discloses moist rales over the lung fields. Roentgenograms disclose irregular bilateral pulmonary shadows. Catheterization of the right heart shows that the pulmonary arterial and capillary pressure is severely increased. The temperature remains normal, unless the condition is complicated by secondary infection. The *diagnosis* is made from the history and the clinical manifestations listed. *Treatment* consists of correcting the cause. Meanwhile, as emergency necessitates, the judicious use of the following is advocated (1) venesection, (2) pressure respiration, (3) drugs such as morphine, atropine, or mercurials (depending upon the cause), and (4) antifoaming agents such as (*a*) ether or ethyl alcohol aerosol or (*b*) silicone in ether or water. The *prognosis* depends upon the cause and the rapidity (and extent) with which the lungs can be cleared of the fluid.

Infarction. —The general features of infarction have already been considered in Chapter 6 (p. 190). The condition usually *occurs* in adults of middle age or beyond, but rarely it may also be encountered in children (Zuschlag). It is prone to develop on the basis of an already impaired pulmonary circulation and is thus generally seen in "cardiac" patients and postoperatively. Its precise *cause* is occlusion of a pulmonary artery and this is, as a rule, accomplished by embolism or thrombosis. *Pathologically* pulmonary infarcts are of varying sizes but usually average about 3 to 4 cm. in greatest diameter (Hampton and Castleman). They are always peripheral in location, are found in any part of either lung with three-quarters occurring in the lower lobes, and are irregular or triangular in outline, with the base occupying the pleural portion. The overlying pleura always discloses a pleuritis which varies from fibrinous to fibrous, depending upon the age of the lesion (Fig. 229). Originally all pulmonary infarcts are red but as they age they become paler and paler. In due course (if the patient survives) they heal by resorption, granulation tissue replacement, and fibrosis and ultimately are represented by simply a fibrous scar or a mass of fibrous tissue. *Histologically* the process passes progressively through the stages of degeneration, necrosis, granulation tissue replacement, and fibrosis (Chapter 6, p. 190). The *complications* are gangrene of the lung (if the infarct is large), pulmonary abscess, and empyema. The initial *clinical manifestations* are generally those of pulmonary embolism and consist of sudden pain, dyspnea, cyanosis, perspiration, rapid respirations, rapid pulse, and drop in blood pressure. The manifestations due to the infarct as such consist of hemoptysis, pleural friction rub, fever, and leuko-cytosis.   The *diagnosis* is made from the clinical manifestations in the pres-ence of an irregular or fan-shaped opacity roentgenographically.   The con-dition may be confused with congestive heart failure, pneumonia, myo-cardial infarction, bronchogenic carcinoma, etc. (Miller and Berry).   *Treat-ment* is generally symptomatic.   Surgical interference is indicated in the presence of complications.   The *prognosis* depends upon the age of the

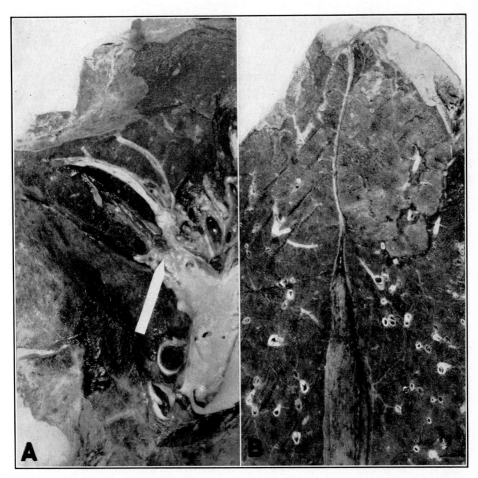

Fig. 229.—Pulmonary infarcts illustrating *A*, an irregularly defined dark red area, vascular thrombus, and fibrinous pleuritis, and *B*, an older, blanching, more sharply defined area with a fibrous pleural reaction.

patient, the cause (embolism or thrombosis), the associated disease process, and the size of the infarct.   When a large pulmonary vessel is suddenly occluded by an embolus an infarct generally does not develop for the pa-tient usually dies within a few seconds.

   Tracheal and Bronchial Obstruction. —The general causes of obstruction of hollow organs have already been outlined in Chapter 6 (p. 224).   Some of the more specific causes of obstruction of the trachea and bronchi are anomalies of the larger vessels, congenital atresia, congenital stenosis, con-genital web, tracheopathia osteoplastica, a variety of chronic inflammations (including nonspecific tracheitis and bronchitis, tracheal scleroma, tuberculosis, syphilis, etc.), a variety of intrinsic (secretions and broncholiths) and extrinsic (almost any small object) foreign bodies, and primary or secondary bronchial tumors (especially carcinoma and adenoma). The *chief complications* are atelectasis, emphysema, bronchiectasis, abscess, and empyema.

Foreign Bodies.—Foreign bodies in the *tracheobronchial tree* are endogenous or exogenous. *Endogenous* foreign bodies consist of (1) *inspissated* plugs of glairy, greenish-gray mucus of putty-like consistency (Shaw), or (2) *broncholiths*. The latter may consist of a progression of the former with deposition of calcium salts but, more commonly, they arise as calcification, and then intrabronchial extrusion, of dead or dying tissue such as seen in areas of necrosis, infarcts, scar tissue, tuberculous lesions, hematomas, and degenerating nerve cells (Schmidt). *Pathologically* they may thus arise within the bronchial lumen, the bronchial wall, or the pulmonary parenchyma. They are usually multiple, variable in size, grayish white, irregular, and hard (Fig. 230*A*). They may remain impacted in the bronchus or they may be coughed up. *Exogenous* tracheal and bronchial foreign bodies are common and varied (Fig. 230*B* and *C*). Any object that is small enough to pass the laryngeal barrier may be lodged in the trachea or bronchi. A few of the many foreign bodies removed bronchoscopically by Clerf are (1) vegetable materials—peanuts, other nuts, seeds, shells, beans, grains of corn, and timothy heads, (2) bones, (3) round objects—coins, discs, and buttons, (4) teeth, (5) safety pins, and (6) miscellaneous—tacks, screws, toys, jacks, etc. The *complications* of foreign bodies in the trachea and bronchi are laryngotracheobronchitis, pneumonia, atelectasis, pulmonary abscess, bronchiectasis, empyema, and subcutaneous and mediastinal emphysema. The *clinical manifestations* are those of the complications, chief among which is dyspnea. The *diagnosis* is made from the history, roentgenograms, and bronchoscopic examination. *Treatment* consists of removal and attention to the complications. The *prognosis* varies with the age of the patient, the nature of the foreign body (peanuts because of their oil worst of all), duration of its sojourn, complications, etc.

Foreign bodies in the *thorax*, other than those in the tracheobronchial tree, almost always gain entrance as a result of external trauma and are thus most common in warfare (Sommer and McColloch). The foreign bodies usually consist of bullets and shell fragments and they may be located in any of the structures including lungs, pleural cavity, mediastinum, and chest wall. The *complications* are pneumonitis, abscess, empyema, embolism hemothorax, pneumothorax, and diaphragmatic hernia. The *clinical manifestations* are sometimes absent but, when present, they are those of the trauma and the complications that develop with pain, hemoptysis, expectoration, and fever leading the list. *Treatment* is variable. Small asymptomatic foreign bodies are generally left alone while the larger ones that are attended by symptoms are removed. The *mortality* rate is recorded as varying from 0.4 to 4.1 per cent.

Microlithiasis.—*Microlithiasis*, also known as pulmonary alveolar microlithiasis, diffuse pulmonary calcification, calcium metastasis, and calcified corpora amylacea, is a disorder characterized by the presence of microscopic concretions within the alveoli of both lungs (Sosman). It was first described by Hartiz in 1918. Through 1957 there were some 46 cases recorded in the literature. The condition, however, is probably considerably more common than these reports would tend to indicate. It *occurs* in no particular race, has been recorded mostly in adults between the ages of 30 to 50 years but is now being recognized in children, has no predilection for either sex, and appears to be distinctly familial. The *cause* is unknown. It is not microbial, industrial, or hormonal in origin. It apparently arises on the basis of deposition of calcium and phosphorous in intra-alveolar pulmonary exudates but the reason for this is not known. One theory is that it constitutes an unusual hyper-immune response. Another is that it is a reflection of a congenital or inborn error of oxygen-carbon dioxide metabolism at the alveolar interface.

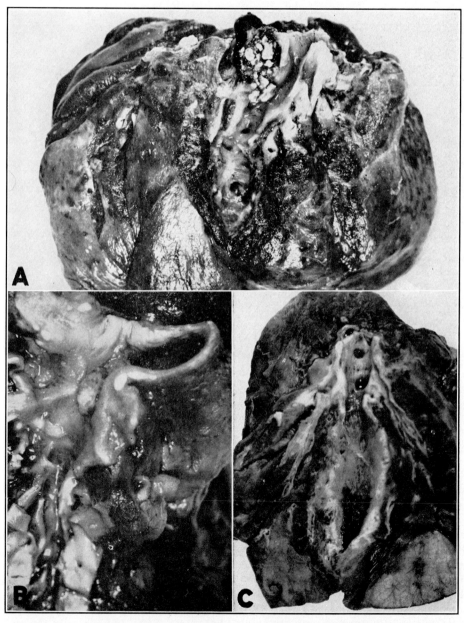

Fig. 230.—Bronchial foreign bodies showing *A*, broncholiths originating in a calcified peribronchial lymph node, *B*, bean, and *C*, pine needles.

The *gross* pathologic changes are confined to the lungs. The pleural surfaces are smooth or covered with adhesions. Immediately beneath the pleura and throughout the parenchyma there are present sand-like or gritty particles. Their concentration is most marked at the bases of the lungs where they may be numerous enough to produce more or less complete consolidation. This may be so great as to necessitate cutting with a saw. The apical portions contain fewer concentrations and often disclose emphysema. The characteristic *histologic* picture is the presence of laminated, often calcified, intra-alveolar concretions that measure 0.2 to 3 mm. in diameter (Fig. 231, *A*). They bear a striking resemblance to corpora amyt

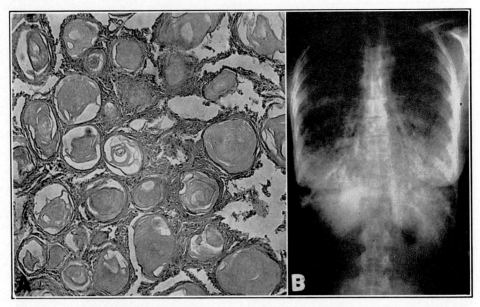

Fig. 231.—Pulmonary alveolar microlithiasis showing *A*, alveoli filled with varisized laminated concretions. × 100, and *B*, a roentgenogram of the chest with bilateral miliary opacities concentrated mostly in the basilar portions of the lungs.

lacea of the prostate (p. 39). They give a positive colloidal iron stain and contain doubly refractile lipids. Chemically, they are composed mostly of calcium and phosphorous, lesser amounts of magnesium, sodium, and iron, and slight amounts of other elements. Occasionally, the alveoli show some fibrosis. More often, however, they are completely normal.

Clinically, most of the patients have shown no manifestations and the disorder has been uncovered during routine roentgenography of the chest. When symptoms do develop they are those of pulmonary insufficiency and consist of shortness of breath on exertion, increasing dyspnea, cyanosis, cough, increased sputum, occasional clubbing of the digits, and cor pulmonale with heart failure. Physical examination of the chest is generally normal. Biochemical studies of the blood, urine, etc. are unrevealing. Roentgenograms of the chest disclose diffuse granular opacities of miliary size most heavily concentrated at the bases and medial portions of the lungs (Fig 231, *B*). The *diagnosis* is made from the roentgenograms and is confirmed by biopsy of the lungs and rarely by finding the concretions in sputum. A differential diagnosis should include any miliary process of the lungs such as tuberculosis, sarcoidosis, fungous infections, pneumoconioses, and miliary tumor metastases. *Treatment* is entirely symptomatic. The *prognosis* is fair, although deaths have been recorded from pulmonary insufficiency 10 to 25 years after discovery of the lesion.

Emphysema.—Emphysema (Gr. = inflation) connotes a swelling or inflation due to the presence of air. As far as the thorax is concerned, it may be divided into two types—pulmonary and mediastinal. *Pulmonary emphysema* consists of an overdistention of the pulmonary alveoli with air. In some cases, it results from partial bronchial obstruction (asthma, tumor, etc.) allowing air to enter the lungs but not to leave, while in other cases no bronchial occlusion is demonstrable. While the cause in the latter

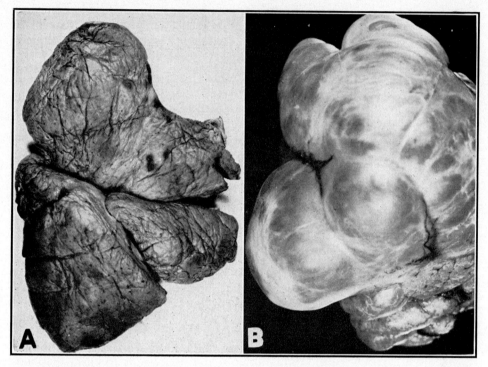

FIG. 232.—Pulmonary emphysema illustrating *A*, diffuse enlargement of the lung with wrinkling of the pleura due to loss of some of the air, and *B*, formation of cysts with air under tension.

group is frequently unknown, the condition, in some cases, has been attributed to chronic cough, loss of elasticity of the lungs, recurrent bronchial infection, bronchospasm, industrial hazards, etc. (Crenshaw and Rowles). *Grossly* pulmonary emphysema may affect a part of a lung, an entire lung, or both lungs (Robertson and James). Most often the involved area is diffusely enlarged, light, dry, soft, and hypercrepitant (Fig. 232*A*). Sometimes, however, the lung parenchyma completely dissolves, producing one or more thin-walled cysts containing air under tension (Fig. 232*B*). Such a lesion has been variously called pneumatocele, cystic emphysema, air cyst, bullous emphysema, emphysematous blebs, and vanishing lung (Dugan and Sampson). *Histologically* uncomplicated emphysema consists simply of dilatation of the alveolar sacs with thinning of the alveolar septa

34

(Hartroft). Rupture of alveoli is a complication and indicates beginning cyst formation. Fully developed cysts or bullæ disclose a wall formed of compressed pulmonary parenchyma without an epithelial or connective tissue lining. The *clinical manifestations* of pulmonary emphysema consist of increasing dyspnea, cough, and asthma-like attacks. *Treatment* consists of removal of the cause if that can be found. Surgical puncture or removal of the cysts is indicated in the cystic variety. The *prognosis* is variable.

Mediastinal emphysema, also known as pneumomediastinum, is the presence of air in the connective tissue of the mediastinum. The *air* may gain *entrance* by way of (1) interstitial tissues of the lungs, (2) fascial planes of the neck, (3) perforation of the tracheobronchial tree and esophagus, and (4) dissection along the retroperitoneal space (Evans and Smalldon). The disorder occurs *in conjunction with* a wide variety of conditions including (1) intense expiratory effort, (2) bronchial occlusion, (3) inflammations of the lungs, (4) pulmonary irritants, (5) wounds of the face, neck, esophagus, tracheobronchial tree, thorax, etc., (6) surgical procedures on the neck and thorax, (7) spontaneously, and (8) pneumothorax and pneumoperitoneum (Towbin). Once in the mediastinum, the air may trek in the direction of any of the routes listed above and, in addition, into the subcutaneous tissues. The *clinical manifestations* are those of increased mediastinal pressure and consist of pain, dyspnea, cyanosis, and obliteration of cardiac dullness. Subcutaneous crepitation may also be elicited. The *diagnosis* is made from the clinical examination and the roentgenographic findings. *Treatment* consists of reassurance. If, however, the pressure continues to increase the air must be removed by way of the thorax or mediastinum and new air must be prevented from entering. The *prognosis* is variable. Of 50 cases reported on by Evans and Smalldon, 18 died.

Atelectasis. —Atelectasis (Gr. = imperfect + expansion) signifies either failure of expansion of the lungs at birth or collapse of the pulmonary parenchyma at any time thereafter. The *cause* of *failure* of *expansion* is some abnormality of the lung parenchyma (such as alveolar dysplasia) or a central nervous system lesion. The cause of *collapse* once the lungs have expanded is either compression from the outside or bronchial obstruction. Compression from the pleural side results from air, fluid, or tumor in the pleural cavity while bronchial obstruction may be due to any one of the many causes listed in a preceding section (p. 525). Of these, probably the most common are accumulations of bronchial secretions in cases of pneumonia and tracheobronchitis and aspiration of foreign material (especially vomitus and blood) postoperatively (Orange, Gans, and Dripps). The mechanism in cases of bronchial obstruction is simply inability of new air to enter and absorption of the air already present in the lungs. *Pathologically* a portion of the lobe, a whole lobe, or an entire lung may be affected (Fig. 208, p. 483). The involved portion is diminished in size, depressed below the surface of the adjacent lung tissue, deep red to cyanotic in color, firm, and noncrepitant. *Histologically* it discloses simply a disappearance of the alveolar spaces and broadening, congestion, and increased cellularity of the alveolar septa. The *complications* are pneumonia, bronchiectasis, and pulmonary abscess. The *clinical manifestations* consist of diminished respiratory expansion, respiratory embarrassment, perhaps cyanosis, anxious expression, loss of resonance, absence of bronchial sounds, homolateral shift of the trachea and mediastinum, and a roentgenographic opacity corresponding to the size of the area involved. Also, radiologically, the causative factors such as an opaque foreign body, tumor, hydrothorax, etc., may be apparent. The *diagnosis* is made from the clinical manifestations and the roentgenographic appearance. *Treatment* consists of removal of the cause. The *prognosis* is good if the lesion is discovered and treated early. Otherwise the condition is followed by the complications already listed.

Irradiation Pneumonitis. — This condition usually results from irradiation of the lung fields during the course of treatment for cancer of the breast, lungs, mediastinum, etc., and, less often, from inhalation of radio-active dusts. The disorder has been willfully produced in experimental animals on many occasions (Bergmann and Graham). *Pathologically* the affected lung tissue may be reduced in size and the pleura may reveal fibrous adhesions. The parenchyma discloses decreased crepitations, an increase in consistency, and a diffuse irregular gray appearance or distinct linear or nodular shadows of fibrosis (Fig. 233*B*). *Histologically* the process is essentially an interstitial pneumonitis (Fig. 233*C* and *D*). The alveoli are thickened first by an increase of connective tissue and a deposition of leukocytes and fibrin and later by an increase of collagenous connective tissue and elastic fibers. The alveolar spaces are diminished in number and size. Some are lined by prominent septal cells and others by a hyaline membrane. The alveolar spaces are empty or disclose an exudate of fibrin and mononuclear cells in varying stages of organization. The bronchial and bronchiolar epithelium reveal degenerative changes and the bronchial cartilages may be calcified. The chief *complication* is reduction in vital capacity. The *clinical manifestations* consist of dry or moderately productive cough, dyspnea, pain in the chest, occasionally fever (due to secondary infection), diminished respiratory excursions on the affected side, impaired percussion, rales, and bronchial breathing. Radiologically the lungs reveal a diffuse haziness which progresses to irregular patchy areas of consolidation that appear to spread from the hilum (Fig. 233*A*). The *diagnosis* is made from a history of irradiation, from the symptoms and signs, and from the roentgen appearance. *Treatment* has been most unsatisfactory. In 1951, Bergmann and Graham performed a pneumonectomy in 2 cases with unilateral irradiation pneumonitis and recorded palliation of symptoms. Generally, however, the disorder progresses and the *results* are poor.

Fistula. — A fistula (L. = pipe) is a tract connecting a hollow organ with another cavity or the exterior of the body. As far as the lower respiratory system is concerned, the communication may be between the (1) trachea and esophagus — *tracheo-esophageal* fistula, (2) bronchus and pleura — *bronchopleural* fistula, (3) bronchus and biliary tree — *bronchobiliary* fistula, (4) pleura and skin — *pleurocutaneous* fistula, and (5) stomach and pleura — *gastropleural* fistula. The *causes* vary with the type of fistula and may be listed as follows: (1) tracheo-esophageal — congenital (Longmire), carcinoma, and tuberculous lymphadenitis, (2) bronchopleural — inflammations (especially abscess, empyema, and tuberculosis), accidental trauma, and postoperative pulmonary resection (Stemmermann), (3) bronchobiliary — trauma and hepatic or subdiaphragmatic infection (Guy and Oleck), (4) pleurocutaneous — trauma or postoperative, and (5) gastropleural — gastric ulcer, diaphragmatic hernia, subdiaphragmatic abscess, thoracentesis, gunshot, echinococcosis, and tumor (Laws).

Hemothorax. — The accumulation of grossly detectable blood in the pleural cavity may occur as a result of some blood dyscrasia, acute or chronic(tuberculous) inflammation, rupture of a pleural adhesion, trauma, tumor (especially hemangioma) of the pleura, or no known cause. If the bleeding is slight, the blood will, in time, be absorbed and leave no after

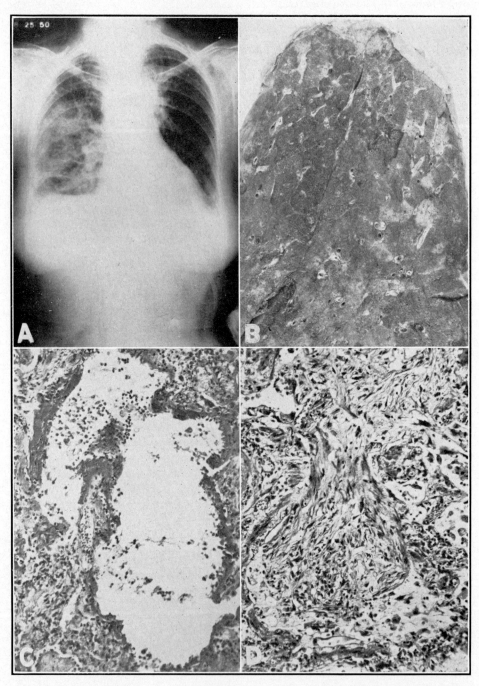

FIG. 233.—Irradiation pneumonitis showing *A*, opacities in the right lung roentgenographically, *B*, irregular fibrosis and areas of consolidation grossly, *C*, hyaline membrane lining a thickened alveolus. × 100, and *D*, fibrosis of the alveolar walls and exudate. × 100.

effects. If it is massive it produces atelectasis and, being too bulky to be absorbed in its entirety, it may undergo secondary infection or organization (Langston and Ogilvie). The latter ultimately results in a dense fibrous plaque or encasement of some or most of the lung.

Pneumothorax. — Pneumothorax (Gr. = air + thorax) is the presence of air or gas in the pleural cavity. It may be produced purposefully (artificial pneumothorax — as in the treatment of tuberculosis) or it may occur accidentally (Mitchell and Rottenberg). Air *enters* the pleural space either from the outside or from the lung itself. The former *occurs* as a result of needle puncture of the thoracic wall (artificial pneumothorax or during aspiration of fluid from the chest), operations on the neck, thoracotomy, or wounds. The latter most commonly occurs in conjunction with pulmonary tuberculosis and localized or generalized pulmonary emphysema. The condition is about eight times as common in males as it is in females and reaches a peak incidence in the early part of the fourth decade of life. It is usually *unilateral* and has no predilection for either side. Since air is space consuming, pulmonary atelectasis is invariably present. In some instances, the condition is *complicated* by bleeding, effusion of serous fluid, or infection. The chief *clinical manifestations* are pain and dyspnea. The *diagnosis* is readily made roentgenographically. *Treatment* (for the pneumothorax as such) consists of release (needle aspiration or thoracotomy) of the entrapped air and is indicated when the condition is bilateral or when air is under tension. The *prognosis* in simple unilateral pneumothorax is excellent while that in bilateral pneumothorax and complicated pneumothorax is guarded. In artificial pneumothorax the outcome is generally that of the underlying tuberculosis.

Trauma. — *Blast injury* of the lungs has already been mentioned in Chapter 6 (p. 224). Similar effects are also produced by blows from *blunt objects* and *nonpenetrating wounds* caused by high velocity missiles (Sealy). The lesions consist of scattered foci of bleeding, larger areas of hemorrhage, pulmonary lacerations, pulmonary consolidation, hemothorax, pneumothorax, and fracture of ribs. Less commonly, there may be rupture of a bronchus or trachea (Kinsella and Henry). Aside from the types of injury already mentioned, *crushing* and *penetrating* wounds of the chest are perhaps even more common (Valle and Cameron). In military life they are caused by penetrating missiles, while in civilian life they are due to automobile accidents, stabbing, or gunshot. The lesions sustained comprise penetration or laceration of the chest wall, fracture of ribs, hemothorax, pneumothorax, pneumonitis, atelectasis, contusion of the lungs, lacerations of the lungs, pulmonary abscess, empyema, and retention of foreign bodies.

Herniation of the Lung. — Herniation of the lung may occur at sites of thoracotomy scars (Baxter), in the cervical region, or, rarely, through the diaphragm (Reinhart). It is seen at all ages and is more prevalent in males than it is in females. The *cause* is weakness of the pleura, fascia, or muscles of the thoracic wall. It may be on the basis of a congenital abnormality, trauma, or disease. The chief *clinical manifestation* is the appearance of a soft, crepitant mass on deep or forced inspiration and its disappearance on expiration. Rarely are there pain, paroxysmal cough, or hemoptysis. *Roentgenograms* generally reveal the presence of air in the herniated mass. *Complications* occur infrequently. They consist of incarceration, strangulation, or inflammation (Chapter 6, p. 225). *Treatment* is surgical repair. The *prognosis* is good.

Hydrothorax. — The general principles underlying the accumulation of serous fluid in the pleural cavities have been considered in Chapter 6 (p. 203). While the etiologic factors vary, the causes of the condition in decreasing order of frequency as listed by Sahn in a series of 103 cases were carcinoma, congestive heart failure, pulmonary infarction, lymphoblastoma, pneumonia, tuberculosis, cirrhosis of the liver, nephrosis, and miscellaneous. Of these, carcinoma and congestive failure accounted for 81 cases.

Hemoptysis. — The spitting or coughing up of blood is a symptom and not a disease. The amount expectorated may be scanty (barely noticeable) or copious and the effects upon the patient may be correspondingly nil or disastrous. Although any disease of the lung may produce hemoptysis, some of the more common causes may be listed as follows: tuberculosis, bronchiectasis, pneumonia, bronchogenic carcinoma, pulmonary abscess, pulmonary infarction, mitral stenosis, pulmonary congestion and edema from whatever cause, and idiopathic (Chaves and Parker).

TUMORS

Orientation. — In this section, tumors of the following structures may be considered in the order listed: (1) lower respiratory system proper, (2) pleura, (3) superior thoracic inlet, and (4) mediastinum.

Tumors of the Lower Respiratory System Proper. — In this category may be included tumors of the trachea, bronchi, and pulmonary parenchyma. Pathologically the growths are as protean as the tissues that compose the lower respiratory system. The lesions may be listed as follows: papilloma, carcinoma, adenoma, fibroma, fibrosarcoma, lipoma, liposarcoma, hemangioma (arteriovenous fistula), hemangio-endothelioma, myoblastoma, leiomyoma, leiomyosarcoma, rhabdomyoma, rhabdomyosarcoma, carcinosarcoma, chondroma, chondrosarcoma, osteoma, osteosarcoma, osteochondroma, neurofibroma, lymphoblastoma, plasmocytoma, and metastatic. Of these, the most common and, therefore, the most important are carcinoma, adenoma, and metastatic tumors. They may be considered briefly in the order mentioned.

Carcinoma. — Primary carcinoma of the lower respiratory system (commonly called carcinoma of the lung or bronchogenic carcinoma) is a malignant tumor of the epithelial cells of the mucosa and, less often, of the submucosal glands of the tracheobronchial tree. While there is still some controversy as to whether carcinoma does or does not arise in alveolar septal cells, the probability is that it does not. Statistics regarding the *incidence* of primary pulmonary carcinoma vary, but it can be safely said that it is one of the top three cancer killers in males (the other two being carcinoma of the stomach and carcinoma of the prostate) — annually accounting for approximately 10,000 deaths in the United States and 4,500 deaths in England (Mason). It constitutes approximately 7 per cent of all cancers of the body (Ariel). While it may occur at all ages from infancy to old age, it is seen mostly beyond the age of forty years. It predominates in males over females in the approximate ratio of 8 to 1 and it is seen in all races. The *cause* is not known but inhalation of dirt, dust, fumes, and gases is considered by many authors to be significant. Among these, smoke (especially that from cigarettes) is considered to be of paramount importance. In this connection, many statistical and clinical studies have been carried out in recent years both in the United States and other countries by reputable clinicans, statisticians, and other scientists and almost all of them have come to the same conclusion—cigarette smoking is an important factor in the genesis of cancer of the lungs (Doll, Ochsner, and Strong). It has been proved repeatedly, for example, that cancer of the lung occurs 5 to 15 times more frequently among cigarette smokers than among nonsmokers and that there is a direct relationship between the incidence of tumor development and the number of cigarettes smoked. *Experimentally*, too, carcinoma of the skin of mice and rabbits has been produced as a result of painting with tars obtained from cigarette smoke and both carcinoma and sarcoma have been produced in rats by direct inoculation of such material into the lungs (Graham, Wynder, and Blacklock). Despite these reports, there is another group of observers, who are equally reputable but definitely in the minority, that holds that there has been no actual increase in cancer of the lung in proportion to other cancers and that mere association of smoking and lung cancer does not necessarily prove a causal relationship (Rigdon). Aside from cigarette smoking, inhalation of carcinogenic metals such as arsenic, uranium ores, chromate, nickel, asbestos, and bituminous substances as encountered in industry, together with air pollution and smog from a variety of sources in large cities, are all considered to be of etiologic significance (Hueper). Thus, while there is no doubt that the controversy regarding smoke and other inhalants as causative factors in carcinoma of the lung will continue, as it has over many decades in the past, in your author's opinion the evidence in favor of such a relationship is overwhelming. Since all people who smoke and all people who live in cities do not, however, develop pulmonary carcinoma there must be other factors entering into the picture. The most important of these appears to be heredity.

Pathologically carcinoma may arise in any portion of the tracheobronchial tree but, of the various subdivisions, is relatively rare in the trachea where, by 1953, there have been less than 200 cases recorded. In the remaining portion of the bronchial tree, the growths are equally distributed between the hilum and the periphery. Any portion of either lung may be affected with no preponderance for either the right or the left side. As a rule, the tumor arises in a single area, although multicentric foci occasionally occur. The *earliest lesion* is indicated by a segmental roughening of the mucosa. The surface is granular, superficially ulcerated, and bleeds readily upon the slightest manipulation. As the lesion enlarges, it grows toward the lumen, into and along the wall, and into the peribronchial parenchyma (Fig. 234). Tumors that protrude into the *lumen* are of variable shapes and sizes. They may be pedunculated or sessile, pink to gray, superficially intact or ulcerated, friable or firm, and measure up to 3 or 4 cm. in diameter, depending upon the size of the bronchus involved. As they enlarge, they gradually encroach upon and, ultimately, completely occlude the bronchial lumen. Tumors that grow *in the wall* are usually firm, gray, and sclerotic. They have a tendency to encircle and thus constrict or completely occlude the lumen and to extend longitudinally along the bronchial tree for 2, 3, or more cm. Tumors that grow in the peribronchial *parenchyma* ultimately assume one of three appearances. They may appear (1) as solid masses of grayish-white, firm, friable tissue that are sharply circumscribed and that completely replace the pulmonary parenchyma, (2) as large, abscess-like cavities with peripheral areas of grayish-white tissue and necrotic excavated centers that communicate directly with adjacent bronchial lumens, or (3) as ill-defined, grayish-white areas of pneumonic consolidation that are indistinguishable from gray hepatization in lobar pneumonia or tuberculous caseous pneumonia.

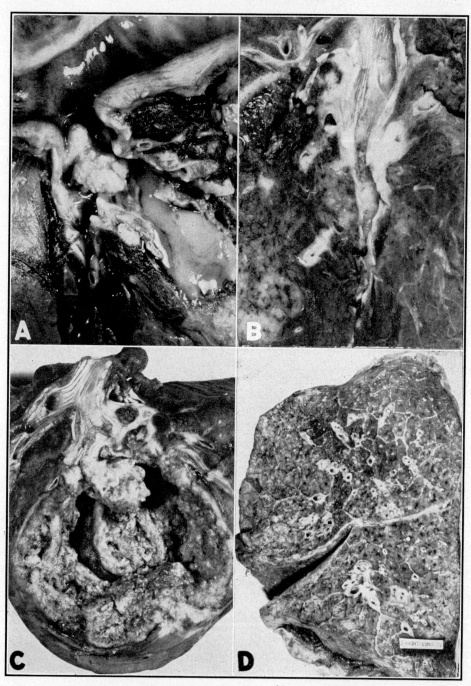

FIG. 234.—Primary carcinoma of the lung illustrating A, a nodular growth protruding into the lumen of a bronchus and causing bronchiectasis distally, B, an infiltrating growth producing diffuse thickening and narrowing of a bronchus, C, a large growth that has become necrotic centrally and drained by a bronchus, and D, a diffuse pneumonic infiltration simulating lobar pneumonia.

Histologically the growths doubtlessly arise from the basal cells of the tracheobronchial mucosa or submucosal glands. Normally, these cells are primitive cells that may proliferate to reproduce their own kind (other primitive cells) or that may differentiate into columnar, cuboidal, or squamous epithelial cells. Thus, it is understandable that when they go awry they may also differentiate into the three main types of cells and hence produce anaplastic carcinoma, adenocarcinoma, and squamous cell carcinoma (Fig. 235). Further, since each of these has as its progenitor a common stem cell, it is not uncommon to find all three varieties of carcinoma not only in the same tumor but actually in a single microscopic field. Of the three tumors, *squamous cell carcinoma* is the most common. Microscopically, as elsewhere, it exists in the form of small or large masses of relatively large, fairly well-defined, polyhedral cells with a moderate amount of eosinophilic cytoplasm and round or oval, hyperchromatic nuclei. Keratinization and pearl formation are frequent in the better differentiated growths but are infrequent or entirely absent in the more highly malignant tumors. *Adenocarcinoma* exists in the form of large or small acini lined with a single layer of columnar or cuboidal epithelial cells. The nuclei are round or oval, hyperchromatic, and usually basilar in position. The cytoplasm is variable in amount. It may or may not reveal vacuoles of secretion. The lumens of the glands may be empty or may contain eosinophilic or basophilic, stringy material. Usually the glands are irregularly distributed throughout the tissues. Sometimes, however, they use the alveolar septa for a scaffolding and thus appear as though they are arising from septal cells. Such tumors have been referred to as *alveolar cell tumor* or *alveolar cell carcinoma*. *Anaplastic carcinoma* is quite variable in its appearance. Sometimes it discloses cells that are definitely of a squamous, columnar, or cuboidal appearance but that do not have the typical formations that these cells normally possess. At other times they form grotesque cells with abundant eosinophilic cytoplasm and sometimes multiple hyperchromatic nuclei. At other times still, they exist as small, round, oval, or somewhat irregular cells with scanty, almost imperceptible cytoplasm and irregular hyperchromatic nuclei. In any case, the cells in anaplastic carcinoma are diffusely distributed in clumps, masses, or singly and do not form any distinct pattern. Usually the underlying architecture is completely replaced with the neoplastic cells. Sometimes, however, they collect within the lumens of the alveoli in a manner similar to the leukocytes in an ordinary pneumonia. In such cases, the alveolar septa remain well preserved. The *stroma* in any of the types of carcinoma of the lung is quite variable. In some instances it is loose and scanty while in others it is collagenous and abundant. It usually discloses an abundant infiltration with plasma cells, lymphocytes, monocytes, and neutrophils.

Carcinoma of the lung *spreads* (1) by direct extension to contiguous portions of the lung and beyond this to the pleura, chest wall, mediastinal structures (recurrent laryngeal nerve, blood vessels, heart, etc.), diaphragm, etc., (2) by air passages to the same or opposite lung, (3) by lymphatics to the pleural, hilar, mediastinal, etc., lymph nodes, and (4) by the bloodstream to the same or opposite lung and throughout the body. With regard to spread of the tumor beyond the lung in which it originates, the frequency of involvement of other organs in decreasing order is regional lymph nodes, adrenal glands, liver, pleura, opposite lung, bones, brain, and the other tissues throughout the body.

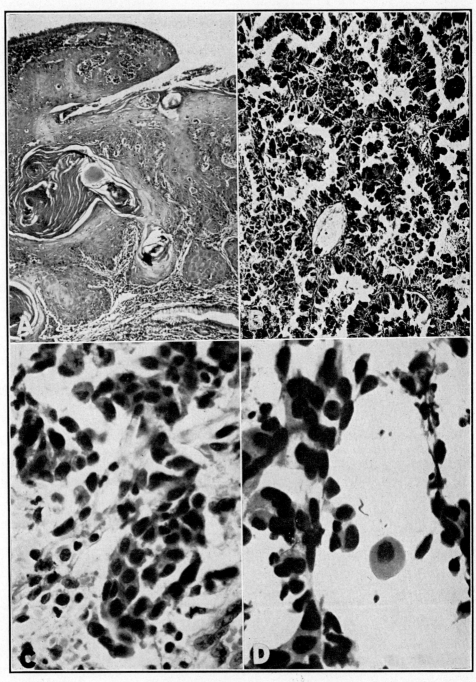

FIG. 235.—Primary carcinoma of the lung showing *A*, masses of keratinizing squamous cells infiltrating the submucosa. × 50, *B*, columnar neoplastic cells lining alveoli (alveolar cell tumor). × 100, *C*, anaplastic cells irregularly infiltrating the parenchyma. × 400, and *D*, neoplastic cells in bronchoscopically removed secretions. × 400.

The *complications* of carcinoma of the lung, aside from extension and metastasis of the tumor, consist of (1) bronchiectasis, (2) pulmonary abscess, (3) hydrothorax or empyema, (4) atelectasis, and (5) emphysema. Most of the *clinical manifestations* are due to the complications just listed. It is for this reason that the condition is often silent in its early stages. In an analysis of 1,000 cases, Mason recorded the following in decreasing order of frequency: cough, pain, dyspnea, lassitude, hemoptysis, loss of weight, fever, wheezing, congestive failure, hoarseness, sputum, clubbing of the fingers, dysphagia, and others. *Radiologically* the following may be noted: tumor mass itself, atelectasis, abscess, obstructive emphysema, or pleurisy. *Bronchoscopically* the tumor may be visualized and a biopsy secured in approximately 30 per cent of cases when the patients initially seek help. In another 20 to 30 per cent there is indirect evidence of tumor in the form of fixation, deformity, etc., of the tracheobronchial tree, but tissue cannot be secured for histologic examination. The *diagnosis* of carcinoma of the lung is arrived at from a consideration of the clinical manifestations, the radiologic findings, the appearance at bronchoscopy, the cytologic examination of bronchoscopically secured secretion or sputum, and, if these fail, the findings at thoracotomy. In connection with diagnosis it might be stated that the cytologic examination of bronchoscopically secured secretions for neoplastic cells should yield positive results in over 85 per cent of cases. A differential diagnosis includes almost any disease of the lungs, especially viral pneumonia, pulmonary infarction, atelectasis, tuberculosis, fungous infection, ordinary bronchiectasis, and pulmonary abscess. The only effective treatment is complete resection of the tumor by way of a pneumonectomy. If this fails, irradiation therapy and chemotherapy may be tried. Neither of these, however, as yet offers any hope of cure. The *prognosis* is poor. In a series of 1,000 cases reported on by Mason, only 353 patients were explorable, 202 were subjected to pneumonectomy, and, of the ones treated surgically, only 62 survived from two months to seven years. In a collected series of 7,815 cases from 10 medical centers in the United States and England, Buchberg found that 2,490 patients were inoperable, 1,239 were resectable, and, of the resectable group, 72 or 5.8 per cent (0.9% of the original 7,815 patients) lived five years or longer. In contrast, of his own series of 443 patients not treated surgically, 2 per cent lived five years or longer. In other words, although pneumonectomy offers the only hope of cure, it has thus far not increased the over-all longevity. In single large series of cases, however, five-year survival rates as high as 6 per cent have been recorded (Ochsner).

Adenoma.—Adenoma of the trachea and bronchi is *also known* as basal cell carcinoma, carcinoid, cylindroma, mixed tumor, adenoid cystic carcinoma, etc. In *frequency* the tumor is second only to carcinoma. It is said to constitute about 12 per cent of all primary pulmonary tumors. It is slightly more common in females than in males and, although it occurs at all ages, it is most frequent in the third decade of life.

Pathologically the tumor is usually located in the main stem or larger bronchi, less often in the trachea, and least often in the smaller bronchi and bronchioles. Classically it exists as a collar button-like structure with a smaller head protruding into the lumen, a constricted neck occupying the wall of the respiratory tube, and a larger base growing into the peritubal tissues (Fig. 236*A*). Sometimes, however, the tumor protrudes entirely into the tracheobronchial lumen. As a rule, the luminal mass is rounded, polypoid, pedunculated, smooth, pink to cyanotic, soft to firm, and easily

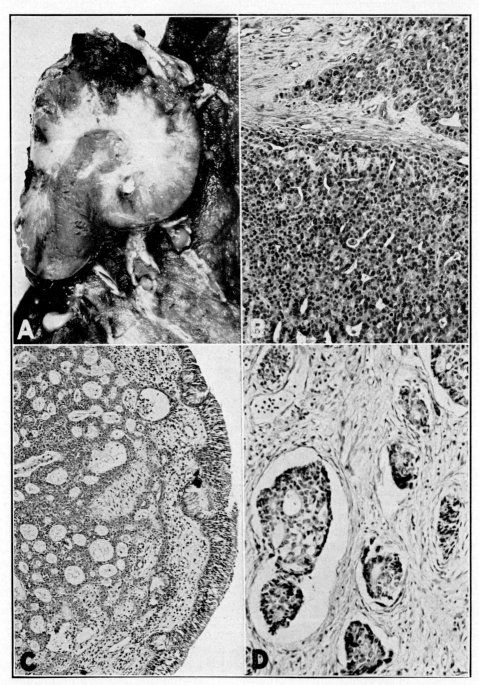

Fig. 236.—Bronchial adenoma illustrating A, a sharply circumscribed tumor involving the bronchial lumen, the bronchial wall, and the peri-bronchial tissue, B, regular cuboidal or poly-hedral cells with an attempt at glandular formation. × 120, C, masses of regular cells with areas of cystic degeneration located in the submucosa. × 375, and D, same tumor shown in C to reveal the regularity of the cells. × 120.

movable at its base. It bleeds readily upon the slightest trauma. The size
varies with the location and the age of the growth, with the average measuring 3 to 4 cm. across. The extraluminal portion is generally sharply circumscribed and similar in appearance to the intraluminal portion. Cut surfaces
may or may not disclose calcified material and bone. *Histologically* most of
the tumors probably arise from the submucosal glands and their ducts. A
few, however, also arise from the basal cells of the overlying mucosa. Characteristically the growth is located in the submucosa. Its two chief components are epithelial cells and stroma. The *epithelial* cells exist in cords,
masses, sheets, glands, and rarely clumps (Fig. 236B, C, and D). The individual cells are monotonously uniform in shape, size, and staining qualities.
They are rounded to cuboidal, usually poorly defined, and of moderate
sizes. The cytoplasm varies in amount but is generally fairly abundant and
lightly eosinophilic. The nuclei are round or oval and evenly stained.
Mitoses are infrequent and hyperchromatism is not apparent. The *stroma*
varies from abundant hyalinized to scanty, loose, and vascular. It usually
contains scattered leukocytes. Occasionally it also contains cartilage, bone,
and bone marrow. These structures, however, appear to be inclusions of
the tracheobronchial tree rather than integral parts of the growth.

As a rule, the neoplasm *spreads* only by local extension. Sometimes,
however, it becomes malignant and then metastasizes to the draining lymph
nodes, mediastinum, pleura, opposite lung, liver, bones, and other areas.

Aside from metastasis, the *complications* consist of tracheal and bronchial
occlusion, pulmonary atelectasis, emphysema, bronchiectasis, and abscess.
The *clinical manifestations* are often of several years' duration. They consist of (1) cough—due to irritation of the bronchial mucosa by the tumor
and the secondary infection, (2) stridor, dyspnea, and wheezing—due to
occlusion of the tracheobronchial lumen, (3) hemoptysis—due to ulceration
of the mass, (4) pain—due to inflammatory pleural involvement, and (5)
fever and other symptoms—due to atelectasis, abscess, and bronchiectasis.
Radiologically the tumor and/or the complications resulting therefrom are
usually apparent. *Bronchoscopically* the tumor is visualized in over 90 per
cent of cases. The *diagnosis* is made from the clinical manifestations,
roentgenographic appearance, and the findings at bronchoscopy. While
destruction of the tumor by local cauterization has been successfully
accomplished, the *treatment* of choice (because many growths are extraluminal and some become malignant) is lobectomy or, if necessary, pneumonectomy. The *prognosis* is good. It is generally conceded that 5 to 10 per
cent of the tumors are or become malignant but even in these, the duration
of life averages about ten years after symptoms first appear.

Metastatic Tumors.—Metastatic neoplasms of the lung are more common than primary growths. They consist both of carcinomas and sarcomas
and may originate in any organ or tissue of the body. The lesions may
affect one or both lungs; they may be single or multiple, and they may
measure from a few millimeters to several centimeters in diameter. *Grossly*
the tumors may be indistinguishable from primary growths (Fig. 237). They
may (1) replace the parenchyma completely, (2) fill the alveolar spaces
and appear like a pneumonia, (3) become necrotic centrally and, upon discharging their contents, resemble an abscess, or (4) penetrate the wall of a
bronchus and protrude into or occlude the lumen. *Histologically* the
neoplasms usually resemble the parent lesions. The distribution of the cells,
however, is similar to that of primary pulmonary tumors. Thus, the cells
may be irregularly arranged, may fill the alveolar spaces similar to leuko-

cytes in pneumonia, or may line the alveolar septa rendering an alveolar cell appearance. The *importance* of metastatic tumors is, of course, their differentiation from primary tumors.

Tumors of the Pleura.—Tumors of the pleura may be secondary or primary. Of the two, *secondary growths* are much more common. They may occur as extensions from adjacent organs (especially the lung) or they may eventuate as a result of metastasis from any organ of the body. Grossly they usually appear as innumerable foci of varying sizes studding both the

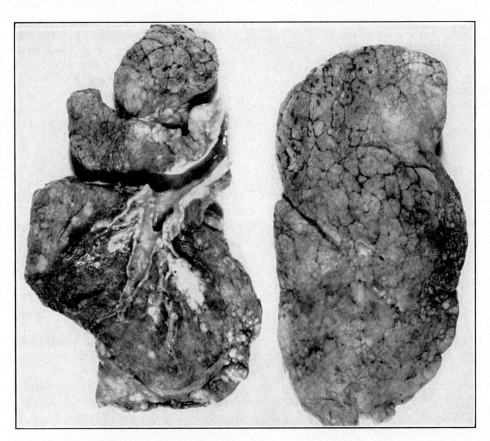

Fig. 237.—Primary carcinoma of a breast with metastasis to a lung. The bronchial, parenchymal, and pleural tumors resemble a primary pulmonary carcinoma.

visceral and parietal surfaces (Fig. 237). Occasionally they form a plaque-like mass that lines the apposing pleural surfaces and encases the lung. Secondary tumors of the pleura are often attended by a hemorrhagic pleural effusion in which neoplastic cells are demonstrable in a high percentage of cases.

Primary growths of the pleura are, in comparison, infrequent. Histologically the normal pleura is composed of connective tissue and elastic fibers covered with a single layer of mesothelial cells. Within the connective tissue are blood capillaries, lymphatic channels, macrophages, lymphocytes, and nerves. Theoretically, therefore, each of these structures should be capable of giving rise to a benign and a malignant tumor. Actually the

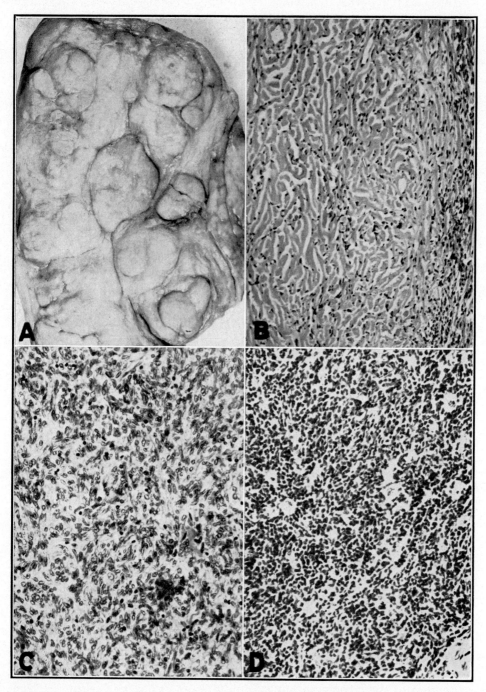

Fig. 238.—Fibroma of the pleura showing A, a solid mass of gray tissue in whorl formation, and B, C, and D, the variable histologic appearance. × 100, × 200, and × 200 respectively.

growths more commonly encountered are mesothelioma, fibroma, neuro-fibroma, hemangioma, lymphangioma, and lymphoblastoma. Of these, mesothelioma and fibroma are the most important. *Mesothelioma*, also called endothelioma, is a tumor composed of the lining cells of the pleura. It may be benign or malignant. Benign growths are usually solitary and circumscribed, while malignant growths consist of numerous small nodules or plaque-like masses that creep along the pleural surfaces. Histologically the neoplasms are quite variable. They consist of cuboidal, columnar, or polygonal cells arranged in glands or cords and supported by dense fibrous tissue. The cytoplasm is moderate in amount and the nuclei are round or oval, deeply stained, and rather uniform. *Fibroma* of the pleura consists of a well-encapsulated, solid mass of dense, gray tissue in whorl formation that resembles a fibromyoma of the uterus (Fig. 238*A*). It is slow growing and often attains a size sufficient to fill an entire hemithorax. Histologically it is quite variable (Fig. 238*B*, *C*, and *D*). Usually it is composed of dense sclerotic fibrous tissue but not infrequently it consists of spindle cells with ill-defined borders, scanty cytoplasm, and oval or elongated nuclei. The latter resemble a sarcoma and, for this reason, the tumor has also been called *giant sarcoma* of the pleura. Despite this appearance, however, the growths remain encapsulated.

Regardless of the type of growth, the *clinical manifestations* in tumors of the pleura are due to pressure upon nerves and collapse of the lung from tumor and/or accumulation of pleural fluid. They consist of pain, dyspnea, orthopnea, and later cachexia. The *diagnosis* is made from the history, roentgen appearance, pleural aspiration, and thoracotomy. *Treatment* in primary growths is surgical excision while in secondary tumors it consists only of palliation. The *prognosis* in primary malignant growths and secondary tumors is poor while that in other growths is good.

Tumors of the Superior Thoracic Inlet. —Tumors located at the base of the neck and superior inlet of the thorax may *originate* (1) as a result of metastasis, especially from the lung, (2) as an extension from an adjacent structure such as the thyroid gland, or (3) locally from a bronchial rest (Herbut and Watson). Histologically, thus, they are quite variable. Regardless of their origin, the neoplasms soon surround and infiltrate the innominate, subclavian, and axillary vessels, the brachial plexus, the vagus nerve, the cervical sympathetic plexus, the vertebral bodies, and the spinal cord (Fig. 239). Accordingly, they produce a chain of *symptoms* and *signs* that is referred to as the *Pancoast syndrome*. In decreasing order of frequency the manifestations consist of (1) presence of a tumor mass and destruction of ribs and vertebræ roentgenographically, (2) Horner's syndrome (enophthalmus, ptosis of the upper eyelid, constriction of the pupil, narrowing of the palpebral fissure, and deficiency of sweating of the face), (3) pain in the shoulder and down the arm, (4) loss of power in the arm and hand, (5) palpable supraclavicular mass, (6) atrophy of the muscles of the arm, (7) cough, (8) dyspnea, (9) hoarseness, (10) edema of the arm, (11) laryngeal paralysis, and (12) hemoptysis. Because of the infiltrative nature of the growth and the structures involved, *treatment* is unsatisfactory and the *prognosis* is poor.

Tumors of the Mediastinum. —Some tumors of the mediastinum are of congenital origin while others are acquired. They occur at all ages but are generally discovered early in adulthood and have no predilection for either sex or any race. *Pathologically* they are as varied as the tissues that compose the mediastinum. They may be classified as follows: (1) from the thymus —

thymoma (p. 984), (2) from connective tissue—fibroma and fibrosarcoma, (3) from vessels—angioma (p. 393), (4) from muscle—myoblastoma, leiomyoma, and rhabdomyosarcoma, (5) from fat—lipoma and liposarcoma, (6) from nerves—neurogenic tumors, (7) from reticulum cells— lymphoblastoma (p. 984), (8) from bony tissue of the thoracic cage—chondroma, osteochondroma, and chondrosarcoma, (9) from congenitally misplaced tissues—cystic masses, (10) from thyroid—adenoma, adeno-

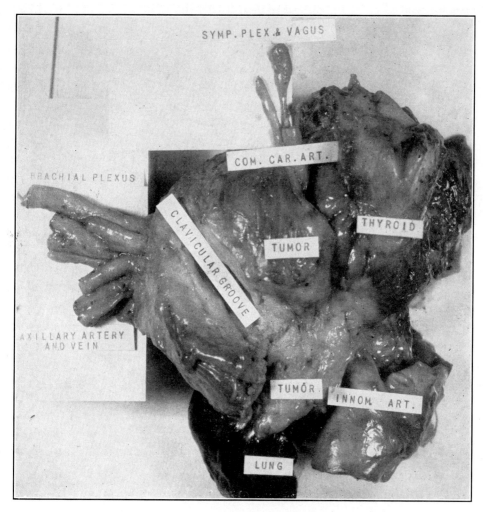

Fig. 239.—Tumor of the superior thoracic inlet producing the Pancoast syndrome.

matous hyperplasia, and carcinoma, (11) from parathyroid glands— adenoma, hyperplasia, and carcinoma, and (12) from distant areas—metastatic tumors. All of the tumors are, of course, space-taking and when they become large enough or when they are strategically located they produce *pressure* upon the following structures: trachea, bronchi, lungs, esophagus, nerves, spinal cord, bones, heart, and vessels. Accordingly they may produce any combination of the following *clinical manifestations*: dyspnea, orthopnea, cough, expectoration, fever, cyanosis, dysphagia, edema, effusion, hoarseness, Horner's syndrome, pain, and erosion. The *diagnosis* is made from the clinical manifestations, the roentgen appearance, and the pathologic examination after removal. *Treatment*, except for lymphoblastoma and metastatic growths, is surgical excision. The *prognosis* is variable. Generally speaking, it is good in connection with benign neoplasms but poor in connection with malignant tumors.

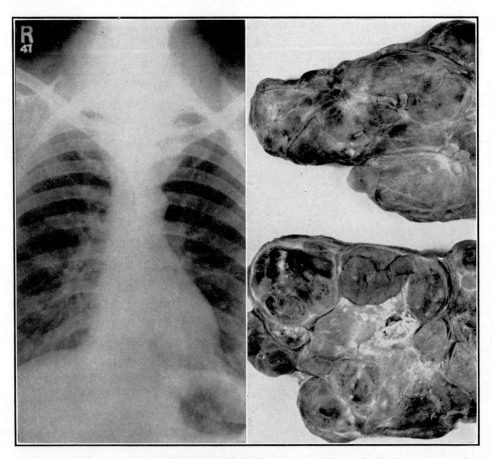

Fig. 240.—Mediastinal thyroid showing, to the left, a symmetrical opacity in the upper portion of the mediastinum and, to the right, a well-encapsulated, lobulated mass of thyroid tissue.

Some of the growths listed above are extremely rare, are identical with similar tumors located elsewhere, and need no further comment; others (as indicated) are discussed elsewhere, and only a few of the more common lesions merit a few additional remarks.

Mediastinal Thyroid.—The most common tumor of the mediastinum is an enlargement of the thyroid. The mass originates from either lobe or from the isthmus and descends inferiorly. It (1) occupies the superior portion of the mediastinum, (2) is usually located anterior to the trachea but occasionally may be situated laterally or even posteriorly, (3) moves vertically on deglutition, and (4) is identical with lesions of the thyroid that are confined to the neck (Fig. 240). Most of the disorders are adenomatous hyperplasias while only a few (less than 4 per cent) are carcinomas.

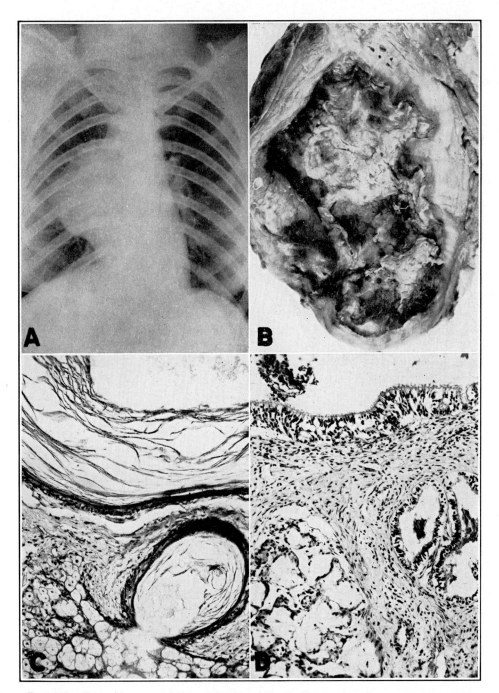

Fig. 241.—Teratoid tumor of the mediastinum illustrating *A*, an opaque tumor protruding into the right lung, *B*, a cystic mass containing hair and sebum, *C*, cyst wall lined with keratinizing squamous epithelium and containing sebaceous glands. × 100, and *D*, another portion of the cyst lined with respiratory epithelium and containing glands lined with columnar epithelium. × 100.

Cystic Tumors. —Cystic tumors of the mediastinum are next in frequency. They consist of (1) pericardial celomic cysts (p. 343), (2) bronchial cysts (p. 457), (3) gastroenteric cysts, and (4) teratoid tumors.

Gastroenteric cysts arise as a result of pinching off and segregation of portions of the foregut. They are usually discovered in the first decade of life, are located in the posterior portion of the mediastinum along the course of the esophagus, may measure 10 to 15 cm. in diameter, and are composed of a smooth muscle wall lined with esophageal, gastric, or enteric mucosa.

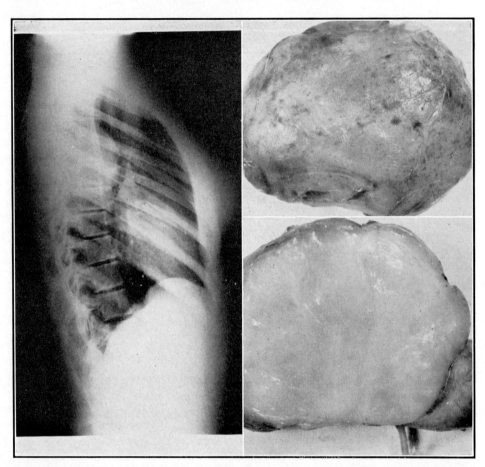

FIG. 242.—Ganglioneuroma showing, to the left, an opacity near the vertebral bodies and, to the right, the external surface (above) and cut surface (below) of the tumor. A nerve is seen entering the lower portion of the lower segment.

Teratoid tumors encompass what were formerly known as epidermoid cysts, dermoid cysts, and teratomas. A teratoid tumor is a potentially or already actually malignant growth composed of tissues derived from ectoderm, entoderm, and mesoderm. The simpler tumors are *cysts* that are filled with keratin, sebum, and hair and that occasionally contain teeth and fragments of bone (Fig. 241). Histologically, they are composed principally of a lining of stratified squamous epithelium beneath which are hair shafts and follicles, sebaceous glands, and sweat glands. The more complex tumors tend to be *solid* and contain, in addition, both entodermal and mesodermal elements (thyroid gland, respiratory epithelium, cartilage, bone, muscle, intestinal mucosa, brain, etc.). A *malignant transformation* (usually a carcinoma) may occur in either the cystic or the solid growths although it is more common in the latter. Anatomically, as far as the mediastinum is concerned, teratoid tumors are generally *located* in the superior portion just beneath the sternum. They may, however, be situated more inferiorly and they may also protrude laterally to involve the lung itself. Their *origin* is not agreed upon. They have been considered to represent (1) inclusions of the skin, thymus, thyroid gland, trachea, and bronchi, and (2) remains of a parasitic fetus.

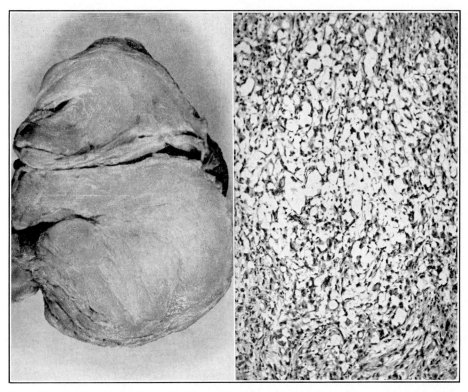

Fig. 243.—Fatty tumor of the mediastinum illustrating, to the left, a well-encapsulated lipoma and, to the right, a liposarcoma of neoplastic lipocytes and lipoblasts. × 100.

Neurogenic Tumors.—Because the mediastinum contains both nerves and nerve ganglia, all types of tumors that are found in the peripheral nervous system may be encountered in this area (Chapter 7, p. 251). Of these, neurofibroma (including neurilemmoma and schwannoma) and neurofibrosarcoma may be located anywhere while ganglioneuroma, neuroblastoma, pheochromocytoma, and pheochromoblastoma are usually seen posteriorly along the vertebræ (that is, along distribution of the sympathetic ganglia). Regardless of the histologic composition (Chapter 29, p. 1013), the growths are usually rounded, well encapsulated, firm, solid, and measure up 15 or 20 cm. in diameter (Fig. 242). Tumors that are located near the vertebræ have a tendency to creep into the spinal canal along the nerve routes and thus produce dumbbell-shaped masses.

Lipomas and Liposarcomas. —Fat tumors of the mediastinum are uncommon. Of the two varieties, lipomas are more frequent than liposarcomas. They may occur in any portion of the mediastinum and may be entirely intramediastinal or may involve also the cervical region, the thoracic wall, or even the subcutaneous tissues. Grossly they are usually well encapsulated, yellowish, and measure as much as 25 cm. in diameter (Fig. 243). Histologically they are composed of mature (in cases of lipoma) and immature (in cases of liposarcoma) fat cells.

REFERENCES

PATHOLOGIC PHYSIOLOGY

AUSTRIAN, R., et al.: Am. J. Med., 11, 667, 1951 (Impairment of Alveolo-Capillary Diffusion).
BALDWIN, E. DE F., et al.: Medicine, 27, 243, 1948 (Pulmonary Insufficiency).
————: Medicine, 28, 1 and 201, 1949 (Pulmonary Insufficiency).
COMROE, J. H., JR: Pulmonary Function in Methods of Medical Research, Chicago, Yearook Publishers, Inc., Vol. 2, 1950.
————: Am. J. Med., 10, 356, 1951 (Pulmonary Function Tests).
DARLING, R., et al.: J. Clin. Invest., 19, 609, 1940 (Intrapulmonary Mixing of Gases).
RICHARDS, D. W.: Pulmonary Fuction in Health and Disease in Cecil and Loeb's Textbook of Medicine, Philadelphia, W. B. Saunders Co., 1951.

CONGENITAL ANOMALIES

ALLBRITTEN, F. R., JR., and TEMPLETON, J.Y., III: J. Thoracic Surg., 20, 749, 1950 (Giant Cysts of the Lung).
BERGSTROM, W. H., et al.: Pediatrics, 6, 573, 1950 (Kartagenar's Triad).
COLE, F. H., et al.: Surg., Gynec. & Obst., 93, 589, 1951 (Aberrant Pulmonary Vessels).
CONWAY, D. J.: A. M. A. Arch. Dis. Child., 26, 504, 1951 (Lung Cysts).
COOKE, F. N., and BLADES, B.: J. Thoracic Surg., 23, 546, 1952 (Cystic Disease of Lungs).
COTTON, B. H., et al.: J. Thoracic Surg., 23, 508, 1952 (Accessory Lung).
DRYMALSKI, G. W., et al.: Am. J. Roentgenol., 60, 403, 1948 (Tracheal Diverticula).
EVANS, W. A., JR.: Am. J. Roentgenol., 62, 167, 1949 (Obstructions Respiratory Tract).
FINDLAY, C. W., JR., and MAIER, H. C.: Surgery, 29, 604, 1951 (Anomalies Pulmonary Vessels).
GANS, S. L., and POTTS, W. J.: J. Thoracic Surg., 21, 313, 1951 (Esophageal Pulmonary Lobe).
GROSS, R. E., and LEWIS, J. E., JR.: Surg., Gynec. & Obst., 80, 549, 1945 (Defect Anterior Mediastinum).
HEALEY, J. E., JR.: J. Thoracic Surg., 23, 433, 1952 (Anomalies Pulmonary Veins).
HEALEY, R. J.: Radiology, 57, 200, 1951 (Bronchogenic Cysts).
HELLER, E. L., et al.: Am. J. Clin. Path., 23, 121, 1953 (Bronchogenic Cysts).
HYDE, L., et al.: Dis. Chest., 19, 190, 1951 (Honey-comb Lungs).
MacMAHON, H. E.: Pediatrics, 2, 43, 1948 (Congenital Alveolar Dysplasia).
MANHOFF, L. J., JR., and HOWE, J. S.: A. M. A. Arch. Path., 48, 155, 1949 (Absence Pulmonary Artery).
MORTON, D. R., et al.: J. Thoracic Surg., 20, 665, 1950 (Lobar Agenesis).
RUBIN, S., and STRATEMEIER, E. H.: Radiology, 58, 552, 1952 (Intrathoracic Meningocele).
TUYNMAN, P. E., and GARDNER, L. W.: A. M. A. Arch. Path., 54, 306, 1952 (Bilateral Pulmonary Aplasia).
WALLACE, J. E.: A. M. A. Arch. Path., 39, 47, 1945 (Bronchial Web).
WYMAN, S. M., and EYLER, W. R.: Radiology, 59, 658, 1952 (Intralobar Sequestration).

DEGENERATIONS

BROWNING, J. R., and HOUGHTON, J. D.: Am. J. Med., 20, 374, 1956 (Idiopathic Hemosiderosis).
CLERF, L. H.: Ann. Otol., Rhin. & Laryngol., 53, 839, 1944 (Tracheopathia Osteoplastica).
DOUB, H. B.: Radiology, 51, 480, 1948 (Pulmonary Calcification).
FORBES, J. J., et al.: Bull. 478, U. S. Dept. Interior, 1950 (Review of Literature on Dust).
FRIEDMAN, P. S., et al.: J. A. M. A., 148, 1418, 1952 (Talc Pneumoconiosis).

HAMLIN, L. E.: J. A. M. A., *139*, 909, 1949 (Pneumoconiosis).
HEATON, T. G.: Canad. M. A. J., *62*, 252, 1950 (Pulmonary Calcification).
HELWIG, E. B.: Military Surgeon, *109*, 540, 1951 (Berylliosis of the Skin).
HEPPLESTON, A. G.: Arch. Indust. Hyg. & Occup. Med., *4*, 270, 1951 (Coal Worker's Pneumoconiosis).
HOFFMAN, I. L., and BELL, H. S.: U. S. Armed Forces M. J., *3*, 689, 1952 (Lipid Pneumonia).
JAFFÉ, F. A.: Am. J. Path., *27*, 909, 1951 (Graphite Pneumoconiosis).
KOVEN, A. L.: Am. Rev. Tuberc., *58*, 55, 1948 (Bagassosis).
LENDRUM, A. C.: J. Path. & Bact., *62*, 555, 1950 (Cardiac Pulmonary Hemosiderosis).
MORGAN, H. G.: Edinburgh M. J., *59*, 261, 1952 (Endogenous Lipid Pneumonia).
SCHAAR, F. E., and RIGLER, L. G.: J. Lancet, *76*, 126, 1956 (Idiopathic Hemosiderosis).
SILVERMAN, F. N.: Am. J. Roentgenol., *64*, 747, 1950 (Pulmonary Calcification).
SOERGEL, K. H.: Pediatrics, *19*, 1101, 1957 (Idiopathic Hemosiderosis).
STOLL, R., *et al.*: A. M. A. Arch. Int. Med., *88*, 831, 1951 (Asbestosis and Carcinoma).
THEODOS, P. A., and GORDON, B.: Am. Rev. Tuberc., *65*, 24, 1952 (Tuberculosis in Anthracosilicosis).
VOLK, W., *et al.*: Am. J. Med., *10*, 316, 1951 (Lipid Pneumonia).
WYATT, J. P.: McManus' *Progress in Fundamental Medicine*, Philadelphia, Lea & Febiger, 1952, p. 277 (Pneumonoconiosis).
WYLIE, W. G., *et al.*: Quart. J. Med., *17*, 25, 1948 (Pulmonary Hemosiderosis).

INFLAMMATIONS
Tracheobronchitis

CALLAHAN, J. A.: J. A. M. A., *147*, 313, 1951 (Fibrinous Bronchitis).
CARDON, L., *et al.*: Ann. Int. Med., *34*, 559, 1951 (Bronchitis).
PRIOR, J. A.: Ohio State M. J., *48*, 310, 1952 (Chronic Bronchitis).

Bronchiectasis

FIELD, C. E.: Pediatrics, *4*, 21 and 231, 1949 (In Childhood).
HERBUT, P. A., and EVERTS-SUAREZ, E. A.: *Advances in Medicine and Surgery*, Philadelphia, W. B. Saunders Co., p. 254, 1952 (Pathogenesis).
JONES, R. S., and COLE, F. H.: Southern M. J., *45*, 101, 1952.
KONWALER, B. E., and REINGOLD, I. M.: Cancer, *5*, 525, 1952 (Carcinoma in Bronchiectasis).
LORENZ, T. H.: Am. J. M. Sci., *221*, 522, 1951.
OCHSNER, A., *et al.*: Surgery, *25*, 518, 1949.
SOUDERS, C. R.: Dis. Chest., *16*, 381, 1949.

Acute Nonspecific Pneumonia

ANDERSON, T.: Edinburgh M. J., *55*, 705, 1948 (Past and Present).
AULD, D.: A.M.A. Arch. Path., *63*, 113, 1957 (Eosinophilic Granuloma).
BARBER, J. M., and GRANT, A. P.: Brit. M. J., *2*, 752, 1952 (Friedländer's).
BLYSTAD, W., *et al.*: Pediatrics, *8*, 5, 1951 (Aspiration Newborn).
BRUCK, E. L.: Dis. Chest., *14*, 73, 1948 (Complications Pneumococcic).
DE, T. D., and ANDERSON, G. W.:Obst. and Gynec. Rev., *8*, 1, 1953 (Hyaline Membrane Disease).
DUBIN, I. N., and KIRBY, G. P.: A. M. A. Arch. Path., *35*, 808, 1943 (Colon Bacillus).
FETTERMAN, G. H., and MORAN, T. J.: Pennsylvania M. J., *45*, 810, 1942 (Food Aspiration).
FLIPPIN, H. F., *et al.*: J. A. M. A., *147*, 918, 1951 (Antibiotics).
GIBSON, M. O. J., and BELCHER, J. R.: Quart. J. Med., *20*, 43, 1951 (Staphylococcic).
GUNN, F. D., and HUNGESTER, W. J.: A. M. A. Arch. Path., *21*, 813, 1936 (Experimental).
HOLOWACH, J., *et al.*: J. Pediat., *41*, 430, 1952 (Friedländer's).
ISRAEL, H. L., *et al.*: New England J. Med., *238*, 205, 1948 (Lobar Pneumonia).
JACKSON, G. G., *et al.*: Ann. Int. Med., *35*, 1175, 1951 (Terramycin).
MELCHER, G. W., JR., *et al.*: J. A. M. A., *143*, 1303, 1950 (Terramycin).
MORAN, T. J.: A. M. A. Arch. Path., *52*, 350, 1951 (Experimental Food Aspiration).
NICHOLSON, H.: Lancet, *2*, 549, 1950 (Suppurative).
PHILLIPS, E.: J. A. M. A., *133*, 161, 1947 (Traumatic).
REIMANN, H. A.: Ann. Int. Med., *33*, 1246, 1950 (Changing Nature).
ROBERTSON, O. H.: J. A. M. A., *111*, 1432, 1938 (Experimental).
ROBERTSON, O. H., and UHLEY, C. G.: J. Clin. Invest., *15*, 115, 1936 (Macrophages in Lobar Pneumonia).
ROMANSKY, M. J., and KELSER, G. A.: J. A. M. A., *150*, 1447, 1952 (Antibiotics).

TREGILLUS, J.: J. Obst. & Gynaec. Brit. Emp., *58*, 406, 1951 (Aspiration Newborn).
VAN BREEMEN, L. L., *et al.*, Am. J. Path., *33*, 769, 1957 (HyalineMembrane Disease).
WEINSTEIN, L., *et al.*: J. Immunology, *67*, 173, 183, and 189, 1951 (Experimental Streptococcic).
WOLLEMAN, O. J., JR., and FINLAND, M.: Am. J. Path., *19*, 23, 1943 (Staphylococcic).
WOOD, W. B., JR., and IRONS, E. N.: J. Exper. Med., *84*, 365, 1946 (Recovery in Pneumococcic).

Allergic Pneumonia

BULLEN, S. T., SR.: J. Allergy, *23*, 193, 1952 (Clinicopathologic Findings in 176 Cases of Asthma).
DERBES, V. J., *et al.*: Am. J. M. Sci., *222*, 88, 1951 (Complications Asthma).
HERBUT, P. A., and KINSEY, F. R.: A. M. A. Arch. Path., *41*, 489, 1946 (Loeffler's Syndrome in Rabbits).
NEMIR, R. L., *et al.*: J. Pediat., *37*, 819, 1950 (Loeffler's Syndrome).
REEDER, W. H., and GOODRICH, B. E.: Ann. Int. Med., *36*, 1217, 1952 (Loeffler's Syndrome).
UNGER, L., and UNGER, A. H.: J. A. M. A., *150*, 562, 1952 (Treatment Asthma).

Tularemia

CORWIN, W. C., and STUBBS, S. B.: J. A. M. A., *149*, 343, 1952.
PULLEN, R. L., and STUART, B. M.: New Orleans M. & Surg. J., *98*, 126, 1945.
STUART, B. M., and PULLEN, R. L.: Am. J. M. Sci., *210*, 223, 1945 (Pneumonia).

Tuberculosis

AMBERSON, J. B., *et al.*: Am. J. Med., *9*, 571, 1950 (Excellent Symposium).
AUERBACH, O.: Am. Rev. Tuberc., *59*, 601, 1949 (Tuberculous Empyema).
CULVER, T. J., *et al.*: J. Thoracic Surg., *20*, 798, 1950 (Tuberculoma).
Diagnostic Standards and Classification of Tuberculosis, 1940 Ed., National Tuberculosis Assoc., New York, 1940.
HARRIS, W. C., and TRENCHARD, H. J.: Tubercle, *33*, 273, 1952 (Congenital).
HILTZ, J. E., *et al.*: Dis. Chest., *20*, 313, 1951 (Tuberculous Tracheobronchitis).
KATZ, J.: Am. Rev. Tuberc., *66*, 651, 1952 (Survival Tuberculous Patients).
LAFF, H. I., *et al.*: J. A. M. A., *146*, 778, 1951 (Bronchial Involvement in Primary).
MACMILLAN, H. A.: A. M. A. Arch. Path., *48*, 377, 1949 (Apical Scars).
MENDENHALL, E., and SHAW, R. R.: J. A. M. A., *148*, 595, 1952 (Treatment).
MIKOL, E. X., *et al.*: Am. Rev. Tuberc., *66*, 16, 1952 (Among Hospital Employees).
MINOR, G. R.: Am. Rev. Tuberc., *48*, 109, 1943 (Hemoptysis).
PUGH, D. L., *et al.*: Tubercle, *33*, 184, 1952 (Tuberculoma).
RICH, A. R.: *Pathogenesis of Tuberculosis*, 2nd Ed., Springfield, Charles C Thomas, 1951.
TSAI, P. I., and BASHE, W. J., JR.: Quart. Bull. Seaview Hospital, *11*, 129, 1950 (Complications Primary).
VEENEKLAAS, G. M. H.: Am. J. Dis. Child., *83*, 271, 1952 (Primary).
WOODRUFF, C. E., and NAHAS, H. C.: Am. Rev. Tuberc., *64*, 620, 1951 (Carcinoma).

Boeck's Sarcoid

JAQUES, W. E.: A. M. A. Arch. Path., *53*, 558, 1952.
LONGCOPE, W. T., and FREIMAN, D. G.: Medicine, *31*, 1, 1952.
RICKER, W., and CLARK, M.: Am. J. Clin. Path., *19*, 725, 1949.

Syphilis

MORGAN, A. D., *et al.*: Thorax, *7*, 1, 1952 (Tertiary Pulmonary).
ROYCE, B. F.: Ann. Int. Med., *33*, 700, 1950 (Pulmonary).
SEGAL, A. J.: A. M. A. Arch. Path., *30*, 911, 1940 (Syphilitic Pulmonary Arteritis).

Plague

HAMPTON, B. C.: Pub. Health Reports, *55*, 1143, 1940.
MEYER, K. F.: Medical Clin. North America, *27*, 745, 1943.

Pertussis

GORDON, J. E., and HOOD, R. I.: Am. J. M. Sci., *222*, 333, 1951.
LaBOCCETTA, A. C., and DAWSON, K. E.: Am. J. Dis. Child., *34*, 184, 1952.

Lees, A. W.: Brit. M. J., *2*, 1138, 1950.
Smith, L. W.: A. M. A. Arch. Path., *4*, 732, 1927.

Interstitial Pulmonary Fibrosis

Anderson, W. A. D.: Dis. Chest., *15*, 337, 1949.
Cox, T. R., and Kohl, J. M.: Am. J. Clin. Path., *22*, 770, 1952.
Rubin, E. H., *et al.:* Ann. Int. Med., *36*, 827, 1952.

Rickettsial Pneumonia

Allen, A. C., and Spitz, S.: Am. J. Path., *21*, 603, 1945.

Viral Pneumonia

Billings, F. T., Jr.: Am. Pract. & Digest of Treatment, *2*, 833, 1951 (Nonbacterial Pneumonias).
Burney, L. E.: J.A.M.A., *164*, 2029, 1957 (Influenza).
Corbett, E. U.: Am. J. Path., *21*, 905, 1945 (Visceral Lesions in Measles).
Finkel, S., and Sullivan, E. H., Jr.: Dis. Chest, *21*, 55, 1952 (Primary Atypical Pneumonia).
Frank, L.: A. M. A. Arch. Path., *50*, 450, 1950 (Varicella Pneumonitis).
Gallagher, H. S.: Am. J. Clin. Path., *22*, 1147, 1952 (Cytomegalic Inclusion Disease of Infancy).
Influenza A Epidemic of 1943: Am. J. Hyg., *48*, 253, 1948.
James, D. G.: J. A. M. A., *151*, 810, 1953 (Primary Atypical Pneumonia).
Lillie, R. D.: A. M. A. Arch. Path., *10*, 241, 1930 (Smallpox and Vaccinia).
Parker, F., Jr., *et al.:* Am. J. Path., *22*, 797, 1946 (Viral Pneumonia).
————: Arch. Path., *44*, 581, 1947 (Primary Atypical Pneumonia).
Pinkerton, H., *et al.:* Am. J. Path., *21*, 1, 1945 (Giant Cell Pneumonia).
Reimann, H. A.: Medicine, *26*, 167, 1947 (Viral Pneumonias).
Thalmann, W. G., *et al.:* J. A. M. A., *144*, 1156, 1950 (Influenzal Pneumonia).
Weinstein, L., and Franklin, W.: Am. J. M. Sci., *217*, 314, 1949 (Pneumonia of Measles).
Wolins, W.: Am. J. M. Sci., *216*, 551, 1948 (Ornithosis).
Wolman, M., *et al.:* Am. J. Dis. Child., *83*, 573, 1952 (Interstitial Giant Cell Pneumonia).

Fungous and Yeast-like Pneumonias

Abbott, J. D., *et al.:* Brit. M. J., *1*, 523, 1952 (Aspergillosis).
Bass, H. E.: J. A. M. A., *143*, 1041, 1950 (Coccidioidomycosis and Histoplasmosis).
Berk, M., and Gerstl, B.: J. A. M. A., *149*, 1310, 1952 (Cryptococcosis).
Bernstein, I. L., *et al.:* Ann. Int. Med., *36*, 852, 1952 (Nocardiosis).
Bonoff, C. P.: Radiology, *54*, 157, 1950 (Blastomycosis).
Cohen, J. R., and Kaufmann, W.: Am. J. Clin. Path., *22*, 1069, 1952 (Cryptococcosis).
Conant, N. F.: Am. Rev. Tuberc., *61*, 690, 1950 (Diagnosis Pulmonary Mycoses).
Forbus, W. D., and Bestebreurtje, A. M.: Military Surgeon, *99*, 653, 1946 (Coccidioidomycosis).
Garrod, L. P.: Tubercle, *33*, 258, 1952 (Actinomycosis).
Good, C. A.: Texas State J. Med., *47*, 817, 1951 (Roentgenology in Fungous Diseases).
Hager, H. F., *et al.:* New England J. Med., *241*, 226, 1949 (Nocardiosis).
Hobby, A. W.: Dis. Chest, *15*, 174, 1949 (Pulmonary Mycoses).
Hodgson, C. H., *et al.:* J. A. M. A., *145*, 807, 1951 (Histoplasmosis).
Kligman, A. M.: *Advances in Medicine and Surgery*, Philadelphia, W. B. Saunders Co., p. 260, 1952 (Pulmonary Fungous Infections).
Littman, M. L., *et al.:* J. A. M. A., *148*, 608, 1952 (Actinomycosis).
Oblath, R. W., *et al.:* Ann. Int. Med., *35*, 97, 1951 (Moniliasis).
Poppe, J. K.: J. Thoracic Surg., *15*, 118, 1946 (Actinomycosis).
Ratcliffe, H. E., and Cook, W. R.: U. S. Armed Forces M. J., *1*, 957, 1950 (Cryptococcosis).
Reid, J. D., Scharer, J. H., Herbut, P. A., and Irving, H.: J. Lab. & Clin. Med., *27*, 419, 1942 (Histoplasmosis).
Robinson, S. S., and Tasker, S.: Ann. West. M. & Surg., *2*, 1, 1948 (Actinomycosis).
Schwartz, J., and Baum, E. L.: Am. J. Clin. Path., *21*, 999, 1951 (Blastomycosis).
Schwartz, J., and Muth, J.: Am. J. M. Sci., *221*, 89, 1951 (Coccidioidomycosis).
Starrs, R. A., and Klotz, M. O.: Arch. Int. Med., *82*, 1, 1948 (Blastomycosis).
Wolff, F. W.: Lancet, *1*, 1236, 1952 (Moniliasis).

Parasitic Infections

CRAIG, C. F., and FAUST, E. C.: *Clinical Parasitology*, 5th Ed., Philadelphia, Lea & Febiger, 1951.
FRENKEL, J. K., and FRIEDLANDER, S.: *Toxoplasmosis*, Federal Security Agency, Pub. Health Service, 1951.
SAWITZ, W. G.: *Medical Parasitology*, New York, The Blakiston Co., 1950.
SULKIN, S. E., and LEVIN, P. M.: Texas State J. Med., *46*, 834, 1950 (Toxoplasmosis).

Pulmonary Abscess

BROCK, R. C.: Guy's Hospital Reports, *96*, 97, 125, and 141, 1947.
DRAKE, E. H., *et al.*: Ann. Int. Med., *35*, 1218, 1951.
JEWETT, J. S., and DIMOND, G. E.: Dis. Chest, *18*, 478, 1950.
LEVINE, L., *et al.*: Dis. Chest, *14*, 218, 1948.
SAMPSON, P. C.: Dis. Chest, *14*, 78, 1948.
TOUROFF, A. S. W., *et al.*: J. Thoracic Surg., *20*, 266, 1950.
WEISEL, W., *et al.*: Am. Rev. Tuberc., *61*, 474, 1950.

Pleurisy

SMITH, E. B.: A. M. A. Arch. Path., *35*, 553, 1943 (Fibrous Pleural Adhesions).

Empyema

BROWN, B., *et al.*: Ann. Int. Med., *24*, 343, 1946.
FRAZIER, C. A., and DAVIS, E.: J. A. M. A., *146*, 247, 1951.
GORDON, B., *et al.*: Am. Rev. Tuberc., *47*, 35, 1943 (Tuberculous).
SELLORS, T. H., and CRUICKSHANK, G.: Brit. J. Surg., *38*, 411, 1951 (Chronic).
SHANK, P. J.: Am. J. Surg., *66*, 224, 1944.

Mediastinitis

ADAMS, R.: J. Thoracic Surg., *15*, 336, 1946.
KORKIS, F. B.: Lancet, *1*, 4, 1952.
NEUHOF, H., and RABIN, C. B.: Am. J. Roentgenol., *44*, 684, 1940.

PHYSICAL DISTURBANCES

BAXTER, M. D., and SHACKELFORD, R. T.: Arch. Surg., *65*, 856, 1952 (Pulmonary Hernia).
BERGMANN, M., and GRAHAM, E. A.: J. Thoracic Surg., *22*, 549, 1951 (Irradiation Pneumonitis).
CAMERON, D. A., *et al.*: Am. J. Surg., *79*, 361, 1950 (Thoracic Trauma).
CHAVES, A. D.: Am. Rev. Tuberc., *63*, 194, 1951 (Hemoptysis).
CLERF, L. H.: Surg., Gynec. & Obst., *70*, 328, 1940 (Tracheobronchial Foreign Bodies).
CRENSHAW, G. L., and ROWLES, D. F.: J. Thoracic Surg., *24*, 398, 1952, (Pulmonary Emphysema).
DRIPPS, R. D., and DEMING, M. V. N.: Ann. Surg., *124*, 94, 1946 (Atelectasis and Pneumonia).
DUGAN, D. J., and SAMPSON, P. C.: J. Thoracic Surg., *20*, 729, 1950 (Giant Pulmonary Blebs).
EVANS, J. A., and SMALLDON, T. R.: Am. J. Roentgenol., *64*, 375, 1950 (Mediastinal Emphysema).
GANS, B.: A. M. A. Arch. Dis. Child., *27*, 254, 1952 (Atelectasis in Children).
GUY, C. C., and OLECK, H. T.: A. M. A. Arch. Surg., *55*, 316, 1947 (Bronchobiliary Fistula).
HAMPTON, A. O., and CASTLEMAN, B.: Am. J. Roentgenol., *43*, 305, 1940 (Pulmonary Infarction).
HARTROFT, W. S.: Am. J. Path., *21*, 889, 1945 (Pulmonary Emphysema Histologically).
HENRY, G. A.: Canad. M. A. J., *64*, 134, 1951 (Rupture Trachea).
KINSELLA, T. J., and JOHNSRUD, L. W.: J. Thoracic Surg., *16*, 571, 1947 (Rupture Bronchus).
LANGSTON, H. T., and TUTTLE, W. M.: J. Thoracic Surg., *16*, 99, 1947 (Hemothorax).
LAWS, J. W.: Gastroenterology, *21*, 351, 1952 (Gastropleural Fistula).
LUISADA, A. A., and CARDI, L.: Circulation, *13*, 113, 1956 (Acute Pulmonary Edema).
LONGMIRE, W. P., JR.: A. M. A. Arch. Surg., *55*, 330, 1947 (Tracheo-esophageal Fistula).

MILLER, R., and BERRY, J. B.: Am. J. M. Sci., *222*, 197, 1951 (Pulmonary Infarction).
MITCHELL, R. S.: Am. Rev. Tuberc., *64*, 127, 1951 (Artificial Pneumothorax).
OGILVIE, A. G.: Thorax, *5*, 116, 1950 (Hemothorax).
ORANGE, R.: Canad. M. A. J., *59*, 531, 1948 (Pulmonary Atelectasis).
PARKER, E. F.: Dis. Chest., *21*, 677, 1952 (Hemoptysis).
REINHART, H. A., and HERMEL, M. B.: Radiology, *57*, 204, 1951 (Cervical Pulmonary Hernia).
ROBERTSON, R., and JAMES, E. S.: Pediatrics, *8*, 795, 1951 (Lobar Emphysema).
ROTTENBERG, L. A., and GOLDEN, R.: Radiology, *53*, 157, 1949 (Spontaneous Pneumothorax).
SAHN, S. H., *et al.*: New England J. Med., *246*, 927, 1952 (Pleural Effusion).
SCHMIDT, H. W., *et al.*: J. Thoracic Surg., *19*, 226, 1950 (Broncholithiasis).
SEALY, W. C.: A. M. A. Arch. Surg., *59*, 882, 1949 (Pulmonary Contusions).
SHAW, R. R.: J. Thoracic Surg., *22*, 149, 1951 (Bronchial Mucoid Impaction).
SOMMER, N. J., JR., and McCOLLOCH, C. S.: Am. J. Surg., *77*, 314, 1949 (Thoracic Foreign Bodies).
SOSMAN, M. C., *et al.*: Am. J. Roentg., *77*, 947, 1957 (Microlithiasis).
STEMMERMANN, G. N., *et al.*: J. Thoracic Surg., *22*, 392, 1951 (Bronchopleural Fistulas).
TOWBIN, M. N.: Ann. Int. Med., *35*, 555, 1951 (Mediastinal Emphysema).
VALLE, A. R., and WATKINS, D. R.: Military Surgeon, *111*, 422, 1952 (Thoracic Wounds).
ZUSCHLAG, E.: Am. J. Dis. Child., *74*, 399, 1947 (Pulmonary Infarction in Children).

TUMORS

ARIEL, I. M., *et al.*: Cancer, *3*, 229, 1950 (Pulmonary Carcinoma).
BLACKLOCK, J. W. S.: Br. J. Cancer, *11*, 181, 1957 (Condensate Cigarette Smoke and Cancer in Rats).
BLADES, B.: Ann. Surg., *123*, 749, 1946 (Mediastinal Tumors).
BRADFORD, M. L., *et al.*: Surg., Gynec. & Obst., *85*, 467, 1947 (Mediastinal Tumors).
BREWER III, L. A., and DOLLEY, F. S.: Am. Rev. Tuberc., *60*, 419, 1949 (Mediastinal Tumors).
BUCHBERG, A., *et al.*: Dis. Chest., *20*, 257, 1951 (Carcinoma of the Lung).
CAYLEY, C. K., *et al.*: Am. J. Dis. Child., *82*, 49, 1951 (Bronchogenic Carcinoma in Children.)
CLERF, L. H., and BUCHER, C. J.: Ann. Otol., Rhin. & Laryngol., *51*, 836, 1942 (Bronchial Adenoma).
CLERF, L. H., and HERBUT, P. A.: J. A. M. A., *150*, 793, 1952 (Diagnosis Pulmonary Carcinoma).
CLERF, L. H., HERBUT, P. A., and NEALON, T. F., JR.: Ann. Otol., Rhin. & Laryngol., *60*, 840, 1951 (Cytologic Diagnosis Carcinoma of the Lung).
CURRERI, A. R., and GALE, J. W.: A. M. A. Arch. Surg., *58*, 797, 1949 (Mediastinal Tumors).
DICK, D.: Edinburgh M. J., *57*, 265, 1950 (Bronchial Adenoma).
DOLL, R.: Advances in Cancer Research, *3*, 1, 1955 (Etiology Lung Cancer).
EHRENHAFT, J. L., and WOMACK, N. A.: Ann. Surg., *136*, 90, 1952 (Bronchial Adenoma).
GIBBON, J. H., JR., *et al.*: J. Thoracic Surg., *17*, 419, 1948 (Carcinoma of Lung).
GODWIN, J. T., *et al.*: J. Thoracic Surg., *20*, 169, 1950 (Intrathoracic Neurogenic Tumors).
GRAHAM, E. A., *et al.*: Cancer Res., *17*, 1058, 1957 (Cigarette Tar and Cancer in Rabbits).
GREGORIUS, F.: Arch. Indust. Hyg. & Occup. Med., *5*, 196, 1952 (Bronchogenic Carcinoma in Chromate Industry).
HERBUT, P. A.: Am. J. Path., *20*, 911, 1944 (Alveolar Cell Tumor).
————: A. M. A. Arch. Path., *41*, 175, 1946 (Metastatic Carcinoma).
HERBUT, P. A., and RAKOFF, A. E.: *Cytologic Diagnosis of Cancer*, Monographs on Surgery, New York, Thomas Nelson & Sons, p. 177, 1951.
HERBUT, P. A., and WATSON, J. S.: A. M. A. Arch. Path., *42*, 88, 1946 (Tumors Thoracic Inlet).
HOCHBERG, L. A.: Am. Rev. Tuberc., *63*, 150, 1951 (Mesothelioma).
HOLLEY, S. W.: Military Surgeon, *99*, 528, 1946 (Bronchial Adenoma).
HUEPER, W. C.: Indust. Med. & Surg., *20*, 49, 1951 (Environmental Lung Cancer).
HUEPER, W. C.: Dis. Chest, *30*, 141, 1956 (Environmental Causes Lung Cancer).
HUTCHISON, H. E.: Cancer, *5*, 884, 1952 (Alveolar Cell Tumor).
MASON, G. A.: Lancet, *2*, 587, 1949 (Carcinoma of the Lung).
McBURNEY, R. P., *et al.*: J. Thoracic Surg., *24*, 411, 1952 (Bronchial Adenoma).
McNAMARA, W. L., *et al.*: A. M. A. Arch. Surg., *55*, 632, 1947 (Pleural Giant Sarcoma).
OCHSNER, A., *et al.*: J. A. M. A., *148*, 691, 1952 (Bronchogenic Carcinoma of the Lung).
OCHSNER, A.: *Smoking and Lung Cancer*, New York, Julian Messner, Inc., 1954.
PANTRIDGE, J. F.: Brit. J. Surg., *37*, 48, 1949 (Carcinoma of the Trachea).

RAMSEY, J. H., and REIMANN, D. L.: Am. J. Path., *29*, 339, 1953 (Bronchial Adenoma).

REID, J. D.: Cancer, *5*, 685, 1952 (Bronchial Adenoma).

REINGOLD, I. M., *et al.*: Am. J. Clin. Path., *20*, 515, 1950 (Necropsies in Bronchogenic Carcinoma).

RIENHOFF, W. F., JR.: Dis. Chest., *17*, 33, 1950 (Carcinoma of the Lung).

RIGDON, R. H.: South. M. J., *50*, 524, 1957 (Smoking and Lung Cancer).

SCHLUMBERGER, H. G.: A. M. A. Arch. Path., *41*, 398, 1946 (Teratoid Tumors Mediastinum).

STOUT, A. P., and HIMADI, G. M.: Ann. Surg., *133*, 50, 1951 (Mesothelioma).

STRONG, F. M., *et al.*: Science, *125*, 1129, 1957 (Smoking and Lung Cancer).

WYNDER, E. L.: Arch. Indust. Hyg. & Occup. Med., *5*, 218, 1952 (Smoking and Cancer of the Lung).

WYNDER, E. L., and WRIGHT, G.: Cancer, *10*, 255 and 431, 1957 (Tobacco Carcinogens).

13

Thyroid Gland

PATHOLOGIC PHYSIOLOGY

Joseph J. Rupp

Normally, the follicle cells of the thyroid gland accumulate iodide and convert it to iodine which, in turn, iodinates a globulin to form *thyroglobulin*. The thyroglobulin is secreted into the follicle where it forms colloid. Colloid is the storage form of the thyroid *hormones*. When the need for thyroid hormones occurs, thyroglobulin is hydrolyzed by a proteolytic enzyme, thereby releasing thyroxine, tri-iodothyronine, mono-iodotyrosine, and di-iodotyrosine. The two mentioned last are coupled by the action of another enzyme to form thyroxine or tri-iodothyronine. Thyroxine results from the coupling of two molecules of di-iodotyrosine while tri-iodothyronine results from the coupling of one molecule of di-iodotyrosine and one molecule of monoiodotyrosine. *Thyroxine* and *tri-iodothyronine* are the circulating thyroid hormones. Normally di-iodotyrosine, monoiodotyrosine, and thyroglobulin are not found in the peripheral circulation. Thyroxine and tri-iodothyronine circulate bound to a protein which is located between alpha 1 and alpha 2 globulin in the electrophoretogram and is referred to as the thyroxine binding protein. Since thyroxine and tri-iodothyronine are precipitated with the proteins, and inorganic iodide is not, the former two are often referred to as the *protein bound iodine* (PBI).

TSH (*thyroid stimulating hormone*) is necessary for the normal function of the thyroid gland. When TSH is absent, the thyroid gland decreases in size and its rate of iodide accumulation, hormone synthesis, and hormone release are depressed. Under such circumstances, the circulating levels of thyroid hormones are insufficient for the maintenance of normal metabolism. For these reasons, hypothyroidism is present in patients with panhypopituitarism. Normally, a reciprocal relationship exists between the pituitary and thyroid glands. Decreased thyroid function results in an increased rate of formation and release of TSH, whereas increased levels of thyroid hormones (as follows ingestion of thyroid extracts) causes a suppression of TSH production. For this reason, exogenous thyroid substances result in atrophy of the thyroid gland and the rate of endogenous hormone production decreases.

An adequate *supply* of *iodide* is necessary for normal thyroid function. When iodide deficiency occurs, the supply of thyroid hormone is maintained by hyperplasia of the thyroid gland. The hyperplasia is a response to increased TSH production and does not occur in the iodide dificient hypophysectomized animal. If iodide deficiency is severe and prolonged, hypothyroidism may develop, but this is an unusual occurrence even in areas where severe iodide deficiency exists. The same kind of hyperplasia which results from iodide deficiency follows the ingestion of agents which interfere with thyroidal iodide metabolism and hormone synthesis. Some of the agents which produce hyperplasia (goiter) by interfering with iodide metabolism are thiocynate, arsenic, antithyroid drugs, resorcinol, sulphonamides, soy bean flour, cobalt, and goiterogens which are present in food and water.

Goiter.—A normally functioning pituitary gland is essential for the development of *nontoxic goiter*. The colloid goiter is the result of repeated bouts of thyroid hyperplasia and hyperinvolution because of iodide deficiency or as the result of the ingestion of agents which interfere with thyroidal iodide metabolism. The hyperinvolution may occur at a time when the cause of the hyperplasia is removed or it may occur even while the cause of the hyperplasia is operating. The cysts which develop contain a pale blue staining colloid which is deficient in iodide and has very little metabolic activity.

Congenital enzymatic defects of the thyroid gland result in the production of inadequate amounts of thyroid hormone. In some cases, iodinated substances which have but little metabolic activity are secreted into the peripheral circulation. In these cases, the abnormal circulating hormone does not maintain growth and *cretinism* is present. Likewise, it does not regulate the pituitary production of TSH which is now secreted in greater than normal amounts. The excessively high levels of TSH cause hyperplasia of the thyroid gland and *goiter* develops. Among the *defects* in *hormone synthesis* found in goiterous cretins are (1) failure of organification of iodide and thus failure of production of iodinated amino acids, (2) production and release into the circulation of metabolically inert iodinated polypeptides, and (3) inability to couple monoiodotyrosine and di-iodotyrosine resulting in thyroxine and tri-iodothyronine not being formed and the iodinated tyrosines being released into the circulation and rapidly excreted in the urine.

Cretinism.—Thyroid hormones are necessary for normal *growth* and differentiation of *bone*. The latter action is a direct one, while the former is mediated through the pituitary growth hormone. In the absence of thyroid hormone, the pituitary production of growth hormone is decreased and the growth of bone as well as of other tissues is impaired. The delayed time of appearance of the epiphyseal centers and failure of bone age to parallel the chronological age are manifestations of delayed bone differentiation as a result of lack of thyroid hormone.

These hormones are also necessary for normal *brain development*, at least in so far as mental capacity is concerned. Since neither thyroxine nor tri-iodothyronine cross the placenta with any facility, the failure of fetal thyroid gland development and the absence of thyroid activity during infancy leads to mental retardation. Such a disturbance is often not correctable by substitution therapy. Should the hormonal deficiency occur later in childhood, mental retardation is less severe and is more completely corrected by replacement of the absent hormones. In addition to the retardation of physical and mental development, cretins have umbilical hernias, pale pasty complexions, large tongues, depressed bone age with epiphyseal dysgenesis, low serum alkaline phosphatase, and, after the first year of life, hypercholesterolemia.

Thyrotoxicosis.—Thyroid hormones regulate metabolism in most of the tissues, excepting the brain, testes, and spleen. The increses in oxidations induced by thyroxine may be mediated by epinephrine rather than by direct action of thyroxine itself. It should be pointed out that there are no qualitative differences in the actions of thyroxine and tri-iodothyronine. The latter is four or five times more potent and although its action starts sooner it is of shorter duration. Most of the *clinical manifestations* of thyrotoxicosis, but not goiter or exophthalmos, can be reproduced by treatment with excessive doses of thyroxine or tri-iodothyronine. In thyrotoxicosis the gland, or a nodule in the gland, is hyperplastic and hyperfunctioning as indicated by the rapid and increased accumulation of radioactive iodine. The circulation levels of the thyroid hormones (PBI) are increased above normal and the oxidative metabolism, as indicated by the basal metabolic rate, is increased. The increase in oxidation results in a faster rate of tissue breakdown, stimulation of the appetite center, and an increase in food intake. Weight loss ensues, however, because food intake is not sufficient to compensate for the tissue lost. The heat produced by the increased oxidation would result in fever, were it not for the accompaning vasodilation and increased sweating. This need for heat loss is responsible not only for the sweating but also the heat sensitivity which are characteristic symptoms of the thyrotoxic patient.

The *cardiovascular changes* are in part a result of changes in heart muscle metabolism and in part a result of the need for increased oxygen supply. The cardiac rate, cardiac output, and pulse pressure increase. The circulation time is decreased and blood volume is increased. Should heart failure occur it is of the high output type and the circulation time is rarely as prolonged as in low output type failure. Auricular fibrillation without evidence of valvular disease or of coronary artery disease is not uncommon in patients with thyrotoxicosis.

The changes in personality, nervousness, hyperirritability, and tremor reflect the influence of the thyroid hormone on the *central nervous system*. The reasons for these changes are not known for, as mentioned above, oxygen consumption of brain is not increased by thyroid hormone.

Thyroxine also increases the activity of the *gastrointestinal tract*, as evidenced by increased frequency of stool and the presence of diarrhea. The *liver* is an important site for the conjugation and excretion of thyroxine and is itself susceptible to changes when thyroid hormone is in excess. Such changes, in patients with thyrotoxicosis, are probably the result of a relative deficiency of essential food factors rather than a result of direct action of thyroxine on the liver.

Hypothyroidism.—Inadequate amounts of thyroid active substances lead to *hypothyroidism* or, when the manifestations are more severe, to *myxedema*. In hypothyroidism, changes opposite to those of hyperthyroidism are present. The patients have hypersomulence, are dull and lethargic, prefer warm weather, and sweat but little. The pulse rate is slow and the circulation time is prolonged. Constipation is the rule. The skin is dry and coarse and nonpitting edema may be present. Acid mucopolysaccharide accumulates in the skin and other tissues. The material acts as a hydrophilic colloid and retains sodium and water. Pericardial effusion, pleural effusion, and ascites may occur. The electrocardiogram shows low voltage with flattening or inversion of T waves throughout. If hypothyroidism is severe and of long standing, myxedematous coma, usually fatal, may occur.

Ophthalmic Changes.—The ophthalmic facet of thyroid disease is the result of accumulation of mucopolysaccharide in the orbit with infiltration of the muscles with this material as well as with lymphocytes. These changes seem to be a result of increased production of a pituitary hormone which is probably not TSH. The same ophthalmologic disorders occur not only in thyrotoxicosis but also in euthyroid patients, and in patients who develop hypothyroidism following treatment for thyrotoxicosis.

Thyroid Carcinoma.—Some thyroid carcinomas are functional, accumulate iodide, and may form and secrete an iodinated polypeptide. Hormone dependency is exhibited by some of these tumors inasmuch as their rate of growth can be increased by TSH or suppressed by exogenous thyroid substances. In some patients with functional thyroid carcinomas, a prolonged inhibition of tumor growth may follow treatment with large doses of radioactive iodine.

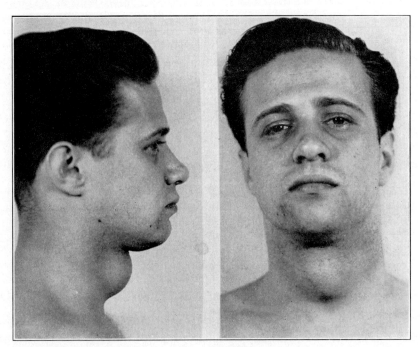

FIG. 244.—Thyroglossal cyst.

Hashimoto's Struma.—This rather uncommon form of thyroid disease is found mainly in women, is usually bilateral, and often results in hypothyroidism. The condition may be the result of autoimmunization with thyroglobulin which has been released into the circulation. Some of the patients have circulation antibodies to human thyroglobulin, and histologic changes suggestive of this type of disorder have been produced in experimental animals by administration of thyroglobulin.

CONGENITAL ANOMALIES

Orientation.—Developmental abnormalities of the thyroid gland may be grouped together under three major headings—(1) thyroglossal remnants, (2) aberrant thyroid tissue, (3) hypoplasia and aplasia, and (4) sporadic familial cretinism with goiter.

Thyroglossal Remnants.—A thyroglossal remnant consists of a cyst, duct, sinus, or fistula that occurs at any point between the foramen caecum at the base of the tongue and the skin above the suprasternal notch (Ward

and Marshall). Since such remnants are developmental in origin, most of
the cases are noted in the first decade of life. They have no predilection for
either sex or any race. A *thyroglossal cyst* occurs as a result of local dilatation of the epithelial-lined remnant. It may measure 6 to 8 cm. in diameter,
is well encapsulated, has a thin fibrous wall, possesses a smooth lining, and
is filled with clear, mucoid, or inspissated material (Figs. 244 and 245*A*). A
thyroglossal duct consists simply of an epithelial-lined tract of varying lengths
and measuring up to 1 cm. in diameter (Fig. 245*C*). A *thyroglossal sinus*

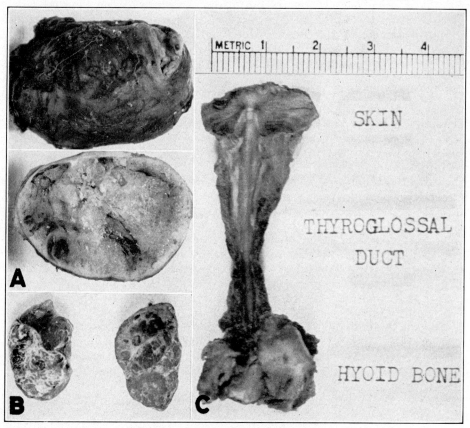

FIG. 245.—Congenital anomalies of the thyroid showing *A*, a thyroglossal cyst filled with
inspissated material, *B*, a removed lingual thyroid, and *C*—a thyroglossal duct.

is a duct that communicates with either the base of the tongue or the skin
of the neck. A *thyroglossal fistula* is a duct that communicates with both
the base of the tongue and the skin of the neck. Regardless of the nature
of the anomaly, its *histologic* composition is similar. The lining cells are
epithelial and may be of a columnar, transitional, or squamous cell variety.
Beyond this is a layer of fibrous tissue that may be infiltrated with leukocytes. The most important *complication* is infection and, if the pus becomes
loculated, an abscess forms. *Clinically* a cyst appears as a swelling; a duct
may be asymptomatic, while a sinus or a fistula is manifested as an opening
through which secretion escapes. Pain, dyspnea, choking sensation, and
redness may occur when infection supervenes. The *diagnosis* is made from

36

the history and clinical manifestation. *Treatment* consists of complete surgical excision (usually necessitating removal of the hyoid bone through which the tract passes). The *prognosis* is excellent.

Aberrant Thyroid Tissue.—Under this heading may be mentioned (1) mediastinal, (2) lingual, and (3) lateral thyroids. As seen in Chapter 12 (p. 546) *mediastinal thyroid* usually consists of an enlargement of either lobe of the thyroid or of the isthmus, with descent into the mediastinum. Sometimes, however, the connection with the main thyroid gland is lost, a portion of a normal thyroid descends into the mediastinum, or the entire thyroid is misplaced in the mediastinum, there being no thyroid tissue whatsoever in the usual location. A *lingual thyroid* connotes the presence of thyroid tissue at the base of the tongue. This may represent simply accessory tissue or, rarely, it may constitute all of the thyroid tissue in the body, there being no thyroid tissue in the usual location. The lesion consists of a circumscribed mass of glistening thyroid tissue that measures as much as 3 or 4 cm. in diameter (Fig. 245 *B*). Histologically the following have been noted: normal tissue, adenoma, adenomatous hyperplasia, hyperplasia, lymphoid aggregates, and, rarely, carcinoma (Timmons). The lesion may be asymptomatic or, because of its location, it may be associated with interference in deglutition or respiration. The diagnosis is made from the symptoms and signs and by using radioactive iodine as a tracer (Crispell). Treatment of choice (if thyroid tissue is present in the usual location) is surgical excision. The prognosis is good. Aside from lingual thyroid, *aberrant thyroid tissue* may be found at any point between the foramen caecum and the skin in the region of the suprasternal notch. *Lateral* (aberrant) *thyroids* consist of thyroid tissue (of a colloid or papillary variety) within lymph nodes located laterally in the cervical region. While the position of the deposits may be explainable on an embryologic arrest of descent of the ultimobranchial bodies, it has been conclusively demonstrated that such deposits represent carcinoma metastasis from a primary tumor in the homolateral lobe of the thyroid gland proper (Wozencraft and Warren). The lesion, therefore, is not a congenital anomaly.

Hypoplasia and Aplasia.—Congenital lack of full development (hypoplasia) or congenital absence of development (aplasia or agenesis) of the thyroid gland results in *cretinism*. Other causes of the disorder are iodine deficiency in the mother, iodine deficiency in infants after birth, destruction of the thyroid by infection during fetal life or in the neonatal period, and pituitary dysfunction (Mullinger and Hurxthal). Cretinism consists of retardation of both physical and mental development. It affects both sexes with equal frequency and is generally apparent before the age of two years. The condition is *characterized by* the following (Mullinger): slow gain in weight; dry, scaly, thick skin; sparse, coarse hair; difficulty in swallowing; obstipation; stunted growth; short, stocky extremities; flatness and broadness of the bridge of the nose; short, underdeveloped nose; delayed dentition; deformity of the teeth; macroglossia; protrusion of the abdomen; pallor and anemia; delayed maturation of bones radiologically; underdevelopment of secondary sex characteristics; listlessness, apathy, drowsiness, and lack of interest in the surroundings; harsh voice, and mental retardation of varying degrees (Fig. 246). *Treatment* consists of administration of thyroxin. Therapy should be started early and maintained in adequate amounts. Even so, the *prognosis* is variable for over one-third of patients (due to impairment of development of brain substance) remain mentally defective (Topper).

Sporadic Familial Cretinism with Goiter. —As the term indicates this condition consists of congenitally acquired cretinism associated with enlargement of the thyroid gland. It is *also known* as nonendemic familial cretinism with goiter, sporadic familial goitrous hypothyroidism, goiter in cretins without iodine deficiency, and goiters in sporadic cretins (Milles,

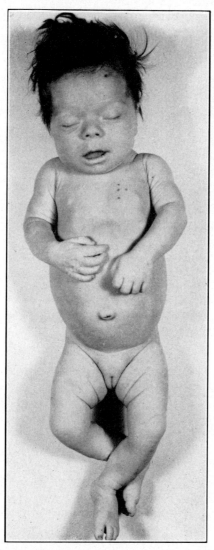

Fig. 246.—Cretinism in a two-month-old infant caused by aplasia of the thyroid gland. Note the broad face, flat nose, enlarged tongue, and protruding abdomen.

Pickering, and Stanbury). It is a *rare* disorder, being only 5 to 10 per cent as frequent as sporadic nongoitrous cretinism. It usually becomes apparent in infants or young children but it has also not been recognized the latter part of the first or the second or even the third decades of life. The disorder represents an inborn error of metabolism, probably transmitted by a recessive autosomal gene. The hypothyroidism and the goiter are *due to* an inadequate synthesis of thyroxine by the thyroid gland, with the thyroid enlargement resulting from excessive secretion of the thyroid stimulating hormone of the pituitary. At least 3 mechanisms are implicated in the arrest of secretion of thyroxine (Stanbury)—(1) thyroid can concentrate trapped iodine from serum but cannot produce iodotyrosines from tyrosyl residues and iodide due to lack of an oxidative enzyme, (2) thyroid cannot couple iodotyrosines into iodothyronines sufficiently rapidly to produce an adequate supply of hormone, due probably to failure of enzymatic coupling, and (3) hormone precursors monoiodothyrosine and deiodotyrosine escape

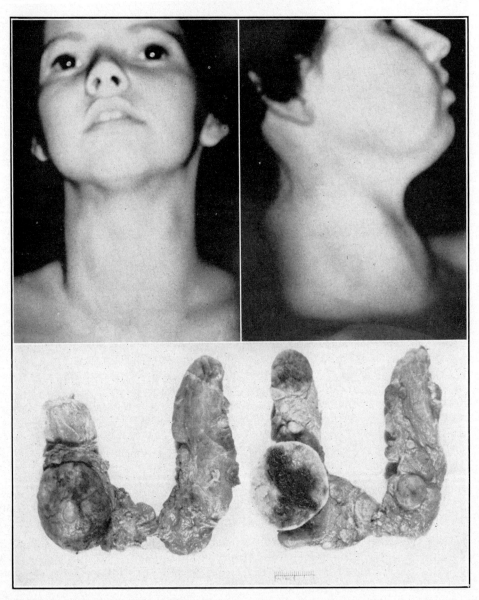

FIG. 247.—Sporadic familial cretinism with goiter showing nodular enlargement of the thyroid gland in an 18 year old girl above and the nodular appearance of the removed organ below.

from the thyroid gland into the blood stream and urine because of lack of
the enzyme dehalogenase. This, of course, leads to iodine deficiency.

The *pathologic* picture depends upon the degree of thyroid deficiency and
the response of the gland to sustained stimulation of the thyroid stimulating
hormone of the pituitary (Pickering). *Grossly* the thyroid gland has weighed
from 40 to 497 grams (Milles). It is nodular and asymmetrical (Fig. 247).
Cut surfaces disclose multiple nodules from a few millimeters to several
centimeters in diameter. They vary in color from ivory to tan or dark
reddish brown and they may or may not show degeneration and hemorrhage.

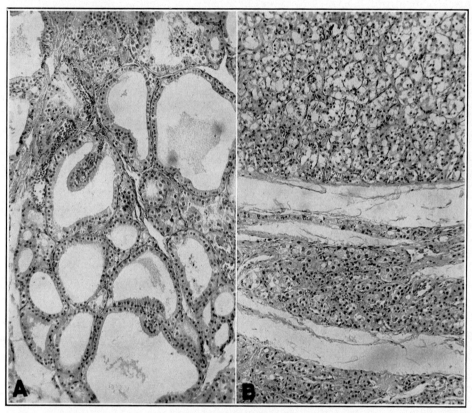

Fig. 248.—Sporadic familial cretinism with goiter, from same case illustrated in Figure 247,
showing *A*, diffuse hyperplasia in one nodule and *B*, embryonal type of adenoma in another nodule
together with irregularity of the adjoining thyroid cells. × 100.

The intermediate tissue is scanty and lacks the beefy appearance of normal
thyroid. *Histologically*, the picture is most varied (Fig. 248). The nodules
are similar to those in nodular hyperplasia (p. 579), with the exception that
the cells are less regular and at times may even be mistaken for carcinoma.
The pattern may thus be one of hyperplasia, fetal adenoma, embryonal
adenoma, or even papillary adenoma. The interlobular tissue is composed
of cords, nests, or follicles of thyroid tissue set in a scanty connective tissue
stroma and distorted by pressure from adjacent nodules. The cells may be
quite irregular with varying amounts of cytoplasm and deeply stained irregular nuclei.

The most important *complications* are stunting of growth and mental retardation. Both of these occur if the disorder starts early in ifancy, if it is severe, and if substitution therapy is not started in time. The *clinical* manifestations are those listed above in connection with hypoplasia and aplasia, with the exception that the thyroid is enlarged and nodular. The blood cholesterol is elevated and the basal metabolic rate is low. There is an increase in uptake of I_{131}, due undoubtedly to secretion of the thyroid stimulating hormone of the pituitary gland. The *diagnosis* is made from an evaluation of the clinical manifestations together with studies such as BMR and I_{131} uptake. *Treatment* consists of administration of thyroid preparations. Thyroidectomy is generally performed when the gland remains enlarged and nodular. The *prognosis* depends upon the severity of the disturbance and the age at which adequate treatment has been instituted.

DEGENERATIONS

Degenerative disorders of the thyroid gland consist of the usual atrophy, parenchymatous degeneration, hydropic degeneration, hyaline and hyaline droplet degeneration, mucoid degeneration, fatty change, fibrosis, calcification, hemosiderin deposition, and necrosis and liquefaction. The changes affect the parenchyma, the stroma, and/or the vessels. They are common because the thyroid gland is continuously in a state of flux—undergoing hyperplasia and involution. The conditions listed, however, are not disease entities but occur in conjunction with other disturbances, especially nodular enlargement. In addition to the retrogressive processes mentioned, there is still another disorder that has been called *amyloid goiter* (Walker). It consists of a diffuse enlargement of the thyroid gland due to permeation of the connective tissue with amyloid. The condition is generally seen as part of secondary amyloidosis.

INFLAMMATIONS

Orientation.—Inflammation of the thyroid gland is known as *thyroiditis*. While there are several classifications in vogue, the disorders may be considered under the following headings: nonspecific thyroiditis, Hashimoto's struma, Reidel's struma, tuberculosis, syphilis, actinomycosis, and Boeck's sarcoid.

Nonspecific Thyroiditis.—Nonspecific thyroiditis may be divided into three groups—acute, subacute, and chronic.

Acute nonspecific thyroiditis is rare, probably because the thyroid (1) is well protected by a fascial covering, (2) has no duct by way of which infection can travel, and (3) has an abundant, profusely anastomosing blood vessel and lymphatic supply (Higbee). The condition *occurs* twice as frequently in females as in males and, although it may be found at any age, it is most common in the third and fourth decades of life. Generally some previous disorder of the thyroid acts as a predisposing *cause*. The precipitating causes are any of the ordinary pyogenic bacteria, especially staphylococci and streptococci (Womack). The source of the infection is an inflammatory focus in any portion of the body, especially the upper respiratory tract and lungs, while the route of infection is usually by way of the bloodstream and, less commonly, by direct extension from adjacent structures. *Pathologically* the process is entirely nonspecific. The initial changes occur in the interacinar stroma and then spread peripherally to involve the capsule. They consist of congestion, edema, and a diffuse permeation with neutrophils. In more severe instances there is complete destruction of tissue with pooling of neutrophils, nuclear fragments, and debris. The process heals by resolution and, in more severe cases, by granulation tissue formation and fibrosis. The most important *complication* is abscess formation (Prioleau). If not treated promptly, the abscess may rupture into the tissues of the neck or into the trachea. Occasionally, when destruction has been severe, enough thyroid tissue may be destroyed to result in hypothyroidism. The *clinical manifestations* are due to tension within the capsule of the thyroid, to pressure upon adjacent structures, and to congestion and edema of the surrounding tissues (Higbee). They may consist of the following: pain, cough, hoarseness, aphonia, dyspnea, dysphagia, and, when abscess develops, chills, fever, and leukocytosis. Physical examination discloses a hard, firm, tender swelling that may be confined to the outline of the thyroid gland or that may involve all the tissues in the anterior portion of the neck. The *diagnosis* is made from a consideration of the history and the clinical findings. *Treatment* consists of antibiotic therapy, surgical drainage (when abscess develops or is impending), and tracheotomy. The *prognosis* in nonsuppurative infections is good, with recovery usually occurring in a week. It is also favorable in cases of suppuration if the condition is recognized and treated early.

Subacute nonspecific thyroiditis means various things to different authors. To some it indicates an inflammation that is similar to acute nonspecific thyroiditis but of lesser intensity (McGavack), to others it connotes a distinct entity that is probably of viral origin (Crile and Westwater), and to others still it signifies an early phase of what ultimately constitutes Riedel's struma. In your author's opinion it seems better to confine the caption to a low-grade nonspecific inflammation caused by the usual pyogenic organisms or to a subsidence of an acute nonspecific thyroiditis. In favor of this are (1) a history of a preceding acute pharyngitis or tonsillitis, (2) clinical findings identical with those of acute nonspecific thyroiditis but of lesser severity, and (3) the presence of a histologic picture similar to that in acute nonspecific thyroiditis but with the addition of eosinophils, plasma cells, lymphocytes, and monocytes.

Chronic nonspecific thyroiditis is a term that is used by some authors to encompass both Hashimoto's struma and Riedel's struma (Womack and Marshall) and by other authors to indicate simply the reactive changes to degenerative process in any goiter (McGavack). In your author's opinion, the term should be restricted to the latter use if for no other reason than that Hashimoto's struma and Riedel's struma constitute specific entities. The changes are usually seen in a thyroid that is the seat of an adenomatous hyperplasia (nodular goiter). They consist of focal or more diffuse areas of degeneration of colloid and epithelial cells together with varying degrees of fibrosis and infiltration with lymphocytes and plasma cells. In older lesions, there may be collagenization of the fibrous tissue with focal areas of calcification.

Hashimoto's Struma.—This condition is commonly known as *struma lymphomatosa* and *lymphomatoid goiter*. It is worldwide in distribution, *occurs* almost exclusively in females, and reaches a peak incidence in patients around fifty years of age (Davison and Craig). The *cause* is unknown. *Pathologically* there is a diffuse uniform enlargement of the entire gland with increases in weight to as much as 340 grams (McGavack). The capsule is intact and glistening. The external surface of the gland is smooth

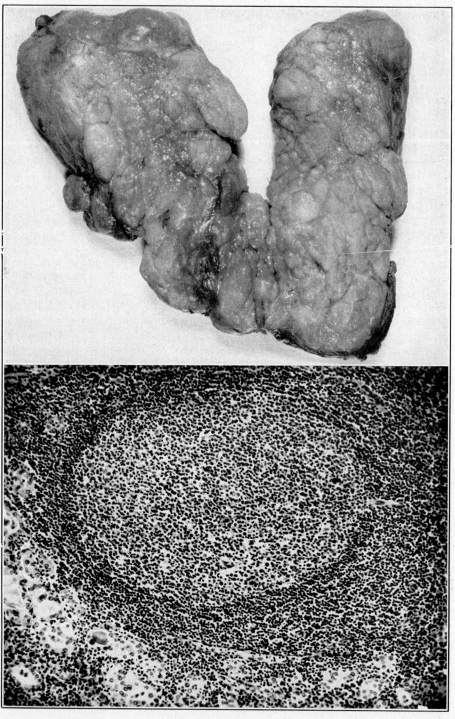

FIG. 249.—Hashimoto's struma illustrating, above, a diffuse enlargement of the gland by lobulated, moderately firm, gray tissue and, below, diffuse lymphocytic infiltration, lymph follicle formation, and atrophy of the thyroid acini. × 100.

or lobulated. The consistency is firm. Cut surfaces disclose a uniform or lobulated replacement of the entire organ by soft to moderately firm, pinkish gray to light brown, homogeneous tissue (Fig. 249). *Histologically* all portions of the gland are affected. The initial changes consist of focal degeneration, atrophy, and ultimately complete disappearance of the colloid, acinar cells, and acini. Concomitantly there is a diffuse, dense, interacinar infiltration with lymphocytes arranged diffusely and in follicle formation (Fig. 249). As the process ages there is a moderate increase of connective tissue. The only noteworthy *complications* consist of spontaneous hypothyroidism (occurring in about one-third of the patients) and pressure upon adjacent structures. The latter, however, is not a prominent feature. *Clinically* the usual symptom is gradual enlargement of the thyroid gland. Occasionally (as a result of pressure) there may be discomfort in the neck, alterations in the voice, choking sensation, and dyspnea but none of these, even when present, is alarming (McGavack). On physical examination, the gland is uniformly enlarged and nontender. The basal metabolic rate is usually slightly below normal. The *diagnosis* is made from the history, physical examination, and, of course, histologically. A differential diagnosis includes any enlargement of the thyroid, especially nonspecific thyroiditis and Reidel's struma. *Treatment* of choice is subtotal or total thyroidectomy. The *prognosis*, as far as ridding the patient of the thyroid enlargement is concerned, is good but about 80 per cent of the patients develop postoperative hypothyroidism.

Riedel's Struma. — Riedel's struma is also called diffuse chronic thyroiditis, ligneous thyroiditis, and chronic fibrous thyroiditis. The conditions variously called pseudotuberculous, granulomatous, giant cell, and de Quervain's thyroiditis should also be included under this caption for, in your author's opinion, they represent simply an early stage of Riedel's struma. The disorder is less common than Hashimoto's struma, *occurs* three to seven times as frequently in females as it does in males, and reaches a peak incidence in patients around forty years of age (Lindsay and Mc-Gavack). The *cause* is unknown but a low-grade bacterial infection has been suspected. *Pathologically* one lobe is involved in approximately one-half of the cases, while the entire gland is affected in the remaining half. Early in the course of the disease the affected part of the gland is only slightly enlarged, and the enlargement is well encapsulated, free of adhesions, pale pink, and moderately firm. Later, as the disorder progresses, the involved area increases several times in size, is poorly encapsulated, forms numerous dense adhesions to adjacent structures, is pale gray with yellowish foci, and becomes stony hard and brittle (Fig. 250). *Histologically* the earliest changes consist of atrophy and degeneration of the acini. The epithelial cells become smaller and disappear and the colloid is depleted and broken up. Frequently small masses of colloid are surrounded by remaining nuclei of the epithelial cells to render formations that resemble giant cells of the Langhans' type (Fig. 250). The resemblance to tuberculosis is further enhanced by the collection of these cells around inflammatory or necrotic foci. In addition to the degeneration there is a diffuse permeation with lymphocytes and a rapid progression of the process through stages of granulation tissue formation with culmination in a homogeneous deposition of dense fibrotic tissue. The chief *complications* are those of compression of adjacent structures in the neck. *Clinical manifestations* consist of the following: (1) stony hard, often painful and tender, focal or diffuse enlargement of the thyroid gland, (2) cough and dyspnea (due to

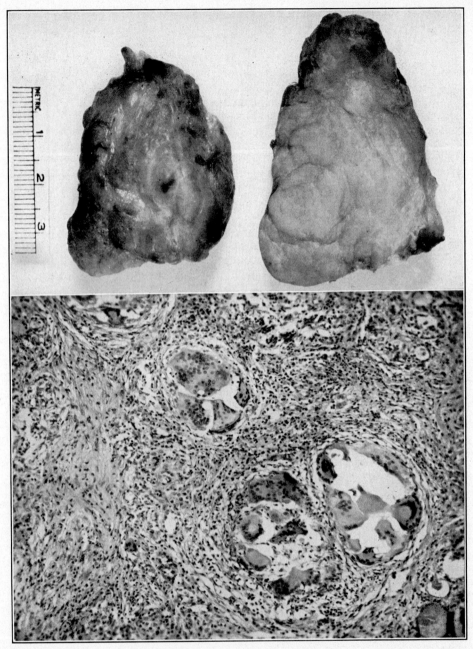

Fig. 250.—Riedel's struma showing, above, diffuse replacement of a portion of the gland by gray sclerotic tissue and, below, diffuse fibrosis, several atrophic acini, and pseudogiant cell formation. × 100.

pressure on the trachea), (3) hoarseness and respiratory stridor (due to involvement of the recurrent laryngeal nerve), and (4) dysphagia (due to pressure on the esophagus). In addition, signs of hyperthyroidism often occur in the early stages. The *diagnosis* is made from the clinical manifestations and histologic examination of removed tissue. The condition is readily confused with carcinoma. *Treatment* consists of surgical removal of the involved part of the gland or the entire gland. Postoperative hypothyroidism and parathyroid tetany develop occasionally. The *prognosis* in general, is good.

Tuberculosis.—Tuberculosis of the thyroid gland is rare (Postlethwait and Berg). It *occurs* at all ages and affects males and females with equal frequency. The condition is usually secondary to tuberculosis elsewhere in the body, especially in the lungs. *Pathologically* the lesions may be of the caseous variety with abscess formation or of the miliary type. The former produce a swelling and often pressure symptoms while the latter are asymptomatic. The *diagnosis* is made histologically. Great care must be taken to differentiate the pseudogiant cells and the pseudotubercles of Riedel's struma from those of tuberculosis. *Treatment* consists of local drainage or thyroidectomy. Generally the *prognosis*, as far as the local condition is concerned, is good.

Syphilis.—Syphilis of the thyroid gland is extremely rare. The lesions may be congenital or acquired and each may consist of diffuse interstitial fibrosis or gummatous formations (McGavack).

Boeck's Sarcoid.—Sarcoidosis of the thyroid gland is even less frequent than syphilis for, by 1951, there were only 4 cases recorded in the literature (Cummins). Clinically the condition is characterized by enlargement of the gland while pathologically the lesion consists of solid tubercles.

PHYSICAL DISTURBANCES

The only noteworthy physical disturbances of the thyroid are those consequent to *thyroidectomy*. They may be listed as follows: (1) removal of too much of the gland resulting in adult hypothyroidism or myxedema, (2) removal of the parathyroid gland eventuating in tetany, (3) severance of one or both recurrent laryngeal nerves causing laryngeal paralysis, (4) hemorrhage, (5) infection, (6) retention of foreign bodies (sponges, instruments, etc.), (7) mediastinal emphysema, and (8) pneumothorax.

Adult Hypothyroidism or Myxedema.—This condition is also known as cachexia thyreopriva or strumipriva (when it follows an operation) and Gull's disease. It is *brought about* primarily by hyposecretion of thyroxin which, in turn, may be secondary not only to thyroidectomy but also to (1) exhausted or "burned out" thyrotoxicosis, (2) thyroiditis, (3) hypofunction of the pituitary gland, (4) primary atrophy of the thyroid, and (5) prolonged use of drugs such as iodine, thiouracil, and potassium thiocyanate. The condition is about one-fifteenth as *common* as toxic goiter and is approximately four to seven times as frequent in females as it is in males. According to McGavack, the *clinical manifestations* may be listed as follows: (1) *psychic*—complacency, drowsiness, lack of initiative, and loss of memory, (2) *nervous system*—numbness and tingling in the extremities, uncertain gait, clumsy motions of the extremities, headache, facial neuralgia, vertigo, tinnitus, hallucinations, and delusions, (3) *weight*—apparent increase due to accumulation of fluid but actually consisting of a depletion of stored fat, (4) *skin*—sensitivity to cold, roughness, dryness, scaliness, absence of sweating, thickening of the dermis by myxedema fluid, secondary inflammation, thickening and brittleness of the nails, and thinning and coarseness of the hair (Fig. 251, *A*) (5) *cardiovascular*—dyspnea, orthopnea, cardiac pain (coronary sclerosis), cardiac failure, and pericardial effusion, (6) *gastrointestinal tract*—constipation, flatulence, anorexia, abdominal pain, nausea, and vomiting, (7) *urinary system*—renal impairment, and (8) *genital system*—suppression of primary sexual activity together with diminution of libido in both sexes, impotence in the male, and sterility and irregular menses in the female. In addition, from the *laboratory standpoint*, there are (1) low basal metabolic rate, (2) anemia from hypoplasia of the bone marrow, (3) low protein bound iodine, (4) hypercholesterolemia, (5) albuminuria and low inulin tolerance, and (6) lowered urinary eleven-oxycorticoids. As stated, most of the disturbances of the various organs are *explainable* primarily on the basis of inadequate amounts of thyroxin. Other factors are imbalance of the autonomic nervous system, interference in absorption of food from the intestines, improper nutrition of the various tissues, and

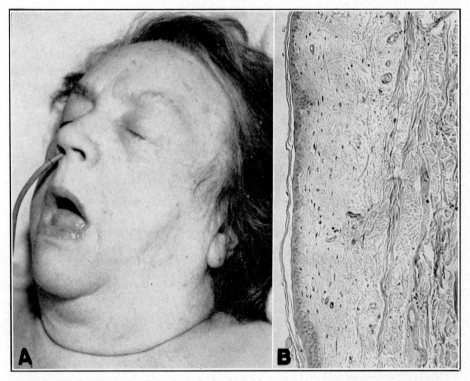

Fig. 251.—Spontaneous myxedema in a woman 50 years old illustrating *A*, thick skin, large tongue, and coarse hair, and *B*, myxedema of the superficial portion of the corium. × 100.

infiltration of the tissues with myxedematous material. This material gives a positive periodic-acid Schiff stain, thus indicating that it contains mucopolysaccharide (Berkheiser). It accumulates in the connective tissue throughout the body and accounts for the increased thickness of the skin, the enlargement of the tongue, enlargement of the heart, and pseudohypertrophy of the striated muscles (Figs. 251 and 252). Coupled with degeneration of both striated and smooth muscles it also accounts for myocardial weakness and failure, skeletal muscle fatigue, and loss of tonicity of the large intestine (Curtis). *Pathologic changes*, aside from those already mentioned, consist of (1) severe generalized arteriosclerosis, (2) hypoplasia of the bone marrow, (3) atrophy of the adrenal cortex, and (4) alterations in the thyroid gland depending upon the cause of decreased thyroid activity.

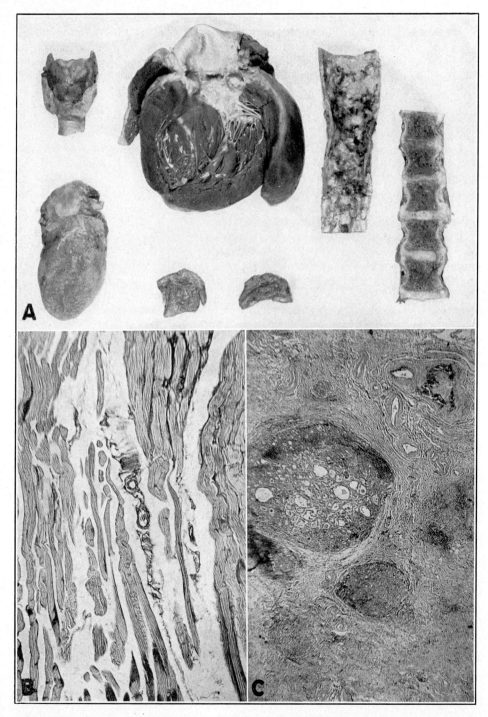

FIG. 252.—Myxedema from the same case shown in Figure 251 illustrating *A*, a small thyroid gland, enlargement of the tongue and heart, atrophy of the adrenals, severe atherosclerosis of the aorta, and dry hypoplastic bone marrow, *B*, myxedema and degeneration of striated muscle. × 50, and *C*, atrophy of thyroid acini along with replacement with fibrous tissue. × 50.

When the condition follows thyrotoxicosis the gland shows remnants of diffuse hyperplasia with the presence of exhaustion cells. When it follows inflammation, stigmata of an inflammatory process remain. When it follows primary atrophy collections of ill-defined acini and foci of degenerating cuboidal cells are found embedded in a dense connective tissue stroma (Bastenie). When it follows drug therapy, similar atrophic and fibrotic changes are encountered.

TUMORS

Orientation.—Under this heading may be considered both true tumors and hyperplasias or tumor-like conditions. While precise classifications are many, most of them differ only in minor details or in the choice of synonyms. For practical purposes the following listing appears to be quite adequate: diffuse hyperplasia, colloid goiter, adenomatous hyperplasia, solitary adenoma, carcinoma, and other tumors.

Diffuse Hyperplasia.—Diffuse hyperplasia of the thyroid gland is a pathologic term used to indicate hypertrophy and hyperplasia of the functioning cells with clinical manifestations of hyperthyroidism. Some of the many *synonyms* are exophthalmic goiter, Graves' disease, and Basedow's disease. The condition *affects* all races, occurs at all ages with the greatest incidence between thirty and sixty years and a peak incidence in the fourth decade, and is four times as frequent in females as it is in males (Bartels and Kingsley). The *cause* of the condition is neurohormonal stimulation. One of the prerequisites for its development appears to be a certain "susceptible constitution"—a high-strung, highly emotional person. The trigger mechanism in such an individual is psychic trauma in the form of grief, pain, fright, infection, puberty, marriage, pregnancy, menopause, change of environment, etc. (McGavack). Any one of these disturbances causes stimulation of the hypothalamus which stimulates the anterior pituitary gland to increase production of thyrotropic hormone and this, in turn, stimulates the thyroid cells to an overproduction of thyroxin. The thyroxin then causes an overstimulation of the various target organs throughout the body, resulting in a chain of symptoms referred to as *hyperthyroidism* or *thyrotoxicosis*. Normally the increased output of thyroxin is sufficient to cause depression of the output of thyrotropic hormone but, under the circumstances outlined, it apparently cannot overcome the powerful stimuli received from the hypothalamus.

Pathologically there is a diffuse uniform enlargement of all portions of the thyroid gland with as much as a two- to threefold increase in its size (Fig. 253). The external surface is well encapsulated, smooth, and glistening. The consistency is normal or only slightly increased over that of normal. Cut surfaces reveal a diffuse, homogeneous replacement of the entire organ with deep red or reddish-brown tissue that lacks the luster of a normal thyroid gland. *Histologically* there is marked variation in the shape and size of the acini (Hellwig). Some are large while others are small (Fig. 253). They are either completely devoid of colloid or they contain varying amounts of granular, watery material that stains only lightly eosinophilic. The lining epithelial cells are usually tall columnar. They are closely packed, have ill-defined borders, disclose lightly eosinophilic, rather granular cytoplasm, and reveal oval, closely packed, hyperchromatic, basilar nuclei. The cells either line the acini in a regular manner or project into their lumens in papillary formations, thus increasing greatly the surface area.

The supporting stroma is scanty and is usually of a loose connective tissue variety. It contains moderate numbers of capillaries and blood vessels and scattered foci of lymphocytes. Sometimes the latter are grouped to form definite lymphoid follicles. The picture in patients who have received pre-

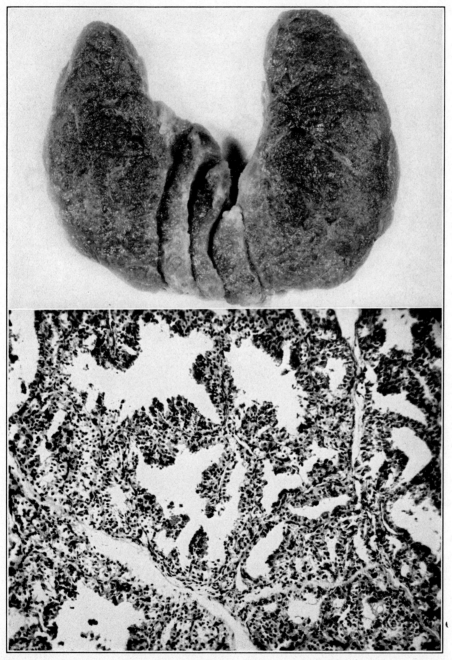

FIG. 253.—Diffuse hyperplasia of the thyroid illustrating, above, a diffuse uniform involvement of the gland with light reddish-brown lusterless tissue and, below, marked hypertrophy and hyper-plasia of the epithelial cells with papillary formations and complete absence of acinar colloid. × 100.

operative thiouracil is similar with the exception that the hypertrophy and hyperplasia are intensified (Fig. 254*A*). Administration of iodine, on the other hand, results in involution of the gland with a tendency of the structures to return to normal (Fig. 254*B*). The acini become more regular; they become filled with densely eosinophilic colloid that often shows scalloping of its borders, and they are lined with epithelial cells that have a tendency to assume a low cuboidal appearance.

The *complications* of diffuse hyperplasia of the thyroid may be listed as follows: (1) cardiac failure—more common in patients with previous or

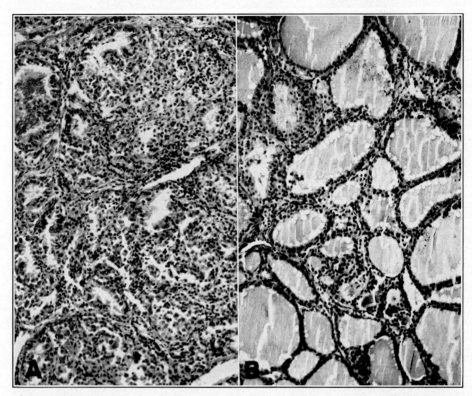

FIG. 254.—Diffuse hyperplasia of the thyroid showing *A*, severe hypertrophy and hyperplasia consequent to thiouracil therapy and *B*, involution (deposition of colloid) consequent to iodine therapy. × 100.

coexisting cardiac disease than in those without such concomitant changes (Griswold and Keating), (2) diabetes mellitus—occurring in about 2 per cent of cases (McGavack), (3) rarely hepatic deficiency—with pathologic changes in the liver characterized by a decrease in weight, fatty change, lymphoid infiltrations in the portal areas, and cirrhosis (Shaffer), (4) thyroid crisis—a severe exaggeration of the usual symptoms and signs precipitated by a variety of stimuli (infection, thyroidectomy, stress, etc.) and often resulting in death (Rives), and (5) carcinoma—developing extremely rarely. The *clinical manifestations* are due to either direct or indirect effect of excessive amounts of thyroxin upon the various target organs of the body. Considered systemically (McGavack) they may be listed as follows: (1) *nutritional*—often no disturbances but if food intake is not maintained there is loss of weight, (2) *nervous* and *mental*—increased irritability resulting in emotional (anger, laughing, or crying) outbursts, perspiration, palpitation, anxiety, manic-depressive disturbances, phobias, and fine tremor of the hands and tongue, (3) *countenance*—flush-faced (when nutrition is good), exophthalmos, widening of the palpebral fissures, infrequency of blinking, lid-lag, difficulty in focusing on near objects, inability to wrinkle forehead, edema of the lids, and (less often) corneal dystrophies, (4) *neck*—diffuse, smooth, nontender, slight to moderate enlargement of the thyroid with rarely a thrill or bruit elicited, (5) *integument*—flushed, hot, moist, soft skin with occasionally increased pigmentation, vitiligo (areas of depigmentation), acne, increased growth of hair (in less severe cases), and alopecia (in more severe cases), (6) *muscles*—weakness due primarily to atrophy of muscle fibers, (7) *cardiovascular*—palpitation, tachycardia, disturbance of rhythm, and anginal pain, and (8) *gastrointestinal*—increased appetite early in the disease with maintenance of weight but anorexia and loss of weight in more severe cases, diarrhea, or constipation. In addition, *laboratory data* of importance are: increased basal metabolic rate, decreased serum cholesterol, decreased liver function tests, decreased glucose tolerance, increased protein bound iodine of blood plasma, osteoporosis roentgenographically, and greater accumulation of radioactive iodine than normal. The *diagnosis* is arrived at by a consideration of the clinical manifestations as listed with special emphasis on emotional disturbances, eye signs, physical examination of the thyroid gland, and elevation of the basal metabolic rate. *Treatment* should be individualized to suit the case at hand (Robertson, Crile, Bartels, and Clark). In general, it consists of (1) administration of radioactive iodine, (2) administration of thiouracil, and (3) thyroidectomy (usually with preoperative administration of iodine and thiouracil). Each of these forms of treatment is, however, not without *danger*. With administration of radioactive iodine there is the possibility of developing carcinoma. The disorder has been produced in rats (Goldberg). Administration of thiouracil may be attended by a variety of toxic effects such as fever, rash, urticaria, arthralgia, granulocytopenia, etc. Because of the intense hyperplasia that follows its use, there is also the danger of the development of carcinoma. Thyroidectomy may be attended by (among other things) thyroid crisis, myxedema, or return of the hyperthyroidism. The *prognosis*, in properly treated patients with therapy instituted early, is usually good.

Colloid Goiter.—A colloid goiter may be defined as a diffuse enlargement of the thyroid gland due to hypertrophy and hyperplasia of the acini and deposition of colloid material. Some of the many *synonyms* are iodine deficiency goiter, subiodic goiter, simple goiter, and endemic goiter (McGavack). The condition *occurs* endemically and sporadically, is worldwide in distribution but is more common in mountainous areas (Alps, Himalayas, Andes, etc.) and also in some lowlying areas (such as the Great Lakes region), affects all races, and is seen at all ages but usually starts before puberty. The principal *cause* is iodine deficiency (Spence, Kimball, and DeCourcy). The deficiency may be absolute in the form of (1) an insufficient amount of iodine in the diet (due to decreased amount in the soil and water), (2) insufficient absorption from the intestine, or (3) presence of other substances that prevent the utilization of iodine. At other times, the deficiency may be relative in the form of an increased demand on the part of the body such as is seen during puberty, pregnancy, lactation, or the menopause. At any rate, decreased availability of iodine results in insufficiency of thyroxin. A low output of thyroxin brings about hyperstimulation of the anterior pituitary gland with increased thyrotropic hormone production

37

and this, in turn, produces hypertrophy and hyperplasia of the thyroid gland (McGavack). When the stimulus persists, the hypertrophy and hyperplasia, for some unknown reason, undergo secondary pathologic changes manifested mainly in the formation of colloid that is poor in iodine and thyroxin. This colloid, also for some unknown reason, is not influenced by the thyrotropic hormone of the anterior pituitary gland and is stored in excessive amounts in the thyroid acini.

Pathologically uncomplicated colloid goiter consists of a diffuse, uniform enlargement of the entire organ. The capsule is intact and smooth and the consistency is moderately increased. Cut surfaces disclose a diffuse, homogeneous, pinkish-brown appearance. *Histologically* the early changes con-

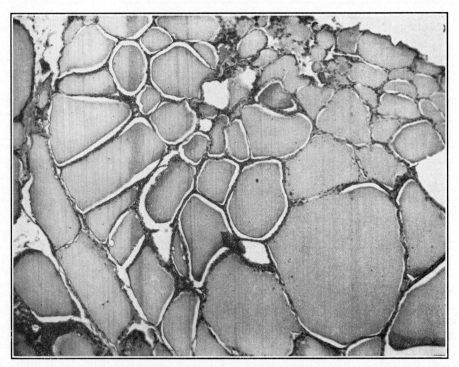

Fig. 255.—Colloid goiter illustrating varisized acini filled with colloid
and lined by low cuboidal epithelium. × 100.

sist of hypertrophy and hyperplasia of the epithelial cells and acini. Later, these changes are reduced to scattered focal areas while the predominating alteration consists of varisized acini filled with eosinophilic colloid and lined by low columnar or cuboidal epithelial cells (Fig. 255). The stroma is scanty and of a loose connective tissue variety and the vessels are inconspicuous.

The *complications* of colloid goiter are hypothyroidism, cretinism, adenomatous hyperplasia, and rarely (usually after many years) carcinoma. *Clinically*, the chief manifestation consists of a diffuse enlargement of the thyroid gland that usually begins about the age of five or six years. There is a steady increase in size until puberty after which there is generally a decline in size of the organ in males and a persistence or an increase in enlargement in females. The basal metabolic rate is usually around −15.

In the more severe endemic areas, the enlargement may produce a sense of fullness in the neck or may cause actual compression of the trachea, esophagus, recurrent laryngeal nerve, sympathetic chain, etc. The *diagnosis* is established by the presence of a diffuse enlargement of the thyroid gland before puberty in an endemic area. The condition may be *treated* and cured by the addition of iodine to the diet.

According to Kimball, the incorporation of 0.01 per cent of potassium iodide to natural salt is sufficient to overcome the deficiency. In long-standing and well-developed cases administration of thyroxin may be necessary. The *prognosis* is generally good.

Adenomatous Hyperplasia.—Adenomatous hyperplasia of the thyroid, also known as nodular goiter, adenoma, cystadenoma, etc., represents simply an advanced stage of colloid goiter (Spence and McGavack). As would be

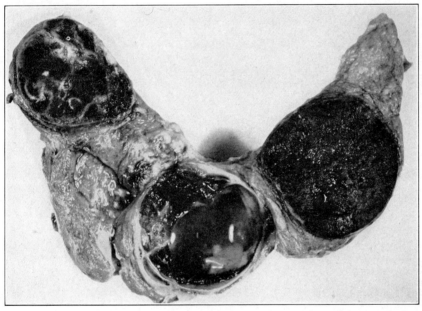

Fig. 256.—Adenomatous hyperplasia of the thyroid gland showing three well-encapsulated nodules—one with moderate hemorrhage, a second with extensive hemorrhage, and a third with liquefaction and cyst formation.

expected, therefore, the geographic distribution is the same as that of colloid goiter. While the condition *occurs* at all ages, it is more common in adults than it is in children. It affects females from seven to ten times as frequently as it does males. The fundamental *cause* of adenomatous hyperplasia of the thyroid is iodine deficiency and the mechanism is similar to that already outlined in connection with colloid goiter.

Pathologically, the thyroid gland is enlarged from slight to that which fills the entire anterior portion of the neck and even overhangs the sternum. Some enlargements, in addition, are directly behind the trachea while others descend into the mediastinum. The external surface is irregularly lobulated, well encapsulated, and usually quite free of adhesions. Cut surfaces disclose a few to many, well-encapsulated nodules of varying sizes and varying appearances (Fig. 256). Younger nodules are ill defined and glistening and blend more or less with the adjacent parenchyma. Older ones are more sharply delineated and are surrounded by a fibrous tissue capsule. From the capsule, fibrous trabeculæ often stream into the central portions of the nodules. Both the capsule and the trabeculæ may contain areas of degeneration and calcification. Some of the encapsulated nodules are composed of light brown, glistening tissue like that in the thyroid proper; some contain variegated, brown, yellow, or gray areas; others disclose varying degrees of hemorrhage, and others still show complete liquefaction. The supporting thyroid parenchyma varies in amount from abundant to that which is scarcely apparent.

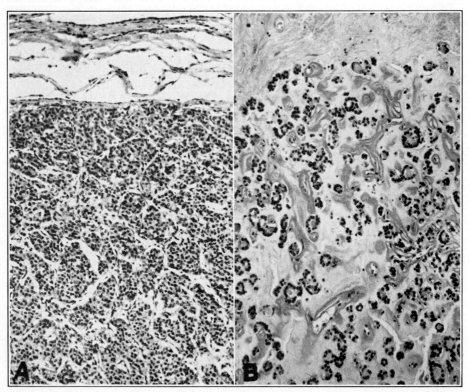

FIG. 257.—Adenomatous hyperplasia of the thyroid illustrating *A*, embryonal adenoma consisting of cords and nests of ill-defined cells with moderate amount of cytoplasm and round nuclei and *B*, fetal adenoma consisting of small acini supported by an abundant dense stroma. Note the fibrous capsule in each instance. × 100.

The *microscopic* appearance varies from nodule to nodule. The variations are readily understandable if the process is looked upon simply as one of hyperplasia and involution (Spence and Lindsay). Hyperplasia comes about as a result of budding from thyroid epithelium, whereas involution represents nothing more than the accumulation of colloid within the proliferated acini. When hyperplasia prevails, the nodule is referred to as embryonal adenoma, fetal adenoma, or papillary adenoma, while when involution prevails it is called colloid adenoma. Frequently, combinations and transitions from one to the other exist in the same thyroid gland and even in the same nodule. *Embryonal adenoma* is generally encountered in early lesions of young patients. It consists of rather uniform appearing, ill-defined, cuboidal cells arranged in clusters or cores with only a slight attempt at acinar formation (Fig. 257A). The supporting stroma is scanty and of a loose connective tissue type. *Fetal adenoma* (microfollicular adenoma) is somewhat more common. It is composed of similar cuboidal cells which, however, form small, round, uniform glands that are devoid of colloid (Fig. 257B). The supporting stroma is usually abundant and collagenous and often resembles colloid itself. *Papillary adenoma* (papillary cystadenoma) is next in frequency. It exists in the form of long or squatty,

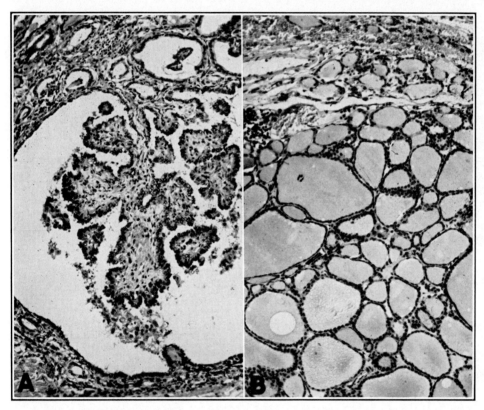

FIG. 258.—Adenomatous hyperplasia of the thyroid showing *A*, papillary adenoma consisting essentially of a small cyst containing a branching stalk of connective tissue covered with a single layer of cuboidal epithelial cells and *B*, colloid adenoma consisting of a capsule of compressed thyroid tissue enclosing acini filled with dense colloid and lined with flattened epithelial cells. × 100.

branching, finger-like projections that generally fill a cyst-like cavity (Fig. 258A). The stroma may be scanty, well vascularized, and of a loose connective tissue variety or it may be more abundant, poorly vascularized, and somewhat collagenous. The covering epithelial cells are generally one layer thick and are cuboidal to columnar. The cell borders are fairly sharply defined; the cytoplasm is moderate in amount and eosinophilic, and the nuclei are round or oval, and hyperchromatic or uniformly stained. Mitoses are few or absent. There is generally no deposition of colloid between the papillæ. *Colloid adenoma* is the most common. It comprises the majority of the nodules in older patients with long-standing goiters. It consists of large or small acini filled with densely eosinophilic colloid and lined by a single layer of low cuboidal or flattened epithelial cells (Fig. 258*B*). The latter contain scanty cytoplasm and round or oval, regular, evenly staining nuclei. Regardless of the type of adenoma, as the nodule enlarges it outgrows its blood supply. This results in degeneration, necrosis, liquefaction, cyst formation, and secondary hemorrhage. Also, irrespective of the histologic structure of the nodule, the thyroid parenchyma adjacent to the nodule first becomes compressed and then undergoes degeneration, fibrosis, and sometimes calcification. Ultimately it forms an encircling capsule.

The *complications* consist of (1) *pressure* on adjacent structures such as the trachea, esophagus, recurrent laryngeal nerve, etc., (2) *thyrotoxicosis* reported as occurring in from 10 to 50 per cent of all nodular enlargements (McGavack), and (3) *carcinoma*. Statistics regarding the incidence of carcinoma in nodular goiter (toxic and nontoxic) vary from 3 to 12 per cent. The types of adenoma that become malignant in decreasing order of frequency are papillary, embryonal, fetal, and colloid. A most distressing fact is that morphologically there is often no detectable difference between the benign and the malignant lesion. So true is this that pathologists more and more are considering all papillary nodules of the thyroid as carcinomatous regardless of their histologic appearance. While invasion of the capsule and the blood vessels is proof positive of the presence of carcinoma, such alterations may not be demonstrable and yet the patient may disclose metastasis from the tumor. *Clinically* the symptoms and signs are those of the complications. In general, they are referable to the enlargement of the thyroid gland, thyrotoxicosis, and pressure. The *diagnosis* is made from the history and physical examination. *Treatment*, because of the high incidence of carcinoma and thyrotoxicosis, consists of thyroidectomy. The *prognosis* is generally good.

Solitary Adenoma.—The only morphologic difference between a solitary adenoma and adenomatous hyperplasia of the thyroid is that in the former there is a single nodule while in the latter there are two or more. Histologically the two conditions are similar. The lesion doubtlessly arises in a manner similar to that of adenomatous hyperplasia. The only reason for mentioning the condition separately is that it is more prone to undergo a malignant transformation than are the nodules in adenomatous hyperplasia. In support of this statement may be quoted statistics by the following authors signifying a cancerous change in adenomatous hyperplasia and solitary adenoma respectively: Crile—5.6 per cent and 24.5 per cent, Hermanson—10.4 per cent and 14.4 per cent, Cerise—12.8 per cent and 19.8 per cent, and Cole—11 per cent and 24 per cent. Because of these experiences, every solitary adenoma of the thyroid gland regardless of its location, size, consistency, etc., should be removed surgically.

Carcinoma.—Primary carcinoma of the thyroid gland is one of the more common cancers of the body. It is said to *constitute* about 1 per cent of all malignant tumors (Hare) and to be found in as high as 6.8 per cent of all thyroidectomies (Dailey). It affects all races, is recorded as being two to eight times more common in females than in males, and is found at all ages. Regarding age distribution, however, 20 per cent of the patients in the series recorded by Dailey were under twenty years of age, while Duff stated that 6.5 per cent of all carcinomas of the thyroid occur in children. The precise *cause* of the lesion is not known. Many authors, however, agree that carcinoma of the thyroid starts in a pre-existing adenoma or adenomatous hyperplasia in over 90 per cent of all cases.

Pathologically primary carcinoma generally originates in the thyroid

proper, although occasionally it may arise in a mediastinal thyroid and rarely
in thyroglossal remnants (Aronoff).   As stated at the beginning of this
Chapter (p. 562), tumors found in the lateral cervical region are now considered by most authors to represent metastatic growths rather than lateral
aberrant thyroids.   The *gross* appearance of the thyroid gland is of no value
in making a precise diagnosis of early carcinoma.   Since, as already stated

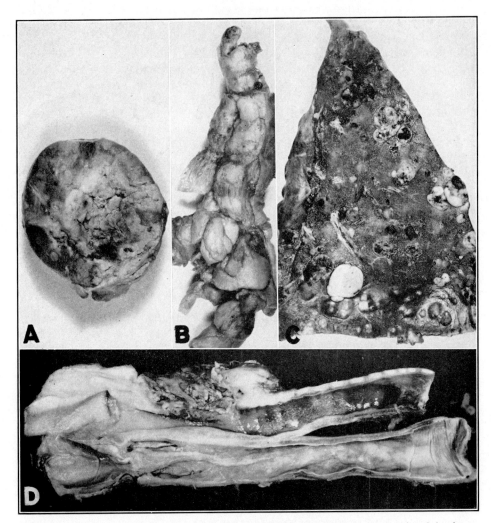

Fig. 259.—Carcinoma of the thyroid illustrating *A*, an apparently encapsulated nodule of gray
tissue showing foci of necrosis, *B*, invasion of the jugular vein by tumor, *C*, metastasis to a lung,
and *D*, extension of cancerous tissue through the larynx and trachea into the airway.

several times, the lesion usually originates in an adenomatous hyperplasia
or a solitary adenoma of the thyroid, the initial changes are indistinguishable
from these two conditions (Fig. 259).   In some instances, features which aid
in distinguishing a carcinoma from the predisposing conditions are increased
firmness, replacement of the glistening colloid appearance by solid pinkish-
gray tissue, and penetration of the capsule of the nodule by the tumor tissue.
As the tumor becomes more extensive, most or all of the thyroid gland may

be replaced with neoplastic tissue, the capsule of the thyroid is penetrated in many areas, and the adjacent structures of the neck become infiltrated. The appearance and consistency of the extensive growths vary greatly from case to case. The entire organ may remain small or it may increase to many times its normal size. The tissue is usually gray or pinkish gray and it may be extremely firm or soft and brain-like.

Histologically many classifications have been proposed. It is well to remember, however, that the thyroid is normally composed of glandular tissue with or without papillary infoldings, depending upon the amount of colloid present. Thus, the basic pattern is that of an adenocarcinoma or a papillary carcinoma and other appearances generally represent simply greater degrees of malignancy of these two fundamental lesions (Fig. 260). *Adenocarcinoma* (follicular, alveolar, or acinar carcinoma) varies considerably in appearance. On the one hand, the tumor resembles closely a colloid adenoma or, for that matter, a normal thyroid and it has thus been called (erroneously) "benign metastasizing goiter." At the other extreme, the tumor is composed of small, ill-formed, irregular glands lined by one, two, or more layers of cuboidal or columnar epithelial cells with ill-defined borders, varying amounts of cytoplasm, and round, oval, or irregular, hyperchromatic nuclei. The lumens of the glands may or may not contain colloid. *Papillary carcinoma* may be relatively pure or may exist in combinations with an adenocarcinoma. When the tumor is less malignant, it is indistinguishable from a papillary adenoma (Fig. 258). As the growth increases in malignancy the papillæ become less distinct, the connective tissue stalks become thin, and the covering epithelium becomes more irregular. It may be one, two, or more layers thick and is composed of cuboidal, columnar, or irregular epithelial cells with indistinct borders, varying amounts of cytoplasm, and hyperchromatic nuclei. When the lesions become highly malignant the basic pattern is completely replaced by clumps, masses, sheets, or individually infiltrating cells with little or no attempt at glandular or papillary formation. Such lesions may be referred to as *diffuse carcinomas* and then further qualified as to *round cell, spindle cell,* or *giant cell,* depending upon the type of cell that predominates. *Round cell carcinomas* are usually composed of rather small, sharply-defined, round cells with a moderate or scanty amount of cytoplasm and round hyperchromatic nuclei. *Spindle cell carcinomas,* as their name suggests, are composed of elongated or spindle cells with a moderate amount of ill-defined, eosinophilic cytoplasm and elongated nuclei. The lesion resembles a sarcoma. In either case, round cell and spindle cell tumors are relatively uniform in appearance. *Giant cell carcinoma,* on the other hand, is composed of polyhedral, often grotesque cells with abundant cytoplasm and single or multiple, hyperchromatic nuclei. In each of the more malignant tumors the stroma is usually scanty or imperceptible. In addition to the histologic types of growths already listed, mention should be made of a squamous cell carcinoma and a Hurthle cell tumor. *Squamous cell carcinoma* is rare and morphologically consists of polyhedral cells similar to a squamous cell carcinoma elsewhere in the body. A *Hurthle cell tumor* is an adenocarcinoma. It is composed of relatively uniform appearing, large, plump, columnar epithelial cells with dense, intensely eosinophilic cytoplasm and round or at most oval, evenly stained, centrally placed nuclei (Fig. 261). The origin of Hurthle cells is not agreed upon. They have been considered to represent oncocytes, postbranchial inclusions, and simply epithelial cells that have undergone a pathophysiologic change. Of these, the last mentioned theory appears to be the most

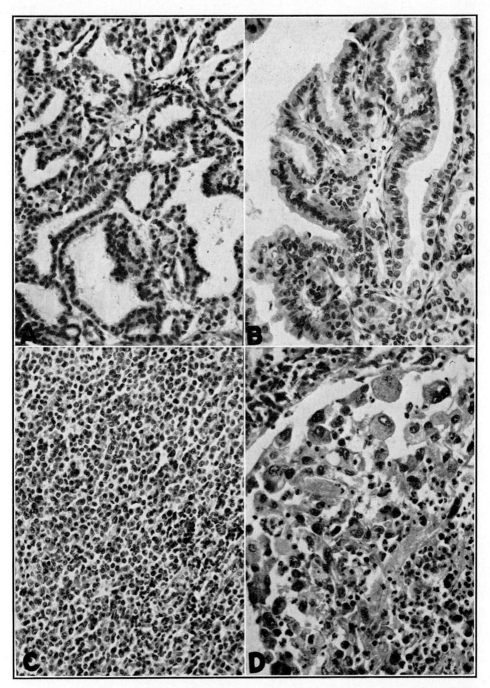

Fig. 260.—Carcinoma of the thyroid showing *A*, a well-differentiated adenocarcinoma with large and small colloid-containing or empty glands lined with a single layer of cuboidal epithelial cells, *B*, papillary carcinoma consisting of thin connective tissue stalks covered with irregular columnar epithelial cells, *C*, diffuse carcinoma of a round cell variety with rather uniform-appearing cells, and *D*, giant cell carcinoma with large sharply circumscribed cells disclosing abundant cytoplasm and hyperchromatic nuclei. Some of the cells have undergone necrosis. × 200.

plausible. Hurthle cell tumors have also been called small alveolar large cell adenocarcinoma, struma postbranchialis, Getzowa tumor, Barbar tumor, and acidophilic adenocarcinoma (Chesky). In closing the microscopic description, it should again be emphasized that carcinomas of the thyroid of low-grade malignancy are morphologically indistinguishable from some adenomatous hyperplasias or solitary adenomas. Thus, aside from regarding all papillary tumors (regardless of their appearance) with suspicion, the pathologist relies heavily upon infiltration of the capsule of the nodule and the capsule of the thyroid gland itself by tumor tissue and upon the presence of tumor cells within blood vessels and lymphatic channels.

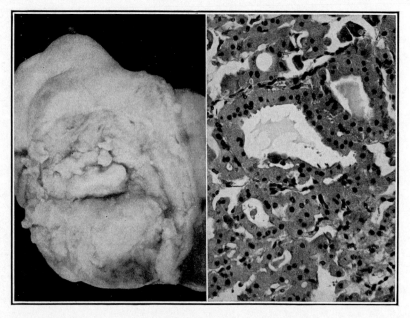

Fig. 261.—Hurthle cell tumor illustrating, to the left, a mass of moderately firm gray tissue and, to the right, large, intensely eosinophilic cells in glandular formation. × 100. (Herbut, *Surgical Pathology*, 2nd Ed., Lea & Febiger.)

Spread of carcinoma of the thyroid is by direct extension, lymphatics, and blood vessels. By direct extension the tumor infiltrates adjacent structures such as muscles, larynx, trachea, esophagus, and larger arteries and veins. By lymphatic channels the growths metastasize first to the deep cervical lymph nodes in relation to the omohyoid muscle and clavicle and then to other lymph nodes in the mediastinum and elsewhere. By blood vessels the tumors metastasize to the lungs, bones, liver, and almost any other tissue and organ of the body.

The *complications* of carcinoma of the thyroid consist of (1) extension of the tumor to adjacent structures, (2) metastasis, and (3) hyperthyroidism. Excessive function of the thyroid gland is said to occur in as high as 33 per cent of all cases of carcinoma (Ward). Some of the hyperthyroidism is due to hyperactivity on the part of the remaining uninvolved thyroid tissue while some is also due to excessive activity on the part of the tumor tissue. The *clinical manifestations* in early carcinoma of the thyroid gland consist simply of single or multiple nodules or, less often, of a diffuse enlargement of the organ. Sometimes, however, the primary lesion may be so small that it is not detectable at all by physical examination or is found only with difficulty. As the lesion increases in size and penetrates the capsule it infiltrates the adjacent tissues and produces symptoms and signs of compression similar to those found in diffuse colloid goiter, adenomatous hyperplasia, or Riedel's struma. The *diagnosis* of carcinoma of the thyroid in the last analysis is made only by histologic examination of removed tissue or belatedly by demonstration of metastasis roentgenographically. It follows, therefore, that every nodular hyperplasia of the thyroid, especially if the nodule is single, should be removed and subjected to most careful microscopic scrutiny. *Treatment* of choice is surgical removal. When the lesion is confined to one lobe, complete removal of the involved lobe and the isthmus together with removal of the lymph nodes on the affected side is considered to be sufficient by many authors. When the lesion is more extensive or bilateral, total thyroidectomy and bilateral neck dissection is indicated. When the tumor cannot be removed surgically or when metastases have occurred, external irradiation or administration of radioactive iodine is indicated. The latter, however, is effective only in cases of adenocarcinoma or papillary carcinoma with good differentiation. The *prognosis* varies greatly. It is better when the lesion is discovered incidentally to a thyroidectomy than it is when the condition is suspected clinically for the obvious reason that the former lesions are usually in an earlier stage of development. In general also, the outlook is better in patients with well-differentiated adenocarcinomas, papillary carcinomas, and Hurthle cell tumors as compared with the more highly anaplastic diffuse carcinomas. Finally, since the lesions in children and young adults are usually of the well-differentiated papillary or adenomatous variety, the prognosis is better in this group than it is in the older age group in which the growths tend to be of a more diffuse nature.

Other Tumors. —Aside from epithelial growths, other *primary tumors* of the thyroid gland are lymphoblastoma, plasmocytoma, hemangio-endothelioma, lipoma, liposarcoma, fibroma, fibrosarcoma, osteoma, osteosarcoma, and teratoma. *Secondary tumors* arise as (1) direct extensions from the larynx, esophagus, or metastatic masses in cervical lymph nodes and (2) metastases from distant areas such as the lung, kidney, and other organs.

REFERENCES

Pathologic Physiology

DeGroat, L. J., et al.: J. Clin. Endocrinol. & Metab., 18, 158, 1958 (Peptide-linked Iodotyrosines and Iodothyronines in Blood of a Patient with Congenital Goiter).

Doniach, D., and Roitt, I. M.: J. Clin. Endocrinol. & Metab., 17, 1293, 1957 (Auto-immunity in Hashimoto's Disease and Its Implications).

Rawson, R. W., and Rall, J. E.: The Endocrinology of Neoplastic Disease, Recent Progress in Hormone Research, New York, Academic Press, Vol. XI, 257, 1955.

Rosenberg, I. N., and Astwood, E. B.: Glandular Physiology and Therapy, 5th Ed., Philadelphia, J. B. Lippincott Co., 1954, p. 258.

Stanbury, J. B., et al.: Endemic Goiter, Cambridge, Mass., Harvard University Press, 1954.

General

Arey, L. B.: Developmental Anatomy, 5th Ed., Philadelphia, W. B. Saunders Co., 1946.

Leblond, C. P., and Gross, J.: J. Clin. Endocrinol., 9, 149, 1949 (Secretion of Thyroxin).

McGavack, T. H.: The Thyroid, St. Louis, C. V. Mosby Co., 1951.

Congenital Anomalies

CRISPELL, K. R., and PARSON, W.: South. M. J., *43*, 945, 1950 (Lingual Thyroid).
HURXTHAL, L. M., and MUSULIN, N.: Am. J. Med., *1*, 56, 1946 (Cretinism).
MARSHALL, S. F., and BECKER, W. F.: Ann. Surg., *129*, 642, 1949 (Thyroglossal Remnants).
MILLES, G.: Am. J. Path., *31*, 997, 1955 (Goiters Sporadic Cretins).
MULLINGER, M., *et al.*: Canad. M. A. J., *66*, 560, 1952 (Cretinism).
PICKERING, D. E., *et al.*: J. Dis. Child., *93*, 510, 1957 (Goiters Sporadic Cretins).
STANBURY, J. B., and McGIRR, E. M.: Am. J. Med., *22*, 712, 1957 (Goiters Sporadic Cretins).
TIMMONS, J. R., and TIMMONS, J. M.: Ann. Surg., *133*, 90, 1951 (Lingual Thyroid).
TOPPER, A.: Am. J. Dis. Child., *81*, 233, 1951 (Cretinism).
WARD, G. E., *et al.*: Surg., Gynec. & Obst., *89*, 727, 1949 (Thyroglossal Remnants).
WARREN, S., and FELDMAN, J. D.: Surg., Gynec. & Obst., *88*, 31, 1949 (Lateral Aberrant Thyroid).
WOZENCRAFT, P., *et al.*: Cancer, *1*, 574, 1948 (Lateral Aberrant Thyroid).

Inflammations

CRAIG, P. E., *et al.*: Am. J. Surg., *84*, 286, 1952 (Hashimoto's Struma).
CRILE, G., JR.: Ann. Int. Med., *37*, 519, 1952 (Thyroiditis).
CUMMINS, S. D., *et al.*: Arch. Path., *51*, 68, 1951 (Boeck's Sarcoid).
DAVISON, T. C., and LETTON, A. H.: J. Clin. Endocrinol., *9*, 980, 1949 (Hashimoto's Struma).
HIGBEE, D.: Ann. Otol., Rhin. & Laryngol., *52*, 620, 1946 (Acute Thyroiditis).
LINDSAY, S., *et al.*: J. Clin. Endocrinol., *12*, 1578, 1952 (Hashimoto's and Riedel's Struma).
MARSHALL, S. F., *et al.*: New England J. Med., *238*, 758, 1948 (Chronic Thyroiditis).
McGAVACK, T. H.: *The Thyroid*, St. Louis, C. V. Mosby Co., 1951.
POSTLETHWAIT, R. W., and BERG, P., JR.: A. M. A. Arch. Surg., *48*, 429, 1944 (Tuberculosis).
PRIOLEAU, W. H.: Surgery, *14*, 871, 1953 (Abscess).
WALKER, G. A.: Surg., Gynec. & Obst., *75*, 374, 1942 (Amyloid Goiter).
WESTWATER, J. O.: California Med., *76*, 66, 1952 (Subacute Thyroiditis).
WOMACK, N. A.: Surgery, *16*, 770, 1944 (Thyroiditis).

Physical Disturbances

BASTENIE, P. A.: J. Am. Geriat. Soc., *1*, 845, 1953 (Spontaneous Myxedema in Aged).
BERKHEISSER, S. W.: J. Clin. Endo. Metab., *15*, 44, 1955 (Adult Hypothyroidism).
CURTIS, R. R., and ARNOLD, W. O.: Med. Cl. N. Am., July, 1127, 1955 (Hypothyroidism).
McGAVACK, T. H.: *The Thyroid*, St. Louis, C. V. Mosby Co., 1951.

Tumors

ARONOFF, B. L.: Am. Surgeon, *18*, 362, 1952 (Papillary Carcinoma in Thyroglossal Cysts).
BARTELS, E. C.: Ann. Int. Med., *37*, 1123, 1952 (Treatment Hyperthyroidism).
BARTELS, E. C., and KINGSLEY, J. W., JR.: Geriatrics, *4*, 333, 1949 (Hyperthyroidism Over Sixty).
BEIRWALTES, W. H.: Ann. Int. Med., *37*, 23, 1952 (Radioactive Iodine Treatment of Carcinoma).
CERRISE, E. J., *et al.*: Surgery, *31*, 552, 1952 (Carcinoma in Nodular Goiter).
CHESKY, V. E., *et al.*: J. Clin. Endocrinol., *11*, 1535, 1951 (Hurthle Cell Tumor).
CLARK, D. E., *et al.*: J. A. M. A., *150*, 1269, 1952 (Radioactive Iodine in Hyperthyroidism).
COLE, W. H., *et al.*: J. Clin. Endocrinol., *9*, 1007, 1949 (Carcinoma in Nodular Goiter).
CRILE, G., JR., and DEMPSEY, W. S.: J. A. M. A., *139*, 1247, 1949 (Nodular Goiter).
CRILE, G., JR., and McCULLAGH, E. P.: Ann. Surg., *134*, 18, 1951 (Treatment Hyperthyroidism).
DAILEY, M. E., *et al.*: Am. J. Med., *9*, 194, 1950 (Carcinoma).
———: Arch. Int. Med., *83*, 382, 1949 (Nodular Goiter).
DeCOURCY, C. D., and DeCOURCY, J. L.: Am. J. Surg., *75*, 661, 1948 (Etiology of Goiter).
DOBYNS, B. M., and MALOFF, F.: J. Clin. Endocrinol., *11*, 1323, 1951 (Carcinoma Treated with Radioactive Iodine).
DUFFY, B. J., JR., and FITZGERALD, P. J.: Cancer, *3*, 1018, 1950 (Cancer in Childhood).
DUNCAN, J. A., *et al.*: West. J. Surg., *60*, 435, 1952 (Carcinoma).
ECKERT, C., and BYARS, L. T.: Ann. Surg., *136*, 83, 1952 (Papillary Carcinoma).
FRAZELL, E. L., and DUFFY, B. J., JR.: Cancer, *4*, 952, 1951 (Hurthle Cell Carcinoma).
GOLDBERG, R. C., and CHAIKOFF, I. L.: A. M. A. Arch. Path., *53*, 22, 1952 (Radioactive Iodine and Thyroid Cancer in Rats).

References

GRISWOLD, D., and KEATING, J. H., JR.: Am. Heart J., *38*, 813, 1949 (Heart in Hyperthyroidism).

HARE, H. F., and SALZMAN, F. A.: Am. J. Roentgenol., *63*, 881, 1950 (Carcinoma).

HELLWIG, C. A.: A. M. A. Arch. Path., *28*, 870, 1939 (Pathology Hyperthyroidism).

HEPTINSTALL, R. H., and PORRITT, A.: Brit. J. Surg., *39*, 433, 1952 (Nodular Goiter in Children).

HERMANSON, L., *et al.*: J. Clin. Endocrinol., *12*, 112, 1952 (Treatment Nodular Goiter).

HORN, R. C., JR., and RAVDIN, I. S.: J. Clin. Endocrinol., *11*, 1166, 1951 (Carcinoma in Youth).

HOWARD, M. A.: West. J. Surg., *59*, 163, 1951 (Carcinoma).

KIMBALL, O. P.: J. A. M. A., *130*, 80, 1946 (Iodized Salt in Endemic Goiter).

LINDSAY, S.: California Med., *71*, 207, 1949 (Pathology Nodular Goiter).

McGAVACK, T. H.: *The Thyroid*, St. Louis, C. V. Mosby Co., 1951.

MILES, G. O., and HARSHA, W. N.: Am. Surgeon, *18*, 117, 1952 (Management Carcinoma).

MURPHY, W. B., and AHNQUIST, G.: A. M. A. Arch. Surg., *35*, 211, 1937 (Fetal Adenoma).

RIVES, J. D., and SHEPARD, R. M.: Am. Surg., *17*, 406, 1951 (Thyroid Crisis).

ROBERTSON, C.: Lancet, *2*, 675, 1948 (Treatment Thyrotoxicosis).

SHAFFER, J. M.: A. M. A. Arch. Path., *29*, 20, 1940 (Liver in Hyperthyroidism).

SPENCE, A. W.: Brit. M. J., *2*, 529, 1952 (Pathogenesis Simple Goiter).

WARD, G. E., *et al.*: Ann. Surg., *131*, 473, 1950 (Carcinoma).

Chapter

14

Parathyroid Glands

PATHOLOGIC PHYSIOLOGY

Joseph J. Rupp

THE parathyroid glands secrete a *hormone*, called *parathormone*, which is of prime importance in the regulation of calcium and phosphorus metabolism. The rate of secretion of the parathyroid hormone is controlled by the levels of serum calcium—increasing when the calcium level decreases and decreasing when the calcium level rises.

When *excessive amounts* of parathyroid hormone are secreted, whether by an adenoma or by hyperplastic glands the clinical condition of *hyperparathyroidism* develops. In this condition the level of serum calcium increases, the level of serum phosphorus decreases, the urinary excretion of calcium and phosphorus increases, and a negative calcium balance is present. The high levels of the hormone decrease the renal tubular resorption of calcium and phosphorus and this, in turn, results in an increased loss of these electrolytes in the urine. These changes in the electrolytes, as well as a direct action of the hormone on bone, mobilize calcium and increase the level of the serum calcium. The loss of the mineral salts from bone causes decalcification, development of bone cysts, osteitis fibrosa cystica, possibly giant cell tumors, resorption of the lamina dura, and pathologic fractures. Any or all of these changes may occur in patients with hyperparathyroidism. The *clinical* manifestations of hyperparathyroidism may be divided into three main groups: osseous, renal, and those resulting from hypercalcemia. The skeletal changes lead to bone pain, bone tenderness, pathologic fractures, and skeletal deformities. When *osseous* changes are present the serum alkaline phosphatase levels are increased. As a result of the increased calcium load excreted by the kidney, renal stones and calcinosis frequently develop. Indeed, the *renal* symptoms are the most common and often the only ones the patient complains of. Should renal insufficiency develop, the electrolyte pattern is modified by uremia in which case the levels of serum phosphorus increase and those of calcium decrease. On the other hand, long-standing renal insufficiency with acidosis leads to excessive loss of calcium in the urine, secondary hyperparathyroidism, mobilization of calcium, and decrease of bone density. When the levels of serum are increased above 13 or 14 mg. per 100 ml. the symptoms of hypercalcemia may develop. These are nausea, vomiting, lethargy, and severe constipation— for the most part the reflection of the atony of the gastrointestinal tract induced by hypercalcemia.

Hyperparathyroidism should be considered in the differential diagnosis in all cases of *renal stones*. To arrive at such, a high index of suspicion is needed, since the changes in electrolytes often are not marked nor persistently elevated.   While the occurrence of *peptic ulcer* or *pancreatitis* in patients with hyperparathyroidism is less frequent than that of renal stone, their association with hyperparathyroidism is greater than mere co-incidence would indicate.   Other *conditions* in which *high levels* of *serum calcium* occur and which must be considered in the differential diagnosis of hyperparathyroidism include Boeck's sarcoid, hypervitaminosis D, multiple myeloma, milk-alkali syndrome, metastatic bone disease, and tumors, especially of the kidney, which sometimes produce hypercalcemia without evidence of bone spread.

The clinical manifestations of *hypoparathyroidism* are those resulting from the low serum calcium levels.   In this condition, whether idiopathic or postoperative, the level of serum calcium is decreased and the level of phosphorus is increased.   The urinary excretion of calcium and phosphorus is decreased.   The major clinical manifestation is increased neuromuscular irritability which may result in tetany.   In children, the occurrence of convulsions as a result of hypocalcemia often leads to an erroneous diagnosis of idiopathic epilepsy.   The hypocalcemia may cause changes in tissues of ectodermal origin resulting in such lesions as cataracts, calcification of the brain, loss of hair, changes in the enamel and loss of teeth, and brittle nails.

Pseudohypoparathyroidism is a condition attended by hypocalcemia, normal-appearing parathyroid glands, and (often) physical and mental retardation.   It results from lack of response of the renal tubules to parathyroid hormone.   The condition should be differentiated from the malabsorption syndrome where hypocalcemia may also be present.

GENERAL CONSIDERATIONS

The parathyroid glands *develop* as thickenings of the third and fourth pharyngeal pouches.   The pair from the third pouches is drawn inferiorly with the migrating thymic tissue to rest at the inferior border of the thyroid gland, while the pair from the fourth pouches remains near the superior border of the thyroid gland.

Departing somewhat from the established outline used in other sections of the book, disorders of the parathyroid glands can perhaps be considered best under the following headings: Congenital Anomalies, Hypoparathyroidism, and Hyperparathyroidism.

CONGENITAL ANOMALIES

Normally there are four parathyroid glands distributed in relation to the thyroid gland.   On each side, one is located inferiorly at the posterolateral border of each lobe in relation to the inferior thyroid artery and the other is located superiorly at the junction of the upper and middle thirds of the thyroid or approximately opposite the lower border of the cricoid cartilage.

Developmental abnormalities consist of (1) variations in *number* of glands — either less than, or more than, four, (2) *aberrant locations* — within the thyroid, anterior to the thyroid, behind the esophagus, within the thymus, and at any level between the upper portion of the neck through the mediastinum to the diaphragm (Buchanan and Staub), and (3) *cysts*.   Cysts of the parathyroid glands are rare (Maxwell).   They occur in the lateral cervical region, may be large enough (10 cm. or more in diameter) to attract clinical attention, are lined by cuboidal epithelium, and contain parathyroid tissue in their walls.

HYPOPARATHYROIDISM

Hypoparathyroidism connotes simply hyposecretion of parathormone and, thus, hypofunction of the parathyroid glands. The condition may *occur* (1) as a result of removal (during thyroidectomy) of the parathyroid glands, leaving insufficient tissue present to take care of the body needs, or (2) idiopathically, that is, of unknown cause but theoretically resulting from congenital hypoplasia or aplasia or from destruction of the glands by hemorrhage or infection. The *incidence* of post-thyroidectomy hypoparathyroidism has decreased precipitously in recent years until, at present, it occurs (in the better clinics) in less than 1.5 per cent of all operations on the thyroid gland (MacBryde). Paralleling operations on the neck, this type of hypoparathyroidism is more common in females than in males and is usually seen after the age of thirty years. The incidence of true idiopathic hypoparathyroidism is difficult to determine but the condition is rare for, by 1952, there were only 52 acceptable cases recorded (Steinberg). It occurs in females as often as in males and the average age of onset is about seventeen years. *Pathologically* normal parathyroid tissue is found in abnormally small amounts or is entirely absent. The *clinical manifestations* are due mainly to a decreased level of calcium in the circulating blood. They consist of (1) tetany (carpopedal spasm) or convulsions—occurring spontaneously or provoked by excitement, exertion, overbreathing, or menstruation, (2) tetanic equivalents—paresthesias, numbness, muscle cramps, or laryngeal stridor, (3) gastrointestinal disturbances—pain, gas, and alternating constipation and diarrhea, (4) psychosis, (5) nervousness, (6) ectodermal changes—bilateral cataracts, brittle hair, loss of hair, and ridged nails and teeth, (7) hypocalcemia (to as low as 3 mgm. per cent) and hyperphosphatemia (to as high as 14 mgm. per cent), and (8) occasionally increased density of bones roentgenographically. The *diagnosis* is made from the clinical manifestations, especially the determination of blood calcium and phosphorus. *Treatment* consists of administration of vitamin D, calcium, and parathormone. The *prognosis* is variable—the morbidity being great but the mortality remaining low.

HYPERPARATHYROIDISM

Hyperparathyroidism signifies hypersecretion of parathormone and, therefore, hyperactivity of the parathyroid glands. The condition is generally divided into two groups—primary and secondary. *Primary* hyperparathyroidism results from primary hyperplasia or neoplasia of the parathyroid glands with excessive production of parathormone. The cause of the condition is not known, although it is thought by some to be the result of direct hormonal stimulation. The disorder is three times as common in females as it is in males and, although it occurs at all periods of life, it is most common between the ages of thirty and sixty years. *Secondary* hyperparathyroidism is a state where the greater than normal production of parathormone results from secondary hyperplasia of the parathyroid glands which, in turn, represents a compensatory response to an increased demand for the hormone on the part of the body. It occurs in cases of rickets, osteomalacia, decreased calcium in the diet, pregnancy, lactation, and chronic disorders of the kidneys (Blackwell). Of these, the most common is chronic glomerulonephritis. In this condition, the diseased kidney is unable to excrete waste endogenous phosphates from the body, resulting instead in their excretion through the intestinal mucosa. This blocks the absorption of calcium from the food which, in turn, results in calcium starvation and mobilization of calcium from the bones by way of hyperactivity and hyperplasia of the parathyroid glands (Hughes and Gislason).

Normally the fundamental cell in the parathyroid glands is the *chief* or *principle cell* (Castleman and Mallory). It gives rise to both the water-clear and the oxyphil cells. The chief cell forms most of the parathyroid gland until puberty. It measures from 6 to 8 microns in diameter, is polyhedral and ill defined, possesses a scanty amount of lightly acidophilic cytoplasm, and discloses a large, round nucleus that occupies approximately one-half of the cell. The *water-clear* cell is present after puberty in some of the glands. It measures from 10 to 15 microns in diameter, is more sharply defined than the chief cell, contains vacuolated or clear cytoplasm, and discloses a pyknotic, eccentric nucleus. The *oxyphil* cell is first noted at puberty and is found in increasing numbers thereafter. It may be pale or dark. The pale oxyphil cell occurs in circumscribed clumps or masses, is polygonal, has sharp borders, discloses dark, finely granular cytoplasm, reveals a round, deeply staining nucleus, and measures from 11 to 14 microns in diameter. The *dark* oxyphil cell usually appears singly near the stroma, possesses indistinct borders, discloses homogeneously dark red cytoplasm and a pyknotic nucleus, and measures from 8 to 10 microns in diameter. The *stroma* in a normal parathyroid gland is of a loose connective tissue variety and contains an increasing deposition of fat from puberty to approximately forty years of age. After puberty the glands are prone to undergo cystic degeneration with the cysts containing granular or eosinophilic material. *Grossly* each parathyroid gland measures approximately $6 \times 4 \times 2$ mm. and weighs about 0.03 grams.

The important *pathologic* changes in the parathyroid glands that occur in connection with hyperparathyroidism have been ably reviewed by Norris, Murphy, Black, Wolner, and others. They consist of adenoma, primary hyperplasia, secondary hyperplasia, and carcinoma. *Adenoma* is usually single but it may be multiple. It accounts for over 80 per cent of all cases of primary hyperparathyroidism. It is four times as common in the lower parathyroids as it is in the upper glands, occurs with equal frequency on either side, and, in about 10 per cent of cases, is aberrant in position. While the size varies up to 4.9 cm. in greatest diameter and the weight to 120 gm., the average diameter is generally less than 1 cm. and the average weight is about 3 gm. The tumor is sharply circumscribed, encapsulated, yellowish brown to tan, and moderately firm. Cystic degeneration and hemorrhage are frequent, while calcification occurs occasionally. Histologically the tumor consists of any one or any combination of relatively normal-appearing, chief, water-clear, or oxyphil cells. Of these, the chief cells usually predominate (Fig. 262) and, only rarely, is the entire tumor composed of oxyphil cells (Fig. 263). The cells are usually arranged diffusely, in sheets, or in strands but occasionally they form papillary processes or glands. The stroma is scanty and devoid of fat and the vascularity is moderate. *Primary hyperplasia* consists of an enlargement of all the glands to a point where the total weight may exceed 65 gm. The glands are poorly encapsulated, grayish white, and soft. They may disclose cysts and hemorrhagic extravasation. Peripheral excrescences, referred to as pseudopods, are commonly seen. Histologically the lesion consists of hyperplasia and hypertrophy of

38

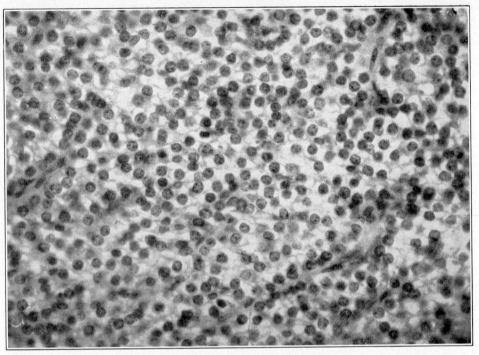

FIG. 262.—Adenoma of the parathyroid gland showing mostly
uniform-appearing chief cells. × 400.

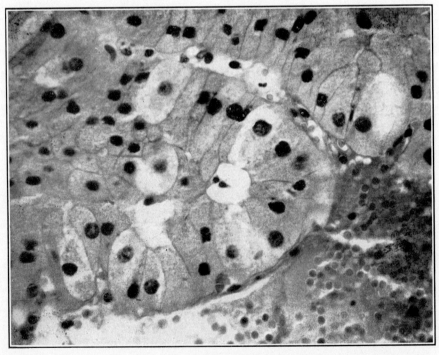

FIG. 263.—Adenoma of the parathyroid gland illustrating mostly large
polyhedral sharply defined oxyphil cells. × 400.

mainly the water-clear cells (Fig. 264). They measure from 10 to 40 microns in diameter, possess vacuolated but occasionally eosinophilic granular cytoplasm, and disclose varisized (usually 6 to 7 microns but occasionally larger) nuclei that are basilar in position. The cells are arranged in compact masses, glands, or pseudoglands. *Secondary hyperplasia* consists of enlargement (but to a lesser degree than in primary hyperplasia) of all the parathyroid glands with, however, a more irregular variation from gland to gland (Black and Fritz). Histologically the stroma and fat of the glands are depleted and the columns of cells are widened. Ultimately the cells consist of masses or sheets. In most of the cases they are composed of normal sized chief and water-clear cells, with little variation in size and

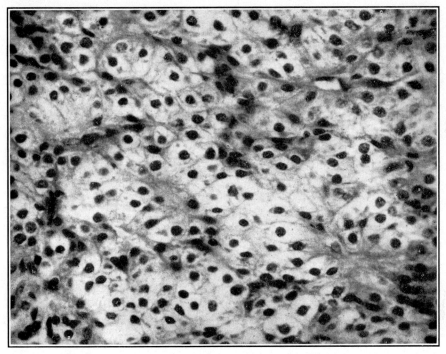

FIG. 264.—Primary hyperplasia of the parathyroid gland
showing large water-clear cells. × 400.

staining qualities (Fig. 265). In severe cases of long standing renal disease the predominating cell may, however, be of the water-clear variety. In either case, islands of oxyphil cells may be more numerous than those in a normal gland from a person of the same age. *Carcinoma* of the parathyroid glands is rare, there having been only 19 cases recorded in the literature by 1950 (Stephenson). Of these 19 cases, 9 were nonfunctioning while 10 were functioning. Histologically the tumors are similar to adenomas except that (1) there is more variation in shape, size, and staining qualities of the cells, (2) mitoses are more numerous, and (3) the capsule, blood vessels, and lymphatic channels are invaded by neoplastic cells. The carcinomas have a tendency to involve adjacent structures of the neck by direct extension and to metastasize to the lungs, the cervical and mediastinal lymph nodes, pleura, kidneys, and other portions of the body.

The *complications* of hyperplasia and neoplasia of the parathyroid glands may be listed as follows: (1) hypercalcemia resulting in decreased irritability of muscles which, in turn, brings about lethargy and weakness, (2) metastatic calcification (p. 64) consisting of: (*a*) deposition of calcium in the lungs, kidneys, myocardium, gastric mucosa, blood vessels, conjunctiva, cornea, etc., and (*b*) formation of calculi in the kidneys, (3) withdrawal of calcium from the bone resulting in the formation of osteitis fibrosa cystica (p. 1251), and (4) tetany developing postoperatively. The *clinical manifestations* are usually of one to twenty or more years' duration (Murphy) but they may be acute and of only a few months' duration (Waife). They

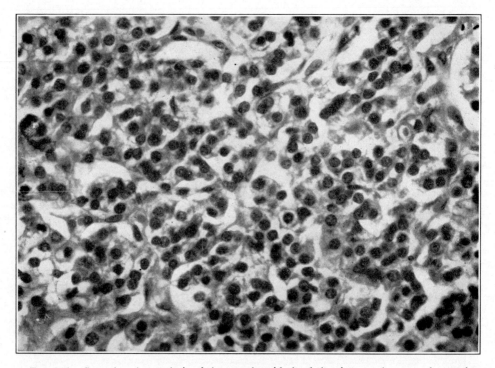

Fig. 265.—Secondary hyperplasia of the parathyroid gland showing mostly water-clear and chief cells but also smaller, darker oxyphil cells. × 400.

are due to the complications listed above and, as such, may be enumerated as follows: (1) weakness, lassitude, easy fatigability, constipation, nausea, vomiting, anorexia, and cramp-like abdominal pain—due to hypercalcemia, (2) renal colic, hematuria, secondary renal infection, and renal insufficiency —due to deposition of calcium in the kidney and to renal calculi (Miller), and (3) pain, fracture, deformities, and roentgenographic changes in the bones (osteitis fibrosa cystica)—due to resorption of calcium. The important laboratory findings are hypercalcemia, hypophosphatemia, and, in the presence of bone destruction, elevated alkaline phosphatase. The *diagnosis* is made from a consideration of the clinical manifestations and the laboratory findings. *Treatment* consists of parathyroidectomy. The *prognosis*, when the condition is discovered and treated relatively early, is generally excellent.

REFERENCES

Pathologic Physiology

ALBRIGHT, F., and REIFENSTEIN, E. C.: *The Parathyroid Glands and Metabolic Bone Disease*, Baltimore, Williams & Wilkins Co., 1948.

HOWARD, J. E.: J. Clin. Endocrinol. & Metab., *17*, 1105, 1957 (Review Calcium Metabolism).

MUNSON, P. L.: Ann. N. Y. Acad. Sc., *60*, 776, 1955 (Parathyroids in Calcium and Phosphorous Metabolism).

REIFENSTEIN, E. C., and HOWARD, R. P.: Glandular Physiology and Therapy, 5th Ed., Philadelphia, J. B. Lippincott Co., 1954, p. 351.

WILKINS, L.: Ann. N. Y. Acad. Sc., *60*, 763, 1955 (Hormones Skeletal Growth).

General

BLACK, B. K., and ACKERMAN, L. V.: Cancer, *3*, 415, 1950 (Tumors).

BLACKWELL, C. C.: Am. J. Surg., *82*, 439, 1951 (Adenoma).

BUCHANAN, L. C.: Am. Surgeon, *18*, 439, 1952 (Hidden Adenoma).

CASTLEMAN, B., and MALLORY, T. B.: Am. J. Path., *11*, 1, 1935 (Pathology in Hyperparathyroidism).

FRITZ, G. E., and BRINES, O. A.: Am. J. Path., *27*, 265, 1951 (Secondary Hyperplasia).

HUGHES, B., and GISLASON, G. J.: J. Urol., *55*, 330, 1946 (Secondary Hyperparathyroidism).

MACBRYDE, C. M.: Surgery, *16*, 804, 1944 (Surgical Hypoparathyroidism).

MAXWELL, D. E., *et al.*: A. M. A. Arch. Surg., *64*, 208, 1952 (Cysts).

MILLER, A., and MITCHELL, J. P.: Brit. J. Urol., *24*, 91, 1952 (Hyperparathyroidism and Renal Calculi).

MURPHY, R., *et al.*: A. M. A. Arch. Int. Med., *89*, 783, 1952 (Primary Hyperparathyroidism).

NORRIS, E. H.: Internat. Abst. Surg., *84*, 1, 1947 (Adenoma).

STAUB, W., *et al.*: A. M. A. Arch. Int. Med., *85*, 765, 1950 (Mediastinal Adenoma).

STEINBERG, H., and WALDRON, B. R.: Medicine, *31*, 133, 1952 (Idiopathic Hypoparathyroidism).

STEPHENSON, H. U., JR.: A. M. A. Arch. Surg., *60*, 247, 1950 (Malignant Tumors).

WAIFE, S. O.: Am. J. M. Sci., *218*, 624, 1949 (Acute Hyperparathyroidism).

WOLNER, L. B., *et al.*: Cancer, *5*, 1069, 1952 (Tumors and Hyperplasia).

Chapter

15

Upper Digestive System

PATHOLOGIC PHYSIOLOGY

M. H. F. FRIEDMAN

THE *principal activities* of the *mouth* and *pharynx* are concerned with the ingestion of food and include taste perception, salivation, and the preliminary phases of deglutition. Of no less importance are the activities concerned with respiration, speech, and defence. Since each of these functions is carried out by interdigitative actions of nearly all the organs comprising the mouth and pharynx, it is understandable why a disorder in one organ is accompanied by impairment in several functions. The absence of teeth resulting in difficulties in mastication and phonation, and edema of the larynx resulting in difficulties in respiration, phonation and deglutition, are common examples.

Speech is perhaps the most sophisticated of the numerous integrated functions exhibited by the human central nervous and neuromuscular systems. Contractions of the diaphragm and intercostal muscles send a column of air from the lungs flowing through the aperture of the glottis over the vocal cords. The intensity of the sound is regulated by the volume of the air blast, while the pitch is regulated by the tension of the vocal cords. The vibrations are amplified by resonators consisting of the mouth, nose, pharynx, trachea, and possibly also paranasal sinuses, which explains the change in voice quality in *coryza*. The sounds which are produced are converted to phonation of speech by the tongue, teeth, lips, and cheeks. *Edema* of the base of the epiglottis and vocal cords (occurring here more readily than elsewhere in the pharynx because of the loose areolar tissue and low tissue turgor) results in *"loss of voice."* *Hoarseness* is also produced by impaired vibrations of the cords as by papillomas or ulceration of the vocal cords.

Taste is a sensory perception due to activation of special chemoreceptors or taste buds which are distributed principally over the tongue and palate but also found on other parts of the mouth and pharynx. Little is known about the physical factors involved except that a substance to be tasted must be in solution. Specific receptors are present for the tastes of sour and salt but sweet and bitter are probably sensed by a common receptor. In addition to the taste buds, the gustatory qualities of a food depend also on tactile receptors in the mouth and on olfaction. The statement that most of the so-called tastes are actually odors is readily borne out by the decreased gustatory discrimination which is experienced during nasal congestion. Normally the sense of taste assists in determining the palatability of a food but the receptors may also be stimulated by certain substances in

(598)

the circulation. The *diabetic* may complain of a sweet taste and the patient with *jaundice* frequently has a "bitter mouth."

Chewing consists of prehension of food and reducing it to size suitable for swallowing. The biting functions of the incisor teeth are made possible by the overbite of the upper jaw. This permits the food to be sheared (as by scissors) and requires less force than would cutting. Biting is impaired when the upper and lower *incisor* surfaces *meet closely* as well as when they are *misaligned*, as in marked protrusion or retrusion of the jaw or in "*buck teeth.*" In such individuals, biting is often substituted by the tearing of the food with the canine teeth which are primarily used for grasping and for defence (*vide* the prominent fangs of the ape).

The role of *mastication* or grinding is performed by the molars. This involves movements of the jaw in three planes, namely, up and down for crushing, protrusion and retraction, and side to side motion for grinding. (The motions of the jaws in the lateral planes are illustrated nicely in cattle during rumination). The jaw movements of mastication may be voluntary but usually are involuntary and comprise reflex rhythmic activities of the jaw extensor and flexor muscles. These are in the nature of reciprocal excitation and inhibition rather analogous to the muscle movements in walking. The simultaneous contraction of all jaw muscles leads to "*lock jaw,*" due to the greater force exerted by the contractors, while paralysis of all muscles results in "*hang-jaw,*" due to gravitational force. In addition to the jaws, mastication also involves movements of the tongue, cheeks, and lips—all coordinated by a *chewing center* located probably in association with the deglutition center.

The comminution of the *food* and its *mixing* with *saliva*, which occurs during chewing, are necessary steps in the formation of a food bolus preparatory to swallowing. These, however, are not the important functions of chewing nor are they essential to the body economy. Perhaps the most important benefits derived from chewing are due to the *secretion* of *gastric* (and possibly also *pancreatic*) *juices* by reflexes elicited from the mouth. The excitation of taste and tactile receptors as well as nasal olfactory receptors promptly provokes a sustained enzyme-rich secretion from the gastric glands. Gastric digestion can thus commence as soon as food reaches the stomach after only a relatively brief interval in the mouth. Reflex gastric secretion is important in the management of patients, especially children, who require alimentation by gastric fistula because of *obstructive* lesions of the *esophagus* (such as lye strictures). The subject is found to maintain a better nutritional state if before and during each gastric feeding he is permitted to chew (and expectorate) foods from which he derives pleasurable gustatory sensations.

Salivary secretion occurs constantly, and apparently spontaneously, but the basal secretory rate is rapidly augmented by buccal reflexes excited by the taste and chewing of food. The cells of the small buccal glands are all mucous cells, those of the parotid gland all serous, while those of the submaxillary and sublingual glands are combinations of the two in varying ratios. The composition of saliva will thus vary with the proportion contributed by the various glands and this will, in turn, depend upon the nature of the stimulus. The basal salivary secretion is important in keeping the mouth and nasopharynx moist and were it not for this the sensitivity of olfactory and taste receptors to environmental gases, including obnoxious fumes, would suffer. Probably the impaired sense of taste found among "*mouth breathers*" is in part due to the dry mouth.

The secretion of *saliva* is exclusively under *nervous regulation*. The nervous influence on salivation is both by ecbolic and hydrelatic stimulation of the alveolar secretory cells and by regulation of blood flow to the glands. The cranial autonomic system (parasympathetic) supplies secretory fibers to the gland cells and dilator fibers to the arterioles. The thoracico-lumbar system (sympathetic) supplies pressor fibers to the myo-epithelial cells which surround certain alveoli and constrictor fibers to the blood vessels. It is evident that on diffuse *sympathetic stimulation*, as in fright, the reduced blood flow to the salivary glands will result in a dry mouth. Contrariwise, *sympathectomy* of the salivary glands results in profuse salivation or paralytic secretion. Due to removal of tonic vasoconstrictor influences, lesions of the cervical sympathetics may be associated by drooling at the mouth.

The usual *stimuli* for *salivary secretion* are the taste and chewing of food and conditioned reflexes established on these responses. The *sight* and *odor* of food or the *sound* of *food* being prepared readily cause watering of the mouth.

The *salivary center*, situated in proximity to the masticatory and degluti- tion centers, integrates secretion with other mouth and throat activities. The *salivary glands* show to a remarkable degree the *phenomenon* of *adaptivity* to the nature of the stimulus. Thus, *acid* placed in the mouth provokes a profuse secretion of watery saliva which serves to dilute the acid and make it less corrosive. Since the parotid gland is entirely serous secreting, most of the acid-stimulated saliva comes from the parotid. In *obstruction* by compression of the *ducts* of the parotid gland, as in *mumps*, the introduction of vinegar or lemon juice into the mouth will give rise to pain due to dis- tention of the duct by the secretion. With drier foods, such as powders or crackers, the secretion is at first watery and then becomes viscous. The watery saliva dissolves much of the dry material while undissolved particles are placed in suspension by the mucus. The mucus further serves to put a coating around hard or sharply-edged particles which might be errosive to the esophageal mucosa.

Secretion of *saliva* may be *provoked* by stimulation of the esophagus, as by distention with a food bolus or foreign body lodged in the esophagus. The saliva, on being swallowed, initiates a new series of peristaltic waves which act to carry the stuck bolus of food into the stomach. This esophago- salivary reflex also is found in the presence of *tumors* of the esophagus and, consequently, all conditions of excessive salivation of unknown cause war- rant investigation with this in mind. Excessive salivation in children too young to talk should also make one alert to the possibility of the presence of a *foreign body*, such as a toy, in the esophagus. Due to esophageal irritation by regurgitated gastric juice salivation may, at times, be quite profuse in patients with peptic ulcer and in others experiencing nausea. *Sialorrhea* of pregnancy, which may be an inherited characteristic, is seen in some women early enough to be the first sign of pregnancy. This should be distinguished from apparent sialorrhea which is due to unswallowed basal secretion which accumulates because of dysphagia.

CONGENITAL ANOMALIES

Developmental malformations of the mouth may best be considered under the structures that compose this part of the digestive system. Accordingly, they may be listed as follows: (A) *Lips:* (1) hare lip—vertical splitting of the lip, affecting most commonly the upper lip, resulting from a failure of

union of the frontonasal and maxillary processes, being unilateral or bilateral, and extending as far as the wing of the nose, (2) macrocheilia—large
lips, (3) microchelia—small lips, and (4) hypertrophy of the frenum labii;
(B) *Jaw:* (1) micrognathia—underdevelopment of both jaws or either
jaw, (2) macrognathia—overdevelopment of both jaws or either jaw, (3)
agnathia—absence of a jaw, (4) retrusion or retraction—location of the jaw
posterior to its normal position, and (5) protrusion or protraction—location
of the jaw anterior to its normal position; (C) *Teeth:* (1) malocclusion, (2)
partial or maleruption, (3) diastema—separation, especially of the incisor
teeth in which case there is also hypertrophy of the frenum labii, (4) supernumary teeth, (5) union of adjacent teeth, (6) megadontism—increase in
size of the crowns and roots of all teeth, (7) microdontism—decrease in
size of the crowns and roots of all teeth, (8) hypoplasia—decrease in size of
some teeth or parts of some teeth, and (9) dysplasia—defective formation;
(D) *Palate:* (1) cleft—frequently associated with hare lip, occurring as a
result of failure of union of the palatal processes, and consisting of a split
in the soft palate or in the soft and hard palates, and (2) atresia of the soft
palate; (E) *Tongue:* (1) macroglossia—enlargement, (2) microglossia—
decrease in size, (3) aglossia—absence, (4) ankyloglossia or tongue-tied—
anchoring of the tongue to the floor of the mouth due to a short or anteriorly shifted frenum, (5) bifid tongue—splitting of the tip due to failure of
union of the two halves of the tongue, (6) absence of papillæ, (7) grooved or
fissured tongue—linear defects generally located longitudinally but also
having side branches, (8) median rhomboid glossitis—diamond-shaped,
nonpapillary area just anterior to the foramen caecum, and (9) geographic
tongue—irregular, map-like denudations of the epithelium; (F) *Opening:*
(1) macrostomia—large mouth and (2) microstomia—small mouth; (G)
Salivary Glands: (1) absence, (2) cysts—single or multiple, of varying sizes,
lined with squamous epithelium, and generally occurring in the parotid
gland, and (3) sialectasis—dilatation of the ducts of generally the parotid
gland and occurring unilaterally or bilaterally; (H) *Branchial Remnants:*
(1) first branchial cleft—uncommon, resulting from maldevelopment of the
first and second branchial arches and/or the first branchial cleft, and consisting of malformations or absence of the auricle (ear), of pre-auricular
tabs and sinuses, and of a sinus high in the neck anterior to the upper end
of the sternocleidomastoid muscle, and (2) second branchial cleft—accounting for most branchial anomalies, usually beginning internally in the
region of the tonsillar fossa, ending in the anterior part of the neck opposite
the hyoid bone, and consisting of *sinuses, fistulas,* and *cysts.* In each of the
last three the epithelial lining is of a stratified squamous, pseudostratified,
or columnar variety and immediately external to the epithelium there is a
mantle of lymphocytes with or without the presence of lymphoid follicles.
One of the complications that may arise is the development of *branchogenic
carcinoma.* Such a lesion, however, is extremely rare and one must be careful to differentiate it from the much more frequent metastatic carcinoma.
In your author's opinion, the following criteria must be met in order to call
a lesion a branchogenic carcinoma: (1) location in the anterior and lateral
parts of the neck opposite the hyoid bone, (2) evidence of branchogenic
remains in the form of an epithelial lining that covers lymphoid tissue, (3)
transition from the epithelial lining to the carcinoma, and (4) no evidence
of any primary tumor elsewhere in the body.

DEGENERATIONS

Degenerations of the mouth are common associates of practically every disorder occurring in this area. Of particular importance perhaps are retrogressive processes found in connection with avitaminosis and industry. *Vitamin deficiency* may bring about (1) cheilosis due to deficiency in riboflavin (p. 61), (2) black hairy tongue due to deficiency in niacin (p. 62), and (3) atrophy of the epithelium as seen in pernicious anemia due to defiiciency in vitamin B_{12} (p. 701). Disorders associated with *industry* may consist of the following (Heacock): (1) abrasions of teeth and mucosa due to substances of relative hardness such as silica, garnet, alundum, silicon carbide, and rouge, (2) decalcification of teeth due to the action of organic and inorganic acids on the calcium and phosphorus of the enamel, (3) caries resulting from the action of factors that cause decalcification or degeneration of organic constituents of the teeth, (4) pigmentation of the enamel due to ingestion of fluorides in drinking water during early childhood and to exposure to heavy metals, (5) pigmentation of the gingivæ resulting from ingestion of minerals such as mercury, bismuth, lead, and nickel, and (6) degenerations due to exposure to materials containing radium.

INFLAMMATIONS

Orientation. —Inflammation of the lips is known as *cheilitis* (Gr. = lip + inflammation), of the gingivæ (gums) as *gingivitis* (L. = gum + inflammation), of the mucosa of the mouth as *stomatitis* (Gr. = mouth + inflammation), of the tongue as *glossitis* (Gr. = tongue + inflammation), of the tonsils as *tonsillitis* (L. = tonsil + inflammation), of the pharynx as *pharyngitis* (Gr. = pharynx + inflammation), and of the parotid gland as *parotitis* or *parotiditis* (Gr. = beside the ear + inflammation). While the inflammations are many, the important ones may be listed as follows: nonspecific stomatitis, noma, gingivitis, Ludwig's angina, tonsillitis, peritonsillar abscess, retropharyngeal abscess, diphtheria, aphthous stomatitis, herpes simplex, foot and mouth disease, Koplick spots, fungous and yeast-like infections, leukoplakia, syphilis, tuberculosis, Boeck's sarcoid (p. 501), leprosy (p. 415), scleroma (p. 414), granuloma inguinale (p. 1112), lymphogranuloma venereum (p. 1112), mumps, and nonspecific inflammation of the salivary glands.

Nonspecific Stomatitis. —Nonspecific stomatitis comprises any inflammation of the mucosa of the mouth that is *caused* by the pyogenic organism that usually compose the oral flora. Predisposing causes are many and include such factors as (1) poor oral hygiene, (2) trauma from toothbrush bristles, firm food particles, or other hard objects, (3) irritants such as tobacco smoke, alcohol, hot foods, etc., and (4) debilitating systemic conditions. The *lesions* consist grossly of discrete or coalescing papules, vesicles, or superficial ulcers and microscopically of a neutrophilic, plasma cell, and lymphocytic response. *Clinically* there is usually some associated pain and there may be excessive secretion of saliva.

Noma. —Noma (Gr. = spreading), also known as cancrum oris and gangrenous stomatitis, is a rare, spreading, gangrenous inflammation of the mouth. It occurs in undernourished children or patients of any age that are debilitated from a chronic disease (Thoma). The disorder is *caused* by organisms usually found in the mouth but with a preponderance of micro-aerophilic or anaerobic strains. The initial *lesion* generally starts in the mucosa of the cheek near the angle of the jaw as a red, board-like infiltration. Soon it softens, breaks down, and ulcerates producing massive destruction of tissue with a foul, putrefactive odor. The *histologic* changes consist of degeneration to complete necrosis of the mucosa and underlying tissues, thrombosis of the vessels, edema, and rather sparse leukocytic infiltration (Eckstein). *Clinically* the condition is associated with fever, prostration, and, in a high percentage of cases, death.

Gingivitis. —Inflammation of the gums may be a simple process of the gingivæ or it may be more extensive and associated with lesions in other portions of the mouth. While the conditions are variously classified they may be conveniently grouped under the following: nonspecific gingivitis, fusospirochaetosis, and gingivitis in systemic diseases.

Nonspecific gingivitis encompasses those inflammations that result from local disturbances with invasion by micro-organisms that are usually present in the mouth. Some of the predisposing factors are (1) faulty hygiene, (2) trauma caused by toothbrush, toothpicks, hard or hot food, carious teeth, etc., (3) senile recession of the gingivæ with atrophy of the alveolar bone, (4) underfunction or understimulation of the gums, and (5) overfunction or overstimulation of the gums (Burket and Thoma). Regardless of the precise etiologic factors, the gingivæ are reddened, swollen, soft, boggy, and ulcerated. They bleed readily upon even the slightest trauma. There may or may not be associated pain.

Fusospirochaetosis (also known as ulceromembranous gingivitis, Vincent's infection, Plaut-Vincent's disease, trench mouth, and phagedenic stomatitis or gingivitis) is an acute to chronic infectious disorder that usually starts in the gingivæ at their junction with the teeth and then spreads to other portions of the buccal mucosa. The condition is seen most often in the adolescent and young adult and is more common in males than in females (Burket). While the precise *causative agents* have not been agreed upon, it is generally conceded that the fusiform bacillus (*Fusiformis dentium*) and Vincent's spirochete (*Borellia vincentii*) are of etiologic significance. *Pathologically* the early lesions consist of punched out ulcerations of the gingival margins and the interdental papillæ. As the condition ages the lesions spread by contiguity and contact to involve the tonsillar mucosa, margins of the tongue, palate, and inner surfaces of the cheeks and lips. The ulcers are bathed in pus, bleed readily upon the slightest trauma, and are usually covered with an easily removable, yellowish-gray membrane. *Clinically* the condition starts suddenly with local pain, sialorrhea, metallic taste, and occasionally systemic reactions in the form of headache, malaise, and fever. The *diagnosis* is made from the appearance of the ulcers and the demonstration of myriads of causative organisms in smears from the lesions. *Treatment* consists of irrigation with solutions of sodium borate, hydrogen peroxide, or similar chemicals. The *prognosis* is good.

Gingivitis may also occur as a result of *systemic disorders*. Some of these consist of (1) hormonal imbalances such as those that accompany pregnancy, menstruation, and the menopause, (2) blood dyscrasias such as purpura, leukemia, agranulocytosis, and hemophilia, (3) vitamin C deficiency, (4) arteriosclerosis, (5) diabetes mellitus, and (6) metallic poisoning such as mercury, arsenic, lead, and bismuth (Thoma and Naish). Except for the metallic poisons (pp. 243 and 244) the lesions are characterized by redness, swelling, bleeding, and irregular superficial ulceration.

Ludwig's Angina. —Ludwig's angina is an acute phlegmonous inflammation of the floor of the mouth caused by the *Streptococcus hemolyticus*

(Thoma). The route of entrance of the organisms is directly through the buccal mucosa, either following trauma or as a result of infection. *Pathologically* all of the tissues of the floor of the mouth, base of the tongue, and even the neck are thickened, reddish, and board-like in consistency. *Histologically* there is edema, a diffuse infiltration with neutrophils, and often thrombosis of the smaller vessels (Fig. 266). In some instances, the process goes on to suppuration. *Clinically* the tongue is elevated and pushed back, the laryngeal mucosa may be swollen, there is obstruction to breathing and swallowing, and the temperature is elevated. *Treatment* consists of administration of antibiotics and, in some instances, of surgical drainage. The *prognosis* in patients treated early and adequately is good.

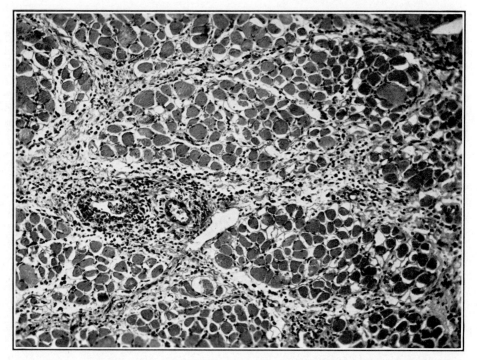

Fig. 266.—Ludwig's angina showing edema of the connective tissue, a diffuse infiltration with neutrophils, and a thrombus of one of the vessels. × 100.

Tonsillitis.—Acute and chronic nonspecific tonsillitis and adenoiditis generally accompany and are similar to acute and chronic nonspecific rhinitis, sinusitis, pharyngitis, and laryngitis (p. 410). *Pathologically* the process consists of hypersecretion of the mucosa, of congestion and edema of the submucosa, and of a leukocytic infiltration of both the mucosa and the underlying tissues. Although *complications* may consist of Ludwig's angina, peritonsillar abscess, and retropharyngeal abscess, and although the tonsils may serve as a focus of infection for the rest of the body, such untoward effects have been greatly overemphasized. Today, with the advent of antibiotic and chemotherapeutic agents, most infections of the tonsils can readily be *controlled* and tonsillectomy is gradually but surely being relegated to obscurity.

Peritonsillar Abscess.—Peritonsillar abscess, also known as quinsy, is a complication of acute tonsillitis. The condition usually occurs in the third decade of life and affects males and females with equal frequency (Capus). The usual *causative* organisms are *Streptococcus hemolyticus* and *Strepto-coccus nonhemolyticus* combined with *Staphylococcus aureus*. *Pathologically* the disorder consists of an acute abscess in the superior peritonsillar area. The lesion (1) is generally filled with thick, gray pus, (2) is well encapsulated, and (3) measures as much as 3 to 4 cm. in diameter. Because of its location the mass bulges downward and medially, encroaching upon the posterior fossa of the mouth and the airway, and pushing the uvula to one side. The more common *complications* consist of cellulitis of the neck, otitis media, retropharyngeal abscess, hemorrhage, cervical lymphadenitis, and erysip-elas. *Clinically* the enlargement produces obstruction of the airway and dyspnea, while the edema and inflammation of the muscles cause dysphagia and trismus. The *diagnosis* is made from a history of tonsillitis followed by a typical cystic swelling in the superior peritonsillar area. *Treatment* con-sists of administration of antibiotics and, when fluctuation occurs, of in-cision and drainage. The *prognosis* is good.

Retropharyngeal Abscess.—As the name indicates, a retropharyngeal abscess is a localized accumulation of pus in the connective tissue between the pharynx and the cervical vertebræ. It is more *common* in infants and young children than it is in adults and has no predilection for either sex. The *causative* organisms are usually the pyogenic bacteria that are ordinarily present in the mouth and nasopharynx. The *pathogenesis* is generally con-sidered to be a breakdown of retropharyngeal lymph nodes that have been infected from inflammation of the nose, pharynx, or occasionally the ears. *Histologically* the process is entirely nonspecific. It consists of a varisized, walled-off mass of pus that protrudes into the pharynx and later into the lateral side of the neck. The chief *complications* are extension retro-esoph-ageally to the mediastinum, rupture into the pharynx with aspiration of pus, and laryngeal edema. *Clinically* there may be dyspnea, dysphagia, swollen cervical nodes, fever, sore throat, cough, and convulsions. The *diagnosis* is made from the history, indirect mirror examination of the pharynx, and forward displacement of the pharynx roentgenographically. *Treatment* consists of administration of antibiotics along with intra-oral or cervical drainage. The *prognosis* is good. The mortality rate in the cases recorded by Weille and DeBlois was 3.7 per cent.

Diphtheria.—Diphtheria (Gr. = membrane) is an acute infectious dis-ease caused by *Corynebacterium diphtheriæ* and transmitted by coughing, sneezing, etc. It affects primarily the pharyngeal and tonsillar mucosa but may also involve the mucosa of the mouth, esophagus, nose, larynx, eyes, and genital tract and may even occur primarily in the skin (Bixby). Once the scourge of the nation, the incidence in the United States has dropped from 106 cases per 100,000 population in 1924 to about 10.7 cases per 100,-000 population in 1944 (Collins). The disease is worldwide in distribution and *occurs* most frequently within the first five years of life (Burket).

Pathologically the lesions appear as irregular, superficial ulcerations cov-ered with a closely adherent gray membrane (Fig. 267). When the latter is removed, bleeding occurs. *Histologically* the membrane consists of a mix-ture of fibrin, leukocytes, bacteria, and necrotic material while the ulcer is composed of nonspecific granulation tissue.

The *complications* consist of (1) suffocation due to aspiration of a dis-lodged membrane, (2) myocarditis due to absorption of powerful exotoxins liberated by the causative organisms (p. 317), and (3) degeneration of peripheral nerves also caused by exotoxins and resulting in paralysis (post-diphtheritic occurring in the third to fifth week of the disease) of the soft palate, eyes, pharynx, diaphragm, and skeletal muscles (Wesselhoeft). The *incubation period* varies from three to five days. The *clinical manifestations* are due to the local lesions and to the powerful exotoxins distributed systemically (toxemia). They consist of sore throat, headache, malaise, fever, vomiting, prostration, dyspnea, dysphagia, rapid pulse, leukocytosis, and (later) paralysis of the striated muscles listed above. The *diagnosis* is made from a history of contact, the appearance of the lesions, and the isolation of *Corynebacterium diphtheriæ*. *Treatment* consists of prevention

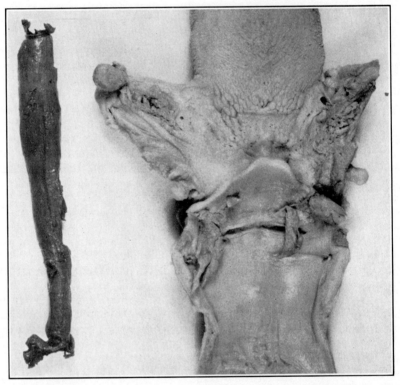

FIG. 267.—Diphtheria illustrating a gray membrane attached to the laryngeal mucosa and (to the left) a membranous cast removed from the larynx and trachea.

by artificial antitoxin. The *prognosis* depends upon the virulence of the organisms and the rapidity with which adequate treatment is started. In the United States, the mortality in 1924 was 8.8 per 100,000 population, while in 1944 it was 0.86 per 100,000 population (Collins).

Aphthous Stomatitis.—Aphthous stomatitis (also known as canker sores and dyspeptic ulcers) consists of a periodic appearance of small vesicles in the mucosa of the mouth (especially the cheeks and lips) and (in women) the mucosa of labia minora, vagina, and cervix. As they age, they rupture and leave small, depressed, punched out, painful ulcers measuring 3 to 4 mm. in diameter (Thoma). The cause is not known. The lesions heal in four to seven days.

Herpes Simplex.—Herpes simplex (also known as a cold sore and a fever blister) is a viral infection that may occur without a preceding or associated disease or that may accompany or follow pneumonia, influenza, coryza, meningitis, sunburn, etc. (Thoma). The condition is referred to as *herpes labialis* when it affects the lips, as *herpetic stomatitis* when it involves the mucosa of other portions of the mouth, and as *herpes progenitalis* when it occurs on the genitals. Following the presence of a localized burning sensation, the *lesions* appear as clusters of small, red papules that soon coalesce and then disclose a collection of clear fluid in their apices. Later the fluid turns milky, dries, and the surface becomes covered with a scaly crust. When this falls off the lesion is healed. *Histologically* the early lesions consist of the formation of intranuclear inclusions (Rivers). Later the epithelial cells of the prickle cell layer are destroyed and separated by edema fluid, thus accounting for the vesicles seen grossly. An occasional *complication* is encephalitis. *Treatment* is unnecessary. The disorder usually clears up in five to seven days but *recurrences* are common.

Foot and Mouth Disease.—This disorder is a viral infection of cloven-footed animals (cattle, pigs, sheep, and goats) that is occasionally transmitted to man as a result of direct contact (Rivers). In man, the incubation period varies from two to eighteen days and the disease is manifested by fever, salivation, and the appearance of vesicles in the mucosa of the lips, mouth, and pharynx, and the skin of the soles and palms. In several days the vesicles rupture leaving irregular ulcers which ultimately heal. Histologically the following changes are seen: hyperkeratosis, intranuclear epithelial inclusions, intra-epithelial vesicles, and neutrophilic infiltration of the subepithelial tissues.

Koplick Spots.—Koplick spots are buccal eruptions that precede the cutaneous manifestations of measles by one to four days (Rivers). They are bilateral, are found in the mucosa of the cheeks near the openings of the parotid ducts, and consist of papules with a bluish-white or occasionally hemorrhagic center mounted on an elevated erythematous base. Histologically there is focal necrosis of epithelial cells and an accumulation of serum.

Fungous and Yeast-like Infections.—Although any of the fungous and yeast-like infections that have been previously considered (pp. 157 and 513) may affect the mouth, tonsils, and pharynx the more common disorders are *moniliasis* (most commonly affecting the tongue when it is known as thrush), *actinomycosis* (usually involving the tonsil, tongue, and cervico-facial region of the face), and *histoplasmosis* (generally causing ulceration of the oropharynx or base of the tongue). The pathologic changes are similar to those already described.

Leukoplakia.—Leukoplakia (Gr. = white + plaque), also known as leukokeratosis and smoker's patch, is a chronic inflammatory, hypertrophic, and degenerative disorder of the buccal (and other) mucous membranes. The condition *occurs* in adults and preponderates overwhelmingly in males (McCarthy). Its *cause* is unknown but, among other things, it has been thought to be due to constitutional factors, avitaminosis, faulty occlusion of teeth, use of tobacco, syphilis, and irritation from such things as carious or rough teeth, habitual biting, hot and spicy foods, betel nut quid, etc. In the mouth the *lesion* occurs on the tongue, palate, lips, and cheeks. Early, it consists of a red, granular, sharply defined, slightly sensitive area. Later, it becomes bluish-white and then white and plaque-like (Fig. 268). In the latter stage, it becomes wrinkled, fissured, indurated, and leathery. *Histologically* the first change consists of a plasma cell and lymphocytic infiltration of the corium. This is followed by hyperkeratosis (excessive keratin deposition on the surface), acanthosis (increase of the prickle cell layer), and hypertrophy of the rete pegs. The chief *complication* is the development of a carcinoma. Such a change is indicated by ulceration and increased induration in a portion of the plaque. *Clinically* the condition is attended by discomfort or pain early in its development and again later when fissures occur. Otherwise it is asymptomatic. The *diagnosis* is made from the gross appearance of the lesion. *Treatment* consists of removal of all irritants. Although excision, electrocauterization, etc., have been advocated by some authors, they are frowned upon by others. The *prognosis* is guarded for the lesions are resistant to treatment and have a great tendency to recur.

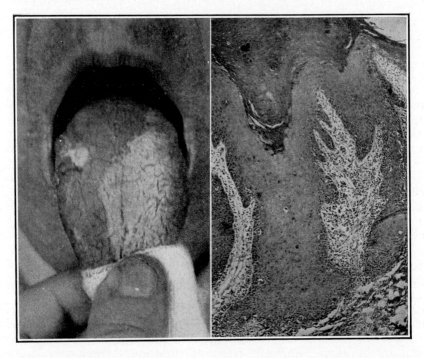

FIG. 268.—Leukoplakia showing (on the left) a white coating of the tongue with a cancerous change in the right margin of the posterior portion and (on the right) hyperkeratosis, acanthosis, and proliferation of the rete pegs. × 25. (From Herbut's *Surgical Pathology*).

Syphilis.—Buccal syphilis may be congenital or acquired (Burket). *Congenital* syphilis is manifested in the mouth in the form of (1) rhagades—linear fissures of the skin arranged perpendicularly to the mucocutaneous junction and being most common in the lower lip and angles of the jaw, (2) *Hutchinson's triad*—comprising: (*a*) hypoplastic, peg-shaped, and centrally notched incisor teeth, (*b*) eighth nerve deafness, and (*c*) interstitial keratitis, and (3) *dentofacial changes*—exhibited essentially as malocclusion that results from lack of proper development of the premaxilla. *Acquired* syphilis may be manifested as: (1) *a chancre*—usually on the lips, tongue, or tonsils, (2) *acute pharyngitis*—seen during the secondary stage, (3) *mucous patches*—slightly raised, grayish-white lesions surrounded by an erythematous base, abounding in spirochetes, seen in the secondary stage, and usually affecting the lips, tongue, tonsils, and pharynx, and (4) *tertiary lesions*—in the form of diffuse ulcerative infiltrations or gummas and located anywhere but most often affecting the tongue and hard palate. The *histologic changes* in syphilis have already been described (p. 178).

Tuberculosis.—Tuberculosis of the mouth is infrequent, being listed as constituting from 0.35 to 3.65 per cent of all tuberculous infections (Burket). Most, if not all, of the lesions are secondary to tuberculosis elsewhere in the body (especially the lungs) and while the route of invasion is generally by way of direct inoculation from infected sputum, some cases doubtlessly arise as a result of hematogenous or lymphogenous spread. Although any part of the mouth may be affected, the *sites* of predilection are the tongue (Titche), tonsils (Bernstein), and pharynx (Szanto). Of the salivary glands,

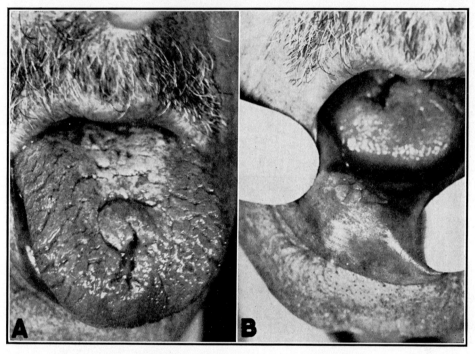

FIG. 269.—Tuberculosis of *A*, the tongue and *B*, the lip from the same patient. Each of the lesions is elevated and irregularly ulcerated.

the parotid is more commonly involved than the others (Berman). *Mucosal lesions*, regardless of their precise location, start as papules which coalesce, break down, and ulcerate (Fig. 269). The ulcers are irregular and of varying sizes. They have raised, undermined, firm edges and gray floors covered with necrotic material. The surrounding tissue is generally indurated so that the lesion is readily mistaken for carcinoma. Histologically the characteristic unit is the tubercle. *Clinically* the ulcers are usually painful. The *diagnosis* is made upon isolating the tubercle bacilli or from biopsy. *Treatment* is that of tuberculosis in general. The local lesions may be removed surgically or by the electrocautery. The *prognosis* depends upon the systemic rather than the local condition of the patient. Once the pulmonary lesions are controlled, the buccal infection usually disappears spontaneously.

39

Mumps.—Mumps, also known as *epidemic parotitis*, is an acute infectious disease of primarily the salivary (especially the parotid) glands *caused* by a virus (Rivers). The *incubation period* is generally eighteen to twenty-one days after exposure. The condition is worldwide in *distribution*, occurs in epidemics in winter and early spring, predominates in children, and affects both sexes.

Pathologically, although any or all of the salivary glands may be affected, the disorder is most common in the parotid gland (Fig. 270). It may be

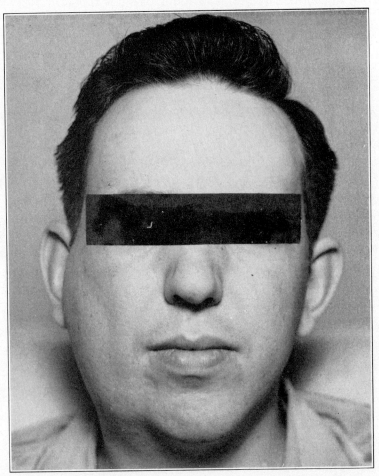

FIG. 270.—Mumps showing a swelling of the right parotid gland.

unilateral or bilateral and when bilateral the swellings may occur simultaneously or in succession. The enlargements are confined to the glands affected, develop rapidly (reaching a maximum within forty-eight hours), are generally large enough to produce noticeable disfigurement, are firm in consistency, and usually disappear in from seven to ten days. The *histologic* change consists of an exudation of serum, fibrin, and neutrophils in the supporting connective tissue of the glands without suppuration. The epithelial cells of the ducts reveal degeneration, necrosis, and neutrophilic infiltration but do not disclose intracellular inclusions. The process heals by resolution.

As a *complication*, similar inflammation may occur in the testes, epididymides, prostate, ovaries, pancreas, spleen, thyroid, kidneys, ear, eye, thymus, myocardium, vulvovaginal glands, mammary glands, and nervous system. Sterility, however, as a result of gonadal involvement is rare. *Clinically* the chief manifestation is swelling. It is usually accompanied by slight fever, malaise, local discomfort, and pain. The last-mentioned is especially noticeable when the patient attempts to eat citrus fruits. The *diagnosis* is generally made from the clinical manifestations and is particularly easy to establish in the presence of an epidemic. The virus, however, can be isolated in the chick embryo and complement fixing antibodies and antihemagglutinins can be demonstrated in the blood. *Treatment* is symptomatic although administration of gamma globulin or convalescent serum is said to decrease the incidence of complications. The *prognosis* is generally excellent. One attack usually confirms lifelong immunity.

Nonspecific Inflammation of the Salivary Glands. — Nonspecific inflammation of the salivary glands is usually confined to the parotid glands and is, at least to begin with, an acute process. Some of the many *synonyms* are acute surgical, septic, gangrenous, suppurative, phlegmonous, necrotic, postoperative, etc., parotitis or parotiditis. The *incidence* is recorded as varying from 1 in 209 to 1 in 3,600 surgical procedures (Coughlin and Gish). The condition is somewhat more common in females than in males, occurs at all ages, and is present in both surgically treated and nonsurgical patients. Although any of the usual pyogenic organisms may *cause* the inflammation, staphylococci by far outnumber all others. The routes of infection are the lymphatics, blood vessels, parotid duct, and direct extension from contiguous structures. Some of the many accompanying or preceding conditions are arteriosclerosis, diabetes mellitus, oral sepsis, nasal pharyngitis, pneumonia, and carcinoma.

Pathologically the process usually develops with great rapidity. The initial changes consist of congestion, edema, and leukocytic infiltration of the ducts, acini, and interacinar tissue. As a result, there is rapid swelling of the gland. Because of the dense fibrous capsule that surrounds the gland and the fibrous trabeculæ that penetrate its substance, the intraglandular tension may be raised to a point where the blood supply becomes occluded and extensive necrosis ensues. The gland may be completely destroyed within a period of twenty-four hours. In less fulminating cases, focal destruction of tissue brings about abscess formation. In either instance, the gland grossly becomes enlarged and firm; the papilla of the duct becomes swollen; sometimes pus can be expressed from the opening of the duct, and the mucosa surrounding the duct discloses hyperemia.

The most important *complication* consists of extension of the inflammation beyond the parotid gland. This generally occurs through three weak spots — (1) along the course of the duct, (2) below and anterior to the styloid process with the pus treking along the stylohyoid muscle and great vessels of the neck, and (3) anterior wall of the external auditory canal with the pus extending to the base of the skull. The *clinical manifestations* consist of dryness of the mouth, sore throat, pain in the angle of the jaw with radiation to the ear, chills, fever to 104° F., and local swelling, edema, redness, and tenderness. The *diagnosis* is made from a history of the predisposing factors as outlined and the local appearance of the lesion. *Treatment* consists of prevention by attention to oral hygiene, maintaining proper hydration, controlling the systemic disorders, etc. Once the condition develops, administration of antibiotics and surgical drainage are indicated.   The overall *prognosis* is usually that of the associated disease. The parotid lesion can generally be controlled.

PHYSICAL DISTURBANCES

Orientation.—Minor physical disturbances of the mouth are frequent. Mention has already been made of trauma to the mucosa from carious teeth, biting, toothpicks, hard food particles, hot and spicy foods, toothbrush bristles, etc.   Such trauma is important for it frequently leads to local or more widespread inflammation. Fractures and dislocations of the jaw are also important, although they are part of the skeletal system and are identical with similar conditions in other osseous tissues of the body.   Three

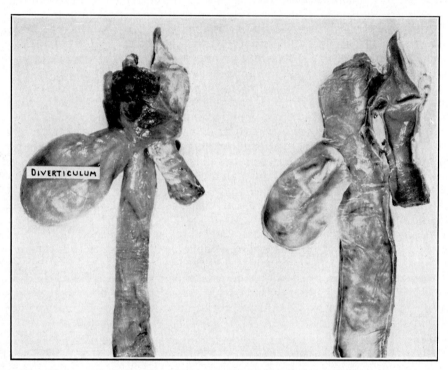

Fig. 271.—Pharyngeal diverticulum showing a large outpocketing originating at the junction of the pharynx with esophagus.

conditions in the category of Physical Disturbances that merit a few separate words are pharyngeal diverticulum, salivary gland calculi, and ranula.

Pharyngeal Diverticulum.—Pharyngeal diverticulum (also known as pharyngo-esophageal diverticulum) is an outpocketing of the wall of the gullet at the junction of the pharynx with the esophagus.   The condition has been recorded as *constituting* 0.11 per cent of all routine barium examinations (Janes).   It is much more common in males than in females and is usually encountered after the age of fifty years.   A predisposing *cause* is an anatomical defect produced by the oblique direction of the inferior constrictor muscle of the pharynx and the horizontal direction of the cricopharyngeus (Negus).   The actual cause is improper coordination of constriction and relaxation of the cricopharyngeus sphincter with contraction of the pharyngeal muscles above this level.   This results in increased intrapharyngeal pressure and herniation of the pharyngeal wall through the weakened area.   Thus the usual *site* of the diverticulum is between the cricopharyngeus and the inferior constrictor muscles (Fig. 271).   The lesion is generally unilateral and, more commonly, on the left side but it may also be bilateral (Buckstein).   The pouch is of varying sizes with measurements as great as 6 to 8 cm. in greatest diameter (Fig. 272).   Its direction is laterally and downward, in which instance it may reach as far as the mediastinum. The ostium is generally wide; the lumen is empty or contains food and fluid; the inner surface is smooth but occasionally may be inflamed or ulcerated, and the wall measures as much as 5 to 6 mm. in thickness.   *Histologically* the inner surface is lined by pharyngeal mucosa and the wall is composed from within out of pharyngeal aponeurosis, scattered longi-

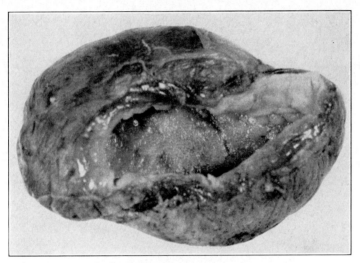

Fig. 272.—Pharyngeal diverticulum illustrating a smooth external surface, a large ostium, an intact (what can be seen of it) inner surface, and an empty lumen.

tudinal and circular muscle fibers, and the buccopharyngeal fascia.   The *complications* are (1) emaciation and dehydration from inability to swallow foods and fluids and (2) aspiration of regurgitated contents.   The *clinical manifestations* consist of difficulty in swallowing first solid and then liquid foods (due to pressure of the diverticulum on the esophagus), regurgitation of food from the pouch, splashing or gurgling sounds in the neck, and emaciation.   The diverticulum can be outlined with ease roentgenographically by using contrast (barium) medium.   The *diagnosis* is made from the history and roentgenographic appearance.   *Treatment* consists of surgical excision. The *prognosis* is excellent.

Salivary Gland Calculi.—Calculi or stones in the salivary glands predominate in males over females in the ratio of 2 to 1 and occur at all ages with an increased *incidence* after adolescence (McKechnie).   The *cause* of their formation is concentration and precipitation of organic salts about food particles, bacteria, necrotic cells, and other debris.   The *sites* of occurrence are submaxillary glands in approximately two-thirds of the cases, parotid glands in one-quarter of the cases, and sublingual glands in the remaining cases.   The reasons for the preponderance in the submaxillary gland are (1) more viscid secretion containing a higher percentage of calcium and phosphates normally produced by these glands, (2) dependent position of the glands as compared with the ostia of the draining ducts, thus accounting for stagnation, (3) more likelihood of foreign particles entering the ducts because of the location of the ductal opening in the floor of the mouth, and (4) normal anatomic angulations of the ducts and constrictions of the lumens from muscular action, both predisposing to stagnation of secretions.   *Pathologically* stones are more commonly found in the ducts

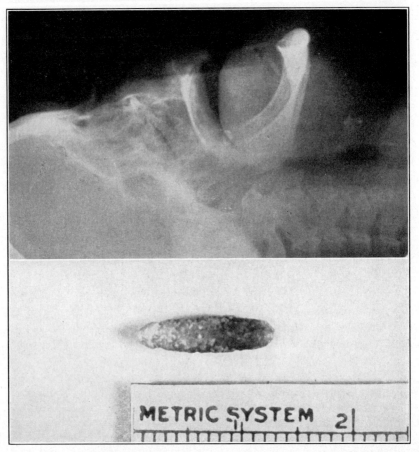

FIG. 273.—Calculus of a submaxillary gland showing both the stone and its appearance roentgenographically.   (Specimen submitted by Dr. Joseph F. McCloskey.)

but occasionally are located within the substance of the gland.   Ductal stones conform to the outline of the duct and are elongated, smooth or rough, and gray to white (Fig. 273).   They usually measure up to 2 cm. in length and 0.6 cm. in diameter.   Calculi found in the gland proper are more irregular and may be larger.   The gland itself generally discloses nonspecific chronic inflammation.   The *complications* consist of suppuration within the gland and extension of the inflammation to produce cellulitis of adjacent tissues.   *Clinically* some of the patients are asymptomatic while others reveal (1) painless swelling of the involved gland, especially at meal time,

(2) pain when the calculus is being extruded, and (3) the usual manifestations of inflammation when infection becomes marked. The *diagnosis* is made from the history, the ability to feel the calculus on gentle palpation, and the readiness with which it is demonstrated roentgenographically (Fig. 273). *Treatment* is surgical removal. The *prognosis* is excellent.

Ranula.—A ranula (L. = frog) literally *means* a cystic tumor in the floor of the mouth. Although the term has been variously used by different authors (Laub) it should be restricted to signify a cyst of the submaxillary or sublingual gland or its duct. It is *caused* by obstruction to the duct. The *cyst* is usually unilateral and thin-walled, measures up to 6 cm. in diameter, and contains clear, milky, or flaky fluid. *Histologically* it is lined with attenuated ductal epithelium resting upon connective tissue cells. *Treatment* is surgical excision. The *prognosis* is good.

TUMORS

Orientation.—Tumors and tumor-like conditions of the mouth and pharynx are extremely varied. Virtually each of the tissues normally present—epithelium, connective tissue, nerves, blood vessels, lymphatics, lymphoid structures (tonsils and adenoids), fat, muscle, bone, and cartilage can give rise to a benign and malignant neoplasm. In addition, such specialized organs as (1) the teeth may give rise to odontogenic tumors, (2) the salivary glands to mixed tumors, papillary cystadenoma lymphomatosum, and Mikulicz's disease and syndrome, and (3) the carotid body (in the neck) to carotid body tumor. In this Chapter, cysts of the floor of the mouth, epulis, tumors of the specialized organs (as listed), and carcinoma only will be considered.

Cysts of the Floor of the Mouth.—Aside from ranula (which has been discussed above) cysts of the floor of the mouth are usually epidermoid or dermoid (Johnston and Korchin). *Epidermoid cysts* are the simpler of the two, being filled with clear, flaky, or sebaceous material and lined by stratified squamous epithelial cells covering a fibrous tissue wall (Fig. 274). They may occur in the midline or laterally and they may arise as congenital epithelial inclusions, as traumatic epithelial occlusions, or as derivatives of the second branchial cleft. *Dermoid cysts* are more complex, being lined by squamous epithelium and containing hair, sebaceous material, bone, and even teeth. They are usually located in the midline and arise as congenital epithelial inclusions. In either case, the cysts may measure as much as 6 to 8 cm. in diameter, may interfere with deglutition, and may become infected. *Treatment* is surgical excision. The *prognosis* is good.

Epulis.—An epulis (Gr. = on + gum) means simply a tumor located on the gum. The lesion may be congenital or acquired. A *congenital epulis* is a benign pedunculated tumor seen predominantly in female infants, located in the region of the incisor teeth, and affecting the maxilla three times as often as the mandible (Custer). It may measure as much as 9 cm. in greatest diameter, is composed of sheets of large polyhedral cells with abundant granular cytoplasm, occasionally encompasses islands of epithelium, and is covered externally with stratified squamous epithelium. The lesion does not recur after *excision* and subsequent dentition is not impaired. An *acquired epulis* is also a benign tumor that is found in relation to a tooth and that originates from the pericementum or the periosteum of the marginal alveolar process (Anderson). In the majority of cases there is a history of preceding injury usually in the form of a carious, a broken

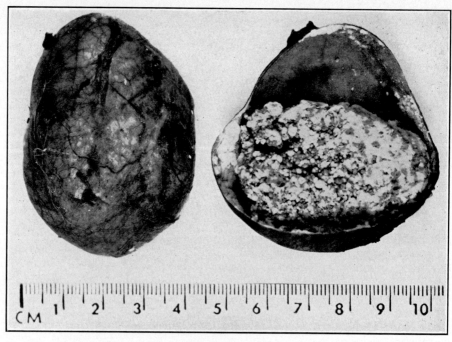

FIG. 274.—Epidermoid cysts of the floor of the mouth illustrating a structure composed of a relatively thin wall and filled with sebaceous material.

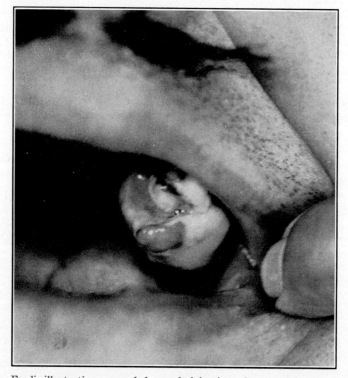

FIG. 275.—Epulis illustrating a rounded mass bulging into the mouth from behind a tooth.

down, or an extracted tooth. *Grossly* the tumors are sessile to pedunculated, usually smooth externally, and may measure as much as 3 cm. in greatest diameter (Fig. 275). *Histologically* they are covered with squamous epithelium and are composed of varying proportions or almost exclusively of connective tissue (fibromatous epulis), vessels (angiomatous epulis), and giant cells (benign giant cell or "sarcomatous" epulis). *Treatment* consists of local excision. If the lesion recurs, a second excision together with extraction of the adjacent tooth may be necessary.

Odontogenic Tumors.—Odontogenic tumors are complex structures derived from dental or potential dental tissue (Thoma). They may be classified as follows: (1) odontogenic cysts consisting of: (*a*) a simple epithelial-lined cyst without remnants of a tooth and (*b*) a more complex structure containing a tooth, a remnant of a tooth, or proliferated elements of a tooth, (2) *adamantinoblastoma* consisting of soft and *enameloma* of calcified tumors of odontogenic epithelium, (3) *odontogenic fibroma* consisting of connective tissue and called *dentinoma* if dentin is produced and *cementoma* if cementum is produced, and (4) *odontogenic mixed tumors* or odontomas composed of both odontogenic epithelium and mesenchyme in various stages of development. Of these, adamantinoblastoma is the most important.

Adamantinoblastoma is also known as adamantinoma, ameloblastoma, multilocular cysts, epithelial odontoma, and fibrocystic disease of the jaw (Davis). It is essentially a benign tumor that arises from the odontogenic tissue or cells with a potentiality for forming tissues of the enamel organ (Robertson). The condition is most *common* from the latter part of the second to the fourth decades of life, affects females about as frequently as males, and occurs in the mandible in almost 90 per cent of cases and in the maxilla in 10 per cent of cases. The *cause* is not known but irritation is apt to play a significant role. *Grossly* the tumors are found within the jaw bone which they have irregularly infiltrated and destroyed to varying extents (Fig. 276*A*). They are ill defined, grayish white, firm, and often cystic. The cysts are filled with amber or more hemorrhagic fluid and may contain unerupted teeth. *Histologically* the tumor is essentially epithelial in nature (Fig. 276*B*). The cell types are basal, columnar, or squamous. Of these, the basal cell variety predominates. Thus, the tumor generally exists as masses, nests, or sheets of polyhedral cells of moderate sizes with ill-defined borders, moderate to slight amounts of lightly basophilic cytoplasm, and round to oval, even staining nuclei. At the periphery the cells tend to be arranged at right angles to the surface and, centrally, they have a tendency to undergo focal degeneration resulting in a pseudoglandular appearance. The stroma is scanty and of a loose connective tissue variety. The *complications* consist of destruction or fracture of the jaw and of a malignant transformation. The latter is said to occur in about 4.5 per cent of cases. Metastases may be found in the cervical lymph nodes, lungs, and bones. *Clinically* the usual manifestations consist of a painless tumor of the jaw of long (usually up to eight years) duration. *Roentgenograms* reveal cystic destruction of the bone (Fig. 276*C*). The *diagnosis* is made from the history, the roentgenographic appearance, and biopsy. *Treatment* consists of surgical excision or amputation of the jaw. The *prognosis* is guarded for recurrences are common.

Mixed Tumors of the Salivary Glands.—Mixed tumors of the salivary glands are primarily benign, slow-growing neoplasms composed essentially of a hyaline or cartilaginous-like matrix in which are embedded actively

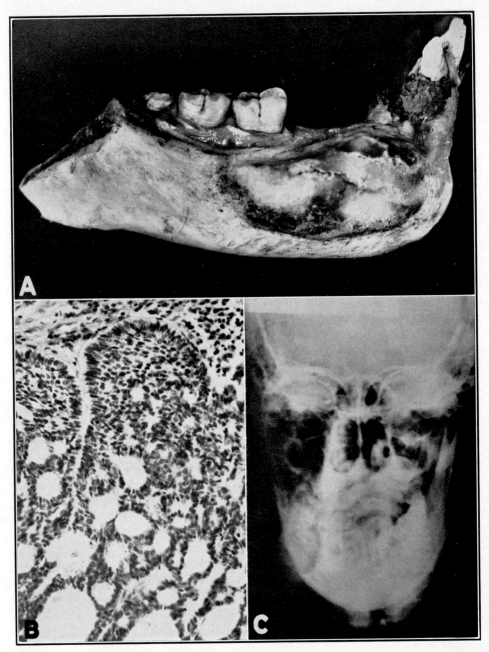

Fig. 276.—Adamantinoblastoma showing *A*, massive destruction of the mandible by a cystic tumor, *B*, typical histologic appearance of basal-like cells.   × 200, and *C*, a roentgenogram illustrating cystic destruction of the right mandible.

proliferating epithelial elements. They *comprise* about 80 per cent of all tumors of these structures, are most common in the sixth and seventh decades of life, and occur approximately equally in both sexes (Kirklin). The *cause* of their formation is unknown. Some of the many *theories* of *origin* hold that the tumors represent a growth of (1) endothelium of lymphatic channels, (2) congenitally misplaced pluripotent cells, (3) ectodermal inclusions from the mouth or skin, (4) notochordal inclusions, (5) branchial cleft remnants, (6) epithelial cells which change in part to resemble cartilage, and (7) epithelial cells that exert a provocative reaction on the connective tissue changing it into a hyaline-like structure (Friedman). In your author's opinion, the last theory mentioned appears to be the most acceptable.

Pathologically most of the tumors occur in the parotid gland while a lesser number are found in the submaxillary and the sublingual glands (Fig.

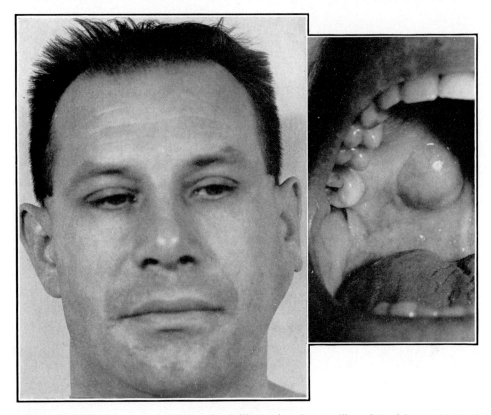

FIG. 277.—Mixed tumors of salivary glands illustrating *A*, a swelling of the left parotid gland and *B*, a rounded enlargement of submucosal glands of the hard palate. (Specimen submitted by Doctor L. M. Tanner).

277). Rarely, they may also arise in the submucosal glands of the oral cavity, especially those of the palate and the lips (Cutler and Cawley). Wherever they are found, they usually exist as sharply defined, seemingly encapsulated, irregularly lobulated, solid or occasionally cystic, gray, cartilaginous-like masses that measure from a few millimeters to 5 cm. or more in diameter (Fig. 278*A*). *Histologically*, as stated at the beginning, they are composed of epithelial cells and stroma (Fig. 278*B* and *C*). The epithelial cells are arranged in masses, sheets, clusters, glands, or individually. They are cuboidal to polyhedral, ill defined, and of moderate sizes. The cytoplasm is fairly abundant and lightly eosinophilic and the nuclei are round to oval, central in position, and evenly stained. Mucoid degeneration with pseudo-

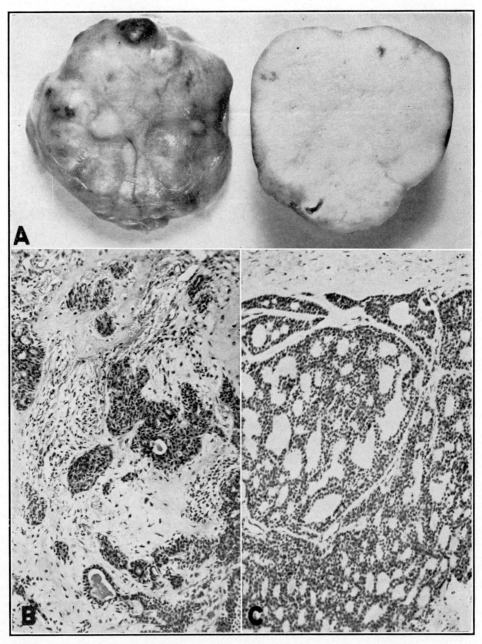

Fig. 278.—Mixed tumor of a salivary gland showing *A*, a well-encapsulated external and a cartilaginous-like cut surface, *B*, epithelial cells arranged in nests and glands and embedded in a fibrous and cartilaginous-like stroma. × 100, and *C*, masses of epithelial cells with foci of degeneration resulting in pseudoglands producing what is often called a cylindromatous appearance (low-grade carcinoma). × 100.

glandular formation is common in tumors that tend to grow in masses or sheets. The stroma is scanty to abundant and varies from loose to fibrous to cartilaginous-like in appearance. Only rarely is there true bone formation (Yates).

The most notable *complication* is a cancerous transformation. Whether such tumors are *cancerous* from the start or whether they represent an actual change in the previously benign growth has not been settled. It is known, however, that the alteration always occurs in the epithelial component and, accordingly, the tumors have been called cylindromas, adenocarcinomas, squamous cell carcinomas, anaplastic carcinoma, muco-epidermoid carcinomas, etc. (Rawson and Kirklin). *Clinically* the only mani-

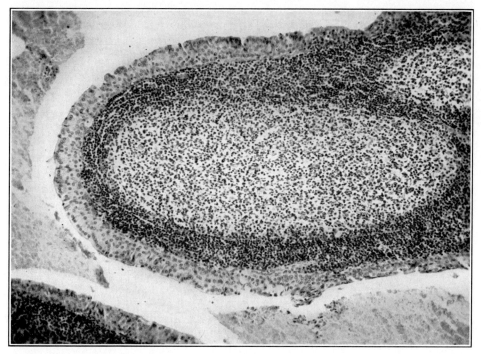

Fig. 279.—Papillary cystadenoma lymphomatosum showing a stroma of lymphoid tissue in papillary formation covered with columnar and basal cell epithelium that discloses intensely eosinophilic cytoplasm.   × 100.

festation is a mass that is slowly (over a period of years) increasing in size. Pain may occur as a result of pressure or ulceration and secondary infection The *diagnosis* is made from the location of the growth, the duration of its presence, and the hardness of its structure. *Treatment* consists of surgical excision. The *prognosis* is guarded for recurrences are common and a malignant transformation may occur.

Papillary Cystadenoma Lymphomatosum.—This tumor, also known as adenolymphoma, oncocytoma, and Warthin's tumor, is a benign lesion that is almost confined to the parotid gland but that, on rare occasions, may be seen in the submaxillary gland (Thompson). It *predominates* in males over females in the ratio of about 7 to 1 and is uncommon before the age of thirty years. While the *cause* of the growth is not known, the most logical explanation for its origin appears to be a neoplastic proliferation of salivary

gland ducts included in lymph nodes with the latter subsequently responding in an inflammatory-like manner. *Grossly* the tumor is unilateral in
over 90 per cent of cases. It is well encapsulated, externally lobulated,
moderately firm to cystic, and usually measures up to 6 cm. in diameter
(Martin). Cut surfaces disclose gray tissue punctuated by many small or
several large cysts filled with chocolate-colored, watery, mucinous, or inspissated material. *Histologically* the cysts are rounded or reveal papillæ.
They are lined by epithelium that discloses one or two luminal layers of
tall columnar cells with eosinophilic cytoplasm and oval nuclei and several
basal layers of smaller, more polyhedral but otherwise similar cells (Fig.
279). Sometimes the epithelium is of a distinct squamous variety. The
stroma is composed of lymphocytes arranged diffusely or in follicles and
containing nests or glands of epithelium similar to that lining the cysts. A
malignant transformation of the stroma into sarcoma and of the epithelial
cells into carcinoma has been recorded but is rare and the cases described
are not altogether acceptable. The only *clinical manifestation* is a tumor
mass. The *diagnosis* is made histologically. *Treatment* consists of surgical
removal. The *prognosis* is excellent.

Mikulicz's Disease and Syndrome.—In 1888 Mikulicz described a disorder characterized grossly by a gradual diffuse symmetrical enlargement of
the lacrimal and all the salivary glands and microscopically by a diffuse
proliferation of round (lymphocytic) cells enclosing epithelial cells arranged
singly, in clumps, or in glands (Jackson and Godwin). The disorder has
since been known as *Mikulicz's disease.* It may *occur* at any age but is most
common in early adulthood to middle age and is more prevalent in males
than in females. The *cause* is unknown. Godwin believes that the condition is similar to or is part of papillary cystadenoma lymphomatosum and
prefers to call it a "benign lympho-epithelial lesion." The *clinical manifestations* consist of enlargement of the lacrimal and salivary glands, narrowing of the palpebral fissures, and (due to lack of salivation) dryness of the
mouth. The *diagnosis* is made from the gross and microscopic appearance.
Treatment in the past has consisted of surgical excision and roentgen therapy.
Recently sulfonamides and antibiotics have been used successfully. The
prognosis is variable. Spontaneous remissions after months or years have
been recorded. *Mikulicz's syndrome* is a clinical entity consisting grossly of
a symmetrical enlargement of the lacrimal and salivary glands similar to
Mikulicz's disease but, pathologically, being due to leukemia, tuberculosis,
Boeck's sarcoid, syphilis, lymphosarcoma, and toxic conditions caused by
such chemicals as lead and iodides (Jackson).

Carotid Body Tumor.—As the name suggests, carotid body tumor is a
neoplasm of a carotid body. A normal carotid body is located at or near the
bifurcation of each common carotid artery (Lahey). It measures about 5
mm. in diameter and consists of an encapsulated nodule of large polyhedral
cells with finely granular cytoplasm and large, oval, hyperchromatic nuclei.
Although there is still some dispute, many authors consider the organ as
part of the chromaffin system. At one time it was thought that the cells of
the carotid body secreted adrenalin and that hyperplasia of the cells resulted in hypersecretion of adrenalin with production of attacks of syncope.
Now, however, it is known that the *clinical* increase in rate and depth of
respirations, a rapid decline of blood pressure, decrease in pulse rate, prolonged periods of cardiac standstill, and fainting (so commonly seen in
patients with carotid body tumors) are due to pressure of the growth on the
carotid sinus (Michie). Other symptoms of hoarseness, Horner's syndrome,

etc., are due to neoplastic invasion of the nerves. The *tumor* is rare, occurs in both sexes, and is most common in middle life (Lewison). It is usually unilateral but may be bilateral and is characteristically located at the bifurcation of the common carotid artery (Fig. 280). The mass is well encapsulated, measures up to 6 cm. in diameter, is moderately firm, compresses or encircles the carotid arteries and adjacent nerves, and is diffusely tan to gray. *Histologically* it is composed of cells that are larger but otherwise similar to those in a normal carotid body (Fig. 280). In rare instances, a malignant transformation has been recorded. In such cases the cells are essentially similar but become quite irregular. The clinical *diagnosis* is

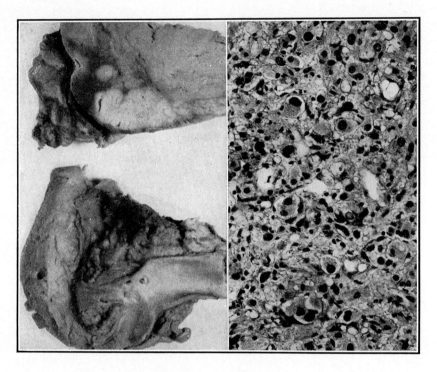

Fig. 280.—Carotid body tumor showing (to the left) a mass of brownish-gray tissue attached to a common carotid artery and (to the right) the histologic appearance consisting of large poly-hedral cells with hyperchromatic nuclei. × 100. (Herbut's *Surgical Pathology*, Lea & Febiger.)

made from the location of the tumor together with a typical history as outlined. *Treatment* consists of surgical excision. During operation, ligation of the carotid arteries to control bleeding or permit removal of the entire growth may be followed by hemiplegia. For this reason the *prognosis* is guarded.

Carcinoma.—In this section on carcinoma of the mouth, certain general characteristics may be considered together after which a few pertinent remarks relative to the various sites of the tumor may be presented. Although there is some variation relative to the different anatomic structures involved, in general carcinoma of the mouth is *seen* about seven to nine times as frequently in males as in females, occurs at almost any age but is most common between forty and seventy years, and is common in white people but is infrequent in Negroes. While the *causes* of carcinoma of the mouth are not known, irritation from biting, trauma, use of tobacco, etc., is thought to play a contributing role by most authors and lesions such as keratosis, leukoplakia, warts, papillomas, chronic fissures, etc., are definitely known to be precancerous. In addition, carcinoma of the lips is more apt to occur in people with thin dry skin and in those whose occupation exposes them to the sun.

Pathologically carcinoma of the mouth is usually single but occasionally may be multiple. Regardless of its precise location the lesion may start as a papule, an ulcer, a fissure, or a blister which crusts and then ulcerates. Fully

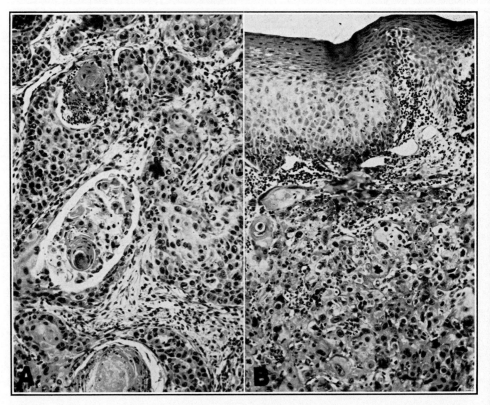

FIG. 281.—Squamous cell carcinoma of the mouth illustrating *A*, a well-differentiated tumor with polyhedral prickle cells and epithelial pearls, and *B*, a more anaplastic growth with great irregularity of the cells that still, however, resemble prickle cells. × 100.

developed lesions are generally flat or fungating. The size varies with the rapidity of growth and the duration of the lesion. In general, the tumor is seldom more than 4 cm. in diameter when the patient first seeks treatment, usually measures less than 1 cm. across, and occasionally may be only 2 or 3 mm. in greatest diameter. In any case, a flat lesion is only slightly (if at all) raised above the surface of the adjacent mucosa, is usually centrally ulcerated, possesses sloping or slightly undermined edges, discloses only a scanty amount of necrotic tissue covering its floor, and reveals an indefinite infiltration of the adjacent tissues by extremely firm, gray, rather friable and bloodless tissue. A fungating growth, as the term suggests, protrudes above the level of the adjacent mucosa. It is usually sessile but occasionally may be somewhat pedunculated, may be covered by an intact mucosa or may reveal irregular superficial ulceration, is composed of extremely firm, grayish-white tissue, and irregularly infiltrates the adjacent tissues at its base. In either case, because of its infiltrative properties, the tumor is firmly anchored to the submucosal structures—a characteristic which helps to distinguish it from a benign lesion. *Histologically* carcinoma of the mouth is generally of a stratified squamous cell variety. Occasionally the lesion may be an adenocarcinoma (arising from the submucosal glands) and only rarely may it consist of a basal cell carcinoma (arising from the basal cells of the mucosa). In addition, a tumor that is found high up in the pharynx may be, on infrequent occasions, a lympho-epithelioma. A squamous cell carcinoma in the mouth, as elsewhere in the body, may run the gamut from a well-differentiated lesion to a poorly differentiated lesion (Fig. 281). A tumor that is well differentiated or one that is of low-grade malignancy consists of strands, masses, or nests of epithelial cells streaming from the mucosa into the submucosa and underlying tissues. The clumps are usually sharply defined, consist of large polyhedral cells of a prickle variety, and may disclose epithelial pearls. Mitoses are present but are not numerous. At the other end of the scale, tumors that are poorly differentiated (high-grade malignancy) consist of masses or single cells that irregularly infiltrate the submucosal structures. In some instances, the cells can still be recognized as of squamous epithelial origin while in others they become so anaplastic that they may resemble a round cell or a spindle cell sarcoma. Between the two extremes there are all gradations. In any case, the stroma is usually moderate in amount, of a rather dense fibrous nature, and infiltrated with plasma cells, lymphocytes, and neutrophils.

Carcinoma of the mouth *spreads* by direct extension, by lymphatic permeation, and by the bloodstream. By direct extension, the lesion involves ever increasing portions of the mucosa, the submucosa, and the subjacent muscle and bone. As a result of such an extension, the involved structures degenerate, become destroyed, and lose their proper function. Spread of the carcinoma by lymphatic permeation is noted primarily in the lymph nodes that drain the particular site of the lesion. As a result of the blockage of some of the lymphatic channels and of the frequent cross anastomosis, however, lymph nodes on the opposite side of the body or in positions normally not draining the affected area may become involved. Clinically it is frequently difficult and sometimes impossible to be certain whether a particular enlargement of lymph nodes is on an inflammatory or a neoplastic basis. As a rule, lymph nodes that are permeated with tumor tissue are more discreet, firmer, and not tender while lymph nodes representing an inflammatory response show the opposite characteristics. Spread of carcinoma of the mouth by the blood vessels is usually a late phenomenon and, in comparison with other methods of spread, is infrequent. The two organs most commonly involved are lung and liver.

The *complications* of carcinoma of the mouth are metastasis, ulceration, hemorrhage, extensive local inflammation, and, occasionally, formation of fistulas. Complications that may arise as a result of irradiation therapy are (1) dryness, scarring, and telangiectasia of the mucosa, (2) radionecrosis of both the soft tissues and adjacent bone, and (3) infrequently, a sarcomatous change in tissues of mesenchymal origin. The only early *clinical manifestation* is a painless pimple, lump, ulcer, or "sore." Local discomfort or pain does not occur until the lesion has become ulcerated or secondarily infected or until it infiltrates the adjacent tissues. As these complications occur, the patient is unable to eat and becomes emaciated. In lesions that

40

are located in the tonsillar area or the pharynx, the patient may complain simply of a sore throat or may first note a mass (metastasis) in the cervical region. The *diagnosis* is made from a careful examination of the lesion and from biopsy. *Treatment* must be individualized to suit the case. Precancerous lesions should be excised surgically. When the lesion is already cancerous it may be removed surgically or destroyed by irradiation. In curable cases, metastases to draining lymph nodes are best treated by surgical excision (Brown). The *prognosis* depends upon the size of the lesion, its duration, the degree of differentiation of its cells, the presence or absence of metastases when the patient is first seen, and the precise location of the growth. In general, the nearer the tumor is toward the lips the better is the outlook and, conversely, the nearer it approaches the pharynx the poorer is the end result. Aside from the generalities just given, a few remarks may be made regarding carcinomas affecting the various anatomic subdivisions of the mouth.

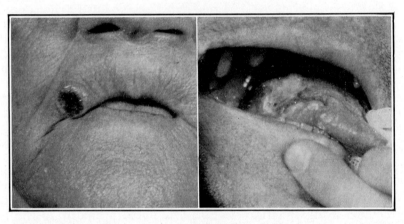

Fig. 282.—Carcinoma (*left*) of the lip showing an elevated, centrally ulcerated, firm mass and (*right*) the lateral border and midportion of the tongue illustrating an irregularly ulcerated, elevated, firm mass. (Herbut's *Surgical Pathology*, Lea & Febiger.)

Carcinoma of the *lips* is the most frequent. The lesion is said to constitute from 4 to 30 per cent of all carcinomas of the body, occurs at the mucocutaneous junction, affects the lower lip in over 90 per cent of cases, is usually single, most commonly consists of a flat ulcer, and is generally of a low grade stratified squamous cell type (Fig. 282). Metastases from the lower lip, as a rule, occur in the corresponding mental, submental, and maxillary lymph nodes; those from the upper lip and from the commissure occur in the corresponding preauricular, postauricular, intraparotid, submaxillary, and submental lymph nodes, while those from the labial midline occur bilaterally to the lymph nodes already listed. The prognosis in carcinoma of the lips, as already stated, is better than in any other portion of the mouth. The over-all five-year survival rates as given by most authors vary from 70 to 90 per cent (Burkell, Ward, Bernier, Cross, and Sharp).

Carcinoma of the *gums* is said to constitute approximately 2.5 per cent of all carcinomas of the body (Martin). The lesions involve both the lower and the upper gums with equal frequency and in decreasing order are most common in the region of the third molar, bicuspid, and canine teeth. Metastases from the lateral external and internal portions of the upper gums are similar to those of the adjacent part of the cheek and affect the corresponding lymph nodes below the angle of the jaw. Metastases from the internal portions of the gum, in addition, affect the corresponding lymph nodes in the retropharyngeal area. Metastases from the lateral external and internal portions of the lower gums affect primarily the submental lymph nodes while metastases from tumors of the gums in the region of the midline involve the lymph nodes already listed but on both sides. The five-year cure rate of carcinoma of the gums is given as about 25 per cent.

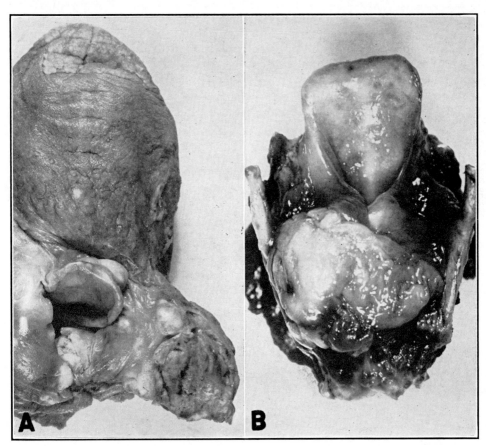

Fig. 283.—Carcinoma of *A*, the right tonsil showing an ulcerating mass and *B*, the hypopharynx illustrating a circumscribed nonulcerating tumor.

Carcinoma of the *tongue* is said to constitute approximately 2 per cent of all cancers of the body. The lesion usually consists of an irregular ulcer with indurated edges and is most frequently located in the lateral border and middle third of the tongue (Fig. 282). The prognosis is better in cases with lesions at the tip of the tongue than in those located closer to the base. The over-all five-year cure rate is usually listed as varying from 25 to 38 per cent (Lyall, Wilson, and Elkins).

Carcinoma in other portions of the *mouth* is said to constitute from 0.6 to 1.43 of all cancers of the body (Hendrick and Mattick). The lesions are most commonly located in the floor of the mouth, have no predilection for either side or for either the anterior or the posterior portion, and are usually of the elevated fungating variety. Metastases usually occur to the sub-lingual, submaxillary, and jugular lymph nodes. They are unilateral when the lesions are located laterally and bilateral when they are located near the midline. The over-all five-year survival rate is usually less than 18 per cent.

Carcinoma of the *tonsils* is said to constitute approximately 1.18 per cent of all cancers of the body. The lesion is usually unilateral, has no predilection for either side, and may involve the anterior pillar, posterior pillar, or the tonsillar fossa. The tumor may be fungating or flat and ulcerating (Fig. 283*A*). The over-all five-year rate is given as approximately 5 per cent (Teloh).

Carcinoma of the *oropharynx* and *hypopharynx* is about as frequent as carcinoma of the tonsils. As already stated, the lesion is usually of a squamous cell variety but, in the upper portion of the oropharynx, it may consist of a lympho-epithelioma. The former tumors are usually fungating and superficially ulcerated (Fig. 283*B*). Lympho-epithelioma, as already stated (p. 431), is frequently so small that it is grossly barely detectable. The five-year cure rate in carcinoma of the hypopharynx is recorded as approximately 6 per cent (Baclesse).

REFERENCES

Pathologic Physiology

BABKIN, B. P.: *Gordon's Dental Science and Dental Art*, Philadelphia, Lea & Febiger, 1938 (Salivary Gland Function).
————: Secretory Mechanism of Digestive Glands, New York, Paul Hoeber Inc., 1950.
BERNSTINE, R. L., and FRIEDMAN, M. H. F.: Obst. & Gynec., *10*, 184, 1957 (Salivation in Pregnancy).
CURRY, J.: *Mechanism of the Human Voice*, London, Churchill, 1939.
MANLY, R. S., and BRALEY, L. C.: J. Dent. Res., *29*, 448, 1950 (Masticatory Efficiency).
MOSHER, H. P.: Laryngoscope, *37*, 235, 1927 (Movements of Tongue).
WANG, S. C.: J. Neurophysiol., *6*, 195, 1943 (Salivary Center).

Congenital Anomalies

BAILEY, H.: J. Internat. Coll. Surg., *8*, 109, 1945 (Parotid Sialectasis).
BURKET, L. W.: *Oral Medicine*, 2nd Ed., Philadelphia, J. B. Lippincott Co., 1952.
MARTIN, H., *et al.*: Ann. Surg., *132*, 867, 1950 (Bronchogenic Carcinoma).
MOORE, T.: Lancet, *1*, 168, 1940 (Cysts of Parotid).
RANKOW, R. M., and HANFORD, J. M.: Surg., Gynec. & Obst., *96*, 102, 1953 (First Branchial Cleft Anomalies).
SEDGWICK, C. E., and WALSH, J. F.: Am. J. Surg., *83*, 3, 1952 (Branchial Anomalies).
THOMA, K. H.: *Oral and Dental Diagnosis*, 3rd Ed., Philadelphia, W. B. Saunders Co., 1949.
WARD, G. E., *et al.*: Western J. Surg., *57*, 536, 1949 (Branchogenic Anomalies).
WEAVER, D. F.: Laryngoscope, *56*, 246, 1946 (Pre-auricular Sinuses).

Degenerations

HEACOCK, L. D.: Indust. Med., *15*, 184, 1946 (Oral Diseases of Occupational Origin).

Inflammations

BERMAN, H., and SEIN, M. J.: Ann. Surg., *95*, 52, 1932 (Tuberculosis Parotid Gland).
BERNSTEIN, D.: A. M. A. Arch. Otolaryng., *44*, 280, 1946 (Tuberculosis Tonsils).
BISHOP, J. M., *et al.*: Lancet, *1*, 1183, 1952 (Acute Sore Throat).
BIXBY, E. W., JR.: A. M. A. Arch. Dermat. & Syph., *58*, 381, 1948 (Cutaneous Diphtheria).
BURKET, L. W.: *Oral Medicine*, 2nd Ed., Philadelphia, J. B. Lippincott Co., 1952.
CAPUS, B.: A. M. A. Arch. Otolaryng., *38*, 210, 1948 (Peritonsillar Abscess).
COLLINS, S. D.: Pub. Health Reports, *61*, 203, 1946 (Diphtheria).
COUGHLIN, W. T., and GISH, D. R.: A. M. A. Arch. Surg., *45*, 361, 1942 (Acute Parotitis).

ECKSTEIN, A.: Am. J. Dis. Child., *59*, 219, 1940 (Noma).

EPHRAIM, H.: Brit. J. Dermat., *61*, 414, 1949 (Moniliasis).

HALL, W. B.: Am. J. Clin. Path., *14*, 215, 1944 (Actinomycosis of the Tonsil).

McCARTHY, F. T.: A. M. A. Arch. Dermat. & Syph., *34*, 612, 1936 (Leukoplakia).

NAISH, J.: The Practitioner, *168*, 127, 1952 (Gingivitis).

PERLSTEIN, W. H.: New England J. Med., *248*, 67, 1953 (Cervicofacial Actinomycosis).

RIVERS, T. M.: *Viral and Rickettsial Infections of Man*, 2nd Ed., Philadelphia, J. B. Lippincott Co., 1952.

SZANTO, P. B., and HOLLANDER, A. R.: Ann. Otol., Rhin. & Laryngol., *53*, 508, 1944 (Tuberculosis Nasopharynx).

THOMA, K. H.: *Oral and Dental Diagnosis*, 3rd Ed., Philadelphia, W. B. Saunders Co., 1949.

TITCHE, L. L.: Am. Rev. Tuberc., *52*, 342, 1945 (Tuberculosis Tongue).

——————: Ann. Otol., Rhin. & Laryngol., *60*, 370, 1951 (Tuberculosis Pharynx).

WEED, L. A., and PARKHILL, E. M.: Am. J. Clin. Path., *18*, 130, 1948 (Histoplasmosis).

WEILLE, F. L., and DeBLOIS, E.: A. M. A. Arch. Otolaryng., *39*, 344, 1944 (Retropharyngeal Abscess).

WESSELHOEFT, C.: Cecil's *Textbook of Medicine*, 8th Ed., Philadelphia, W. B. Saunders Co., 1951, p. 188 (Diphtheria).

WHITMAN, L., *et al.*: J. A. M. A., *131*, 1408, 1946 (Herpes Simplex Encephalitis).

Physical Disturbances

BUCKSTEIN, J., and REICH, S.: J. A. M. A., *144*, 1154, 1950 (Pharyngeal Diverticula).

JANES, E. C.: Canad. M. A. J., *66*, 255, 1952 (Pharyngo-esophageal Diverticula).

LAUB, G. R.: A. M. A. Arch. Otolaryngol., *41*, 300, 1945 (Ranula).

McKECHNIE, R. E.: West. J. Surg., *59*, 153, 1951 (Calculi Salivary Glands).

NEGUS, V. E.: Brit. J. Surg., *38*, 9, 1950 (Pharyngeal Diverticula).

Tumors

ANDERSON, B. G.: A. M. A. Arch. Surg., *38*, 1030, 1939 (Acquired Epulis).

BACLESSE, F.: J. A. M. A., *140*, 525, 1949 (Carcinoma Hypopharynx).

BERNIER, J. L., and CLARK, M. L.: Military Surgeon, *109*, 379, 1951 (Carcinoma Lip).

BROWN, J. B., and McDOWELL, F.: Ann. Surg., *119*, 543, 1944 (Metastatic Carcinoma Neck).

BURKELL, C. C.: Canad. M. A. J., *62*, 28, 1950 (Carcinoma Lip).

BYARS, L. T., and ANDERSON, R.: Am. Surgeon, *18*, 386, 1952 (Cancer Oral Cavity).

CAWLEY, E. P., and WHEELER, C. E.: A. M. A. Arch. Dermat. & Syph., *66*, 340, 1952 (Mixed Tumor Lip).

CROSS, J. E., *et al.*: Surg., Gynec. & Obst., *87*, 153, 1948 (Carcinoma Lip).

CUSTER, R. P., and FUST, J. A.: Am. J. Clin. Path., *22*, 1044, 1952 (Congenital Epulis).

CUTLER, M.: Am. J. Roentgenol., *61*, 82, 1949 (Mixed Tumors Palate).

DAVIS, E. D. D.: Lancet, *2*, 862, 1952 (Adamantinoblastoma).

ELKINS, H. B.: Am. J. Roentgenol., *68*, 81, 1952 (Carcinoma Tongue).

FRIEDMAN, E. A.: A. M. A. Arch. Otolaryngol., *56*, 277, 1952 (Origin Parotid Tumors).

GODWIN, J. T.: Cancer, *5*, 1089, 1952 (Benign Lympho-epithelial Lesion Parotid).

HENDRICK, J. W.: Am. Surgeon, *18*, 1092, 1952 (Carcinoma Tongue and Floor Mouth).

JACKSON, A. S.: A. M. A. Arch. Surg., *63*, 99, 1951 (Mikulicz's Disease and Syndrome).

JOHNSTON, W. H.: Ann. Otol., Rhin. & Laryngol., *51*, 917, 1942 (Cysts Floor Mouth).

KIRKLIN, J. W., *et al.*: Surg., Gynec. & Obst., *92*, 721, 1951 (Parotid Tumors).

KORCHIN, L.: U. S. Armed Forces M. J., *2*, 289, 1951 (Dermoid Cyst Floor Mouth).

LAHEY, F. H., and WARREN, K. W.: Surg., Gynec. & Obst., *92*, 481, 1951 (Carotid Body Tumors).

LEDLIE, E. M., and HARMER, M. H.: Brit. J. Cancer, *4*, 6, 1950 (Cancer Mouth).

LEWISON, E. F., and WEINBERG, T.: Surgery, *27*, 437, 1950 (Carotid Body Tumors).

LYALL, D., and SCHETLIN, C. F.: Ann. Surg., *135*, 487, 1952 (Cancer Tongue).

MARTIN, H.: Am. J. Surg., *54*, 765, 1941, (Carcinoma Gums).

——————: A. M. A. Arch. Surg., *44*, 599, 1942 (Tumors of the Palate).

MARTIN, H., and EHRLICH, H. E.: Surg., Gynec. & Obst., *79*, 611, 1944 (Papillary Cyst-adenoma Lymphomatosum Parotid).

MATTICK, W. L., *et al.*: Surgery, *31*, 575, 1952 (Carcinoma Floor Mouth).

MICHIE, W., and SIMPSON, R. G.: Edinburgh M. J., *59*, 443, 1952 (Carotid Body Tumor).

NEW, G. B., and CHILDREY, J. H.: A. M. A. Arch. Otolaryngol., *14*, 596, 1931 (Tonsillar and Pharyngeal Tumors).

RAWSON, A. R.: Cancer, *3*, 445, 1950 (Tumors Salivary Glands).

ROBINSON, H. B. G.: A. M. A. Arch. Path., *23*, 831, 1937 (Adamantinoblastoma).

SHARP, G. S., *et al.:* J. A. M. A., *142*, 698, 1950 (Carcinoma Lip).

TELOH, H. A.: A. M. A. Arch. Surg., *65*, 693, 1952 (Carcinoma Tonsil).

THOMA, K. H.: Internat. Abst. of Surgery, *67*, 522, 1938 (Tumors of the Mouth and Jaws).

———————: *Oral and Dental Diagnosis*, 3rd Ed., Philadelphia, W. B. Saunders Co., 1949.

THOMA, K. H., and GOLDMAN, H. M.: Am. J. Path., *22*, 433, 1946 (Odontogenic Tumors).

THOMPSON, A. S., and BRYANT, H. C., JR.: Am. J. Path., *26*, 807, 1950 (Papillary Cystadenoma Lymphomatosum Parotid).

WARD, G. E., and HENDRICK, J. W.: Surgery, *27*, 321, 1950 (Carcinoma Lip).

WILSON, J. L., and BRIZZOLARA, L. G.: Ann. Surg., *136*, 964, 1952 (Carcinoma Tongue).

YATES, P. O., and PAGET, G. E.: J. Path. & Bact., *64*, 881, 1952 (Salivary Gland Tumor).

Chapter

16

Esophagus

PATHOLOGIC PHYSIOLOGY

M. H. F. FRIEDMAN

THE *esophagus* serves as a conduit of food from the mouth and pharynx to the stomach and plays an important role in swallowing. The apparently simple act of *swallowing* involves one of the most complicated series of reflexes studied. There is no unanimity on all aspects but the picture can be described best as occurring in *three phases*. In the *first* or *buccal phase*, which is entirely voluntary, the mouth is closed and the tongue, moving against the hard palate, presses food towards the pharynx. With the assistance of the myohyloid and other muscles, the food on reaching the base of the tongue is shot rapidly backward. The piston-like action of the base of the tongue exerts a pressure of about 20 cm. H_2O on the food bolus so that it is delivered forcibly through the fauces into the pharynx. On passing over the base of the tongue, the food bolus excites sensory mechano-receptors, located there as well as in the pillars of the fauces and the pharyngeal wall. This initiates the reflex of the *second* or *pharyngeal phase* of deglutition. This phase is purely involuntary and cannot be initiated without mechanical excitation of the sensory receptors. Furthermore, once initiated this phase cannot be arrested voluntarily. A person making swallowing movements in the absence of food does so by excitating these sensory receptors with saliva. Swallowing is therefore understandably difficult if the mouth is dry or the back of the throat has been painted with a local anesthetic. The second phase of swallowing consists of a number of reflex activities occurring both concurrently and in rapid succession. The mouth is still closed and the base of the tongue is against the palate so that additional closure of the nasopharynx effectively seals off the pharynx from the outside. The anterior wall of the laryngeal pharynx moves forward along with the larynx and hyoid bone, thus increasing the capacity of the pharynx. The larynx is brought up against and under the base of the tongue and epiglottis so that food can pass over or on either side of the larynx. The true and false vocal cords are approximated and respiration is inhibited. The enlarging of the pharynx creates a negative pressure of about 35 cm. H_2O so that the food bolus is literally aspirated into the pharyngo-esophagus. It is at this point that the *third* or *esophageal phase* of swallowing ensues. This phase too is purely involuntary. The esophagus relaxes and a peristaltic wave engulfs and carries the food to the cardiac sphincter. When liquid is swallowed in a rapid series of gulps the esophagus remains relaxed so that the fluid flows by gravity into the stomach in a stream. Solid foods, however, are carried along only by peristaltic waves.

Aspiration of *food* into the *trachea* may occur as the result of failure of the glottis to close. This occurs in *injuries* to the *pharynx*, especially when the afferent pharyngeal branches of the vagus are affected so that inspiration is not inhibited, and in *brain* injuries affecting the deglutition centre.

A series of *supplemental propulsive contractions* may occur as the result of local stimulation of the esophagus when the primary peristaltic wave which is initiated by the swallowing is not strong enough to sweep the food bolus into the stomach. Secondary peristalses are due to vagovagal esophageal reflexes while tertiary peristalses are due to myenteric reflexes. Since the upper third of the esophagus is composed of striated muscle it becomes completely paralyzed after extrinsic denervation, but the lower esophagus will still respond to a distention stimulus because of the intrinsic innervation. *Paralyses* of the thoracic esophagus as the result of lesions to the extrinsic nerves are correspondingly rare.

Dysphagia, or difficult swallowing, results from impaired motility of the esophagus and failure of the cardio-esophageal sphincteric mechanism to relax. The more serious of the esophageal dysfunctions is that of *cardio-spasm* or *achalasia*. This disorder involves not only the sphincteric mechanism but also most of the esophagus as well. Basically, achalasia is a neuromuscular dysfunction due to relative or absolute absence of intramural ganglion cells. In the milder cases, propulsive activity of the esophagus is usually present but the distention pressures required to elicit the propulsive response are much higher than normal. The esophagus may be hypertrophied and not relax well. Later, the esophagus may become greatly dilated (mega-esophagus), thin walled, and redundant. Peristaltic waves start well in the pharnygo-esophagus but become shallow ineffectual waves when they reach the lower thoracic portion of the tube. Whether or not food will be passed into the gastric cardia will depend upon the degree of dilatation, the effectiveness of the secondary and tertiary peristaltic waves, and the adequacy of gastro-esophageal relaxation.

Dysphagia due to *spasm* of the *thoracic esophagus* may be a transitory condition observed in nervous states, especially in children. In diffuse spasm of the esophagus the peristalsis may be normal in the cervical segment but is replaced by an exaggerated mass contraction of the thoracic esophagus. Unlike achalasia, in this type of dysphagia the sphincteric mechanism functions normally.

Pyrosis or *"heartburn"* is a subjective burning sensation experienced by ulcer patients and is associated with regurgitated acid gastric juice. The pain probably is not due to direct chemical irritation of pain nerve fibers as was once believed, but results from the increased muscle tension and spasm which is inititated by the acid juice. The pain may be duplicated by other means which give rise to strong esophageal contractions or spasm.

Like the buccopharyngeal secretions, the *secretion* from the *esophagus* is under nervous regulation only. The secretion is an alkaline mucus without enzymatic activity and its principle function is the lubrication of the food bolus in transit to the stomach. Prolonged stimulation of the esophageal glands leads to secretion of a serous fluid when the mucous glands become exhausted. This is seen when there is continued mechanical stimulation by a foreign body in the esophagus.

CONGENITAL ANOMALIES

Orientation.—Developmental abnormalities of the esophagus may be: (1) primary in the esophagus and affect the esophagus alone or the esophagus along with other structures or (2) primary in adjacent structures and affect the esophagus secondarily (Holinger). They may be listed as follows: (1) absence, (2) duplication, (3) atresia, (4) webs, (5) stenosis, (6) short esophagus, (7) tracheoesophageal fistula, and (8) obstruction by vascular ring. Each of these may now be briefly considered in the order mentioned.

Absence.—Complete absence of the esophagus is extremely rare. The upper part of the gastrointestinal tract ends in a pouch of the hypopharynx while the stomach is completely sealed off below the diaphragm.

Duplication.—Duplication of the esophagus may exist in the form of (1) gastro-enteric cysts—cystic structures located in the mediastinum (p. 548) and (2) tubular duplications. The latter are of varying lengths, are located parallel to the esophagus, anatomically duplicate the normal esophagus, may be entirely separated from the esophagus and stomach or may be connected with the esophagus above by a fibrous cord and with the stomach below by a regular luminal opening, and are subjected to the same disorders as the esophagus proper (Langston and Butler). In rare instances the duplication may communicate with the small intestine (Davis).

Atresia.—Atresia (complete occlusion of the lumen) of the esophagus as an isolated anomaly of the esophagus alone is rare. The occlusion is usually single, varies in length, is generally located near the vicinity of the tracheal bifurcation, and is associated with an otherwise relatively normal esophagus above and below the affected segment (Fig. 284). The clinical manifestations are similar to those in atresia associated with tracheoesophageal fistula.

Webs.—Webs of the esophagus are rare. They may be single or multiple and consist of partial transverse partitions or shelves covered on each surface with mucosa.

Stenosis.—Congenital stenosis of the esophagus means narrowing of the lumen of the gullet. It may occur at any level but is most common opposite the tracheal bifurcation, varies in length from 1 to 10 cm., consists either of a fibrous thickening of the wall or of a failure of the lumen to epithelialize, and is attended by an increasing inability to swallow first solids and then even liquids.

Short Esophagus.—A congenitally short esophagus is relatively common. The lesser than normal length of the esophagus does not permit the stomach to descend to its normal position below the diaphragm and, as a result, a portion of it is retained above the diaphragmatic opening (Sinclair and Rennie). The condition is attended by stenosis at the gastro-esophageal junction (Holinger) and ulceration of the supradiaphragmatic gastric mucosa. The lesion should be differentiated from hiatal or diaphragmatic hernia (p. 894).

Tracheo-esophageal Fistula.—A congenital fistula between the esophagus and trachea results from failure of complete closure of the laryngotracheal groove that separates the esophagus from the trachea and larynx in early embryonic development. The condition is relatively common, the incidence having been recorded as about 1 in 2,500 births (Bigger). It is almost confined to newborn infants (Potts) but cases have been recorded in adults (Berman). The ostium between the esophagus and the trachea is virtually always found at or just above the bifurcation of the trachea. It may be the only anomaly present or it may be associated with stenosis, atresia, or complete absence of a segment of the esophagus at this level. In cases of segmental esophageal atresia or absence, the upper segment of the esophagus ends blindly in over 90 per cent of cases while the lower segment bears the fistulous opening. In less than 10 per cent of cases, the reverse is true. The *clinical manifestations* are due to starvation and to aspiration pneumonia from regurgitation of food from the upper segment of the esophagus. The *diagnosis* is made from the history and the presence of air in the stomach roentgenographically. *Treatment* consists of surgical reconstruction of the digestive pathway. The *prognosis* is good if the diagnosis is made early and proper treatment instituted before complications occur.

Obstruction by Vascular Ring. — Pressure on the esophagus (and trachea) may occur as the result of a double aortic arch, a right-sided aortic arch with a left ligamentum arteriosum, or a posterior right subclavian artery (Gross). These lesions have already been discussed in Chapter 9 (p. 355).

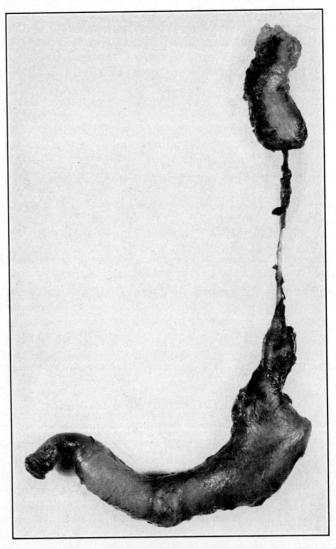

Fig. 284.—Congenital atresia of the midportion of the esophagus. The defective segment of the gullet is represented by a fibrous cord.

DEGENERATIONS

Orientation.—Degenerative processes in the esophagus are common but, as in most other organs of the body, they are incidental to other specific conditions or diseases. Two disorders that may be mentioned here (although they are not strictly speaking degenerations as such) are changes in scleroderma and the Plummer-Vinson syndrome.

Esophagus in Scleroderma.—Scleroderma is a transitory inflammatory but definitively degenerative systemic disorder with the most outstanding

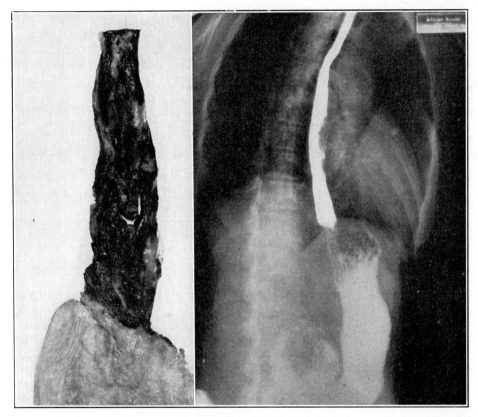

Fig. 285.—Scleroderma showing, to the left, perforation of the esophagus and hemorrhage after an attempted esophagoscopy and, to the right, two defects in the central portion and constriction at the esophagogastric junction roentgenographically.

changes affecting the skin (p. 1076). In the *esophagus* the following alterations may be noted (1) fibrosis and collagenization of the submucosa near the cardia, (2) hyperplastic changes in the arterioles, and (3) irregular superficial ulcerations of the mucosa with surrounding plasma cell, lymphocytic, and neutrophilic infiltration (Kaisch). *Clinically* the esophageal symptoms consist of: (1) difficulty in deglutition—due to the diffuse increase of sclerotic connective tissue, with resulting constriction of the esophagus and loss of peristalsis, and (2) burning sensation and pain—caused by inflammation and ulceration that are consequent to the sclerotic changes. *Roentgenographically* the characteristic alterations consist of diffuse or focal dilatation above an area of constriction that is due to spasm and/or fibrosis

(Fig. 285). The *diagnosis* is made from an association of the esophageal manifestations with those in other organs, especially the skin. *Treatment* is that of the disease in general together with esophageal dilatation when obstruction becomes marked (Olsen). The over-all *prognosis* is not good.

Plummer-Vinson Syndrome.—This syndrome was first described as consisting of a primary inability to swallow solid foods as a result of neurosis followed, in time, by anemia, glossitis, splenomegaly, and achlorhydria (Kernan). Subsequent reports on whether the esophageal condition is caused by neurosis, neuromuscular incoordination, or organic changes are quite divergent (Cordray). From a few instances in which examination of the *esophagus* was made it has become evident that in some, inflammation of the esophagus may be present, while in others, actual obstruction may occur as a result of elevation of folds of the mucosa, hyperkeratosis of the epithelium, and degeneration of the muscle. *Clinically* there are dysphagia, cracks in the corner of the mouth, soreness of the tongue, and manifestations consequent to anemia. The condition is virtually confined to women in the fifth decade of life. *Treatment* is mostly symptomatic including dilatation of the esophagus when constriction is marked. The *prognosis* is fair to good.

INFLAMMATIONS

Orientation.—Inflammation of the esophagus is known as *esophagitis* (Gr. = to carry + food + inflammation). Some of the many varieties of inflammation of the esophagus are acute esophagitis, peptic ulcer, typhoid esophagitis, diphtherial esophagitis, esophagitis in scarlet fever, fungous and yeast-like esophagitis, leukoplakia, granulomatous esophagitis, tuberculosis, and syphilis. The lesions in *typhoid fever*, *diphtheria*, and *scarlet fever* are usually incidental findings in an otherwise gravely ill patient; *leukoplakia* is identical with a similar lesion on the tongue and other mucosal surfaces (p. 607), while *fungous* and *yeast-like* esophagitis (moniliasis, actinomycosis, histoplasmosis, etc.) are the same as the corresponding infections in other organs (pp. 157 and 513). The remaining lesions merit a few separate remarks.

Acute Esophagitis.—Acute esophagitis, also known as acute ulcerative esophagitis, is a *common* finding at autopsy in newborn or older infants and in adults who have been previously operated upon for a nonesophageal condition. It has been recorded in as high as 17 per cent of all infants (Gruenwald) and 7 per cent of all adults (Olsen) coming to autopsy. The predisposing *cause* appears to be shock. In this condition the submucosal vessels become congested. The resulting stasis leads to impaired nutrition and this, in turn, causes degeneration, ulceration, and then invasion of the mucosa by bacteria normally present in the esophageal lumen. The *site* of predilection is the lower end of the esophagus just above the cardia. The *lesions* are usually multiple and consist of (1) irregular, deep red to cyanotic, blotchy areas of congestion, (2) superficial erosions of varying sizes and configurations, (3) irregular ulcers that may extend all the way to the periesophageal tissues, and (4) ulcerations with marked phlegmonous infiltration of the adjacent esophageal tissues. *Histologically* the inflammation is entirely nonspecific, consisting of congestion, edema, and an infiltration with neutrophils, plasma cells, and lymphocytes. The *complications* are hemorrhage and perforation with periesophagitis and mediastinitis. *Clinically* the patient may complain of "heart burn," "sour stomach," epigastric discomfort, etc., but the complaints are usually minor and the condition generally remains unsuspected. The *diagnosis* is, as a rule, made at autopsy. The disorder probably exists in many other patients but *heals* completely upon recovery from the associated illness.

Peptic Ulcer of the Esophagus. —The term peptic ulcer of the esophagus is usually reserved for clinically recognizable acute or chronic ulcers of the lower portion of the esophagus that occur on the basis of ectopic gastric mucosa, a short esophagus, hiatal or diaphragmatic hernia, or an operative esophagogastric anastomosis (Radish, Potter, Harman, Cleaver, and Ripley). The condition *occurs* in middle-aged and older people of both sexes. The *causes* (aside from the local alterations listed above) are thought to be similar to those of peptic ulcer in the stomach and duodenum (p. 664). The *lesion* may be single or multiple and is usually located in the lower

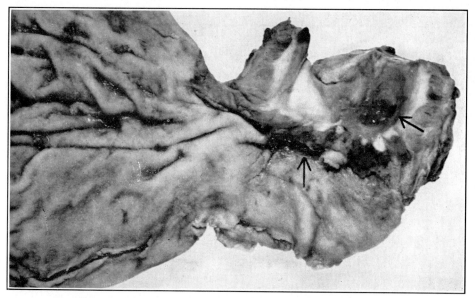

FIG. 286.—Peptic ulcer of the lower portion of the esophagus (upper arrow) and the first portion of the stomach (lower arrow).

portion of the esophagus just above the esophagogastric junction (Fig. 286). *Grossly* the ulcer is of varying size and is clean-cut. It is rounded or irregular, has sloping or undermined edges, discloses a clean floor, and reveals a gray base located at the muscle coats or periesophageal tissues. *Histologically* it shows an acute to chronic nonspecific inflammatory reaction. The *complications* consist of hemorrhage, perforation, or cicatricial stenosis. The *clinical manifestations* consist mainly of pain, hematemesis, and dysphagia. The *diagnosis* is made from the history, roentgenographic findings, esophagoscopy, and biopsy. *Treatment* is not standardized, consisting of both a medical regimen and surgical intervention. The *prognosis* is guarded.

Granulomatous Esophagitis. —Nonspecific granulomatous (regional) esophagitis is a chronic inflammation of the esophagus of unknown cause (Franklin). It is characterized by increasing dysphagia, an obstructive lesion in the middle portion of the esophagus that is readily demonstrable roentgenographically, and histologic changes that are similar to those in regional enteritis (p. 709).

Tuberculosis.—Tuberculosis of the esophagus is probably less frequent than tuberculosis of any other organ of the body (Guggenheim). Any portion of the esophagus may be affected with the *site* of predilection depending upon the *route* of invasion and the predisposing factors. Thus (1) infection as a result of extension from the pharynx involves the upper part of the esophagus, from the vertebra any portion, and from the mediastinal lymph nodes the midportion at the level of the bifurcation of the trachea, (2) infection at the site of a pre-existing lesion or stricture results in a lesion in the part of the esophagus thus affected, while (3) infection by the blood or lymphatic stream may produce a lesion in any portion of the organ. Of these, extension from mediastinal tuberculous lymph nodes is the most common (Fig. 287). In such instances, the lymph nodes show caseation

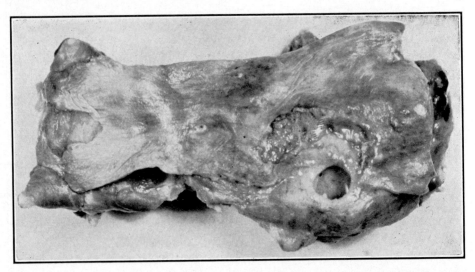

Fig. 287.—Tuberculosis of the esophagus resulting from a periesophageal tuberculous ulcer which, in turn, resulted from periesophageal tuberculous lymphadenitis. The lesion in the esophagus consists of an ulcer that communicates by a round opening with the periesophageal abscess.

with or without calcification and liquefaction. The caseous material then spreads to produce a periesophageal abscess which secondarily involves the esophagus or spreads directly to the esophageal wall. In either case, the esophageal *lesion* ultimately consists of an ulcer with varying numbers of adjacent tubercles and varying degrees of fibrosis. When the latter is abundant, stenosis may result. *Clinically* the symptoms are those of esophageal obstruction. The *diagnosis* is made from esophagoscopy and biopsy. *Treatment* is that of tuberculosis in general and of local dilatation or surgical resection when the obstruction becomes severe. The *prognosis*, as a rule, is not good.

Syphilis.—Syphilis of the esophagus is rare, for by 1950 the literature contained records of only 75 cases (Hudson). The clinically recognized disease occurs in the tertiary stage and the *lesion* consists of either a diffuse inflammatory reaction or of a gumma. Each lesion is prone to ulceration and fibrosis with resulting esophageal obstruction. The *symptoms* are those of esophageal obstruction but when perforation into the trachea occurs there may also be cough, expectoration, and hemoptysis. The *diagnosis* is made from the history, positive serologic tests for syphilis, roentgenography, esophagoscopy, and biopsy. *Treatment* consists of the usual antisyphilitic measures but when fibrotic obstruction is severe, esophagectomy may be necessary. The *prognosis* is good.

PHYSICAL DISTURBANCES

Orientation. —In this section the following unrelated conditions may be conveniently considered in consecutive order: diverticulum, cardiospasm, chemical burns, varices, foreign bodies, fistulas, rupture, and dysphagia.

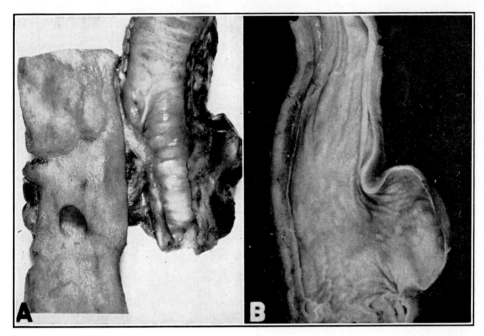

Fig. 288.—Diverticula of the esophagus showing *A*, a traction diverticulum of the midportion of the organ and *B*, a pulsion diverticulum of the supradiaphragmatic portion.

Diverticulum. —Diverticulum of the esophagus, as in any other organ, is an outpocketing of its wall. It may be *located* at the junction of the pharynx and esophagus (p. 612), in the midportion of the esophagus, or in the lower portion (DeBakey). A diverticulum in the *midportion* of the *esophagus* is generally located opposite the tracheal bifurcation and because it arises as a result of contraction of an adherent, chronically inflamed (usually tuberculous) lymph node it is commonly referred to as a *traction diverticulum* (Katz). The condition generally occurs in persons past the age of fifty years. The diverticulum is, as a rule, single and located in the anterior wall of the esophagus, is conical or triangular in shape, has a wide ostium, is directed horizontally or upward, and measures only from 2 to 4 cm. in greatest diameter (Fig. 288*A*). A diverticulum in the lower portion of the esophagus is often referred to as an *epiphrenic* or a *supradiaphragmatic diverticulum*. Since it arises as a result of pressure from the esophageal lumen on a weak spot in the wall it is also known as a *pulsion diverticulum*

(Kausel and Goodman). The diverticulum is usually single, is located posterolaterally and directed inferiorly, has a wide ostium, consists of all the layers of the esophagus except the outer muscular coat, and may measure as much as 8 cm. or more in diameter (Fig. 288B). *Complications* are rare in diverticula of the midportion of the esophagus but are common in those located above the diaphragm. They may consist of ulceration, hemorrhage, stenosis, and perforation. *Symptoms* are often absent in diverticula of the midportion of the esophagus but are usually present in those located more inferiorly. They may consist of pain, dysphagia, and hematemesis. The *diagnosis* is made roentgenographically and esophago-scopically. *Treatment* consists of surgical excision. The *prognosis* is good.

Cardiospasm.—Cardiospasm may be defined as a nonorganic stenosis of the distal portion of the esophagus (Olsen). Some of the many *synonyms* are achalasia, mega-esophagus, idiopathic dilatation of the esophagus, diffuse dilatation of the esophagus, and preventriculosis. The condition *occurs* at any age after the second decade and is more common in females than it is in males. The *cause* is unknown. At one time or another the following have been considered to be of etiologic significance: deformity of the liver tunnel through which the esophagus passes, periesophageal fibrosis, incoordination of the diaphragmatic crura, phrenospasm, and degenerative changes in Auerbach's plexus resulting in incoordination of muscular contractions and relaxations (Kay).

Pathologically the spasm is localized to a short segment of the esophagus at the cardia, measuring from 1 to 5 cm. in length. Above this level there is marked dilatation, lengthening, and tortuosity of the esophagus. The lumen is filled with food and fluid; the mucosa is gray, smooth, and may be superficially ulcerated, and the wall is usually thick and rigid but occasionally it may be thin. *Histologically* the mucosa may be intact and relatively normal or hyperkeratotic but occasionally it may be superficially ulcerated. The rest of the wall shows acute to chronic diffuse inflammation that predominates in the submucosa and the serosa (Cross). The circular and longitudinal muscles, especially in areas of thickening, reveal moderate to marked fibrosis, while Auerbach's plexus discloses inflammation, fibrosis, and loss of ganglion cells.

The *complications* consist of loss of weight, aspiration pneumonia, pulmonary fibrosis, pulmonary tuberculosis, bronchiectasis, and (as a result of esophageal dilatation) hemorrhage and rupture of the esophagus (Andersen and Olsen). *Clinically* the duration of symptoms varies from one to many years. The condition is characterized by increasing dysphagia followed in time by regurgitation (due to esophageal obstruction) and paroxysmal coughing (as a result of spilling of the contents into the respiratory tract). The *diagnosis* is made from the history and the characteristic dilatation seen roentgenographically when barium is used as the contrast medium. *Treatment* consists of dilatation of the constricted segment or (in more severe cases) some type of operative procedure aimed at removing the obstruction. The *prognosis* is fair to good. Following dilatation of the esophagus the results are favorable in about 75 per cent of cases while following surgical intervention (because the cases are more advanced) the results are less favorable.

Chemical Burns.—Many chemicals, when swallowed accidentally or for suicidal purposes, may produce burns of the esophagus. Accidental burns *account for* over 80 per cent of cases, are almost exclusively seen in children, and are most common in boys. Some of the many *chemicals* listed by Uhde are lye, lysol, bichloride of mercury, phenol, iodine, formaldehyde, silver salts, sulphuric acid, hydrochloric acid, lactic acid, chlorox, nitric acid, acetic acid, chromic acid, oxalic acid, copper sulfate, ammonia, wood-staining compounds, caustic dyes, and chloroform (see also p. 242). Of these, lye still leads the list, accounting for about two-thirds of all cases.

Pathologically, regardless of the chemical, the areas affected are the mouth, pharynx, and the anatomic and physiologic narrowings of the esoph-

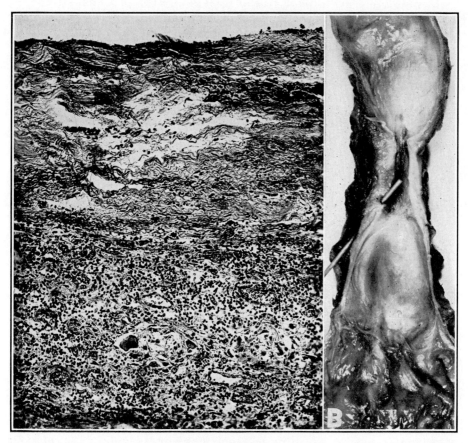

Fig. 289.—Lye burn of the esophagus illustrating *A*, complete denudation of the mucosa filling of the floor of the ulcer with fibrinous and necrotic material, and intense leukocytic infiltration of adjacent tissues. × 100, and *B*, stricture of the midportion of the esophagus with perforation resulting from an attempt at dilatation with a bougie. The expansion of the segment of the esophagus distally was produced by stuffing the lumen with cotton to accentuate the stricture.

agus. These are located at the level of the left bronchus, the region of the cricopharyngeus, and the esophagogastric junction. The appearance of the early lesion varies somewhat with the chemical but once the initial stage is passed there is little or no difference. Since a *lye* burn is the most common it merits a few separate words. At twenty-four hours the mucosa is edematous and often superficially ulcerated. The ulcers are covered with a brownish-gray exudate or slough and are surrounded by an intense leukocytic reaction (Fig. 289*A*). Within one to two weeks, their beds are covered with granulation tissue that is rich in capillaries and possesses a tendency to bleed readily. At approximately six weeks the granulation tissue is replaced with fibrous tissue and a stricture begins to form (Fig. 289*B*).

The *complications* consist of hemorrhage, perforation with periesophagitis and periesophageal abscess formation, esophageal obstruction, pulmonary disorders from aspiration of esophageal contents, and impaction of a foreign body in the esophagus at or above the point of constriction. *Clinical manifestations* consist of pain, frothy secretion in the pharynx, stridor (due to pressure of a dilated esophagus) and symptoms and signs resulting from the complications listed. The *diagnosis* is made from a history of swallowing the chemical, the appearance of the lesions in the mouth and pharynx elicited by direct examination, and the appearance of the lesions in the

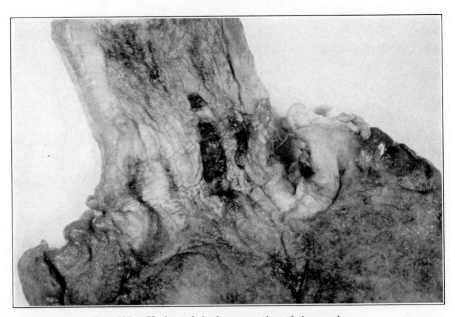

FIG. 290.—Varices of the lower portion of the esophagus.

esophagus as seen at the time of esophagoscopy. While *treatment* is variable, it is the concensus that neutralization of the chemical should be carried out immediately and that dilatation of the esophagus should be performed as necessary to prevent the formation of a stricture or to reestablish the lumen if stricture does occur. Recently cortisone has been advocated to prevent stricture formation (Rosenberg). The *prognosis* is fair to good.

Varices.—Varices (L. = dilated veins, arteries, or lymphatic channels) of the esophagus usually connote dilatation of the submucosal veins and occur in conjunction with portal hypertension (p. 831). The condition generally occurs in adults and the *incidence* parallels that of the *causative* factors. The latter may be listed as (1) intrahepatic—consisting of portal cirrhosis, thrombosis of hepatic veins, primary or secondary tumor of the liver, and hepatic abscess, (2) extrahepatic—consisting of thrombotic or other occlusions of the portal vein, or (3) idiopathic (Linton and Garrett). While the usual *site* of dilatation is the portion just above the esophagogastric junction, occasionally the cervical area may be affected (Palmer). *Grossly* the lesions are seen as prominent, dilated, serpiginous, deep blue channels coursing beneath the mucosa in a longitudinal fashion (Fig. 290). They contain fluid or clotted blood. *Histologically* they consist of dilated but otherwise relatively normal venous channels. The most common and most important *complications* are rupture and hemorrhage. The *clinical manifestations* consist of sudden, usually massive, hematemesis. The diagnosis is made from the history and the visualization of the dilatations esophagoscopically and roentgenographically. *Treatment* is principally that of the primary disease. Locally, balloon tamponade and, in some cases, surgical ligation have been advocated. The over-all late *prognosis* is usually poor, for death comes sooner or later as a result of hemorrhage.

Foreign Bodies. — Foreign bodies of the esophagus are more commonly seen in children than in adults. The *objects* are most variable. Those listed by Boyd, in a study of 400 cases, are coins, safety pins, buttons, thumb tacks, marbles, jacks, whistles, magnifying glasses, broken glass, fish bones, food, plastic toys, and pins. The usual *site* of lodgment is at the level of the cricoid for most objects (except a large bolus of food) go on into the stomach once they pass this barrier. The *complications* are (1) erosion and ulceration of the mucosa, (2) perforation with periesophagitis, mediastinitis, fistulous tract formation, and hemmorrhage, (3) esophageal fibrosis and stenosis, and (4) traction diverticulum from contraction of the periesophageal fibrous tissue. The *clinical manifestations* consist of vomiting, dysphagia, coughing, choking, and excessive salivation. The *diagnosis* is made from the history, roentgenography, and esophagoscopy. *Treatment* is esophagoscopic removal. The *prognosis* is excellent provided the sojourn is short and the object is removed skillfully. Otherwise, the complications listed may occur.

Fistulas. — An esophageal fistula may connect the esophagus with the tracheobronchial tree, mediastinum, pleura, pericardium, or skin (Abbott). Of these, one connecting the esophagus with the *respiratory tract* is most common. The communication usually occurs between the esophagus and trachea or the esophagus and the left bronchus. The *causes* are (1) congenital anomalies — esophageal atresia with tracheo-esophageal fistula (p. 633), (2) inflammations — peptic ulcer of the esophagus, fungous and yeast-like infections of the esophagus, tuberculous esophagitis, and syphilis of the esophagus, (3) physical disturbances — diverticulum, cardiospasm, chemical burns, trauma, and foreign bodies, and (4) tumors — especially carcinoma of the esophagus and, less often, carcinoma of the trachea or bronchus (Clagett). The most important *complication* is chronic pneumonitis (with its complications) from aspiration of esophageal contents (Levine). *Clinically* the following may be noted: increasing dysphagia, sudden cough and choking upon eating, expectoration of purulent sputum and occasionally blood, and fever. The *diagnosis* is made from the history, roentgenograms (not using barium for it is irritating to the respiratory tract), bronchoscopy, and esophagoscopy. *Treatment* resolves itself to eradicating the causative agent and restoring the passageway. The *prognosis* is that of the etiologic factor.

Rupture. — Rupture or perforation of the esophagus may occur spontaneously, as a result of previous disease, or as a result of trauma. By *spontaneous rupture* is meant perforation of the esophagus without preexisting disease and in the absence of direct mechanical trauma. Whether this is possible is still debatable. At any rate, the mechanism is stated as consisting of sudden increase of intraesophageal pressure as a result of (1) the forcing of gastric contents into the esophagus during vomiting, (2) defecation, (3) lifting heavy weights, and (4) induction of or recovery from anesthesia (Ware and Small). *Rupture* as a result of a *previous disease* may occur in conjunction with almost any one of the disorders of the esophagus listed in this Chapter (Gay). Of these, inflammations and tumors associated with ulceration are the most common. *Traumatic perforation* occurs as a result of the swallowing of foreign bodies, passing of bougies, and esophagoscopy (Figs. 289 and 291). The most common sites of perforation are at the levels of normal anatomic and physiologic constrictions and at (or in)

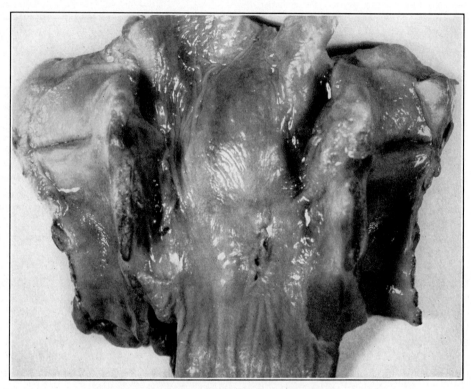

FIG. 291.—Perforation of the esophagus at the level of the cricoid as a result of injudicious esophagoscopy.

areas of organic stenosis. The *complications* are hemorrhage, mediastinal emphysema, periesophagitis, periesophageal abscess, fistulous tract formation, and the untoward effects of these complications. The *clinical manifestations* consist of pain, vomiting, shock, and the symptoms and signs of the complications listed. The *diagnosis* is made from the history, roentgenography, and esophagoscopy. *Treatment* consists of removal of the cause and suturing of the perforation. The *prognosis* depends upon the etiologic factor and the promptness with which therapy is instituted.

Dysphagia.—Dysphagia (Gr. = ill + to eat) means difficulty in swallowing. It is, of course, a symptom and not a disease. It may be on an organic or a functional basis. *Organic* causes of dysphagia constitute virtually all of the organic disorders that have been listed or discussed in this Chapter on the Esophagus. They may, of course, be classified under Congenital

Anomalies, Degenerations, Inflammations, Physical Disturbances, and Tumors. *Functional* causes of dysphagia consist of globus hystericus, diffuse spasm of the esophagus, and cardiospasm (McMahon).

TUMORS

Orientation.—Tumors and tumor-like conditions of the esophagus are quite common. They occur at all ages. Some are congenital while others are acquired, but the precise *etiologic agents* are not known. *Pathologically* virtually all of the tissues present in the normal esophagus (and sometimes tissues occurring as a transformation of normal cells or tissues not normally present) may give rise to benign and malignant neoplasms. They may be listed as follows: carcinoma, papilloma, adenoma, polyp, cyst, myoma, leiomyoma, rhabdomyosarcoma, fibroma, fibrosarcoma, myxofibroma, neurofibroma, lipoma, hemangioma, osteochondroma, and melanoblastoma. In addition, secondary tumors from distant areas also occur. Histologically the tumors are identical with similar growths elsewhere in the body. The *complications* of benign neoplasms are those of obstruction while the complications of malignant growths are those of obstruction and metastasis. The most outstanding *clinical manifestations* are dysphagia, mediastinal discomfort, and loss of weight. Later there is complete esophageal obstruction. The *diagnosis* of tumor may be made from the history, roentgenograms, and esophagoscopic appearance but a definitive diagnosis can be made only by biopsy. *Treatment* consists of excision or esophageal resection. The *prognosis* in benign tumors is good, while that in malignant tumors is fair to poor. Since carcinoma of the esophagus is about 100 times as common as all other growths put together it alone merits a few separate words.

Carcinoma.—Carcinoma of the esophagus, as a tumor of the digestive tract, is outnumbered in *frequency* only by carcinoma of the stomach and carcinoma of the large bowel. Although it may be found at any age beyond thirty years it is most common in the fifth and sixth decades of life (Merendino). It is recorded as predominating in males over females in an approximate ratio of 5 to 1. Not only is the *cause* unknown but even speculation regarding the etiologic agents is wanting.

Pathologically the most common sites of the growth, in decreasing order of frequency, are middle third, lower third, and upper third of the esophagus. While the early lesion doubtlessly starts as a small papule or ulcer, such changes are rarely seen for, by the time a correct diagnosis is made, the tumor is already well advanced. Fully developed growths may assume one of three forms with transitions from one to the other (Fig. 292). The most common is a diffuse infiltrating variety in which the wall is permeated for varying depths and over varying lengths. With the penetration there is gradual stenosis of the lumen until the passageway is almost completely or completely obliterated. The second most common variety is the ulcerating type. Such a tumor ulcerates as it penetrates until ultimately the entire central portion may be eaten away and the wall perforated. The least common variety is the fungating papillary type. Such a growth protrudes into the lumen as a large, usually sessile, bulky mass that may or may not show secondary superficial ulceration. In any case, the tumor is gray, firm, friable, and ill defined from the adjacent tissues. As it outgrows its blood supply it discloses yellowish foci of necrosis. *Histologically* carcinoma of the esophagus is usually of a squamous cell type of low or intermediate

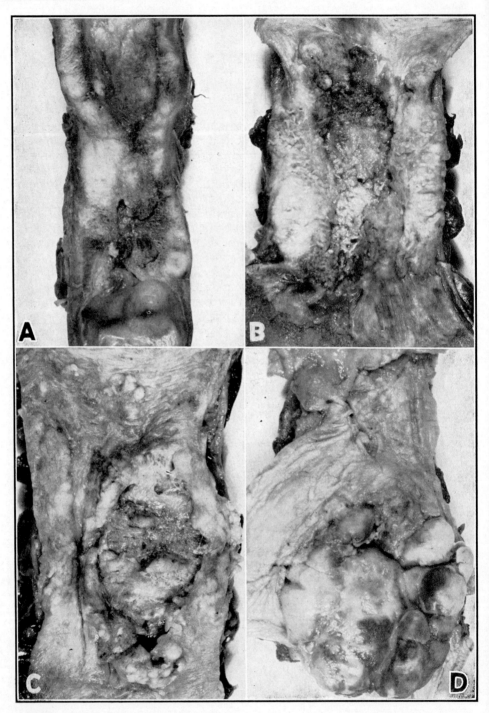

FIG. 292.—Carcinoma of the esophagus showing *A* and *B*, infiltrating stenotic lesions, *C*, an ulcerating tumor, and *D*, a fungating mass.

grade malignancy (Fig. 293A). As such, the tumor exists in the form of sheets, rounded masses, or single cells that infiltrate the submucosa, the musculature, and the periesophageal tissues. As in other locations of the body, the cells are large, polyhedral, and sharply or ill defined. The cytoplasm is moderate to abundant in amount and densely eosinophilic, and the nuclei are round, oval, or irregular and hyperchromatic. Epithelial pearl formation is generally abundant and mitoses may be numerous. In approximately 5 per cent of cases, carcinoma of the esophagus is of a gland-

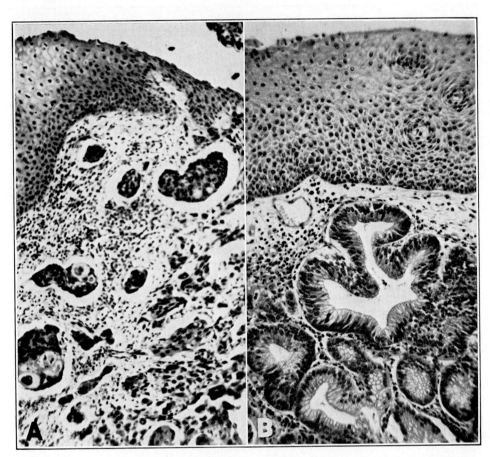

Fig. 293.—Carcinoma of the esophagus illustrating A, a squamous cell carcinoma with clusters of keratinizing squamous cells invading the submucosa and penetrating the lymphatics, and B, an adenocarcinoma with columnar cells in glandular formation invading the submucosa. × 100.

ular variety (Fig. 293B). As such, the cells are generally columnar or tall cuboidal, sharply defined, and arranged in more or less typical glands. The cytoplasm is moderate in amount and eosinophilic and the nuclei are oval and basilar in position. Some of the tumors secrete varying amounts of mucoid material. On extremely rare occasions, the tumor may consist of both a carcinoma and a sarcoma and is then referred to as a carcinosarcoma (Ende).

Carcinoma of the esophagus *spreads* by (1) direct extension to involve the aorta, bronchus, trachea, heart, and other mediastinal structures, (2) by the lymphatics to involve other portions of the esophagus, especially the mucosa (Figs. 292C and 293A) and to the mediastinal lymph nodes, and (3) by the bloodstream to involve the lungs, liver, adrenal glands, kidneys, pancreas, and almost every other organ of the body (Raven).

Aside from metastasis, the *complications* of carcinoma of the esophagus are starvation, dehydration, perforation, fistulous tract formation (Fig. 294), and pulmonary suppuration. In addition, it must be remembered

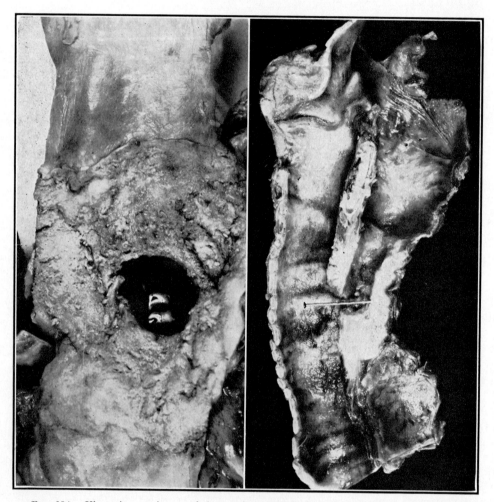

FIG. 294.—Ulcerating carcinoma of the esophagus producing a tracheo-esophageal fistula.

that patients with carcinoma of the esophagus are usually in the older age bracket and that they may possess many other disorders that are not directly or even indirectly related to the tumor. *Clinically* the most common manifestations consist of dysphagia (first to solids and then to fluids), pain, vomiting, and regurgitation (Merendino and Parker). In addition, as the lesion advances, there are frequently cough, hemoptysis, weakness, hematemesis, melena, anorexia, hoarseness, etc. The *diagnosis* is arrived at from the history, the roentgenographic appearance of a barium-filled esophagus, and biopsy. *Treatment* of choice is surgical resection with esophagogastric anastomosis (Brewer). In nonresectable lesions, palliative procedures consist of irradiation, gastrostomy, or some sort of thoracic shunt (Ravitch). The *prognosis* is poor for the over-all five-year survival rate is less than 1 per cent. The average expectation of life after the diagnosis has been made varies from two to twelve months.

REFERENCES

Pathologic Physiology

BOSMA, J. F.: Physiol. Rev., *37*, 275, 1955 (Deglutition, Pharyngeal Stage).
CREAMER, B., *et al.*: Gastroenterol., *34*, 782, 1958 (Esophageal Motility).
FLOOD, C. A., *et al.*: Gastroenterol., *34*, 410, 1958 (Achalasia).
TEMPLETON, F. E.: X-*ray Examination of Stomach*, Chicago, Univ., Chicago Press, 1944 (Esophagus Radiology).
WINKELSTEIN, A.: Med. Clin. N. America, *28*, 589, 1944 (Cardiospasm).

Congenital Anomalies

BERMAN, J. K., *et al.*: J. Thoracic Surg., *24*, 493, 1952 (Esophagobronchial Fistula in Adults).
BIGGER, I. A.: Ann. Surg., *129*, 572, 1949 (Tracheo-esophageal Fistula).
BUTLER, C. L., and ENDE, M.: A. M. A. Arch. Path., *49*, 605, 1950 (Double Esophagus with Carcinoma).
DAVIS, J. E., and BARNES, W. A.: Ann. Surg., *136*, 287, 1952 (Duplications Alimentary Tract).
GROSS, R. E., and NEUHAUSER, E. B. D.: Pediatrics, *7*, 69, 1951 (Compression Esophagus by Vascular Anomaly).
HOLINGER, P. H., *et al.*: Ann. Otol., Rhin. & Laryngol., *60*, 707, 1951 (Anomalies).
LANGSTON, H. T., *et al.*: A. M. A. Arch. Surg., *61*, 949, 1950 (Esophageal Duplications).
POTTS, W. J.: J. Thoracic Surg., *20*, 671, 1950 (Tracheo-esophageal Fistula).
RENNIE, J. B., *et al.*: Brit. M. J., *2*, 1443, 1949 (Short Esophagus).
SINCLAIR, W. J.: A. M. A. Arch. Surg., *62*, 557, 1951 (Congenitally Short Esophagus).

Degenerations

CORDRAY, D.: Ann. Otol., Rhin. & Laryngol., *49*, 160, 1940 (Plummer-Vinson Syndrome).
KERNAN, J. D.: A. M. A. Arch. Otolaryngol., *32*, 662, 1940 (Plummer-Vinson Syndrome).
KISCH, A. M.: Am. J. Digest. Dis., *16*, 405, 1949 (Esophageal Lesions in Scleroderma).
OLSEN, A. M., *et al.*: A. M. A. Arch. Int. Med., *76*, 189, 1945 (Esophageal Lesions in Scleroderma).

Inflammations

CLEAVER, E. E.: Am. J. Digest. Dis., *10*, 319, 1943 (Peptic Ulcer).
FRANKLIN, R. H., and TAYLOR, S.: J. Thoracic Surg., *19*, 292, 1950 (Granulomatous Esophagitis).
GRUENWALD, P., and MARSH, M. R.: A. M. A. Arch. Path., *49*, 1, 1950 (Acute Esophagitis in Infants).
GUGGENHEIM, A., *et al.*: Am. Rev. Tuberc., *46*, 577, 1942 (Tuberculosis).
HARMAN, J. B.: Brit. M. J., *1*, 941, 1952 (Esophagitis).
HUDSON, T. R., and HEAD, J. R.: J. Thoracic Surg., *20*, 216, 1950 (Syphilis).
OLSEN, A. M.: Surg., Gynec. & Obst., *86*, 372, 1948 (Esophagitis).
POTTER, W. H., *et al.*: New York State J. Med., *51*, 1924, 1951 (Peptic Esophagitis).
RADISH, M. H., and KERTZNER, B.: Gastroenterology, *18*, 579, 1951 (Peptic Ulcer).
RIPLEY, H. R., *et al.*: Surgery, *32*, 1, 1952 (Esophagitis after Esophagogastric Anastomosis).

Physical Disturbances

ABBOTT, O. A.: J. Thoracic Surg., *14*, 382, 1945 (Fistulas).
ANDERSEN, H. A., *et al.*: J. A. M. A., *151*, 608, 1953 (Cardiospasm).
BOYD, G.: Canad. M. A. J., *64*, 102, 1951 (Foreign Bodies).
CLAGETT, O. T., *et al.*: Surg., Gynec. & Obst., *82*, 87, 1946 (Fistulas).
CROSS, F. S.: Surgery, *31*, 647, 1952 (Cardiospasm).
DEBAKEY, M. E.: J. A. M. A., *150*, 1076, 1952 (Diverticula).

GARRETT, N., JR., and GALL, E. A.: A. M. A. Arch. Path., *55*, 196, 1953 (Varices without Cirrhosis).

GAY, B. B., JR.: Am. J. Roentgenol., *68*, 183, 1952 (Perforations).

GOODMAN, H. I., and PARNES, I. H.: J. Thoracic Surg., *23*, 145, 1952 (Epiphrenic Diverticulum).

KATZ, H. L.: Am. Rev. Tuberc., *65*, 455, 1952 (Traction Diverticula).

KAUSEL, H. W., and LINDSKOG, G. E.: Dis. Chest., *21*, 334, 1952 (Epiphrenic Diverticulum).

KAY, E. B.: J. Thoracic Surg., *22*, 254, 1951 (Cardiospasm).

LEVINE, I.: J. A. M. A., *151*, 995, 1953 (Broncho-esophageal Fistula and Pneumonitis).

LINTON, R. R.: Ann. Int. Med., *31*, 794, 1949 (Varices).

McMAHON, J. M.: Am. Pract., *3*, 744, 1952 (Functional Dysphagia).

OLSEN, A. M., *et al.*: J. Thoracic Surg., *22*, 164, 1951 (Cardiospasm).

PALMER, E. D.: Am. J. Digest. Dis., *19*, 375, 1952 (Varices Cervical Esophagus).

ROSENBERG, N., *et al.*: A. M. A. Arch. Surg., *63*, 147, 1951 (Lye Strictures and Cortisone).

SMALL, A. R., and BOYD, L. J.: Am. J. Digest. Dis., *19*, 73, 1952 (Rupture).

UHDE, G. I.: Ann. Otol., Rhin. & Laryngol., *55*, 795, 1946 (Chemical Burns).

WARE, G. W., *et al.*: A. M. A. Arch. Surg., *65*, 723, 1952 (Spontaneous Rupture).

Tumors

BREWER L. A. III,: West. J. Surg., *60*, 1, 1952 (Carcinoma).

CHI, P. S. H., and ADAMS, W. E.: A. M. A. Arch. Surg., *60*, 92, 1949 (Benign Tumors).

CORNELL, A., *et al.*: Gastroenterology, *15*, 260, 1950 (Cysts).

ENDE, N., *et al.*: Am. J. Roentgenol., *65*, 227, 1951 (Carcinosarcoma).

ENGELKING, C. F., *et al.*: A. M. A. Arch. Otolaryngol., *52*, 150, 1950 (Benign Tumors).

GIBBON, J. H., JR., *et al.*: J. A. M. A., *145*, 1035, 1951 (Carcinoma).

GOLDMAN, J. L., *et al.*: J. A. M. A., *149*, 144, 1952 (Adenocarcinoma).

McPEAK, E., and ARONS, W. L.: A. M. A. Arch. Path., *44*, 385, 1947 (Adenoacanthoma).

MERENDINO, E. A., and MARK, V. H.: Cancer, *5*, 52, 1952 (Carcinoma).

————: Surg., Gynec. & Obst., *94*, 110, 1952, (Carcinoma).

PARKER, E. F., *et al.*: Ann. Surg., *135*, 697, 1952 (Carcinoma).

RAVEN, R. W.: Brit. J. Surg., *36*, 70, 1948 (Carcinoma).

RAVITCH, M. M., *et al.*: J. Thoracic Surg., *24*, 256, 1952 (Carcinoma).

SCHAFER, P. W., and KITTLE, C. F.: J. A. M. A., *133*, 1202, 1947 (Leiomyoma).

Chapter

17

Stomach

PATHOLOGIC PHYSIOLOGY

M. H. F. FRIEDMAN

ALTHOUGH *reservoir* capacity probably is the most important function of the *stomach*, the pathophysiology of gastric disease is mainly referable to dysfunctions of gastric *secretion* and *motility*. Symptoms due to absence of *storage capacity* are evident only following surgical removal of the stomach and are quite different from those found in patients with a completely non-functioning stomach. After total *gastrectomy* the *dumping syndrome* which is associated with rapid filling of the small intestine frequently may be quite marked, while in extensive atrophic *gastritis* and *gastric atony* the symptoms are due to gastric retention and impaired evacuation.

The role of the esophagus in the filling of the stomach has been referred to in Chapter 16, page 631. The question of a distinct *sphincter* muscle at the *esophago-cardiac junction* still remains to be settled. The consensus is that the sphincteric action at this junction is not due to a single specific anatomic unit but to the interplay of several para-esophageal attachments. The sphincteric mechanism is relaxed very readily by slight pressure from the esophageal side but can withstand high pressures from the gastric side. When intragastric pressure builds up to the extent of forcibly overcoming sphincteric resistance, the sudden release of gas constitutes the "*belch*." The major function of the cardiac sphincteric mechanism is to prevent regurgitation into the esophagus of acid gastric contents. *Esophagitis* and *peptic ulceration* of the esophagus may result from chronic gastric reflux. In *hiatal hernias*, particularly those due to a congenitally short esophagus, the supradiaphragmatic esophago-cardiac sphincteric mechanism is chronically patent and erosive lesions are common.

The *empty stomach* shows periodic *bouts* of *activity* which increase in intensity, though not duration, the longer the period of fasting. Peristaltic waves originate at a rate of about three per minute in the cardiac region and course over the stomach toward the duodenum. A progression of waves of about 30 minutes' duration is succeeded by a relatively quiescent period of one or two hours' duration to be followed once again by a phase of activity. Subjective sensations of hunger are associated with the more powerful contractions and hence these are usually called "*hunger contractions*." Interdigestive periodic contractions are also exhibited by the duodenum usually concomitant with those occurring in the stomach. In the healthy person it is probable that the associated gastric and duodenal contractions are experienced as "*hunger pangs*" while in the patient with duodenal ulcer they constitute the *ulcer pains*. Gastroduodenal motor activity in the ulcer patient may be particularly strong in the early morning hours and at this

time give rise to severe pains. Both the gastric and duodenal hunger contractions and the accompaning hunger sensations are readily inhibited by
sipping water or smoking. This inhibition is the basis for the relief from
ulcer pain which the patient obtains from even small amounts of food.

On food being swallowed there is, for a brief interval, a decrease in *gastric
tonus* and cessation of gastric contractions. The lowered tonus is an accommodation reflex of receptive relaxation which permits filling of the stomach
without increasing the intragastric pressure. Soon after the meal is ingested,
the tonus returns and a new kind of peristaltic motor activity begins. The
peristalses of digestion differ from the interdigestive peristalses in that the
waves begin with regular frequency at the corpus rather than cardia, they
progress at a steady rate towards the pylorus, and they continue uninterrupted until the stomach is empty.

The phasic pressure generated by the peristaltic wave together with the
basal intragastric pressure due to muscle tonus establish a *pressure gradient*
between the stomach and duodenum. Emptying of the stomach is regulated
almost entirely by this pressure gradient. To correct a common misconception it must be emphasized that normally the state of the pyloric sphincter has little control over gastric evacuation. If the intragastric pressure
is low, as in gastric atony, then gastric evacuation does not occur even though
the sphincter is also relaxed. The failure of the stomach to empty after
vagectomy is due to exactly this condition. The *pyloric sphincter* probably
is closed only a small fraction of the time. The major role of the pyloric sphincter
is to regulate retrograde flow. In this, the sphincter acts in a manner similar
to the cardiac sphincter. When the intraduodenal pressure rises, regurgitation of duodenal contents into the stomach is prevented by closure of the
sphincter.

Spasm of the *pylorus* probably occurs infrequently. What is usually
diagnosed as pylorospasm is most often a state of low gastric tonus. Barium
which is found radiographically to have remained in the stomach is often
erroneously interpreted as being due to spasm of the pyloric muscle. More
often, this indicates an inadequate pressure gradient due to *gastric atony*
and is readily recognized as such from the absence of peristaltic movements.
When pylorospasm does occur, as in *infants*, it appears to involve the myenteric ganglion cells of the muscle and may be differentiated from retention
due to low gastric tonus by the presence of vigorous antral peristalisis.
Similarly, in gastric retention due to pyloric obstruction, the dilated stomach
is not atonic but exhibits strong peristaltic movements.

Gastric evacuation time is also affected by *stomach shape*, being longer in
the fish-hook or J-shaped than in the steer-horn shaped stomach. This
reflects the influence of body habitus. In addition, the larger the meal, the
coarser its composition, and the greater the fat content the longer will it
remain in the stomach. The effects of fat are largely due to the formation
by the intestinal mucosa of *enterogastrone* which acts to inhibit both gastric
mobility and secretion.

Stimulation of the *vagus nerve* generally causes increase in tonus and motor
activities of the stomach, and decrease in tonus or relaxation of the pyloric
sphincter. *Sympathetic stimulation* usually has the opposite effects. Lest,
however, this be interpreted as evidence for the view that gastric motor
dysfunctions are due to autonomic imbalance, it should be pointed out that
the two autonomic effector systems are synergistic rather than antagonistic,
and that the effect of either nervous system is determined by the metabolic
state of the gastric musculature. In inflammatory disease processes involv-

ing the muscle, belladonna sometimes may have a mild to moderate spasmic rather than spasmolytic effect. The vagus exerts a tonic effect on the gastric musculature as may be evident from the acute atony which develops after vagectomy. Tonus of smooth muscle, however, is myogenic in origin and ultimately gastric tonus may return to near normal.

The motor activities of the stomach, and hence *emptying time*, can also be influenced by the *emotional state* of the patient. In acute episodes of fear there is delay in the gastric evacuation. The associated thoracico-lumbar (or sympathetic) discharge and adrenal gland secretion is evident from blanching, pupil size, etc. On the other hand, in chronic emotional states, such as anger and resentment, there is hypermotility and rapid stomach emptying. Direct inspection of the stomach at this time shows the gastric mucosa to be reddened and engorged with blood.

Vomiting is a complicated process in which many somatic and visceral structures participate in a co-ordinated manner through regulation by a medullary vomiting center. So-called *"central vomiting"* may be induced by direct mechanical stimulation of the center (as by increased intracranial pressure) or indirectly following administration of drugs (such as emetine, apomorphine, morphine, or digitalis) by excitation of one or more closely allied chemo-receptor trigger zones in the brain (forebrain, hypothalamus, and other areas). *"Peripheral vomiting"* is initiated by reflexes from nearly all body structures but most usually these originate in the gastrointestinal tract and other abdominal viscera. *Motion* (sea) *sickness* is due to visceral and labyrinthine stimulation of the vomiting center. One may consider vomiting a self-perpetuating process to the extent that the odor of vomitus is a potent stimulus for vomiting. *Retching* is distinguished from vomiting in that no gastric contents are expelled.

The principal *stimuli* for *reflex vomiting* are gastrointestinal irritation (as by mustard) and disention of bowel loops. The afferent pathways of such reflex vomiting are chiefly along vagal fibers but undoubtedly afferents in sympathetic trunks also participate. The chief force for the act of vomiting is derived from the abdominal muscles and diaphragm and not, as erroneously assumed, from the stomach. The esophagus, cardiac sphincter, and stomach are relaxed and the thorax becomes fixed with the glottis closed. Then the diaphragm descends with concurrent sudden contraction of the abdominal muscles. The pyloric sphincter is usually closed but in extensive vomiting it may be relaxed and associated with reverse peristalsis of the intestine. The presence of stool in the vomitus indicates participation of the large bowel in this reverse gradient of transfer.

In man, the *gastric glands* at *birth* are potentially able to secrete acid of relatively high concentration. Gastric secretion occurs spontaneously even before the first meal is taken but a small percentage of children fail to secrete acid during the first year of life and it is probable that most of these will remain achlorhydric. The incidence of true achlorhydria increases with age and reaches a plateau of about 10 per cent by the sixth decade.

The gastric glands in the *adult* human secrete continously even in the absence of discernible stimuli. This continuous basal or interdigestive secretion is augmented by appropriate stimuli such as food and psychic phenomena. In the healthy individual the volume of fasting secretion which can be recovered by morning is usually less than 50 ml. It is usually believed that basal gastric hypersecretion is a characteristic of the patient with duodenal ulcer. Single aspirations of the stomach or serial intermittant aspirations certainly show that more gastric juice may be recovered from the ulcer patient. This, however, frequently reflects the degree of gastric retention in the ulcer patient (due to pyloric stenosis, etc.) rather than a true over-activity of the secretory elements.

Gastric secretion is dependent (as indeed are all digestive secretions) on an adequate blood flow to provide the water in which the electrolytes and enzymes are dissolved. The gastric mucosa is fed by blood from a vast mucosal capillary bed which is derived from numerous arteries with many freely interanastamotic connections. The arrangement is such as to best supply the mucosa with the tremendous quantities of blood required for active secretion without depriving at the same time the circulatory needs of nonsecretory elements. The intramural blood supply from several sources readily explains the resumption of secretory functions after external devascularization of large segments of the stomach. In extensive impairment of *blood flow* to the secretory glands, however, as in edema of the stomach, there is a marked reduction in acid secretion. The lability of the gastrointestinal circulation is also a feature well adapted for homeostasis. The blood supply to the digestive tract in periods of stress may readily be shifted to muscular and nervous tissue which have more urgent needs for adequate maintenance of blood flow. This accounts in part for the reduced digestive activities and impaired absorption which occurs in stress situations and also for the complaint of dyspepsia, etc. in tense individuals.

The mechanism by which *acid* is *formed* and secreted by the *parietal cell* remains unknown. Normally, the parietal cell is indefatigable as long as the supply of water is maintained. The energy requirements for the secretory process are relatively high so that interference with parietal cell metabolism by antimetabolites and disease produce achlorhydria quite readily. In contrast to the parietal cells, the *chief cells* which secrete *pepsin* and the *mucus-secreting* surface *epithelial cells* are readily exhaustable. The near identity of the chemical structures of both pepsin and the mucin which is secreted by the neck cells suggests that the neck cells serve as precursors in the histogenesis of the chief cells. If true, this would explain why, even in the achlorhydria of pernicious anemia, the gastric juice contains pepsin and mucus.

The concentration of the *hydrochloric acid* secreted by the *parietal cell* is constant at 170 milli-equivalents per liter. Each cell always secretes at its maximal rate so that variations in the volume of juice formed are due to variations in the number of secreting parietal cells. The term *"hyperacidity"* is a misnomer for a condition which actually reflects inadequate neutralization of larger volume of acid. More properly, it should be designated *"hyper-secretion."* The *lowered acidity* usual in gastritis and frequent in gastric cancer similarly is explained by a reduction in the number of parietal cells which can participate in the secretory process.

The *properties* and *functions* of the *gastric acid* and *pepsin* are well known and require no comment here. The chemical properties of mucus, such as its high viscosity, adhesiveness, absorptive powers, and alkalinity show that it is ideally suitable for counteracting gastric irritants. When, however, such protection by the mucus layer which closely surrounds the epithelium fails to be adequate, then the response of the mucous cells themselves constitutes a second line of defence. The cells become themselves detached from the epithelium to enter into interaction with the irritant. Epithelial surfaces so denuded show remarkable regenerative powers and may appear normal in a matter of hours. Whether failure in such protection against dietary carcinogens is involved in gastric cancer is problematic.

Gastric secretion is under both *nervous* and *humoral control*. The secretory fibers to the parietal, peptic, and mucous cells are carried only in the *vagus*. No direct inhibitory fibers for secretion are present but *sympathetic stimulation* may depress secretion indirectly through reduction in volume flow of blood to the glands. Hypoglycemia induced by insulin excites the central nervous system, including the vagus centers, and hence provokes gastric secretion. Since insulin-induced hypoglycemia does not excite secretion after the vagi have been cut, the *insulin test* can be used to determine the thoroughness of a *vagotomy* operation for peptic ulcer. *Histamine* is the most potent known stimulus for the parietal cells. Unlike vagus stimulation, histamine has no effect on pepsin secretion. In trauma due to muscle crush or skin burns the associated gastric hypersecretion and perforating acute gastric ulcer sometimes is seen probably due to histamine released by the injured tissues.

The *secretion* of *gastric juice* can best be described as occurring in three *phases*, designated by the chief site of action of the secretory stimulus. The *initial reflex phase*, often called the cephalic or psychic phase, occurs promptly after food is taken into the mouth and is provoked by the tastes and odors of the foods. The secretion of this phase is of high peptic activity and in man may account for more than half of the total volume of acid secreted in response to a meal. The secretion is purely nervous in origin and is readily abolished by vagectomy. The *second* or *pyloric phase* is initiated by contact of the food with the mucosa of the pyloric antrum. Either distention of the antrum or certain chemical constituents of the food provoke the elaboration of a gastric hormone called gastrin. Gastrin has the specific property of stimulating the parietal cells of the corpus and fundus. The acid secretion from the pyloric phase is absent following resection of the pyloric antrum. The *third* or *intestinal phase* of gastric secretion is the weakest. It probably accounts for only about 15 per cent of the acid secreted following a meal and is due in part to an intestinal gastrin, in part to intestinal gastric reflexes, and in part to the secretogogue action of absorbed digestion products.

Fats and *fatty foods* have the property of *depressing gastric secretion* when acting from the intestine. This inhibition is due to the elaboration of the intestinal hormone *enterogastrone*. The secretory depression seen in ulcer patients maintained on milk and cream mixtures is based on this rational. When, however, too much fat is ingested, there is a biophasic action in that the inhibition is followed by a subsequent phase of augmented acid secretion. This rebound secretion of acid results from formation of gastrin by the fatty acids which are regurgitated into the antrum. In ulcer patients particularly the rebound effects from fat ingestion may become distressing because of the sustained secretion of acid.

Autoregulatory mechanism of both extragastric and intragastric origin come into play to regulate the acidity of the gastric contents which enter the duodenum and also to control the rate of acid secretion by the parietal cell. The alkaline mucus and other nonparietal secretions of the stomach dilute and partially neutralize the acid and a similar effect is exerted by the regurgitated succus entericus and the draining salivary and esophageal secretions. There is evidence that, in addition, the acidity is reduced by a process in which hydrogen ions diffuse from the gastric lumen back into the plasma, to be replaced by an equivalent amount of other anions (chiefly sodium) which diffuse into the gastric lumen. The low acidity of the accumulated gastric contents found in pyloric obstruction may in part be explained on this basis.

Under certain conditions *hydrochloric acid* in the stomach or duodenum has a pronounced *inhibitory effect* on the rate of gastric secretion. Furthermore, acid in contact with the antrum inhibits the release of gastrin and hence gastric secretion is depressed. The necessary condition for this inhibitory action of acid in the intestine is an intestinal pH level below 4.0. Since normally in the intestine pH values below 3.5 are rare, it is apparent that this is in the nature of an emergency mechanism brought into play when the acidity of the duodenum is at potentially damaging concentrations. The nature of this mechanism remains obscure. Deficiency or dysfunction of the mechanism may be a factor for the continuous hypersecretion of gastric juice seen in some patients with active ulcer symptoms.

More theories have been advanced for the *etiology* of *peptic ulcer* than for any other disease of the digestive system and the subject is still a controversial matter. Bacterial, toxic, digestive, congenital, nutritional, and allergic factors are only a few of the many factors which have been implicated. Common to these theories is the belief that the various factors bring about defects in the mucosal integrity by adversely affecting the innervation and blood supply to the mucosa. Animal experimentation has shown that these factors may produce mucosal erosions and ulcerations but it must be emphasized that spontaneous healing of the lesions occurs nearly always as soon as the insulting agent is removed. Furthermore, the experimental ulcer resembles the ulcer found in man only superficially. The present-day concept is that the integrity of the gastrointestinal mucosa is maintained by a balance between ulcerogenic factors and reparative factors and that this balance is a constitutional characteristic. The ulcerogenic factors (such as vascular spasm, hypermotility, hypersecretion, etc.) probably are in constant operation but do not express themselves as frank ulcers unless the mucosa is deficient in the protective mechanisms of tissue healing and repair.

In *ulcer treatment* attention has been focused chiefly on reducing the influence of the ulcerogenic factors. Neutralization of the acidity and depression of acid secretion and motility by drugs (belladonna, ganglionic blockading agents) or surgery (vagectomy) are methods most commonly employed to reduce the influence of ulcerogenic factors. Recently, however, attempts at ulcer therapy have been instituted which leave acid secretion unaffected but aim at stimulating the reparative processes by substitution therapy with gastrointestinal tissue extracts. Results are still equivocal.

There is no evidence that benign gastric ulcer is different from duodenal ulcer except for characteristic differences in the acid secretion patterns. In *duodenal ulcer*, as discussed above, there is usually a marked hypersecretion, especially in the interdigestive period, while in *gastric ulcer* acid secretion may be normal but more often is depressed. The provocative question is what this difference indicates. The view that unneutralized acid secretion contributes to the maintenance of ulcer chronicity but probably is not responsible for ulcer pathogenesis may hold for duodenal ulcer but obviously is not applicable to gastric ulcer. There is evidence for the concept that the hypersecretion in duodenal ulcer and the hyposecretion in gastric ulcer result from the ulcer and are not causal factors. Throughout the gastrointestinal tract, local irritation usually results in a decrease in the serous fluid and an increase in the mucous secretions. For example, in gastritis, whether atrophic or hypertrophic, there is an increased secretion of mucus and the gastric glands may even be replaced by intestinal mucous secreting glands. Similarly, irritation of an intestinal loop soon results in the local secretion of small amounts of fluid with high mucus content. Quite different however, are the effects on glandular secretion of irritant stimuli applied at a point removed distally. There is the general rule that gastrointestinal irritation results in profuse secretion of fluid from the glands above or cephalad to the point of stimulation. An example (already referred to) is the esophago-salivary reflex in which stimulation of the esophagus results in profuse secretion of the salivary glands. Another well-known example is the greatly increased secretion of fluid from a segment of intestine cephalad to a point of obstruction. In each the augmented fluid production is a purposive response to remove irritants from lower regions by a "washing away" effect. The ulcer in the duodenum similarly serves as a point of stimulation of increased fluid secretion from the gastric glands. This is consistent with clinical experience that eradication of the ulcer is followed by a lowered basal secretory rate. Since most of the fluid secreted by the stomach is hydrochloric acid there may be initiated a vicious circle. The continued excitation of the pariental cells by the focus of irritation in the duodenum may result in hyperplasia with consequently potentially more acid secreted. According to some pathologists, in duodenal ulcer there is an absolute increase in the number of parietal cells, and hyperplasia has also been produced experimentally by stimulation of parietal cells at high rates of secretion for many weeks.

The basis of *pain* originating in a lesion of the stomach is essentially the same as that of the rest of the gastrointestinal tract and will be considered in detail in the section on the Small Intestine, Chapter 18, page 691.

GENERAL CONSIDERATIONS

In this Chapter on the Stomach the disorders will be discussed under the usual five major categories of disease processes. Before proceeding with the dissertation, however, it may be profitable (because the terminology is often confusing) to review briefly the various subdivisions of the normal stomach. In general, the stomach is more or less J-shaped. Its junction with the esophagus is called the *cardiac orifice*, while its junction with the duodenum is known as the *pyloric orifice*. The *lesser curvature* connects the two orifices superiorly and to the right, while the *greater curvature* connects them inferiorly and to the left. A niche near the distal portion of the lesser curvature is known as the *incisur angularis*, and a line drawn perpendicularly across the stomach from this angulation divides the organ into a larger proximal portion called the *body* and a smaller distal portion referred to as the *pylorus*. The portion of the body that lies above a horizontal line drawn at the junction of the left side of the esophagus with the stomach is called the *fundus*, while that which approaches the cardiac orifice is known as the *cardia*. The pylorus, in turn, is divided into a proximal *pyloric vestibule* and a distal *pyloric antrum* by a transverse line (the sulcus intermedius) directed at right angles to the stomach starting about midway between the incisur angularis and the pyloric orifice.

CONGENITAL ANOMALIES

Orientation.—Some congenital anomalies of the stomach are common while others are rare and some are attended by grave consequences while others are of little significance. The important lesions may be listed as follows: variations in size, variations in position, duplication, faulty development, hypertrophic pyloric stenosis, webs, inclusions, and diverticulum.

Variations in Size.—Normally the size of the stomach varies with its state of contraction or relaxation, the amount of food it contains, and the size of the individual concerned. Beyond this, however, the organ may be larger than normal—*macrogastria* (Gr. = large + stomach) or smaller than normal—*microgastria* (Gr. = small + stomach).

Variations in Position.—Normally the stomach lies in the upper part of the abdomen just beneath the left costal margin, the diaphragm, and the quadrate and left lobes of the liver. An *inferior* displacement to the rim of the pelvis or even into the pelvis is generally an acquired condition that is, as a rule, associated with an inferior displacement (*visceroptosis*) of other abdominal viscera. Its *superior* displacement into the mediastinum or thoracic cavity may be acquired, as in the case of diaphragmatic hernia, or congenital, as in the case of a congenitally short esophagus (p. 633). A superior displacement is usually partial but it may be complete (thoracic stomach). The former is particularly prone to the development of ulcers and neither, of course, escapes other diseases such as carcinoma, etc. (Pack). Another rare abnormality in position is a mirror image transposition as seen in *situs inversus*.

Duplication.—Duplication of the stomach consists of cysts found in relation to the esophagus or the stomach and called *gastroenteric cysts* (p. 548) or of linear *tube-like structures* found in the same areas and communicating with these organs by one or two ostia (Barbosa). In either case, the wall is composed of one or two layers of smooth muscle lined with gastric (and less often enteric) mucosa and the lumen is filled with fluid or is empty. The duplication may produce symptoms by virtue of obstruction of the normal alimentary tract, distention of the duplication, or vascular occlusion of either structure.

Faulty Development.—The most common faulty development of the stomach as a whole consists of an *absence* of the *fundus*, while the most common faulty development of a portion of the stomach consists of a *failure* of the *musculature* to completely invest the circumference of the organ (Herbut and Ross). The latter abnormality is of special interest for it produces a weak spot in the wall of the stomach which readily leads to perforation and, if not attended to promptly, to peritonitis and death.

Hypertrophic Pyloric Stenosis.—This condition consists of a hypertrophy of the pyloric sphincter along with an element of spasm. It is a congenital condition *affecting* (generally first-born) males in about 85 per cent of cases and usually occurring during the third week of postnatal life (Wood) but occasionally being found in adults (Kleitsch). The *cause* of the condition is doubtlessly a hereditary defect in the genes, for the abnormality has been recorded in twins, relatives, and successive generations (Powell and Carter). *Pathologically* there is hypertrophy and hyperplasia of the circular muscle of the pyloric ring (Rheinlander) resulting in a firm sausage-shaped swelling that measures up to 2 cm. in diameter and 2 to 3 cm. in length. The mucosa is thrown into folds and the lumen is completely obliterated. To begin with, there is no inflammation but eventually the submucosa discloses edema and leukocytic infiltration. The *complications* are obstruction, loss of weight, emaciation, and dehydration. *Clinically* the outstanding manifestations are vomiting without anorexia and with constipation followed by the other complications listed (Wood). The *diagnosis* is made from the history, careful physical examination (with palpation of the tumor), and roentgenographic appearance (Astley). *Treatment* consists of surgical severance of the muscle coats from the serosa to the submucosa along the long axis of the duodenum. The *prognosis* is excellent. The mortality rate should not exceed 2 per cent.

Webs.—The occurrence of a web or diaphragm with a central perforation has been described at the pyloric sphincter but is extremely rare (Rota). Pathologically it consists simply of a mucosal fold. The lesion, of course, produces obstruction which clinically is indistinguishable from any other obstruction at the pylorus.

Inclusions.—There are two types of inclusions in the stomach wall—gastrointestinal and pancreatic *Gastrointestinal*. inclusions consist of incorporations of gastrointestinal glands in the musculature along with hypertrophy and hyperplasia of the latter. The lesion thus is similar to adenomyosis of the uterus. It occurs in the region of the pylorus and may be the cause of pyloric obstruction. *Pancreatic* inclusions are fairly common, there being recorded about 150 cases up to 1951 (Benner). The condition represents an abnormal congenital misplacement of pancreatic tissue. *Pathologically* the rest is located within 5 to 6 cm. of the pylorus, may be found between any of the layers of the stomach, measures from a few millimeters to 6 cm. in diameter, and frequently shows ulceration of the overlying mucosa. *Histologically* it is composed of normal pancreatic tissue and is accompanied by hypertrophy and hyperplasia of the supporting muscle and inflammation of the adjacent tissues. The *complications* consist of the formation of diverticula of the stomach wall, ulceration of the mucosa, and pyloric obstruction. *Clinical manifestations* are those of the complications. The *diagnosis* can be made with certainty only upon histologic examination of removed tissue. *Treatment* is surgical excision. The *prognosis* is excellent.

Diverticulum.—Diverticula of the stomach are relatively common for, by 1949, there were at least 242 cases *recorded* (Brown). The incidence, however, as given by different authors varies from 1 in 833 to 1 in 3,661 roentgenographic examinations. The condition is more *common* in females than it is in males and while it is found at all ages, the peak incidence appears to be in the sixth decade. The *cause* is some weakness in the wall of the stomach. *Pathologically* diverticula may be divided into two groups—congenital and acquired. *Congenital* diverticula are due to a congenital weakness in the gastric wall, are almost always located in the cardia, and are generally composed of all the layers of the stomach wall. *Acquired* diverticula are caused by an acquired weakness of the gastric wall (inflammation, tumor, etc.), are located predominantly in the cardia but may be found in any portion of the stomach, and are composed of all or only some of the layers of the stomach wall. Regardless of the type of diverticulum, the ostium is usually wide and the size is seldom greater than 6 × 3 cm. The recorded *complications* are mucosal ulcer, hemorrhage, twisting of the diverticulum with obstruction, and (rarely) carcinoma. *Clinically* most diverticula are asymptomatic. A minority are attended by manifestations similar to peptic ulcer, cholecystitis, etc. The *diagnosis* is made roentgenographically (with the aid of barium) and, less often, gastroscopically. *Treatment* consists of surgical excision. The *prognosis* is excellent.

DEGENERATIONS

Degenerations of the stomach, as elsewhere, are extremely common but represent accompaniments of other disease processes rather than distinct disorders. *Parenchymatous degeneration* and *autolysis* (due to cellular enzymes and gastric juice) are seen in every stomach that is not fixed immediately upon removal from the body or upon death of the patient. In fact, autolysis in the cadaver may be of sufficient degree to cause conplete perforation of the stomach wall and spilling of the gastric contents into the peritoneal cavity. The condition may be differentiated from a perforated ulcer by the absence of a leukocytic reaction at the edge of the gastric defect and on the peritoneum. Other degenerative processes that have already been mentioned are *metastatic calcification* of the mucosa of the fundus (p. 64) and *mucoid degeneration* of any portion of the mucosa (p. 43).

INFLAMMATIONS

Orientation. —Inflammation of the stomach is known as *gastritis* (Gr. = stomach + inflammation). The more important lesions may be listed as follows: catarrhal gastritis, phlegmonous gastritis, emphysematous gastritis, allergic gastritis, chronic gastritis, peptic ulcer, granulomatous gastritis, tuberculosis and syphilis.

Catarrhal Gastritis. —Catarrhal gastritis is generally a mild inflammation of the stomach in which the epithelial cells of the mucosa are irritated to hypersecretion and ultimately degeneration (Fig. 43, p. 132). As a result, the inner surface of the stomach is covered with an excessive amount of slimy mucus. There is concomitant neutrophilic infiltration of the mucosa and submucosa but the degree of the infiltration is generally not great. The condition is usually caused by the ordinary pyogenic organisms and mild chemical irritants.

Phlegmonous Gastritis. —Phlegmonous gastritis is an acute fulminating, pyogenic infection of the wall of the stomach characterized especially by intense inflammation of the submucosa (Stenstrom). A similar condition in the small intestine is called *acute phlegmonous enteritis*, and one in the large intestine is known as *acute phlegmonous colitis* or *cecitis*. The disorder *occurs* in adults and is slightly more common in men than in women. The *causative* agents are bacteria, most often streptococci and less often staphylococci, pneumococci, and other pyogenic organisms. The predisposing factors appear to be oral or pulmonary abscesses, septicemia, exanthemata, alcoholism, gastric operations, gastric foreign body, and such gastric lesions as ulcer and carcinoma. *Pathologically* there is usually a diffuse but occasionally more focal thickening of all the layers of the stomach with particular prominence of the submucosa. The wall may measure 3 cm. or more across and is soft and boggy. The mucosa is generally intact, may be covered with an exudate, and may disclose petechiæ or ecchymosis. The process is, as a rule, sharply delineated by the cardiac and pyloric orifices. *Histologically* the disorder is characterized by extensive congestion, edema, and leukocytic infiltration. These alterations affect all the layers but are especially prominent in the submucosa. The *complications* are gastric abscess (Parsonnet), peritonitis, and septicemia or toxemia. *Clinically* the following are usually present: severe epigastric pain, vomiting, epigastric tenderness, rapid pulse, elevated temperature, leukocytosis, and shock (Miller). The *diagnosis* is generally made at autopsy for the clinical manifestations are not distinctive. *Treatment* consists of administration of antibiotics and drainage of the gastric wall if localization is found at the time of operation. The *prognosis* is poor, for in the recorded cases the mortality rate has been about 90 per cent.

Emphysematous Gastritis.—Emphysematous gastritis is nothing more than phlegmonous gastritis that is caused by gas-producing organisms (Henry). The most common of these is *Clostridium welchii* but other organisms such as the colon group, proteus, and staphylococci may also, on occasion, produce gas. Grossly bubbles of gas can be seen and felt within the wall of the stomach. They can also be identified in roentgenograms of the abdomen.

Allergic Gastritis.—Allergic gastritis is an infrequent inflammation of the stomach (Doniachi). The disorder occurs in adults and is apparently *caused* by some sensitizing agent which, however, has been elusive. *Pathologically* the lesion appears to be confined to the pyloric antrum with possible extension to the duodenum. It consists grossly of a diffuse thickening of the wall and microscopically of edema and marked eosinophilic infiltration of the mucosa, submucosa, and muscle coats. Arteritis is minimal. The *clinical manifestations* consist of intermittent abdominal pain unrelated to meals but associated with melena and hematemesis, eosinophilia, and retention of barium roentgenographically. *Treatment* has consisted of partial gastrectomy when the lesion was mistaken for carcinoma. The *prognosis* appears to be good for the condition tends to resolve spontaneously.

Chronic Gastritis.—While much has been written on the topic of chronic gastritis, little has been agreed upon. For our purposes, the condition may be defined as a chronic low-grade inflammatory disorder affecting primarily the mucosa. Its *incidence* is difficult to ascertain for in some communications it is recorded as rare while in others it is said to be seen in almost every adult. Generally, the frequency is stated as being between 12 and 40 per cent of all people studied gastroscopically (McGlone). It is twice as common in males as it is in females and usually occurs after the age of thirty years (Ross). The *causes* are undoubtedly diverse. Some of the more important etiologic factors may be listed as follows: (1) irritants—poisons alcohol, coffee, highly seasoned foods, etc., (2) hematogenous toxins, (3) mechanical contraction of the stomach, (4) nervous mechanism similar to that seen in peptic ulcer, and (5) allergic reactions to various materials (Curtis).

Pathologically the process is usually diffuse but occasionally it may be localized to the antrum, cardia, or other portions of the stomach. Although there are various classifications, the disorder is usually divided into two varieties—atrophic and hypertrophic (Larson). In *atrophic gastritis* the mucosa is pale, thin, and gray. The rugæ are greatly decreased in depth and width and sometimes are completely erased, leaving a smooth flat surface. Because of the thinness of the mucosa, the submucosal vessels are clearly seen coursing beneath the surface. Superficial erosions and hemorrhages are frequent. *Hypertrophic gastritis* consists of a marked increase in depth, width, and number of rugæ (Fig. 295*A*). The entire wall of the stomach is thus greatly increased in thickness. The mucosa is often covered with thick mucus and the tendency to superficial erosions and hemorrhages is less frequent than it is in the atrophic variety. *Histologically* the mucosa in *atrophic gastritis*, as would be expected, is exceedingly thin (Fig. 295*B*). The normal epithelial cells (parietal, etc.) are replaced with mucus-secreting cells of an intestinal type. In some instances, even Paneth cells are identi-

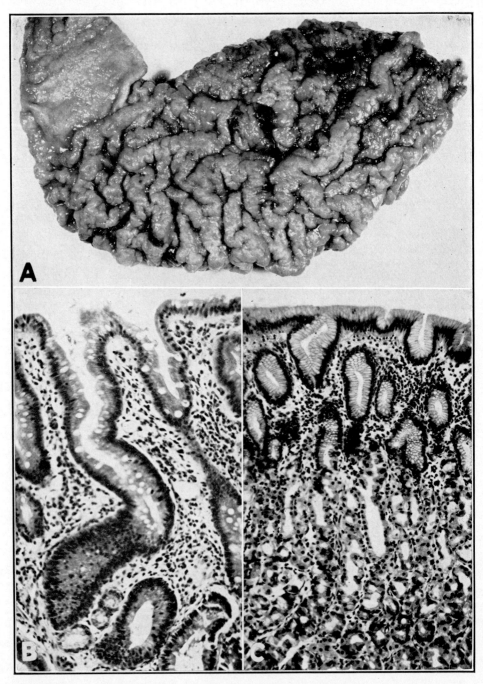

FIG. 295.—Chronic gastritis showing *A*, the hypertrophic variety with prominent deep rugæ,
B, the atrophic variety with an intestinal type of epithelium and an increase of plasma cells and
lymphocytes, and *C*, the hypertrophic variety with enlargement of the glands in corkscrew-like
fashion. × 100.

fiable. Sometimes the mouths of the glands become occluded forming
cystic spaces filled with watery or mucoid material. The muscularis mucosa
and submucosa disclose a moderate increase of fibrous tissue and throughout
both the mucosa and the submucosa there is an increase in lymphocytes and
plasma cells. In *hypertrophic gastritis* the mucosa, as would be expected, is
many times the normal thickness. The glands are also of an intestinal
type but because of their hypertrophy they are arranged in a corkscrew-like
fashion (Fig. 295C). The fibrosis and lymphocytic and plasma cell infiltration are similar to those in the atrophic variety.

The *complications* of chronic gastritis consist of (1) hemorrhage from
superficial erosions, (2) definite peptic ulcer formation in a small percentage
of cases, and (3) development of carcinoma. The incidence of carcinoma
developing upon a chronic gastritis is difficult to determine. Some authors
state that chronic gastritis, particularly of the atrophic variety (especially
that which is seen in pernicious anemia) definitely predisposes to carcinoma
and conversely that carcinoma is much more frequent in such stomachs
than it is in normal ones (Kennedy). Other authors, however, state that
there is no relationship between the two and that the incidence of carcinoma in patients with gastritis is no greater than it is in those without
such an inflammation. The *clinical manifestations* are nonspecific. They
may consist of epigastric distress, burning or aching sensation not relieved
by alkalis or bland foods, anorexia, nausea and vomiting, loss of weight,
weakness, lethargy, constipation, anemia, etc. The degree of *gastric acidity*
also varies. In some patients it is normal, in others it is elevated, and in
others still it is decreased. The *diagnosis* is made from the appearance of
the lesions gastroscopically and, when possible, from biopsy. *Roentgenograms* show a prominent rugal pattern roentgenographically in cases of
hypertrophic gastritis (Vaughan) but reveal nothing characteristic in cases
of atrophic gastritis. *Treatment* is both medical and surgical. The former
consists of the avoidance or removal of the irritant (whenever that is possible) and, in general, is like that of peptic ulcer. The administration of
vitamin B complex has been reported to have a salutary effect (Berry).
Surgical treatment consists of partial gastrectomy and is indicated when (1)
there is persistent bleeding, (2) the distress does not respond to the medical
regimen, (3) a differentiation from carcinoma cannot be made, and (4) when
there is obstruction (Palumbo). The *prognosis* is variable. Some patients
respond well to medical treatment, while others do well after surgical
intervention. Since, however, the patients are usually in the older age
group, many die of unrelated disorders.

Peptic Ulcer.—A peptic ulcer may be *defined* as an ulceration of the
mucosa of that part of the gastrointestinal tract that is bathed by gastric
(peptic) juices. The term generally includes gastric and duodenal ulcers
but actually also encompasses ulcers of the lower portion of the esophagus
and of the jejunum at the site of a gastroenterostomy. Although peptic
ulcers *occur* at all ages from infancy (Gillespie) to old age (Mulsow), the
most common age period is from twenty-five to fifty years. The disorder
is more common in males than it is in females, being recorded as two to
eight times as frequent in the former as in the latter (Smith and Doig).
Clinically recognizable ulcers are from three to ten times as common in the
duodenum as they are in the stomach and occur simultaneously in the
duodenum and stomach in approximately 10 per cent of all ulcer patients
(Weiss). *Geographically* the incidence of peptic ulcer is highest in Denmark
and Great Britain, is intermediate in the United States, Switzerland, South

China, Gold Coast, and Brazil, and is rare or practically unknown in Japan, Himalayan India, Rhone Valley, Bavarian Alps, Siam, and French Morocco. In the United States it is said to occur in from 5 to 12 per cent of the entire population. While there have been many theories attempting to explain the *causes* of peptic ulcers, the etiologic factors may be conveniently listed under three headings—constitutional predisposition, increased vulnerability of the mucosa, and local irritation. *Constitutionally* the ulcer patient is apt to be a long, lean, underweight individual with a narrow chest, narrow costal angle, depressed diaphragm, wrinkles about the mouth, high arched palate, long face, and a long neck. He is highly emotional, high-strung, and a perfectionist, being subjected to anxiety, stress, frustration, and resentment. Since all persons with a constitution such as that just outlined do not develop peptic ulcers, the aforesaid physical and mental makeup merely prepares the soil for other factors. One of these is *increased vulnerability* of the *gastric mucosa.* This is brought about by: (1) a vascular disturbance in the form of vasospasm, arteriosclerosis, thrombosis, embolism, congestion, and stasis of blood, (2) increased activity or spasm of the gastric muscles, and (3) avitaminosis. The second factor that acts in the presence of a constitutional predisposition is *local irritation.* This is due to many factors, among which are hyperchlorhydria and increased pepsin production (induced by slight stimuli by way of the vagus nerves), spicy or hot foods, alcohol, drugs, smoking, foreign bodies, etc. As a result of clinical observations and experimental work (with ACTH, cortisone, etc.) the *fundamental mechanism* responsible for peptic ulceration may be outlined rather simply. Any stress from any cause stimulates the pituitary gland to increased ACTH production which is responsible for an acceleration of secretion of cortical hormones by the adrenal cortex and these, in turn, bring about an increase in gastric secretion and higher values for pepsinogen and hydrochloric acid (Stone, Woldman, and McDonnell). The increase in pepsinogen and hydrochloric acid, together with the other factors listed above, finally produces ulceration of the mucosa.

Pathologically, as already stated, unless otherwise qualified the term peptic ulcer connotes ulceration of the stomach and first portion of the duodenum. In the stomach, the most common *locations* of the ulcers in decreasing order of frequency are (1) the anterior surface, posterior surface, and lesser curvature of the body in almost two-thirds of the cases, (2) the pylorus in almost one-third of the cases, and (3) the greater curvature of the body and the fundus in the remaining few cases (Fig. 296). In the duodenum it is the posterior wall of the first portion within 2 or 3 cm. of the pylorus that is most commonly affected. In either organ the ulcers may be acute or chronic. *Acute ulcers* in the stomach are usually multiple while those in the duodenum are generally single. They are of irregular shapes and sizes but, as a rule, do not cover a large area. When they measure 2 or 3 cm. in length, for example, they are usually only 5 or 6 mm. wide. In any case, they are sharply defined, usually possess overhanging undermined edges, disclose a rough floor covered with necrotic gray material, and penetrate any depth from the muscularis mucosa to and through the serosa. *Chronic ulcers* measure on an average up to 1.5 cm. in diameter but occasionally may measure as much as 3 or 4 cm. across. They are usually round or oval and more punched out and regular than are acute ulcers. The mucosa approaching the ulceration generally appears relatively normal. The edges are sloping, steep, or slightly undermined. The floor is usually clean and devoid of debris. The base is composed of dense sclerotic fibrous

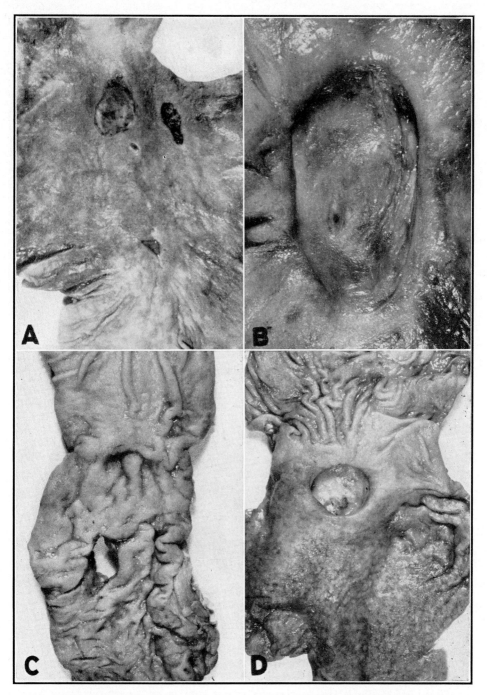

FIG. 296.—Peptic ulcers illustrating *A*, four irregular acute ulcers of varying configurations in the mucosa of the lesser curvature, *B*, a large chronic ulcer with smooth sloping and undermined edges with an eroded vessel near the center of the floor, *C*, an acute irregular duodenal ulcer that has perforated the posterior wall, and *D*, a chronic rounded duodenal ulcer with smooth undermined edges and a clean gray floor.

tissue and is located at any level from the submucosa to the serosa. In either acute or chronic ulcers the excavation causes erosion of vessels as it advances. If the vessels are previously thrombosed, they are simply removed along with the other tissues. If, however, they are not occluded massive hemorrhage results. Also, as the process advances through the wall, the inflammatory reaction in the adjacent tissues produces an adherence of the gastric or duodenal wall to organs that appose these structures. Thus, when the excavation reaches the serosa it is still sealed off by the adhesions that have previously formed. In such cases, however, spread of infection beyond the confines of the ulceration is apt to produce perigastric and periduodenal abscesses. In some instances, the surrounding inflammatory reaction is insufficient to produce adhesions with adjacent organs and the perforation, upon reaching the peritoneal cavity, results in localized or diffuse peritonitis. *Histologically* the theme is destruction and loss of normal tissues with surrounding nonspecific inflammation (Fig. 297). In *acute ulcers* the process is more fulminating and the reaction is, as would be expected, acute. The depth of the ulceration varies from the muscularis mucosa to the serosa. The edges are almost always undermined and both the edges and the base disclose the following zones from within out: (1) exudation composed mostly of neutrophils and fibrin, (2) necrosis consisting of debris and nuclear fragmentation, (3) granulation tissue consisting of capillaries, fibroblasts, and scattered leukocytes, and (4) beginning cicatrization. Because of the acuteness of the process, however, sometimes the zones of exudation blend, the zone of granulation tissue discloses extensive congestion and edema, while the zone of cicatrization is ill defined. In *chronic ulcers* the four zones as enumerated are usually more definite. Because of the duration of the process the zone of granulation tissue formation is generally quite broad and the zone of cicatrization is the most prominent. In the chronic process the base of the ulcer is almost always at the level of the muscle coats or the serosa. The vessels in the granulation tissue and cicatricial zones show fibrosis of the walls and thrombotic occlusions of their lumens (Key).

The *complications* of peptic ulcers are hemorrhage, penetration of the wall, pyloric obstruction, and carcinomatous transformation. *Hemorrhage* occurs in from 9 to 38 per cent of hospitalized patients (Chinn). It results from erosion of vessels in the floor and base of the ulcer. Depending upon the size of the vessel and the ability or inability of thrombi to form, bleeding may be single or repeated and slight or massive (Higgins and Binder). *Penetration* of the ulcer is said to occur in 1 out of every 4 patients. As already stated above, it may result in abscess formation in association with adjacent organs, in fistulous tract formation with the gallbladder or colon, and in perforation with generalized peritonitis (Bonar, Glenn, Mikal, and Burbank). Perforation is about five times more common in duodenal ulcers than it is in gastric ulcers. *Obstruction* of the *pylorus* results from cicatricial contraction at the point of ulceration, from edema superimposed upon the ulceration, or from both. The question of a *carcinomatous transformation* is quite controversial (Waugh, Lampert, Brown, Smith, and Allen). As far as the duodenum is concerned, such a complication is unimportant for, although it does occur, the incidence is so low that for practical purposes it is nonexistent (Geever). In the stomach, various estimates are that from 1 to 20 per cent of chronic gastric ulcers become malignant. In your author's opinion, the lower figure is probably correct. One of the chief difficulties of arriving at any statistics is the inability to

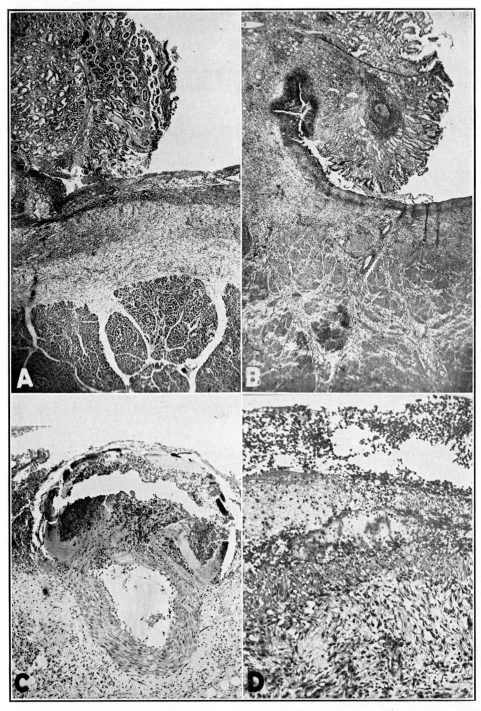

Fig. 297.—Peptic ulcer showing *A*, an acute duodenal ulcer with an undermined edge and edema but little fibrosis of the base. × 5, *B*, a chronic gastric ulcer with an undermined edge and extensive fibrosis of the base. × 5, *C*, the base of an acute ulcer disclosing essentially a zone of necrosis overlying a broad zone of edema and leukocytic infiltration with an eroded vessel at the junction of the two. × 100, and *D*, the base of a chronic ulcer disclosing, from above down, a zone of exudation, necrosis, granulation tissue, and fibrosis. × 100.

differentiate clinically an ulcerating carcinoma from a benign ulcer that ultimately becomes cancerous. It is probable that most benign chronic ulcers remain as benign ulcers and that most cases that are considered to be benign ulcers with carcinomatous transformations are carcinomas from the start. While attempts have been made to distinguish one from the other from the location and size of the lesion (lesions located on the greater curvature or in the fundus or those that measure more than 2 cm. in diameter being considered as more probably malignant than benign), such criteria may be all right for a series of cases but in any individual case they are of little or no significance. Even pathologically it may be difficult to distinguish a benign ulcer that has become cancerous from an ulcerated carcinoma. In general, one appears justified in speaking of a cancerous change in a chronic ulcer when (1) there is definite evidence of the existence of a chronic ulcer (with the four layers as indicated, extension to the muscle coats, and the vascular changes enumerated) for a prolonged period together with (2) definite evidence of carcinomatous transformation and cancerous infiltration at the margins of the ulcer (Brown).

Clinically some peptic ulcers are more or less asymptomatic and are discovered during routine roentgenography of the upper gastrointestinal tract. Most ulcers, however, are attended by some combination of the following clinical manifestations: pain, tenderness in the epigastrium, nausea and vomiting, dizziness, weakness, flatulence, melena, hematemesis, loss of appetite, and loss of weight. The *pain* is generally located somewhere in the epigastrium. It is paroxysmal in type, dull, aching, or burning. When the ulcer is located in the stomach it occurs shortly after meals, for the empty stomach does not protect against the action of gastric juices. When the ulcer is located in the duodenum, there is usually no pain for several hours after a meal because the food, as it leaves the stomach, protects the duodenal mucosa. In general, the pain is relieved by foods that have good acid-combining properties or by the ingestion of antacids (Weiss and Rossien). From the *laboratory* standpoint, patients with peptic ulcers almost always disclose hyperchlorhydria and hypersecretion of gastric juices. The *diagnosis* of peptic ulcer is made from the history, from roentgenograms and fluoroscopic examination using barium as contrast medium, and from gastroscopy (Connell and Russell). *Treatment* must be individualized to suit the case. In general, it is dividable into medical and surgical. Medical treatment consists of rest, removal of emotional stresses, bland foods, antacids, vitamins, etc. (Weiss, Rivers, Rossien, Stone, and Sandweiss). Surgical treatment consists of partial gastrectomy, vagotomy (Jordan and Pollock), simple suture of the rupture, etc. (Allen, Thorek, Dragstedt, and Wangensteen). It is generally agreed that duodenal ulcer is primarily a medical problem but opinions regarding gastric ulcer are not unanimous. Most internists believe that a medical regimen is worthy of a trial, while most surgeons think that surgical intervention is the treatment of choice. This decision is based on the fact that it is impossible to distinguish clinically a benign gastric ulcer from an ulcerating gastric carcinoma. The *prognosis* depends upon the duration of the disease, the complications that arise, the delay in treatment of the complications, the faithfulness of carrying out the treatment on the part of the patient, etc. In general, the over-all prognosis is good. Recurrences and complications, however, are common.

Granulomatous Gastritis. —This condition is identical with, and usually accompanies, regional enteritis (p. 709). It affects not only the *stomach* but also the *duodenum* (Comfort). *Pathologically* the wall of the gut is thickened, edematous, and indurated. The mucosa is irregularly ulcerated and between the ulcers the islands of normal mucosa become hypertrophied and polypoid (Fig. 298). Stenosis of the distal portion of the stomach and of the duodenum may occur as a result of fibrosis. *Histologically* the early lesion consists of edema of the wall and infiltration with neutrophils. Later, mononuclear cells dominate the scene and their arrangement in clusters with peripheral giant cells gives the disease a tubercle-like appearance. *Clinically* the following may be present: upper abdominal distress, loss of weight and strength, nausea and vomiting, diarrhea, steatorrhea, gastric retention, macrocytic anemia, hypolipemia, hypoproteinemia, hypocalcemia, hypothrombinemia, and a flat glucose tolerance curve. *Roentgenographically* there is disturbed gastric motility and sometimes obstruction and dilatation. The *diagnosis* can be suspected from the clinical and

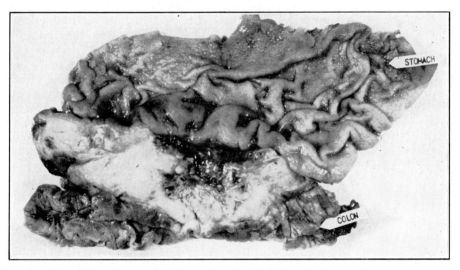

FIG. 298.—Granulomatous gastritis illustrating an ulceration of the gastric mucosa, extensive infiltration of the wall with gray tissue, and adherence of the serosa of the colon.

roentgen findings when both the stomach and duodenum are affected, but it can be made with certainty only upon pathologic examination of the specimen. In the majority of the recorded cases, *exploratory laparotomy* was performed to determine what the condition was, but no further procedures were carried out. The *prognosis* is guarded for the condition tends to persist and to undergo exacerbations and remissions.

Tuberculosis.—Tuberculosis of the *stomach* may be associated with tuberculosis of the duodenum and is usually secondary to tuberculous infection of the lungs. The condition is rare with the recorded *incidence* varying from 0.02 to 0.21 per cent of routine autopsies and from 0.36 to 2.3 per cent of autopsies on patients with pulmonary tuberculosis (Gaines). The *cause* is, of course, *Mycobacterium tuberculosis.* The routes of invasion are (1) mucosal, (2) bloodstream, (3) lymphatic channels, and (4) continuity from adjacent (lymph nodes) structures (Ostrum). *Pathologically* the *ulcerative* type of lesion is the most common. The ulcer may be single or multiple, is of varying sizes and configurations, and is usually located between the incisura and pyloric sphincter on the lesser curvature. The next most commonly encountered lesion is the *hypertrophic* type. This consists of a tumefaction of the wall of the stomach with a tendency to contraction and ulceration. It is readily mistaken for carcinoma. Less frequent and less important types of inflammation are *miliary, focal nodular*, and *diffuse gastric*. The lymph nodes draining the affected portions are generally involved by the tuberculous process. *Histologically* the lesions are similar to those in other organs (p. 167). The *complications* consist of perforation and sinus or fistulous tract formation. *Clinically* there are pain after meals, loss of weight and strength, vomiting, and (in about one-half of the cases) a palpable epigastric mass. *Roentgen* findings are those of benign ulcer or carcinoma. The *diagnosis* is generally made at operation or postmortem. *Treatment* is surgical resection. The *prognosis* is that of the tuberculosis in other organs. As far as the local lesion is concerned, it is good.

Syphilis.—The topic of syphilis of the stomach is quite confused. The inflammation is uncommon, being recorded as occurring in from none in 1,300 to 4 per cent of 200 syphilitic patients (Palmer). The *chancre* has not been recorded. In *early* or *secondary* syphilis the lesion generally consists of a superficial catarrhal gastritis. The process is most marked in the distal half of the stomach and consists of patches of excessive mucoid secretion covering an edematous, hyperemic, superficially eroded mucosa. Histologically the mucosal cells show excessive secretion and the mucosa, submucosa, and occasionally the deeper layers disclose a nonspecific plasma cell and lymphocytic infiltration. In *tertiary* syphilis, the lesions are also generally located in the distal half of the stomach, especially in the pyloric antrum. Fundamentally they may be of three varieties—infiltrative, ulcerative, and tumorous (Palmer). *Infiltrative* lesions consist of an ill-defined velvety swelling of the mucosa and of diffuse thickening of the wall, especially the submucosa (Williams and Kimmelstiel). The mucosa is generally intact but it may be superficially ulcerated and it usually discloses a disappearance of the rugæ. *Ulcerative* lesions are multiple, irregular, serpiginous, and superficial but extensive in surface area. The edges are sloping rather than undermined and the centers of the ulcers often contain islands of intact mucosa. The floor is covered with a gray membrane that is loosely adherent to the underlying tissues. *Tumorous* lesions are generally considered to be variants of infiltrative lesions in which the process is more localized. Gummas, however, have been described (Willeford). The swelling is ill defined and the mucosa may or may not be ulcerated. Histologically, regardless of the gross appearance, tertiary lesions are usually of a diffuse granulomatous type but, as already stated, gummas are rarely encountered (p. 178). The *clinical manifestations* are nonspecific. They may consist of pain, loss of weight, vomiting, and a palpable epigastric mass. The *diagnosis* is made from a history of syphilis, the presence of syphilitic lesions elsewhere, the gastroscopic appearance of the mucosa, the presence of a tumor or ulcers roentgenographically, and positive serologic tests. *Treatment* is that of syphilis in general. The *prognosis* is good.

PHYSICAL DISTURBANCES

Orientation.—Physical disturbances of the stomach constitute a heterogeneous collection of unrelated conditions. Some of the more important disorders may be listed as follows: fistula, hemorrhage, chemical burns, foreign bodies, interstitial emphysema, perforation, mucosal prolapse, intussusception, volvulus, and obstruction.

Fistula.—As elsewhere in the body, a fistula of the stomach connects the lumen of this organ with the lumen of another organ or the skin. The *causes* are generally congenital anomalies, degenerations, inflammations, physical disturbances, and tumors. The more common fistulas are *gastropleural* (p. 531), *gastrojejunal* (usually purposeful and surgical), *gastrocutaneous*, *gastrobiliary*, and *gastrojejunocolic*. Of these, the last mentioned is probably the most important. It is virtually confined to middle-aged adults and is more common in males than in females. While, on rare occasions, the *cause* may be carcinoma of the stomach or colon, intestinal tuberculosis, or trauma, most of the cases are due to perforation of a (marginal) stomal jejunal ulcer (peptic ulcer of the jejunum at the site of a gastroenterostomy) into the colon (Tartakoff and Vaughn). Stomal jejunal ulcers are said to occur in from 3 to 15 per cent of all gastroenter-

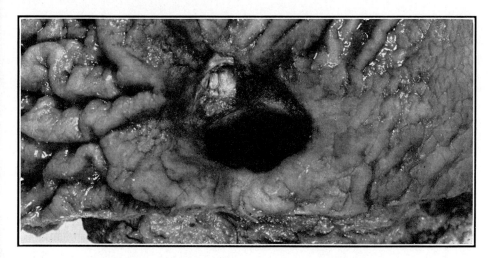

Fig. 299.—Stomal ulcer at the site of a gastroenterostomy.

ostomies and about 12 per cent of these perforate into the colon. *Pathologically* the transverse colon becomes adherent to the gastrojejunal anastomosis and the stomal ulcer ultimately perforates into the large bowel, producing a communication between the stomach, jejunum, and colon (Figs. 299 and 300). As a result of the flow of fecal material into the stomach and small bowel, the jejunum and ileum become secondarily infected. The outstanding *complication* is rapid and severe loss of weight. *Clinically* the development of the fistula varies from one to forty years after the gastroenterostomy. The findings consist of (1) pain—most marked during the stomal ulcer period and abating once the fistula develops, (2) tenderness—at the point of ulceration, (3) diarrhea—severe and due not so much to shunting of the food from the stomach to the colon as to increased peristalsis of the small bowel from irritation by fecal material that enters from the colon, (4) foul odor to the breath—due to fecal eructation, (5) loss of weight, hypoproteinemia, and anemia—resulting from inability to digest and absorb food, and (6) demonstration of a fistula roentgenographically after a barium enema. The *diagnosis* is made from the history and roentgenograms. *Treatment* consists of surgical excision of the affected portion of the stomach, jejunum, and colon. The *prognosis* is good in cases of noncancerous fistulas but is generally poor in neoplastic ones.

Hemorrhage.—The escape of blood into the stomach or duodenum is a symptom and not a disease. A few of the many *causes* may be listed as follows: (1) ulcerations of the stomach and duodenum—gastritis, peptic ulcer, carcinoma, and benign tumor, (2) varices, (3) blood dyscrasias—splenic anemia, leukemia, hypoplastic anemia, hemolytic anemia, and purpura, (4) infectious diseases—malaria, yellow fever, and cholera, (5) diseases of the lung and heart—producing failure of the circulation and

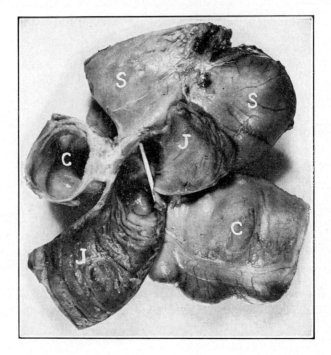

FIG. 300.—Gastrojejunocolic fistula showing *S*, stomach, *C*, colon, and *J*, jejunum. The applicator is inserted into the stomach and colon. (Herbut's *Surgical Pathology*.)

increase of venous pressure, (6) trauma to the abdomen—penetrating and nonpenetrating injury, and (7) foreign bodies (Meyer and Crohn). Of these, *ulcerations* and *varices* account for well over 90 per cent of all cases. The *bleeding* may be single or repeated and slight or massive. The *clinical manifestations* are (1) hematemesis (vomiting of blood), (2) melena (passage of blood in the stools), (3) anemia (generally due to repeated loss of blood), and (4) shock (resulting from rapid and massive loss of blood). *Treatment* depends entirely on the cause of the bleeding. The *prognosis* also depends on the etiologic factor but, in addition, it varies with the type (capillary, artery, or vein) and size of the vessel affected.

Chemical Burns.—Although most ingested chemicals will produce retrogressive changes in the stomach if they are taken in sufficient amount and in high enough concentration, the most important compounds are alkalies and acids (Baker and Strode). In general, *alkalies* are of extreme im-

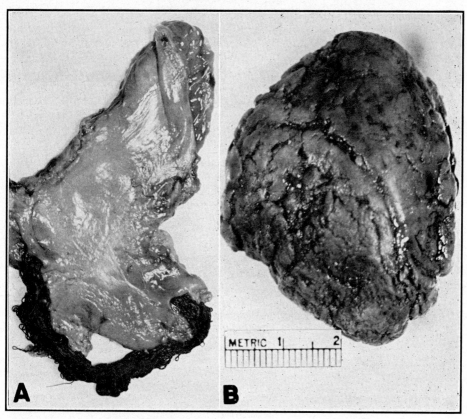

FIG. 301.—Foreign bodies illustrating *A*, string wound around the circuit produced by a gastroenterostomy and *B*, a phytobezoar.

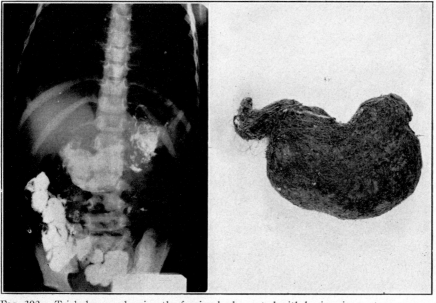

FIG. 302.—Trichobezoar showing the foreign body coated with barium in a rotengenogram and the ball of hair itself.

43

portance as far as the esophagus is concerned (p. 640) but are of lesser importance as far as the stomach is concerned because in the latter they are neutralized by the gastric juice. *Acids*, on the other hand, are not neutralized and are, therefore, permitted to exert their full effect. The most common acids are sulphuric acid and hydrochloric acid. *Pathologically* there are superficial burns of the mouth and esophagus but the stomach shows the maximum effect. The lesser curvature and pyloric antrum are more severely involved than other portions of the stomach. Early, the mucosa is discolored brown to black in cases of sulphuric acid poisoning and white in cases of hydrochloric acid poisoning. Later the affected areas slough and irregular nonspecific ulcers are formed. In time, they heal by granulation tissue formation and cicatrization. When the stomach is empty and the amount and concentration of the acid is great, the entire thickness of the wall of the stomach may be eroded. The *complications* are (1) perforation early after ingestion and (2) cicatricial pyloric obstruction after healing has

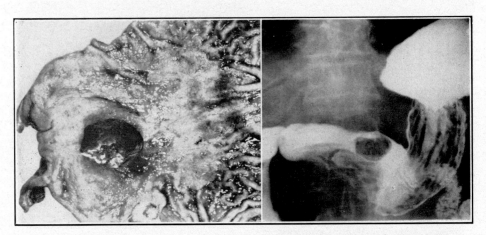

Fig. 303.—Gallstone impacted at the pylorus with its roentgenographic appearance.

occurred. The immediate *clinical manifestations* consist of (1) burning pain in the mouth, esophagus, and upper abdomen, (2) vomiting, (3) thirst, (4) difficulty in swallowing, and (5) symptoms and signs of shock. Late manifestations consist of pyloric obstruction. The *diagnosis* is made from the history and the symptoms and signs. *Treatment* consists of neutralization of the acid by ingestion of an alkali, combating shock, and surgical attention to the complications as they develop. The *prognosis* is fair to good. In acute stages, death may result from shock or perforation of the stomach and peritonitis.

Foreign Bodies.—Foreign bodies of the stomach (and intestines) are swallowed by accident or by design (Cannaday). The former occur mostly in children, less often in adults, and occasionally in jugglers. The latter are found in mentally unbalanced or frankly insane people of all ages. The objects are usually varied consisting, among others, of nails, needles, knife blades, spoons, coins, buttons, matches, toothpicks, bones, gallstones, string, and bezoars (Figs. 301, 302, 303). *Bezoars* (Persian = antidote or counterpoison) in contrast to other objects are concretions that are formed in the stomach or intestines. They are usually classified according to their component parts as (1) *trichobezoars* or *hairballs*—the most common and composed essentially of ingested hair, (2) *phytobezoars*—composed chiefly of fruit fibers, vegetable fibers, seeds, and skins of fruits and vegetables, (3) *trichophytobezoars*—composed of mixtures of hair, fruits, and vegetables, and (4) *firmer concretions*—as a rule composed of shellac and found in painters (Hurwitz). Bezoars are usually large and conform to the outlines of the organs in which they lie. In general, *foreign bodies*, regardless of the type, produce *symptoms* by virtue of obstruction, inflammation, ulceration, or perforation of the gastrointestinal tract. The *diagnosis* is made from the history, roentgenographic appearance (especially in cases of radiopaque bodies), and the findings at operation. *Treatment* consists of surgical removal if the object does not pass out with the feces. The *prognosis* is good.

Interstitial Emphysema.—This condition has been described in connection with gastroscopy (Fierst). When air is pumped into the stomach (for purposes of visualizing the mucosa) it may enter the perivascular spaces at points of erosion or ulceration, trek along the course of the vessels to the serosa, and then produce serosal blebs which rupture and cause pneumo-

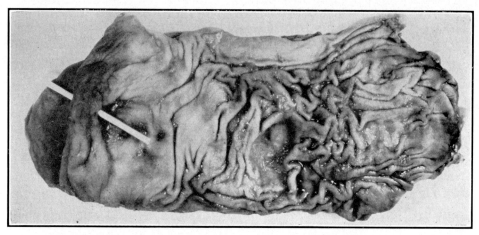

Fig. 304.—Mucosal prolapse into the duodenum with a perforated ulcer (containing the applicator) in the mucosal fold. (Specimen submitted by Doctor W. V. McDonnell.)

peritoneum. The lesion in the stomach is referred to simply as interstitial gastric emphysema.

Perforation.—Perforation or rupture of the stomach connotes a focal loss of continuity of the gastric wall. It may be caused by (1) congenital anomalies—defect in the musculature of the stomach, (2) degenerations—erosions as a result of stasis of blood or terminal enzymatic and peptic digestion, (3) inflammations—especially peptic ulcer, (4) physical disturbances—particularly chemical burns, foreign bodies, instrumentation (during esophagoscopy or gasoscopy), and trauma (penetrating or non-penetrating) from without, and (5) tumors—ulcerating malignant growths, both carcinoma and sarcoma (Shellito and Wolf).

Mucosal Prolapse.—Mucosal prolapse of the stomach means a redundancy and protrusion of its mucosa usually through the pyloric (Lichstein) or rarely through the cardiac orifice (Feldman). The *causes* of the redundancy are inflammation and hypertrophy of the mucosa. The *force* is reverse peristalsis in the case of the cardiac orifice and forward peristalsis in the case of the pyloric orifice. *Pathologically* the process consists simply of a redundant fold of mucosa containing a core of muscularis mucosa and submucosa (Fig. 304). The *complications* that may occur are esophageal or pyloric obstruction and ulceration of the protruding mucosa. The ulcer, in turn, may cause hemorrhage or a through-and-through perforation of the fold. The *clinical manifestations* consist of bouts of epigastric distress associated with nausea and vomiting. The *diagnosis* is made roentgenographically (after ingestion of barium) from the appearance of a mushroom-like defect. *Treatment* is primarily medical. If, however, (1) symptoms are not relieved, (2) obstruction or hemorrhage occurs, or (3) the lesion cannot be differentiated from a tumor, surgical resection is indicated. The *prognosis* is good.

Intussusception. —Intussusception (L. = within + to receive) means a telescoping of one portion of the stomach into: (1) the stomach—*gastrogastric*, (2) the duodenum—*gastroduodenal*, (3) the jejunum (following a gastroenterostomy)—*gastroenteric*, or (4) the esophagus—*gastroesophageal* (Hobbs). In contrast to mucosal prolapse, the invaginating portion (intussusceptum) consists of the entire thickness of the gastric wall from the mucosa to the serosa inclusive. The *cause* is generally some form of pedunculated tumor which is carried along by peristaltic waves. The *clinical findings*, etc., are similar to those enumerated under Mucosal Prolapse above.

Volvulus. —Volvulus (L. = to turn about) is a twisting of the stomach about itself or about its cardiac orifice in a clockwise or anticlockwise direction (Bazzano and Russell). The condition may be divided into two types— *total* or *acute* in which the whole stomach rotates and *partial, chronic,* or *intermittent* in which one portion of the stomach twists upon another. The predisposing *causes* of total volvulus are unknown for sure but are thought to be due to relaxed gastric ligaments, ptosis, and faulty peritoneal attachment of the duodenum. The predisposing causes of partial volvulus may be diaphragmatic hernia, peptic ulcer, benign and malignant tumors, hourglass stomach, perigastritis, and perigastric adhesions. The precipitating causes in either case may be overfilling of the stomach, reverse peristalsis, vomiting, hiccoughs, and mechanical torsion after body movements. *Pathologically*, as rotation exceeds 180°, the twisting is attended by occlusion of the blood supply, necrosis, and rupture of the stomach. It is also attended by obstruction of the pyloric and cardiac orifices. Depending upon the acuteness and completeness of the torsion, the *clinical manifestations* consist of recurrent attacks of indigestion, epigastric pain, nausea, vomiting, and shock. *Treatment* is surgical, usually entailing the unwinding of the twist and the correction of the predisposing cause if that can be found. The *prognosis* is good.

Obstruction. —Obstruction of the stomach usually occurs at its narrowest portion—the pyloric orifice or antrum. It may be caused by virtually every disorder mentioned or discussed in the foregoing pages. Some of the more important etiologic factors are (1) congenital—hypertrophic pyloric stenosis, webs, and diverticulum, (2) inflammations—peptic ulcer, granulomatous gastritis, tuberculosis, and syphilis, (3) physical disturbances— chemical burns, foreign bodies, mucosal prolapse, intussusception, and volvulus, and (4) tumors—any benign or malignant tumor strategically located. In addition to the above, another frequent cause of *gastroduodenal obstruction* (of an acute variety) is external pressure on the third portion of the duodenum (where it crosses the aorta) by the *superior mesenteric* *artery.* In such cases, predisposing factors are emaciation, ptosis, short mesentery, and lordosis of the lumbar spine (Beck).

TUMORS

Orientation.—Tumors and tumor-like conditions of the stomach are quite varied. They may be listed as follows: polyp, carcinoid, carcinoma, fibroma, fibrosarcoma, myxosarcoma, leiomyoma, leiomyosarcoma, rhabdomyosarcoma, lipoma, liposarcoma, neurofibroma, neurofibrosarcoma, hereditary hemorrhagic telangiectasia, hemangioendothelioma, lymphoblastoma, plasmocytoma, osteosarcoma, chondrosarcoma, adenomyoma, teratoid tumor, and secondary tumors. Regardless of the type, all tumors produce relatively similar clinical manifestations and the various growths can be differentiated from each other only histologically. Most of the lesions mentioned are extremely rare with only the following three being frequent enough to merit separate consideration: smooth muscle tumors, polyps, and carcinoma.

Smooth Muscle Tumors.—Smooth muscle tumors of the stomach are dividable into two groups—leiomyoma (benign) and leiomyosarcoma (malignant). Leiomyomas have been recorded as *occurring* in as high as

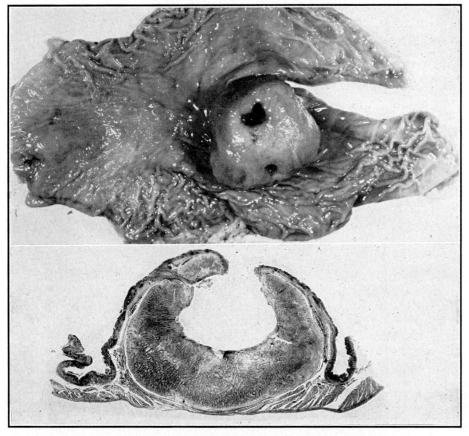

Fig. 305.—Leiomyoma of the stomach showing, above, a submucosal mass with two excavations and, below, a sharply circumscribed tumor with central ulceration.

46 per cent of random autopsies and 39.9 per cent of all benign symptomatic gastric tumors, while leiomyosarcomas have been recorded as comprising about 10 per cent of all gastric sarcomas (Cole).   Smooth muscle
tumors affect both sexes with equal frequency and, although they are found
at all ages, they are most common between forty and seventy years. *Pathologically* the tumors originate in the muscle coats of the stomach, and,
regardless of whether they are benign or malignant, the gross appearance is
more or less similar (Fig. 305).   The lesions may affect any part of the
stomach but predominate in the distal third, are generally single, protrude
into the lumen more often than beneath the serosa, usually measure from
2 to 5 cm. in diameter, and are well encapsulated, firm, and light brown to

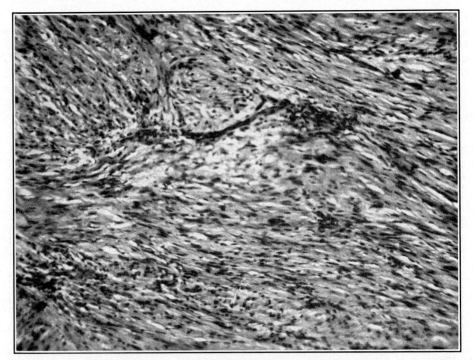

Fig. 306.—Leiomyoma of the stomach illustrating interlacing
bundles of smooth muscle fibers.   × 100.

gray.   The intraluminal growths have a tendency to undergo central or
eccentric ulceration and excavation.   Occasionally the benign growths may
undergo calcification.   *Histologically* leiomyomas are composed of interlacing bundles of quite regular and normal appearing smooth muscle
fibers (Fig. 306).   The cells in leiomyosarcoma are similar except that they
exhibit a decrease in the cytoplasmic nuclear ratio and more irregularity of
the nuclei.   In some cases, the cells become rounded and quite bizarre.
Leiomyosarcomas, as a rule, are much more vascular and have a greater
tendency to undergo cystic degenerations than do leiomyomas.   Leiomyosarcomas spread, by way of metastasis, to the regional lymph nodes, liver,
and other sites.   The chief *clinical manifestations* are due to ulceration and
hemorrhage and consist of hematemesis, melena, anemia, and weakness.   In
addition, the following may be present: indigestion, epigastric pain, evidence

of pyloric obstruction, and a palpable tumor in the epigastrium. The *diagnosis* is made from the clinical manifestations, visualization of the tumor gastroscopically, and the appearance of a tumor with a central depression roentgenographically. *Treatment* consists of surgical excision. The *prognosis*, even in most cases of leiomyosarcoma, is good.

Polyps.—As elsewhere, a gastric polyp means simply a finger-like projection of tumor tissue from the mucosa into the lumen. Although, theoretically, it may consist of any of the tissues that constitute the normal gastric wall, actually it has come to mean a benign pedunculated epithelial

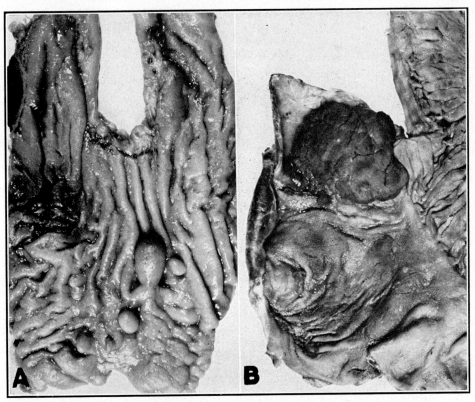

Fig. 307.—Adenomatous polyps of the stomach showing *A*, at least five small pedunculated mucosal masses and *B*, a large fungating mucosal tumor.

overgrowth. A better designation is *epithelial* or *adenomatous polyp*, *papilloma*, or *adenoma*. The condition has been recorded as *occurring* in from 1.6 to 2 per cent of all gastroscopies and from 0.25 to 0.7 per cent of all autopsies (Yarnis and Hardt). While it may occur at all ages, it is most frequent beyond the sixth decade of life and is about as common in males as it is in females (Carey). Although the precise *cause* is unknown, atrophic gastritis is said to be present in as high as 90 per cent of cases. *Pathologically* single polyps occur as frequently as multiple polyps. While any portion of the mucosa may be involved, that which is most frequently affected is the distal third (Fig. 307). The initial lesion exists as a sessile protrusion of the mucosa. As it ages, it becomes elongated and pedunculated and ultimately it measures on an average of from 1 to 3 cm. in length and 0.5 to

2 cm. in diameter. The surface may be superficially ulcerated and is pinkish gray. The consistency is moderately firm and the mass is freely movable at its attachment with the mucosa. *Histologically* the lesion consists of a stalk of connective tissue covered with hyperplastic columnar epithelial cells in glandular formation (Fig. 308). The epithelial cells do not invade the core or the base of the polyp. The *complications* are ulceration, hemorrhage, rarely intussusception, and carcinomatous transformation. The incidence of carcinoma in adenomatous polyps is recorded as varying from 6 to 51 per cent. *Clinically* bleeding and abdominal pain or epigastric distress are the most characteristic symptoms. In addition, there may be anorexia, loss of weight, weakness, and vomiting. Achlorhydria is present

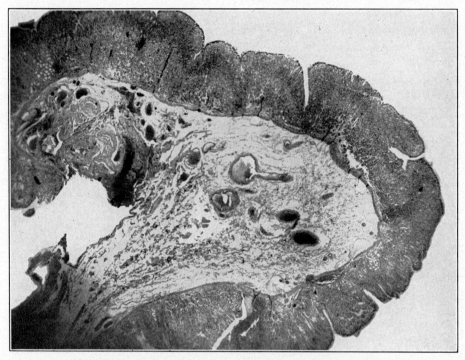

Fig. 308.—Adenomatous polyp of the stomach illustrating a core of edematous connective tissue covered with hyperplastic mucosa. × 7.

in about 90 per cent of cases. *Roentgenographically* the lesions are seen as rounded, smooth, filling defects while gastroscopically they appear as freely movable, usually pedunculated masses. The *diagnosis* is made from the history and roentgenographic and gastroscopic findings. *Treatment* of choice consists of local excision or partial gastrectomy. The *prognosis* is generally good.

Carcinoma.—Carcinoma of the stomach is one of the most *common* cancers of the entire body, accounting for an estimated 28,000 deaths annually in the United States (Pack). While it may *occur* at any age it is most common between forty and seventy years and it affects males twice as frequently as females (Jemerin and Swynnerton). The precise *cause* of carcinoma of the stomach is unknown. Aside from a constitutional predisposition (which appears to be the basis for the development of all cancers) the following have been often suggested as being of etiologic significance (Jemerin): dietary factors, infection, irritation from food, gastric ulcer (Beattie and p. 663), atrophic gastritis, polyps, pernicious anemia (Norcross), and achlorhydria (Comfort).

Pathologically carcinoma of the stomach is generally considered to be of unicentric origin, although there is evidence to indicate that in a certain number of cases it may start in multiple foci (Collins). It may be found in any portion of the stomach. In about two-thirds of the cases it is located

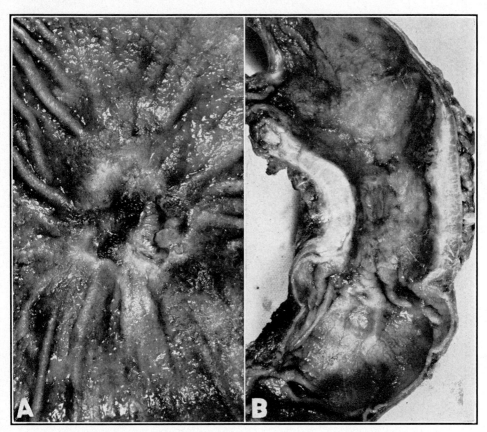

Fig. 309.—Carcinoma of the stomach showing *A*, a superficially ulcerated lesion and *B*, a diffusely infiltrating tumor of the linitis plastica variety.

in the pylorus, in about one-fifth in the body, in about one-eighth in the cardia, and in the remaining cases in more than one anatomic subdivision. *Grossly* recognizable lesions may generally be divided into three groups — ulcerating, infiltrating, and polypoid (Figs. 309 and 310). *Ulcerating* lesions may be indistinguishable from an ordinary gastric ulcer (p. 663). They may measure from a few millimeters to many centimeters in diameter, may be superficial or deeply penetrating, and may be sharply circumscribed. As a rule, however, they differ from benign ulcers in that the edges are more sloping, the normal rugæ of the stomach disappear at some distance from the crater, and the edges are considerably firmer. *Infiltrating growths* (generally referred to as *linitis plastica*) may involve only a small segment of the stomach or may affect the entire organ. In either case, the involved wall is greatly thickened and rigid. The different layers of the stomach are separated by tumor tissue and are thus more prominent than normal. This is especially true of the submucosa and the serosa. The mucosa is usually intact and the rugæ are erased. In the more extensive tumors the capacity of the stomach is greatly reduced with the entire organ forming a long, narrow, unyielding tube (so-called *leather-bottle stomach*). *Polypoid* or

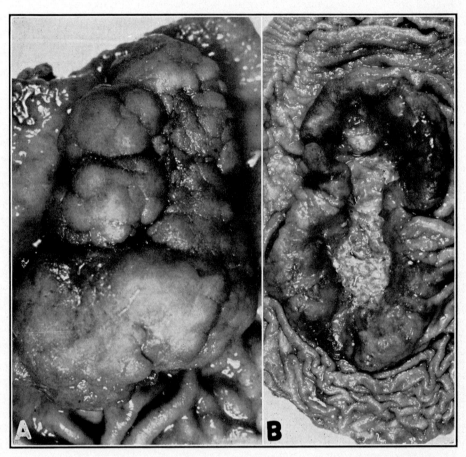

FIG. 310.—Carcinoma of the stomach illustrating *A*, a fungating, nonulcerating growth and *B*, a fungating tumor with central ulceration.

fungating tumors are less common than either the ulcerating or the infiltrating type. The growths are generally sessile, may be relatively flat or considerably elevated, and may measure 4 to 6 cm. or more in diameter. The surface is, as a rule, composed of fine, rough projections and has frequently been likened to the surface of a cauliflower. Usually it is superficially eroded but sometimes it may disclose a deep central ulceration. *Histologically* carcinoma of the stomach is basically an adenocarcinoma (Figs. 311 and 312). As in other organs of the body, it shows varying degrees of differentiation from a low-grade to a high-grade malignancy. Low-grade tumors are composed of varisized glands lined by cuboidal or columnar epithelial cells. The cells borders are usually indistinct; the cytoplasm is moderate in amount and eosinophilic, and the nuclei are oval, hyper-chromatic, and basilar in position. Droplets of secretion may or may not be present in the luminal portions of the cells. Tumors of high-grade malignancy are so pleomorphic and primitive that they can scarcely be recognized as of gastric origin. In some instances, they consist of relatively small, round cells with scanty cytoplasm and round, deeply stained nuclei, thus possessing a strong resemblance to lymphoblasts. In other cases, the cells are larger, more irregular, and more polyhedral. They present a

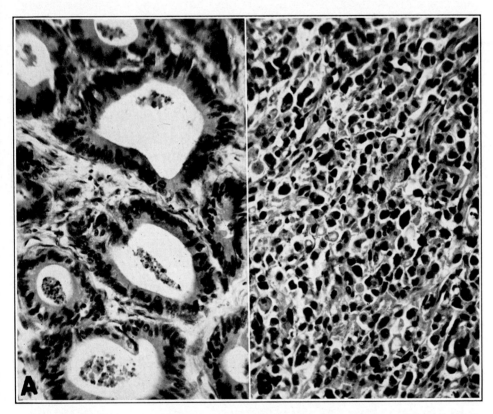

FIG. 311.—Carcinoma of the stomach showing A, an adenocarcinoma with well-formed glands lined by columnar epithelium, and B, an anaplastic carcinoma with single cells permeating the muscle. × 200.

moderate amount of eosinophilic cytoplasm and round, oval, or irregular hyperchromatic nuclei. Between the two extremes there are all gradations and combinations. Some tumors, usually referred to as *mucinous car-cinomas*, are attended by considerable secretion of mucin and actually mucoid degeneration of the epithelial cells. When the secretion is moderate in amount, the cytoplasm of the neoplastic cells becomes distended with round vacuoles and the nucleus is pushed aside in a crescentic manner thus forming what has been referred to as *signet ring cells*. When the secretion is more abundant, the cells burst and become destroyed, leaving the mucus to accumulate in large amounts both around the epithelial cells and between the cells of the supporting stroma. In any case, the *stroma* may be scanty, of a loose connective tissue type, and well vascularized or it may be abundant, more collagenous, and poorly vascularized. It always discloses varying degrees of leukocytic infiltration with the leukocytes consisting mainly of plasma cells, lymphocytes, and mononuclear cells.

Carcinoma of the stomach *spreads* by (1) contiguity to the peritoneum, adjacent portions of the gastric mucosa, pancreas, liver, and spleen, (2) by lymphatics to the lymph nodes of the lesser and greater curvature, liver hilum, aorta, mediastinum, and the left supraclavicular region, and (3) by the blood vessels to the liver, lungs, bones, and almost every other organ and tissue of the body (Brown). The question of drop metastasis through the peritoneal cavity to the pelvic organs, especially the *ovaries*, has re-

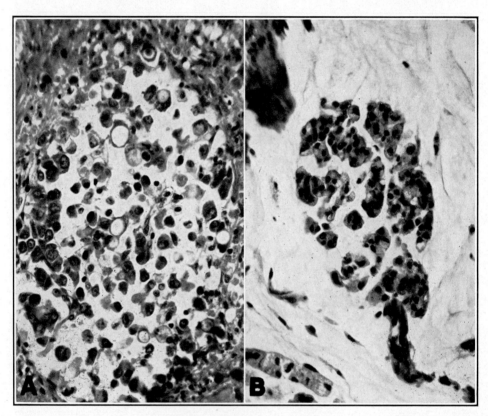

Fig. 312.—Carcinoma of the stomach illustrating *A*, anaplastic carcinoma of the signet ring variety. × 200, and *B*, a mucinous carcinoma with clusters of cells surrounded by an abundant amount of mucinous material. × 200.

ceived considerable attention. While at one time it was thought that carcinoma of the stomach (and for that matter carcinoma of the rest of the intestinal tract) became implanted on the surface of the ovaries whence it extended into their substance (*Kruckenberg tumor*), it is now generally conceded that ovarian involvement occurs by way of retroperitoneal lymphatic channels and blood vessels.

The *complications* of carcinoma of the stomach are gastric obstruction, gastric ulceration with hemorrhage or perforation (Mayo), and metastasis. *Clinically*, it is asymptomatic for varied and probably prolonged periods. Symptoms usually begin when there is ulceration, obstruction, tumefaction, or rigidity of the gastric wall (Jemerin).   They may consist of various combinations of the following: indigestion, epigastric pain, loss of weight, weakness, anorexia, vomiting, melena, constipation or diarrhea, dysphagia, and hematemesis (Swynnerton and Pack).   Physical examination is essentially negative in the early stages of the disease.   The *laboratory findings* consist of hypochromic anemia, demonstration of blood in the stool in 75 per cent of cases, and achlorhydria or hypochlorhydria in over 80 per cent of cases.   *Roentgenographically* a mucosal defect and impairment in motility of the stomach are generally demonstrable.   *Gastroscopically* the tumor can actually be visualized in over three-quarters of the cases and a gastroscopic biopsy may be obtained in as high as 10 per cent of cases. *Cytologic examination* of gastric secretions is thought to be of value by some authors (Cooper and Papanicolaou) but to be of questionable value by others.   Your author's experience supports the latter contention.   The *diagnosis* is usually made from the clinical manifestations (especially epigastric distress), roentgenography, gastroscopy, and gastroscopic biopsy when possible.   The only effective *treatment* is total or subtotal gastrectomy (Boyce).   The over-all *prognosis* is quite poor.   In general, it may be stated that the stomachs in only from 30 to 50 per cent of patients are resectable and that the five-year survival of patients thus treated is around 20 per cent.   The over-all five-year survival rate is usually less than 6 per cent.

REFERENCES

Pathologic Physiology

BABKIN, B. P.: *Secretory Mechanism of Digestive Glands*, New York, Paul Hoeber Inc., 1950 (Gastric Secretion Nervous Control).

BORISON, H. L., and WANG, S. C.: Pharmacol. Rev., *5*, 193, 1953 (Vomiting).

BROBEK, J. R.: New York Acad. Sci., *63*, 44, 1955 (Appetite).

HOLLANDER, F.: A.M.A. Arch. Int. Med., *93*, 107, 1954 (Mucous Barrier).

IVY, A. C., *et al.*: Peptic Ulcer, Philadelphia, Blakiston Co., 1950 (Experimental Ulcer Pathology).

QUIGLEY, J. P., and LOUCKES, M. S.: Gastroenterol., *19*, 533, 1951 (Gastric Evacuation After Vagotomy).

SANDWEISS, D. J., *et al.*: Nocturnal Gastric Secretion, Gastroenterol., *7*, 38, 1946 (Gastric Secretion in Ulcer).

THOMAS, J. E., and FRIEDMAN, M. H. F.: Sandweiss' *Peptic Ulcer*, Philadelphia, W. B. Saunders, 1951 (Gastrointestinal Secretions).

THOMAS, J. E.: Physiol. Rev., *37*, 453, 1957 (Gastric Emptying).

TYLOR, D. B., and BARD, P.: Physiol. Rev., *29*, 311, 1949 (Motion Sickness).

Congenital Anomalies

ASTLEY, R.: Brit. J. Radiol., *25*, 342, 1952 (Radiology Infantile Pyloric Stenosis).

BARBOSA, J. DEC.: J. A. M. A., *149*, 1552, 1952 (Duplication).

BENNER, W. H.: Surgery, *29*, 170, 1951 (Aberrant Pancreas).

BROWN, C. H., *et al.*: Gastroenterology, *12*, 10, 1949 (Diverticula).

CARTER, C. O., and SAVAGE, T. R.: A. M. A. Arch. Dis. Child., *26*, 50, 1951 (Pyloric Stensosis in Cousins).

HERBUT, P. A.: A. M. A. Arch. Path., *36*, 91, 1943 (Congenital Defect Musculature Stomach).

KLEITSCH, W. P.: A. M. A. Arch. Surg., *65*, 655, 1952 (Hypertrophic Pyloric Stenosis in Adults).

PACK, G. T., *et al.*: J. Thoracic Surg., *23*, 593, 1952 (Cancer in Thoracic Stomach).

POWELL, B. W., and CARTER, C. O.: A. M. A. Arch. Dis. Child., *26*, 45, 1951 (Pyloric Stenosis in Twins).

RHEINLANDER, H. F., and SWENSON, O.: J. Pediat., *41*, 314, 1952 (Congenital Hypertrophic Pyloric Stenosis).

ROSS, M., *et al.*: J. A. M. A., *146*, 1313, 1951 (Neonatal Rupture Stomach).

ROTA, A. N.: A. M. A. Arch. Path., *55*, 223, 1953 (Pyloric Diaphragm).
WOOD, E. C., and SMELLIE, J. M.: Lancet, *2*, 3, 1951 (Congenital Hypertrophic Pyloric Stenosis).

Inflammations

ALLEN, A. W.: Rev. Gastroenterol., *16*, 13, 1949 (Gastroduodenal Ulcer).
BERG, M.: Am. J. Digest. Dis., *16*, 35, 1949 (Experimental Peptic Ulcer).
BERRY, L. H., and COLE, T. J.: J. A. M. A., *138*, 485, 1948 (Atrophic Gastritis).
BINDER, M., and PAUL, J. T.: Am. J. Digest. Dis., *19*, 278, 1952 (Bleeding Peptic Ulcer).
BONAIR, A. A., and LIVINGSTONE, D. J.: Glasgow M. J., *33*, 1, 1952 (Perforated Peptic Ulcer).
BROWN, C. H., et al.: Gastroenterology, *22*, 103, 1952 (Gastric Ulcer and Carcinoma).
BURBANK, C. B., and ROE, B. B.: New England J. Med., *247*, 424, 1952 (Perforation Peptic Ulcers).
CHINN, A. B., and WECKESSER, E. C.: Ann. Int. Med., *34*, 339, 1951 (Hemorrhage Peptic Ulcer.
COMFORT, M. W., et al.: Am. J. M. Sci., *220*, 616, 1950 (Granulomatous Gastritis).
CONNELL, F. G.: Am. J. Digest. Dis., *16*, 55, 1949 (Duodenal Ulcer).
CURTIS, W. S.: Radiology, *59*, 317, 1952 (Review Literature Chronic Gastritis).
DOIG, R. K., and WOOD, I. J.: M. J. Australia, *1*, 602, 1952 (141 Cases Gastric and Duodenal Ulcer).
DONIACHI, I., and McKEOWN, K. C.: Brit. J. Surg., *39*, 247, 1951 (Eosinophilic Gastritis).
DRAGSTEDT, L. R.: Rev. Gastroenterol., *19*, 286, 1952 (Surgical Aspects Peptic Ulcer).
FORRESTER-WOOD, W. R.: Brit. J. Surg., *37*, 278, 1950 (Hypertrophic Gastritis).
GAINES, W., et al.: Radiology, *58*, 808, 1952 (Tuberculosis).
GEEVER, E. F., and FAWCETT, N. W.: Am. J. Digest. Dis., *18*, 61, 1951 (Duodenal Ulcer and Carcinoma).
GILLESPIE, J. B., and BLISS, H. E.: A. M. A. Arch. Pediat., *68*, 361, 1951 (Peptic Ulcer in Childhood).
GLENN, F., and HARRISON, C. S.: A. M. A. Arch. Surg., *65*, 795, 1952 (Perforation Peptic Ulcer).
HENRY, G. W.: Am. J. Roentgenol., *68*, 15, 1952 (Emphysematous Gastritis).
HIGGINS, A. R., and BARTON, H. C., JR.: Gastroenterology, *17*, 353, 1951 (Hemorrhage Peptic Ulcer).
JORDAN, S. M., et al.: Gastroenterology, *22*, 295, 1952 (4,076 Cases Peptic Ulcer with Vagotomy).
KENNEDY, T. J.: Radiology, *59*, 367, 1952 (Diagnosis Gastritis).
KEY, J. A.: Brit. M. J., *2*, 1464, 1950 (Blood Vessels in Gastric Ulcer).
LAMPERT, E. G., et al.: Surg., Gynec. & Obst., *91*, 673, 1950 (Gastric Ulcer and Carcinoma).
LARSON, L. W., and KLING, R. R.: Radiology, *59*, 371, 1952 (Pathology Gastritis).
McDONNELL, W. V., and McCLOSKEY, J. F.: Ann. Surg., *137*, 67, 1953 (Peptic Ulcers Complicating Surgery).
McGLONE, F. B.: Radiology, *59*, 358, 1952 (Clinical Aspects Gastritis).
MIKAL, S., and MORRISON, W. R.: New England J. Med., *247*, 119, 1952 (Perforation Peptic Ulcer).
MILLER, E., and NUSHAN, H.: Am. J. Roentgenol., *67*, 781, 1952 (Phlegmonous Gastritis).
MULSOW, F. W.: Am. J. Digest. Dis., *16*, 383, 1949 (Peptic Ulcer in the Aged).
OSTRUM, H. W., and SERBER, W.: Am. J. Roentgenol., *60*, 315, 1948 (Tuberculosis Stomach and Duodenum).
PALMER, E. E.: Am. J. Syph., *33*, 481, 1949 (Syphilis).
PALUMBO, L. T., et al.: Ann. Surg., *134*, 259, 1951 (Hypertrophic Gastritis).
PARSONNET, V., et al.: A. M. A. Arch. Path., *51*, 76, 1951 (Gastric Abscess).
POLLOCK, A. V.: Lancet, *2*, 795, 1952 (1,524 Cases Peptic Ulcer and Vagotomy).
RIVERS, A. B.: Rev. Gastroenterol., *16*, 18, 1949 (Peptic Ulcer).
ROSS, J. R., et al.: Gastroenterology, *22*, 205, 1952 (Sequelæ of Gastritis).
ROSSIEN, A. X.: Rev. Gastroenterol., *16*, 34, 1949 (Treatment Peptic Ulcers).
RUSSELL, W. A., et al.: Radiology, *51*, 790, 1948 (Roentgen Findings Gastric Ulcer).
SANDWEISS, D. J., and SUGARMAN, M. H.: Rev. Gastroenterol., *19*, 271, 1952 (Medical Aspects Peptic Ulcer).
SMITH, F. H., and JORDAN, S. M.: Gastroenterology, *11*, 575, 1948 (600 Cases Gastric Ulcer).
STENSTROM, J. D., and HOEHN, G. H.: Canad. M. A. J., *64*, 317, 1951 (Phlegmonous Gastritis).
STONE, C. T.: J. A. M. A., *150*, 1655, 1952 (Nature Peptic Ulcer).
VAUGHAN, W. W., et al.: Radiology, *56*, 813, 1951 (Enlarged Gastric Rugæ).
WANGENSTEEN, O. H.: J. A. M. A., *149*, 18, 1952 (Gastric Resection Peptic Ulcer).

WAUGH, T. R., and CHARENDOFF, M. D.: Ann. Int. Med., *37*, 534, 1952 (Gastric Ulcer and Carcinoma).
WEINSTEIN, V. A., and COLP, R.: Surgery, *32*, 96, 1952 (Gastrojejunal Ulcer).
WEISS, S., *et al.*: Rev. Gastroenterol., *16*, 336, 1949 (Peptic Ulcer).
WILLEFORD, G., *et al.*: Pediatrics, *10*, 162, 1952 (Gumma).
WILLIAMS, C., and KIMMELSTIEL, P.: J. A. M. A., *115*, 578, 1940 (Syphilis).
WOLDMAN, E. E.: J. A. M. A., *149*, 984, 1952 (Peptic Ulcers and Stress Syndrome).

Physical Disturbances

BAKER, L., and SPELLBERG, M. A.: J. A. M. A., *150*, 442, 1952 (Acid Burns).
BAZZANO, J. J., and HOOD, T. K.: Ann. Surg., *135*, 415, 1952 (Volvulus).
BECK, W. C.: A. M. A. Arch. Surg., *52*, 538, 1946 (Acute Gastroduodenal Obstruction).
CANNADAY, J. E.: Ann. Surg., *94*, 218, 1931 (Foreign Bodies).
CROHN, B. B.: J. A. M. A., *151*, 625, 1953 (Hemorrhage).
FELDMAN, M.: Am. J. M. Sci., *222*, 54, 1951 (Mucosal Prolapse into Esophagus).
FIERST, S. M., *et al.*: Ann. Int. Med., *34*, 1202, 1951 (Interstitial Gastric Emphysema).
HOBBS, W. H., and COHEN, S. E.: Am. J. Surg., *71*, 505, 1946 (Intussusception).
HURWITZ, S., and MCALENNEY, P. F.: Am. J. Dis. Child., *81*, 753, 1951 (Bezoars).
LICHTSTEIN, J., and ASHER, L. M.: J. A. M. A., *151*, 720, 1953 (Mucosal Prolapse).
MEYER, K. A., and STIGMANN, F.: Surg. Clin. North America, *24*, 29, 1944, (Hemorrhage).
RUSSELL, J. Y. W.: Brit. J. Surg., *38*, 17, 1950 (Volvulus).
SHELLITO, J. G., and RIVERS, A. B.: Gastroenterology, *12*, 919, 1949 (Perforation).
STRODE, E. C., and DEAN, M. L.: Ann. Surg., *131*, 801, 1950 (Acid Burns).
TARTAKOFF, J.: Rev. Gastroenterol., *17*, 810, 1950 (Gastrojejunocolic Fistula).
VAUGHN, A. M., *et al.*: Am. J. Surg., *78*, 99, 1949 (Gastrojejunocolic Fistula).
WOLF, N. J.: New York State J. Med., *36*, 1539, 1936 (Rupture).

Tumors

BEATTIE, A. D., and MORONEY, M. J.: Brit. J. Cancer, *6*, 215, 1952 (Ulcer Cancer).
BOYCE, F. F.: J. A. M. A., *151*, 15, 1953 (Carcinoma).
BROWN, C. H., and KANE, C. F.: Gastroenterology, *22*, 64, 1952 (Carcinoma).
CAREY, J. B., and HAY, L. J.: Gastroenterology, *14*, 280, 1950 (Polyps).
COLE, J. W., and BARRY, F. M.: Am. J. Surg., *79*, 524, 1950 (Smooth Muscle Tumors).
COLLINS, W. T., and GALL, E. A.: Cancer, *5*, 62, 1952 (Multicentric Carcinoma).
COMFORT, M. W.: Ann. Int. Med., *34*, 1331, 1951 (Gastric Acidity and Carcinoma).
COOPER, W. A., and PAPANICOLAOU, G. N.: J. A. M. A., *151*, 10, 1953 (Cytologic Diagnosis of Cancer).
ELLIOTT, G. V., and WILSON, H. M.: A. M. A. Arch. Int. Med., *89*, 358, 1952 (Mesenchymal Tumors).
HARDT, L. L., *et al.*: Gastroenterology, *11*, 629, 1948 (Polyps).
JEMERIN, B. E., and COLP, R.: Surg., Gynec., & Obst., *95*, 99, 1952 (Carcinoma).
MARSHALL, S. F., and MEISSNER, W. A.: Ann. Surg., *131*, 824, 1950 (Sarcoma).
MAYO, H. W., JR., and POSTLETHWAIT, R. W.: Am. Surg., *17*, 103, 1951 (Perforated Carcinoma).
MOLNAR, G. D., and MACKENZIE, W. C.: Canad. M. A. J., *67*, 313, 1952 (Leiomyosarcoma).
NORCROSS, J. W., *et al.*: Ann. Int. Med., *37*, 338, 1952 (Pernicious Anemia and Carcinoma).
PACK, G. T.: J. Thoracic Surg., *23*, 593, 1952 (Statistics Carcinoma).
PACK, G. T., and MCNEER, G.: Surgery, *24*, 769, 1948 (End Results in Cancer).
PALMER, E. D.: Am. J. Digest. Dis., *17*, 186, 1950 (Sarcomas).
RABINOVITCH, J., *et al.*: Am. J. Surg., *80*, 550, 1950 (Sarcomas).
————: A. M. A. Arch. Surg., *58*, 529, 1949 (Benign Epithelial Tumors).
RAGINS, A. B., and COHEN, H.: Am. J. Surg., *80*, 192, 1950 (Intrinsic Lesions).
STATE, D., *et al.*: J. A. M. A., *142*, 1228, 1950 (Early Diagnosis Carcinoma.)
SWYNNERTON, B. F., and TRUELOVE, S. B.: Brit. M. J., *1*, 287, 1952 (Carcinoma).
WEINBERG, F. S.: Am. J. Digest. Dis., *18*, 45, 1951 (Achlorhydria and Carcinoma).
YARNIS, H., *et al.*: J. A. M. A., *148*, 1088, 1952 (Polyps).

Chapter

18

Small Intestine

PATHOLOGIC PHYSIOLOGY

M. H. F. FRIEDMAN

THE principle *functions* of the *small intestine* are those dealing with motor activities, secretion, and absorption. Secondary functions are of an endocrine nature which relate to humoral regulation of digestive processes and also in the regulation of water balance. The symptoms of pathophysiology of the small intestine include pain, nausea and vomiting, diarrhea or constipation, and distention, and reflect disorders in these functions.

The *normal motor activities* of the small intestine consist of local rhythmic segmenting movements and of spreading peristaltic waves. The segmentation serves to pass the contents backward and forward within an area of a few centimeters. This acts to keep the contents churned or stirred, and affords a mechanical means for increasing the surface presented for enzymatic digestion and absorption. Peristaltic waves begin at the pylorus and proceed at a steady rate along the intestine for a distance of about 50 centimeters before dying out. The intestinal contents are kept moving along by other waves which originate at various points of the small intestine and so ultimately reach the colon. Normally, reverse peristalses are absent from the small intestine but in the presence of irritation, particularly if the locus is in the upper regions, reverse peristalses may be initiated. These frequently are associated with vomiting and obviously constitute a means of defence. Another mechanism of defence operating to remove an intestinal irritant is a rapidly moving peristaltic wave which may sweep over the whole intestine and which has been designated as a *peristaltic rush*. Peristaltic rushes are characteristic of *diarrhea*.

With each phasic wave of gastric evacuation about 2 to 4 ml. of liquid and semisolid *contents* are *passed* into the *duodenum*. There is each time a momentary receptive relaxation of the duodenum as part of an accommodation reflex so that intraduodenal pressure is not raised by the filling. Apparently, in the *"dumping syndrome"* this reflex is absent and may be responsible in part for the symptoms of overdistention.

The *filling* of the *small intestine* occurs at a constant rate as long as digestible food can be evacuated from the stomach. A *test meal* begins to appear in the duodenum within 15 minutes if it is liquid and 30 minutes if it is solid. The mouth to terminal ileum transit time is between one and one-half to three hours but the terminal ileum is rarely empty before the sixth hour. No correlation has been found between the length of the small intestine and the transit time so that children do not necessarily fill their colon more frequently than do adults. The rate of emptying of the ileum

(688)

normally depends upon the state of intestinal tonus, degree of fullness of the colon, and the composition of the meal.

Reflexes which *control intestinal transit* have an important bearing on the symptoms due to motor dysfunctions. On distention of the stomach there are normally initiated reflex peristalses of the small and large bowel. In diseases of the terminal ileum these reflexes may account for pain in the lower abdomen occurring as soon as food is eaten and long before it reaches the affected region of intestine. One may speak of a *law* of *excitatory* and *inhibitory intestinal motor gradients* to account for other symptoms. This, briefly stated, is that motor activity is inhibited in the intestine proximal to the point of stimulation but is accelerated in regions distal to the point.

The *duodenal glands* of the area extending from the pyloric orifice to the pancreatic papilla secrete mucus from the glands of Brunner. Significantly, the distribution of these glands is limited to the region which first receives the gastric contents. Furthermore, the major potent secretory stimulus is acid gastric juice. An autoregulatory mechanism for the protection of the duodenal cap by secretion of acid-binding mucus is thus provided. This may form the basis for *hypertrophy* of the region of the glands of Brunner which has been described in some patients with gastric hypersecretion.

The *rest* of the *small intestine* normally *secretes* smaller quantities of mucus but in inflammatory processes the mucus flow may be prodigeous. In *regional enteritis* there is hyperplasia of the mucosa occurring in patches with an absolute increase in the number of Paneth cells. The normal secretory stimuli include acid and mechanical distention. The former acts by liberation of the hormone *enterocrinine* from the intestinal mucosa, while the latter acts by myenteric reflexes. Extrinsic nerves supply few secretory fibers to the glands but the increase in blood flow to the intestine following sympathetic denervation results in a profuse *"paralytic" secretion*.

Other than the diarrheas due to *rush peristalses*, the important *motor dysfunctions* which give rise to symptoms are those associated with impaired intestinal transit which is found in *obstructions*. In organic obstructions the continuity of the bowel lumen is interrupted either acutely as by strangulation, or chronically as by a tumor mass or cicatricial tissue of a healed ulcer. The digestive secretions which accumulate proximal to the site of obstruction distend the bowel to act as an effective distention stimulus for further secretion. When the intraluminal pressure reaches the capillary pressure, the blood supply to the bowel becomes inadequate and gangrene occurs.

Bowel spasm as a cause of functional obstruction is rare. More prominent and more serious is the interference with transit through the intestine which is due to absence of peristaltic waves. In *adynamic ileus*, following abdominal surgery, a segment of intestine becomes paralyzed. The reasons for this are still unknown but probably the intramural ganglion cells are involved. Contents of the proximal parts of the intestine are propelled into the atonic segment and here accumulate. Weak peristalses may be set up by the distention stimulus but these are ineffectual as a propulsive force. As in organic obstruction, the distention may inaugurate further secretion.

Absorption of the *digestion products* of a *meal* occurs almost entirely from the small intestine. Except for alcohol and certain drugs which may be absorbed from the mouth and stomach, all other materials are taken up through the intestinal villi. (Steroid hormones, cardiac glycosides, and other drugs which may be inactivated by the liver but exhibit transbucal absorption, can bypass the liver and exert therapeutic effects when given sublingually). While absorption may take place from the whole of the small intestine it normally occurs most actively from the upper segment. The intestine, however, shows remarkable adaptability should the total absorptive surface be reduced. The fair to good nutritional state of some patients who have had all but 12 to 18 inches of the small intestine resected, as for ileitis, attest to this. The intestinal content reaching the terminal ileum is essentially a liquid suspension of feces from which all absorbable nutrient matter has already been removed. In cases of rush peristalses involving the small bowel, however, there may not have been enough time for food digestion products to be absorbed. In such diseases of *malabsorption*, nutritional deficiencies become evident.

Few of the *factors regulating intestinal absorption* are understood but at least two mechanical factors are intestinal motility and movements of the villi. The intestinal movements constantly make available new surfaces for absorption, while the intestinal villi exert a "pumping" action to force materials along into the lacteals and portal capillaries. In the bowel which has been *denervated*, or in which motor activities of the muscle and villi have been depressed, as by *drugs* such as atropine or in *nutritional deficiency* states, absorption of all foodstuffs is markedly reduced.

Some substances exhibit the phenomenon of *selective* or preferential *absorption* in comparison with others of identical molecular weight. Thus, dextrose is two to ten times as readily absorbed as is fructose but the reasons for this are still conjectural. Furthermore, some substances, such as dextrose, are absorbed at a constant rate apparently independent of the concentration in the intestine.

Carbohydrate and *protein digestion* occurs chiefly in the duodenum and jejunum and the end products of degradation are absorbed as soon as formed. Cellulose is degraded to absorbable dextrose and fructose in the intestine of certain animals by bacterial action but such bacteria are absent from the human bowel. For this reason, raw vegetables and medicinal cellulose preparations remain undigested and form "bulk laxatives" to stimulate peristalsis. Native proteins are absorbed only after enzymatic degradation to amino acids and the view that they are absorbed unaltered from the intestine with eroded or hemorrhagic mucosal surface is fallacious. Indeed, in the intestine with erosions of the mucosal surface absorption of all substances is depressed rather than enhanced. Whereas aqueous soluble materials (sugar, amino acids, and salts) are absorbed through the portal channels of the villi, most of the fat absorption occurs by way of the lymphatic lacteals. The loss of villi in erosive lesions accounts for the reduced absorption.

The hydrolyzed *dietary fat* passes through the epithelial cell membrane either as a fatty acid complex or as a finely emulsified neutral fat complex. A process of reconversion occurs within the epithelial cell so that most of the fat leaving through the lacteal is neutral fat. The so-called *postprandial lipemia* is due to the absorbed lipid droplets or chylomicrons entering the systemic circulation by way of the thoracic duct lymph. The relation of fat absorption to *gastrointestinal* and *systemic diseases* is of great importance. The greater part of ingested lipid and lipid-soluble substances are taken up by the thoracic duct and hence metabolic alterations, including detoxification, by the liver are bypassed. The possibility therefore exists, for example, that the deposition of lipid-like substances, such as cholesterol, in the arterial intima is a matter of abnormal chylomicron size, and that a disease such as atherosclerosis is primarily a matter of intestinal dysfunction rather than a disturbance in the arterial wall. *Impaired fat absorption*, whether due to pancreatic or biliary tract disease, diarrhea, or reduced absorptive surface following very extensive intestinal resection, is early a cause for concern because of inadequate absorption of fat-soluble vitamins A, D, E, and K. Evidence that some of these are essential for maintaining the integrity of the intestinal absorptive epithelium suggests that *malabsorption* readily establishes a vicious cycle and, for this reason, such diseases are among the most difficult to treat.

Dietary iron, which is chiefly in the ferric form, must first be reduced to the ferrous form by the acid gastric juice to be absorbed from the intestinal tract. For this reason, nutritional iron anemia may develop following gastrectomy or may be seen in patients with achlorhydria. Normally, the intestinal tissue is saturated with iron in the form of ferritin so that absorption is limited to only a few milligrams of iron daily. When equilibrium between depot iron and plasma iron is upset, as in chronic anemia or hemorrhage, iron absorption from the intestine is greatly increased but restitution of depot iron occurs more slowly than depletion. Serum iron levels may, therefore, remain low for some time before a dietary regimen can exert a corrective effect.

Gases in the gastrointestinal tract which give rise to distention and bloatting, particularly in biliary tract disease and in paralytic ileus, are derived from four major sources: swallowed air, bacterial action, chemical action, and diffusion from the blood stream. The proportions of gas derived from each source vary with the disease but most important clinically is the swallowed air. This accounts for the distention in nursing infants and adults with faulty eating habits and also in some cigarette smokers who ingest tobacco smoke as well as inhale it. *Aerophagia*, or air gulping, is especially common in certain nervous individuals and is frequently indulged in because of the "gratifying sensations of belching" which ensue. Diffusion of gas from the blood stream into the bowel accounts for the cramps experienced at high altitudes and is similar to the "bends" following rapid decompression of deep sea divers. Probably the gas accumulated in an atonic bowel loop is, in part, of such origin. The belching and passage of flatus in ulcer patients is probably in part due to carbon dioxide liberated from the bicarbonate of pancreatic juice by gastric hydrochloric acid and, in part, due to carbon dioxide liberated from certain foodstuffs, particularly starches. Peristaltic waves passing over an intestinal loop filled with gas are heard as *borborygmi* or intestinal noises which become higher pitched as the loop becomes more distended.

Pain has been defined as an unpleasant sensation induced by noxious stimuli and overlaid with psychologic and emotional reactions. The benefits from pain are in the nature of alarm signals and automatic avoidance reactions. *Visceral pain* differs from pain in most somatic structures in that the only adequate stimulus is tension of the viscus muscle such as is produced in distention. *Pain elsewhere* may be induced by nearly all kinds of stimuli of adequate intensity (cutting, burning, etc.) but to these the *bowel* is insensitive. The *peritoneum*, however, and especially the parietal peritoneum, is sensitive to chemical and mechanical stimuli and to this is due the pain of peritonitis. Peritoneal irritation, even if not consciously felt as pain sensations, may give rise to reflexes elsewhere. Reflex muscle spasm from peritoneal stimulation may be noted in the abdominal rigidity of peritonitis. Localization of visceral pain is usually poor but with recurrence the patient soon learns to localize the site quite accurately. Thus, the position of a renal calculus passing down the ureter may be well localized after several episodes and the pain in acute appendicitis focuses attention on a narrowly delineated area.

The *mechanism* of *gastrointestinal pain* is not well understood but is probably due to local ischemia within the muscle in spasm. In a bowel with an inflammatory process the threshold to stimuli is lowered. What would normally result in a peristaltic wave or increase in tonus may in the inflamed bowel result in spasm and occlusion of the blood supply. Probably all bowel pain, including ulcer pain, originates in *muscle spasm*. Acid introduced directly into the normal duodenum results in peristaltic activity but in the ulcerated duodenum the acid evokes a greater degree of muscle contraction, particularly of that segment bearing the ulcer site. The concept that ulcer pain is due to excitation of sensory nerve fibers in the denuded ulcer area is therefore incorrect. Atropine and also ganglionic blocking agents will abolish the ulcer pain by depressing motor activity even though acid still bathes the ulcer area. The afferent fibers carrying pain sensations from the abdominal viscera course with the sympathetic nerves. The peptic ulcer patient who has been subjected to bilateral vagectomy may still experience pain of upper abdominal origin but in the patient subjected to sympathectomy, the viscera may be silent. For this reason, acute bowel ulceration and perforation may occur without warning in a patient who has had a sympathectomy for hypertension.

The *vomiting* characteristic of intestinal irritation and obstruction has been discussed in Chapter 17, page 653 dealing with the Stomach. *Nausea*, frequently a prelude to retching or vomiting, may be due to traction of the distended loop on the mesenteric pedicle.

GENERAL CONSIDERATIONS

This Chapter on the Small Intestine will include dissertations not only on diseases that affect the duodenum, jejunum, and ileum directly, but also on some of the disorders of adjacent structures (as for example mesenteric cysts) that are indirectly concerned with this portion of the digestive tract. Contrarily, some lesions (as for example duodenal ulcer, bezoars, superior mesenteric artery obstruction of the duodenum, etc.) that have been described in connection with the stomach shall be omitted. The pathologic processes, as elsewhere, may be discussed under the usual five general groups of diseases—Congenital Anomalies, Degenerations, Inflammations, Physical Disturbances, and Tumors.

CONGENITAL ANOMALIES

Orientation.—Congenital anomalies of the small intestine are many, varied, and frequently multiple. Some of the more important maldevelopments may be considered under the following headings: obstructive lesions, omphalomesenteric duct abnormalities, tubular duplications, diverticula, mesenteric cysts, and duodenal cysts.

Obstructive Lesions.—The important developmental obstructive lesions of the small intestine are congenital volvulus, congenital adhesions, and stenosis and atresia. *Congenital volvulus* is due to inadequate fixation of the midgut and the mesentery to the posterior wall. The small intestine and ileocecal region of the gut are anchored only at the entrance of the superior mesenteric artery, are allowed free movement, may readily undergo torsion about the axis of the attachment, and may thus produce volvulus and obstruction

(Fig. 339*A*, p. 728) (Spencer). *Congenital adhesions* consist of adventitious peritoneal bands and reflections that traverse and constrict the third part of the duodenum, the duodenojejunal junction, or the first part of the jejunum (Spencer). *Stenosis* and *atresia* consist respectively of incomplete or complete failure of canalization of the small intestine (Fig. 313). The occlusion may occur anywhere in the small bowel, may be single or multiple, and may consist of a fold, a perforated or nonperforated diaphragm, a fili-

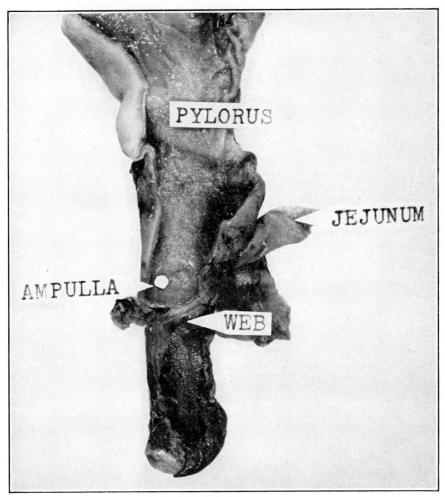

FIG. 313.—Incomplete canalization of the duodenum showing a transverse fold or web obstructing the lumen. A duodenojejunostomy had been performed.

form stricture, a fibrous cord attached to blindly ending segments of the intestine, or a completely separated blind end of gut (Swenson, Kautz, and Dyson).

Omphalomesenteric Duct Abnormalities.—In embryonic life, the omphalomesenteric duct (vitelline duct) connects the yolk sac with the midgut by way of the umbilicus (Thiel). As the embryo develops, the duct gradually becomes atretic and ultimately completely disappears. Abnormally it may persist in its entirety or in part and, accordingly, may account for

the following abnormalities: (1) *entero-umbilical* (ileo-umbilical) *fistula*—
resulting from complete patency and connecting the umbilicus with the
ileum at a point approximately 50 cm. proximal to the ileocecal valve
(Scalletar and Brown), (2) *fibrous cord*—resulting from atresia but failure
of absorption and also extending from the umbilicus to the ileum, (3)
cysts of midportion—resulting from obliteration of the proximal and distal
ends but with persistence of the patency in the midportion (Thiel), and
(4) *Meckel's diverticulum*—resulting from persistence of the proximal portion
only. Of these, the most important is Meckel's diverticulum. Its *incidence*
is generally recorded as varying between 1 and 2.5 per cent of the population
with the occurrence in males being twice that in females (Jay and Merritt).

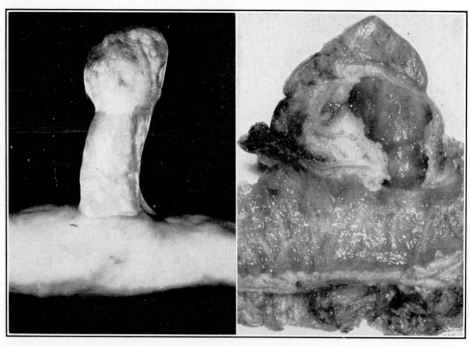

Fig. 314—Meckel's diverticula showing, to the left, an unopened, elongated outpocketing and,
to the right, an opened, somewhat squattier sac that resembles the wall of the attached ileum.

Pathologically the diverticulum is located in the antemesenteric border of
the ileum about 50 cm. proximal to the ileocecal valve. It appears simply
as a blindly ending segment of small intestine arranged perpendicularly to
the long axis of the ileum and measuring from 3 to 5 cm. in length (Fig.
314). The ostium of the diverticulum is widely patent and the wall is
composed of all the layers normally found in the small bowel. As a rule,
the mucosa is of an ileal variety but in from 15 to 25 per cent of all cases
and from 60 to 70 per cent of symptomatic cases, it discloses heterotopic
gastric, duodenal, jejunal, or colonic mucosa or pancreatic tissue. Of these
gastric mucosa and pancreatic tissue are the most common. The *complications* are obstruction with mucocele, peptic ulceration, hemorrhage, perforation, intussusception, volvulus, diverticulitis, fistula, and tumor (Fig. 315)
(Thomas). The *clinical manifestations* are those of the complications,
generally mimicking the symptoms and signs of duodenal ulcer, appendi-

citis, peritonitis, or intestinal obstruction. The *diagnosis* is usually established at operation (or postmortem) for the clinical manifestations are not distinctive enough for a definitive evaluation. *Treatment* is entirely surgical, consisting of simple excision or segmental resection of the ileum. The *prognosis* is, as a rule, excellent.

Tubular Duplications.—Tubular duplications of the small intestine, as the caption suggests, consist of formations of accessory segments of the small bowel (Jay and Moore). They are *located* along the mesenteric border of any portion of the small intestine but are usually single, measure as much as 20 to 25 cm. in length, may or may not be connected with the lumen of the adjacent bowel, and generally resemble the small bowel, both grossly and microscopically. Sometimes, however, the mucosa may resemble that of other than the adjacent bowel. The blood supply is, as a rule, shared with

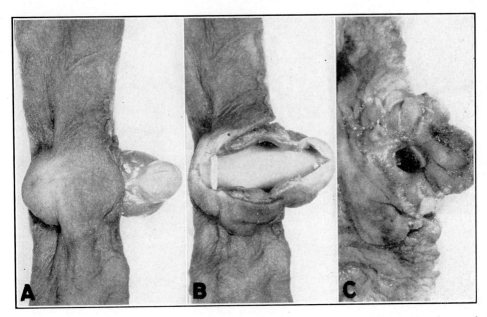

Fig. 315.—Complications of Meckel's diverticulum illustrating A and B, a closed and opened mucocele and C, a peptic ulcer at its base.

the corresponding segment of normal bowel. The *clinical manifestations* are generally those of intestinal obstruction, peptic ulcer, or inflammation and, among others, may consist of abdominal pain, nausea and vomiting, melena, and anemia. *Treatment* is surgical excision. The *prognosis* is good.

Diverticula.—Diverticula of the small intestine are of two varieties—congenital and acquired. *Congenital diverticula* are those that occur as a result of some developmental abnormality of the gut. Some represent a persistence of fetal structures (Meckel's diverticulum) while others represent simply a local rounded duplication of the gut. The former are found along the antemesenteric border, while the latter are located at the attachment of the gut with the mesentery. The wall of a congenital diverticulum is composed of all the layers present in the normal bowel wall. *Acquired diverticula* develop after birth and arise as a result of some weakness in the bowel wall. This weakness usually exists at the entrance of the vessels into the wall. In the jejunum and ileum the diverticula are, therefore, always located along the mesenteric attachment (Ritvo, Radcliffe, and Mayo). In the duodenum, they may be located in any portion of the concavity but they are most frequent in the second part of the organ just medial to the ampulla of Vater (Ferguson and Patterson). Regardless of which portion of the gut is affected, the diverticula may be single but are more often multiple, usually measure 2 to 4 cm. in greatest diameter, are generally connected to the bowel by a large ostium, and disclose a wall that is similar to that of the gut at the point of origin with the exception that the muscle coats are defective or entirely absent (Figs. 316 and 317). The *incidence* of diverticula of the small bowel is recorded as varying from less than 1 per cent to as high as 22 per cent of all autopsies and/or roentgen examinations (Patterson). In general, they occur with decreasing fre-

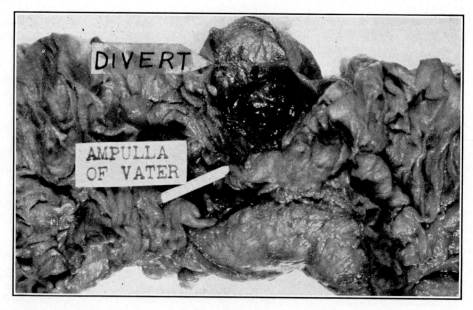

Fig. 316.—Duodenal diverticulum located medial to the entrance of the common bile duct into the duodenum.

quency proximodistally so that they are most common in the duodenum and least common (rare) in the ileum. The *complications* are infection, ulceration, perforation, and hemorrhage. *Clinically* diverticula of the small intestine are usually asymptomatic. When manifestations do develop they are entirely nonspecific and are indistinguishable from those of peptic ulcer, cholecystitis, or a host of other upper abdominal diseases. The *diagnosis* is made roentgenographically and at operation. *Treatment* is operative only when clinical manifestations are severe or when complications develop. Otherwise it is symptomatic and medical. The *prognosis* is good.

Mesenteric Cysts.—As this caption suggests, mesenteric cysts are simply cysts that are located within the mesentery, that is, between the root and the free border and between the two folds of peritoneum (Blackmun). They do not constitute a single entity but comprise rather a heterogeneous collection of cystic masses grouped together because of a common anatomic location. Some of the many types of cysts as *classified* by Peterson (Oberhelman) are as follows: (1) those arising from embryonic remnants and sequestrations—serous, chylous, sanguineous, and dermoid, (2) those of intestinal origin—sequestrations of the bowel and pinched-off diverticula, (3) those arising from urogenital organs—germinal epithelium, ovary, wolffian body, and müllerian duct, and (4) pseudocysts—infective (hydatid or tuberculous) and neoplastic (degeneration of tumors). Thus, as would be expected, the *pathologic* appearance varies with the cause and type of cyst. In general, however, the cysts are single or multiple, encroach upon or obstruct the lumen of the gut as they enlarge, vary in size from a few to many centimeters, possess a wall that is paper thin or measures 2 to 3 cm. across, and are filled with chylous, clear, or bloody fluid. The chief *complication* is intestinal obstruction. The *clinical manifestations* are, therefore, those of obstruction and consist of pain, vomiting, alternating

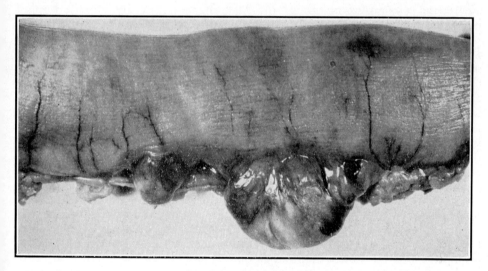

Fig. 317.—Jejunal diverticula located at the attachment of the jejunum with the mesentery.

diarrhea and constipation, anorexia, and loss of weight. The *diagnosis* is generally made at operation for, preoperatively, a mesenteric cyst may mimic an ovarian cyst, fibromyoma of the uterus, retroperitoneal tumor, etc. *Treatment* of choice is surgical excision. The *prognosis* is generally good.

Duodenal Cysts.—Duodenal cysts are of enterogenous origin, *developing* on the same basis as duplications of the intestine or congenital diverticula (Shallow). They are *rare* and are usually encountered before the age of fifteen years. *Pathologically* they are attached to the wall of some part of the duodenum, measure from 2 to 12 cm. in diameter, are composed of all the layers seen in a normal duodenum, and are filled with *clear*, pale, thin, or mucoid fluid. The *clinical manifestations* are those of duodenal obstruction. Sometimes pressure on the common bile ducts results in jaundice. The *diagnosis* in the recorded cases has been made only at operation. *Treatment* consists of surgical excision. The *prognosis* is guarded for the recorded mortality is 50 per cent.

DEGENERATIONS

Orientation. —Degenerations of the small intestine are common but, as elsewhere, are usually accompaniments of other disease processes. Thus, for example, *atrophy* is seen in a variety of conditions, notably above a point of obstruction, *parenchymatous degeneration* is virtually always present regardless of the disease, *hyaline degeneration* occurs frequently in chronic inflammatory processes, *amyloidosis* is seen in the more severe cases of secondary amyloid disease, *mucoid degeneration* is an accompaniment of certain mild inflammations and occasionally of tumors, and *steatorrhea* (Gr. = fat + to flow or the presence of excess fat in the stools) is the result of improper enzymatic hydrolysis, emulsification, and absorption of intestinal fat. Aside from these generalities, the following conditions may be considered briefly: Malabsorption syndrome sprue, celiac disease, and intestinal lipodystrophy.

Malabsorption Syndrome. —The *malabsorption syndrome* may be considered as a complex metabolic disorder characterized by impaired small intestinal absorption of various dietary substances including fat, protein, iron, folic acid, vitamin B_{12}, and ascorbic acid (Adlersberg and Oxenhorn). It may be divided into two groups—primary and secondary. *Primary malabsorption syndrome* encompasses those conditions in which there is no obvious gross, or for that matter even undisputed microscopic, pathologic alteration. It includes nontropical sprue, tropical sprue, celiac disease, and idiopathic steatorrhea. *Secondary malabsorption syndrome* encompasses conditions attended by manifestations similar to those in the primary group but arising secondary to removal of large segments of small intestine or to disorders attended by definite pathologic changes as seen in regional enteritis, lymphosarcomatosis, intestinal lipodystrophy, etc.

Sprue. —The term sprue (Dutch = herpetic stomatitis) means a sore mouth and the disorder thus called is doubtlessly named after one of the prominent features of the disease. The condition is *characterized* by asthenia, loss of weight, abdominal distention, steatorrhea, flat glucose tolerance curve, osteoporosis, hypocalcemia sometimes leading to tetany, hypoproteinemia, edema, anemia, atrophic glossitis, and stomatitis (Bjerkelund and Preuss). General manifestations such as asthenia, loss of weight, etc., are likened to those in Addison's disease and are *explainable* on the basis of adrenal cortical deficiency (Rivas). Steatorrhea results from improper hydrolysis, emulsification, and absorption of fat, with the fat content of dried stool varying from 40 to 80 per cent as compared with a normal 5 to 10 per cent. The cause of steatorrhea is unknown although disturbances of lipolytic activity of the pancreas, rapid intestinal passage, disturbances in resynthesis of fat, mechanical obstruction of mesenteric lymphatics, intestinal dysfunction as a result of infection, etc., have been considered as of etiologic significance. The flat glucose tolerance curve is due to impaired absorption of glucose from the intestine which, in turn, results from adrenal cortical insufficiency. The latter also accounts for osteoporosis and hypocalcemia. Hypoproteinemia and edema may be due to an increased demand for materials necessary for erythropoiesis, although it must be confessed that a satisfactory explanation is wanting (Stefanini). The anemia may be of a microcytic hypochromic or a macrocytic hyperchromic variety. It is due to the unavailability of folic acid. In sprue, folic acid is liberated by the gastric enzymes but it cannot be utilized because it is either improperly absorbed or is destroyed in the fermented intestinal contents. Atrophic glossitis and stomatitis are probably due to lack of the vitamin B₂ complex. Thus, the varied symptoms and the *causes* of the disorder are due to a variety of factors chief among which appear to be adrenal cortical deficiency, unavailability of folic acid, and avitaminosis. Although the disease is called *tropical sprue* when it occurs in the tropics and nontropical sprue when it occurs in temperate climates, such a delineation is unnecessary for the two conditions are identical.

Pathologically the findings are disappointing. The lesions in the mouth are similar to those in ordinary avitaminosis (p. 92). The bone marrow shows the anemia as mentioned. The intestinal tract, in uncomplicated cases, discloses neither gross nor microscopic alterations. Atrophy of intestinal mucosa, inflammation, ulceration, petechial hemorrhages, and

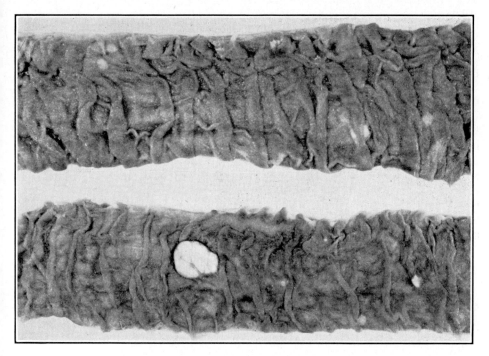

Fig. 318.—Intestinal lipodystrophy showing many small and several larger collections of fat in the mucosa.

thinning of the wall, are thought by some to represent characteristic changes (Butterworth) but by others are thought to be terminal and coincidental (Preuss).

The *clinical manifestations* have been referred to above. The *diagnosis* is made on the basis of the clinical findings with particular significance being attached to the presence of steatorrhea (bulky, liquid, tan-colored, and—upon stirring—crackling stools), anemia, and *roentgen findings.* Roentgenographic examination reveals dystonia, loss of variability of the mucosal pattern with eventually only circular folds present, and the presence of sausage-shaped masses and flocculation of barium within the lumen. *Treatment* consists of substitution liver and vitamin therapy. The *prognosis* is variable. Spontaneous remissions are common.

Celiac Disease.—Celiac or coeliac (Gr. = belly) disease is a condition in infants and children characterized essentially by distention of the abdomen and steatorrhea. Although there are still some differences of opinion, the disorder is doubtlessly analogous to sprue (Anderson and Sheldon).

Intestinal Lipodystrophy.—Intestinal lipodystrophy, also known as intestinal lipogranulomatosis and Whipple's disease, is a rare intestinal disorder characterized by sprue-like manifestations (Pemberton, Hendrix, and Upton). It is virtually confined to males of a mean age of about fifty years. The *cause* is unknown. *Pathologically* the mucosa of the jejunum and ileum contains scattered circumscribed deposits of fatty material that vary in diameter from less than a millimeter to 1 cm. (Fig. 318). The smaller deposits are nonelevated but the larger ones protrude into the lumen in a polypoid manner. The mesentery is thick, yellow, and rubbery. The contained lymph nodes, especially those near the bowel and opposite the mucosal deposits, are enlarged, firm, yellowish, and spongy. *Histologically* the dominant features are dilatation of the lacteals and the presence of macrophages filled with fat (Fig. 319). The lacteals are readily visualized in the submucosa while the fat-laden foam cells are seen in the mucosa and the mesenteric lymph nodes. Usually the cells are arranged diffusely but sometimes they are grouped in clusters to form pseudotubercles. As the fat deposits are increased, the cells disintegrate and the fat accumulates in larger globular masses. About the periphery of these, giant cells of the foreign body type are frequently seen. *Clinical manifestations* consist of indigestion, gaseous distention of the abdomen, diarrhea, loss of weight, progressive asthenia, and general debility (Pemberton). There are, in addition, steatorrhea, moderate anemia, achlorhydria, increase in the fat content of the stool to as high as 80 per cent, and relatively normal roentgenographic studies of the bowel. The *diagnosis* is usually made at postmortem for the condition, clinically, is virtually indistinguishable from sprue. *Treatment* is unsatisfactory. The *prognosis* is poor.

INFLAMMATIONS

Orientation.—Inflammation of the small intestine as a whole is referred to as *enteritis* (Gr. = intestine + inflammation) while inflammation of the duodenum is known as *duodenitis*, of the jejunum as *jejunitis*, and of the ileum as *ileitis*. Although enteritis may be variously categorized, the following *classification* encompasses most of the important diseases: acute duodenitis, simple ulcer, acute ulcerative enteritis, acute phlegmonous enteritis, periarteritis nodosa, enteritis necroticans, diarrhea of infants, food poisoning, typhoid and paratyphoid fever, regional enteritis, tuberculosis, fungous and yeast-like enteritis and colitis, and parasitic infections. *Acute phlegmonous enteritis* is identical with acute phlegmonous gastritis which has already been discussed (p. 660), while the enteric lesions in *periarteritis nodosa* have been mentioned in connection with the description of periarteritis nodosa as a disease entity (p. 370). The remaining conditions may now be referred to briefly.

Acute Duodenitis.—Acute duodenitis is a nonspecific acute inflammation of the duodenum. The condition *occurs* at all ages and is probably much commoner than the few reports in the literature would tend to indicate (Kirklin and Gillespie). The *cause* is unknown, although the etiologic agents are considered to be similar to those in peptic ulcer. In the recorded cases, particular stress has been laid upon allergy and a highly emotional constitution. *Pathologically* the mucosa discloses a diffuse or focal redden-

ing with occasional superficial erosion but no definite ulceration. The wall
is not indurated and is relatively normal to palpation. The serosa discloses a hyperemic stippling. *Histologically* the mucosa shows little or no
loss of epithelial structures although, as grossly, it may occasionally be
superficially denuded. The submucosa and the rest of the wall reveal
varying degrees of congestion, edema, and leukocytic exudation that predominates in lymphocytes, plasma cells, and occasionally eosinophils. The
chief recorded *complication* is frank duodenal ulcer. The *clinical manifestations* resemble those of uncomplicated peptic ulcer but are usually of a
milder degree. *Roentgenographically* there is increased irritation of the

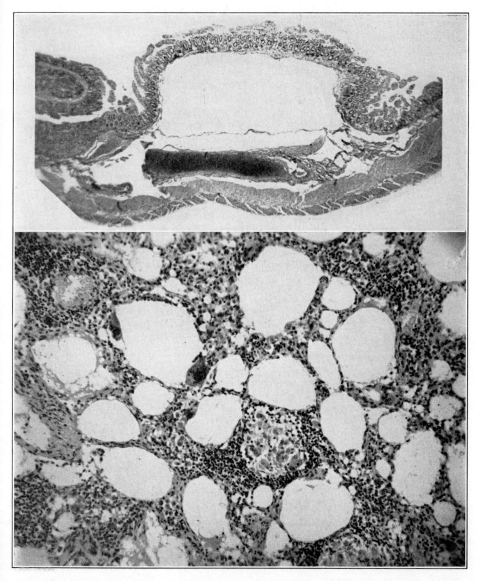

Fig. 319.—Intestinal lipodystrophy illustrating, above, a dilated submucosal lacteal. × 7, and,
below, foam cells, pseudotubercles, vacuoles, and foreign body giant cells in a mesenteric lymph
node. × 100.

duodenum manifested by spasticity and hypermotility. In addition, the mucosal pattern is coarse and irregularly reticulated. The *diagnosis* is made from the clinical manifestations, the roentgenographic appearance, and the findings at operation. *Treatment* is essentially similar to that in peptic ulcer. The *prognosis* is good for the response to treatment is generally rapid. Recurrences, however, do occur and occasionally, as already stated, frank ulcers may develop.

Simple Ulcer. —Under the heading of simple or primary ulcer has been described an acute to chronic ulcer of the jejunum or ileum that differs from peptic ulcer in that it is not bathed by gastric juice. The condition is *rare* for up to 1948 there have been only 130 cases recorded in the litera-

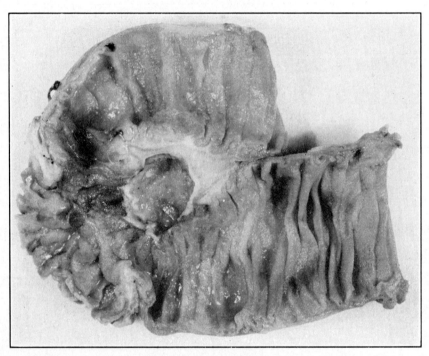

Fig. 320.—Simple ulcer of the jejunum showing a punched-out, clean-cut defect extending to the serosa and causing kinking of the bowel.

ture (Evert). The incidence at the Mayo Clinic has been 1 in 100,000 patients registered. The lesion predominates in males in the ratio of 3 to 1 and it occurs at all ages. The *cause* is unknown although infection, trauma, and vascular occlusion have been mentioned as of etiologic significance.

Pathologically most ulcers are solitary, although occasionally multiple lesions have been described. When there is more than one lesion present, the ulcers have a tendency to group in small collections of two or three. In the recorded cases, about one-third of the lesions were located in the jejunum and approximately two-thirds were found in the ileum. Any portion of the circumference of the bowel may be involved with no preponderance in any one area. As a rule, the ulcer measures up to 1 or, at most, 2 cm. in diameter, is rounded and punched-out, has a smooth gray floor, discloses little undermining of its edges, and extends all the way to or through the serosa (Fig. 320). When the ulcer is acute it is attended by little fibrosis but when it is chronic it may be accompanied by marked cicatrization, adhesion formation, and distortion of the bowel lumen. The draining mesenteric lymph nodes are usually enlarged. *Histologically* the ulcer is entirely nonspecific and resembles closely a peptic ulcer.

The *complications* are perforation, bleeding, and obstruction. Perforation may result in peritonitis, abscess, and fistulous tract formation. Bleeding

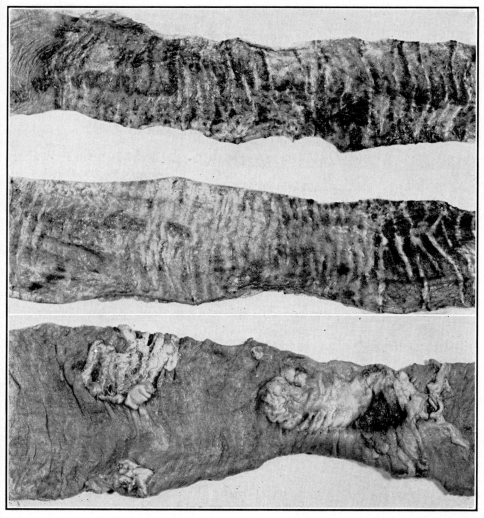

FIG. 321.—Acute ulcerative enteritis disclosing, in the upper two segments of bowel, marked congestion and superficial ulceration and, in the lower segment, several irregular ulcers covered with gray pseudomembranes.

is generally massive and is indicated by the passage of blood in the stool. Obstruction occurs from cicatricial stenosis and/or kinking of the bowel from peritoneal adhesions. *Clinically* the manifestations are generally those of the complications that arise but, in the absence of complications, they mimic those of peptic ulcer when the lesions are proximally located and those of appendicitis when they are distally located (Evert and Kim). The *diagnosis* is usually made at the time of laparotomy or autopsy for the manifestations are not distinctive. Occasionally the ulcer may be demonstrated roentgenographically (Creighead). *Treatment* is entirely surgical. The operation of choice is resection of the segment of the bowel involved but in the presence of perforation and an extremely ill patient simple closure of the opening may be indicated. The *prognosis* is guarded for the mortality in the recorded cases has been as high as 66 per cent (Shea).

Acute Ulcerative Enteritis. —This condition, also known as *acute pseudo-membranous enterocolitis*, is a nonspecific acute inflammatory disease that affects not only the small bowel but also the colon and sometimes the esophagus and even the stomach (p. 636). It *occurs* with equal frequency in males and females and has been described in patients of all ages. It has been recorded in connection with the following: (1) postoperative state, (2) neoplastic obstruction of the intestines, (3) cardiac disease, and (4) infection such as septicemia, pneumonia, etc. (Kleckner). In searching for more specific common denominators the ultimate causative factors appear to be (1) circulatory collapse with the pathogenesis being vascular dilatation, stasis, impaired nutrition, degeneration, necrosis, and ulceration (Penner) and/or (2) staphylococcic infection (Newman, Johnston, Turnbull, and Lepley). The latter is almost always due to an antibiotic rsistant, coagulase-positive, hemolytic *Staphylococcus aureus*. As would be expected, therefore, the wide use of broad spectrum antibiotics in recent years has brought about a sharp increase in the number of cases due to staphylococcic infection.

Pathologically the gastrointestinal tract shows diffuse congestion, swelling, and often petechial erosion of the mucosa. In addition, the jejunum, ileum, and/or colon disclose numerous or few, superficial or deep uclers that measure from a few millimeters to several centimeters in greatest diameter (Fig. 321). The ulcers are irregular in distribution and configuration. The borders are often undermined; the floor may be clean or may be covered with a loosely adherent, gray, brown, hemorrhagic, or green membrane, and the base is located at any point between the mucosa and the serosa. The segment of the bowel in the region of the ulcerations is usually dilated and the mucosa is more congested than that of the adjacent portions of the bowel. Occasionally the affected segment shows distinct infarction. *Histologically* the mucosa discloses erosion or frank ulceration (Fig. 322). The tissue surrounding the defect reveals marked congestion and edema together with varying degrees of neutrophilic, plasma cell, and lymphocytic infiltration. Microscopically, as grossly, the lesion may extend all the way through the serosa. Because of the acuteness of the process there is virtually no fibroblastic proliferation.

Aside from shock and renal impairment, the most important *complication* is perforation with resulting peritonitis. *Clinically* the manifestations, in decreasing order of frequency, are circulatory collapse, abdominal pain, vomiting, fever, abdominal distention, and diarrhea (Dixon). The *diagnosis* is usually made at postmortem although, with increasing awareness of the condition, it can be suspected from a history of the predisposing causes listed above together with the clinical manifestations. *Treatment* is essentially the treatment of shock—both as a preventive and a curative measure together with the use of antibiotics that will inhibit *Staphylococcus aureus*, when this is the causative agent. The *prognosis* is guarded for the mortality rate (at least in the recorded cases) has been greater than 90 per cent.

Enteritis Necroticans. —Enteritis necroticans is an acute fulminating infection of the small intestine that is similar to lamb dysentery and "struck" (Patterson). It is *caused* by *Clostridium welchii* with the route of infection being directly through the mucosa. *Pathologically* the bowel shows severe congestion with areas of mucosal erosion and superficial necrosis that measure as much as 4 cm. in diameter. The outstanding feature, however, is the presence of mucosal and submucosal gas crepitations. *Histologically* the erosions and ulcers disclose congestion, edema, severe nonspecific leuko-cytic infiltration, and numerous blunt, gram-positive bacilli. The adjacent bowel reveals simple air sacs. The *complications* are shock culminating in death, and cicatricial stenosis in some of the patients that recover. *Clinically* there is usually an acute onset with violent abdominal pain localized

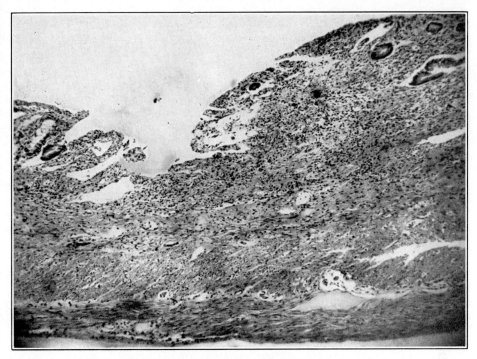

Fig. 322.—Acute ulcerative enteritis illustrating a superficial mucosal defect with surrounding edema and neutrophilic infiltration. × 50.

to the left of the umbilicus, nausea and vomiting, abdominal rigidity, and shock. In the absence of immediate (twenty-four hour) death there are also bloody diarrhea, fever, increased sedimentation rate, leukocytosis, and urinary retention. The *diagnosis* is usually made at laparotomy or post-mortem. *Treatment* in recorded cases has consisted of supportive measures and, in a few cases, of surgical resection. The *prognosis* is guarded for the mortality rate is high.

Diarrhea of Infants.—Diarrhea of infants, also known as infantile diarrhea, diarrhea of the newborn, and viral diarrhea, is, of course, a symptom and not a disease. It is so called because the etiologic agent in most instances is unknown. The condition *occurs* with suddenness and, because of its contagiousness, is the bane of the hospital nursery. It is most prevalent in infants up to six months of age. Although, as stated

45

above, the precise *cause* is unknown in most instances, there are doubt-lessly a variety of agents that produce the disorder (Trussell). In approx-imately one-half of the 456 cases studied by Alexander, the patients dis-closed infections of the respiratory tract, ear, skin, etc. Whether these, however, had anything to do with the intestinal disorder is not definitely known. Also, in connection with etiology, Buddingh has isolated a virus (from mouth washings and stools) of infants with stomatitis followed by diarrhea and has, therefore, shown that some of the cases at least are of viral origin. Regardless of the causative agents, the spread of the infection is doubtlessly directly from person to person. The incubation period is unknown. *Pathologically* what changes are present are confined to the small intestine. In some cases the bowel appears relatively normal. In others, the lumen contains greenish, watery material with an abundant amount of mucus. The mucosa is swollen and hyperemic, sometimes disclosing pinpoint hemorrhages with central ulceration. *Histologically* the changes are entirely nonspecific, consisting of congestion, edema, focal epithelial necrosis, and infiltration of the mucosa and submucosa with neutrophils. The chief *complication* is dehydration. The *clinical mani-festations* consist of (1) diarrhea with from four to twelve loose greenish stools daily composed mostly of mucus and containing flecks of blood, and (2) a mild stomatitis in about three-quarters of the cases. The latter is often minimal and easily overlooked unless careful inspection of the buccal mucosa is made. The *diagnosis* is made entirely from the history and the appearance of the stools. *Treatment* consists of prevention by way of ter-minal sterilization of the formula with nipple and cap attached, carrying out isolation techniques once the disorder occurs, and combating dehydra-tion by parenteral administration of fluid (Trussell and Alexander). The *prognosis* is good provided treatment is instituted early. In different out-breaks the mortality rates have varied from 0 to 50 per cent.

Food Poisoning.—The caption "food poisoning" literally indicates any poison ingested with or as food. As such, it includes (1) *chemicals* such as arsenic, bichloride of mercury, chloral hydrate, etc., that are intentionally or accidentally added to food, (2) *poisonous plants* such as snakeroot, certain mushrooms, water hemlock, fava bean, etc., (3) *contaminated animals* such as encountered occasionally in shellfish (mussel poison) and a variety of other fish, and (4) *microbial* (Dack). Of these, microbial poison-ing is perhaps the most important and is usually considered synonymous with food poisoning unless otherwise specified. Although most microbes are poisonous if ingested in adequate amounts, those that are usually asso-ciated with food poisoning are *Staphylococcus*, *Clostridium botulinum*, and *Salmonella*.

Staphylococcus food poisoning is the most common. It is *caused* by a toxin formed in the food before ingestion. The *conditions necessary* for such poisoning are (1) contamination with an enterotoxin-producing *Staphylo-coccus*, (2) suitable food (such as ham pie, meats, cream puffs, cheeses, custards, milk, sandwiches, etc.) in which the organisms can grow, and (3) suitable environmental temperature for a sufficient period to allow the organ-isms to multiply and produce their toxins. *Pathologically* there are no spe-cific or constant changes other than a mild gastroenteritis. The *clinical manifestations* appear in from one to six hours after ingestion of contam-inated foods. They consist of salivation, nausea, vomiting, retching, abdominal pain, diarrhea, with or without blood and mucus, headache, muscle cramps, sweating, fever, and prostration. The *diagnosis* is made from a history of several people developing similar symptoms after ingesting similar food, by culturing the food, or by reproducing the disorder in a rhesus monkey by feeding or injecting the animal with the filtrate of the cultures. *Treatment* consists of emptying the stomach of the food ingested and combating shock. The *prognosis* is good for recovery is usually complete in from one to three days.

Poisoning by *Clostridium botulinum* is known as *botulism*. Like *Staphylococcus* food poisoning, botulism is also *caused* by toxin formed in the food before ingestion. Improperly preserved meats and home-canned fruits and vegetables are usually the responsible foods. *Pathologically* the only important recorded changes are thrombi in meningeal veins in patients dying after forty-eight hours. The *clinical manifestations* appear in from twelve to thirty-six hours but may not become apparent for several days. They affect the gastrointestinal tract and central nervous system. *Gastrointestinal* symptoms consist of nausea, vomiting, diarrhea followed by constipation, and abdominal distress and burning. *Central nervous system* manifestations consist of muscular weakness, dyplopia, blepharoptosis, mydriasis, loss of pupillary reflex to light, photophobia, nystagmus, vertigo, difficulty in swallowing, pharyngeal paralysis, and, in severe cases, death in respiratory failure from two to twenty-six days. The *diagnosis* is made from the history, swelling of the can in which the food is packed, production of "limber-neck" in chickens fed the contaminated food, and the injection of antitoxin protected and unprotected mice with a saline extract of the contaminated food. The former will not develop botulism while the latter will. *Treatment* consists of administration of botulinum antitoxin, maintenance of fluid balance, and prevention of aspiration pneumonia. The *prognosis* is guarded for the mortality is about 65 per cent.

Although often incriminated, *Salmonella* accounts for only a small number of food poisoning outbreaks. Unlike the other types of poisoning already mentioned, in this group the organisms are ingested with the food and must multiply in the intestine before they produce ill effects. The condition, therefore, is, in reality, an infection. Although there are many species of organisms in the group the most common offenders are *Salmonella enteriditis*, *Salmonella typhimurium*, *Salmonella newport*, and *Salmonella thompson*. *Pathologic* changes are minimal, consisting at most of a mild inflammation of the gastrointestinal tract. *Clinically* the incubation period is usually twelve to twenty-four hours. The condition is often ushered in with a headache and chill and these are followed by nausea, vomiting, abdominal pain, diarrhea, muscular weakness, faintness, and prostration. The *diagnosis* is made upon isolating the organisms either from the food or stool. *Treatment* is symptomatic. The *prognosis* is good with the mortality rate being less than 1 per cent.

Typhoid and Paratyphoid Fever. — Typhoid and paratyphoid fever, often referred to collectively as *enteric fever*, may be considered together for the disorders are caused by related organisms and are attended by similar clinical manifestations and pathologic changes. The *incidence* of the disease has declined precipitously in the United States in the last fifty years, from thousands of cases in 1900 to a mere 2,515 cases in 1950 (Turner). The steady decline has been due entirely to enforcement of stringent public health measures. While formerly the disease occurred in dreaded epidemics in the late summer weeks now it occurs only sporadically. The *cause* of typhoid fever is *Salmonella (Eberthella) typhosa*, while the cause of paratyphoid fever is *Salmonella paratyphi*. Each is a gram-negative motile rod that can be differentiated fron other intestinal gram-negative rods by carbohydrate fermentation and from each other by agglutination reactions. The *source* of the infection is ingestion of fecally contaminated materials (Beeson). The organisms are discharged in the excreta of a person with active disease or a carrier and are then transferred to food (milk, salads, etc.) by fingers or flies and to water by sewage contamination. With the food they pass through the stomach, are picked up by the plasma cells of the intestinal lymphoid patches and mesenteric lymph nodes, multiply in these areas, are discharged into the lymphatic channels, gain entrance into the bloodstream, and are disseminated throughout the body (Adams). The organisms can be readily recovered from the bloodstream during the

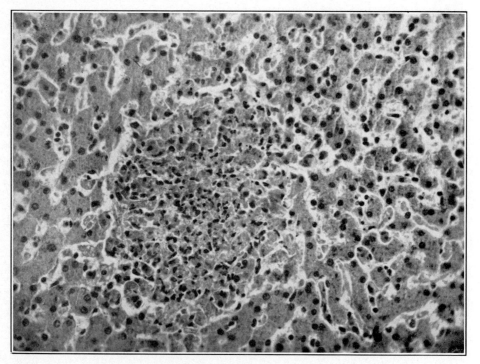

Fig. 323.—Typhoid fever showing a circumscribed nodule of
mononuclear cells in the liver. × 200.

first week of the disease, from the sternal marrow from the first to the fifth week of the disease, from the stool after the third or fourth week of the disease, and from the urine during the third and fourth weeks. After the second week, antibodies begin to appear in the bloodstream and their demonstration in increasing titers over 1:80 (Widal reaction) is definite evidence of infection.

Pathologically the disorder is essentially a disease of the reticuloendothelial system and, as such, affects primarily the intestines, lymph nodes, spleen, liver, and bone marrow (Mallory). Regardless of the organ involved, the process is characterized by focal proliferation of large, actively phagocytic, mononuclear cells and later by necrosis (Fig. 323). The cells not only contain bacteria but they also disclose ingested fragments of leukocytes, erythrocytes, and tissue cells. In the *intestines* the lesions affect Peyer's patches and solitary lymph follicles. During the first week of the disease the lymphoid structures become enlarged and more conspicuous than normal. During the second and third weeks ischemic necrosis occurs and ulcers are formed. The ulcers conform to the anatomic configuration of the intestinal lymphoid structures. They are sharply defined, have slightly undermined edges, disclose clean floors, and show a base at any point between the submucosa and serosa. After the third week, healing occurs by regeneration of the lymphoid patches and follicles and re-epithelization from the adjacent mucosa. Scarring does not occur. The *mesenteric lymph nodes*, *spleen*, and *liver* are enlarged and these structures along with the *bone marrow* may show tiny gray foci macroscopically. These foci, of course, represent mononuclear cell proliferation with necrosis. In addition to the inflammatory changes, the liver, heart, and kidneys disclose parenchymatous degeneration and the striated muscle reveals Zenker's degeneration.

The *complications* consist of the following: (1) intestinal hemorrhage, perforation, and peritonitis (Keen), (2) cholecystitis which often becomes chronic and serves as a focus of infection rendering the victim a carrier (Mallory), (3) osteomyelitis affecting especially the flat bones such as the sternum, ribs, and vertebræ with the infection becoming manifested up to twenty years or more after the original attack of the disease, (4) pyelonephritis, (5) bronchopneumonia (Neva), (6) arthritis, and (7) vascular thrombosis. The *clinical manifestations* are quite variable depending upon the mildness or severeness of the process (Beeson). The incubation period is from ten to twelve days and the onset is gradual. The symptoms and signs may consist of the following: malaise, headache, remittent fever, nonproductive cough, anorexia, nausea, vomiting, constipation (early), diarrhea (later), abdominal distention, epistaxis, sweats, chills, dulled sensorium, delirium (typhoid state), palpable spleen (second week), rose spot rash (second to third week), rales in the lungs, slow pulse, anemia, leukopenia, and occasionally albuminuria. Some of these manifestations are explainable on local involvement of the various organs and tissues while others are explainable on the basis of a generalized toxemia. The *diagnosis* is made from (1) the clinical manifestations, (2) the isolation of the causative organisms, from the blood, feces, etc., as outlined under *"cause"* above, and (3) specific agglutination reactions of the blood after the second week. *Treatment* consists of the administration of chloromycetin which apparently is specific (Turner). Other than this, the care of the patient is symptomatic. The *prognosis*, unlike formerly, is good for if the patients are treated early and adequately, virtually all of them should recover.

Regional Enteritis.—Regional enteritis is an acute to chronic granulomatous inflammation of primarily the ileum and jejunum. It is also known as segmental enteritis, cicatrizing enteritis, regional ileitis, terminal ileitis, and Crohn's disease. A similar condition in the large intestine is called *regional colitis*. While the exact *incidence* is difficult to determine, it may be stated with assurance that the condition represents one of the most common diseases of the small intestine. It seems to predominate in the temperate and northern climates and is rather rare in Southern United States, Central America, and Coastal South America (Bockus). It occurs in all races and, while it may occur at any age, it is most common in the third and fourth decades of life. It is slightly more frequent in males than in females. The *cause* remains undetermined. At one time or another the following, however, have been considered to be of etiologic significance: viruses, animal parasites, bacteria, constitutional predisposition, external violence, nutritional deficiency, endocrine disturbance, allergy, and mesenteric lymphadenitis (Bockus).

The *pathologic* changes have been admirably described by Rappaport and Warren. As already stated, the disorder affects primarily the ileum and jejunum although it may also affect the cecum and colon. In the small intestine it is most common in the terminal portion of the ileum (Fig. 324). The length of the segment affected varies anywhere from 5 to 80 cm. or more. In general, the disease may be divided into two stages—acute and chronic. The *acute stage* is usually seen by the surgeon but, because surgical excision is contraindicated, it is rarely encountered by the pathologist. Characteristically the affected segment is sharply demarcated from the rest of the bowel. The serosa is intensely congested and of a reddish-purple hue. It is dull and frequently covered by a fibrinopurulent exudate. The wall is thickened, edematous, and pliable. The mucosa, especially opposite the mesenteric attachment, discloses irregular ulcers that measure as much

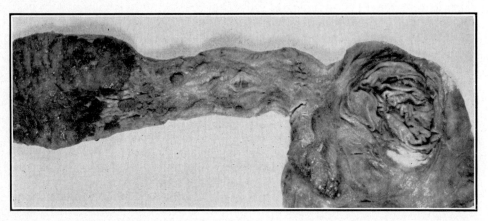

FIG. 324.—Regional enteritis illustrating segmental involvement of the terminal portion of the ileum with sharp demarcation from normal bowel proximally, contraction and fibrosis of the affected segment, ulceration of the mucosa, and polypoid hypertrophy of the remaining islands of mucosa. The lesion also extends into the ascending colon.

as 1 cm. in diameter. *Histologically* the outstanding change consists of edema that is most prominent in the submucosa and the serosa. The ulcers are nonspecific, consisting of a disruption of the mucosa with a diffuse mononuclear and neutrophilic infiltration of the floor and base (Fig. 325*A*). In the rest of the wall the exudative cells are mostly of a mononuclear variety. In the *chronic stage* the serosa remains dull and hyperemic. It is covered with a fibrinous or fibrinopurulent exudate or discloses numerous fibrous adhesions matting the segments of the bowel to each other and to adjacent structures. Frequently also the serosa discloses numerous pinpoint grayish-white nodules that histologically are composed of aggregations of lymphocytes. The transition between the affected and normal bowel is abrupt. The wall of the affected segment is greatly thickened, fibrotic, and unyielding. The lumen is reduced in caliber. The mucosa discloses irregular, coalescing, map-like ulcerations with clean floors and bases extending as far as or beyond the serosa. Between the ulcerations, the mucosa undergoes polypoid enlargement. The ileocecal valve is usually hypertrophied. The lesions in the large bowel are generally less severe than those in the small intestine and consist essentially of mural thickening and ulceration without stenosis. The mesentery is generally thickened, edematous, and rather rigid. The lymph nodes are enlarged in approximately two-thirds of the cases. *Histologically* the affected mucosa discloses (1) a reduction of goblet cells and an increase of Paneth cells, (2) complete ulceration in focal areas, and (3) hyperplasia of the islands of mucosa between the ulcers. Early ulcers disclose the defects to be filled with neutrophils and nuclear fragments. Later these are replaced by granulation tissue and ultimately by fibrous tissue. The latter, as healing becomes complete, is eventually covered with a single layer of atrophic columnar epithelium.

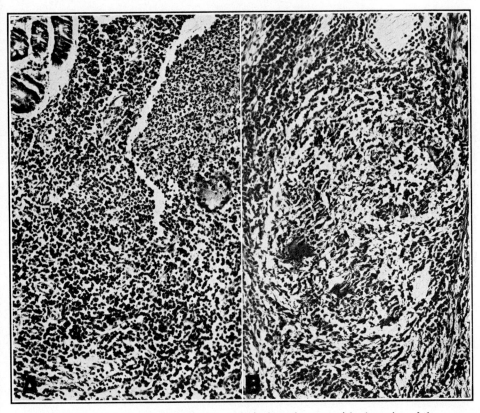

Fig. 325.—Regional enteritis showing *A*, a relatively early stage with ulceration of the mucosa and dense leukocytic infiltration and *B*, granulomas composed of epithelioid cells and occasional giant cells. × 100.

Throughout the rest of the wall there is marked edema with dilatation of the lymphatic channels and a nonspecific inflammatory or granulomatous reaction. The nonspecific inflammation consists of a diffuse infiltration of primary monocytes and lymphocytes, with the lymphocytic cells often aggregated in small circumscribed foci. The granulomatous reaction consists essentially of a focal mononuclear or epithelioid cell proliferation with scattered peripheral giant cells (Fig. 325*B*). In some instances the lesion thus resembles tuberculosis, while in others it mimics that of Boeck's sarcoid. The mesenteric lymph nodes disclose lymph stasis, chronic inflammation, and granulomas similar to those seen in the bowel.

The *complications* consist of intestinal obstruction and perforation of the bowel. The latter leads to (1) abscess formations, (2) fistulas and sinuses that affect other loops of the large and small bowel, the urinary bladder, and (when preceded by laparotomy) the abdominal wall and anus, and (3) peritonitis as a result of direct perforation or perforation by way of an abscess, sinus, or fistula (Gow). *Clinically* the symptoms and signs are quite variable but generally consist of combinations of the following: abdominal pain, loss of weight, diarrhea, vomiting, nausea, fever, blood in the stool, anorexia, constipation, abdominal tenderness, palpable abdominal mass, cutaneous (abdominal wall or anal) fistulas, visible peristalsis, anemia, and leukocytosis (Rappaport). *Roentgenographically* the lesion may be demonstrated as a linear, string-like stenosis of varying lengths in over 90 per cent of cases. The *diagnosis* is made from a consideration of the clinical manifestations and the roentgenographic appearance. *Treatment* is primarily surgical, especially in the presence of complications, but symptomatic medical therapy is also indicated in selective cases (Garlock and Bockus). The *prognosis* is guarded for exacerbations and remissions occur over periods of many years.

Tuberculosis. — Tuberculosis of the intestines, as tuberculosis of the stomach, is generally secondary to tuberculosis of the lungs (Kornblum). On rare occasions, however, it may be primary, in which case it is of the bovine type (Schaffner). The condition may *occur* at all ages but, since it is generally seen in cases of advanced pulmonary tuberculosis, it is most frequent in young adults. *Pathologically* any part of the small or large bowel may be affected but the most common site is the ileocecal region (Brown). The organisms are capable of penetrating an intact mucosa and usually do so in the area overlying Peyer's patches or lymphoid follicles. From here they spread to the serosa and mesenteric lymph nodes. The initial lesion consists of tubercles that are readily identifiable both in the mucosa and the serosa. With coalescence of the mucosal and submucosal tubercles, ulcerations follow. Subsequently the lesions remain as penetrating undermined ulcers or, with fibrosis supervening, as a thick, indurated, conglomerate, hyperplastic mass (Fig. 326). The latter is grossly readily mistaken for carcinoma. Regardless of the type of lesion, healing ultimately occurs by resolution and fibrosis. The draining mesenteric lymph nodes are virtually always affected. The *complications* consist of (1) intestinal obstruction as a result of stenosis, kinks, or adhesions, (2) perforation, (3) acute nonspecific or tuberculous peritonitis, and (4) focal abscesses (Brown). The *clinical manifestations* are extremely varied and consist of anorexia, nausea and vomiting, bouts of diarrhea alternating with constipation, and abdominal pain (Schaffner). *Roentgenographically* there are intestinal hypermotility, failure of the cecum or ascending colon to retain barium, spastic filling defects in the ascending colon, segmentation of coils of small intestine, and abnormal retention of barium in ileal loops. The *diagnosis* is made from the clinical manifestations and the roentgenographic studies. *Treatment* is that of tuberculosis in general with particular emphasis on antibiotic and chemotherapeutic agents (Kallqvist). The *prognosis* is that of the disease in the lungs.

Fungous and Yeast-like Enteritis and Colitis. — Virtually any fungous or yeast-like infection that attacks other portions of the body may also be found in the small and large intestines. There are only two infections, however, that are important — actinomycosis and histoplasmosis. *Actinomycosis* is generally localized to the ileocecal region and involves the

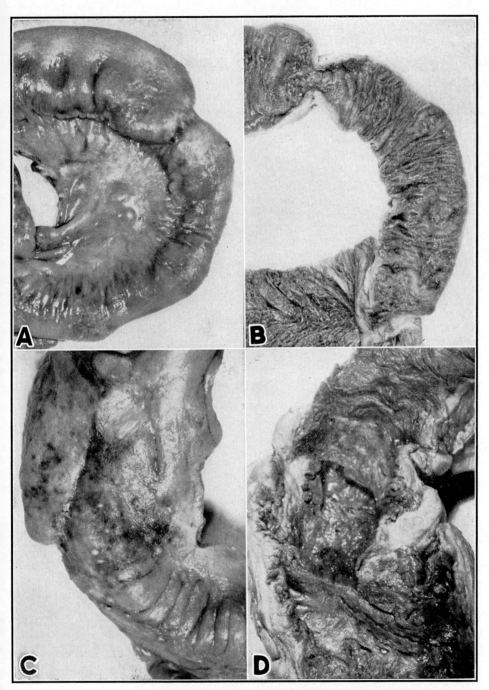

Fig. 326.—Intestinal tuberculosis illustrating *A* and *B*, external and longitudinal section of a constricting lesion of the lower portion of the ileum, *C*, serosal tubercles of the ileum, and *D*, a hypertrophic lesion with ulceration at the junction of the cecum and ascending colon. Note the enlarged mesenteric lymph nodes in specimen *A*.

terminal ileum, cecum, and appendix. Pathologically it produces extensive ulceration, fibrosis, and fistulous tracts and may affect all the adjacent tissues including the abdominal wall. The histologic changes are similar to those found elsewhere (p. 515). Clinically the disorder may be mistaken for appendicitis or carcinoma. Treatment of choice is surgical excision. The prognosis is poor. Since *histoplasmosis* is a disease of the reticulo-endothelial system it is the lymphoid patches and follicles of the intestines that are primarily involved. The lesions, therefore, are most common in the ileo-cecal area. Grossly they consist of irregular ulcers that penetrate the wall for varying depths and that are attended by varying degrees of fibrosis. The histologic reaction is similar to that in other organs (p. 513). As a rule, the intestinal involvement is only part of a systemic infection.

Parasitic Infections.—Although there are many parasites that gain entrance into the small intestine, the more important ones, from a medical standpoint, are *Giardia lamblia, Chilomastix mesmeli, Ascaris lumbricoides, Necator americanus, Ancylostoma duodenale, Strongyloides stercoralis, Hymenolepis nana, Taenia saginata, Taenia solium,* and *Diphyllobothrium*

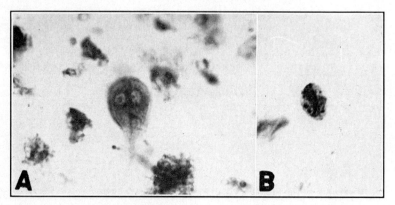

Fig. 327.—*Giardia lamblia* showing *A*, a ventral view of a trophozoite, and *B*, a cyst with four nuclei. × 1380.

latum (Sawitz and Craig and Faust). The parasites and the lesions which they produce may be considered in the order listed.

Giardia lamblia is a protozoan flagellate that exists in a trophozoite and a cystic stage. The trophozoite is pear-shaped, with the anterior end being rounded, and measures about 14 × 7 microns (Fig. 327). Its dorsal portion is convex; its ventral portion contains an ovoid cavity that serves as a sucking disc, and its flagella are eight in number, being divided into anterior, middle, ventral, and caudal pairs. The cysts are ovoid bodies measuring 10.5 × 7.4 microns and contain from two to four nuclei. Trophozoites exist in the small intestine (especially the duodenum) where they may produce irritation, abdominal discomfort, and mild diarrhea. The organisms are discharged in formed stool as cysts and in this stage are transmitted to another host as contaminants of food and water. The diagnosis is made by identifying trophozoites in liquid stool or duodenal drainage and cysts in formed stool.

Chilomastix mesneli is a protozoan flagellate that exists in both a trophozoite and a cystic stage. The trophozoite is ovoid or pear-shaped and measures about 13 × 7 microns. The body possesses a spiral groove, a cytostome (mouth), an anterior nucleus, three anterior flagella, and one posterior flagellum (Fig. 328). The cyst is lemon-shaped and measures about 8.5 × 5 microns. It consists of a distinct wall, a single anterior nucleus, and a structure that represents the remains of a cytostome. The organisms inhabit both the small and large intestines but are most numerous in the cecum. They may produce diarrhea, although this pathogenic property has never been absolutely proved. Trophozoites are discharged in liquid stool but only cysts are present in formed stool. The cysts serve as a source of food contamination and reinfection. The diagnosis is made by microscopic identification of the organism in the stool.

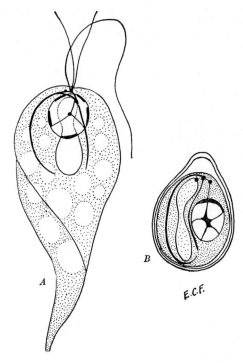

FIG. 328.—*Chilomastix mesneli* illustrating *A*, a trophozoite and *B*, a cyst.
(Craig and Faust, *Clinical Parasitology*, Lea & Febiger.)

Ascaris lumbricoides is a common round worm of worldwide distribution. The worms are cylindrical with the females measuring from 20 to 35 cm. in length and the males from 15 to 31 cm. (Fig. 329). The anterior end is blunt and is provided with three lips. The posterior end is tapering and, in males, is curved ventrally. Ova are deposited by the female at the rate of approximately 200,000 a day and are passed out with the feces. Fertilized ova are ovoid and measure about 60 × 42 microns. They are surrounded by a thick transparent shell covered with a coarse, brown, albuminoid outer layer. Their centers are composed of coarse granules. The unfertilized ova are more elongated and do not disclose the outer coating. Under favorable atmospheric conditions, embryos develop within the ova in from nine to thirteen days. These are then swallowed with food or water and larvæ, measuring about 0.25 mm. in length, are liberated from the shells by the action of intestinal juices. The larvæ penetrate the intestinal mucosa and are carried through the mesenteric lymphatics and venules and the heart to the lungs. They then enter the alveoli and bronchi, are swallowed with the sputum, and develop into adult worms in the small intestine. In the lungs the larvæ produce hemorrhage and, in sensitive individuals, eosinophilic infiltrations. The latter account for some of the cases of Loeffler's syndrome (p. 483). In the intestine they may entangle themselves in such a manner as to produce obstruction of the bowel. Also, absorption of toxic products of live or dead worms may result in generalized

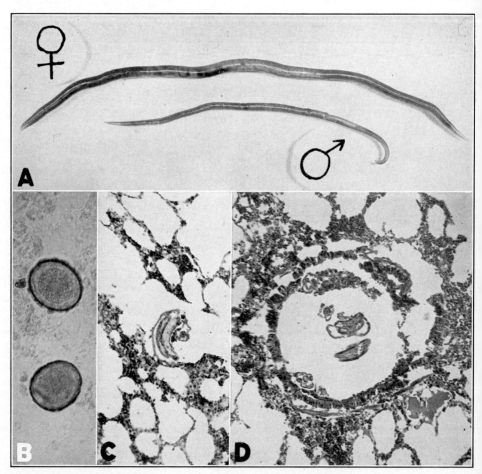

FIG. 329.—*Ascaris lumbricoides* showing *A*, an adult female and male worm, *B*, fertilized ova. × 200, *C*, migrating larvæ in the pulmonary parenchyma. × 100, and *D*, migrating larvæ in a bronchiole. × 100.

toxemia and the utilization of food by the worm may deprive the patient of necessary nutrition. The diagnosis is usually made by identifying ova in the stool or, after a vermifuge, the finding of the worms themselves.

Necator americanus is a *hookworm* that is found in Southern United States, Caribbean Islands, Central America, North and South America, Central and Southern Africa, South Asia, Melanesia, and Polynesia. The adult worm is cylindrical with the female measuring about 10 × 0.4 mm. and the male about 8 × 0.3 mm. (Fig. 330). Anteriorly it possesses a mouth with

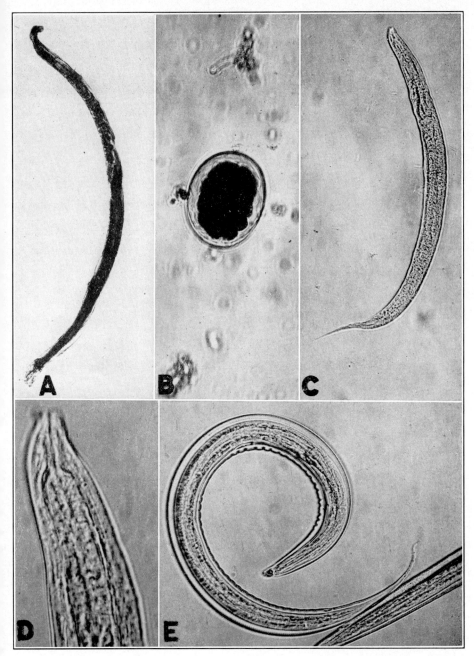

Fig. 330.—*Necator americanus* illustrating *A*, an adult male worm, *B*, an ovum. × 400, *C*,
rhabditiform larva, *D*, anterior end of rhabditiform larva, and *E*, filariform larva.

a ventral and a dorsal pair of semilunar plates. Posteriorly the female is
cone-shaped while the male possesses a bursa with a pair of copulatory
bristles each tipped with a barb. The ova are oval and measure about
70 × 38 microns. They disclose a thin hyaline shell and, by the time they
are evacuated from the body, they are in the two to eight segmentation
stage or, in constipated stool, in the tadpole stage. The ova hatch in moist,

warm soil in from one to two days releasing rhabditiform larvæ that measure about 250 × 17 microns. These larvæ can be distinguished from those of *Strongyloides stercoralis* by the presence of a long narrow buccal chamber. At about eight days the mouth closes and the larvæ become transformed into filariform larvæ. The filariform larvæ penetrate the skin of man producing what is referred to as "ground itch" and then migrate by way of the blood to the lungs whence they are swallowed with the sputum. In the small intestine they develop into adult worms and attach themselves to the mucosa. In the lungs they cause hemorrhages and pneumonitis. In the small bowel they (1) produce irritation and diarrhea and (2) by sucking blood, a microcytic hypochromic anemia and ultimately hypoproteinemia. The diagnosis is made by identifying the ova and/or rhabditiform larvæ in the stool.

Ancylostoma duodenale or the *"Old World"* hookworm is found in the Far East, Northern Africa, and Southern Europe. Adult male worms measure about 9 × 0.45 mm. while adult female worms measure approximately 12 × 0.1 mm. (Fig. 331). They differ from those of *Necator americanus* in

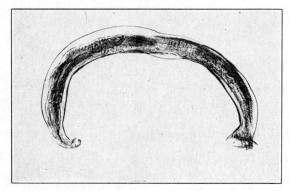

Fig. 331.—*Ancylostoma duodenale* showing an adult male worm.

that the mouth possesses two pairs of teeth rather than chitinous plates and the ova measure about 60 × 40 microns. Otherwise the life cycle, clinical manifestations, etc., are similar to those of *Necator americanus*.

Strongyloides stercoralis is a round worm that is particularly prevalent in warm climates but that also occurs in temperate climates and is worldwide in distribution. The basic life cycle is in the soil. The male worm is fusiform, measuring approximately 0.7 mm. in length and possessing a pointed, ventrally curved tail. The female is approximately 1 mm. long and has a bicornuate uterus that is filled with ova. The discharged ova contain partially developed embryos that hatch in the soil in a few hours. The resulting rhabditiform larvæ are similar to those of *Necator americanus* except that the buccal cavity is short and narrow (Fig. 332). The larvæ then moult and develop into adult worms or, when conditions are unfavorable, they develop into filariform larvæ. These are twice as long as rhabditiform larvæ, measuring approximately 500 microns in length and possessing a blunt, posterior extremity. They are infective for man, penetrating the skin and being carried by the blood to the lungs where they develop into adolescent worms. Here they gain entrance into the bronchioles and bronchi and are swallowed with the sputum. The female, having been fertilized

during its sojourn in the lungs, burrows into the mucosa of the small intestine where it matures and begins to deposit ova. The ova hatch rhabditiform larvæ which are passed in the stool or develop into filariform larvæ.
The latter, in turn, are also excreted in the stool or may penetrate the mucosa of the colon or the skin of the anus and thus reinfect the host. Pathologically, inflammation at the point of cutaneous entrance is present in the
form of a petechial rash attended by pruritis. During the stage of migration
eosinophilia develops. The sojourn in the lungs is attended by focal hemorrhages and, in some instances, by pneumonic infiltrations. In the intestines
there is sufficient irritation to cause mucous diarrhea and sometimes mucosal
ulceration. The diagnosis is made by finding larvæ in the stool or in
duodenal drainage.

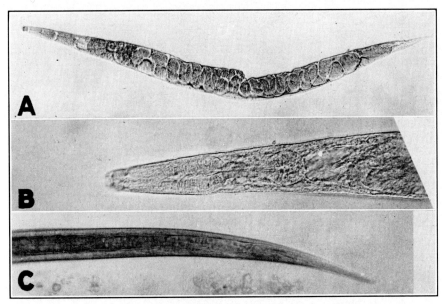

FIG. 332.—*Strongyloides stercoralis* illustrating *A*, a rhabditiform larva. × 100, *B*, the head
of a rhabditiform larva. × 400, and *C*, blunt tail of a filariform larva. × 60.

Hymenolepis nana or the *dwarf tapeworm* is worldwide in distribution,
being prevalent in warmer climates. The entire worm measures about 32
mm. in length (Fig. 333). The scolex is rhomboid in shape, has four suckers,
and possesses a terminal rostellum with twenty to thirty hooklets. The
proglottids increase in maturity and size from the neck to the posterior
end. The ova are discharged by disintegration of terminal proglottids.
They are rounded, measure about 40 microns in diameter, and disclose from
without in a thin shell, a gelatinous membrane, and a hexacanth larva with
three pairs of hooklets. The ova are passed in the feces and, without the
medium of an intermediate host, are infective for man. When swallowed
with infected food they hatch in the small intestine, liberating hexacanth
larvæ which, in turn, develop into cysticercoid larvæ. These mature into
adult worms and the latter become attached to the intestinal mucosa. The
usual clinical manifestations are abdominal cramps and diarrhea although
in children there may also be irritability and convulsions. The diagnosis is
based on the identification of ova in feces.

Tænia saginata or the *beef tapeworm* is worldwide in distribution and is the commonest tapeworm in the United States. It is usually less than 10 meters in length (but may be longer) and possesses about 1000 to 2000 proglottids (Figs. 334 and 335). The head measures approximately 1.5 mm. in diameter, has a concave apical portion, and is provided with four suckers. Beyond the head the proglottids pass progressively through immature, mature, and gravid stages. The gravid proglottids possess a uterus with from fifteen to twenty lateral ramifications on each side. The ova are

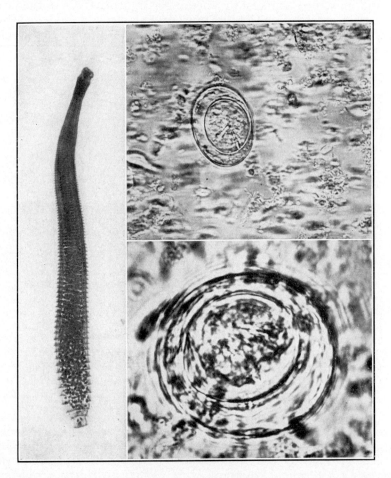

FIG. 333.—*Hymenolepis nana* showing, to the left, the entire worm and, to the right, two ova each with a concentrically fibrillated membrane and central hooklets. × 400 and 900.

rounded, measure about 38 microns in diameter, are buff to brown, and consist externally of a thick rim with radial striations and internally of a hexacanth embryo with three pairs of hooklets. The adult worm lives in the small intestine of man. Gravid proglottids are passed in the feces but occasionally they disintegrate in the colon and ova are liberated. In either case, the ova are ingested by cattle and the hexacanth embryos are liberated in the intestine. They then penetrate the mucosa and are carried by the bloodstream to the muscles. In the muscles they develop into cysticerci which are transmitted to man in insufficiently cooked beef. They are liberated in the small intestine of man and grow into adult worms. Clinically *Tænia saginata* may produce diarrhea and, as a result of the worms feeding on intestinal contents, loss of weight. The diagnosis of tæniasis is made from identification of ova and *Tænia saginata* is differentiated from *Tænia solium* by the fact that it contains more than thirteen lateral uterine segments.

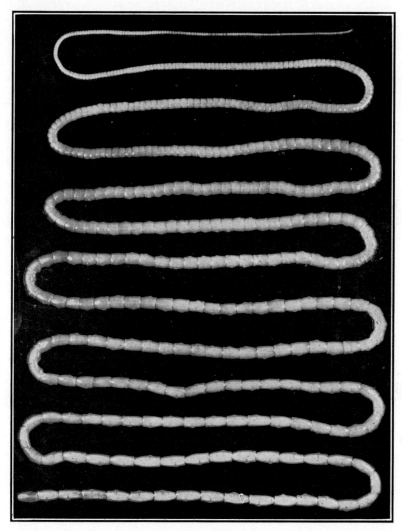

Fig. 334.—*Tænia saginata* illustrating the head, neck, and many remaining segments.

Tænia solium or the *pork tapeworm* is worldwide in distribution but is much less frequent in the United States than is *Tænia saginata*. The usual length is from 2 to 7 meters. The scolex is approximately 1 mm. in diameter and possesses four suckers and an apical rostellum with a double row of hooklets (Fig. 336). The proglottids pass consecutievly through immature, mature, and gravid stages. The gravid proglottid has a uterus with from seven to thirteen lateral branches. The ova are indistinguishable from those of *Tænia saginata*. Gravid proglottids and occasionally ova are passed in the feces and the ova are ultimately ingested by pigs. In the intestine of the pig, hexacanth embryos are freed and, after penetrating the mucosa, are carried to the muscles by the bloodstream. Here they develop into cysticerci in which stage they are infective for man if the pork is improperly cooked. Once such pork is ingested by man the cysticerci are liberated, become attached to the intestinal mucosa, and grow into adult worms. The ova of *Tænia solium* are also infective for man and, accordingly, cysticerci may be found in most of the tissues of the body including muscle, eye, and brain. The clinical manifestations, due to adult worms, consist of occasional diarrhea and loss of weight. Cysticercosis is attended by local inflammatory reactions and the symptoms, of course, vary with the tissues affected. Involvement of the brain may be accompanied by convulsions. The diagnosis

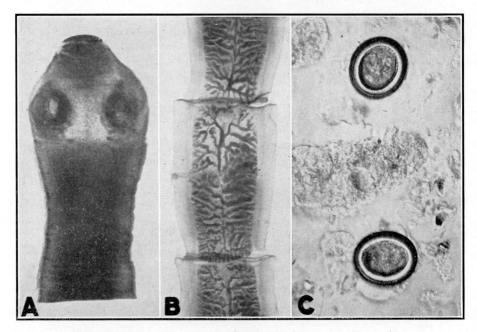

Fig. 335.—*Tænia saginata* showing *A*, a scolex. × 40, *B*, gravid proglottids. × 7, and *C*, ova. × 400.

of tæniasis is made by identifying the ova and *Tænia solium* infection is differentiated from *Tænia saginata* infection by the fewer number of uterine segments in the former.

Diphyllobothrium latum or the *broad fish tapeworm* is found in countries with fresh water lakes. The adult worm is ivory colored and measures from 3 to 10 meters or more in length. The scolex measures about 1×2.5 mm. and possesses a ventral and a dorsal sucker. The proximal proglottids are immature while the more distal ones are mature and gravid. The uterus of the gravid proglottid is coiled and rosette-like in appearance. The ova are ovoid and operculated and measure about 70×45 microns (Fig. 336C). The adult worm lives in the small intestine of man and other fish-eating animals. The eggs are discharged in the feces and upon reaching fresh water release ciliated hexacanth embryos. The embryos are ingested by crustaceans where they develop into procercoid larvæ. Crustaceans harboring the larvæ are then eaten by carnivorous fish (in North America, pike and pickerel) and, in their muscle, the larvæ develop into sparganum larvæ. These (as well as procercoid larvæ) are infective for man when the fish (or crustaceans) are insufficiently cooked. After ingestion, larvæ are liberated in the intestines of man where they grow into adult worms. Clinically infection with *Diphyllobothrium latum* is attended by abdominal discomfort, diarrhea, and macrocytic hyperchromic anemia. The diagnosis is made from identification of ova in the stool or, after treatment, the passage of proglottids and even the scolex.

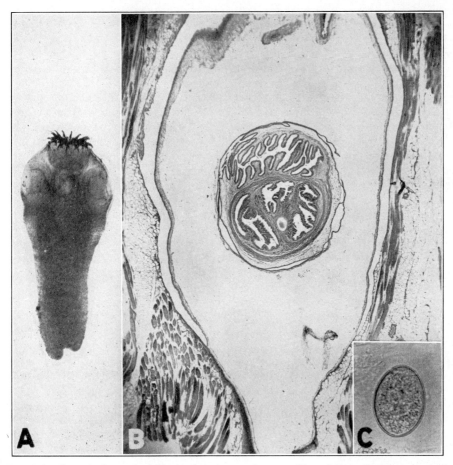

Fig. 336.—Intestinal parasites illustrating *A*, a scolex.   × 40, and *B*, a cysticercus.   × 5 of *Tænia solium*, and *C*, an ovum of *Diphyllobothrium latum* with the operculum distinctly visible. × 300.

PHYSICAL DISTURBANCES

Orientation.—Some of the more important conditions of the small intestine in this category are fistulas, foreign bodies (p. 674), intestinal pneumatosis, perforation, irradiation changes (p. 233), mesenteric thrombosis, intussusception, volvulus, and obstruction.

Fistulas.—Fistulas of the small intestine may connect any portion of the duodenum, jejunum, or ileum with (1) other portions of the small bowel (enteroenteric, jejuno-ileal, etc.), (2) the stomach (gastrojejunal, etc.), (3) the colon (enterocolic, jejunocolic, etc.), (4) the gallbladder and/or the bile ducts (cholecystoduodenal, choledochoduodenal, etc.), (5) the skin (enterocutaneous, jejunocutaneous, etc.), (6) the urinary bladder (entero-vesical, ileovesical, etc.), and (7) other hollow organs such as the uterus, fallopian tubes, etc. Of these, the most common spontaneous fistulas (that is, not man-made) are those connecting some portion of the extrahepatic biliary system with the duodenum (Brown, Tate, and Kredel). In general, the *causes* of fistulas of the small intestine are (1) congenital anomalies — patency of the omphalomesenteric duct, (2) inflammations — peptic ulcer, cholecystitis, etc., (3) physical disturbances — erosions of gallstones or other foreign bodies, operative, penetrating or blunt trauma, etc., and (4) tumors —malignant neoplasms of either the small intestine or of other organs with which it forms the fistula.

Intestinal Pneumatosis. — This condition (also known as pneumatosis cystoides intestinorum hominis, abdominal gas cysts, intestinal emphysema, gas cysts of the intestine, etc.) consists of the presence of multiple gas-filled sessile pedunculated cysts affecting the gastrointestinal tract (Koss, Thoma, and Sherwin). While only 250 (approximately) cases had been recorded by 1952, the condition is probably more common than these reports tend to indicate. The disorder *occurs* at all ages but is most common in the fourth and fifth decades and affects males four times as frequently as females. The most common *cause* is some defect (such as an ulcer, tumor, etc.) in the gastrointestinal mucosa which allows air to be forced into the tissues and dissect along the tissue planes. In some cases the cysts may be formed by gas-producing bacteria. *Pathologically* the sites of involvement in decreasing order of frequency are ileum, cecum, ascending colon, jejunum, duodenum, and retroperitoneal tissues. Grossly the cysts are multiple, occur singly or in clusters, possess thin walls, are filled with gas, and measure as much as 5 cm. in diameter. The gas is composed of nitrogen 70 to 90 per cent, oxygen 3 to 20 per cent, and carbon dioxide 0 to 15 per cent. Histologically the centers consist of empty spaces while the walls are composed of connective tissue or are endothelial-lined. In some cases there is a peripheral inflammatory reaction of giant cells, monocytes, and lympho-cytes. The chief *complication* is intestinal obstruction. The *clinical manifestations*, unless obstruction occurs, are generally those of the under-lying disease with pneumatosis being an accidental finding. The cysts are readily visualized roentgenographically. *Treatment* of the cysts as such, in cases discovered at operation, has consisted of partial resection of the bowel for, in some instances, the cysts tend to persist and progress if left untouched. The *prognosis*, as far as the cysts are concerned, is good.

Perforation. — Perforation of the small intestine may occur in a pre-viously diseased or a previously normal bowel. Some of the conditions that cause or predispose to perforation are (1) congenital anomalies — obstruc-tion, (2) degenerations — stasis of blood (in shock) followed by erosion, (3) inflammations — duodenal ulcer, simple ulcer of other portions, acute ulcerative enteritis, typhoid and paratyphoid fever, regional enteritis, and tuberculosis, (4) physical disturbances — foreign bodies, mesenteric throm-bosis, volvulus, other intestinal obstructions, and trauma, and (5) tumors — ulcerating carcinoma. Of these, *trauma* is one of the more important agents. It may be *penetrating*, in which case the object (bullet, knife, etc.) perforates the bowel directly or it may be *nonpenetrating*, in which cases there is no interruption of continuity of the abdominal wall. In the latter the trauma consists of any blunt blow such as that sustained in an auto accident, fight, football game, etc. (Bosworth and Cohn). In penetrating trauma any portion or portions of the bowel may be involved. In nonpenetrating trauma the sites of perforation in decreasing order of frequency are jejunum, ileum, and duodenum. They may be single or multiple and intraperitoneal or retroperitoneal. The chief *complications* are hemorrhage, shock, abscess, and peritonitis. The *clinical manifestations* differ accordingly. The *diagnosis* can generally be made readily by demonstrating free air in the

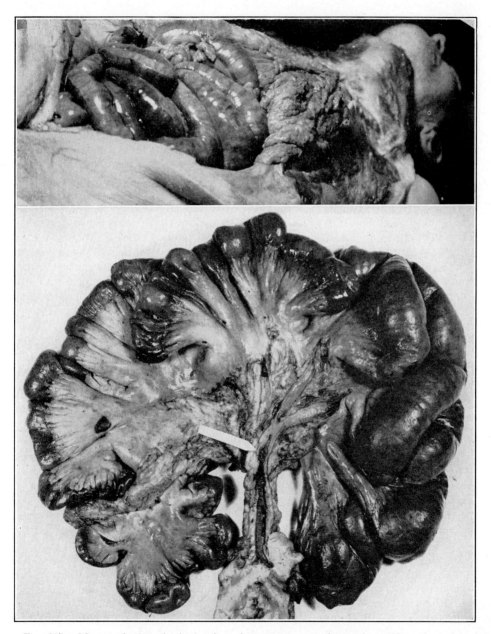

FIG. 337.—Mesenteric thrombosis showing, above, gangrenous loops of small intestine covered with a fibrinopurulent exudate and, below, thrombosis of the superior mesenteric artery and gangrenous small intestine.

peritoneal cavity. *Treatment* is immediate surgical intervention. The *prognosis* is guarded for mortalities up to 50 per cent have been recorded.

Mesenteric Thrombosis.—Mesenteric thrombosis actually means thrombosis of the mesenteric arteries and/or veins. It *occurs* at all ages but is most common in the fifth and sixth decades of life and it affects males twice as frequently as females. The causes consist of (1) pressure on the vessels from the outside such as seen in hernia, volvulus, trauma, etc., (2) changes within the walls of the vessels consisting essentially of arteriosclerosis and infection of both the arteries and the veins, and (3) disturbances in the lumens of the vessels comprising embolism on the arterial side (from thrombi in the heart, aorta, or pulmonary veins) and primary thrombosis on the venous side (occurring as a result of slowing of the circulation as in heart disease and portal hypertension, change in the clotting mechanism, etc.) (McCollum, North, and McClune). The *pathologic changes* in the bowel depend upon the size of vessel or vessels involved, the number of vessels affected, the acuteness of the process, and the degree of occlusion. On the arterial side, the main or larger branches of the superior mesenteric artery are usually affected while on the venous side, the occlusions are generally multiple and in the more terminal ramifications (Fig. 337). In cases of *sudden occlusion* the affected segment of bowel undergoes successively contraction, relaxation, and infarction. Infarction is indicated by segmental swelling, red to black discoloration, increased friability, dulling of the serosa, and escape of blood into the lumen. The demarcation from the normal bowel is generally sharp. The mesentery is thick, indurated, and doughy. The peritoneal cavity discloses moderate amounts of transparent, sticky, blood-tinged fluid. In cases of *gradual* and *incomplete* occlusion there are varying degrees of congestion, edema, exudation, ecchymosis, and ulceration (Rives). The chief *complications* of mesenteric thrombosis are shock, intestinal obstruction, and peritonitis. The *clinical manifestations* vary with the suddenness and completeness of the occlusion (Rives). They may consist of severe abdominal pain, nausea, vomiting, shock, abdominal distention, first active and then absent peristalsis, initially constipation or diarrhea, later constipation, and, in acute cases, leukocytosis. The *diagnosis* is made from the clinical manifestations although roentgen findings of diffuse dilatation of the small bowel and the presence of free fluid in the peritoneal cavity are also suggestive. *Treatment* consists of surgical resection of the affected portion of the bowel. The *prognosis* is poor for the mortality is usually greater than 80 per cent.

Intussusception.—Intussusception of the small intestine *occurs* more commonly in infants and children than it does in adults. In the former group it is most frequent in the first year of life (Ravitch). The *cause* in infants and children is frequently difficult to determine. Some of the theories advanced to explain the origin are hypertrophied Peyer's patches, ileocecal neuromuscular dysfunction, excessive catharsis, transition from a liquid to a solid diet, etc. (Gross). Only rarely are the mechanical factors present that are found to be the cause of intussusception in adults. These consist generally of a polypoid tumor (any type) and rarely of Meckel's diverticulum (Brown). *Pathologically* the most common area affected is the ileocecal region with the small bowel invaginating through the ileocecal valve into the colon (ileocolic). Invaginations of one portion of the small bowel into another are next in frequency (Fig. 338). Usually the invagination is in a forward direction but rarely it may be retrograde (Thorek). The leading point or invaginating segment is called the intussusceptum, while the receiving segment is referred to as the intussuscipiens. The intussusceptum may be of varying lengths extending even to the anus. The chief *complications* are intestinal obstruction and infarction. Accordingly, the *clinical manifestations* consist of severe colicky abdominal pain, cough, nausea, vomiting, blood in the stool, at first diarrhea then constipation, abdominal distention, fever, increased peristalsis early and absence of peristalsis later, a palpable abdominal mass, and leukocytosis. The *diag-*

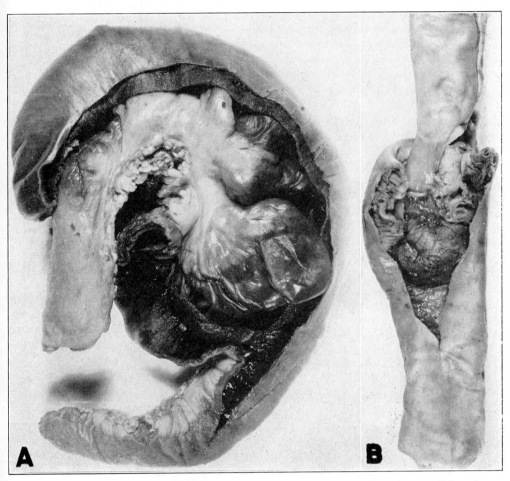

Fig. 338.—Intussusception illustrating *A*, an invagination of one portion of the small intestine into another without a tumor at the leading point and *B*, a similar invagination with a metastatic pedunculated rhabdomyosarcoma at the tip of the intussusceptum.

nosis is generally made from the clinical manifestations alone. *Treatment* is surgical intervention with release of the invagination and correction of the cause or resection of the affected segment in cases of gangrene. The *prognosis*, as far as the intussusception is concerned, is fair to good for recent mortality rates are recorded as low as 3 per cent.

Volvulus.—Volvulus (L. = to turn about) of the small intestine *means* simply a twisting of the bowel with resulting obstruction. The recorded *incidence* is about 10 per cent of all cases of obstruction of the small intestine (Moretz). The condition occurs at all ages but predominates slightly in infants. The *mechanism* of its formation is fixation of one part of the gut in the presence of normal or abnormally great freedom of motion of another portion (McKechnie). Some of the *predisposing factors* are Meckel's diverticulum, long mesentery (p. 692), congenital bands, and postoperative adhesions. Gaseous distention is an aggravating factor. *Pathologically* any part of the small gut may be affected but the most common site is the ileum (Fig. 339*A*). Aside from obstruction of the lumen of the intestine, the chief *complication* is gangrene of the wall from vascular occlusion. The *clinical manifestations* are those of obstruction. *Treatment* is detorsion, correction of the cause, and resection of the bowel if necessary. The *prognosis* is guarded for mortality rates as high as 50 per cent have been recorded.

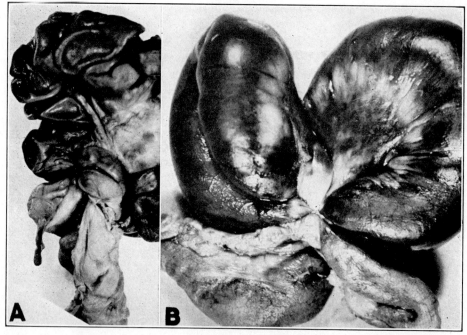

Fig. 339.—Intestinal obstruction showing *A*, a volvulus about the root of the mesentery with infarction of most of the small bowel and *B*, strangulation of loops of small bowel by an adhesive band.

Obstruction. —The *causes* of obstruction of the small intestine may be listed as follows: (1) congenital—adhesions, stenosis, atresia, mesenteric cysts, and Meckel's diverticulum, (2) inflammations—paralytic ileus from peritonitis, stenosis from cicatricial narrowing of the lumen, and adhesions, (3) physical disturbances—incarcerated or strangulated hernia, foreign bodies (such as gallstones, bezoars, etc.), meconium ileus, volvulus, intussusception, mesenteric thrombosis, and parasitic (massing of parasites such as *Ascaris lumbricoides*), and (4) tumors—encroaching upon the lumen as a fungating or stenosing mass or producing volvulus, intussusception, etc. The *pathologic changes* differ according to the cause of the obstruction (Fig. 339). In simple obstruction the lumen at the point of involvement is partially or completely occluded, that distally is collapsed, and that proximally is generally greatly dilated. In addition, the lumen proximal to the point of occlusion contains varying amounts of (often hemorrhagic) fluid.

The intestinal wall in this area may be greatly thinned or thickened, congested, and edematous. It may or may not reveal mucosal erosions and/or ulcerations. In more complex obstructions such as those occurring in connection with mesenteric thrombosis, volvulus, or hernia, the affected loop of bowel may be gangrenous and the vessels leading to these areas are thrombotic. The chief *complications* consist of (1) dehydration and acidosis from vomiting and (2) shock from absorption of toxic products. The *clinical manifestations* are variable depending upon the acuteness or chronicity of the process, the site of obstruction, the degree of occlusion, the presence or absence of gangrene, etc. In general, they consist of combinations of the following: abdominal pain (of varying intensity, nature, etc.), constipation or obstipation, vomiting, dehydration, shock, abdominal distention, abdominal muscular rigidity, abdominal tenderness, palpable abdominal mass, fever, and leukocytosis. The *diagnosis* is made from the history and physical examination. Roentgenographic examination discloses gaseous distention of the small bowel with fluid levels. *Treatment* is surgical relief of the obstruction. The *prognosis* depends upon the causative factor, the age of the patient, the duration of the process, the rapidity of its development, etc. Over-all mortality rates as high as 20 per cent have been recorded in large series of cases.

TUMORS

Orientation. — Tumors of the small intestine are relatively infrequent (Joergenson, Olson, Shallow, and Weinberg). The lesions may be benign or malignant and, of the two, the latter of course are the more serious. Malignant tumors are said to *constitute* 0.098 per cent of all malignant growths in the body. It has also been recorded that from 1.4 to 8.9 per cent of all gastrointestinal carcinomas and that 60 per cent of all intestinal sarcomas are located in the small bowel. While the sex distribution varies somewhat from tumor to tumor, in general, neoplastic involvement of the small bowel is about twice as frequent in males as it is in females. It *occurs* in all races and is most frequent after the age of thirty years. The *cause* is unknown although inflammation has been considered to be of definite etiologic significance.

Pathologically, virtually every tissue that is normally present in the small intestine may give rise to both a benign and a malignant tumor. The lesions may be listed as follows: polyp, carcinoid, carcinoma, fibroma, fibrosarcoma, leiomyoma, leiomyosarcoma, lipoma, liposarcoma, hereditary hemorrhagic telangiectasia, hemangioma, lymphangioma, neurofibroma, neurofibrosarcoma, neuroma, lymphoblastoma, and secondary tumors. In general, carcinoma appears to be more common in the upper portion of the small intestine while other malignant tumors are more common in the lower portion. Benign growths occur with equal frequency in the duodenum and ileum and are more common in these locations than they are in the jejunum.

The *complications* of tumors of the small intestine are obstruction by simple encroachment upon the lumen, intussusception, volvulus, hemorrhage, and perforation with peritonitis. The clinical *symptoms* and *signs* are due to small bowel obstruction, bleeding, perforation, peritonitis, and obstruction of the biliary tract. The more important manifestations, in decreasing order of frequency, are loss of weight, pain, nausea and vomiting, anorexia, jaundice, weakness, constipation, diarrhea, melena, hematemesis, fever, gas or bloating, hiccoughs, and pruritus (Joergenson). The *diagnosis* is made from the clinical manifestations, the demonstration of blood in the stool, and the roentgenographic appearance using barium as contrast medium. The only effective *treatment* is surgical resection. The *prognosis* is generally good in benign tumors but is fair to poor in malignant tumors. In the latter, the operative mortality has been recorded as high as 50 per cent and the five-year survival rate as less than 5 per cent. The *causes* of *death* in cases of malignant tumor are recurrent disease with obstruction and metastasis, postoperative pneumonia, peritonitis, pulmonary embolism, postoperative bleeding, postoperative evisceration, and infarction of the bowel. Aside from the general characteristics, a few separate words may be said about the more common lesions.

Polyps.—As in other portions of the body, a polyp of the small intestine simply connotes a finger-like projection of tissue into the lumen. Generally, however, the proliferated tissue is mucosal epithelium and unless otherwise specified the term polyp is synonymous with adenoma or adenomatous polyp. The lesion may be located in any portion of the small intestine but is most common in the duodenum and ileum and is least frequent in the jejunum (Fig. 340*A* and *B*). The lesion may be single of multiple and sessile or pedunculated (Olson and Roberts). While there is considerable variation in size with measurements ranging from a few millimeters to 6 or 8 cm. in greatest diameter, the majority of lesions measure less than 1 cm. across (Camp). As a rule, the growths are pinkish-gray, moderately firm, and superficially ulcerated. Histologically they are composed of cuboidal or columnar cells in glandular formation covering a thin stalk of well-vascularized connective tissue.

Polyposis and Mucocutaneous Pigmentation.—As the caption indicates, polyps of the small intestine may be associated with melanin pigmentation of the mucocutaneous junctions, especially the lips and mouth (Bartholomew). The condition is also referred to as the *Peutz-Jeghers syndrome*— after Peutz who described the combination of polyp and pigmentation in 1921 and Jeghers who reviewed the literature in 1949. The *incidence* of the disorder is probably greater than the reports (75 cases through 1957) in the literature would tend to indicate. It has been described at all ages, equally between males and females, and in many races. The *cause* of the association is not known but the syndrome is definitely familial. *Pathologically* the polyps have been located mostly in the small bowel, although they have also involved the stomach and the large intestine. They have varied in number from one to many, in shape from sessile to pedunculated, and in size from less than one to 7 cm. or more. *Histologically* they are composed of columnar or cuboidal cells in glandular formation covering thin stalks of connective tissue. The most common *complications* are intussusception and hemorrhage. A malignant transformation is said to have occurred in as high as 20 per cent of cases. The chief *clinical manifestations* are blood in the stool and recurring episodes of abdominal pain (due to intestinal obstruction). The *diagnosis* is made from the history (especially familial occurrence), the oral pigmentation, and the demonstration of intestinal polyps roentgenographically. *Treatment* consists of surgical removal of the intestinal growths. The *prognosis* is good if treatment is instituted before a malignant transformation occurs.

Smooth Muscle Tumors.—Smooth muscle tumors of the small intestine are next in frequency to polyps, there having been about 210 cases recorded by 1951 (Cherry). Most of the lesions are located in the jejunum; a few are found in the duodenum, and only rarely are they found in the ileum

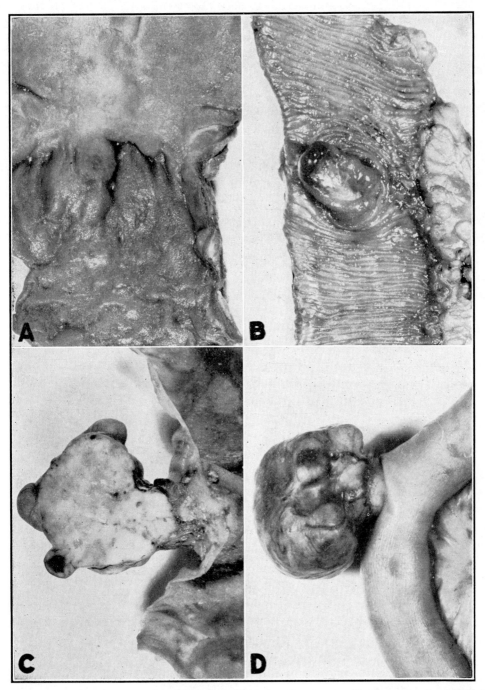

FIG. 340.—Benign tumors of the small intestine illustrating *A*, a sessile adenomatous polyp of the duodenum, *B*, a more pedunculated adenomatous polyp of the jejunum, *C*, a subserosal leiomyoma of the jejunum, and *D*, a subserosal neurofibroma of the jejunum.

(Olson). The tumors start in the smooth muscle of the bowel and protrude intraluminally, extraluminally, or in both directions (Fig. 340C). Generally they measure less than 6 cm. in diameter. They are well encapsulated, moderately firm, diffusely grayish white, and sharply circumscribed. Smaller tumors are solid. Larger tumors have a tendency to undergo central necrosis, hemorrhage, and liquefaction. Histologically the growths are definitely of two varieties—benign and malignant—although it is sometimes difficult to distinguish one from the other. In general, they are composed of elongated, ill-defined, spindle cells with moderate amounts of

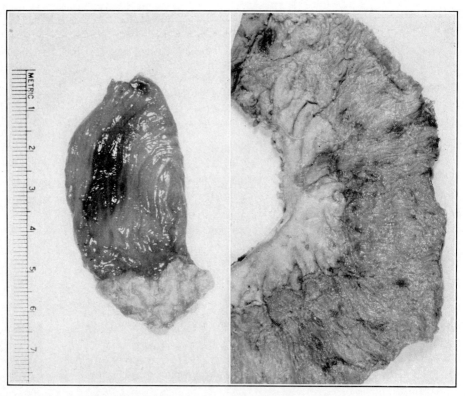

FIG. 341.—Hereditary hemorrhagic telangiectasia illustrating two pieces of small bowel with irregular, ill-defined, hemorrhagic areas in the mucosa.

eosinophilic cytoplasm and elongated, evenly stained nuclei. The malignant growths (leiomyosarcoma) reveal more irregularity of the nuclei, giant cell formation, and hyperchromatism in contrast to the usual regularity of the benign (leiomyoma) tumors.

Fibroma.—According to Olson, fibromas of the small intestine are only slightly less frequent than polyps or smooth muscle tumors. Like leiomyomas, they may protrude intraluminally or extraluminally although the latter is more frequent. The tumors are sharply circumscribed, grayish white, and firm. They measure as much as 10 cm. in diameter. A myxomatous change, detected both grossly and microscopically, is of frequent occurrence. Histologically the tumors are composed of young or collagenous connective tissue cells.

Neurofibroma.—Neurofibroma (also known as neurilemmoma and schwannoma) is a rare tumor of the small intestine, for only 20 operative cases have been reported on up to 1949 (Smith). The tumors arise from the nerve sheaths and, like leiomyomas or fibromas, protrude either intraluminally or extraluminally (Fig. 340D). They can be distinguished from the two neoplasms just mentioned only by the fact that, histologically, they reveal pallisading of the nuclei. Neurofibromas may occur as solitary tumors of the small bowel or may be found in conjunction with similar growths in other portions of the body.

Lipoma.—A lipoma of the small intestine is a benign tumor composed of adult fat cells. It occurs with increasing frequency proximodistally, being least common in the duodenum and most common in the ileum. The growth is usually located in the submucosa, is generally pedunculated, measures as much as 5 cm. in diameter, and is a frequent cause of intussuseption.

Angioma.—Angiomas of the small intestine are relatively rare, constituting about 6 per cent of all benign tumors of the small bowel, 3.4 per cent of all tumors of the small intestine, and 0.3 per cent of all gastrointestinal neoplasms (Rickham). Infrequently the lesion is a lymphangioma. This growth is yellowish gray in appearance, may be single or multiple, and measures as much as 6 cm. in diameter (Puppel). Histologically it is composed of endothelial-lined spaces filled with lymph. *Hereditary hemorrhagic telangiectasia* (Figs. 341 and 342) is probably next in frequency. The lesions are usually multiple and consist of ill-defined, hemorrhagic, mucosal and submucosal areas composed of dilated, thin-walled capillaries. The intestinal lesions generally represent only part of a systemic disorder (p. 393). *Hemangioma* is the most common angiomatous tumor of the small bowel. The lesion may be single or multiple and the individual tumor may measure as much as 5 cm. in diameter. Histologically it is composed either of endothelial-lined capillary or cavernous spaces filled with blood. Hemangioma is important because the overlying mucosa frequently ulcerates with resulting massive hemorrhage. A malignant vascular tumor (*hemangioendothelioma* or *hemangiosarcoma*) of the small bowel is extremely rare and when it does occur the tumor is probably malignant from the start rather than representing a sarcomatous transformation of a previously benign growth.

Carcinoma.—Carcinoma of the small intestine occurs with decreasing frequency proximodistally, being most common in the duodenum and least common in the ileum (Pridgen and Shallow). In the duodenum the tumors are usually located at or in the vicinity of the ampulla of Vater (Fig. 343). Such growths, of course, encroach upon the lumen of the biliary tree and produce jaundice (Miller). In the rest of the intestine there is no particular predisposition for any specific area. Regardless of the location, the tumor may be fungating, ulcerating, or diffusely infiltrating (Fig. 344). The *fungating* growths protrude into the lumen of the bowel in a cauliflower-like fashion. They are pinkish gray, rather soft, and superficially ulcerated. They may produce obstruction of the bowel simply by encroaching upon the lumen or may serve as the starting point for an intussusception. *Ulcerating* growths protrude slightly if at all above the surface of the adjacent mucosa and differ from simple ulcers in that the edge and base are composed of firm gray tissue. These tumors may produce obstruction of the bowel by constriction of the lumen and they may also penetrate through the serosa and result in peritonitis. *Diffusely infiltrating* growths permeate along the

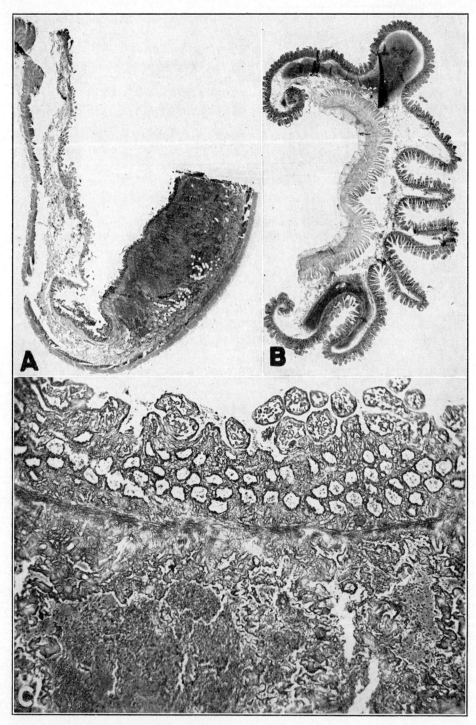

FIG. 342.—Hereditary hemorrhagic telangiectasia disclosing *A* and *B*, focal submucosal hemorrhages.   × 5, and *C*, dilated submucosal capillaries filled with blood.   × 100.

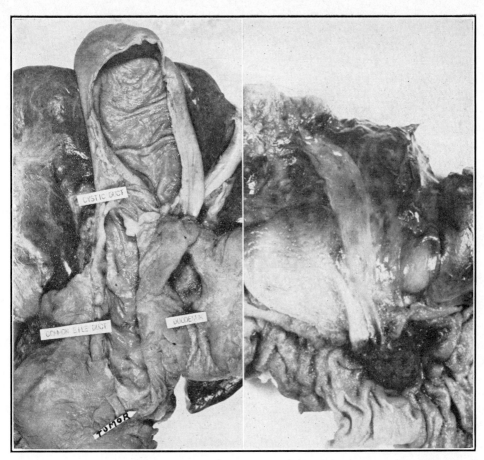

Fig. 343.—Carcinoma of the ampulla of Vater showing, to the left, an infiltrating growth with marked dilatation of the biliary system proximally and, to the right, a papillary tumor.

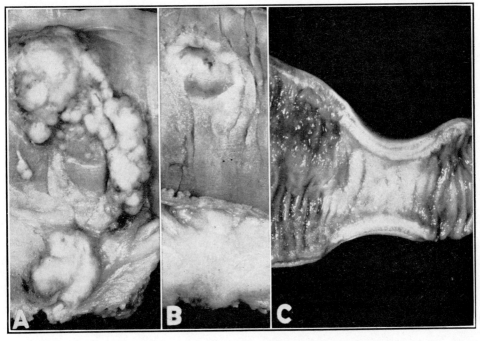

Fig. 344.—Carcinoma of the jejunum and ileum illustrating *A*, a fungating growth, *B*, an ulcerating tumor, and *C*, a diffusely infiltrating neoplasm.

(735)

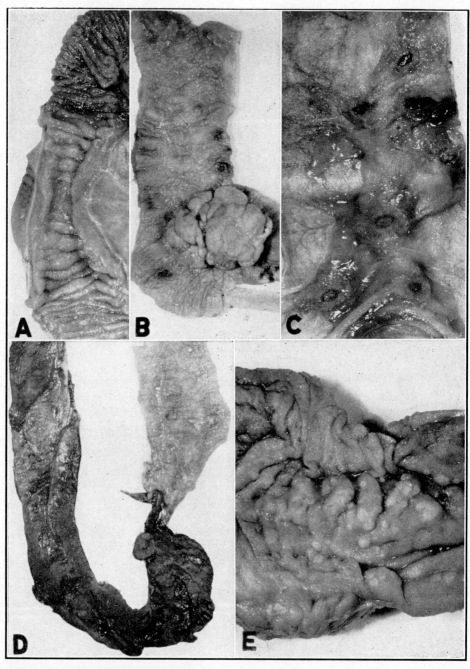

Fig. 345.—Malignant tumors of the small intestine showing A, an infiltrating reticulum cell sarcoma, B, a fungating lymphosarcoma, C, lymphoid leukemia with ulceration, D, a metastatic melanoblastoma which produced intussusception and gangrene of the bowel wall, and E, metastatic bronchogenic carcinoma affecting the mucosa.

various planes of the bowel wall. The mucosa generally remains intact, although it may be superficially ulcerated; the submucosa is prominent, and the serosa is likewise thickened with neoplastic tissue. As the tumor infiltrates it also constricts causing segmental obliteration of the lumen of the bowel. Regardless of the specific type of growth, the tumor is usually single although on rare occasions it may be multiple (Feldman). *Histologically* carcinoma of the small intestine is identical with carcinoma of the stomach (p. 682). Of the various types of growths, well-differentiated adenocarcinoma and anaplastic carcinoma account for most of the cases while signet ring or mucinous carcinoma accounts for but only a few cases.

Lymphoblastoma.—Lymphoblastoma of the small intestine may be primary or may represent simply a local manifestation of a generalized process (Marcuse). The lesions may be single but are frequently multiple. Usually they exist in the form of a diffuse permeation of the entire wall over segments of varying lengths. The mucosa remains intact; the submucosa is greatly thickened; the muscular coat is undisturbed, and the serosa is prominent (Fig. 345*A*). Superficial ulceration is sometimes noted. Less frequently, the tumor protrudes into the lumen in a papillary fashion (Fig. 345*B*). Finally, in cases of leukemia, the lesions are multiple, correspond to the distribution of Peyer's patches or lymphoid follicles, and are ulcerative (Fig. 345*C*). Histologically the tumors consist of lymphocytes or lymphoblasts (lymphosarcoma), reticulum cells (reticulum cell sarcoma), a variety of leukocytes together with giant cells (Hodgkin's disease), or leukemic cells (lymphoid, myeloid, or monocytic).

Plasmocytoma.—This is a rare tumor, there having been only a few cases recorded (Esposito). The lesion may affect any portion of the small intestine, is single or multiple, may form part of a generalized process or be primary, and consists of rather regular appearing plasma cells.

Secondary Tumors.—Secondary tumors of the small intestine may affect any portion of the bowel. In the duodenum they arise more commonly as direct extensions from adjacent structures such as the pancreas, stomach, bile ducts, and retroperitoneal lymph nodes. In the jejunum and ileum they occur most frequently as a result of metastasis to the mucosa and submucosa (Fig. 345*D* and *E*). The primary tumors may be located anywhere in the body with melanoblastoma perhaps leading the list (Herbut and Manges). Usually the lesions are multiple. They may be sessile or pedunculated and generally they measure up to 1 or 2 cm. in diameter. As all pedunculated growths, they have a propensity to cause intussusception.

REFERENCES

Pathologic Physiology

AGAR, W. T., *et al.*: J. Physiol., *121*, 255, 1953 (Amino Acid Absorption).
ALVAREZ, W. C.: *An Introduction to Gastroenterology*, 4th Ed., New York, Paul Hoeber Inc., 1948 (Intestinal Motility).
BINGHAM, J. R., *et al.*: Gastroenterol., *15*, 18, 1950 (Intestinal Pain).
CORI, F. C.: Physiol. Rev., *11*, 143, 1931 (Sugar Absorption).
FRAZER, A. C.: Physiol. Rev., *26*, 103, 1946 (Fat Absorption).
GROSSMAN, M. I.: Physiol. Rev., *30*, 33, 1950 (Gastrointestinal Hormones).
THOMAS, J. E. and FRIEDMAN, M. H. F.: Sandweiss' *Peptic Ulcer*, Philadelphia, W. B. Saunders, 1951, Chapter III (Intestinal Functions).
WRIGHT, R. D., *et al.*: Quart. J. Physiol., *30*, 73, 1940 (Intestinal Secretion).
YOUMANS, W. B.: *Nervous and Neurohumoral Regulation of Intestinal Motility*, New York, Interscience Pub., 1949.

47

Congenital Anomalies

BLACKMUN, R. L.: Am. J. Surg., 77, 371, 1949 (Mesenteric Cysts).
BROWN, K. L., and GLOVER, D. M.: Am. J. Surg., 83, 680, 1952 (Persistent Omphalomesenteric Duct).
DYSON, R.: J. Lancet, 71, 174, 1951 (Congenital Duodenal Obstruction).
FECHER, M. P., et al.: Ann. Surg., 135, 555, 1952 (Ileal Duplications).
FERGUSON, L. H.: Am. Surg., 18, 1121, 1952 (Duodenal Diverticulum).
GLASIER, P., and CORBETT, A. J.: Am. J. Surg., 83, 9, 1952 (Duodenal Diverticula).
JAY G. D., III, et al.: A. M. A. Arch. Surg., 61, 158, 1950 (Meckel's Diverticulum).
KAUTZ, F. G., et al.: Radiology, 46, 334, 1946 (Congenital Duodenal Obstruction).
MAYO, C. W., et al.: Ann. Surg., 136, 691, 1952 (Jejunal Diverticulitis).
MERRITT, W. H., and RABE, M. A.: A. M. A. Arch. Surg., 61, 1083, 1950 (Meckel's Diverticulum).
MOORE, T. C., and BATTERSBY, J. S.: Surg., Gynec. & Obst., 95, 557, 1952 (Duplications).
OBERHELMAN, H. A., and CONDON, J. B.: A. M. A. Arch. Surg., 57, 301, 1948 (Mesenteric Cysts).
PATTERSON, R. H., and BROMBERG, B.: Ann. Surg., 134, 834, 1951 (Duodenal Diverticula).
RADCLIFFE, J. W., et al.: New England J. Med., 242, 387, 1950 (Jejunal Diverticula).
RITVO, M., and VOTTA, P. J.: Radiology, 46, 343, 1946 (Diverticula).
SCALETTAR, H. E., et al.: J. Pediat., 40, 310, 1952 (Entero-umbilical Fistula).
SHALLOW, T. A., et al.: Surgery, 21, 532, 1947 (Duodenal Cysts).
SPENCER, R.: Surg., Gynec. & Obst., 95, 568, 1952 (Intestinal Obstruction in Newborn).
SWENSON, O., and LADD, W. E.: New England J. Med., 233, 660, 1945 (Congenital Anomalies)
THIEL, J. M.: Am. Surgeon, 18, 826, 1952 (Meckel's Diverticulum).
TOMAS, H. O.: Surgery, 32, 667, 1952 (Myosarcoma Meckel's Diverticulum).

Degenerations

ADLERSBERG, D.: J. Mount Sinai Hosp., 24, 177, 1957 (Malabsorption Syndrome).
ANDERSON, C. M., et al.: Brit. J. Radiol., 25, 526, 1952 (Celiac Disease).
ANDERSON, C. M., et al.: Lancet, 1, 836, 1952 (Celiac Disease).
BJERKELUND, C. J., and HUSEBYE, O. W.: Am. J. Digest. Dis., 17, 139, 1950 (Steatorrhea).
BUTTERWORTH, C. E., and PEREZ-SANTIAGO, E.: Ann. Int. Med., 48, 8, 1958 (Jejunal Biopsy Sprue).
HENDRIX, J. P., et al.: A. M. A. Arch. Int. Med., 85, 91, 1950 (Intestinal Lipodystrophy).
OXENHORN, S., et al.: Ann. Int. Med., 48, 30, 1958 (Malabsorption Syndrome).
PEMBERTON, J. DEJ., et al.: Surg., Gynec. & Obst., 85, 85, 1947 (Intestinal Lipodystrophy).
PREUSS, J.: Am. Pract., 3, 400, 1949 (Sprue).
RIVAS, F. D., et al.: J. A. M. A., 150, 647, 1952 (Sprue).
SHELDON, W., and LAWSON, D.: Lancet, 2, 902, 1952 (Celiac Disease).
STEFANINI, M.: Gastroenterology, 11, 50, 1948 (Sprue).
UPTON, A. C.: Am. J. Clin. Path., 22, 755, 1952 (Intestinal Lipodystrophy).

Inflammations

ADAMS, J. W., JR.: Am. J. Path., 15, 561, 1939 (Intracellular Bacilli in Typhoid Fever).
ALEXANDER, M. B.: Brit. M. J., 2, 973, 1948 (Infantile Diarrhea).
BEESON, P. B.: Cecil's Textbook of Medicine, 8th Ed., Philadelphia, W. B. Saunders Co., p. 200, 1951 (Typhoid Fever).
BOCKUS, H. L.: J. A. M. A., 127, 449, 1945 (Regional Enteritis).
BROWN, L., and SAMPSON, H. L.: Intestinal Tuberculosis, 2nd Ed., Philadelphia, Lea & Febiger, 1930.
BUDDING, H. J.: South. M. J., 39, 382, 1946 (Viral Diarrhea of Infants).
CRAIG, C. F., and FAUST, E. C.: Clinical Parasitology, 5th Ed., Philadelphia, Lea & Febiger, 1951.
CREIGHEAD, C. C.: Am. J. Surg., 84, 47, 1952 (Benign Ulcer).
DACK, G. M.: Food Poisoning, Revised Edition, Chicago, University of Chicago Press, 1949.
DIXON, C. F., and WEISMANN, R. D.: S. Clin. North America, 28, 999, 1948, (Acute Pseudomembranous Enterocolitis).
EVERT, J. A., et al.: Surgery, 23, 185, 1948 (Nonspecific Ulcers).
GARLOCK, J. H., et al.: Gastroenterology, 19, 414, 1951 (Results Regional Enteritis).
GILLESPIE, J. B., and DUKES, R. E.: Pediatrics, 6, 601, 1950 (Duodenitis).
GOW, J. G., and WALSH, A.: Brit. J. Surg., 39, 445, 1952 (Perforation in Regional Enteritis).

JOHNSTON, J. H., *et al.*: Surgery, *39*, 975, 1956 (Pseudomembranous Enterocolitis).
KALLQVIST, I.: Am. Rev. Tuberc., *64*, 430, 1951 (Chemotherapy Tuberculosis).
KEEN, W. K.: *The Surgical Complications and Sequels of Typhoid Fever*, Philadelphia, W. B. Saunders Co., 1898.
KIM, Y., and KIM, B.: West. J. Surg., *60*, 606, 1952 (Nonspecific Ulcerative Ileitis).
KIRKLIN, B. R.: Am. J. Roentgenol., *31*, 581, 1934 (Duodenitis).
KLECKNER, M. S., JR., *et al.*: Gastroenterology, *21*, 212, 1952 (Pseudomembranous Enterocolitis).
KORNBLUM, S. A., *et al.*: Am. J. Surg., *75*, 498, 1948 (Tuberculosis).
LEPLEY, D., and SMITH, M. B.:A.M.A. Arch. Surg., *75*, 377, 1957 (Staphylococci Enterocolitis).
MALLORY, F. B.: J. Exper. Med., *3*, 611, 1898 (Histology Typhoid Fever).
MALLORY, T. B., and LAWSON, G. M., JR.: Am. J. Path., *7*, 71, 1931 (Typhoid Cholecystitis).
NEVA, F. A.: Ann. Int. Med., *33*, 83, 1950 (Pneumonia in Typhoid Fever).
NEWMAN, C. R.: Ann. Int. Med., *45*, 409, 1956 (Pseudomembranous Enterocolitis).
PATTERSON, M., and ROSENBAUM, H. D.: Gastroenterology, *21*, 110, 1952 (Enteritis Necroticans).
PENNER, A., and DRUCKERMAN, L. J.: Gastroenterology, *11*, 478, 1948 (Enterocolitis).
RAPPAPORT, H., *et al.*: Military Surgeon, *109*, 463, 1951 (Pathology Regional Enteritis).
SAWITZ, W. G.: *Medical Parasitology*, New York, The Blakiston Co., 1950.
SCHAFFNER, V. D.: Canad. M. A. J., *57*, 561, 1947 (Tuberculosis).
SHEA, P. C., JR.: J. A. M. A., *146*, 1490, 1951 (Nonspecific Ulcer).
TRUSSELL, R. E.: New York State J. Med., *49*, 2789, 1949 (Diarrhea of the Newborn).
TURNBULL, R. B.: J.A.M.A., *164*, 756, 1957 (Staphylococcic Enteritis).
TURNER, O. E.: Pennsylvania M. J., *56*, 360, 1953 (Typhoid Fever).
WARREN, S., and SOMMERS, S. C.: Am. J. Path., *24*, 475, 1948 (Regional Enteritis).

Physical Disturbances

BECKER, W. F.: Surg., Gynec. & Obst., *95*, 472, 1952 (Acute Adhesive Ileus).
BOSWORTH, B. M.: Am. J. Surg., *76*, 472, 1948 (Nonpenetrating Trauma).
BROWN, C. H., and MICHAELS, A. G.: Surgery, *31*, 538, 1952 (Intussusception in Adults).
BROWN, R. B., *et al.*: Ann. Surg., *132*, 913, 1950 (Duodenal Fistula).
COFFEY, R. J., and WILLOX, G. D.: Am. Surg., *18*, 286, 1952 (Gallstone Obstruction).
COHN, I., JR., *et al.*: Am. J. Surg., *84*, 293, 1952 (Nonpenetrating Trauma).
COLLER, F. A., and BUXTON, R. W.: J. A. M. A., *140*, 135, 1945 (Acute Obstruction).
GROSS, R. E., and WARE, P. F.: New England J. Med., *239*, 645, 1948 (Intussusception in Childhood).
HURWITT, E. S., and ARNHEIM, E. E.: Am. J. Dis. Child., *64*, 443, 1942 (Meconium Ileus).
KOSS, L. G.: A. M. A. Arch. Path., *53*, 523, 1952 (Intestinal Pneumatosis).
KREDEL, F. E.: Am. Surg., *17*, 99, 1951 (Duodenocolic Fistula).
LAUFMAN, H., and DANIELS, J.: A. M. A. Arch. Surg., *62*, 365, 1951 (Strangulated Hernia).
McCOLLUM, W. T.: Ann. Int. Med., *37*, 579, 1952 (Mesenteric Thrombosis).
McCUNE, W. S., *et al.*: Ann. Surg., *135*, 606, 1952 (Mesenteric Thrombosis following Trauma)
McKECHNIE, R. E.: West. J. Surg., *59*, 375, 1951 (Volvulus).
McLAUGHLIN, C. W., JR., and COE, J. D.: A. M. A. Arch. Surg., *64*, 541, 1952 (Obstruction in Infancy).
MORETZ, W. H., and MORTON, J. J.: Ann. Surg., *132*, 899, 1950 (Volvulus).
NEMIR, P., JR.: Ann. Surg., *135*, 367, 1952 (Obstruction).
NORTH, J. P., and WOLLENMAN, O. J., JR.: Surg., Gynec. & Obst., *95*, 665, 1952 (Venous Mesenteric Occlusion).
RAVITCH, M. M., and McCUNE, R. M., JR.: J. Pediat., *37*, 153, 1950 (Intussuseption in Infants).
RIVES, J. D.: Military Surg., *103*, 348, 1948 (Mesenteric Vascular Occlusion).
SHERWIN, B., and MESSE, A. A.: Ann. Surg., *136*, 893, 1952 (Intestinal Pneumatosis).
TATE, R. C., and SHAW, H.: Am. Surgeon, *18*, 443, 1952 (Duodenal Fistula).
THOMA, G. W., and HENNIGAR, G. R.: Am. J. Clin. Path., *22*, 765, 1952 (Intestinal Pneumatosis).
THOREK, P., and LORIMER, W. S., JR.: J. A. M. A., *133*, 21, 1947 (Retrograde Intussusception).

Tumors

BARTHOLOMEW, L. G., *et al.*: Gastroenter., *32*, 434, 1957 (Polyposis and Mucocutaneous Pigmentation).
BOTSFORD, T. W., and SEIBEL, R. E.: New England J. Med., *236*, 684, 1947 (Benign and Malignant Tumors).

CAMP, O. B., and LESSER, A.: Ann. Surg., *136*, 1034, 1952 (Polyps).
CHERRY, J. W., and HILL, R. L.: A. M. A. Arch. Surg., *62*, 580, 1951 (Leiomyoma).
CLIFFORD, W. J.: Am. Surg., *18*, 1164, 1952 (Reticulum Cell Sarcoma).
ESPOSITO, J. J., and STOUT, A. P.: Am. J. Roentgenol., *53*, 33, 1945 (Plasmocytoma).
FELDMAN, M.: Am. J. Digest. Dis., *20*, 1, 1953 (Multiple Carcinomas).
HERBUT, P. A., and MANGES, W. E.: A. M. A. Arch. Path., *39*, 22, 1945 (Melanoblastoma).
JOERGENSON, E. J., and WEIBEL, L. A.: California Med., *75*, 395, 1951 (Tumors).
LUNN, G. M.: Brit. J. Surg., *40*, 5, 1952 (Carcinoma Duodenum).
MARCUSE, P. M., and STOUT, A. P.: Cancer, *3*, 459, 1950 (Lymphosarcoma).
McGUFF, P., *et al.:* Surg., Gynec. & Obst., *86*, 273, 1948 (Endometriosis).
MILLER, E. M., *et al.:* Surg., Gynec. & Obst., *92*, 172, 1951 (Carcinoma Ampulla of Vater).
OLSON, J. E., *et al.:* Ann. Surg., *134*, 195, 1951 (Benign Tumors)
PRIDGEN, J. E., *et al.:* Surg., Gynec. & Obst., *90*, 513, 1950 (Carcinoma).
PUPPEL, I. D., and MORRIS, L. E., JR.: A. M. A. Arch. Path., *38*, 410, 1944 (Lymphangioma).
RICKHAM, P. P.: Brit. J. Surg., *39*, 462, 1952 (Hemangioma).
ROBERTS, S. M., *et al.:* Radiology, *59*, 409, 1952 (Adenoma).
SHALLOW, T. A., *et al.:* Am. J. Surg., *69*, 372, 1945 (Malignant Tumors).
SHALLOW, T. A., *et al.:* Surgery, *27*, 348, 1950 (Carcinoma Duodenum).
SMITH, J. R., and MacNAUGHTON, E. A.: Canad. M. A. J., *60*, 399, 1949 (Neurofibroma).
WEINBERGER, H. A., and PALTAUF, R. M.: Surgery, *24*, 35, 1948 (Tumors).

Chapter

19

Appendix

PATHOLOGIC PHYSIOLOGY

M. H. F. FRIEDMAN

ALTHOUGH disease of the vestigial organ called the vermiform appendix has been the known or suspected cause of death since historical times, very little is known about its *functions*. In animals, such as the rabbit, the appendix is a large glandular structure similar in many respects to the cecum and like it is utilized in digestion. In man, however, the appendix apparently has no known utilitarian functions. In the healthy adult the capacity of the lumen is less than 1 ml. Normally, its glands secrete about 2 ml. of fluid daily at a relatively high secretory pressure. The fluid is a clear serous liquid containing some dissolved mucin but without digestive activity. Numerous bacteria may be present but these normally are not pathogenic. When the lumen at the cecal-appendiceal junction is obstructed, the accumulated secretion may distend the organ. Whether or not this distention results in occlusion of the circulation is uncertain but the organ soon becomes devitalized. While the normal appendix can withstand intralumenal pressures of several hundred centimeters of water, in gangrene the appendix ruptures readily with just slight tension.

GENERAL CONSIDERATIONS

The vermiform (worm-like) appendix or vermix (Fr. = *vermi*form + append*ix*) is a long narrow tube that originates from the apex of the cecum and is directed into the pelvis, behind the ileum and mesentery, or behind the cecum. Its average dimensions are 8×0.5 cm. Structurally it is similar to the large intestine except that the submucosa contains a continuous layer of lymphoid cells in follicle formation. This layer is particularly prominent in infancy and youth and decreases in quantity after the twentieth year. In man and higher anthropoid apes the organ represents an undilated segment of the gut and is thus a vestigial structure.

CONGENITAL ANOMALIES

Developmental malformations of the appendix are infrequent and, as a rule, unimportant. They may consist of the following: (1) *hypoplasia*—an organ so diminutive that it can scarcely be recognized as an appendix, (2) *hyperplasia*—an increase in size of the appendix to 20 cm. or more in length, (3) *agenesis*—complete absence of the organ, being recorded as occurring in as high as 0.006 per cent of postmortem examinations, 0.25 per cent of cadaver dissections, 0.0009 per cent of appendectomies, and 0.0005 per cent of hospital admissions (Collins), (4) *duplication*—consisting of partial or complete formation of a second organ arising from a single or a double cecum (Menten), (5) *ectopic mucosa*—complete investment of the external surface by a mucosa (Mahrburg), and (6) *diverticula*—outpocketings or evaginations of the mucosa. The *incidence* of *diverticula* of the appendix is recorded as varying from 0.08 to 2.8 per cent (Ladin). They occur at all ages with the greatest number in the third and fourth decades of life and are twice as frequent in males as they are in females. Diverticula of the appendix may be divided into two groups—congenital and acquired (Wilson). *Congenital* diverticula are developmental in origin and disclose all the layers of the normal appendix. *Acquired* diverticula usually arise as a result of inflammatory weakening of the muscle of the wall and an increase of intraluminal pressure beyond a point of obstruction. They lack the muscular component of the wall. In either case, the outpocketings are single or multiple, are generally found in the mesenteric border, and measure up to 2 cm. in greatest diameter. The chief *complication* is inflammation. The *clinical manifestations* are those of acute appendicitis. *Treatment* is surgical removal of the entire appendix. The *prognosis* is good.

DEGENERATIONS

The only important degenerative disorder of the appendix is *mucocele* (L. = mucus + tumor). It may be *defined* simply as an accumulation of excessive amounts of mucoid material within the lumen of the appendix. The condition is relatively *common*, there having been about 500 cases

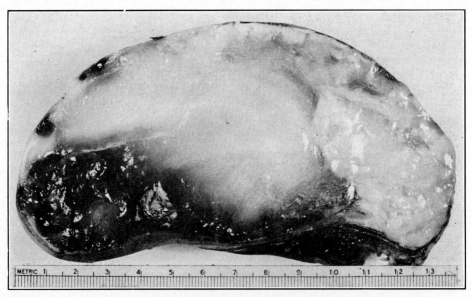

FIG. 346.—Mucocele of the appendix showing an organ filled and distended with slimy mucoid material.

recorded by 1948 (Probstein). It generally occurs in adults and affects both sexes with equal frequency. It is usually *caused* by partial to complete obstruction of the appendix in the absence of bacterial invasion. The obstruction is most frequently on an inflammatory basis but sometimes it is produced by such lesions as carcinoid, mucosal polyp, and endometriosis (Hilsabeck). In rare instances, the appendiceal lumen is patent, but the ascending colon discloses carcinoma or some other obstruction. *Experimentally* mucocele of the appendix may be produced at will in rabbits and dogs by washing the lumen with saline and ligating the organ at its base. *Pathologically* the appendix may measure as much as 20 cm. or more in diameter (Fig. 346). When small, it retains its normal shape but as it increases in size it becomes globular and irregular. The serosa is smooth; the wall usually measures up to 5 mm. in thickness, and the lumen is filled with slimy, clear, mucoid material. Sometimes (7.8% of recorded mucoceles) the mucoid material contains globoid bodies that measure 2 to 3 mm. in diameter and that resemble frog eggs (Probstein). This condition is referred to as *myxoglobulosis*. The bodies consist of central inspissated pseudomucin or cellular debris to which mucus and mucin become adherent. *Histologically* early lesions disclose hypersecretion and degeneration of epithelial cells. Later, however, most of the epithelial cells become destroyed so that the mucoid material rests directly upon an inner lining of fibrous tissue. The rest of the wall shows an attenuation of the layers and a slight infiltration with plasma cells and lymphocytes. The chief *complication* is rupture with the production of pseudomyxoma of the peritoneum. The *clinical manifestations* may be those of appendicitis or the lesion may be essentially asymptomatic and discovered (usually considered as carcinoma of the cecum) during the course of roentgenographic gastrointestinal studies. *Treatment* is surgical excision. The *prognosis* is good unless rupture and pseudomyxoma of the peritoneum are present.

INFLAMMATIONS

Orientation.—Inflammation of the appendix is known as appendicitis. While there are many varieties of inflammation, the more important lesions may be listed as acute appendicitis, chronic appendicitis, appendix in measles, granulomatous appendicitis, tuberculosis, and parasitic appendicitis.

Acute Appendicitis.—Under the heading of acute appendicitis are included all acute inflammations of the appendix caused by the ordinary pyogenic organisms. The *incidence* of the condition varies somewhat with the age of the patient. It is rare in infancy and old age and is most common in the second and third decades of life (Carp, Benson, and Snyder). It also varies somewhat with the sex. Until puberty, it is as frequent in males as it is in females; between the ages of fifteen and twenty-five it is twice as common in males as it is in females, and after the age of twenty-five there is a gradual decline in males with the incidence ultimately being equal in both sexes (Bohrod). The *causes* of acute appendicitis are predisposing and precipitating. The *predisposing* causes consist of obstruction of the lumen and/or injury to the mucosa (Bohrod). Some of these factors are lymphoid hyperplasia, fecal contents, fecaliths, parasites, kinks, adhesive bands, tumors, and foreign bodies such as toothpicks, thorns, seeds, etc. (Fig. 349*A*). *Precipitating* causes are bacteria that are normally found in the intestines. Generally they consist of colon bacilli and streptococci (Moloney).

Pathologically the initial changes consist of congestion and edema of the serosa (Fig. 347). The vessels become prominent and their minute ramifications are readily discernible. As the lesion ages, an exudate composed

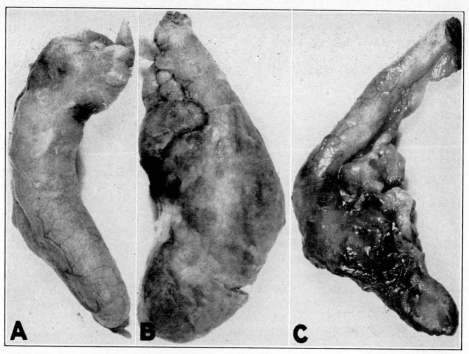

FIG. 347.—Acute appendicitis illustrating *A*, dilation of the capillaries in the distal half and a purulent exudate in the proximal half, *B*, an abundant fibrinopurulent exudate covering the entire organ, and *C*, gangrene of the distal portion with perforation.

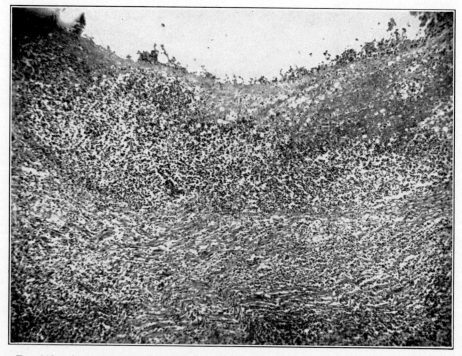

FIG. 348.—Acute appendicitis showing complete ulceration of the mucosa and congestion, edema, and neutrophilic infiltration of the rest of the wall. × 50.

of varying amounts of purulent material and fibrin, appears on the surface causing the serosa to become dull and rather opaque. The consistency of the entire organ becomes increased and the wall as a whole becomes thickened resulting in a two- to threefold increase of the diameter of the organ. Concomitantly, the lumen generally becomes filled with light brown to gray, purulent material mixed with feces. As the lesion progresses still further, focal areas of necrosis appear and, upon coalescing, result in frank gangrene. At any time from the purulent to the gangrenous stage, the wall may become so weakened that frank perforation occurs causing a direct communication between the lumen of the organ and the peritoneal cavity.

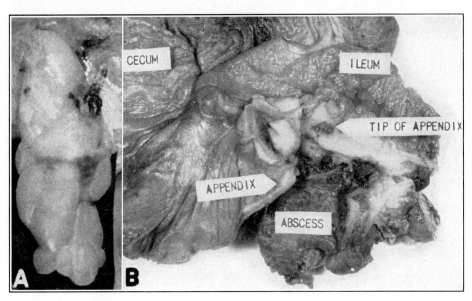

FIG. 349.—Complications of appendicitis disclosing *A*, perforation
with an intraluminal toothpick and *B*, an abscess.

The different names applied to the inflammation are merely descriptive of the stage and severity of the process. Thus (1) *acute appendicitis* refers simply to congestion, edema, and minimal leukocytic infiltration, (2) *acute purulent* or *suppurative appendicitis* connotes an inflammation in which there is an abundant exudate that permeates and covers the organ, and (3) *acute gangrenous appendicitis* means simply an acute inflammation that is attended by gangrene. *Histologically* the changes are entirely nonspecific (Figs. 348 and 351). The initial changes consist of congestion, edema, and neutrophilic infiltration. The degree of each of these changes varies so that in one organ the prominent feature may be dilatation of the capillaries, in another edema, and in still another intense permeation with neutrophils. As a rule, the alterations occur in sequence with congestion coming first and neutrophilic infiltration appearing as the process ages. In time, the latter may be severe enough to overshadow most of the normal components of the appendiceal wall. In such cases, the mucosa is generally ulcerated and the submucosa, muscle coat, and serosa reveal varisized areas of complete destruction. Aside from these more or less orthodox changes, there are some cases in which only vascular lesions are noted. In general, these are similar to the changes seen in periarteritis nodosa (p. 230) but, unlike in this condition, the lesions are localized to the appendix for removal of the organ is not followed by manifestations in other areas of the body (Gordon). In any case, the process in acute appendicitis either progresses to result in the complications listed below or spontaneous recovery ultimately occurs. The latter is accomplished by ordinary resolution and, in cases where tissue has actually been destroyed, by fibrous tissue replacement.

The *complications* of appendicitis are many (Avent, Rhoads, Milliken, and Welborn). They may be listed as follows: (1) *peritonitis*—localized to the ileocecal region or generalized, (2) *abscess*—said to occur in from 4 to 8 per cent of cases of suppurative appendicitis and occurring in the ileocecal region, retrocecally, subdiaphragmatically, or in the pelvis (Fig. 278*B*), (3) *intestinal obstruction*—caused by paralytic ileus early in the course of the disease and by adhesive bands late in the course of the disease, (4) *pylephlebitis*—said to occur in from 0.09 to 0.82 per cent of cases of suppurative appendicitis, (5) *wound infection*—seen in cases of suppuration but occurring less frequently now with the advent of antibiotics and chemotherapeutic agents, and (6) *fistulas*—connecting the appendiceal lumen with the skin of the abdominal wall, the lumen of the bowel, or the lumen of the urinary bladder. The *clinical manifestations* are often not characteristic at the two extremes of life but at any age they usually consist of some combination of the following: abdominal pain (umbilical, right lower quadrant, or pelvic), nausea, vomiting, fever, rigidity of the abdominal muscles, tenderness (especially rebound) over McBurney's point, rectal mass or tenderness, and leukocytosis. The *diagnosis* is generally made from the following: eliciting a careful history, the finding of tenderness in the right lower quadrant upon abdominal or rectal examination, and demonstrating an increasingly high leukocytic count of the peripheral blood. *Treatment* consists of the administration of antibiotics and chemotherapeutic agents and of appendectomy. The *prognosis* in recent years is good, with the overall mortality being less than 1 per cent. The improvement in the mortality rates has doubtlessly been due to earlier diagnosis, antibiotic and chemotherapeutic agents, better anesthesia, and more liberal use of intravenous fluids (Gilmour). The *causes* of *death* are attributable to the complications listed together with shock and, occasionally, unrelated (heart) diseases (Slattery).

Chronic Appendicitis.—Literally, chronic appendicitis means an infiltration of the appendix with plasma cells, lymphocytes, and monocytes. Actually, however, such changes are rarely encountered so that the caption has come to indicate a clinical syndrome characterized by recurrent attacks of vague abdominal pain in the right lower quadrant, occasional nausea and vomiting, changes in bowel habits, low-grade fever, and slight leukocytosis. Although, in some cases, these manifestations may be due to other conditions (as for example ovarian lesions in females) in many cases they are probably of appendiceal origin. In the latter group the most constant changes in the appendix consist of fibrous obliteration of the lumen and proliferation of nerve fibers and bundles within the fibrous stroma. Pathologically the lesion has been referred to as *neuroma* (because histologically it appears similar to an amputation neuroma) while clinically the condition has been called *neuroappendicopathy* (Isaacson).

Appendix in Measles.—During the prodromal stages of measles there may be epigastric or right lower quadrant pain, nausea, vomiting, and fever (but an absence of leukocytosis) and the appendix may, therefore, be removed because of a diagnosis of ordinary appendicitis. Histologically such an appendix discloses characteristic multinucleated giant cells in the hyperplastic lymph follicles of the submucosa (Mulligan). The cells are only of moderate sizes, are ill defined, and contain scanty cytoplasm with from four to eight piled up, round, hyperchromatic nuclei (Fig. 350). The lesion is an incidental finding and the progress of the disease is unaltered by its presence.

Granulomatous Appendicitis.—This term has been applied to a granulomatous mass found in conjunction with a perforated retrocecal or retroileal appendix (Musgrove). The area of inflammation consists of fibrous tissue permeated with small abscesses, may measure as much as 12 cm. in diameter, and encroaches upon the lumen of the large or small bowel.

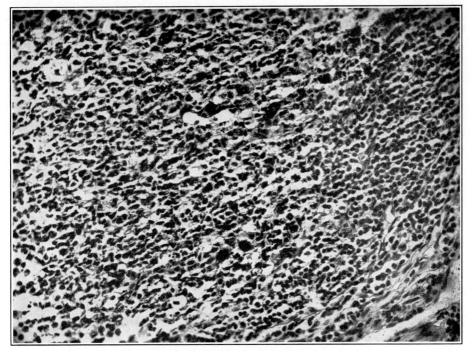

FIG. 350.—Appendix in measles showing several multinucleated giant cells in a hyperplastic submucosal lymph follicle. × 200.

Histologically it discloses a background of fibrous tissue containing acute and chronic abscesses, foam cells, and focal collections of foreign body giant cells. Treatment consists of hemicolectomy. The *prognosis* is good.

Tuberculosis.—Tuberculous appendicitis is infrequent but not rare, for over 200 cases have been reported on up to 1951 (Jaffe). The *incidence* has been recorded as varying from 0.11 to 0.3 per cent of all appendices seen in the laboratory with an equal distribution between males and females and an age distribution between the twentieth and fiftieth years. The *cause* is *Mycobacterium tuberculosis* and the condition is usually secondary to pulmonary or (in the female) genital tuberculosis. In a few instances, however, a primary focus has not been demonstrated. *Grossly* the appendix appears normal or is indistinguishable from ordinary appendicitis. Close inspection, however, may disclose serosal tubercles. *Histologically* the characteristic change consists of tubercle formation with involvement of any part of the wall but with prevalence of the lesion in the submucosa. In addition, in patients operated upon, there is frequently an accompanying nonspecific inflammation of the organ. In the recorded cases *complications* have been few, consisting essentially of postoperative fecal fistula. In symptomatic patients the *clinical manifestations* are indistinguishable from those in other types of appendicitis. *Treatment* is appendectomy. The *diagnosis* is made pathologically. The *prognosis* in patients operated upon has been good.

Parasitic Appendicitis.—Some of the more common parasites that may involve the appendix are *Endamoeba histolytica*, *Ascaris lumbricoides*, *Trichocephalus trichiurus*, and *Enterobius vermicularis*. Since all of these parasites are primarily inhabitants of either the small or the large intestine and since they only incidentally affect the appendix they are considered in Chapters 18 (p. 714) and 20 (p. 769).

PHYSICAL DISTURBANCES

Orientation.—The only three conditions in this category that are worthy of a few comments are fecaliths, intussusception, and fistulas.

Fecaliths.—A fecalith (Gr. = feces + stone) is a concretion or stone formed around a nucleus of fecal material. The *incidence* of radiopaque calculi in recorded cases of acute appendicitis is approximately 5 per cent, while the incidence of fecaliths in routine examination of all appendices has been listed as high as 80 per cent (Laforet). The condition usually occurs in adults and affects both sexes with equal frequency. The fundamental *cause* is impaired appendiceal drainage. This results in stasis, inspissation of contents, irritation, and increased secretion of mucus. The mineral salts in the mucus then precipitate around the nucleus of fecal material to produce the calculus (Chapple). *Pathologically* the stones may be single or multiple and large or small. The largest calculi on record have measured as much as 4 cm. in diameter and have weighed as much as 13.5 gm. (Chapple). Multiple calculi tend to be faceted while single calculi are usually oval shaped. In either case, they tend to conform to the lumen of the organ. The external surface is smooth and light brown and the consistency is firm to hard. Cut surfaces disclose a lamellated appearance with granules of calcium irregularly distributed (Fig. 351). In general, chemical analyses have disclosed the mineral portion to consist of calcium and magnesium phosphate while the other materials consist of vegetable pulp, mucus, and bacteria (Chapple). The *complications* consist of (1) simple erosion through the appendiceal wall with production of peritonitis and (2) a diffuse, nonspecific inflammation of the wall of the organ (Lowenberg). The *clinical manifestations* are usually those of acute appendicitis but occasionally may consist simply of colic. The *diagnosis* is made clinically only when the calculi are demonstrable roentgenographically. This may be accomplished in simple roentgenograms of the abdomen or following the use of a contrast medium (Laforet). A differential diagnosis from a roentgenographic standpoint consists of ureteral calculus, renal calculus, calcified mesenteric lymph nodes, gallstone, phlebolith, enterolith, and foreign body. *Treatment* is appendectomy in both symptomatic and in asymptomatic (as a prophylactic measure) cases. The *prognosis* is good.

Intussusception.—Intussusception of the appendix is rare (Allman). It may *occur* at all ages but is most frequent in the middle of the second decade of life. The *causes* are probably variable with the following having been mentioned as of etiologic significance: intestinal parasites, fecaliths, increased amount of lymphoid tissue, contracted sphincter at the base of the appendix, inflammation of a segment of the appendiceal wall, and tumors. In any case, each of the above listed conditions acting as a foreign body brings about increased peristalsis and this, in turn, produces an inversion of the organ. *Pathologically* the lesion may consist of (1) an invagination of the appendix into the appendix, (2) an invagination of the appendix into the cecum, or (3) an invagination of the appendix into the cecum and an

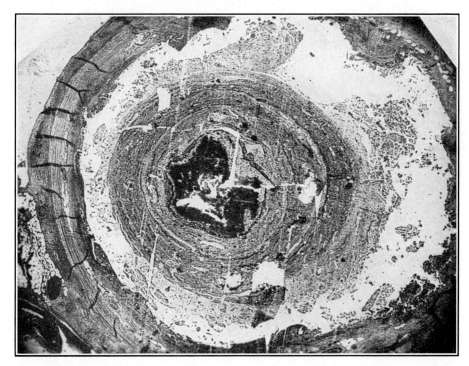

Fig. 351.—Fecalith in the appendix, illustrating a concentrically lamellated and irregularly calcified body filling the lumen. The wall of the appendix reveals extensive acute inflammation. × 7.

invagination of the cecum into the colon (compound type). The *complications* are gangrene of the organ and peritonitis. The *clinical manifestations* of simple intussusception consist of (1) intermittent, cramp-like, abdominal pain, (2) nausea and vomiting, (3) blood in the stool, (4) increase in pulse rate, and (5) slight increase in fever. The *diagnosis* is generally made at operation. *Treatment* consists of reduction of the intussusception (in cases of the compound type) and appendectomy. The *prognosis* in general is good although a mortality rate of 14.8 per cent has been recorded in connection with intussusception of the compound variety.

Fistulas.—An appendiceal fistula may connect the appendix with the peritoneal cavity (appendicoperitoneal), the skin (appendicocutaneous), the urinary bladder (appendicovesical) or the ileum (appendico-ileal). The condition almost always results from an inflammation of the appendix and may arise as a direct extension of the inflammation or secondarily by way of an appendiceal abscess. The clinical manifestations and prognosis obviously vary with the type of fistula. Treatment is surgical intervention.

TUMORS

Orientation.—Tumors or tumor-like conditions of the appendix are infrequent. While they may *occur* at any age, most are seen between the third and sixth decades of life. In the over-all, there is no preponderance in either sex or any race. The cause of the growths, as in other portions of the body, is unknown. *Pathologically* the tumors are quite varied. While theoretically they may arise in any of the tissues composing the wall of the appendix the lesions that have been described are polyp, carcinoid, carcinoma, leiomyoma, leiomyosarcoma, fibrosarcoma, myxosarcoma, angioma,

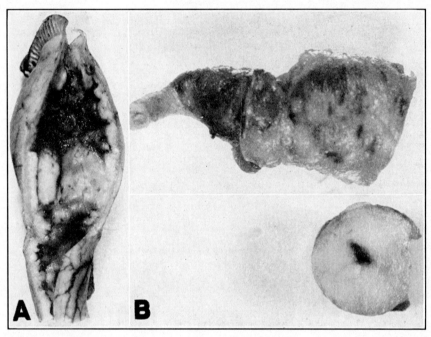

Fig. 352.—Tumors of the appendix, showing *A*, an adenomatous polyp and *B*, a lymphosarcoma with the external surface above and the cut surface below. (Specimen submitted by Doctor R. L. Breckenridge.)

hemangioendothelioma (hemangiosarcoma), neuroma, neurofibroma, lymphoblastoma, and secondary tumors (endometriosis, carcinoma, etc.). The *complications* consist of (1) obstruction of the lumen of the appendix with the production of mucocele or inflammation, (2) the untoward effects of any inflammation of the appendix (p. 743), (3) intussusception, and (4) metastasis in cases of malignant tumors. The *clinical manifestations* are those of the complications. Since inflammation is the most common complication the symptoms and signs are generally similar to those in acute appendicitis. In many instances, however, they consist simply of vague abdominal discomfort, occasional nausea and vomiting, change in bowel habits, etc. Finally, the lesion is often entirely asymptomatic. The *diagnosis* is generally made pathologically after the organ has been removed. *Treatment*

consists of appendectomy. The *prognosis* is variable. It is good in
benign tumors and poor in malignant ones. In addition to the aforesaid
general remarks, a few separate words may be made in connection with
polyp, smooth muscle tumors, carcinoid, carcinoma, and lymphoblastoma.

Polyp.—The term appendiceal polyp generally refers to a finger-like
projection of glandular tissue and is, therefore, synonymous with adenomatous polyp and adenoma. The condition is rare and is usually found
before the age of forty years (Martineau). The favorite location is the
midportion of the appendix. The lesion may be single or multiple and each
polyp generally measures not more than 0.5 × 3.0 cm. (Fig. 352*A*). The

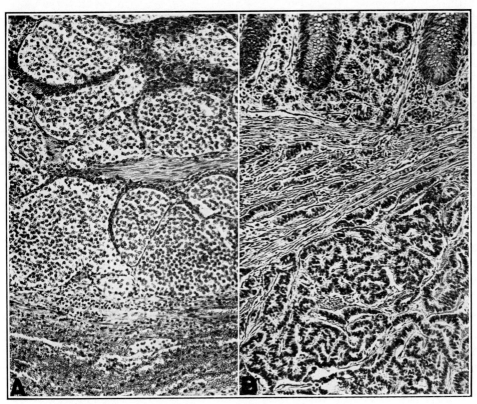

FIG. 353.—Carcinoid showing *A*, a solid variety of tumor in an appendix
and *B*, a glandular type of growth in a rectum. × 100.

external surface is smooth, nonulcerative, and pink; the consistency is
soft, and the pedicle is narrow or sessile. Histologically the polyp is composed of a core of connective tissue covered with regular appearing but
hyperplastic appendiceal glands. Malignant transformations have been
recorded but are infrequent.

Smooth Muscle Tumors.—These tumors are also rare, being estimated as
occurring in 0.0024 per cent of all appendectomies (Iovetz-Tereshchenko).
They are less frequent in the appendix than in any other part of the gastrointestinal tract. About 75 per cent of appendiceal smooth muscle tumors
are benign (leiomyomas) while 25 per cent are malignant (leiomyosarcomas).
The lesions may be single or multiple and may measure from a few millimeters to 9 cm. in greatest diameter. Grossly they are sharply circum-

scribed, pinkish gray, and firm. Histologically the benign growths are composed of elongated, ill-defined cells with a moderate amount of cytoplasm and elongated, evenly stained nuclei. The malignant growths disclose more cellularity and greater variations in nuclear appearance.

Carcinoid.—A carcinoid tumor is also referred to as an *argentaffinoma*. Although the lesion may be found at any age, two-thirds of the patients are less than thirty years old. The *cause* of the tumor is not known, but its origin from silver-positive (argentaffin) Kulchitsky cells situated in the bases of the crypts of Lieberkuhn throughout the gastrointestinal tract has been definitely established (Foreman). The cells and the tumors are most numerous in the appendix (90% of all cases), the incidence of the tumors being recorded as varying from 0.16 to 0.5 per cent of all appendectomies (Hyman). Other sites of involvement in decreasing order of frequency are ileocecal region, jejunum, duodenum, colon, and stomach (Reid). In the *appendix* the tumor characteristically occurs near the tip of the organ and usually measures up to 2 cm. in diameter. It is homogenous, yellow or yellowish gray, fairly sharply circumscribed but not encapsulated, and moderately firm. Primarily it is located in the submucosa, but it has a tendency to infiltrate the other coats of the organ and to extend into the mesentery. In other portions of the *gastrointestinal tract* the tumor is often multiple, is submucosal in location, and protrudes into the lumen in a sessile or pedunculated fashion. As a rule, it measures less than 1 cm. in diameter, is fairly sharply circumscribed, and may penetrate outwardly but usually leaves the mucosa intact. *Histologically* most of the tumors are composed of nests, columns, or masses of uniform-appearing polyhedral cells (Fig. 353*A*). The cell borders are indistinct; the cytoplasm is moderate in amount and lightly eosinophilic, and the nuclei are round to oval, sharply defined, and stippled with deeply staining chromatin. Nucleoli are usually prominent. Less frequently the tumors are composed of cuboidal or columnar cells in glandular formation (Fig. 353*B*). The cell borders are more distinct than in the solid variety and the cytoplasm is more eosinophilic. The nuclei are round or oval and basilar in position. In either case, the stroma is generally abundant and of a collagenous variety. It exhibits little or no leukocytic infiltration. As a rule, the solid tumors are argentaffin-positive but the glandular growths, especially those of the rectum, are argentaffin-negative. The most important *complication* of carcinoids is a malignant transformation. The incidence of such a change is difficult to determine but up to 1952 there were over 400 cases recorded in which metastasis occurred (Foreman). Since it is virtually impossible to tell from the histologic appearance which tumors will and which will not metastasize, some authors consider all carcinoid tumors as carcinomas of low-grade malignancy. This is especially true of the lesions found in locations other than the appendix. In this regard there is general agreement that the appendiceal lesions rarely become frankly malignant while almost 40 per cent of extra-appendiceal tumors become cancerous (Pearson). Even in the malignant growths, however, metastasis is generally limited to the draining lymph nodes and liver.

Syndrome of Malignant Carcinoid.—While many of the carcinoid tumors, as described above, produce manifestations referable mainly to obstruction of the lumen of the gastrointestinal tract or associated inflammation, some, especially the malignant ones, produce manifestations referable to their secretion of a hormone—*serotonin*. Such a picture has been referred to as the *syndrome* of *malignant carcinoid, carcinoid flushing syndrome*, and the *Thorson-Biörck syndrome* (Mattingly). *Serotonin* (5-hydroxytryptamine) is a vasoconstrictor substance found normally in small amounts (0.1 to 0.3 micrograms/cc.) in blood (Borges). Its formation occurs in two steps. The first of these occurs in the liver. Here the amino aicd tryptophane with the addition of a hydroxyl group forms a new amino acid 5-hydroxytryptophane. The second step occurs in the wall of the gut, as well as in the liver, kidney, and brain. It consists of the loss of carbon dioxide from the amino acid with the formation of serotonin. In completing its metabolism, serotonin is inactivated by an amine oxidase (found in most tissues of the body) producing an inactive excretory product 5-hydroxyindoleacetic acid which is excreted normally in the urine in amounts varying from 2 to 9 mg./24 hours. *Pharmacologically*, among other things, serotonin acts on smooth muscle to produce vasoconstriction, intestinal paralysis, and bronchospasm and it also is capable of inducing local fibrous tissue proliferation.

The *source* of *serotonin* in the *gastrointestinal tract* is the enterochromaffin system. In 1953, Lembeck demonstrated large amounts of serotonin in *carcinoid tumors*. In 1954, Thorsen *et al.* described a *syndrome* associated with metastasizing malignant carcinoid tumors consisting clinically of cyanotic flushing, fluctuations in blood pressure, diarrhea, and asthma and pathologically by right-sided endocardial fibrosis and valvulitis together with bronchial constriction. They suggested that the syndrome may be due to serotonin and later actually produced the manifestations by administering this compound. Subsequently it was shown that the blood of patients with this syndrome contains a high level of serotonin and, concomitantly, that the urine contains an excessive amount of the inactivation product of serotonin, namely, 5-hydroxyindoleacetic acid. These original observations and suggestions have been quickly substantiated by numerous subsequent reports and the syndrome has thus been well established. Through the urinary determination of 5-hydroxyindoleacetic acid, a simple and accurate procedure is now available for the diagnosis of a tumor which hitherto could be recognized only as a result of associated complications of intestinal obstruction or inflammation.

Carcinoma.—Although carcinoma of the appendix is recorded as being rare (French and McCampbell), there have been at least 116 cases reported on in the literature up to 1951 (Sillery). The condition usually *occurs* at an older age period than does carcinoid, being found most commonly in the fifth and sixth decades of life. *Pathologically* the lesion is similar to carcinoma of other portions of the gastrointestinal tract (Fig. 354). The usual location is at the base of the appendix but any part of the organ may be affected. The growths are either polypoid or infiltrative and ulcerative. As they increase in size they distend the lumen of the appendix or infiltrate its wall. In the latter instance, the neoplastic tissue penetrates the serosa and extends into the adjoining tissues, especially the cecum, colon, and mesentery. *Histologically* the tumors are primarily of a glandular variety with varying degrees of differentiation from well-formed glands to single cells aimlessly infiltrating the tissues which they contact (Fig. 355). In some instances the cells disclose an abundant secretion of mucus. Thus, the lesions are identical with those seen in the stomach, small intestine, and large intestine (p. 682). Although *metastasis* may be widespread it is more often confined to the mesenteric and para-aortic lymph nodes and liver. The *prognosis* is better than it is in carcinoma of the ileum or right side of the large bowel, mainly because symptoms are produced earlier and the lesion can be completely removed.

48

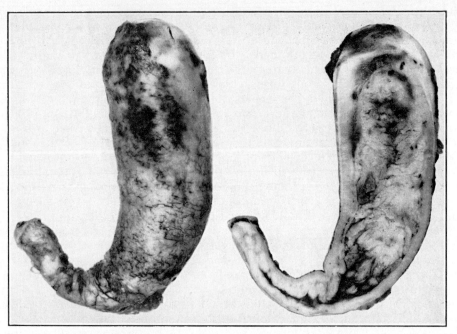

FIG. 354.—Carcinoma of the appendix illustrating enlargement of the distal three fourths of the organ, to the left, and filling and distention of the lumen by tumor along with infiltration of the wall, on the right.

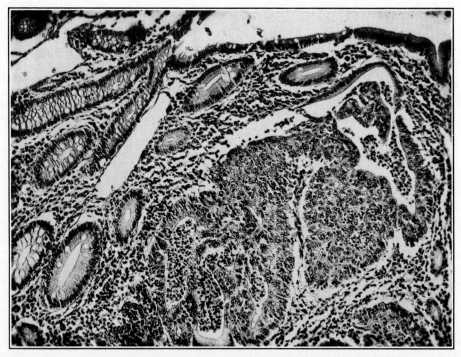

FIG. 355.—Adenocarcinoma of the appendix illustrating neoplastic cells in glandular formation. × 100.

Lymphoblastoma. —Lymphoblastoma accounts for about three-quarters of all cases of sarcoma of the appendix. The two types of lymphoblastoma most commonly encountered are *lymphosarcoma* (Knox) and *giant follicular lymphoblastoma* (Morehead). While the lesions may be primary in the appendix, the local tumors usually represent only part of a systemic disease. The appendix may be focally or diffusely affected with the neoplasm grossly consisting of a circumferential infiltration with grayish-white, rather soft tissue (Fig. 352*B*). The over-all diameter may be increased manifold; the serosa remains intact; the muscle coats may be conspicuous or entirely obscured, and the lumen is virtually completely occluded or at least greatly reduced in caliber. *Histologically* the changes are those of lymphoblastoma in lymph nodes or other tissues (p. 745). In general, the *prognosis* is poor for the patients usually die of systemic involvement.

REFERENCES

Congenital Anomalies

COLLINS, D. C.: Am. J. Surg., *82*, 689, 1951 (Agenesis).
LADIN, P.: A. M. A. Arch. Surg., *62*, 514, 1951 (Diverticula).
MAHRBURG, S.: A. M. A. Arch. Path., *44*, 578, 1947 (Ectopic Mucosa).
MENTEN, M. L., and DENNY, H. E.: A. M. A. Arch. Path., *40*, 345, 1945 (Duplication).
WILSON, R. R.: Brit. J. Surg., *38*, 65, 1950 (Diverticula).

Degenerations

HILSABECK, J. R., *et al.:* Am. J. Surg., *84*, 670, 1952 (Mucocele).
PROBSTEIN, J. G., and LASSAR, G. N.: Ann. Surg., *127*, 171, 1948 (Myxoglobulosis).

Inflammations

AVENT, C. H., *et al.:* Surgery, *27*, 862, 1950 (Ruptured Appendix).
BENSON, C. D., *et al.:* A. M. A. Arch. Surg., *64*, 561, 1952 (Appendicitis in Infants).
BOHROD, M. G.: Am. J. Clin. Path., *16*, 752, 1946 (Pathogenesis Acute Appendicitis).
CARP, L., and ARMINIO, J. A.: Am. J. Surg., *83*, 773, 1952 (Appendicitis in Old Patients).
GILMOUR, I. E. W., and LOWDON, A. G. R.: Edinburgh M. J., *59*, 361, 1952 (Acute Appendicitis).
GORDON, B. S.: A. M. A. Arch. Surg., *62*, 92, 1951 (Arteritis in Appendix).
ISAACSON, N. H., and BLADES, B.: A. M. A. Arch. Surg., *62*, 455, 1951 (Neuroappendicopathy).
JAFFE, F. A.: Am. Rev. Tuberc., *64*, 182, 1951 (Tuberculosis).
MILLIKEN, N. K., and STRYKER, H. B., JR.: New England J. Med., *244*, 52, 1951 (Pylephlebitis and Appendicitis).
MOLONEY, G. E., *et al.:* Brit. J. Surg., *38*, 52, 1950 (Appendicitis).
MULLIGAN, R. M.: A. M. A. Arch. Path., *37*, 61, 1944 (Appendix in Measles).
MUSGROVE, J. E., and DOCKERTY, M. B.: A. M. A. Arch. Path., *50*, 427, 1950 (Granulomatous Appendicitis).
PATTON, G. D.: Am. J. Surg., *84*, 215, 1952 (Chronic Appendicitis or Painful Ovary).
RHOADS, J. E., and DARROW, R. P.: Pennsylvania M. J., *54*, 435, 1951 (Complication Appendicitis).
SLATTERY, L. R., *et al.:* A. M. A. Arch. Surg., *60*, 31, 1949 (Acute Appendicitis).
SNYDER, W. H., JR., and CHAFFIN, L.: A. M. A. Arch. Surg., *64*, 549, 1952 (Appendicitis in Infants).
WELBORN, M. B.: Am. J. Surg., *83*, 176, 1952 (Appendiceal Abscess).

Physical Disturbances

ALLMAN, D. D., *et al.:* J. A. M. A., *149*, 1133, 1952 (Intussusception).
CHAPPLE, C. F.: Brit. J. Surg., *38*, 503, 1951 (Fecalith).
LAFORET, E. G., *et al.:* Am. J. Roentgenol., *65*, 867, 1951 (Fecalith).
LOWENBERG, R. I.: Ann. Surg., *130*, 975, 1949 (Fecalith).
SHALLOW, T. A., *et al.:* Am. J. Surg., *71*, 423, 1946 (Fistula).

Tumors

Borges, F. J. and Bessman, S. P.: Ann. Int. Med., *46*, 425, 1957 (Malignant Carcinoid Syndrome).

Foreman, R. C.: Ann. Surg., *136*, 838, 1952 (Carcinoid).

French, W. E.: Am. Surg., *18*, 313, 1952 (Carcinoma).

Hyman, R. M.: Am. J. Surg., *79*, 569, 1950 (Tumors).

Iovetz-Tereshchenko, N. N.: Lancet, *1*, 903, 1950 (Leiomyoma).

Knox, G.: A. M. A. Arch. Surg., *50*, 288, 1945 (Lymphosarcoma).

Mattingly, T. W.: Med. Ann. Dist. Col., *25*, 239 and 304, 1956 (Malignant Carcinoid Syndrome).

Martineau, P. C., *et al.*: J. A. M. A., *149*, 1548, 1952 (Adenomatous Polyps).

McCampbell, B. R., and Dickinson, E. H.: U. S. Armed Forces M. J., *3*, 125, 1952 (Carcinoma).

Morehead, R. P., and Woodruff, W. E.: A. M. A. Arch. Path., *40*, 51, 1945 (Giant Follicular Lymphoblastoma).

Pearson, C. M., and Fitzgerald, P. J.: Cancer, *2*, 1005, 1949 (Carcinoid).

Reid, D. R. K.: Brit. J. Surg., *36*, 130, 1948 (Argentaffinoma).

Sillery, R. J.: J. A. M. A., *147*, 854, 1951 (Carcinoma).

Chapter

20

Large Intestine

PATHOLOGIC PHYSIOLOGY

M. H. F. FRIEDMAN

THE most important *function* of the *colon* is the reabsorption of electrolytes
and water from the ileal contents which have remained in the small intestine
after all nutrient material has undergone absorption. Little else other than
water and salts is absorbed from the colon, a point to be remembered when
considering rectal feeding of the debilitated patient. In the healthy person
on a normal diet there is little in the stool which represents unabsorbed
food material. The role of the colon as an organ for excretion of toxins
has been grossly exaggerated. In poisoning with heavy metals, however,
appreciable excretion of the metal by the colonic mucosa takes place.

Filling of the *cecum* and *colon* appears to be a continuous process. Even
in the fasting state the small intestine contains mucus and epithelial debris
suspended in the secretions from the upper digestive tract. An advancing
peristaltic wave in the terminal ileum carries from about 1 to 5 ml. of liquefied material towards the cecum. This is discharged into the cecum only if
the phasic pressure of the ileum is greater than that of the large bowel. The
ileo-cecal sphincteric mechanism acts to close and prevent regurgitation of
colonic fecal contents whenever the pressure gradient is reversed. In extensive vomiting, however, this may be relaxed to permit retrograde flow of
fecal matter by reverse peristalsis.

The ileal contents which pass into the large bowel slowly accumulate in
the cecum. The *mechanism* responsible *for progression* into the colon is not
well known. Perhaps haustral contractions and possibly also a difference
in pressures due to tonus changes move the material along to the colon.
In the colon, the material moves forward by shallow peristaltic waves, and
then moves backward for a small distance. Except in the spastic colon,
the backward movement in man is not due to antiperistalsis but the exact
mechanism is still not known. The backward and forward movement results
in constant stirring of the fluid mass and dehydration until ultimately the
more concentrated material reaches the descending colon. The stimulus
for progression from here will depend principally on mechanical distention.

The passage of liquid stool in *diarrhea* is almost wholly an activity of the
colon while the evacuation of formed stool involves the abdominal muscles
and diaphragm as well. In diarrhea the rush peristalses sweep from the
ileum over the colon and sigmoid to the rectum. The internal sphincter is
relaxed reflexly and the propulsion may be forceable enough to overcome
the external sphincter. On the other hand, in the process of *stool formation*
the intraluminal pressure in the descending colon is gradually built up by
the distention of the accumulated contents to a point which causes reflex

mass contraction of the whole descending colon. Though sometimes erroneously called mass peristalses, it differs from true peristalses in that the whole section of involved colon is contracted simultaneously rather than by a progressive wave of constriction. The process of *stool extrusion* consists of shortening of the rectum by contraction of the longitudinal muscle layer and lifting of the anal ring by contraction of the levator ani, accompanied by active relaxation of the internal sphincter. The force for extrusion of the stool comes from the increased intra-abdominal pressure developed by the descent of the diaphragm and contraction of the abdominal muscles.

Distention of the colon which arouses a mass contraction is devoid of accompanying *sensory perceptions*. The sensation of need to *defecate* arises from distention of the rectum which otherwise in health is empty. Irritation of the rectum gives rise to tenseness because the evoked sensations are mistaken for the presence of stool.

Following ingestion of a meal there is initiated a gastrocolic reflex. The evacuation of the colon which occurs on gastric distention is seen in the infant during or soon after feeding. The ready inhibition of this reflex by conditioning is the basis for bowel training. Poor toilet habits account for most *constipations*. Suppression of the defecatory reflex leads to accumulation of fecal material in the colon, which becomes harder as it undergoes dehydration. Ultimately, the stool becomes too hard and too large to be passed without pain so that attempts to evacuate are failures.

The *cathartic action* of certain agents is based on the foregoing. Peristaltic rush activity which is extensive and powerful enough to evacuate the bowel may be initiated by mucosal irritation of either the colon or the whole intestine (*e.g.*, cascara and castor oil). Fatty acids are potent bowel irritants and the effectiveness of soapsud enema is due to the formation of fatty acids from the administered soap. So-called bulk cathartics increase intestinal motility by mechanical distention of the bowel. Distention results from prevention of intestinal absorption of fluid either through the osmotic activity of nonabsorbable salts (magnesium sulfate and saline cathartics) or swelling of hydrophilic colloid by water retention (psyllium seed, bran). Since constipation is most often due to improper diet and poor toilet habits the use of cathartics is analogous to whipping a tired horse to improve his performance. Serious functional and organic changes, such as erosions of the colonic mucosa, spastic colitis, and systemic effects due to calcium deficiency, may result from indiscriminate use of cathartics. In particular, cathartics used in appendicitis or intestinal obstruction may cause rupture by increasing the tension in a weakened intestinal wall.

Secretion of *mucus* by the colon is a continuous process but the rate is greatly augmented by mechanical stimuli. The adhering mucus is particularly effective as a coating against erosive injury by hardening stool. Probably the mucous-secreting glands, particularly in the sigmoid colon, are continuously being destroyed and rapidly regenerated. In *ulcerative colitis* the disease process usually begins in the rectum and extends up the colon while during remission the reverse order is followed. In a matter of a few days, the colon mucosa again may look entirely normal even though the rectal mucosa is still ulcerated or friable. Although the statement that secretions from the colonic glands are under both parasympathetic and sympathetic control needs re-examination, there can be little question that secretion is readily influenced by higher nervous activity. The profuse mucus secreted in *mucous colitis* is partly psychogenic and partly due to coexisting bowel hypermotility acting as a mechanical stimulus.

GENERAL CONSIDERATIONS

In this Chapter on the Large Intestine the more important disorders of the cecum, colon, rectum, and anus will be included. Conditions such as acute ulcerative colitis, tuberculosis, fungous and yeast-like enteritis and colitis, gastrojejunocolic fistula, carcinoid, etc., that also affect other portions of the gastrointestinal tract will be omitted for they have already been discussed in Chapters 17, 18, and 19. As in other sections of the book, the diseases may be divided into Congenital Anomalies, Degenerations, Inflammations, Physical Disturbances, and Tumors.

CONGENITAL ANOMALIES

Orientation.—Developmental malformations of the large intestine are many and important. The more common abnormalities may be listed as follows: anomalies of rotation, duplication, cysts, megacolon, diverticula, imperforate anus, congenital fistulas, and anal ducts.

Anomalies of Rotation.—Normally, as the large intestine re-enters the abdominal cavity, the cecum is carried to the right and inferiorly and becomes fixed to the posterior abdominal wall in the right iliac and hypogastric regions. Abnormally, as a result of faulty anchorage or rotation, the following may be encountered: (1) *mobile cecum*—when the entire ileocecal region fails to become attached to the posterior abdominal wall allowing unrestricted mobility, (2) *transposition of the large intestine*—when rotation occurs to the left instead of to the right, resulting in location of the cecum in the left iliac and hypogastric regions, the ascending colon on the left, the transverse colon in the usual position, and the descending colon, sigmoid colon, and rectum on the right, (3) *retroposition of the transverse colon*—when the transverse colon rests behind the stomach, duodenum, and small intestine, and (4) *interposition of the transverse colon*—when it is located inferior to the diaphragm and superior to the liver, stomach, and spleen.

Duplications.—Duplications of the colon are rare (van Zwalenburg). The more common anomalies consist of *segmental* duplications (in reality congenital diverticula) wherein a segment of the colon of variable length lies between the root of the mesentery and the normal bowel. The duplicated segment communicates with the colon by a single ostium and is interposed between the vessels supplying the colon. The less common anomalies consist of *complete* duplications of the entire colon. Generally there are two large intestines but there may be three. The duplications start in the terminal ileum and parallel each other all the way to the anus. At the anus one or both of the bowels may open into the perineum, may end blindly, or may open into the urinary bladder. Complete duplication is generally accompanied by duplication of the urethra and bladder and is a result of early twinning. *Treatment* is surgical correction. The *prognosis* depends upon the extent of the abnormalities.

Cysts.—Enterogenous (of gastrointestinal origin) cysts of the large intestine *arise* either as a pinching off of a congenital diverticulum or as an isolation of groups of cells during the stage of recanalization of the gut (Custer). The condition is *rare*. The most common *location* is the ileocecal region and the least common site is the rectum. The *cyst* may be located in the wall of the gut or between the gut and its mesentery. It may measure as much as 12 cm. in diameter and is usually filled with mucoid material. Its wall consists of all the layers of the bowel. The lesion produces intestinal obstruction by encroaching upon the lumen of the gut. *Treatment* is surgical excision. The *prognosis* is good.

Megacolon.—Megacolon is also referred to as *idiopathic congenital megacolon* and *Hirschsprung's disease.* The condition is *rare* but nevertheless it has been estimated as occurring once in every 9,000 cases (Whitehouse). The lesion is most common in the first two decades of life and affects males five times as frequently as females. In the past, the *cause* has been attributed to mechanical obstructions such as valves, local aplasia, torsion of the gut, and kinking of the bowel, but careful studies have been negative in this respect (State). More recently, histologic examinations of the bowel wall have shown the absence of ganglion cells in the myenteric plexuses of the rectosigmoid junction. This abnormality results in the failure of transmission of peristaltic waves distal to the affected segment thus producing a functional obstruction at the junction of the sigmoid colon and rectum.

Pathologically the anus and rectum are relatively normal. At the junction of the rectum with the sigmoid, the bowel wall consists of a narrowed segment that measures from 2 to 4 cm. in length. Proximal to this point the colon is greatly dilated, elongated, and redundant. The bowel wall is as much as ten times the normal thickness; the mucosa is superficially ulcerated, and the lumen is filled with soft or impacted fecal material. *Histologically* the following changes are noted: an absence of ganglion cells in the myenteric plexus at the rectosigmoid junction, nonspecific mucosal ulcerations, and varying degrees of chronic colitis.

The usual *complications* are fecal impaction with obstruction of the bowel, perforation of the ulcers with resulting peritonitis, and volvulus of the redundant loops of bowel. The *clinical manifestations* may consist of the following: (1) vomiting and bouts of diarrhea alternating with constipation during the first few months of life, (2) abdominal distention, (3) almost no spontaneous evacuation of the bowel, (4) history of use of laxatives and enemas since birth, (5) stunting of growth and failure to gain weight, (6) weakness, (7) headache, (8) loss of energy, (9) anemia, (10) thin, pale, weak abdominal wall, and (11) a doughy sensation and masses upon abdominal palpation (Whitehouse). The *diagnosis* is made from a consideration of the clinical manifestations as listed together with the radiologic demonstration (by the use of a barium enema) of a narrow rectosigmoid junction (Swenson). A differential diagnosis should include other obstructions (stenosis, aplasia, imperforate anus, constipation, tumors, etc.) that produce dilatation of the colon. *Treatment* is generally considered to be surgical. It consists of resection of the narrow segment at the rectosigmoid junction together with as much colon proximally as shows no peristalsis and of an anastomosis of the remaining sigmoid colon with the rectum (State) or simply surgical removal of the distal portion of the sigmoid colon and the rectum with anastomosis of the proximal portion of the sigmoid colon to the anus (Swenson). The *prognosis* in patients treated surgically is good. In the absence of adequate therapy, the morbidity is high and the complications listed may occur at any time.

Diverticula.—Diverticula of the large intestine consist of evaginations of the wall of the gut. The presence of more than two diverticula is known as *diverticulosis* and the presence of a superimposed infection is known as *diverticulitis.* The over-all *incidence* is approximately 5 per cent of the general population (Geist). The condition is as frequent in males as it is in females and occurs most commonly in the fifth and sixth decades of life

(Smith and McGowan). The *causes* vary with the type of diverticula. *Congenital* diverticula are due to abnormalities of recanalization of the lumen of the large bowel, while *acquired* diverticula result from herniation of the mucosa through weak spots in the muscle of the wall. Most diverticula of the large intestine are of the acquired variety.

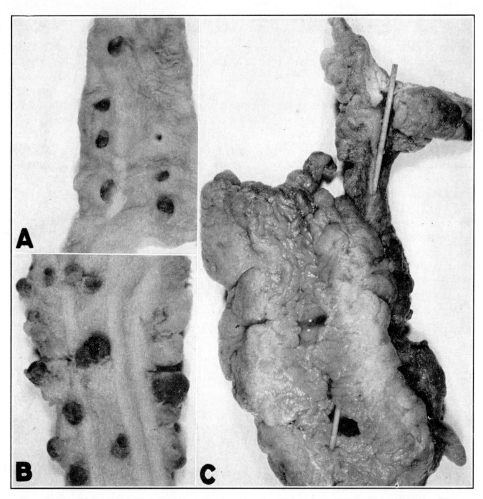

Fig. 356.—Diverticula of the colon showing *A*, the mucosal surface with two rows of linear evaginations, each possessing a wide ostium, *B*, the serosal surface with the evaginations between the tæniæ coli, and *C*, inflammation with a cutaneous fistula.

Pathologically the distribution of the evaginations is approximately as follows: cecum 1.7 per cent, ascending colon 5 per cent, transverse colon 7 per cent, descending colon 8 per cent, sigmoid colon 75 per cent, and rectum 4 per cent (Case). In the cecum the diverticula are often solitary but in the rest of the bowel they are usually multiple. The latter occur in a linear fashion between the taeniæ coli (Fig. 356). Regardless of the precise location, most diverticula of the large intestine measure from 1 to 2 cm. in greatest diameter. The communicating ostia are usually broad, although the mucosa may be redundant and folded over so that the openings are not always readily discernible. The mucosa lining the diverticula is continuous with that of the adjacent bowel. The lumen may be empty or it may be filled with soft fecal material or fecal concretions. *Histologically* congenital diverticula disclose all the layers of the bowel wall, while acquired diverticula present a partial or complete absence of the muscle coats.

The chief complications are (1) *diverticulitis*—occurring in approximately 15 per cent of all cases and manifested by marked thickening, induration, and ulceration of the bowel wall with formation of adhesions, (2) *obstruction* —due to inflammatory thickening of the wall, (3) *perforation*—resulting in *abscess* formation or *peritonitis*, (4) *fistulous tract formation*—the tract occurring between the bowel and some other abdominal viscera (usually urinary bladder) or the skin of the abdominal wall, (5) *hemorrhage*—as a result of concomitant mucosal ulceration (Horner). *Clinically* diverticula are symptomatic only when infection and other complications listed above occur. Thus, the symptoms and signs usually mimic those of acute appendicitis (left-sided when the left portion of the bowel is affected) or those of obstruction (generally mistaken for carcinoma). A *diagnosis* of diverticula can be made with certainty only upon demonstrating the evaginations roentgenographically (using barium as a contrast medium) or at the time of operation. A differential diagnosis in lesions affecting the cecum should include appendicitis, carcinoma, tuberculosis, and actinomycosis while that in lesions of other portions of the large intestine usually includes only carcinoma. *Treatment* is unnecessary unless complications arise. In the presence of the latter, surgical intervention in the form of ileostomy, colostomy, or resection is indicated. The *prognosis* is generally good. Most patients should recover.

Imperforate Anus.—Imperforate anus means a failure of establishment of the patency of the anal canal. Actually this represents only one of a group of congenital anomalies in this area. For the sake of convenience, all of them may be included in this section. It has been estimated that the *incidence* is approximately 1 in 5,000 births (Moore). Males are affected as frequently as females. Failure of perforation of the anorectal septum accounts for imperforate anus, while failure of the urorectal septum to descend completely accounts for the associated fistulas (Bacon). The precise *causes* of these imperfections of development, however, are unknown.

Pathologically the following malformations of the rectum and anus have been established: (1) stenosis of the rectum or anus with a hind gut otherwise patent, (2) an anus represented merely by a dimple and a blindly ending rectum riding high in the pelvis or extending to the perineum, and (3) an interruption of the rectum with a blindly ending pouch above connected with the sigmoid colon and a blindly ending pouch below communicating with the patent anus. In over one-half of the cases, a fistulous tract connects the blindly ending segment of the hind gut with the urinary or female genital tract (Moore).

The *complications* consist of obstruction of the bowel, rupture of the bowel and peritonitis, and urinary tract infection. In the absence of an adequate fistulous tract the *clinical manifestations* are those of low bowel obstruction with abdominal distention and vomiting. In the presence of fistulas there is usually noted the passage of gas and feces by way of the vagina or the urinary tract. The *diagnosis* is made by inspecting the anus and digitally examining the anus and rectum. *Treatment* is surgical correction. The *prognosis* is guarded for the mortality may exceed 40 per cent. *Death* in untreated cases is due to the complications listed above, to loss of fluids and electrolytes, or to pneumonia from aspiration of vomitus.

Congenital Fistulas.—Congenital fistulas of the large intestine are confined to the rectum and, as stated above, occur in connection with abnormalities of the rectum and anus. They may be single or multiple and they connect a blindly ending rectum with the urinary bladder, urethra, perineum, and (in the female) vagina (Moore). The chief *clinical manifestations* are the passage of gas and feces by way of the urethra, perineum (other than the anus), or vagina. The only effective *therapy* is surgical correction. The *prognosis* depends more upon the associated rectal and anal abnormalities than upon the fistula as such.

Anal Ducts.—In as high as 50 per cent of human anal canals, ducts can be seen to originate in the anal (usually posterior) crypts and extend downward and outward to and beyond the external sphincter (Kratzer and Hill). They are generally lined by transitional or squamous epithelium but occasionally the lining cells are columnar and of a mucus-secreting variety. The ducts are important because they may become infected and lead to the formation of abscesses, sinuses, or fistulas.

DEGENERATIONS

Degenerative lesions of the large intestine, as of the small intestine (p. 698), are common but are virtually always associated with other disease processes. Included in the group of degenerations is a condition called *melanosis coli* (p. 81). It is an innocuous, brown to black (melanin) pigmentation of the mucosa of the large bowel and appendix and is important only in so far as its recognition as an entirely benign process is concerned.

INFLAMMATIONS

Orientation.—Inflammation of the colon is known as *colitis*, of the cecum as *cecitis*, of the sigmoid colon as *sigmoiditis*, and of the rectum as *proctitis* (Gr. = rectum + inflammation). As would be expected (because of the length of the large bowel and the constant exposure to trauma and infection) the inflammations are frequent and varied. The more important ones may be listed as follows: acute phlegmonous colitis and cecitis (p. 660), acute pseudomembranous enterocolitis (p. 704), uremic colitis, mucous colitis, bacillary dysentery, cholera, ulcerative colitis, regional colitis (p. 709), tuberculosis (p. 712), fungous and yeast-like colitis (p. 712), nonspecific granuloma, oleogranuloma, parasitic infection, and anal inflammation. Some of these diseases, as indicated, have already been referred to in other parts of the book. The remaining conditions may now be considered in the order listed.

Uremic Colitis.—Frequently, in the terminal stages of uremia there is a nonspecific inflammation and ulceration of the colon that is called *uremic colitis*. Sometimes the small bowel is also affected and the lesion is referred to as *uremic enterocolitis*. The transverse colon is involved most commonly and most severely (Fig. 357). The lesions vary in degree from focal petechiæ to extensive ulcers. The latter are superficial, irregular, and often linearly arranged opposite the taeniæ coli. They may be bare or covered with a pseudodiphtheritic gray membrane. The histologic changes consist of acute denudations of the mucosa, the presence of a membrane composed of fibrin and debris, and edema and leukocytic infiltration of the tissues surrounding the defects.

Mucous Colitis.—This term is reserved for a neurogenic condition of the large bowel characterized chiefly by hyperirritability and hyperspasticity of the colon and excessive secretion of mucus in the stool (Gauss). The disorder *occurs* in the third and fourth decades of life and affects females five times as frequently as males. It is seen in high-strung people and is *caused* by psychoneurotic states including anxiety states, adjustment problems, submerged fear complexes, guilt feeling, inadequacy, etc. The *pathologic* changes are observed only sigmoidoscopically for the patients

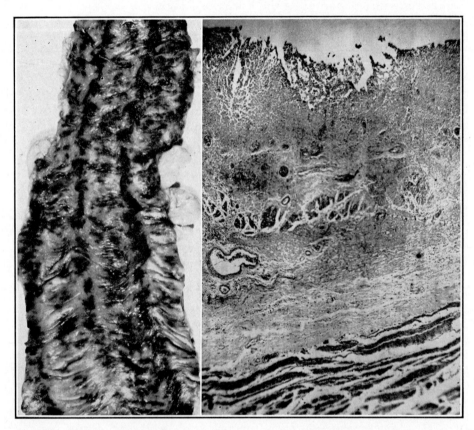

Fig. 357.—Uremic colitis showing, to the left, acute linear ulcerations and severe congestion of the mucosa of the colon and, to the right, ulceration of the mucosa and rather extensive inflammation of the exposed tissues. ✕ 25.

never die of the disease. In the early stages the mucosal capillaries are engorged and prominent and the mucosa is covered with glairy mucus. In intermediate stages the mucosa is diffusely hyperemic. The vascular markings are obscured. The surface is drier and the mucus is more tenacious and appears in patches. In later stages, the mucosa is thin and pale, is again covered with mucus, and discloses pinpoint ulcerations. The chief *clinical manifestations* are mucus in the stool, abdominal pain (localized or diffuse), constipation, flatulence, tender and rope-like descending colon, and spasm of the colon demonstrable roentgenographically. The *diagnosis* is made from the history, the clinical manifestations, and the sigmoidoscopic appearance. *Treatment* is psychiatric. The *prognosis* is guarded for recurrences are common and the morbidity is high.

Bacillary Dysentery.—The term dysentery (Gr. = difficult + intestine) is nonspecific and connotes simply a disorder of the colon attended by frequent bowel movements with blood and mucus in the stool. The caption bacillary dysentery signifies an inflammation of the colon by *Shigella dysenteriæ*, *Shigella paradysenteriæ*, and *Shigella sonnei* (Macumber). These are gram-negative, non-motile bacilli that are distinguishable from each other and from other gram-negative intestinal bacilli by carbohydrate fermentations and antigenic reactions. The disease is worldwide in *distribution* occurring in endemic and epidemic forms and being transmitted by way of contaminated food and water.

Pathologically, not only is the entire colon usually affected but the small intestine is involved in about two-thirds of the cases. As in typhoid and paratyphoid fever, the lymphoid structures first disclose hypertrophy and then ulceration. As the latter progresses the ulcers extend beyond the confines of the lymphoid tissue producing widespread confluent denudations of most of the mucosa. The ulcers are superficial, sharp, and not undermined. They rarely extend into the muscle layers and, in about one-half of the cases, are covered with a gray pseudodiphtheritic membrane. *Histologically*, as grossly, the ulcers are nonspecific. The defects extend to the muscle layers but the leukocytic infiltrations (consisting of neutrophils, lymphocytes, and monocytes) often proceed to the serosa. The edges of the ulcers are not undermined. In older, more extensive lesions, granulation tissue may project from the floors of the defects. Healing occurs by resolution, fibrosis, and re-epithelization.

The *complications* comprise toxicity, dehydration, electrolytic imbalance, and fibrous stricture of the colon with resultant intestinal obstruction. The *clinical manifestations* consist of combinations of diarrhea, abdominal cramps, blood and mucus in the stool, fever, vomiting, tenesmus, nausea, chills, and convulsions. A definitive *diagnosis* is made by isolating the causative organisms from the stool. *Treatment* is symptomatic together with administration of antibiotics (Garfinkel). The *prognosis* is variable with the recorded mortality ranging between 1 and 50 per cent.

Cholera.—Cholera (Gr. = bile) is an acute infectious disease characterized by severe diarrhea, dehydration, and shock-like state. It occurs endemically, epidemically, and pandemically in Eastern Asia and India (Mackie and Strong). The *causative* organism is the *Vibrio choleræ*—a gram-negative, actively motile, ærobic, comma-shaped bacillus that grows readily on ordinary media. It produces a powerful endotoxin (liberated upon disintegration of the organism) that is responsible for the desquamation of the epithelial cells and the toxic symptoms. The route of the infection is ingestion of contaminated food and water and the sources of the organisms are healthy human carriers, infected persons during the incubation period, and patients with the disease.

Pathologically, the morphologic changes are rather disappointing. The chief intestinal alterations are found in the lower part of the ileum. They consist of simply a diffuse congestion of the bowel wall with superficial desquamation of the epithelial cells. The lumens of the small and large intestines contain either rice water stool or brownish fluid material with a foul odor. The tissues of the rest of the body are characteristically dry, sticky, and dark in color. The blood within the cardiovascular system is dark red, jelly-like, and viscid. The bladder is devoid of urine and the renal changes are those of toxic nephrosis (p. 814). The chief *complications* are dehydration, hemoconcentration, and uremia. The *clinical manifesta-*

tions are due to absorption of endotoxins and to dehydration. The disease is generally divided into the following four stages: (1) *incubation stage*—of three to four days' duration, (2) *evacuation stage*—characterized by an abrupt onset of purging diarrhea (with rice water stool), vomiting, muscle cramps, hemoconcentration, cyanosis, and fever to 102° F., (3) *algid* or *collapse stage*—characterized by complete exhaustion with almost complete cessation of circulation (unobtainable pulse and blood pressure and faintly audible heart sounds), rapid and shallow respirations, hypothermia, uremia, coma, and often death, (4) *reaction stage*—characterized by lessening of symptoms and ultimately recovery. The *diagnosis* is readily made from the clinical manifestations during an epidemic but in all cases a definitive diagnosis is made by isolating the *Vibrio choleræ* either in smears of stool or on culture media. *Treatment* is symptomatic with chief emphasis on prevention of dehydration and restoring the electrolytic balance. The *prognosis* is guarded for in epidemics the average mortality is about 50 per cent.

Ulcerative Colitis.—Ulcerative colitis is commonly *known* as chronic ulcerative colitis, nonspecific ulcerative colitis, and colitis gravis. It is a relatively common disorder that occurs in the third and fourth decades of life, affects both sexes with approximately equal frequency, and is found in most races with perhaps a slight preponderance in Hebrews (Sloan and Warren). The specific *cause* remains unknown. The more important of the many theories proposed to explain its origin are as follows: (1) *infections*—due to streptococci, colon bacilli, organisms of the bacillary dysentery group, and a virus, (2) *allergy*—consisting of sensitivity to various foods, (3) *dietary deficiencies*—especially avitaminosis, and (4) *psychosomatic factors*—high-strung personality, emotional upset, etc. (Bassler). Of these, the last mentioned appears to be the most plausible.

Pathologically any part of the large intestine along with the terminal portion of the small intestine may be affected. In a study of 109 cases, Warren noted an involvement of the following portions of the intestinal tract in decreasing order of frequency: sigmoid colon, descending colon, transverse colon, rectum, ascending colon, cecum, and ileum. In the early stages the mucosa is hyperemic and moist, is covered with blood and mucus, and discloses petechiæ. The ulcers vary from punctate defects to large, irregular, coalescing craters involving most of the mucosa (Fig. 358). Usually they are irregularly scattered throughout the mucosa but sometimes they are arranged in three or four longitudinal rows that may be located directly opposite the tæniæ coli. As a rule, they penetrate only to the submucosa but occasionally they may extend into and through the muscle layers. The mucosa between the ulcers becomes hypertrophied and pseudopolypoid and the wall, in time, becomes thickened to as much as 2 cm. It is friable and somewhat contracted and discloses edema of its serosa. The *histologic* changes are not specific. The ulcers are generally surrounded by granulation tissue that contains plasma cells, lymphocytes, monocytes, and eosinophils. The vessels may disclose necrosis, inflammation, and thrombosis. The mucosa between the ulcers discloses hypertrophy with prominence of the underlying submucosal lymph follicles. As the lesions age, the muscle coast become hypertrophied. Ultimately, healing occurs by resolution, fibrosis, and re-epithelization. The wall, however, becomes permanently thickened.

The more important *complications* listed by Sloan in a study of 2,000 cases are as follows: (1) polyposis—19.4 per cent, (2) stricture—11.1 per cent, (3) anal infection—6 per cent, (4) carcinoma—5.4 per cent, (5) perforation of the bowel with or without fistulous tract formation—4.3 per cent, and (6) massive hemorrhage—1.1 per cent. Other complications consist of malnutrition, hepatic disorders (fatty change, necrosis, and cirrhosis), pyelonephritis, pancreatic dystrophy, thrombosis, focal necrosis of the skin, and arthritis (Warren and Brown). The more important *clinical manifestations* consist of diarrhea with blood and mucus in the stool, abdominal cramps or pain, tenesmus, fever, weakness, tachycardia, malnutrition, and mental abnormalities (Warren). The *diagnosis* is made from the clinical manifestations, sigmoidoscopic examination, roentgenographic barium enema studies, and ruling out other conditions (parasitic,

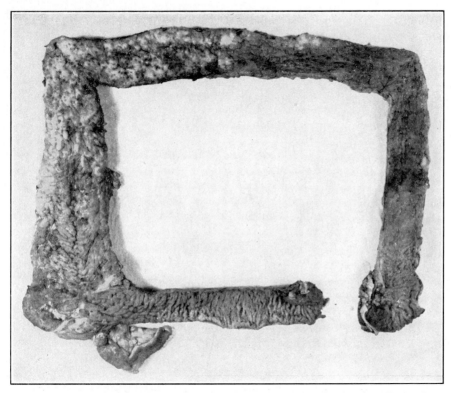

Fig. 358.—Chronic ulcerative colitis disclosing involvement of the entire colon and terminal ileum with irregular ulcers in all stages of development.

etc.) by examination of the stool (Sloan). *Treatment* is primarily medical, consisting of dietary management, sedation, psychotherapy, and administration of antibiotics (Paulley). Surgical treatment, in the form of colectomy, should be performed only in patients in whom severe complications develop (Brown). The *prognosis* is guarded for the disease is characterized by prolonged remissions and a tendency to relapse. Still, the over-all prognosis is good for in a study of 2,000 patients Sloan recorded a ten-year or longer survival in 71 per cent of cases. Most of the *deaths* occur within the first year with the usual causes being pneumonia, peritonitis, perforation of the bowel, metastatic abscess, pulmonary embolism, and cancerous transformation.

Nonspecific Granuloma.—This condition consists of a piled up mass of colonic granulation tissue in varying stages of fibrosis and necrosis (Rankin).

Its *cause* is irritation by a foreign body (inspissated feces, fishbone, ligatures, abdominal trauma, etc.) and the presence of a low-grade bacterial (staphylococcic, colon bacillus, etc.) infection. When the bacteria are staphylococci, the condition is referred to as *botryomycosis* or *staphylococcic actinophytosis* (Kimmelstiel). *Pathologically* the lesion may affect any segment of the large bowel but is more common in the cecal area. It generally involves all of the coats of the gut but, in its thickest portion, extends into the pericolonic tissues (Fig. 359). In over-all size it may measure 15 cm. or more in diameter. It is composed of a mass of granulation and fibrous tissue permeated with multiple, intercommunicating abscesses

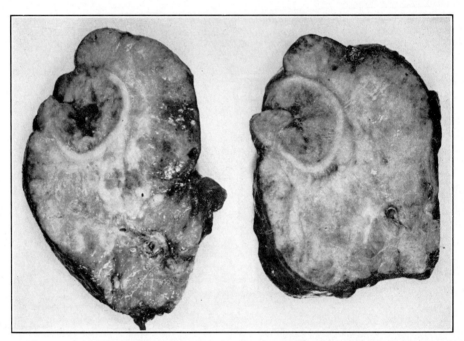

Fig. 359.—Cross section of a nonspecific granuloma of the sigmoid colon demonstrating massive colonic and pericolonic permeation with sclerotic fibrous tissue containing irregular abscesses.

that may contain actinomycotic-like granules. The lumen of the bowel is usually encroached upon and the mucosa is often ulcerated. *Histologically* the mass consists of collections of lymphocytes, plasma cells, monocytes, and neutrophils often containing peripheral giant cells of the foreign body type and surrounded by masses of dense collagenous fibrous tissue. When frank abscesses occur they are apt to contain circumscribed bodies composed centrally of clumps of bacteria and peripherally of club-like excrescences or a hyaline membrane. The chief *complication* is intestinal obstruction. The *clinical manifestations* consist of bouts of abdominal discomfort or pain, constipation, loss of appetite, loss of weight, anemia, and a palpable tumor mass. Roentgenographically a filling defect that is indistinguishable from that produced by carcinoma is readily demonstrable. The *diagnosis* can be made only pathologically. *Treatment* is surgical excision. The *prognosis* is good.

Barium Sulfate Granuloma.—A *barium sulfate granuloma*, as the term suggests, is a tissue reaction to barium sulfate (Mendeloff and Kay). Two sources of barium and its salts in man are (1) inhalation in miners and lithopane industry and (2) ingestion from usage in diagnostic gastrointestinal roentgenography. The former accounts for a benign form of *pneumoconiosis* called *baritosis* while the latter produces inflammatory lesions in the esophagus, stomach, appendix, large bowel, or *peritoneum*. When the *gastrointestinal tract* is intact the barium sulfate passes through innocuously but when it is abraded, ulcerated, or perforated the material escapes into the tissues where it produces a granulomatous reaction (Fig. 360). The

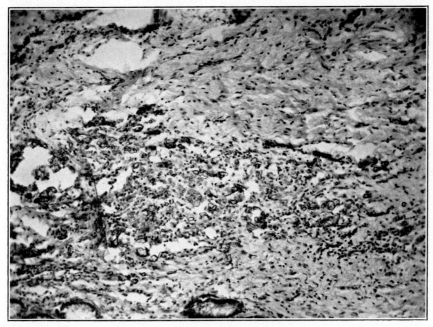

FIG. 360.—Barium sulfate granuloma in the wall of the colon showing crystals surrounded by leukocytes and fibroblasts. × 100.

most characteristic feature of the lesion is the presence of pale, yellow, amorphous crystals of barium sulfate which can be seen with both ordinary and polarized light. They are surrounded by fibroblasts and histiocytes and fewer numbers of plasma cells and lymphocytes. Occasionally, foreign body giant cells are also present but tubercle formation does not occur.

Oleogranuloma.—This is usually a rectal tumor-like mass of granulation and fibrous tissue that *arises* as a result of (1) intrahemorrhoidal injection of sclerosing solutions containing olive, mineral, or cottonseed oil as an excipient or (2) intrarectal instillation of warm petroleum postoperatively (Susnow). *Pathologically* the lesion resembles a nonspecific granuloma (see preceding section) with the exception that foam cells together with droplets of oil surrounded by foreign body giant cells are seen microscopically. The chief *complication* is rectal obstruction. The *clinical manifestations* consist of a sense of weight or pain in the pelvis together with increasing constipation. The *diagnosis* may be made from the history and rectal examination. *Treatment* is surgical excision. The *prognosis* is good.

Parasitic Infections.—The more important parasites that may be considered in connection with the large intestine are *Endamœba histolytica*,

49

Endamœba coli, Balantidium coli, Enterobius vermicularis, Trichocephalus trichiurus, Schistosoma mansoni, Schistosoma japonicum, and *Schistosoma hæmatobium* (Sawitz, and Craig and Faust).

Endamœba histolytica is a protozoa of worldwide distribution. It exists both in a trophozoite and a cystic stage (Fig. 361*A* and *B*). *Trophozoites* measure from 18 to 25 microns in diameter. They disclose a peripheral clear ectoplasm and a central granular endoplasm. The latter contains a round nucleus with a centrally placed karyosome and sometimes erythrocytes. When the amebæ are degenerating the endoplasm may also contain vacuoles and bacteria. Movement is by means of pseudopodia and multiplication occurs by binary fission. *Cysts* are round structures measuring

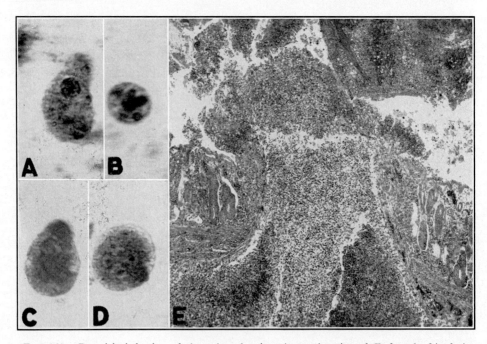

Fig. 361.—Parasitic infection of the colon showing *A*, trophozoite of *Endamœba histolytica*, *B*, cyst of *Endamœba histolytica*, *C*, trophozoite of *Endamœba coli*, *D*, cyst of *Endamœba coli* each × 1380, and *E*, an amebic ulcer of the mucosa of the colon with distinctly undermined edges. × 10.

from 3.5 to 20 microns in diameter. The wall is refractive. The cytoplasm is granular and, depending upon the stage of development, discloses two to four nuclei that are similar to those in the trophozoite stage. The less mature cysts contain rod-like chromatoidal bodies, the nature of which remains undetermined. *Man* becomes *infected* by ingesting food or water contaminated with cysts. The latter pass through the stomach, shed their covering in the small intestine, and are carried to the cecum, sigmoid colon, and rectum as trophozoites. In these areas the trophozoites attach themselves to the mucosa, dissolve the epithelial cells by liberating proteolytic enzymes, and, by means of their own motility, penetrate to the submucosa. Here they multiply and concomitantly dissolve adjacent tissues to produce small, essentially sterile abscesses. In time, the abscesses reach the surface resulting in the formation of ulcers with undermined edges (Fig. 361*E*)

Once the surface is penetrated the ulcers become secondarily infected and are then permeated with numerous neutrophils and other leukocytes. The dissolution of submucosal tissue is also accompanied by erosion of veins enabling the trophozoites to enter the venous channels and produce abscesses in the liver and, less commonly, other organs of the body. Cysts of *Endamœba histolytica* are found in formed stool but trophozoites are present only in liquid stool. The *incubation period* varies from a few days to years. The *clinical manifestations* are similar to those in bacillary dysentery (p. 765). The *diagnosis* is made by identifying the organisms in the stool or in smears or biopsies of the mucosa of the colon (Fig. 362). *Treatment* consists of administration of combinations of carbarsone, diodoquin, viofrom, and emetine hydrochloride. The *prognosis* in general is good.

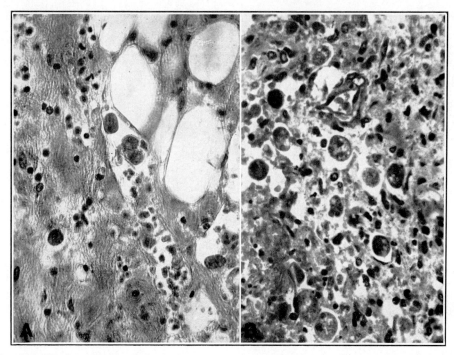

Fig. 362.—Endamoeba histolytica in *A*, a smear and *B*, a biopsy of the mucosa of the colon. × 400.

Endamœba coli is also an intestinal protozoa and exists in both the trophozoite and cystic stage (Fig. 361*C* and *D*). *Trophozoites* measure from 20 to 30 microns in diameter, are sluggishly motile, contain food vacuoles and bacteria, and possess a single nucleus with a coarsely granular membrane and an eccentric karyosome. The *cysts* measure from 10 to 30 microns in diameter, disclose from one to eight (occasionally sixteen) nuclei and may reveal chromatoidal bodies. The life cycle is similar to that of *Endamœba histolytica* but the organisms feed on intestinal contents, do not invade the mucosa, and are not pathogenic.

Balantidium coli is an intestinal protozoa of man, monkey, and pig and is worldwide in distribution. *Trophozoites* measure approximately 75 × 55 microns (Fig. 363*A*). They are ovoid, are covered with cilia, disclose a lateral cytostome (mouth), reveal food and two contractile vacuoles, and contain a large kidney-shaped macronucleus with an adjacent small round micronucleus. *Cysts* measure about 15 microns in diameter, possess a doubly refractile membrane, and contain a macronucleus embedded in granular cytoplasm (Fig. 363*B*). The *life cycle* is similar to that of *Endamœba histolytica*. Trophozoites may live in the lumen of the large intestine off the fecal contents or they may penetrate the mucosa, producing

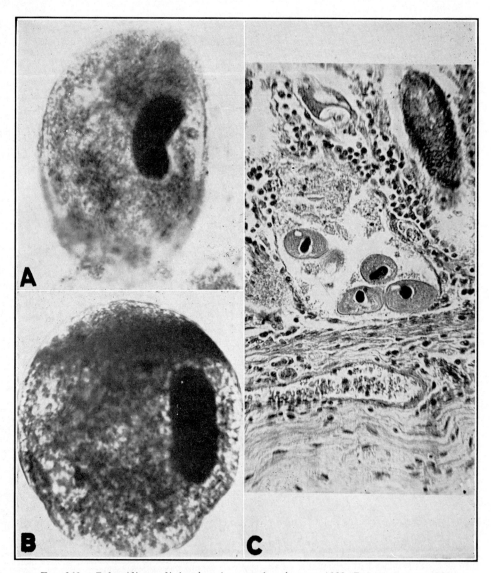

FIG. 363.—*Balantidium coli* showing *A*, a trophozoite. × 1380, *B*, a cyst. × 1380, and *C*, trophozoites in the depths of the mucosa. × 300.

colonic lesions and clinical manifestations similar to those in amebiasis (Fig. 363*C*). The *diagnosis* is made by finding trophozoites in liquid stool and cysts in formed stool. There is no specific *treatment*. The *prognosis* is good for the infection usually disappears spontaneously in due course.

Enterobius vermicularis (*pinworm*) is a common round worm of worldwide distribution but more common in warm climates. The *female* measures 8 to 13 mm. in length and has an attenuated tail while the *male* measures 2 to 5 mm. in length and has a curved tail (Fig. 364*A* and *B*). Each lacks an oral cavity but possesses a buccal capsule with three labia and a pair of lateral alæ. The adult worms inhabit the cecum, terminal ileum, and appendix, attaching themselves to the mucosa by the buccal capsule. The females remain here until they become gravid, at which time they migrate

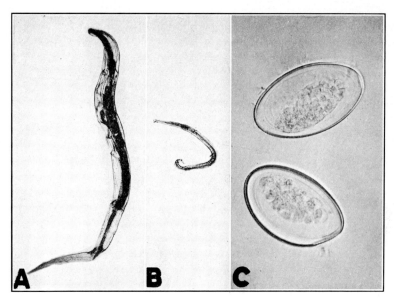

Fig. 364.—*Enterobius vermicularis* illustrating *A*, a female worm, *B*, a male worm, and *C*, ova. × 100.

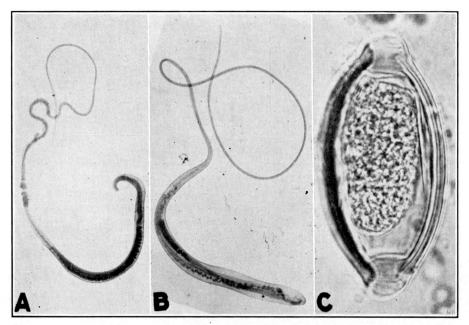

Fig. 365.—*Trichocephalus trichiurus* showing *A*, a male worm, *B*, a female worm, and *C*, an ovum. × 1380.

to the anus and perineum and deposit ova in the sinuous tracts of this region. The *ova* are ovoid and measure about 55 × 25 microns (Fig. 364C). They possess an outer hyaline shell and contain an embryo. From the anus and perineum the ova are carried to the mouth by the fingers, hatch in the jejunum, and develop into adult worms in the ileocecal portion of the gut. The usual *clinical manifestations* consist of perianal itching. Occasionally the worms may produce mild intestinal irritation and diarrhea or may cause symptoms of appendicitis. The *diagnosis* is made by identifying the worms or ova microscopically. The latter can be picked up from the anus or perineum by applying Scotch tape to the integument. *Treatment* consists of oral administration of medicinal gentian violet or quinacrine hydrochloride. The *prognosis* is good.

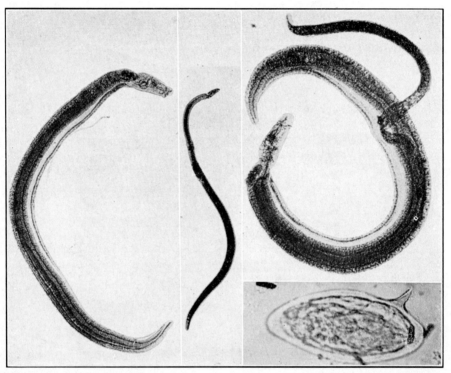

FIG. 366.—*Schistosoma mansoni* disclosing an adult male and female worm, an adult male and female worm in the copulatory state, and an ovum with a lateral spine. × 300.

Trichocephalus trichiurus is a round worm of worldwide distribution but more common in moist warm climates. The worms measure from 30 to 50 mm. in length, are attenuated in their anterior three-fifths, and are fleshy in their posterior two-fifths (Fig. 365A and B). The male can readily be differentiated from the female by its curved posterior portion. The worms live in the ileocecal region of the gut where the fertilized female deposits about 6,000 ova a day. The ova are barrel-shaped, measure about 50 × 22 microns, and possess bipolar, plug-like prominences (Fig. 365C). They are passed in the feces in the unsegmented stage, requiring an outside sojourn of about three weeks before developing embryos. The embryonated eggs are infective for man, are swallowed as contaminants of food and water, hatch in the small intestine, develop into adult worms, and repeat the cycle. The *clinical manifestations* are few, consisting of diarrhea and vague abdominal discomfort. Rarely the worms may block the appendix and cause symptoms of appendicitis. The *diagnosis* is made by finding the ova in the stool. *Treatment* consists of oral administration of *leche de higueron* or ferric ammonium citrate. The *prognosis* is good.

Schistosoma mansoni is a blood fluke that is prevalent in Africa and tropical America. The *male* worm measures from 6.4 to 9.9 mm. in length, is covered with integumentary tubercles, possesses two suckers, and exhibits a longitudinal ventral gynecophoral canal for holding the female during copulation and oviposition (Fig. 366). The *female* is long and slender, measures 7.2 to 14 mm. in length, discloses few and small integumentary

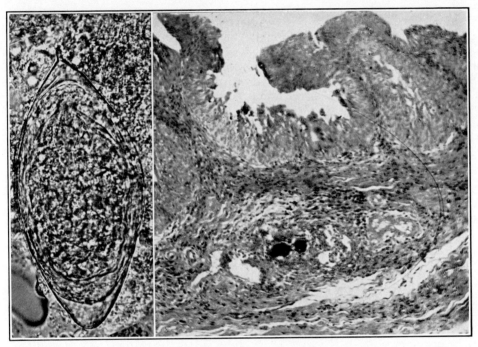

FIG. 367.—*Schistosoma hæmatobium* illustrating an ovum with a terminal spine. × 400, and a granuloma beneath the mucosa of the bladder. × 100.

tubercles, possesses small suckers, and has complicated genitals. The *ova* measure about 150 × 55 microns, have a brownish transparent shell, and disclose a lateral spine. The *mature worms* are found in the mesenteric venules draining the large bowel and, less commonly, in the branches of the superior mesenteric vein, the vesical veins, and the intrahepatic veins. The ova are deposited in the venules and either break through the venous walls into the tissues or the lumen of the large intestine or are carried by the blood into the liver. In the tissues and liver they produce frank abscesses or granulomas similar to those caused by *Schistosoma hæmatobium* (Fig. 367). The granulomas consist of collections of neutrophils, eosinophils, and giant cells and, later, of fibroblasts. The abscesses and granulomas of the bowel break through the mucosa producing ulcers. By the time the ova are discharged in the feces they are mature and hatch when the feces reaches water, producing miracidia. After a sojourn in appropriate snails, the miracidia are transformed into cercariæ. These are infective for man, penetrate the skin, develop into metacercariæ, and are carried through the heart and lungs to all tissues of the body. Only those metacercariæ that reach the mesenteric vessels survive. They are carried to the liver where they mature and then migrate against the current to the tributaries of the portal vein, especially those of the large bowel. The *clinical manifestations* are those of (1) dysentery (due to ulceration of the large intestine), (2) pneumonitis (due to migration of metacercariæ through the lungs), (3) pylephlebitis and cirrhosis of the liver (due to the lodgment of organisms and ova in the portal system), and (4) hypochromic microcytic anemia (due to the feeding of the worms on the blood). The *diagnosis* is made by identifying ova in the stool or in a piece of tissue from the ulcer removed sigmoidoscopically. *Treatment* consists of administration of antimony compounds. The *prognosis* is good in early or lightly infected cases but is poor in advanced cases, especially in the presence of cirrhosis.

Schistosoma japonicum is confined to the Far East and affects not only man but also dogs, cats, mice, and cattle. The male worms measure 12 to 20 mm. in length and the female worms measure approximately 26 mm. in length. The ova measure about 85 × 60 microns and possess a faint terminal spine that ordinarily is invisible. The life cycle, clinical manifestations, etc., are similar to those in *Schistosoma mansoni*.

Schistosoma hæmatobium produces vesical schistosomiasis or bilharziasis. The male worms measure from 10 to 50 mm. in length and the female worms measure about 20 mm. in length. The ova measure about 140 × 50 microns and possess a terminal spine (Fig. 367). The life cycle is similar to that of *Schistosoma mansoni* with the exception that the adult worms ultimately lodge in the vesical and paravesical veins and the ova are discharged in the urine. Thus, granulomas are produced in the urinary bladder (Fig. 367) and the local clinical manifestations are vesical rather than rectal.

Anal Inflammation.—Inflammation of the anus is often accompanied by inflammation of the integument of the adjacent perineum and inflammation of the lower portion of the rectum. Since this area of the body is constantly bathed by bacteria-laden feces, is near the genitals (especially in the female), and is often subjected to trauma, the inflammations are varied and frequent. The ordinary *venereal diseases* are syphilis, gonorrhea, chancroid, granuloma inguinale, and lymphogranuloma venereum (Ault). Each of these is considered in appropriate places in the text. Other inflammations are generally grouped according to the lesions they produce rather than according to the causative agents (Cantor and Smith). Thus, inflammation of the crypts of Morgagni is called *cryptitis* and inflammation of the papillæ is known as *papillitis*. An *anal ulcer* or *fissure* is a radial tear or crack in the skin of the anus extending downward from the pectinate line. A *sinus* is a straight or sinuous tract with one end communicating with the anus or lower portion of the rectum and the other end extending into the adjacent tissues. A *fistula* is similar to a sinus but with both ends of the tract communicating with the anus, rectum, other hollow organs, or skin. An *abscess* is a localized collection of pus that does not communicate with the anus, rectum, or skin. Abscesses in this area are classified according to their anatomic locations as *perianal, perirectal, ischio-anal, ischiorectal, infralevator, supralevator*, etc. Regardless of the type of inflammation, the *predisposing causes* are anal crypts, anal glands, and trauma from hard fecal material. The *precipitating causes* are bacteria. Most often they consist of bacilli of the colon group and of streptococci but any pyogenic organisms may be involved. *Mycobacterium tuberculosis* (originating in a primary focus elsewhere in the body) is an infrequent cause accounting for less than 10 per cent of all cases (Jackman). The most important *clinical manifestations* are exquisite pain and tenderness. The *diagnosis* is made by (1) external and proctoscopic examination, (2) bacteriological studies, and (3) biopsy. *Treatment* is surgical excision or incision with administration of antibiotics. The *prognosis* is generally good.

PHYSICAL DISTURBANCES

Orientation.—In this section the following unrelated conditions may be included: fistulas, foreign bodies, pneumatosis (p. 724), perforation, intussusception, volvulus, infarction appendices epiploicæ, obstruction, rectal prolapse and procidentia, hemorrhoids, melena, and coccydynia.

Fistulas.—Fistulas of the large intestine may connect any portion of the large bowel with an adjacent hollow organ or skin (Wyndham, Mayfield, Gorsch, and Lichtman). The organs secondarily affected are the urethra, bladder, ureter, renal pelvis, vagina, uterus, fallopian tube, appendix, small intestine, stomach, gallbladder, bile duct, peritoneal cavity, pleural cavity, and bronchi. The fistulas are named after the structures connected as, for example, recto-urethral, rectovesical, sigmoidovesical, ureterocolic, rectovaginal, gastrojejunocolic, etc. The usual *causes* are (1) *congenital anomalies*—present in connection with the rectum and lower urinary and genital tracts (p. 762), (2) *degenerations*—found in conjunction with obstructive and other disorders of the bowel, (3) *inflammations*—seen especially in connection with appendiceal abscess, diverticulitis, tuberculosis, actinomycosis, etc., (4) *physical disturbances*—encompassing such conditions as foreign body, trauma, irradiation necrosis, and hernias, and (5) *tumors*— usually carcinoma and occurring primarily in the large intestine or in other organs such as the vagina, cervix, uterus, urinary bladder, stomach, etc.

Foreign Bodies.—Foreign bodies gain entrance into the large intestine by being swallowed or by being inserted from below. Some of the diverse objects that have been encountered are snuff box, whisky glasses, mortar pestle, ox horn, electric light bulbs, ink bottle, petroleum jelly bottle, cold cream jar, lemon, apple, chicken bones, glass tube, portion of a broom handle, pig's tail, Seven-up and other bottles, and a tool box containing a piece of gun barrel, a screwdriver, two hack saws, a boring syringe, a file, several coins, thread, and tallow (Macht). The chief *complications* are trauma to the mucosa and bowel wall, ulceration, inflammation, hemorrhage, perforation, and intestinal obstruction. The *clinical manifestations* are those of the complications. The *diagnosis* is made from the history, symptoms and signs, roentgenographic studies, and proctosigmoidoscopic examination. *Treatment* is removal, either surgical or by way of the lumen of the bowel. The *prognosis* in general is good.

Perforation.—By perforation of the large bowel is meant any complete and, for the most part, sudden loss of continuity of the bowel wall. The lesions may be divided into spontaneous and traumatic. *Spontaneous* perforations occur as a result of some pathologic change in the bowel wall and are unassociated with trauma (Woodruff). They may be located in the bowel wall (usually limited to the cecum) proximal to a point of obstruction (p. 224) or they may be found at the site of the disease process. The latter includes such disorders as diverticulitis, carcinoma, ulcerative colitis, dysentery, tuberculosis, and simple ulcers. Rarely, spontaneous perforation occurs without any obvious cause (Weinstein). In civilian life *traumatic* perforations occur as a result of (1) blunt blows such as sustained in automobile accidents, falls, kicks, high dives, etc., or (2) penetrating wounds such as encountered in connection with foreign bodies, instrumentations, stabbings, and shootings. In military life they may also result from blunt blows but they are due most often to penetration of bullets, missiles, or other products of firearms (Roettig). *Pathologically* any portion of the bowel wall may be affected with the exact site or sites, size, and appearance of the lesion varying with the causative agent. The *complications* are shock, hemorrhage, peritonitis, fecal fistulas, cicatricial stenosis, abdominal adhesions, and concomitant injury to other organs. The more important *clinical manifestations* are abdominal pain, vomiting, trauma, abdominal distention and rigidity, absence of peristaltic sounds, elevated pulse rate, slight fever, low blood pressure, anemia (in cases of hemorrhage), and external wounds (in cases of trauma). The *diagnosis* is made from the history, clinical manifestations, and the finding of gas roentgenographically in the peritoneal cavity. *Treatment* consists of operative repair and the administration of antibiotics. The *prognosis* is variable depending upon the cause, extent of the lesion, presence or absence of associated injuries, rapidity of treatment, etc. The over-all mortality rate is about 20 per cent.

Intussusception.—The most common site of intussusception of the large intestine is in the ileocecal region with the lower portion of the ileum protruding into the cecum and ascending colon (p. 726). Intussusception of large intestine into large intestine is rare due chiefly to the absence of a long mesentery. While a colocolic invagination may occur (Jacobson) the most common lesion is a sigmoidorectal intussusception (Granet). Unlike in the small intestine, most instances of the latter lack a mucosal tumor as the predisposing cause. Instead the *pathogenesis* appears to be (1) abnormal mobility of the sigmoid colon due to its long mesentery, (2) fixation of the rectum and rectosigmoid by the pelvic and sacral fascias, and (3) the relatively narrow caliber of the sigmoid as compared with the large caliber of the rectum. Once the *invagination* is under way its progress is enhanced by repeated straining on the part of the patient. In advanced cases the telescoping may be of such a degree that the intussusceptum appears at the anus. The *complications* are (1) partial to complete intestinal obstruction, (2) gangrene with ultimate sequestration of the intussusceptum and autoanastomosis of the segments of gut affected, and (3) cicatricial stenosis at the site of the autoanastomosis. The *clinical manifestations* consist of a sense of incomplete evacuation of the bowel, constipation, passage of glairy or bloodstained mucus, dull pain, or flatulence. The *diagnosis* is established by roentgenographic and proctosigmoidoscopic studies. *Treatment* in chronic cases of sigmoidorectal intussusception with partial obstruction is reduction by enema, sedation, and maintenance of adequate bulk of stool by administration of hydrophilic preparations. Treatment in acute cases or chronic cases with complete obstruction is surgical reduction and, if necessary, resection. The ultimate *prognosis* is generally good.

Volvulus.—Volvulus of the large intestine is uncommon, especially in the United States where the diet is low in residue (Michel). It occurs most frequently in the sigmoid colon (about 90% of cases), less commonly in the cecum (less than 10% of cases), and only rarely in the transverse colon. The condition is found in patients of an average age of between fifty and sixty years, is about twice as common in males as it is in females, and has no predilection for any particular race (except in so far as diet is concerned). The disorder *arises* as a result of excessive motility of the affected part of the bowel due to a long and freely movable mesentery, increase in length of the intestinal loop, and close proximity of points of fixation at each end of the intestinal loop. *Pathologically* the twist may be clockwise or counter-clockwise and is generally significant only after it rotates more than 180° (Dean). The *effects* upon the bowel consist of obstruction of the lumen and strangulation from occlusion of the blood supply. The latter results in gangrene of the bowel, perforation, and peritonitis. In most cases there is a previous *history* of episodes of crampy abdominal pain, constipation, and local distention. Sooner or later an acute volvulus occurs and is ushered in with (1) sudden severe crampy abdominal pain, (2) inability to pass feces or flatus, (3) nausea and vomiting, (4) abdominal distention and tenderness, and (5) fever, shock, etc., when complications occur. The *diagnosis* is made from the history and clinical manifestations. *Treatment* consists of surgical detorsion or, if necessary, resection. The *prognosis* is guarded for mortality rates as high as 59 per cent have been recorded (Dean).

Infarction Appendices Epiploicæ.—The appendices epiploicæ are serosal covered collections of fat located in one to three rows between the tæniæ coli and measuring from a few millimeters to 15 cm. in length (Rosenbaum). They are more conspicuous in obese people, especially those who have recently lost weight. Their function is to act as protective agents in a manner similar to the omentum. *Pathologically* they may be subjected to inflammation, torsion, and carcinomatous implantation. Of these, *torsion* is the most common and, therefore, the most important. The *cause* remains obscure although increase in length of the veins as compared with the arteries, inflammation, adhesions, and mechanical factors in conjunction with hernia are thought to be of etiologic significance. The *complications* of torsion are gangrene, fibrosis, and detachment with formation of fatty and fibrous foreign bodies in the peritoneum. The *clinical manifestations* are those of appendicitis. The *diagnosis* is usually made at laparotomy. *Treatment* consists of surgical excision after the abdomen has generally been opened under a mistaken diagnosis. The *prognosis* is good.

Obstruction.—Obstructive lesions of the large intestine are protean with virtually every known disease process being capable of participating. Some of the more important *causes* may be listed as follows: (1) *congenital anomalies*—enterogenous cysts, megacolon, diverticula (inflamed), and imperforate anus, (2) *inflammations*—ulcerative colitis, regional colitis, tuberculosis, fungous and yeast-like colitis, nonspecific granuloma, oleo-granuloma, parasitic infection, and lymphogranuloma venereum, (3) *physical disturbances*—foreign bodies, intussusception, volvulus, herniation, and fecal impaction, and (4) *tumors*—especially carcinoma. The path-ologic changes, complications, etc., are similar to those outlined in connec-tion with obstruction of the small intestine (p. 728).

Rectal Prolapse and Procidentia.—While there is some confusion in terminology, *rectal prolapse* generally means a protrusion of the rectal mucosa through the anus, while *rectal procidentia* refers to a protrusion of all the layers of the rectal wall (Smith). The *causes* are (1) age—between one and five years due to immaturity of the pelvic organs and debilitating diseases and in elderly adults due to emaciation and lack of muscle tone, (2) anatomic factors—absence of sacral curve, loose perirectal tissues, high position of pelvic organs, vertical position of rectum, and elongation of the mesocolon, (3) constitutional factors—any disorder causing general muscular relaxation, (4) mechanical factors—those that drag the rectum down such as hemorrhoids, polyps, and cancer, (5) traumatic factors—any injury to the anal sphincter, and (6) increased intra-abdominal pressure. *Pathologically* the mucosa protrudes in a convex fashion. It is deep red, is covered with mucus, bleeds readily, may be superficially ulcerated, and discloses folds radiating from a central axis. Generally it protrudes more in an attempt at or after defecation and recedes completely or only partially after the act has been completed. The *clinical manifestations* consist of protrusion of a red mass after straining or defecation, discomfort or pain especially upon sitting down, excessive secretion of mucus, bleeding, and constipation. The *diagnosis* is made from the history and the appearance of the lesion. The most effective *treatment* is surgical excision of the redundant tissue. The *prognosis* is fair to good.

Hemorrhoids.—Hemorrhoids (Gr. = blood + to flow), also known as piles, are varicosities of the hemorrhoidal plexuses of veins. Although they may *occur* at any age they are by far most frequent in the third and subsequent decades of life (Gorsch). They are found in from 3 to 5 per cent of the entire population and are more common in males than in females in the ratio of 5 to 4. Some of the more important *etiologic factors* are (1) heredity—a congenital deficiency in the supporting tissue coupled with similar environmental, dietary, and occupational circumstances, (2) anatomic—upright position, lack of valves in the hemorrhoidal veins, and looseness of the hemorrhoidal plexuses, and (3) local—chronic infection, constipation, tumors, increased intra-abdominal pressure, increased venous pressure (as in heart failure and cirrhosis of the liver), etc.

Pathologically hemorrhoids are generally divided into three groups—external, internal, and mixed (Smith). *External hemorrhoids* are varicosities of the plexus of the inferior hemorrhoidal vein and are located below the anorectal line. Often (but erroneously) included in this group are anal papilloma and lipomatous or connective tissue polyps. *Internal hemorrhoids* are varices of the plexus of the superior hemorrhoidal vein and are located above the anorectal line. *Mixed hemorrhoids* are varices of the plexus of both the inferior and the superior hemorrhoidal veins. In any case, true hemorrhoids (varicosities) exist as one or more, deep red to cyanotic, soft, sessile or pedunculated, bulbous, polypoid swellings that may measure as much as 2 cm. in diameter. They are soft (unless thrombosed), are covered with intact or superficially eroded mucosa, and protrude from the anus, especially upon straining. *Histologically* they are composed essentially of dilated, thin-walled, venous channels filled with blood and generally surrounded by plasma cells, lymphocytes, monocytes, and neutrophils. The covering epithelium may be of a squamous variety (external hemorrhoids) or of a columnar type (internal hemorrhoids).

The *complications* are thrombosis, ulcerations, hemorrhage (slight to marked and repeated), and infection. The *clinical manifestations* are those of the complications and consist of various combinations of a protruding mass, pain, tenderness, constipation, tenesmus, pruritus, bleeding (especially after a bowel movement), and anemia. The *diagnosis* is made from the history and physical examination. The only effective *treatment* is active intervention in the form of injection with sclerosing solutions or surgical excision. The *prognosis* is usually good.

Melena.—Melena (grossly visible dark red or black blood mixed with stool) is a symptom and not a disease. The *causes* with the *frequency* of occurrence in a study of 293 patients by Thompson were as follows: (1) esophageal—varices 9.2 per cent, carcinoma 0.7 per cent, and adenomatous polyp 0.3 per cent, (2) gastric—carcinoma 7.8 per cent, hiatus hernia 1.7 per cent, acute alcoholism 1.4 per cent, sarcoma 0.3 per cent, and atrophic gastritis 0.3 per cent, (3) gastroduodenal—ulcer 29.7 per cent, (4) enteric—diverticulitis 1.4 per cent, duodenal polyp 0.3 per cent, and nonspecific enteritis 0.3 per cent, (5) colonic—bacterial dysentery 21.5 per cent, carcinoma 8.5 per cent, ulcerative colitis 5.5 per cent, uremic colitis 3.1 per cent, nonspecific colitis 0.3 per cent, diverticulitis 3.8 per cent, intussusception 1.4 per cent, polyposis 1.0 per cent, and stricture 0.8 per cent, and (6) miscellaneous—carcinoma of the pancreas, 0.3 per cent, carcinoma of the prostate 0.3 per cent, and splenomegaly 0.3 per cent.

Coccydynia.—Coccydynia (Gr. = coccyx + pain) means pain in the coccyx and neighboring region and is thus a symptom and not a disease. Some of the more important *causes* as outlined by Thiele are (1) infection—anal, cervical, prostatic, and epididymal, (2) trauma to the coccyx—as seen in falls, pregnancy, parturition, prolonged rides, and bumps on furniture, (3) surgical—after various surgical procedures in the anorectal region, and (4) miscellaneous—spinal cord tumor and herniated disc. To these may be added neurosis, neuritis, and myositis.

TUMORS

Orientation.—Tumors and tumor-like conditions of the large intestine and anus may *occur* at all ages but are most frequent in middle-aged and older adults. They are found in all races and have no over-all predilection for either sex. The *causes*, aside from heredity, are unknown. Chronic inflammation may predispose to some benign tumors and these, in turn, may then become malignant but a known inflammation certainly does not precede all (or, for that matter, even most) neoplasms. *Pathologically* most of the tissues normally found in the bowel wall may give rise to both a benign and a malignant tumor. The more important lesions may be listed as follows: teratoid tumors, polyps, carcinoid (p. 752), carcinoma, smooth muscle tumors, lipoma, liposarcoma, angioma, hemangioendothelioma, fibrosarcoma, neurogenic sarcoma, lymphomatous tumors, carcinoma of the colon and rectum, carcinoma of the anus, melanoblastoma, and secondary tumors. The chief *complications* are intestinal obstruction, hemorrhage, ulceration and perforation, abscess formation, peritonitis and (in cases of malignant tumors) metastasis. The *clinical manifestations* are those of the complications with combinations of the following (depending somewhat on the location and type of tumor) leading the list: melena, constipation, tenesmus, diarrhea, generalized abdominal pain, mucus in the stool, decreased caliber of stool, weakness, rectal fullness, local pain, urinary tract symptoms, abdominal distention, alternating diarrhea and constipation, anorexia, nausea and vomiting, anemia, and abdominal mass (Postlethwait). The *diagnosis* is made on the basis of the clinical manifestations, demonstration of the lesion roentgenographically (barium studies), proctosigmoidoscopic examination and biopsy, and laparotomy. *Treatment* consists of surgical excision. The *prognosis* varies with the type of lesion. It is good in benign growths and fair in malignant tumors. In addition to the general remarks just concluded, a few separate words may be said in connection with some of the more important neoplasms.

Teratoid Tumors. — This group comprises presacral lesions that have been called epidermoid cysts, dermoid cysts, and teratomas. The growths are *uncommon*, there having been about 27 cases recorded in the literature up to 1950 (Bonsar). The ages of the patients have varied from three weeks to fifty-eight years and females have outnumbered males in the ratio of 4 to 1. The lesions are of developmental *origin* but their exact pathogenesis is as difficult to explain as it is in other teratoid tumors (p. 383). *Pathologically* the growths occur between the sacrum and rectum, are cystic, contain hair and sebum but may be filled with purulent material, and usually measure up to 5 or 6 cm. in diameter. Histologically most of them are lined by squamous or ciliated epithelium and disclose epidermal appendages in their walls. Some are more complex and also contain entodermal and mesodermal elements. The chief *complication* is perineal fistulous tract formation.

Polyps. — What has been said regarding polyps, polyposis, papilloma, and adenoma in connection with the stomach (p. 679) also applies to the large intestine. The presence of numerous polyps is referred to as *polyposis* and since the latter condition is hereditary (Boehme) the caption *hereditary* or *familial polyposis* is often used. The *incidence* of polyposis is recorded as about 0.04 per cent of all patients examined proctoscopically (Schantz), while the incidence of solitary or scattered polyps is given as about 17 per cent of all patients examined (Enquist) and up to 17.2 per 10,000 hospital admissions (Sandusky). *Pathologically* the distribution of single or scattered polyps is approximately as follows: rectosigmoid 81 per cent, descending colon 13 per cent, transverse colon 5 per cent, and ascending colon 1 per cent (Klein). In diffuse polyposis the entire large bowel is generally affected. Grossly, most polyps are pedunculated, measure not more than 4 × 1 cm., possess a bulbous tip, are tan to gray, disclose an intact or at most a superficially eroded surface, and are freely movable at the base (Fig. 368*A*, *C* and *D*). Sometimes single polyps are more sessile and, rarely, they may cover a segment of mucosa that measures 8 to 10 cm. in diameter (Fig. 368). Such lesions are usually found in the rectum, are generally centrally ulcerated, and are referred to as *diffuse papillomatous polyps* or *diffuse papillomas* (Fisher). As pedunculated polyps they are, however, limited to the mucosa and do not infiltrate the underlying tissues. *Histologically* (adenomatous) polyps are composed of a core of well-vascularized connective tissue often permeated with plasma cells and lymphocytes and covered with regular but hyperplastic columnar epithelial cells in glandular formation (Fig. 368*E*). A malignant transformation is said to occur in about 15 per cent of all cases (Binkley). It is characterized by the usual alterations in shape, size, and staining qualities of the cells and although it may occur in any part of the growth it is most common at the tip or at the base. Of the two sites the latter is more readily diagnosed but is also more ominous for the cells are closer to the bowel wall and penetrate it more quickly.

Smooth Muscle Tumors. — Smooth muscle tumors may occur in any part of the gastrointestinal tract but are least common in the large bowel. The distribution in the cases studied by Anderson was stomach 65 per cent, small intestine 25 per cent, colon 3 per cent, and rectum 7 per cent. About one-half of the tumors found in the colon and rectum are benign (leiomyoma) while the other half are malignant (leiomyosarcoma). The neoplasms arise

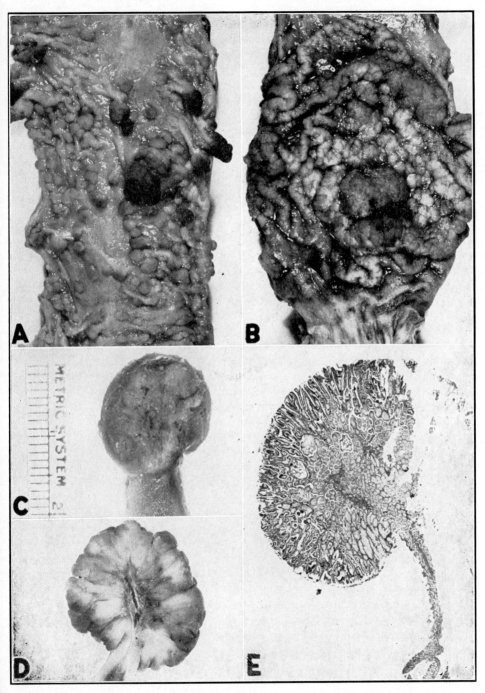

F‍IG. 368.—Adenomatous polyps of the large intestine showing *A*, numerous small sessile and pedunculated growths, *B*, a large spreading mass referred to as diffuse papilloma, *C* and *D*, surgically resected pedunculated polyps, and *E*, a photomicrograph of a small growth with a slender pedicle. × semigross.

in the muscle coats, measure up to 12 cm. or more in diameter, protrude intraluminally or extraluminally (Fig. 369*A*) and, histologically, are identical with similar tumors in the stomach (p. 677).

Lipoma.—Benign fatty tumors of the large intestine are infrequent, there having been about 152 cases recorded in the literature up to 1950 (Cavanaugh). In decreasing order of frequency they affect the transverse

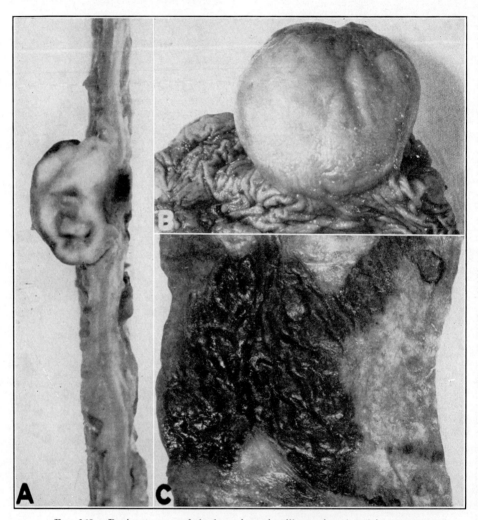

Fig. 369.—Benign tumors of the large intestine illustrating *A*, a leiomyoma, *B*, a lipoma, and *C*, a diffuse hemangioma.

colon, cecum, descending colon, sigmoid colon, ascending colon, splenic flexure, hepatic flexure, and rectum. They arise in the submucosa, protrude into the lumen, measure up to 8 or 10 cm. in diameter, and are composed of adult fat cells (Fig. 369*B*).

Angioma.—Vascular tumors of the large intestine are rare and consist essentially of hemangiomas (Babcock and Jaques). They vary in size from barely detectable to many centimeters in diameter, occur mostly in the submucosa and only rarely in the serosa and muscle coats, are single or multiple, and may be flat, pedunculated, or infiltrating (Fig. 369*C*). Histologically they are cavernous or capillary in type. The outstanding clinical manifestation is repeated hemorrhage into the lumen of the bowel.

Lymphomatous Tumors.—Lymphomatous tumors of the large intestine may be malignant (lymphosarcoma, reticulum cell sarcoma, Hodgkin's disease, giant follicular lymphoblastoma, and leukemia) or benign. The former are uncommon, affect any portion of the large intestine, and are identical with similar tumors in the small intestine (p. 737). The latter, known as *benign lymphoma* or as *benign lymphoid hyperplasia*, are common, are seen at all ages, usually occur in the anorectal region, exist as polypoid projections that are readily mistaken for hemorrhoids or adenomatous polyps, are composed of solid collections of lymphoid cells or lymph follicles, and are entirely benign (Garnet, Barba, and Heller). Their chief importance lies in the fact that, by the unwary, they may be readily confused with malignant lymphoblastoma.

Carcinoma of the Colon and Rectum.—Carcinoma of the colon and rectum is one of the more common lesions in the body, accounting for an estimated 8 per cent of all cancers. It is much more frequent than sarcoma of the colon and rectum, outnumbering the malignant mesodermal growths by a ratio of about 200 to 1 (Dunavant). Although carcinoma of the large bowel may *occur* at any age, it is usually seen after the age of forty years and is most common in the sixth and seventh decades of life (Busar and Spear). In the over-all it has no particular predilection for either sex, but in individual series of cases a slight preponderance in males has been recorded. Although nothing definite is known with regard to *cause*, many authors think that most if not all carcinomas of the large bowel arise from adenomatous polyps (Bacon). It has also been stated that chronic ulcerative colitis precedes carcinoma in about 2 per cent of cases (Shands). *Pathologically* more than one-half of the lesions occur distal to the rectosigmoid junction. In a series of 478 cases reported on by Busar, the distribution was as follows: distal to the rectosigmoid 57.7 per cent, sigmoid 13.6 per cent, descending colon 9.4 per cent, cecum 6.9 per cent, ascending colon 4.6 per cent, transverse colon 3.8 per cent, hepatic flexure 3.2 per cent, and splenic flexure 1.7 per cent. In other reports, essentially similar figures are recorded. Usually the lesion is single but in 7.5 per cent of cases multiple foci are found (Bacon). As in other portions of the gastrointestinal tract the tumors, grossly, are essentially of three varieties—fungating, ulcerating, and diffusely infiltrating (Fig. 370). *Fungating* growths are sessile, protrude into the lumen in a cauliflower-like fashion, may be superficially ulcerated, and may measure as much as 8 cm. in diameter and 3 to 4 cm. in depth. They affect the mucosa and submucosa early in the course of the disease and spare the muscle coats and serosa until the lesions are advanced. *Ulcerating* tumors penetrate the wall early in the course of their development and as they do so they cause an excavation that may extend all the way through the serosa. As the latter is approached, the tumor has a tendency to adhere to adjacent structures and thus ultimately produce fistulous tracts or abscesses. When the perforation occurs into the free peritoneal cavity, peritonitis results. *Infiltrating* growths permeate the wall of the gut circumferentially and over varying distances longitudinally. The mucosa may remain, for the most part, intact or may be superficially ulcerated. The neoplastic cells spread along the submucosa and serosa, thus causing marked accentuation of the different layers of the bowel wall. Some infiltrating tumors produce segmental narrowing of the gut. Others result in the forma-

50

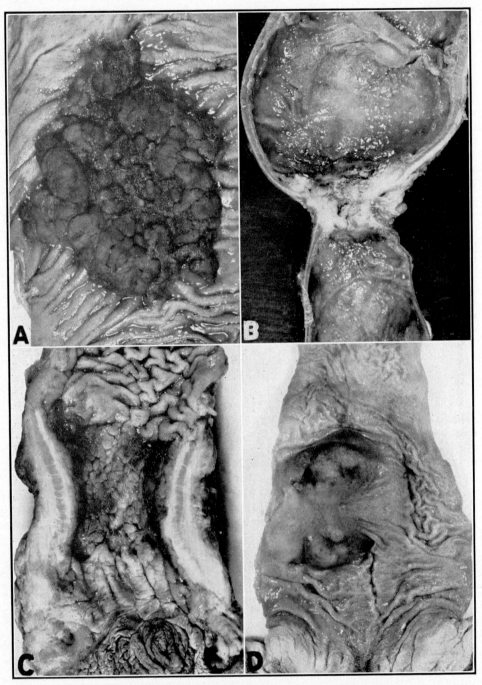

FIG. 370.—Carcinoma of the colon and rectum showing *A*, a polypoid tumor, *B*, an infiltrating and constricting growth, *C*, a diffusely infiltrating neoplasm, and *D*, an ulcerating lesion.

tion of ring-like constrictions and are referred to as napkin ring-like tumors. *Histologically* carcinoma of the colon and rectum is almost always an adeno-carcinoma with cellular types of differentiations being identical with those in the stomach (p. 680). Carcinoma of the colon and rectum *spreads* by direct extension through the wall of the gut to involve the vagina, uterus, fallopian tubes, ovaries, prostate, seminal vesicles, urinary bladder, small intestine, large intestine, stomach, and any other organ or tissue that it may contact (Knight and Taylor). In the gut itself it has a tendency to spread both proximally and distally so that neoplastic cells may be found in any of the layers (between the tissue cells or within lymphatic channels)

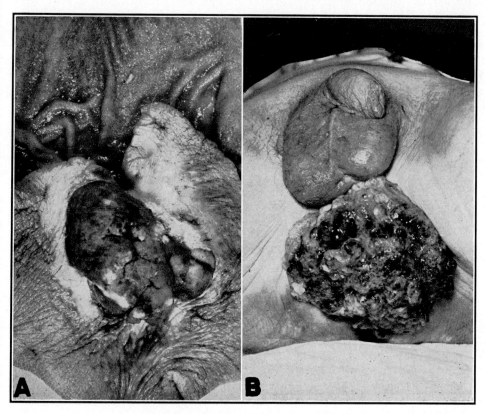

FIG. 371.—Carcinoma of the anus illustrating *A*, an ulcerating, and *B*, a fungating tumor.

as far as 7 or 8 cm. from the tumor (Connell). Spread by lymphatic channels and blood vessels generally occurs to the following organs: regional lymph nodes, liver, peritoneal cavity, lungs, bones, distant lymph nodes, and skin (Busar). The *prognosis* in cases of carcinoma of the colon and rectum is better than in cases of carcinoma of any other portion of the gastro-intestinal tract. The five-year survival rates are generally recorded as varying between 25 and 57 per cent (Busar and Spear).

Carcinoma of the Anus.—Primary carcinoma of the anus is either of a squamous or basal cell variety. *Squamous cell carcinoma* is the commoner of the two. Most patients are in the sixth decade of life and females are somewhat more frequently affected than males (Binkley). The lesions may originate in any part of the anal canal or the immediately adjacent skin but are most common posteriorly. While they may be polypoid they are usually ulcerating with the ulcers disclosing raised sloping edges and gray, rather clean floors (Fig. 371). The areas immediately surrounding the defects, both laterally and basally, are permeated with gray, firm, indurated neoplastic tissue that is ill defined and not encapsulated. Histologically the tumors are composed of keratinizing squamous cells that are generally moderately well differentiated. Spread is by direct extension to adjacent structures, by the bloodstream to distant areas, and by the lymphatics to the draining lymph nodes. Tumors that are located distal to the muco-cutaneous junction metastasize to the inguinal lymph nodes while those located proximal to this point metastasize to the perirectal and para-aortic nodes. The five-year survival rate is recorded as high as 41.5 per cent. *Basal cell carcinoma* of the anus is rare, there having been only a total of 9 cases recorded up to 1949 (Lott). The tumor is usually ulcerating and is distinguishable from squamous cell carcinoma only by biopsy.

Melanoblastoma.—Melanoblastoma (malignant melanoma) always arises in the skin of the anal canal (Raven). Lesions that occur in the rectum are secondary and represent merely upward extensions of the anal growths. The pathologic characteristics and clinical behavior are identical with similar growths in the skin of other portions of the body. The tumors are highly malignant.

Secondary Tumors.—Secondary tumors of the large intestine occur as a result of direct extension of malignant growths from adjacent organs such as (1) the prostate, urinary bladder, female genital tract, etc., to the rectum and sigmoid colon and (2) the stomach, small intestine, and gallbladder to the transverse colon, etc. Less commonly, they occur as a result of metastasis from the skin (melanoblastoma), breast, stomach, gallbladder, etc., to portions of the large intestine that are not in direct contact with the organs in which the tumor has originated. In either case, secondary tumors are important because they may mimic primary growths and because the prognosis (especially in metastatic neoplasms) is poor.

REFERENCES

Pathologic Physiology

Almy, T.: New York Acad. Sci., *58*, 398, 1954 (Constipation).
Code, C. F., *et al.*: New York Acad. Sci., *58*, 317, 1954 (Colon Motor Activities).
Douglas, D. M. and Mann, F. C.: Am. J. Digest. Dis., *6*, 434, 1939 (Gastrocolic Reflex).
Wolff, H. G., *et al.*: Tr. Am. Physicians, *62*, 192, 1949 (Emotions and Large Bowel).

Congenital Anomalies

Bacon, H. E., and Sherman, L. F.: A. M. A. Arch. Surg., *64*, 331, 1952 (Malformations Anus and Rectum).
Case, T. C., and Shea, C. E., Jr.: Am. J. Surg., *85*, 134, 1953 (Diverticulitis Cecum).
Custer, B. S., *et al.*: Ann. Surg., *124*, 508, 1946 (Enterogenous Cysts).
Geist, D. C.: Rev. Gastroenterol., *20*, 56, 1953 (Diverticulitis Cecum).
Hill, M. R., *et al.*: A. M. A. Arch. Path., *47*, 350, 1949 (Anal Ducts).
Horner, J. L.: Gastroenterology, *21*, 223, 1952 (Diverticulitis Colon).
Kratzer, G. L.: Am. J. Surg., *79*, 32, 1950 (Anal Ducts).
McGowan, F. J., and Wolff, W. I.: Gastroenterology, *21*, 119, 1952 (Diverticulitis Colon).
Moore, T. C., and Lawrence, E. A.: Surgery, *32*, 352, 1952 (Malformations Anus and Rectum).
Smith, D. W.: Am. Surg., *18*, 986, 1952 (Diverticulitis Colon).
State, E.: J. A. M. A., *149*, 350, 1952 (Megacolon).

SWENSON, O.: Pediatrics, *8*, 542, 1951 (Megacolon).
VAN ZWALENBURG, B. R.: Am. J. Roentgenol., *68*, 22, 1952 (Duplication).
WHITEHOUSE, F., *et al.:* Gastroenterology, *1*, 922, 1943 (Megacolon).

Inflammations

AULT, G. W.: Am. J. Syph., *21*, 430, 1937 (Venereal Disease of Anus and Rectum).
BASSLER, A.: Am. J. Digest. Dis., *16*, 275, 1949 (Ulcerative Colitis).
BROWN, C. H., *et al.:* Gastroenterology, *14*, 465, 1950 (Treatment Ulcerative Colitis).
BROWN, M. L., *et al.:* Am. J. Digest. Dis., *18*, 52, 1951 (Complications Ulcerative Colitis).
CANTOR, A. J.: *Ambulatory Proctology*, 2nd Ed., New York, Paul B. Hoeber, Inc., 1952.
CRAIG, C. F., and FAUST, E. C.: *Clinical Parasitology*, 5th Ed., Philadelphia, Lea & Febiger, 1951.
GARFINKEL, B. T., *et al.:* J. A. M. A., *151*, 1157, 1953 (Antibiotics in Bacillary Dysentery).
GAUSS, H.: Am. J. Digest. Dis., *13*, 213, 1946 (Mucous Colitis).
JACKMAN, R. J., and DUIE, L. A.: J. A. M. A., *130*, 630, 1946 (Anal Fistula).
KAY, S.: A.M.A. Arch. Path., *57*, 279, 1954 (Barium Sulfate Granuloma).
KIMMELSTIEL, P., and ODEN, P. W.: A. M. A. Arch. Path., *27*, 313, 1939 (Botryomycosis).
MACKIE, T. T., *et al.: Manual of Tropical Medicine*, Philadelphia, W. B. Saunders Co., p. 108, 1945 (Cholera).
MACUMBER, H. H.: A. M. A. Arch. Int. Med., *69*, 624, 1942 (Bacillary Dysentery).
MENDELOFF, J.: Am. J. Cl. Path., *26*, 155, 1956 (Barium Sulfate Granuloma).
PAULLEY, J. W.: Gastroenterology, *16*, 566, 1950 (Ulcerative Colitis).
RANKIN, F. W., *et al.: The Colon, Rectum, and Anus*, Philadelphia, W. B. Saunders Co., p. 203, 1932.
SAWITZ, W. G.: *Medical Parasitology*, New York, The Blakiston Co., 1950.
SLOAN, W. P., JR.: Gastroenterology, *16*, 25, 1950 (2,000 Cases Ulcerative Colitis).
SMITH, F. C.: *Proctology for the General Practitioner*, 4th Ed., Philadelphia, F. A. Davis Co., 1948.
STRONG, R. P.: Stitt's *Diagnosis, Prevention, and Treatment of Tropical Diseases*, 7th Ed., New York, The Blakiston Co., p. 590, 1944 (Cholera).
SUSNOW, D. A.: Am. J. Surg., *83*, 496, 1952 (Oleogranuloma).
WARREN, S., and SOMMERS, S. C.: Am. J. Path., *25*, 657, 1949 (Ulcerative Colitis).

Physical Disturbances

DEAN, D. L.: Ann. Surg., *136*, 319, 1952 (Volvulus Cecum).
DEAN, G. O., and MURRY, J. W.: Ann. Surg., *135*, 830, 1952 (Volvulus).
GORSCH, R. V.: Rev. Gastroenterol., *18*, 806, and 859, 1951 (Hemorrhoids).
————: Rev. Gastroenterol., *19*, 640, 1952 (Anorectal Fistula).
GRANET, E.: Rev. Gastroenterol., *19*, 478, 1952 (Intussusception).
JACOBSON, G., *et al.:* Am. J. Roentgenol., *68*, 198, 1952 (Intussusception).
LICHTMAN, A. L., and MCDONALD, J. R.: Surg., Gynec. & Obst., *78*, 449, 1944 (Fecal Fistula).
MACHT, S. H.: Radiology, *42*, 500, 1944 (Foreign Bodies).
MAYFIELD, L. H., and WAUGH, J. M.: Ann. Surg., *130*, 186, 1949 (Fistulas from Diverticulitis).
MICHEL, M. L., and MCCAFFERTY, E. L., JR.: South. Surg., *14*, 525, 1948 (Volvulus Colon).
ROETTIG, L. C., *et al.:* Ann. Surg., *124*, 755, 1946 (War Wounds).
ROSENBAUM, D., and KISSINGER, C. C.: Am. J. M. Sci., *219*, 427, 1950 (Infarction Appendices Epiploicæ).
SMITH, F. C.: *Proctology for the General Practitioner*, 4th Ed., Philadelphia, F. A. Davis Co., 1948.
THIELE, G. H.: Am. J. Surg., *79*, 110, 1950 (Coccydynia).
THOMPSON, H. L., and MCGUFFIN, D. W.: J. A. M. A., *141*, 1208, 1949 (Melena).
WEINSTEIN, M., and ROBERTS, M.: J. A. M. A., *149*, 1016, 1952 (Spontaneous Perforation).
WOODRUFF, M. F. A.: Ann. Surg., *135*, 221, 1952 (Spontaneous Perforation).
WYNDHAM, N.: Brit. J. Surg., *36*, 175, 1948 (Fistula).

Tumors

ANDERSON, P. A., *et al.:* Surgery, *28*, 642, 1950 (Myomatous Tumors).
BABCOCK, W. W., and JONAS, K. C.: Am. J. Surg., *80*, 854, 1950 (Hemangioma).
BACON, H. E., and LAURENS, J.: A. M. A. Arch. Surg., *62*, 705, 1951 (Metastatic Carcinoma).
BACON, H. E., and TAVENNER, M. C.: Am. J. Surg., *83*, 55, 1952 (Multiple Cancers Colon and Rectum).
BARBA W. P. II,: J. Pediat., *41*, 328, 1952 (Benign Lymphoma).

BINKLEY, G. E.: Am. J. Surg., *79*, 90, 1950 (Epidermoid Carcinoma Anus).

BINKLEY, G. E., *et al.:* J. A. M. A., *148*, 1465, 1952 (Adenomas and Carcinoma).

BOEHME, E. J.: Ann. Surg., *131*, 519, 1950 (Familial Polyposis).

BONSAR, G. M., *et al.:* Brit. J. Surg., *37*, 303, 1950 (Epidermoid Cysts).

BUSAR, J. W., *et al.:* Cancer, *3*, 214, 1950 (Carcinoma Large Bowel).

CAVANAUGH, H. N.: Am. J. Surg., *80*, 860, 1950 (Lipoma).

CONNELL, J. F., JR., and ROTTINO, A.: A. M. A. Arch. Surg., *59*, 807, 1949 (Retrograde Spread Carcinoma).

CRON, S. D., *et al.:* Gastroenterology, *17*, 194, 1951 (Squamous Cell Carcinoma Rectum).

DUNAVANT, D., and GILLESPIE, C. E.: South. Surg., *15*, 916, 1949 (Sarcoma Rectum).

ENQUIST, I. F., and STATE, D.: Surgery, *32*, 696, 1952 (Polyps).

FISHER, E. R., and CASTRO, A. F.: Am. J. Surg., *85*, 146, 1953 (Diffuse Papillomatous Polyps).

GARLOCK, J. H., and KLEIN, S. H.: A. M. A. Arch. Surg., *59*, 1289, 1949 (Ten-year Studies Carcinoma Colon and Rectum).

GRANET, E., *et al.:* Am. J. Surg., *80*, 311, 1950 (Lymphoma).

HELLER, E. L., and LEWIS, H. H., JR.: Am. J. Path., *26*, 463, 1950 (Benign Lymphoma).

JAQUES, A. A.: Am. J. Surg., *84*, 507, 1952 (Hemangioma).

KLEIN, R. R., and SCARBOROUGH, R. A.: A. M. A. Arch. Surg., *65*, 65, 1952 (Adenomatous Polyps).

KNIGHT, C. D., *et al.:* Surg., Gynec. & Obst., *95*, 220, 1952 (Carcinoma Rectum Females).

LOTT, B. E., and ALEXANDER, C. M.: Ann. Surg., *130*, 1101, 1949 (Basal Cell Carcinoma Anus).

POSTLETHWAIT, R. W.: Ann. Surg., *129*, 34, 1949 (Malignant Tumors).

RAVEN, R. W.: Am. J. Surg., *79*, 85, 1950 (Melanoblastoma Anus).

SANDUSKY, W. R., and PARSONS, J. R., JR.: Ann. Surg., *135*, 818, 1952 (Adenomatous Polyps).

SCHANTZ, G. H.: Gasteroenterology, *13*, 430, 1949 (Polyposis).

SHANDS, W. D., *et al.:* Surg., Gynec. & Obst., *94*, 302, 1952 (Carcinoma and Ulcerative Colitis).

SPEAR, H. C., and BRAINARD, S. C.: Ann. Surg., *134*, 934, 1951 (Carcinoma Large Bowel).

TAYLOR, E. R., *et al.:* Surg., Gynec. & Obst., *96*, 193, 1953 (Carcinoma Colon into Urinary Bladder).

Chapter

21

Liver and Biliary System

GENERAL CONSIDERATIONS

Since the liver and biliary system are closely related embryologically, anatomically, and physiologically the diseases of these organs may be considered together in a single Chapter. Because, however, the pathologic disturbances of each of these component portions are numerous, and in order to preserve a certain degree of continuity of thought the dissertation may be conveniently divided into two parts—first the Liver and then the Biliary System.

LIVER

PATHOLOGIC PHYSIOLOGY

W. Paul Havens, Jr.

Normal hepatic cells have a wide diversity of metabolic functions and, in addition, certain excretory activities. These are facilitated by the great permeability of hepatic sinusoids for protein and by the phagocytic activities of their lining Kupffer cells (Popper and Schaffner). The *excretory functions* of the liver are primarily concerned (1) with the transfer of bilirubin from the blood through the hepatic cells and into the biliary canaliculi, (2) with the subsequent formation of bile, and (3) with the excretion of certain exogenous substances such as bromsulphalein, a dye widely used as a test of hepatic function. The *metabolic functions* include (1) the metabolism of carbohydrates, fats, proteins, enzymes, vitamins, minerals, water, bile acids, and pigments, and (2) the detoxification of certain endogenous or exogenous noxious materials. Through common metabolic pathways in the liver, *carbohydrates*, *fats*, and *proteins* may apparently be converted into each other. In carbohydrate metabolism, the liver is primarily active in producing glycogen from monosaccharides, storing it, and breaking it down into glucose for release to the blood. The metabolism of neutral fats, phospholipids, and cholesterol is mediated in large measure by the liver through control of intestinal absorption of fats by the secretion of bile acids and by the synthesis and storage of various lipids and their distribution throughout the body. Both anabolic and catabolic aspects of protein metabolism are carried on and the nucleus of the hepatic cell exercises an important role in synthesis (Brachet). The liver is the site of production of *albumin, fibrinogen*, and alpha and beta *globulins* (Miller and Bale). Its role in the production of gamma globulin is thought to be small, although it is believed to participate. The *catabolic activity* of the liver is manifested by the breakdown of proteins to amino acids, their deamination, and the subsequent formation of urea. Numerous *enzymes* are present in hepatic cells, and they are intimately associated with the various processes connected with the metabolism of carbohydrates, fats, and proteins. The storage of some *vitamins* and the alteration of others are functions of hepatic cells and, conversely, the functions and structure of the liver may be changed by alterations in the metabolism of certain vitamins, particularly members of vitamin B complex. Considerable quantities of various *minerals*, including sodium, potassium, calcium, phosphorus, iron, and copper, as well as smaller amounts of trace elements, such as cobalt, manganese, magnesium, and zinc, are present in the liver. Certain of these, such as phosphorus and manganese, are intimately related to carbohydrate and enzyme metabolism, while the role of others, such as sodium and potassium, is apparently nonspecific. By virtue of being the largest storage place for *iron* in the body, the liver is important in the metabolism of this metal and, conversely, may be affected by changes in it. The handling of *water* is, in part, a function of the liver, probably largely through the neutralization of extrahepatic antidiuretic substances. *Bile acids* are produced in hepatic cells, entering the blood and bile, and from the latter are taken up eventually in the enterohepatic circulation and re-excreted in the bile. Normally, few or no bile acids pass into the urine. *Bilirubin* is formed in the reticulo-endothelial cells during the course of degradation of hemoglobin. It appears in the blood, passes through the Kupffer cells and hepatic cells, and is excreted into the bile. On the basis of the *diazo reaction*, a differentiation has been made between *two types* of *bilirubin* —(a) one minute direct bilirubin commonly defined as bilirubin that has passed through the Kupffer and hepatic cells, and (b) the indirect reacting bilirubin representing the fraction that has not passed through these cells. Although the significance of this is controversial, it is of clinical importance in a differential diagnosis (Watson). Bilirubin is normally not found in the urine. The main pathway of excretion is into the bile and eventually into the gastrointestinal tract where it is broken down into mesobilirubinogen and stercobilinogen. These return to the liver by the enterohepatic circulation with only small amounts excreted in the urine. *Porphyrins* make up another group of substances of which coproporphyrin is an important member. It has two isomers: (a) coproporphyrin I, a by-product of hemoglobin synthesis, and (b) coproporphyrin III, a stage in the formation of hemoglobin. Both are excreted normally in the bile and in the urine. Among the more important metabolic functions of the liver is the *transformation* of endogenous or exogenous *noxious substances* into harmless ones. A variety of pathways are available, including degradation (as with opiates), oxidation (as in the inactivation of certain steroid hormones), and conjugation with organic or inorganic acids (as in the combination of benzoic acid with glycine to make hippuric acid).

It is not unusual that the *liver shares* in the untoward effects of such *generalized body experiences* as acute infections, shock, and anesthesia, resulting frequently in mild *impairment* of *metabolic* or *excretory functions* that are not detectable clinically. Of greater importance are the functional changes that take place when the liver is directly involved in various *pathologic conditions.* In *acute necrosis* of the liver, as occurs in viral hepatitis, the emphasis is on the changes in metabolic function, although excretory function is also sharply impaired. In contrast, when complete or partial *obstruction* occurs somewhere along the course of the common bile duct or when intrahepatic obstruction is present, excretory function is primarily impaired and metabolic activity may remain essentially normal for a considerable period, although eventually changes occur particularly if ascending infection occurs in the biliary tract. When the liver is involved in chronic disease, as in *chronic hepatitis* or *cirrhosis*, evidence of impairment of both metabolic and excretory functions occurs and the emphasis is determined by the phase of disease and degree of necrosis and regeneration. Of interest also are those situations in which the liver is involved with *infiltrative disease*, such as lymphoblastoma, fatty change, primary or metastatic cancer, and sarcoidosis. Under these circumstances, disorders of excretory function are frequently the first to appear, followed subsequently by metabolic derangement.

There are available a large number of *laboratory tests* to measure hepatic functions although few of them determine only the functions of the liver. In contrast to tests of renal and pancreatic function that are, in a sense, organ specific, the tests used to measure hepatic function, with few exceptions, reflect the interaction of functions of the liver and other organs. These tests are vastly different in degree of sensitivity, and, in addition, a large part of the liver must be involved before evidence of dysfunction becomes available. Despite these drawbacks, they are of great value clinically from the standpoints of diagnosis and prognosis.

In *acute necrosis* of the liver, as in viral hepatitis, a number of changes in metabolic and excretory functions occur before the appearance of jaundice. The one minute direct serum bilirubin is increased, bilirubin appears in the urine, the excretion of intravenously injected bromsulphalein is impaired, the urinary urobilinogen increases, and the serum transaminase is sharply increased. Clinical jaundice need not occur but, when it does, it is reflected by increases in both one minute direct and the indirect serum bilirubin. The cephalin flocculation, thymol turbidity, and zinc turbidity tests become positive, reflecting changes in serum proteins, with diminution and qualitative alteration of the serum albumin and increases in the beta and gamma globulins, particularly the latter. Mild increases in serum alkaline phosphatase and serum iron occur. The total serum cholesterol is usually normal although the capacity to esterify it is frequently reduced. Impairment of conversion of benzoic acid to hippuric acid is found and diminution of prothrombin time that fails to respond to the parenteral administration of vitamin K is not unusual. As regeneration and healing occur, jaundice wanes, the serum transaminase and alkaline phosphatase, the prothrombin time, and the ratio between esters and total cholesterol return to normal. Bilirubin disappears from the urine before clinical jaundice is completely gone and the discrepancy between this and its early appearance in the urine before the total serum bilirubin was abnormal suggests some alteration in renal threshold for bilirubin during the course of disease. When the serum bilirubin becomes normal, or shortly thereafter, the excretion of bromsulphalein also returns to normal. The various flocculation and thymol turbidity tests remain positive often for several weeks and reflect the persistent changes in globulins, particularly the increased gamma globulin. The exact significance of this is not understood and it is not known whether the prolonged increase in gamma globulin represents antibody to virus or to some product of hepatic necrosis. If abnormally high amounts of gamma globulin are present after six months in a patient who has had viral hepatitis, the possibility of chronic hepatitis must be considered. When hepatic necrosis is severe, the total cholesterol is reduced, the serum potassium is increased, amino-aciduria with leucine and tyrosine occurs, and spontaneous hypoglycemia or hypoglycemia following intravenous infusions of glucose is not unusual.

In *chronic hepatic disease*, such as portal cirrhosis, it is not unusual to find patients with normal hepatic tests who, on biopsy of the liver, are revealed to have a highly organized cirrhosis with broad bands of fibrous tissue surrounding nodules of parenchymal cells, with little or no evidence of active hepatic cellular degeneration. From this extreme extends a wide degeneration and regeneration, infiltration, and mesenchymal response. A most sensitive test of cellular damage is the capacity to excrete bromsulphalein and this may be abnormal when other tests are normal. In general, as the disease progresses the serum albumin is diminished and the beta and gamma globulins are increased. The flocculation tests are frequently positive, reflecting these alterations. The prothrombin time is reduced, as are the cholesterol-ester ratio and the vitamin E content of the plasma. The serum bilirubin may be increased or normal. Impairment of capacity to neutralize certain extrahepatic antidiuretic substances results in retention of sodium and water and failure to inactivate estrogens is believed to potentiate the appearance of spider naevi.

The liver may be involved in a variety of *neoplastic* or *granulomatous* processes such as sarcoidosis, tuberculosis, syphilis, brucellosis, and others. Depending on the degree of involvement, impaired excretion of bromsulphalein and mild to moderate increases in serum alkaline phosphatase are sensitive indicators of cellular damage, although circulatory impairment may contribute to this in metastatic disease. Alterations in proteins with diminution in albumin and increase in globulins, occur frequently in granulomatous disease, particularly in sarcoidosis (Shay). Increases in serum bilirubin are uncommon. Sufficient fatty change of the liver may also occur to cause increase in serum bilirubin and alkaline phosphatase, abnormal retention of bromsulphalein in the blood, and diminished glucose tolerance, reflecting cellular damage. Impairment of sinusoidal circulation too may account for a part of the diminished excretion of bilirubin and of bromsulphalein. Circulatory disorders causing chronic passive congestion of the liver may also result in impaired excretion of bromsulphalein and bilirubin to a degree that appears out of proportion to the cellular damage.

Cholestasis, resulting in *jaundice*, occurs as a result of extrahepatic obstruction of the common bile duct or of intrahepatic obstruction of the biliary tract by an infiltrative process. In addition, intrahepatic cholestasis occurs in cholangiolitic hepatitis, probably as a result of damage to the ductules. This may be caused by sensitizing substances such as arsenicals or chlorpromazine and at times it appears to be a form of viral hepatitis, occurring at the outset of disease or at any time in the course of it. Characteristically, functional alterations early in the course of disease are similar in cholestasis of extrahepatic and intrahepatic origin. Bilirubin is present in the urine but urobilinogen is usually reduced. The serum proteins and the flocculation and turbidity tests are normal early. The serum transaminase is normal or mildly increased. The total serum cholesterol and alkaline phosphatase are sharply increased due to obstruction and, in the latter, doubtless to increased production by proliferated ductules. The prothrombin time may become reduced but responds to the parenteral administration of vitamin K. Where cholestasis due to extrahepatic obstruction has existed for a considerable period of time or if ascending infection is present, evidence of hepatic cellular degeneration occurs, with alterations in the serum proteins and with positive cephalin flocculation and thymol turbidity tests. If intrahepatic cholestasis persists as a result of the development of chronic cholangiolitic hepatitis, there may occur a considerable increase in gamma globulin with a positive zinc turbidity test. In occasional patients with this disease, the serum lipids increase to large amounts and xanthomatous deposits appear in the skin.

Jaundice may also be caused by increased production of bilirubin due to *excessive hemolysis.* The increase is in the indirect fraction with a normal one minute direct serum bilirubin. Bilirubin is usually absent from the urine, urobilinogen is increased in the feces and, at times, in the urine. Anemia is frequently present and reticulocytosis is common.

CONGENITAL ANOMALIES

Orientation. — Developmental malformation of the liver may consist of (1) *agenesis*—failure of development, (2) *absence of a lobe*—usually the left (Merrill), (3) *hypoplasia*—decrease in size, (4) *hyperplasia*—increase in size, (5) *Riedel's lobe*—a flat, tongue-shaped, posterior enlargement of the right lobe, (6) *transposition*—as seen in *situs inversus* and consisting of a mirror image transference of the entire organ, with the right lobe on the left side and the left lobe on the right side, (7) *Cruveilhier-Baumgarten disease,* and (8) *cysts.* Of these, only the two mentioned last merit a few additional words.

Cruveilhier-Baumgarten Disease. — This *disease* consists primarily of a congenitally patent umbilical vein resulting in shunting of large amounts of blood from the portal vein to the epigastric vein in the abdominal wall (Miller). It is attended by a small cirrhotic liver, enlarged spleen, distended abdominal veins transmitting a thrill or murmur, and leukopenia. A similar group of lesions, except that they are associated with portal cirrhosis and secondary recanalization of the umbilical vein, is referred to as *Cruveilhier-Baumgarten syndrome.*

Cysts. — Cysts of the liver may be congenital, inflammatory (parasitic), traumatic, and neoplastic (Comfort, Stock, and Kerekes). Of these, *congenital* cysts are the most important from the point of view of our present discussion. Although developmental in origin, they are usually not *detectable* until after the age of thirty years. They have no predilection for any race and they affect females four to five times as frequently as males. *Pathogenetically* they arise as a result of segmentation, degeneration, and dilatation of the bile ducts and in over one-half of the cases are associated with similar cysts in the kidneys. Occasionally cysts are also found in the pancreas and the spleen. *Pathologically* the cysts may be single or multiple (Fig. 372). When many are present the condition is referred to as *polycystic disease.* Single cysts may measure up to 30 cm. or more in diameter, multiple cysts (but still a few in number) are generally smaller, while the cysts in polycystic disease do not, as a rule, measure more than 1 to 2 cm. across. In any case, the walls are usually thin; the inner lining is smooth; the lumen is single or partitioned, and the fluid is clear and serous. *Histologically* the wall is composed of connective tissue and is lined by a single layer of columnar, cuboidal, or attenuated epithelial cells (Fig. 373). The *clinical manifestations* vary greatly from none to a mass and discomfort or pain in the region of the liver. The *diagnosis* is made peritoneoscopically or at laparotomy. A differential diagnosis should include cirrhosis, parasitic cysts, and tumors. *Treatment* consists of doing nothing surgically (especially in polycystic disease), of surgical excision (when the lesion is superficial and pedunculated), or of marsupialization. The *prognosis* is good for the condition as such does not generally contribute to the death of the patient.

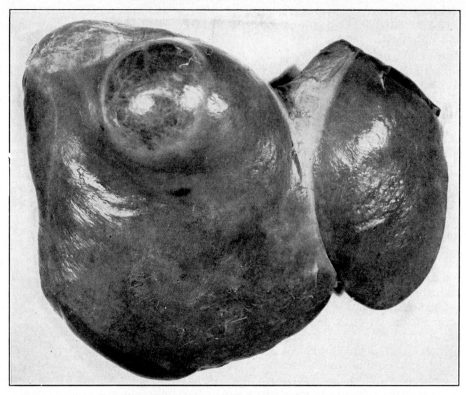

FIG. 372.—Congenital cyst of the right lobe of the liver.

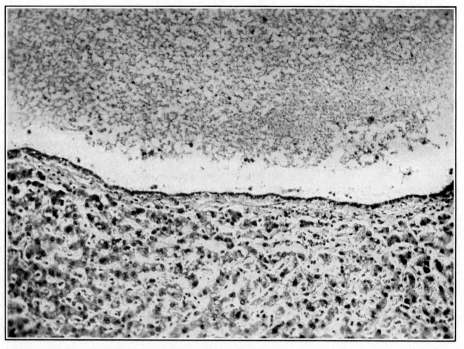

FIG. 373.—Serous cyst of the liver showing precipitated material in the lumen and a connective tissue wall lined with attenuated epithelial cells.

DEGENERATIONS

Orientation. —Since the liver is a central organ intercepting all food and noxious agents absorbed by the gastrointestinal tract and bathed by the systemic arterial blood, it is subjected to a great variety of degenerative disorders. As discussed in Chapter 4 (p. 29), most of these consist of atrophy, parenchymatous degeneration, hydropic degeneration, hyaline droplet degeneration, amyloidosis, disturbances in carbohydrate metabolism, fatty change, lipoid storage, dystrophic calcification, and pathologic pigmentation including hemosiderin, bilirubin, ciroid, and malarial pigment. In the liver, as in other organs of the body, the degenerations listed represent local changes rather than diseases and, as such, can be seen in a variety of

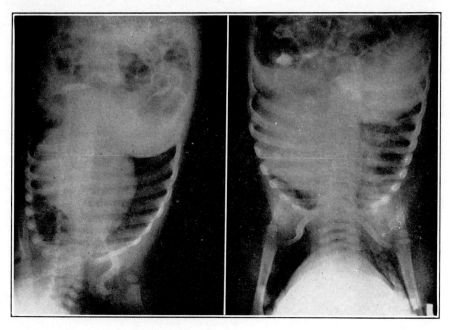

FIG. 374.—Glycogen storage disease showing marked enlargement of the heart roentgenographically.

pathologic states. Aside from the morbid alteration just referred to there are two groups of specific disease processes that may be considered in this section—glycogen storage disease and cirrhosis.

Glycogen Storage Disease. —The general principles involved in carbohydrate metabolism have been outlined in Chapter 4 (p. 45). Normally large stores of glycogen are present in muscle and liver. The glycogen in muscle is used in emergencies when enough sugar cannot be obtained from the blood, while that in the liver is used to supply the blood and all other tissues with glucose. Abnormally, as a *result* of deficiency of glucose-6-phosphatase (Cori), glycogen fails to be converted into glucose and is stored in unusually large amounts in the liver, kidneys, and heart (Fig. 374). The condition is known as *glycogen storage* or *von Gierke's disease*. It is seen in infants and children and is hereditarily transmitted. *Pathologically* the organs affected are greatly enlarged with the parenchymatous cells (muscle

cells of the heart, hepatic cells of the liver, and epithelial cells of the convoluted tubules of the kidneys) distended with glycogen (Figs. 375 and 376).
Because the glycogen is not utilizable, fats are improperly metabolized and,
as a result of both of these circumstances, the following *disturbances* occur:
increased sensitivity to insulin, hypoglycemia during fasting, little response
(elevation) in blood sugar levels upon administration of adrenalin, prolonged
hyperglycemia without glycosuria after ingestion of glucose, and excessive
formation of ketone bodies with the presence of acetone and diacetic acid
in the urine (van Creveld).

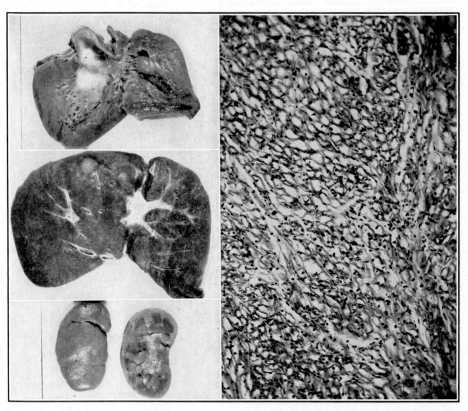

Fig. 375.—Glycogen storage disease illustrating, to the left, enlargement of the heart, liver, and
kidney and, to the right, marked glycogen vacuolization of the myocardial fibers.   × 100.

Cirrhosis.—Cirrhosis (Gr. = orange-yellow) of the liver is a pathologic
change characterized essentially by: (1) degeneration, atrophy, and disappearance of hepatic cells, (2) the presence of mild to moderate inflammation, (3) increase of connective tissue, (4) regeneration of hepatic cells, and
(5) extensive or minimal proliferation of bile ducts.   As would be expected
in the presence of so many variables, the ultimate pathologic picture depends upon which of these combinations initiates the process or prevails.
Accordingly there are numerous, and often overlapping, classifications.   For
our purposes, the following listing appears to encompass most of the important disorders: portal cirrhosis, Wilson's disease, pigmentary cirrhosis,
obstructive biliary cirrhosis, infective biliary cirrhosis, xanthomatous biliary
cirrhosis, postnecrotic cirrhosis, and cardiac cirrhosis.

Portal Cirrhosis.—Portal cirrhosis (Laennec's cirrhosis, atrophic cirrhosis, diffuse nodular cirrhosis, multilobular cirrhosis, alcoholic cirrhosis, or hobnail liver) is by far the most common type of cirrhosis. The condition is worldwide in *distribution* but varies greatly from country to country, being most common in the Orient and least common in Northwestern European Russia. In Chile it constitutes 1.71 per cent of all hospital admissions and 8.5 per cent of all autopsies (Armaz-Cruz) and in our Institution it comprises about 2 per cent of all autopsies (Herbut). Although it may be found in patients of all ages, it prevails in those between thirty and sixty years of age. It affects males two to three times as frequently as

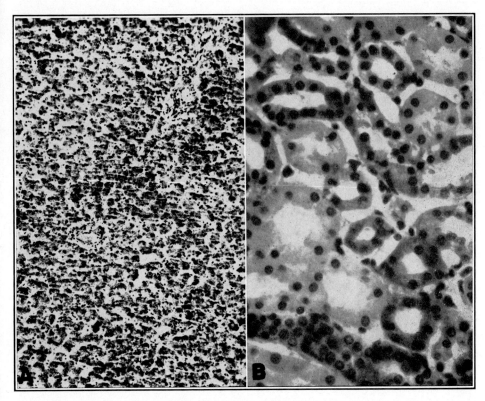

FIG. 376.—Glycogen storage disease showing *A*, a liver filled with glycogen-positive granules. Best's carmine stain. × 100, and *B*, renal tubules filled with similar material. Best's carmine stain. × 400.

females. While a great deal has been written in the past regarding the *cause* of portal cirrhosis it is now generally accepted, as a result of both animal experimentation and investigations of the disease in man, that the disorder arises as a result of a deficiency of protein and vitamin B complex in the diet (Olsen). It is also generally agreed that alcoholism is a common accompaniment, but that alcohol exerts its effect indirectly by way of nutritional deficiency. In addition to the circumstances just noted, there must also be a constitutional susceptibility or an organ vulnerability. If this were not so, the reason one person develops cirrhosis while another, under similar or worse circumstances, does not acquire the disease would remain unexplained.

Pathologically the entire liver is diffusely involved in all cases. Early in the course of the disease the organ is generally enlarged and may weigh as much as twice normal. The surface is smooth; the consistency is firm; the color is light brown or yellowish, and cut surfaces may or may not reveal increased lobular markings. As the lesion advances the liver becomes smaller and smaller until it may shrink to as little as one-half the normal size. Concomitantly both external and cut surfaces become more and more nodular until the entire substance consists of circumscribed irregular protrusions that usually measure up to 1 cm. in diameter and that are sur-

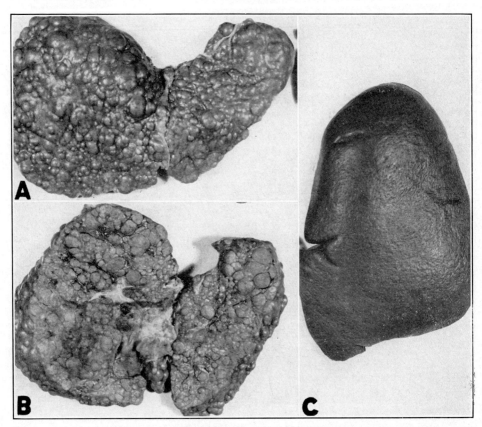

FIG. 377.—Portal cirrhosis of the liver illustrating *A* and *B*, typical nodularity of the external and cut surfaces and *C*, marked enlargement of the spleen.

rounded by depressed bands of grayish-white fibrous tissue (Fig. 377). The hepatic nodules may appear light brown, yellowish (due to deposition of fat), or lemon yellow or green (due to permeation with bile). The consistency, as would be expected, is greatly increased. As the normal hepatic lobules disappear and new irregular ones are formed, there occurs (1) a reduction of the total vascular bed of the liver, (2) obstruction to the portal circulation, and (3) an anastomosis between the portal and hepatic vessels resulting in shunting of the blood with bypassing of the hepatic parenchyma (Popper). As a result of these changes there develops (1) chronic passive congestion of the abdominal organs with moderate to marked enlargement of the spleen, congestion and edema of the mucosa of

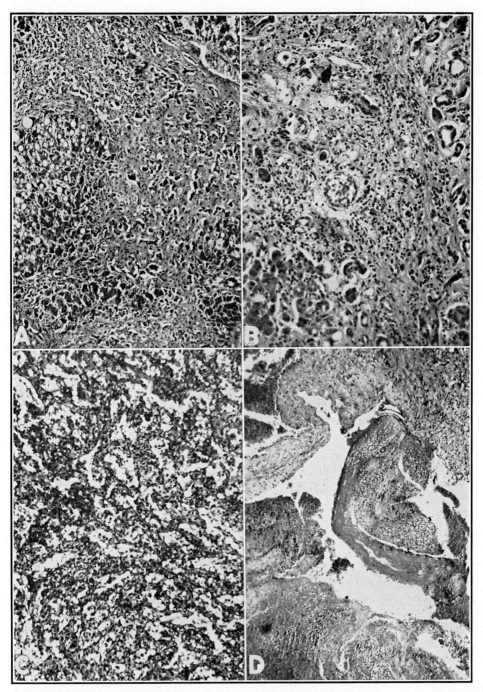

FIG. 378.—Portal cirrhosis showing *A*, distorted hepatic lobules, fatty change in some of the cells, marked portal fibrosis, and extensive bile duct proliferation.   × 50, *B*, another portal radicle with similar changes.   × 100, *C*, spleen with prominently dilated sinusoids.   × 100, and *D*, a ruptured esophageal varix.   × 50.

51

the gastrointestinal tract, ascites, and edema of the lower extremities, and
(2) establishment of collateral circulations, especially at the junction of the
esophagus with the stomach (p. 642). Because of the reduction of the functioning hepatic parenchyma and because of the vascular bypassing of the
parenchyma that does remain, there is a failure of inactivation of the estrogens by the liver and this, in turn, may result in testicular atrophy, spider
nevi of the skin, erythema of the palms, and gynecomastia (Marrione,
Bean, and Glass). *Histologically* the changes encountered consist of varying
degrees of the following: (1) fatty change, atrophy, gradual disappearance,
and occasionally necrosis of the periportal portions of the hepatic lobules,

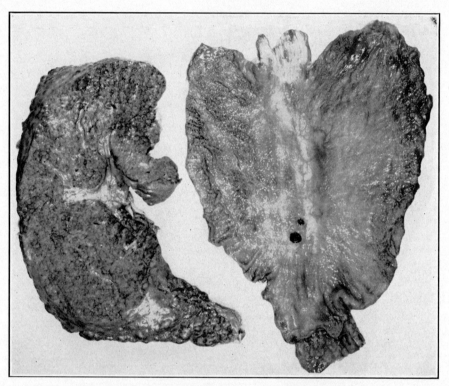

FIG. 379.—Two acute gastric ulcers on the lesser curvature of the stomach occurring as a
complication of portal cirrhosis.

(2) irregular regeneration of the hepatic parenchyma with the formation
of pseudolobules, that is, lobules in which the architecture is not arranged
in radiating cords and in which there is no central vein, (3) connective
tissue proliferation in the portal areas, (4) marked proliferation of the
bile ducts, and (5) varying degrees of (but usually minimal) permeation
with plasma cells, lymphocytes, monocytes, and occasional neutrophils
(Fig. 378).

The chief *complications* are (1) ascites and edema (contributed to by an
accompanying hypoproteinemia which, in turn, is due in part to a decreased
ability of the liver to synthesize albumin, (2) acute gastric ulcer (Fig. 379),
(3) rupture of esophageal varices with gastroesophageal hemorrhage, (4)
hepatic insufficiency (cholemia), and (5) primary hepatic carcinoma developing in from 3.2 to 5.6 per cent of cases (Warren). *Clinically* there is generally

a prolonged asymptomatic latent period followed by a variety of manifestations that vary from case to case (Armaz-Cruz, Ricketts, and Douglass).
The more important of these include anorexia, nausea, vomiting, abdominal
distention, abdominal pain, hematemesis, melena, edema of the lower extremities, jaundice, loss of weight, diarrhea, ascites, spider nevi of the skin,
splenomegaly, hemorrhoids, slight fever, palpable hard nodular liver, vari-
variable liver function tests (normal or abnormal), leukopenia, anemia, and
hypoproteinemia.   Although many attempts have been made to correlate

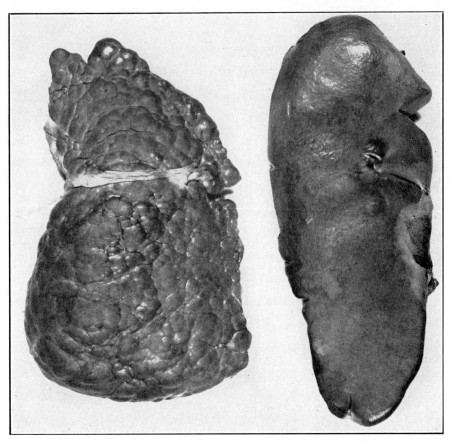

Fig. 380.—Wilson's disease in a woman 19 years old showing the usual type of portal cirrhosis
and a tremendously enlarged spleen.

the clinical findings with the degree of histologic change, it is the concensus
that no constant association exists (Post).   The *diagnosis* is made from
(1) a history of alcholism and dietary deficiency, (2) the clinical manifestations, (3) aspiration biopsy of the liver, and (4) peritoneoscopy with biopsy.
Treatment is both medical and surgical.   Among other things, it includes a
high protein and high carbohydrate diet, administration of vitamins
(especially choline and methionine), paracentesis, and portacaval or spleno-
renal anastomosis in cases of portal hypertension (Portis).   The *prognosis*
is variable.   It is better in asymptomatic than it is in symptomatic patients
and is progressively worse in the presence of hematemesis, ascites, and jaun-

dice. The five-year survival rate in a study of 444 patients by Douglass was 19.6 per cent.

Wilson's Disease.—Wilson's disease, also known as *hepatolenticular degeneration*, consists of degeneration of the lenticular nuclei of the brain and an ordinary type of portal cirrhosis of the liver (Fig. 380). The former accounts for a group of central nervous system *manifestations* that includes masked facies or a fixed smile, tremor, semiflexed postural state, slow movements, contractures, athetoid movements, rigidity, dysarthria, dysphagia, and psychic changes (Sweet and Homberger). The disorder usually *occurs* in the second and third decades of life and preponderates in males. The *cause* is unknown although the condition is familial and may be related to erythroblastosis fetalis (Craig and Campbell).

Pigmentary Cirrhosis. Pigmentary cirrhosis, also known as *hemochromatosis* and *bronze diabetes*, consists of a triad of (1) portal cirrhosis of the liver, (2) hemosiderosis, and (3) diabetes mellitus. Although some authors have captioned cases as hemochromatosis in which diabetes has been absent, such cases rightfully do not fall in this category. The term *endogenous hemochromatosis* is used for cases in which the source of the hemosiderin is not readily apparent while the term *exogenous hemochromatosis* is applied when the source of the iron is excessive administration by mouth or hemolysis of erythrocytes following repeated transfusions (Frumin). Hemochromatosis is relatively *rare*. Warren reported an incidence of 20 cases (0.33%) in a series of 6,048 autopsies and Marble recorded an incidence of 0.6 per cent in a series of 30,000 cases of diabetes mellitus. Over 90 per cent of the cases occur in males and the disorder is usually found in the fourth and later decades of life. While much has been written regarding the *cause* and *pathogenesis* of hemochromatosis, the following explanation appears to be as good as any: (1) *portal cirrhosis*—due to dietary deficiency like any other portal cirrhosis, (2) *hemosiderosis*—in endogenous hemochromatosis resulting from (*a*) abnormal absorption of iron from the diet due to breaking of the epithelial barrier consequent to vitamin A deficiency and (*b*) abnormal retention of iron by the tissues due to an inborn error of metabolism, and in exogenous hemochromatosis resulting from simple excessive flooding of the tissues with iron, and (3) *diabetes mellitus*—due to heredity and/or perhaps an alloxan-like substance acting on the islets of Langerhans (Herbut).

Pathologically all of the organs but especially the skin, mucous membranes, liver, pancreas, spleen, abdominal lymph nodes, and mucosa of the intestinal tract appear dark reddish brown or bronze due to a deposition of hemosiderin (Figs. 381 and 382). The *liver* shows typical portal cirrhosis with, in addition, extensive deposition of hemosiderin and hemofuscin in the hepatic cells, Kupffer cells, fibrous tissue, and bile duct epithelium (Fig. 383*A* and *B*, and Plate I, facing p. 66). The *pancreas* discloses an increase of fibrous tissue between the lobules, between the acini, and within the islets of Langerhans (Fig. 383*C*). Hemosiderin is deposited in the connective tissue, macrophages, islet cells, and ductal epithelial cells (Fig. 383*C*). The *spleen* reveals changes similar to those in cases of portal cirrhosis with, in addition, deposition of hemosiderin in the connective tissue and macrophages. The *lymph nodes*, especially of the upper abdomen, also show extensive hemosiderin deposition but reveal considerably less fibrosis than does the liver, pancreas, or spleen. In the *skin* hemosiderin is deposited within the sweat glands, connective tissue and blood vessels of the corium, and basal cells of the epidermis (Marble). The basal layer of the epidermis also contains an increase of melanin.

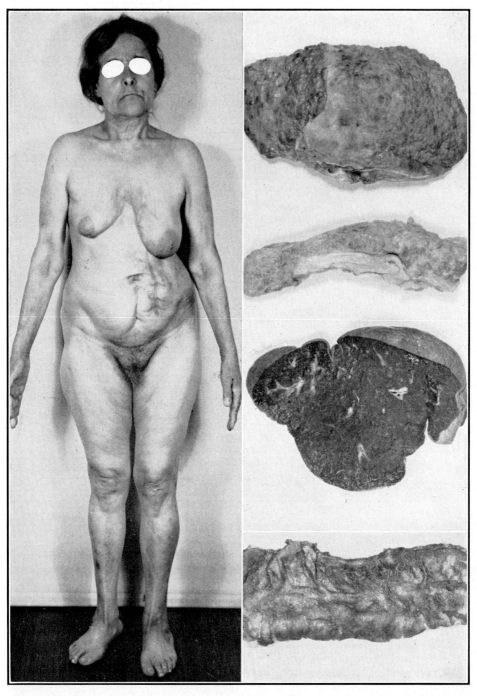

FIG. 381.—Hemochromatosis disclosing, to the left, a diffuse bronzing of the skin in a white woman and, to the right, cirrhosis of the liver, pigmentation of the pancreas, enlargement of the spleen, and pigmentation of the intestinal mucosa.

The *complications* of hemochromatosis are the same as those of ordinary portal cirrhosis of the liver (p. 799) and diabetes mellitus (p. 874). It might be pointed out, however, that the incidence of primary carcinoma of the liver is even higher than it is in cases of ordinary portal cirrhosis, the recorded figures varying from 11.5 to 42.9 per cent (Warren). The chief *clinical manifestations* are those of portal cirrhosis of the liver (p. 802) and diabetes mellitus (p. 874). In addition, of course, there is present the reddish-brown discoloration of the skin and mucous membranes already referred to (Fig. 381). The *diagnosis* of hemochromatosis is made from the

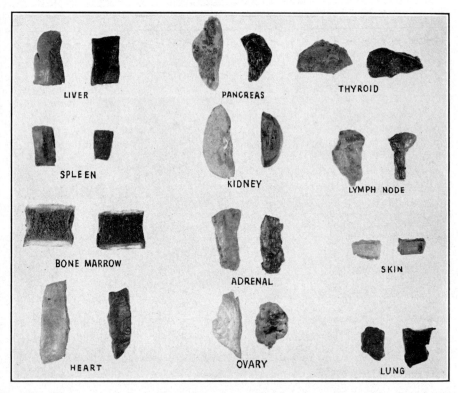

Fig. 382.—Pigmentary cirrhosis illustrating a brown discoloration and a positive Prussian blue reaction of portions of various organs.

clinical manifestations of pigmentation of the skin and mucous membrane, cirrhosis of the liver, and diabetes mellitus, together with demonstration of iron deposits in a biopsy of the skin. *Treatment*, on the whole, is unsatisfactory. The portal cirrhosis and diabetes are treated by dietary and other means (pp. 803 and 874). Treatment of hemosiderosis in exogenous hemochromatosis is prevention, while that recently suggested in endogenous hemochromatosis is repeated phlebotomy (Warthin). The ultimate *prognosis* is poor. The average survival after the diagnosis is made is less than six years (Marble). The usual *causes* of *death* are hepatic insufficiency, carcinoma of the liver, rupture of esophageal varices, diabetic coma, and infection (pneumonia, peritonitis, etc.).

Obstructive Biliary Cirrhosis.—Obstructive biliary cirrhosis, also known as secondary biliary cirrhosis, develops as a result of partial prolonged or

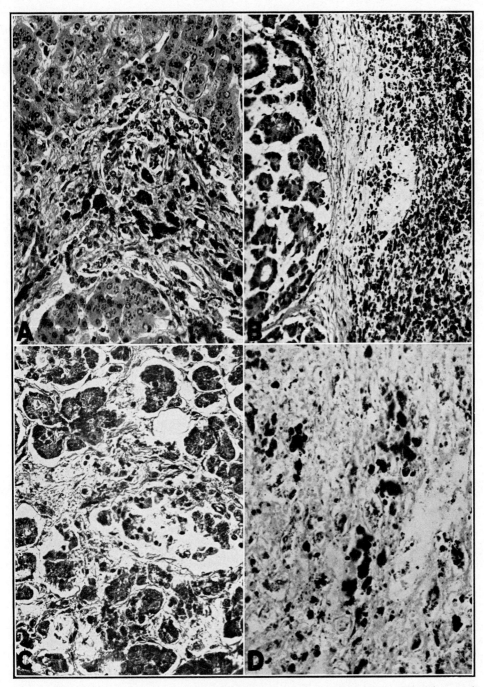

FIG. 383.—Hemochromatosis showing *A*, periportal fibrosis, bile duct proliferation, and deposition of hemosiderin in the portal area and hepatic cells. × 200, *B*, an area of fibrosis with hemosiderin deposition and primary carcinoma of the liver. × 100, *C*, fibrosis and hemosiderin deposition in the pancreas. × 200, and *D*, hemosiderin in the pancreas (iron stain). × 200.

repeated obstruction of the extrahepatic bile ducts. It is second in frequency to portal cirrhosis, occurs at all ages, and has no predilection for either sex. Some of the *causes* of obstruction are congenital atresia of the bile ducts, chronic pancreatitis (head of the pancreas), inflammatory stricture of the extrahepatic bile ducts, biliary calculi, carcinoma of the head of the pancreas, benign and malignant tumors of the bile ducts, and compression of the bile ducts from without by enlarged (usually metastatic carcinomatous) lymph nodes. *Pathologically* the liver is usually enlarged, yellow to green, firm, and finely (rather than coarsely) nodular. It cuts

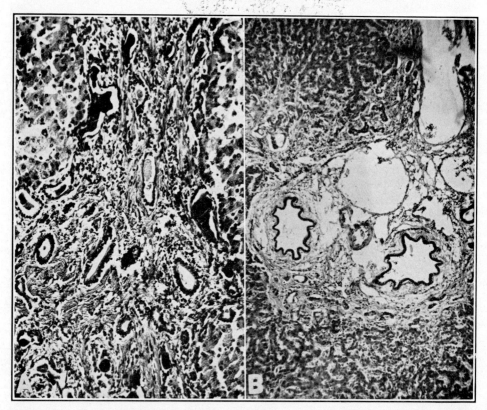

FIG. 384.—Obstructive biliary cirrhosis illustrating *A*, marked proliferation of connective tissue and bile ducts in a portal area with a sprinkling of leukocytes and a few bile casts within the ducts. × 100 and *B*, dilatation of bile ducts and an increase of connective tissue also in a portal radicle. × 50.

with increased resistance, with the cut surfaces disclosing an accentuation of the lobular pattern because of an increased prominence of the portal radicles. The bile ducts may be dilated and filled with excessive amounts of bile. The *histologic* changes vary somewhat with the stage of the disease (Fig. 384). One of the earliest changes is the appearance of lymphocytes, a few plasma cells, and occasional neutrophils where the bile canaliculi join the bile ducts (Moschcowitz). Simultaneously there is edema of the connective tissue of the portal radicles, beginning fibroblastic and capillary proliferation, and beginning proliferation of bile canaliculi. As the process becomes more chronic, bile ducts increase in number and often show both dilatation and papillary infoldings and the fibrous tissue becomes more prominent and collagenous. The hepatic lobules adjacent to the portal radicles reveal degeneration, fatty change, and disappearance and, in time, regeneration of hepatic cells. Ultimately the architecture is so deranged that the histologic appearance is indistinguishable from that of ordinary portal cirrhosis. The usual *complications* consist of increasing jaundice and hepatic insufficiency. The cirrhosis rarely progresses to the point where esophageal varices develop. Carcinoma of the liver may occur but is considerably less frequent than it is in portal cirrhosis. *Clinically* (aside from local manifestations of discomfort, dyspnea, etc.) the following are usually noted: jaundice, itching, pale stool, dark urine, low urobilinogen in the stool, and elevated serum levels of bilirubin, alkaline phosphatase, and total lipids (Ahrens). The *diagnosis* is usually made from the clinical manifestations and is confirmed at laparotomy. *Treatment* consists of relieving the obstruction surgically. The *prognosis* depends upon the cause and the duration of the condition before operation.

Infective Biliary Cirrhosis.—This type of cirrhosis occurs as a result of low-grade chronic persistent or recurring inflammation of the portal radicles of the liver with no involvement of the extrahepatic biliary system. It has *also* been *known* as primary biliary cirrhosis, cholangiolitic biliary cirrhosis, pericholangiolitic biliary cirrhosis, chronic intrahepatic obliterating cholangitis, nonobstructive cholangitic biliary cirrhosis, intrahepatic cholangitic biliary cirrhosis, Hanot's biliary cirrhosis, and cholangitis lenta (Ricketts). The condition *occurs* at all ages and affects both sexes with equal frequency. The *causative factors* are generally bacteria (streptococci, staphylococci, etc.) or viruses, with the condition being recorded as secondary to viral hepatitis, chronic ulcerative colitis, rheumatoid arthritis, etc. (Ricketts and Watson). At this point it should be pointed out, as stated at the beginning of this section, that the infection must be of a low-grade nature for, if it is fulminating, large portions of the liver are destroyed and the ultimate picture is that of post-necrotic cirrhosis rather than of biliary cirrhosis. *Pathologically* the liver grossly is similar to that in obstructive biliary cirrhosis with the nodularity being fine in contrast to the coarse nodulations in portal cirrhosis and to the deep crevasses and large lobules in postnecrotic cirrhosis. *Histologically* the primary lesion consists of infiltration of the portal radicles with lymphocytes, plasma cells, monocytes, and neutrophils, with the proportion of the various leukocytes varying from case to case (Fig. 385). Later there is proliferation of bile ducts, fibrosis, disappearance of the hepatic parenchyma in the portal areas, and ultimately regeneration of the liver lobules producing a picture that is indistinguishable from that of portal cirrhosis. The bile ducts are not dilated. Bile casts are prominent in the bile canaliculi but are not seen in the larger bile ducts of the portal radicles. The chief *complications* consist of jaundice and hepatic insufficiency although occasionally portal hypertension does develop. *Clinically* the following are present: long-standing pruritus and jaundice (of months' and years' duration), hepatomegaly, splenomegaly, good nutritional status, and increased levels of bilirubin, alkaline phosphatase, and cholesterol (Ahrens). The *diagnosis* is made from the clinical manifestations aided by laparotomy and biopsy. *Treatment* is empirical. The ultimate *prognosis* is poor.

Xanthomatous Biliary Cirrhosis.—This type of cirrhosis consists simply of infective biliary cirrhosis of long standing associated with generalized, palmar, or facial cutaneous xanthomatosis (Ahrens, Ricketts, and Miller). It occurs mostly in females in the third and fourth decades of life and has occasionally been recorded as familial. A characteristic finding is elevation of serum lipids.

Postnecrotic Cirrhosis.—Under this heading may be included those cases in which there is a diffuse necrosis of the liver followed by fibrosis and regenerative hyperplasia. The condition has also been called *toxic cirrhosis*, *chronic yellow atrophy*, and *nodular hyperplasia* of the liver (Yazigi). The disorder is relatively uncommon because the patients usually die from the acute diffuse necrosis of the liver before the fibrotic and regenerative changes can take place. The condition may *occur* at any age and has no predilection for either sex. The *causes* of the original necrosis are diverse

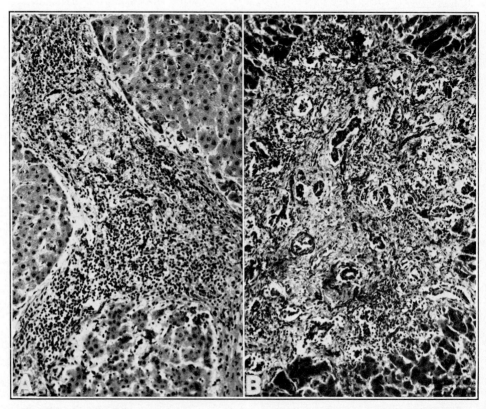

Fig. 385.—Infective biliary cirrhosis disclosing *A*, extensive lymphocytic and, to a lesser extent, monocytic and plasma cell infiltration of a portal radicle and *B*, leukocytic infiltration fibrosis and bile duct proliferation also in a portal radicle. × 100.

including inflammations such as viral hepatitis (Lucké), syphilis, etc., and chemicals such as arsenic, chloroform, carbon tetrachloride, sulfonamides, cincophen, etc. *Pathologically* the liver is generally reduced in size (sometimes greatly) and is grossly irregular (Fig. 386*A*). It is composed of large varisized masses of regenerated hepatic parenchyma that, in themselves, may be secondarily nodular. The consistency is firm and the color varies from dark reddish brown to yellow or green (due to jaundice). The masses are separated by depressed broad or narrow bands of dense fibrous tissue. The *histologic* picture varies with the area examined (Fig. 386*B* and *C*). The regenerated masses consist of regular hepatic cells irregularly arranged. Portal radicles are present but central veins and the radiating pattern of the

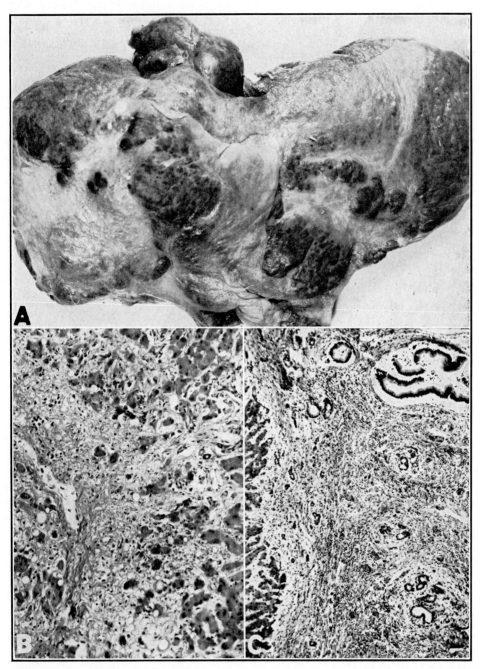

FIG. 386.—Postnecrotic cirrhosis showing *A*, massive scarring and irregular lobulation of the liver, *B*, fibrosis with permeation of the connective tissue between the hepatic cells. × 100, and *C*, also extensive fibrosis with lymphocytic infiltration and bile duct proliferation. × 50.

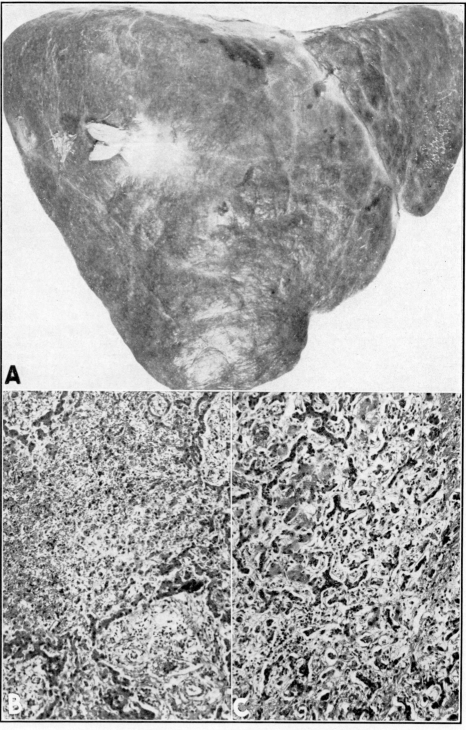

Fig. 387.—Cardiac cirrhosis illustrating *A*, granularity and fine nodularity of the liver, *B*, severe early lesion with virtually complete disappearance of the hepatic cells, and *C*, later lesion with extensive fibrosis and regeneration of the hepatic parenchyma. × 100.

cords are lacking. In other areas there is massive deposition of connective tissue that (1) penetrates into and separates the hepatic cells, (2) contains a sprinkling of lymphocytes, and (3) discloses moderate degrees of bile duct proliferation. The *complications* consist of jaundice, ascites, hemorrhage from esophageal varices, and hepatic failure. The *clinical manifestations* include jaundice, dyspepsia, vomiting, chills, intermittent fever, pain in the right upper quadrant, slight splenomegaly, and anemia. The *diagnosis* may be made clinically from the history, symptoms, and signs but, more often, is accomplished at the time of peritoneoscopy, laparotomy, or necropsy. *Treatment* is symptomatic except in cases of portal hypertension when it is surgical. The *prognosis* is poor, for death usually occurs within a few months after the diagnosis is made.

Cardiac Cirrhosis.—This condition stems from prolonged passive hyperemia (congestion) of the liver consequent to cardiac failure (p. 193). *Grossly* the liver may be larger than normal but is generally reduced in size (Kotin). The edges are somewhat rounded; the capsule is smooth; the external surface is granular or pebbled; the consistency is increased, and cut surfaces disclose an accentuation and irregularity of the lobular markings (Fig. 387*A*). *Histologically* the earliest lesion is that of a "nutmeg" liver (Fig. 69) consisting of dilatation of the central veins and sinusoids, narrowing of the liver cords, and disappearance of the centralmost hepatic cells (Moschcowitz). Ultimately the cellular necrosis extends toward the periphery of the lobule (Fig. 387*B*). As it does so, the remaining framework condenses and proliferates resulting in diffuse central lobular fibrosis (Fig. 387*C*). With the disruption of the vascular system, new "central" veins and tributaries are formed and the latter unite with sprouts from the portal vessels. Concomitantly the remaining peripherally located hepatic cells undergo fatty change, atrophy, and disappearance and the portal connective tissue and bile ducts proliferate in a manner similar to that in portal cirrhosis. Because of the vascular derangement, portal hypertension develops in advanced cases. The *complications* and *clinical manifestations* are primarily those of the cardiac disease but, as the process in the liver advances, they are also those of cirrhosis (consisting essentially of jaundice and hepatic insufficiency). The *diagnosis* is usually not made clinically for the cardiac condition dominates the scene. *Treatment* is primarily directed toward the heart condition but should also consist of proper attention to the diet. The *prognosis* is poor, with death resulting from both the cardiac and the hepatic lesions.

INFLAMMATIONS

Orientation.—Inflammation of the liver is known as *hepatitis*. While there are many types of hepatitis, the following disorders only need be mentioned: abscess, tuberculosis, Boeck's sarcoid, syphilis, Weil's disease, viral hepatitis, and parasitic hepatitis.

Abscess.—Unless otherwise specified, abscess of the liver connotes a localized suppurative infection due to ordinary pyogenic organisms. The condition is *uncommon*, affects both sexes, and has no predilection for any age. Although the *causative organisms* are quite varied, those most commonly found are colon bacilli, streptococci, and staphylococci (Flynn). The routes of invasion are (1) portal vein and its tributaries in cases of inflammation and ulceration of the appendix, large intestine, small intestine, and stomach (see pylephlebitis p. 379), (2) hepatic arteries in cases of osteomyelitis, furuncles, bacterial endocarditis, acute infection of the respiratory tract, etc., (3) directly from infections in contiguous organs comprising disorders such as cholecystitis, subdiaphragmatic abscess, empyema, etc., (4) trauma, either penetrating (bullet or stab wound) or nonpenetrating (blunt blow), and (5) unknown but thought to belong to undetectable lesions in the gastrointestinal tract or inapparent distant foci. Of all these, the most common route is that by way of the portal vein and the *localization* of the abscesses in the liver depends upon whether the primary infection drains into the superior or inferior mesenteric vein. The former produces abscesses in the right lobe of the liver while the latter produces abscesses in the left lobe (Kinney). *Grossly* the liver is usually considerably enlarged and the abscesses are almost always multiple (Fig. 388*A*). They are irregularly distributed, are generally sharply circumscribed, vary in color from gray to yellow to green (depending upon the causative organism), and measure up to 2 cm. in diameter. *Histologically* they appear similar to all pyogenic abscesses with a lumen containing debris and neutrophils and a wall composed of granulation tissue (Fig. 388*B*). As the lesion ages the granulation tissue is converted into scar tissue (Fig. 388*C*) and this may completely replace the abscess (if it is small) or may permanently wall off the destroyed tissue (if it is large). Some of the recorded *complications* are (1) septicemia, (2) rupture of the abscess into the peritoneal cavity, vena cava, pericardium, etc., and (3) pulmonary infarction. The usual *clinical manifestations* consist of fever, chills, pain, sweating, anorexia, loss of weight, weakness, nausea, vomiting, hepatic tenderness and enlargement, jaundice, leukocytosis, and elevation and immobility of the diaphragm roentgenographically. The *diagnosis* is made from a consideration of the clinical manifestations and is confirmed by peritoneoscopy or exploratory laparotomy. *Treatment* consists of prevention by attention to the predisposing infections and of antibiotic and chemotherapy. Once hepatic abscesses have been formed, surgical drainage may be indicated. The *prognosis* in the past has been extremely grave with the mortality rates reaching as high as 95 per cent. Currently, with the advent of antibiotic and chemotherapeutic agents, it is immeasurably improved (Flynn and Michel).

Tuberculosis. —Tuberculosis of the liver is relatively common with the recorded *incidence* ranging from 50 to 80 per cent of all patients dying of pulmonary tuberculosis (Leader). The condition is more common in children than it is in adults and predominates in races (such as Negroes) having a marked susceptibility to tuberculosis. The *cause* is, of course, *Mycobacterium tuberculosis* and the infection is always secondary to tuberculosis elsewhere in the body, especially lungs, lymph nodes, and bones. *Pathologically* the lesions are essentially of three types—miliary, focal, and cholangiolitic. Of these, *miliary tuberculosis* is the most common. As elsewhere, the lesions consist of numerous, sharply circumscribed, gray foci scattered throughout the hepatic parenchyma and measuring not more than 1 or 2 mm. in diameter (Fig. 389*A*). Histologically they consist of soft or hard tubercles scattered irregularly throughout the hepatic parenchyma (Fig. 389*B*). That the lesions sometimes tend to resorb and disappear spontaneously is indicated by the occasional presence of only scattered foci of a similar nature that have been completely calcified (disseminated tuberculosis). *Focal tuberculosis* generally exists in the form of multiple (but occasionally solitary) conglomerate tubercles that produce either tumor-like masses (tuberculomas) or frank abscesses. The latter may be composed of caseous material or more commonly may be filled with pus. In the latter instance, they are difficult to differentiate from ordinary pyogenic

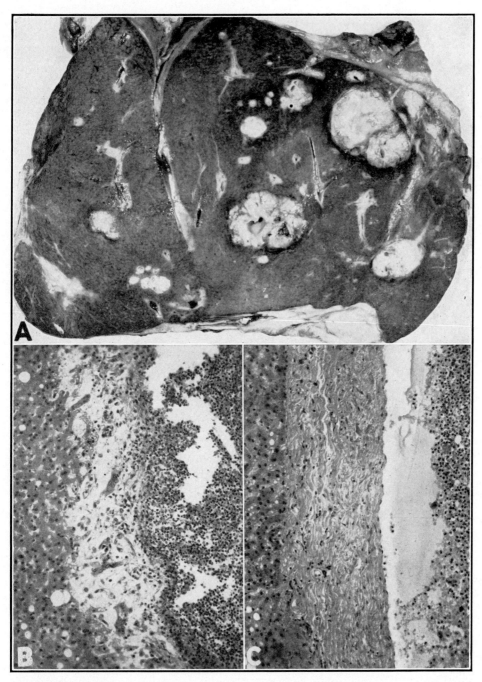

FIG. 388.—Hepatic abscesses showing *A*, multiple varisized but sharply circumscribed lesions, *B*, an acute process with neutrophils, nuclear fragments, and debris centrally and granulation tissue peripherally. × 100, and *C*, a chronic process with the wall composed of collagenous connective tissue. × 100.

abscesses. Histologically these lesions consist of conglomerate masses of hard or soft tubercles, or of caseous material or frank pus surrounded by tuberculous granulation tissue. *Cholangiolitic tuberculosis* consists of multiple abscesses distributed along the ramifications of the bile ducts. They contain either caseous material or pus and, histologically, are similar to the lesions in focal tuberculosis. *Clinically* tuberculous abscesses, whether focal or cholangiolitic in distribution, may be attended by fever, enlargement of the liver, and chills. Jaundice rarely occurs. The *diagnosis* of hepatic tuberculosis is usually made at postmortem but occasionally it is made at laparotomy. The lesions should be differentiated from pyogenic

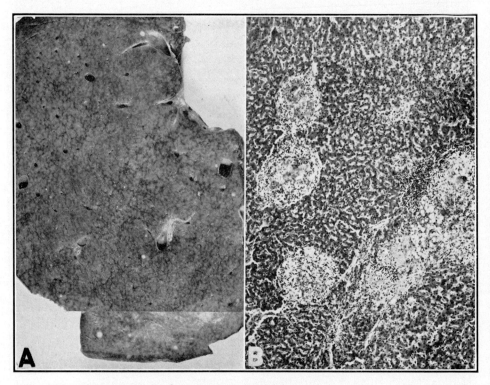

Fig. 389.—Miliary tuberculosis of the liver illustrating *A*, sharply circumscribed gray foci scattered throughout the liver and *B*, several tubercles irregularly distributed in the hepatic parenchyma. × 50.

abscesses, tumors, and gummas. *Treatment* is that of tuberculosis in general. The *prognosis* is usually poor for the condition, as a rule, represents a terminal event.

Boeck's Sarcoid.—The topic of Boeck's sarcoid, in general, has been discussed in the Chapter on the Lungs (p. 501). It is sufficient to mention here that (1) of all organs affected, the liver is involved about fifth in frequency, (2) the organ may or may not be palpably enlarged, (3) the diagnosis can be readily confirmed by needle aspiration biopsy, (4) the histologic changes are similar to those in other organs, (5) derangements of liver function tests do occur, (6) the total serum protein and gamma globulin are elevated, the serum albumin is reduced, and the albumin-globulin ratio is reversed, (7) serum lipid fractions are normal, (8) serum

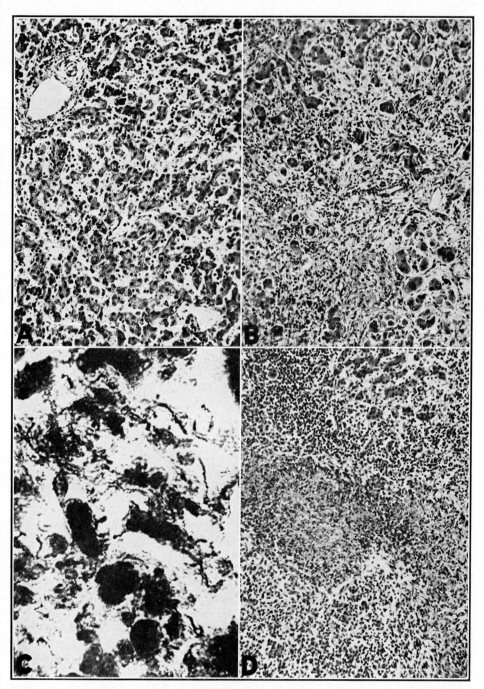

Fig. 390.—Syphilis of the liver showing *A*, an arrest of development in the form of lack of radiation of the liver cords and the presence of hematopoietic foci. × 100, *B*, diffuse interstitial infiltration with plasma cells, lymphocytes and fibroblasts. × 100, *C*, *Treponema pallidum* in a section of the liver stained by the Levaditi method. × 900, and *D*, a miliary gumma. × 100.

alkaline phosphatase is occasionally elevated, and (9) the prognosis is that of the disease in general (Shay).

Syphilis.—Syphilis of the liver may be divided into three groups—early syphilis, late syphilis, and portal cirrhosis in a syphilitic patient (Hahn). *Early syphilis* encompasses both congenital syphilis and early (secondary) acquired syphilis. The most common hepatic lesion in congenital syphilis is an arrest of development. This is manifested by failure of the liver cords to arrange themselves in a radiating pattern and by a persistence of hematopoiesis (Fig. 390*A*). The less frequent lesion in congenital syphilis and the lesion in early acquired syphilis is diffuse interstitial inflammation (Fig. 390*B* and *C*). Generally this consists of an intercellular infiltration with plasma cells and lymphocytes, fibroblastic proliferation, and secondary degeneration and disappearance of hepatic cells—in other words, a diffues syphilitic cirrhosis. Sometimes, however, the lesions are more circumscribed, undergo necrosis, and constitute miliary gummas (Fig. 390*D*). In either case, the liver swarms with *Treponema pallidum* (Fig. 390*C*). The *incidence* of actual syphilitic inflammation of the liver in patients with early syphilis has been calculated as 0.24 per cent in a series of 33,825 patients (Hahn). The chief *clinical manifestation* is jaundice. The *diagnosis* is made by finding jaundice in a patient with a history and other manifestations of syphilis followed by rapid response to antisyphilitic therapy. The *prognosis*, as far as the liver changes are concerned, is generally good.

Late syphilis encompasses tertiary syphilis and is manifested in the liver in the form of a gumma. The lesion may be single or multiple and consists of a sharply circumscribed, grayish-white, rubbery area of necrosis that may measure 16 cm. or more in over-all diameter (Fig. 391*B*). Histologically it is composed of diffuse necrosis (but without destruction of elastic fibers of the stroma) surrounded peripherally by fibroblasts, epithelioid cells, plasma cells, and lymphocytes (p. 178). As the areas of inflammation heal, they become replaced with dense, stellate, fibrous tissue scars which, in turn, transform the liver into an irregularly crevassed, multilobulated structure known as *hepar lobatum* (Shapiro and Symmers). The *incidence* of late syphilis has been calculated as 4.9 per cent in a series of 1,165 patients with late syphilis (Hahn). The condition has no predilection for any race, is somewhat more common in males than in females, and is usually seen between the ages of thirty and fifty years. When the liver is only slightly affected, the condition is asymptomatic but when it is extensively involved the *clinical manifestations* and *course* are the same as those in portal cirrhosis (p. 799).

There is no doubt that *portal cirrhosis*, similar to any other portal cirrhosis (Fig. 391*A*), can occur in a *syphilitic patient*, but whether such a lesion results from dietary insufficiency or whether it is caused by *Treponema pallidum* still remains unanswered (Hahn). The former appears to be the case for the following reasons: (1) the cirrhosis is identical with that seen in ordinary portal cirrhosis, (2) the incidence of this type of cirrhosis among syphilitics is about the same as the incidence of portal cirrhosis in nonsyphilitics, (3) portal cirrhosis has not been recorded in a syphilitic patient less than thirty years of age, and (4) portal cirrhosis almost never occurs in conjunction with definite syphilis of the liver.

Weil's Disease.—Weil's disease is an acute febrile spirochetal infection that is *also known* as leptospirosis, spirochetal jaundice, and leptospiral infection. It is worldwide in *distribution* and is common in the United States where over 300 cases have been recorded up to 1950 (Reid). It is found in people of all ages and affects both sexes. The *cause* is *Leptospira icterohæmorrhagiæ*—a tightly coiled, thin, flexible spirochete that has hooked ends and that measures from 7 to 14 microns in length and 0.25 to 0.3 micron in width (Fig. 392*A*). The organism naturally infects rats and the excreta of rats act as a source of infection for man. The spirochete enters man by way of an abrasion of the skin or mucous membrane or, rarely, by way of a rat bite. Most of the cases in man occur in sewer workers, tunellers, fishermen, miners, slaughterhouse workers, swimmers

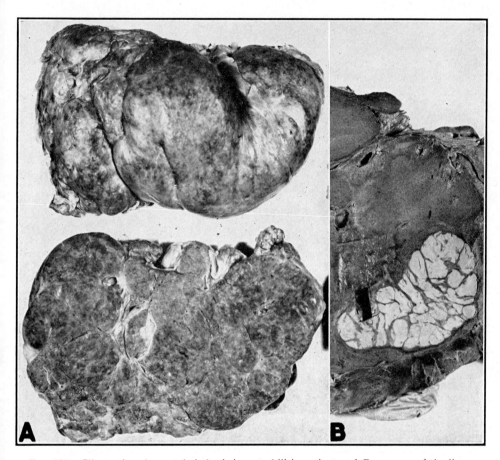

Fig. 391.—Illustrating *A*, portal cirrhosis in a syphilitic patient and *B*, gumma of the liver.

in rat-infected waters, etc. Another spirochete—*Leptospira canicola*—is carried by the dog and produces a disease in man that is virtually identical with Weil's disease (Reid).

Pathologically the initial infection in man is a septicemia with the causative organisms being distributed throughout the tissues of the body. Two of the outstanding features are hemolysis of erythrocytes and increased capillary fragility. These alterations result in a hemorrhagic diathesis that involves mucous membranes, lungs, muscles, and most other tissues of the body. The changes in the liver vary greatly from no involvement to severe necrosis. In most cases, however, the following are noted: degeneration of the hepatic cells, intralobular bile stasis, infiltration of leukocytes in the

portal areas, fatty change in the hepatic cells, and at least focal necrosis.
The kidneys reveal the typical changes of acute toxic nephrosis (p. 1064).
The lungs disclose widespread bilateral hemorrhages and, in some instances,
patchy pneumonia. The striated muscles reveal hemorrhages grossly and
degeneration, disruption of the fibers, erythrocytic extravasation, and
leukocytic infiltration microscopically (Fig. 392 B). The causative spirochetes may be readily demonstrated (by means of silver impregnation) in
the tubules and interstitial tissue of the kidneys and in the liver (Fig.
392 A).

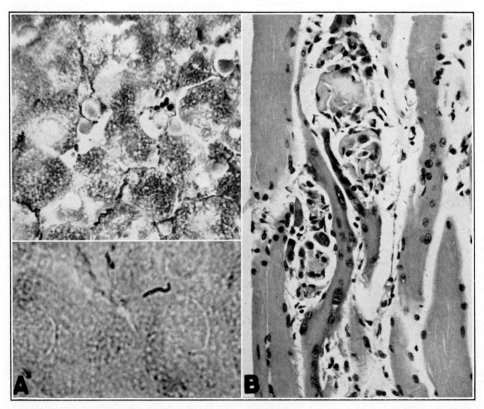

Fig. 392.—Weil's disease disclosing A, *Leptospira icterohæmorrhagiæ* in Levaditi-stained sections
of the liver. × 1350 and B, degeneration, hemorrhage, and leukocytic infiltration in striated
(calf) muscle. × 200.

The chief *complications* occur as part of the disease and consist of hemorrhages, jaundice, pneumonia, and uremia. *Clinically* some infections are so
mild that they may escape notice while other infections are severe. After
an incubation period of from four to twelve days the following manifestations occur rather suddenly: chills, fever, fatigue, weakness, malaise, frontal
headache, muscle pain, anorexia, nausea, vomiting, petechiæ, epistaxis,
hemoptysis, gastrointestinal bleeding, subconjunctival hemorrhages, jaundice (50% of cases), hepatomegaly, tenderness of the liver, leukocytosis,
hematuria, oliguria, anuria, and depressed liver function tests (Leibowitz,
Reid, and Chinn). Convalescence is protracted. The *diagnosis* is made
from a consideration of the following: (1) history, (2) clinical manifestations,
(3) isolation of the causative organisms from the blood during the first

week and from the urine after the seventh day by dark field examination or
by inoculation of guinea pigs, (4) culture of the spirochetes on special
media, (5) positive complement fixation tests, and (6) positive agglutination
tests from the ninth day on using a formalin-killed suspension of spirochetes
as the antigen (Reid). *Treatment* is still unsatisfactory, with convalescent
serum being used in severe cases. Antibiotics are ineffective (Hall). The
prognosis is variable but in the over-all good. The recorded mortality rates,
as a rule, vary between 2.5 and 9.4 per cent (Hall). The usual cause of
death is uremia.

Viral Hepatitis.—There are three viral infections of the liver—yellow
fever, infectious hepatitis, and serum hepatitis—that are caused by different
viruses but that may be considered together because they have many
features in common. *Yellow fever* is caused by the yellow fever virus and is
transmitted to man by the *Aedes ægypti* mosquito (Soper). The virus is one
of the smaller pathogenic viruses, is destroyed by temperatures above 55° C.
and many chemicals, may be preserved for years in a thoroughly desiccated
vacuum stored at low temperature, is culturable only in the presence of
living cells, is pathogenic for Rhesus monkeys by way of extraneural inoculation and for white mice by way of intracerebral inoculation, and
produces lasting immunity in man. Yellow fever is a tropical disease that
currently prevails in South America and Africa. It occurs at all seasons of
the year but is particularly common during the rainy season. *Infectious
hepatitis* is also known as epidemic hepatitis, catarrhal jaundice, and non-
spirochetal infectious jaundice (Mallory). It is the naturally occurring
form of viral hepatitis in which, however, the virus as such has not yet been
isolated. The agent is infectious by mouth, is recoverable in feces, and is
spread by person to person contact although it may be borne by water or
food (Havens, Farquhar, and Kaufmann). The incubation period of the
naturally occurring disease is unknown but when the condition is spread by
syringe or needle it is from sixteen to thirty days. It occurs both endemically and epidemically, is most common in autumn and early winter, and
was the scourge of World War II. In civilian life it is more common in
children than in adults in the ratio of 3 to 2 and is also seen in infants
(Traisman). *Serum hepatitis*, also known as homologous serum hepatitis,
is a form of viral hepatitis that is transmitted from person to person by
receiving serum or some other product of human blood parenterally (Havens,
Greenlee, and Lesses). The incubation period varies from fifty to one hundred and fifty days, with an average of ninety days. The virus may exist
in the bloodstream of the host for long periods of time without causing any
obvious illness. Both infectious hepatitis and serum hepatitis are worldwide in distribution.

The *pathologic* changes are similar regardless of the type of virus causing
the infection. For descriptive purposes, the hepatic alterations may be
divided into three groups—fulminating cases, subacute cases, and nonfatal
cases. In *fulminating* cases, with death occurring within two weeks, the
liver usually weighs between 600 and 1400 gm. (Mallory). The surface is
smooth or finely wrinkled; the consistency is soft and flabby; hemorrhages
may be seen in the subcapsular area and throughout the cut surface, and
the color varies from reddish-brown, to purple, to yellowish green (Fig.
393). Histologically there is a uniform destruction of hepatic cells (Fig.
394*A*, *B* and *C*). The necrosis usually starts in the central area and advances toward the periphery. In some instances, only a portion of the
lobule is destroyed while in others, all but a fringe of peripheral cells or all

the cells are completely destroyed. The necrotic cells are rapidly removed, leaving the underlying reticulum readily apparent. The portal and inter-lobular areas contain varying degrees of infiltration with monocytes, plasma cells, lymphocytes, neutrophils, and eosinophils. Phagocytes laden with brown pigment are scattered here and there. There is usually no evidence of regeneration of the hepatic cells but bile duct proliferation is apparent. Aside from the changes in the liver, fulminating cases may dis-close ascites, congestive splenomegaly, acute toxic nephrosis, degeneration of the ganglion cells of the brain, and occasionally gastroenteritis. In *subacute* cases, death usually occurs in from twenty to fifty days (Lucké and

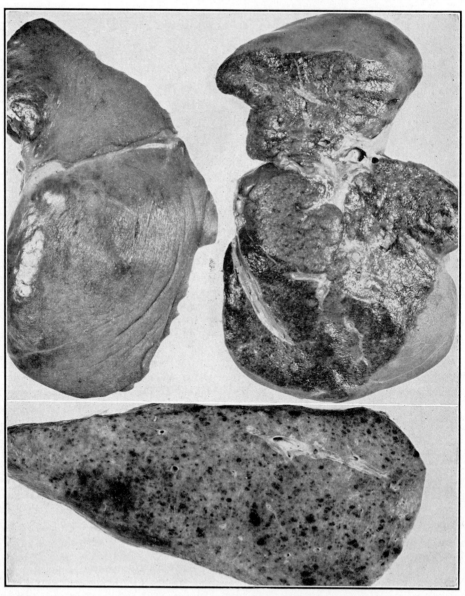

FIG. 393.—Viral hepatitis showing, above, the wrinkled external and blotchy cut surfaces and, below, diffuse small and large hemorrhages.

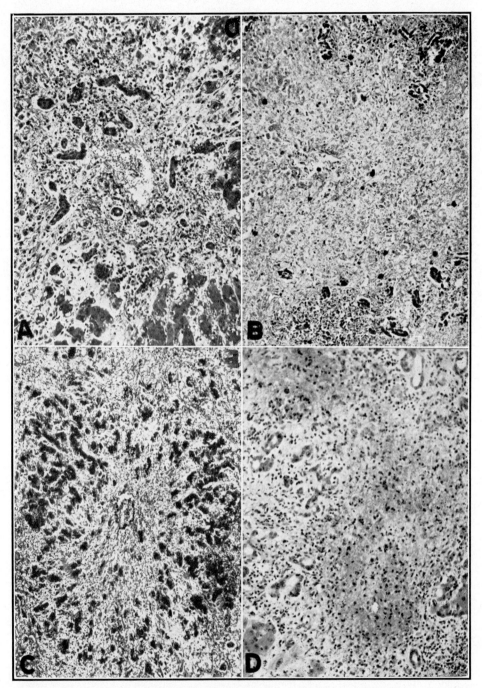

FIG. 394.—Viral hepatitis illustrating *A* and *B*, extensive necrosis and disappearance of hepatic cells and slight leukocytic infiltration in cases of fulminating disease. × 100, *C*, preservance of the underlying reticulum. × 50, and *D*, necrosis of hepatic cells, leukocytic infiltration, bile duct proliferation, and beginning fibrosis in a case of subacute disease. × 100.

Mallory). The liver, as in the fulminating cases, weighs between 600 and 1400 grams. Grossly it is generally obviously deformed and consists of depressed stellate scars that encircle large and small areas of regenerated hepatic parenchyma. Histologically the following changes are usually seen: disappearance of hepatic cells, condensation of the reticulum, engorgement of the sinusoids, proliferation of bile ducts, leukocytic (monocytic, lymphocytic, plasma cells, eosinophilic, and neutrophilic) infiltration in the portal areas, increase of portal connective tissue, irregular regeneration of hepatic cells, and stasis of bile within the canaliculi (Fig. 394D). In other words, the changes in subacute viral hepatitis constitute a healing phase of the acute fulminating disease and are identical with what has been described as post-necrotic cirrhosis (p. 810). Knowledge of the changes in *nonfatal* cases of viral hepatitis has been possible because of needle aspiration biopsy (Mallory and Keller). In such cases, the portal areas contain monocytes, lymphocytes, and occasionally eosinophils and plasma cells (Fig. 395). From these areas, the leukocytes have a tendency to spread into the peripheral portions of the hepatic lobules. The lobules disclose the following: swollen reticuloendothelial cells containing ingested bile pigment and fat, collection of mononuclear cells about clumps of necrotic hepatic cells, disruption of the lobular pattern by enlargement of some and shrinkage of other liver cells, disruption and focal condensation of reticulum, ballooning of some of the hepatic cells, proliferation of hepatic cells as a result of both mitotic and amitotic division, some bile stasis, and the formation of Councilman bodies. These bodies have originally been described in connection with yellow fever but have subsequently been found in other cases of hepatic necrosis. They represent parenchymatous hepatic cells that have reacted to injury. They consist of round, homogenous, intensely eosinophilic, hyaline bodies that may or may not contain a pyknotic or fragmented nucleus. Although they arise in the hepatic cords, they are extruded from the columns into the sinusoids. As previously stated, nonfatal cases of viral hepatitis in which the infection either recurs or smoulders may terminate as infective biliary cirrhosis (p. 809).

The *complications* of viral hepatitis are hepatic insufficiency, recurrence of the disorder, predisposition to secondary infection, uremia, and post-necrotic or biliary cirrhosis. While the *clinical manifestations* vary considerably from case to case, they usually consist of some combination of the following: anorexia, nausea, vomiting, dark urine, lassitude, malaise, fatigue, epigastric discomfort or pain, fever, pruritus, chills, headache, diarrhea, jaundice, and enlargement and tenderness of the liver (Sborov). From the laboratory standpoint, positive thymol turbidity, cephalin flocculation, and zinc turbidity tests are important in differentiating jaundice due to viral hepatitis from that due to extrahepatic obstruction. The *diagnosis* of viral hepatitis is readily made during the course of an epidemic but is more difficult to arrive at otherwise. In general, the following are of importance: history, clinical manifestations, laboratory data, and needle aspiration biopsy of the liver. The best *treatment* is prevention. In the case of yellow fever, this consists of destroying the *Aedes ægypti* and cleaning up its breeding places. In the case of serum hepatitis, proper sterilization of syringes and needles is mandatory. Ultraviolet irradiation of serum and other blood products is no guarantee against transmission of the virus (Greenlee) and convalescent gamma globulin is also not effective as a protective agent (Drake). When the disease has been acquired, treatment is symptomatic and, among other things, consists of absolute bed rest and

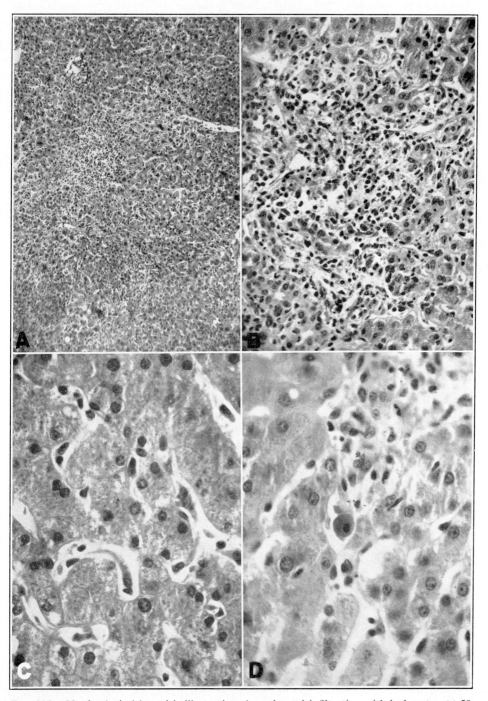

FIG. 395.—Nonfatal viral hepatitis illustrating A, periportal infiltration with leukocytes. $\times$ 50, B, a higher magnification of a portal area permeated with leukocytes. $\times$ 200, C, swollen reticuloendothelial cells. $\times$ 400, and D, a Councilman body. $\times$ 400.

a diet high in protein and carbohydrate and as much dairy fat as the patient can eat. The *prognosis* is generally good, for the mortality rate among Army personnel is about 0.4 per cent (Mallory). In civilian life, however, the mortality in infectious hepatitis has been recorded as being as high as 4.8 per cent and in serum hepatitis as high as 34 per cent (Steele).

Parasitic Hepatitis.—The important parasitic infections of the liver are caused by *Schistosoma* (p. 775), *Endamœba histolytica*, flukes, and *Echinococcus granulosus*.

Endamœba histolytica usually produces ulcerations in the large intestine (p. 770), but sometimes organisms enter the tributaries of the portal vein and cause *amebic abscesses* of the liver. The *incidence* of this complication varies with the material studied (Ochsner). In a collected series of 5,211 fatal cases of amebiasis 36.6 per cent had liver abscesses, while in clinical cases the recorded percentages have varied between 0.12 per cent and 22.6 per cent. Amebic abscesses of the liver affect males in about 90 per cent of cases and generally occur in patients between the ages of twenty and fifty years. *Pathologically* the number of abscesses in a single case is variable although usually the lesion is single and the right lobe is affected more often than the left. The size varies from a few millimeters to 20 cm. in diameter. Early, the wall is thin, is scarcely visible, and discloses a shaggy inner surface. Later, it is composed of dense fibrous tissue of varying thickness. The contents vary with the stage of the disease. Early in the process the lumen contains viscid, glairy, transparent material while later, as a result of escape of blood, the contents consist of chocolate-colored or brown material that has been frequently likened to anchovy or chocolate sauce. When secondary infection supervenes, the contents become purulent. *Histologically* the process consists essentially of liquefaction necrosis and characteristically discloses little or no leukocytic infiltration. The *complications* consist of (1) secondary infection with pyogenic organisms and (2) extension or rupture of the abscess into one of the viscera with the development of peritonitis, empyema, etc. The *clinical manifestations* consist of hepatic pain and tenderness, fever, hepatic enlargement, weakness, loss of weight, diarrhea, chills, nausea and vomiting, and jaundice. Roentgenographically the diaphragm is raised and immobile. The *diagnosis* is made from the clinical manifestations and isolation of *Endamœba histolytica* from the stool. *Treatment* is that employed in amebiasis in general, together with aspiration of the abscess in noninfected cases and open surgical drainage in infected cases. The *prognosis* is variable, depending upon the multiplicity of the hepatic lesions, the presence or absence of complications, and the type of therapy employed. The mortality rate in 181 cases reported on by Ochsner was 16 per cent.

There are two important liver *flukes*—*Fasciola hepatica* and *Clonorchis sinensis* (Craig and Faust, and Sawitz). *Fasciola hepatica* is commonly known as the sheep-liver fluke and produces sheep-liver rot. As would be expected, the infection is prevalent in sheep raising countries. The *organism* is flat and more or less leaf-shaped (Fig. 396A). It measures 30 mm. in length and 13 mm. in breadth. The anterior end is conical and possesses an oral and a ventral sucker. Most of the rest of the organism is composed of a digestive tract and male and female genital organs. The adult worm lives in the bile passages of the liver and the ova are passed by way of the bile in the feces. The *ova* are oval, operculated, and measure about 140 by 75 microns (Fig. 396B). They mature in the water in from nine to fifteen days and upon hatching liberate *miracidia* (Fig. 396C). These invade snails where they develop into cercariæ. Upon leaving the snails, the cercariæ encyst on blades of grass, develop into metacercariæ, and are thus infective for sheep and occasionally man. When ingested, the metacercariæ penetrate the intestinal mucosa, enter the liver, and find their way to the bile ducts (Fig. 396D). Here they produce obstruction, bile duct proliferation, leukocytic infiltration, fibrosis, and even abscesses. The *clinical manifestations* consist of pain, coughing, vomiting, fever, diarrhea, abdominal rigidity, eosinophilia, leukocytosis, and anemia. The *diagnosis* is made by

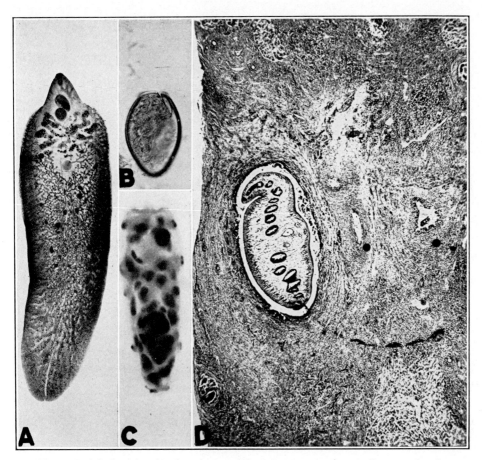

Fig. 396.—*Fasciola hepatica* showing *A*, an adult worm. × semigross, *B*, operculated ovum. × 200, *C*, miracidia. × 40, and *D*, the lesion in the liver. × 100.

finding the ova in the feces or biliary drainage. *Treatment* is unsatisfactory but emetine hydrochloride has been used. The *prognosis* depends upon the severity of the hepatic infection.

Clonorchis sinensis, commonly known as the Chinese liver fluke, is limited to the Far East. The *adult worm* lives in the bile passages, is flat and transparent, possesses an attenuated anterior end with an oral sucker, discloses coarsely branching testes posteriorly, and measures 18 × 4 mm. (Fig. 397*A*). The ova are operculated, often show a protrusion of the shell at the end opposite the operculum, and measure 31 × 15 microns. The ova are discharged in the feces and hatched in fresh water, liberating miracidia. The latter are ingested by snails where they develop into cercariæ. The cercariæ attach themselves to fish and develop into meta-cercariæ which are infective for man. After excystment in the small intestine, the organisms migrate to the liver by way of the lumen of the ampulla of Vater and extrahepatic bile ducts. The *pathologic* alterations in the liver are similar to those caused by *Fasciola hepatica* with the changes frequently severe enough to produce cirrhosis (Fig. 397*B*). The *clinical*

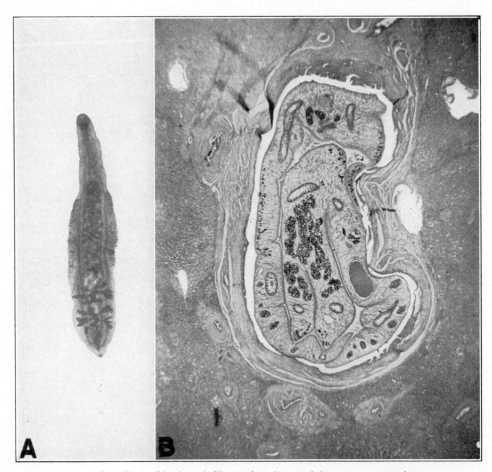

FIG. 397.—*Clonorchis sinensis* illustrating *A*, an adult worm. × semigross and *B*, the lesion in the liver. × 50.

manifestations are those of fascioliasis and, in more severe cases, of cir-rhosis. The *diagnosis* is made by finding ova in the stool or biliary drainage. *Treatment* consists of administration of choloquine or medicinal gentian violet. The *prognosis* is good in light infections but poor in heavy infections.

Echinococcus granulosis is a tapeworm that causes echinococcosis or hydatid disease. It is common in sheep raising countries. The *adult worm* is found only in the small intestine of carnivorous animals such as dogs, wolves, and foxes. It measures from 3 to 5 mm. in length, discloses three proglottids (immature, mature, and gravid) and possesses a pyriform scolex that has four suckers and a crown of hooklets (Fig. 398*A*). The *ova*, dis-

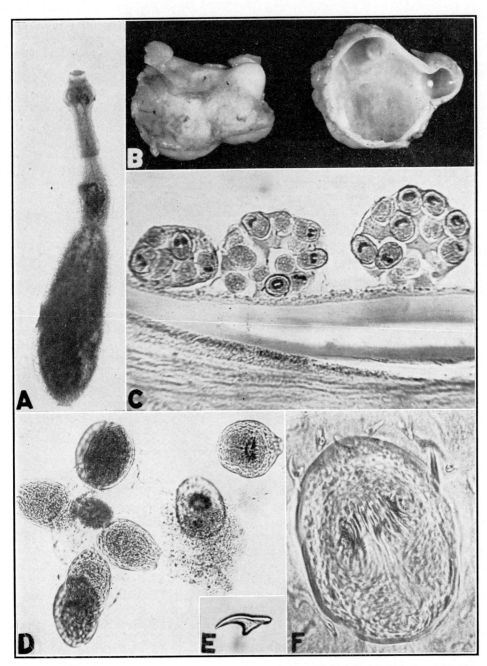

Fig. 398.—*Echinococcus granulosis* showing *A*, an adult worm. × 40, *B*, an external and a cut surface of a small cyst, with two daughter cysts in the latter, *C*, the wall of a cyst composed, from within out, of lumen, "brood capsules," germinal layer, chitinous layer, and adventitious layer. × 75, *D*, hydatid sand with eight scolices. × 200, *E*, typical anvil-shaped hooklet. × 400, and *F*, a scolex with a double row of hooklets. × 400.

charged in the feces of carnivorous animals, are identical with those of *Tænia solium* and *Tænia saginata* (p. 720). Upon ingestion by herbivorous animals such as sheep, pigs, and cattle the ova hatch in the intestine. The emerging *hexacanth larvæ* penetrate the intestinal mucosa and are carried to most of the tissues of the body. Here they form hydatid larvæ and these are infective for carnivorous animals, thus repeating the cycle. As a result of accidental contamination, *man* sometimes replaces herbivorous animals as the intermediate host. Here hexacanth larvæ are carried to the liver and thence to the lungs, heart, kidneys, bones, and most other tissues of the body. Wherever they are deposited, they may develop into hydatid larvæ. These grow slowly, ultimately producing typical *cysts* that may measure as much as 20 cm. or more in diameter (Fig. 398*A*). The cysts are surrounded by an adventitious layer (composed of inflammatory cells and fibroblasts) derived from the host and consist of an outer chitinous laminated layer and an inner germinal layer (Fig. 398*C*). The germinal layer produces cell buds ("brood capsules") which become vacuolated, develop scolices, and may become surrounded by a laminated membrane to produce daughter cysts. The mother cyst is filled with yellowish fluid which contains "hydatid sand." This consists of detached "brood capsules," daughter cysts, scolices, and hooklets (Fig. 398*D*). A hooklet is typically anvil-shaped and measures from 15 to 25 microns in greatest diameter (Fig. 398*E*). The scolex is pear-shaped, measures about 150 × 160 microns, and discloses a central double row of interlocking hooklets (Fig. 398*F*). The *clinical manifestations* vary with the organ affected and are due to the presence of a space-taking lesion and/or rupture with spilling of the contents. The *diagnosis* is made from the typical gross appearance of the cyst and especially from the microscopic identification of scolices and/or hooklets. Complement fixation and skin sensitivity tests are also of distinct value clinically. The *treatment* of choice is surgical excision. The *prognosis* is fair to good. Many of the smaller cysts become completely calcified.

PHYSICAL DISTURBANCES

Orientation.—In this section, the following unrelated conditions of the liver may be mentioned: passive hyperemia (p. 193), infarction, Chiari's disease, portal hypertension, trauma, and chemical necrosis.

Infarction.—Because of a dual blood supply, infarction of the liver is uncommon. The condition may *occur* at any age and in either sex. The *cause* is occlusion of the hepatic artery, hepatic veins, portal vein, or combinations of these vessels (Woolling, Losner, and Rosenbaum). Among others, the condition may be seen in connection with carcinoma of the gallbladder, gallstones, cholecystitis, tumors of the stomach and small intestine, inflammations of the stomach and small intestine, cardiovascular diseases, periarteritis nodosa, abdominal operations, etc. *Pathologically* the more common lesion is the atrophic *red infarct* of *Zahn*. This consists of a triangular or irregular deep reddish-brown, sharply demarcated area that usually measures less than 3 cm. in diameter. Histologically it discloses only dilatation and engorgement of the sinuses and atrophy of the hepatic cells. The less common lesion is the *true infarct* (Fig. 399). Depending upon the number and sizes of the vessel affected, true infarcts may be single or multiple and may be so small that they are barely visible or so large that they virtually involve the entire liver. The affected area is usually sharply demarcated, irregular in outline, reddish brown to yellowish gray, and soft.

Histologically it consists of a central area of partial or complete necrosis of all elements surrounded by a zone of nonspecific inflammation. The lesion tends to heal by resolution, regeneration of hepatic cells and bile ducts, and fibrosis. The chief *complication* is hepatic coma. *Clinically* there may be high fever, jaundice, oliguria, azotemia, and coma. The *diagnosis* is made at operation or postmortem. There is no satisfactory *treatment*. The prognosis in recorded cases has been poor, death having occurred in all.

Chiari's Disease.—The condition known by this name was recognized as endophlebitis of the hepatic veins by Chiari in 1899 (Armstrong). The entity consists of an acute or gradual occlusion of the hepatic veins of a

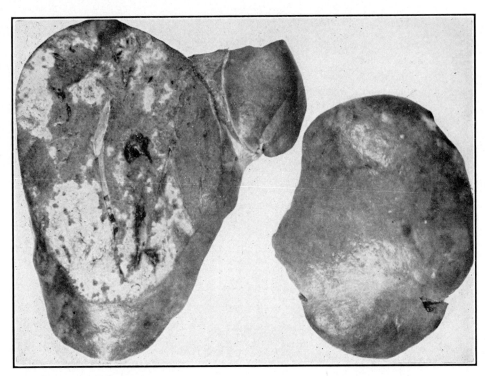

Fig. 399.—Infarction of the liver disclosing many irregular but sharply circumscribed, yellowish-gray areas. The cause was complete acute thrombosis of the portal vein. (Specimen submitted by Dr. Joseph Stasney.)

degree sufficient to produce hepatic failure but of a degree insufficient to cause infarction of the liver. Some of the recorded *causes* of the venous occlusion are primary thrombosis and thrombophlebitis, local and general infection, stasis, systemic disease, polycythemia vera, anomalous venous development, and neoplasm. *Pathologically* collateral circulations may be established in cases that develop gradually. The liver discloses central lobular degeneration and necrosis, hyperemia of the sinusoids, and replacement fibrosis. The spleen is generally enlarged.

Portal Hypertension.—Portal hypertension, also known as *Banti's syndrome* or *disease*, is a syndrome characterized by congestive spleno-megaly, secondary anemia, leukopenia, thrombocytopenia, esophageal varices, and attacks of gastrointestinal bleeding (Blakemore). The *cause* is obstruction to the flow of blood through the portal vein. The obstruction may be (1) intrahepatic and almost always due to cirrhosis, or (2) extra-hepatic and due to (*a*) a congenital extension of the normal thrombotic process that obliterates the umbilical vein and ductless venosis, or (*b*) acquired thrombosis or extramural pressure from inflammation or tumor (Welch). Occasionally cirrhosis of the liver and thrombosis of the portal vein may exist in the same case (Fig. 400). *Pathologically* the *liver*, in cases of intrahepatic block, discloses the changes ordinarily encountered in cirrhosis (p. 800) but, in cases of extrahepatic block, it is generally normal. The

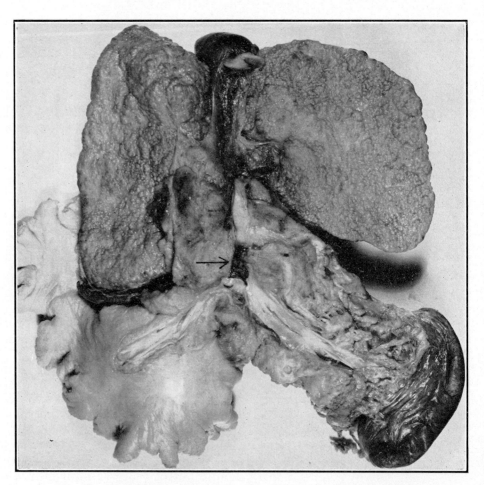

Fig. 400.—Portal hypertension illustrating cirrhosis of the liver, thrombosis of the portal vein (arrow), and congestive splenomegaly.

spleen is enlarged to several times the normal size. At first it discloses simply passive congestion. Later, as the process becomes chronic, it reveals hemorrhages with focal deposits of hemosiderin and surrounding fibroblastic proliferation—the so-called siderotic nodules. An outstanding change in cases of portal hypertension is a development of *collateral circulations*. They occur in the following areas: cardio-esophageal, anorectal, umbilical, and retroperitoneal where peritoneally uncovered abdominal viscera is attached to the abdominal wall. The chief *complications* of portal hypertension are ascites and gastrointestinal bleeding. The *clinical manifesta-*

tions are those outlined in the opening sentence of this paragraph. The *diagnosis* is made from the history and the clinical findings. *Treatment* is surgical by way of a portacaval shunt, that is, an anastomosis between the portal and caval systems of veins. The veins usually used are portal vein to the vena cava or splenic vein to the left renal vein (Fig. 401). The *prognosis* in untreated patients with gastrointestinal hemorrhages is poor with 50 to 80 per cent of them being dead within one year after their first hemorrhage. Surgical treatment is curative in cases of extrahepatic block but is only palliative in cases of intrahepatic block. In Blakemore's series the one-month to seven-year survival in patients operated upon was 95 per cent in 40 cases of extrahepatic obstruction and 82.2 per cent in 90 cases of intra-hepatic obstruction.

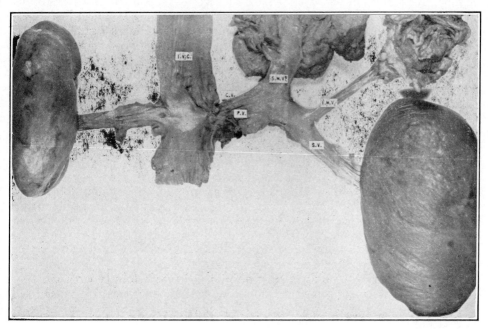

Fig. 401.—Portal hypertension showing the portal vein anastomosed to the stump of the left renal vein. Note the congestive splenomegaly.

Trauma. —Trauma to the liver may be direct or indirect. *Direct* trauma is due to a penetrating injury such as that caused by a knife, bullet or shrapnel, broken ribs, etc. *Indirect* trauma is due to nonpenetrating forces such as crushing injuries (especially those sustained in automobile accidents), falls, and blows. The *incidence* of trauma to the liver in military life is considerably greater than that in civilian life. In general city hospitals, the liver is found to be traumatized once in approximately every 1,200 injuries and in three-quarters of the cases in which intra-abdominal organs are injured (Wright). The injury may occur at all ages and affects males three times as often as females. *Pathologically, penetrating* injuries vary with the type of object producing the disturbance. They may be single or multiple and usually extend considerably deeper into the hepatic substance than the external wound tends to indicate. *Nonpenetrating* injury is usually manifested in the form of an irregular stellate crack (Wright). The defect may be small or may measure as much as 20 cm. in length and depth. The

53

right lobe is involved about six times as frequently as the left; the dome is more commonly involved than other portions, and the lesions may be multiple. Regardless of the size of the laceration, hemorrhage is always present. Bleeding may occur under the capsule of the liver, into the peritoneal cavity, or in both areas. It may be slight or massive. In deeper lacerations the blood is mixed with escaping bile. The chief *complication* of trauma to the liver is bleeding. In addition, associated lesions in other organs of the abdominal, thoracic, and even cranial cavities are common. *Clinically* trauma to the liver is generally associated with some combination of the following: abdominal pain and distention, abdominal tenderness and muscle spasm, shock, nausea, anemia, and leukocytosis (Sawyer). The *diagnosis* is often made with difficulty. It is established on the basis of the history, clinical manifestations, peritoneoscopy, exploratory laparotomy, and postmortem. The advocated *treatment* consists of combating the shock and stopping the bleeding surgically. Surgical procedures used are quite varied (Papen). The *prognosis* is guarded for the recorded mortality rate is as high as 100 per cent. In general, the outlook is considerably better in patients treated surgically than it is in those treated conservatively. In a series of 40 cases reported on by Papen, the mortality rate was 81.8 per cent in patients not operated upon, while it was 38.9 per cent in patients subjected to operation.

Chemical Necrosis. —Some of the numerous chemicals that may produce necrosis of the liver are chloroform, carbon tetrachloride, trichlorethylene, dichlorbenzene, diphenyl chloride, chlorinated naphthalenes, chlorinated phenols, toluylene-diamine, dinitrotoluylene, aliphatic thiocyanates, unsaturated aliphatic hydrocarbons (such as tropene), arsphenamine, cinchophen, phosphorus, mercury, bismuth, alloxan, sulfonamides, tannic acid, extracts of certain algæ, and certain poisonous mushrooms. In addition as, already seen, hepatic necrosis may be caused by dietary deficiency (p. 799) and bacterial or viral infection (p. 821). *Pathologically* the necrosis may be divided into two groups—zonal and massive (Mallory). *Zonal necrosis* connotes destruction of only a portion of the hepatic lobule with the necrosis being similar in each of the lobules affected. It is usually caused by single and small doses of the chemicals listed. Grossly the liver may appear normal or it may disclose tiny areas of yellowish or reddish discoloration in each of the hepatic lobules. Histologically the process is entirely nonspecific, being characterized by (1) degeneration and necrosis of the liver cells, (2) hemorrhagic extravasation, (3) leukocytic infiltration, (4) maintenance of the normal stromal architecture, (5) fatty and other degenerative changes in the remaining hepatic cells, and (6) rapid regeneration of the liver cells in patients that survive. The distribution of the necrosis is (1) center of the lobule, (2) periphery of the lobule, (3) midzonal portion of the lobule, and (4) combinations of these. While certain chemicals may affect a certain portion of the hepatic lobule (as for example, carbon tetrachloride —center and phosphorus—periphery) such a relationship does not always hold. In patients that survive the immediate effects, the liver either undergoes complete resolution and restitution to normal or it becomes cirrhotic. The latter resembles infective biliary cirrhosis (p. 809) but is frequently referred to as arsenic cirrhosis, carbon tetrachloride cirrhosis, etc. *Massive necrosis* is caused by (1) massive, (2) repeated, or (3) small doses in sensitized individuals of the chemicals and substances listed. Pathologically the changes are identical with those seen in fulminating viral hepatitis (p. 824) In patients that survive the immediate effects, the liver undergoes regeneration and fibrosis producing what is referred to as postnecrotic cirrhosis (p. 810).

TUMORS

Orientation. — Tumors of the liver are dividable into two main groups — secondary and primary. Of these, secondary tumors are common while primary tumors are relatively rare. In this general discussion, unless otherwise specified, reference will be made only to the latter. Although the *incidence* of primary tumors of the liver varies with the type of growth, the over-all figures recorded in the literature range from 0.12 to 0.5 per cent of all autopsies (Warvi). They occur in all races, both sexes, and at all ages. The specific *causative agents* are unknown but heredity doubtlessly plays a role. Added factors that have been recorded are congenital cellular rests, prolonged chemical or other irritation of hepatic cells, cirrhosis, and avitaminosis. *Pathologically*, as already mentioned, the lesions may be secondary or primary. Primary tumors of the liver consist of adenoma, hamartoma, carcinoma, hemangioma, lymphangioma, endothelioma, mixed tumors, lymphoblastoma, and other sarcomas (mostly fibrosarcoma). The *complications* are cachexia, jaundice, ascites, and hepatic insufficiency. *Clinically* benign tumors are often asymptomatic but when large or strategically located they produce symptoms and signs similar to those of malignant (primary or secondary) growths. In malignant neoplasms there is usually a combination of the following: anemia, loss of weight, weakness, palpable tumor in the region of the liver, jaundice, pain, fever, vomiting, edema of the legs, ascites, fixed diaphragm, and enlargement of the liver (Warvi). Hepatic function tests are usually of little value in the evaluation of any given case. The *diagnosis* is made from (1) the clinical manifestations, (2) aspiration biopsy, and (3) peritoneoscopy or laparotomy with removal of tissue for microscopic study. The only effective *treatment* is surgical excision. The *prognosis* varies with the type of lesion. In benign growths it is generally good while in malignant tumors it is poor. Aside from the general considerations just concluded, a few separate words may be said concerning the following growths: hamartoma, hemangioma, mixed tumors, primary carcinoma, and secondary tumors.

Hamartoma. — A hamartoma (Gr. = error + tumor) is a benign tumor composed of tissues normally present in an area but arranged in irregular fashion (Levenson). Hamartoma of the liver is usually seen in infants or children, is generally encapsulated, varies in size to as much as 20 cm. in diameter, may be single or multiple, and is composed of mixtures of adult appearing connective tissue, blood vessels, hepatic cells, and bile ducts.

Hemangioma. — Small hemangiomas of the liver are frequent while large hemangiomas are uncommon. Only 84 cases of the latter have been recorded in the literature up to 1952 and of these 72 have been resected surgically (Wilson). The lesions occur at all ages with the greatest incidence in the third and fourth decades of life. *Pathologically* they affect the left lobe more commonly than the right, may measure as much as 20 cm. in diameter, are usually spongy and filled with blood grossly, and are composed of cavernous spaces microscopically (Fig. 402). The chief *clinical complication* is rupture with fatal intraperitoneal hemorrhage.

Mixed Tumors. — A mixed tumor of the liver is one composed of cells originating in more than one germinal layer. It has also been called embryonal tumor, teratoma, carcinosarcoma, and according to the elements it contains such as carcino-osteochondromyxosarcoma, etc. (Milman). The tumor is rare, there having been only 27 cases recorded by 1951. In this group, two-thirds of the cases occurred in children under eight years of age and males predominated over females in the ratio of 3 to 2. *Pathologically* the tumors contain epithelial elements in more or less glandular formation. The majority, in addition, contain adult or embryonal connective tissue and a few also disclose primitive or adult muscle, cartilage, and even bone. Grossly the growths are single or multiple and, in the recorded cases, have predominated in the right lobe. Most of the cases reported on were considered to be malignant.

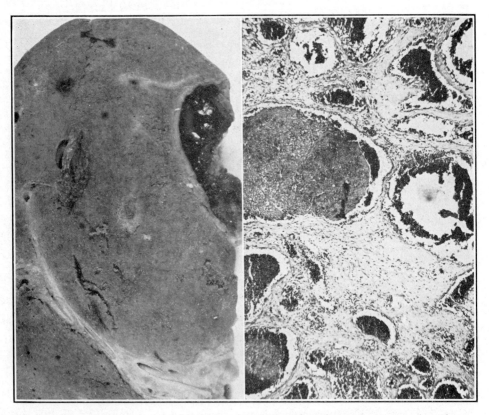

Fig. 402.—Hemangioma of the liver showing, to the left, a dark red spongy and cystic mass and, to the right, cavernous spaces filled with blood. × 50.

Primary Carcinoma.—Primary carcinoma of the liver may *occur* at any age from birth to the ninth decade but is most common in the sixth decade of life (Bigelow and Warvi). Males are affected more commonly than females in the approximate ratio of 2 to 1. The disease is more frequent in the Orient than in Europe and America, due probably to a greater incidence of cirrhosis of the liver in the Far East (Galluzi). *Pathologically* the cases may be divided into three groups—hepatic cell type, bile duct type, and a mixture of the two (Ripstein and McNamara). Of these, the *hepatic cell type* is the most common, accounting for about two-thirds of all cases (Fig. 403). Such a tumor has also been called a hepatoma. This term, however, is confusing unless it is further qualified as to benign or malignant. Only the latter, of course, is synonymous with hepatic cell carcinoma. Histo-

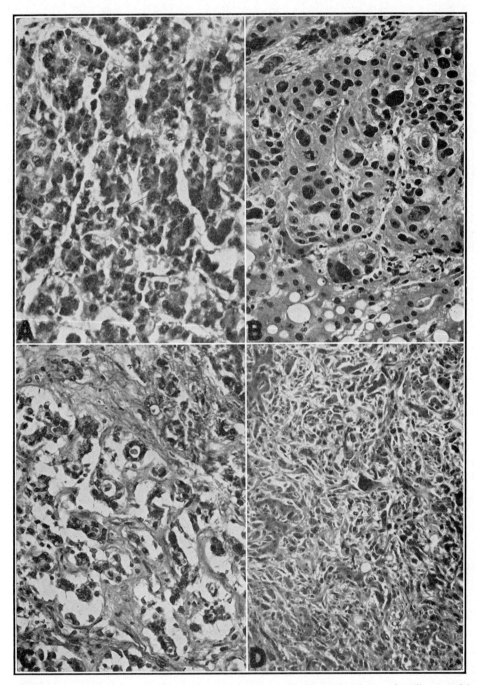

FIG. 403.—Carcinoma of the liver illustrating *A*, a well-differentiated hepatic cell type with rather regular appearing cells arranged in cords. × 200, *B*, a more malignant hepatic cell type with considerable irregularity in the appearance of the cells. × 100, *C*, a bile duct type with an attempt at bile duct formation. × 100, and *D*, a mixed cell type with the cells resembling those seen in a sarcoma. × 100.

logically the cells show varying degrees of differentiation from those that
resemble relatively normal appearing liver cells to those that are quite
irregular. Even the latter, however, can generally be readily recognized as
of liver cell origin. The cells vary in size from those approaching normal to
those several times normal. The borders are often indistinct; the cytoplasm is abundant and more or less homogeneous or diffusely granular, and

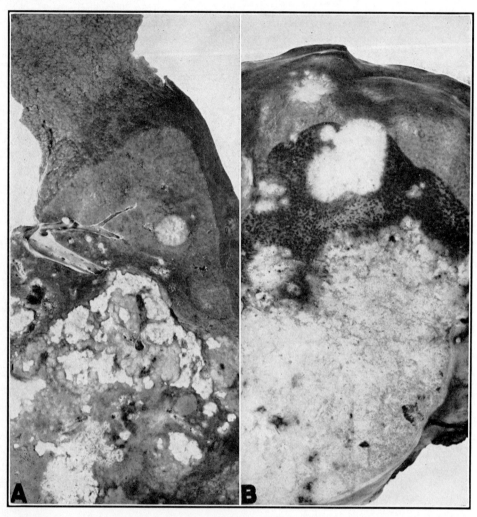

FIG. 404.—Primary carcinoma of the liver disclosing *A*, a hepatic cell type of tumor with
considerable necrosis of the neoplastic tissue. The liver also shows cirrhosis, and *B*, bile duct
type with most of the tumor viable. This liver does not reveal cirrhosis.

the nuclei are single or multiple, regular in the more benign growths but
quite irregular in the more malignant tumors, and usually hyperchromatic.
The supporting stroma within the tumor proper is generally scanty and of a
loose connective tissue variety. A *bile duct type* of carcinoma accounts for
almost one-third of the cases. The tumor has also been called a cholangioma
but, as in the case of hepatoma, when the term cholangioma is used it should
be further specified as to whether it is benign or malignant. It is only the

malignant variety that is synonymous with bile duct carcinoma. The characteristic feature of this type of growth is a proliferation of regular or irregular cuboidal cells tending to reproduce bile ducts. The cytoplasm is moderate in amount and may be vacuolated. The nuclei are round or irregular and hyperchromatic. The supporting stroma is generally more abundant than it is in the hepatic cell type of tumor and usually reveals more collagenous material. *Mixed cell type* of carcinoma is one that is

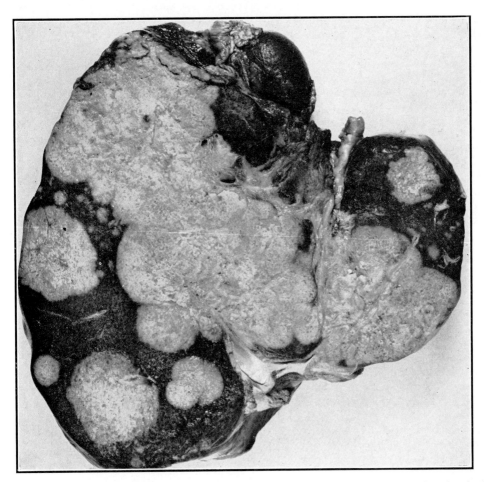

FIG. 405.—Secondary carcinoma of the liver from a primary growth in the colon. Grossly, the tumor is indistinguishable from the primary bile duct carcinoma illustrated in Figure 404B. The liver does not disclose cirrhosis.

composed of both hepatic and bile duct types of cells or that is so poorly differentiated that the tumor cannot be dubbed as either one or the other. In the more malignant growths the cells are quite irregular and may even resemble those of a sarcoma. *Grossly* primary carcinoma of the liver, whether of a hepatic cell or the bile duct type, may consist essentially of a single mass with satellite nodules about the periphery or of numerous varisized nodules scattered throughout the hepatic parenchyma (Fig. 404). The tumors are usually convex externally with often a central umbilication, appear light reddish brown to gray, are moderately firm to hard, and show

varying degrees of necrosis and hemorrhage (Fig. 404). In adults, the uninvolved hepatic parenchyma shows distinct cirrhosis in from 46 to 100
per cent of cases of hepatic cell carcinoma and in about 50 per cent of cases
of bile duct carcinoma (Warvi). In children, however, cirrhosis of the liver
is rarely seen (Bigelow). Primary carcinoma of the liver *spreads* to other
portions of the liver by direct extension and by metastasis. Metastasis also
occurs to other organs of the body, especially in the more malignant growths.
The structures most commonly involved are liver, hilar lymph nodes,
lungs, bones, spleen, adrenals, kidneys, pancreas, peritoneum, pleura, and
brain (Sanford and Strong). The *prognosis* in carcinoma of the liver is
poor for death usually occurs within four months after the diagnosis is
established. Recently *surgical resection* has been performed more and more
frequently but the efficacy of such treatment has yet to be proved.

Secondary Tumors.—Secondary tumors of the liver are far more frequent than primary tumors. The recorded incidence of primary carcinoma
as compared with metastatic cancers varies from 1 in 20 to 1 in 64.5 (Warvi).
While some of the growths arise as a result of direct extension from organs
such as the gallbladder, stomach, pancreas, diaphragm, etc., most of the
tumors are metastatic by way of the blood vessels or lymphatic channels.
The primary growth may occur in any of the tissues or organs of the body
(including the skin) and the most frequent type of tumor is carcinoma.
Grossly the lesions are indistinguishable from those in primary carcinoma
(Fig. 405). Cirrhosis of the unaffected portions of the liver, however, is
generally absent. Histologically the tumors mimic the primary growths.

BILIARY SYSTEM

PATHOLOGIC PHYSIOLOGY

M. H. F. Friedman

The major *activities* of the *gallbladder* are those concerned with the conservation of bile and its retention until used in digestive processes. The
processes involved include those of concentration, storage, and evacuation
of the bile. An additional activity, the secretion of a mucin by the gallbladder epithelium ("white bile"), may be concerned primarily with maintenance of mucosal integrity.

The *importance* of the *gallbladder* in the body economy is not clarified by
the fact that it is absent in some species but is present in certain other
closely allied species. Thus, a gallbladder is wanting in the white rat,
pocket gopher, and camel but is present in the mouse, guinea pig, and
dromedary. No distinct correlations between diet, the total bile secretion,
and the presence or absence of a gallbladder have been established. In
species without a gallbladder, the continuously secreted bile flows directly
into the duodenum and the ducts are not enlarged to act as a compensatory
reservoir. Following *cholecystectomy* in man, the common duct may be
found later to have become dilated but it is doubtful that this represents
development of a compensatory reservoir. It is most probable that post-
cholecystectomy duct dilation constitutes evidence of restrictive bile outflow.

During *filling*, the gallbladder shows accommodation by relaxation so that
bile pressure remains constant with increasing bile volume content. By
this important feature the intravesicular pressure is maintained lower than

the hepatic duct pressure so that hepatic bile is literally aspirated into the gallbladder. Whether the accommodation of relaxation is due to active lengthening of the fibromuscular coat or to passive lengthening by inhibition of tonus is not known. Until recently, it had been assumed that liver bile, secreted at a pressure of about 300 mm. bile, was routed into the gallbladder only when the *sphincter* of *Oddi* was closed. Closure of the sphincter of Oddi, however, as a condition for gallbladder filling is a misconception not supported by experimental evidence. The major regulating factor for filling is a gradient of pressures in which the gallbladder pressure is lower than the hepatic duct pressure, and the common duct pressure is intermediate between these. Such is the case normally during filling but these relations are altered during emptying (see below). Following cholecystectomy, the common duct pressure is constantly high because the pressure-lowering action of the gallbladder is no longer available. Gallbladder filling will occur even when the sphincter of Oddi is kept permanently patent by an indwelling catheter. To permit this, the pressure gradient between hepatic duct and gallbladder is maintained by the *common duct* itself exerting a *sphincter-like action* at some distance above the sphincter of Oddi. No special muscular apparatus has been demonstrated at this point, but the dynamics of bile flow clearly point to such a sphincteric action, rather than the sphincter of Oddi, as being involved in maintaining the necessary filling pressure gradients. The foregoing of course does not mean that artificially-induced contraction of the sphincter of Oddi does not enhance bile filling. To produce better gallbladder contrast a common practice of the radiologist is to administer a drug which produces sphincter spasm so that, among other things, all the liver bile enters the bladder.

The helical *valves* of *Heister* apparently do not function as a pressure-regulating device but instead serve to lend structural support to the cystic duct when traction is exerted by the full dependent gallbladder.

Bile concentration is achieved in the gallbladder by transfer of fluid and electrolyte across the mucous membrane and lymphatics. The light yellow liver bile thus becomes deeper yellow or yellow green the longer the time allowed for concentration in the gallbladder. While in the gallbladder, the bile may become ten to fifteen times as concentrated as liver bile with respect to bile pigment but it does not become hypertonic because the osmotically active electrolytes are absorbed along with the water. Since the gallbladder may hold as much as a 24 hour output of hepatic bile it is apparent that *hepatic duct* obstruction will lead to jaundice earlier than will *common duct obstruction.*

Of great clinical significance is the *ratio* of *bile* to *cholesterol.* Normally, the water-insoluble cholesterol is held in solution as a cholesterol-bile acid complex but at bile acid:cholesterol ratios smaller than 10:1 the cholesterol tends to come out of solution. When reabsorption of bile acid from the gallbladder occurs at a greater than normal rate, this ratio may be lowered to 4:1 or even 2:1 with consequent precipitation of the cholesterol as "*gravel*" or "*stones.*" The reason for formation of calcium stones is not known but an infectious process of the gallbladder wall may be involved. Numerous small stones are more effective in producing obstruction and colic due to duct obstruction than is a solitary stone which is too large to enter the duct. For this reason, single stones may remain in the gallbladder "silent" and symptomless for many years.

The *concentration capacity* is a function of the *mucosa.* This function may be compromised by inflammatory disease in which event the gallbladder bile may be found to be thick and viscid. Under these circumstances, radiopaque material excreted by the liver cannot be concentrated adequately to permit radiographic visualization of the gallbladder. When the gallbladder is filled with bile which is not being concentrated, there is in effect a condition not unlike cholecystectomy in that liver bile is not conserved but goes directly into the intestine.

Though denied by earlier investigators, it is now firmly established that the thin *musculature* of the gallbladder is capable of *contraction* with a force sufficient to evacuate the bile. The older view that gallbladder evacuation occurs only passively, due to relaxation of a sphincter, is not tenable. Vagus stimulation and parasympathomimetic drugs contract the gallbladder both *in vitro* and *in situ*. Stimuli which normally cause gallbladder contraction act from the intestine. The most potent *cholagogues* are fats and acid but protein is also effective. These substances initiate *enterocholecystokinetic reflexes* but possibly more important is the evacuation due to the formation of the hormone *cholecystokinin*. This is the basis for the so-called *Boyden fat meal* used to demonstrate the emptying of the radiographically visualized gallbladder.

Evacuation of the *gallbladder* begins in response to adequate stimulation from the intestine. Two types of motor activities are exhibited—rhythmic waves of local contractions which are superimposed on larger mass contractions and increases in tonus of the whole bladder wall. Intestinal stimuli, such as acid or fat, cause prompt reflex emptying movements. After a period of five to twenty minutes the initial neurogenic contractions come to be replaced by contractions due to the hormone cholecystokinin. The prompt emptying response of the gallbladder to intestinal instillation of fat is absent after vagal denervation, but the slower sustained contractions due to the formation of cholecystokinin persist. Probably total evacuation is a rare occurrence but the frequent emptying and refilling, together with the peristaltic-like movements, keep the bile stirred up enough to minimize layering or sedimenting. The fact that in some patients intravenous administration of a purified cholecystokinin preparation will contract the gallbladder when a fat meal fails to do so, may well demonstrate that the basis for motor dysfunction of the gallbladder can be of intestinal rather than biliary origin.

Vagal stimuli and the hormone cholecystokinin, both of which act to contract the gallbladder, also act simultaneously to *relax* the *sphincter* of *Oddi*. With the sphincter relaxed, the force generated by the contracting gallbladder musculature is less than the secretory pressure of the liver, and consequently the bile flows into the duodenum. When, however, the sphincter is in spasm or there is obstruction at the ampulla, the developed bile pressure may be great enough to force the material into the intrahepatic duct system with possible serious consequences to liver functions. The intrahepatic biliary ducts can be visualized radiographically by the administration of morphine to constrict the sphincter, together with a fat meal to cause the gallbladder to expel its concentrated radiopaque contents.

It has been noted that the principal factor regulating normal filling and emptying of the gallbladder is a pressure gradient which is properly directed, and is not the state of tonus of the sphincter of Oddi. A relaxed sphincter neither prevents filling nor is it, as such, the cause of emptying of the gallbladder. The question then may well be raised, "What is the main *function* of the *sphincter* of *Oddi?*" All recent evidence points to this sphincter as normally preventing regurgitation of duodenal contents into the extra-

hepatic biliary system. When the intraduodenal pressure exceeds the intraductal pressure, the sphincter of Oddi is reflexly closed. Fats in the intestine
lower the intestinal tonus at the same time as they cause contraction of the
gallbladder and relaxation of the sphincter. This demonstrates the fine
integration between various parts of the biliary tract and intestine. In
the absence of such synergism we have biliary dyskenesia.

CONGENITAL ANOMALIES

Orientation.—Developmental malformation of the gallbladder and
extrahepatic bile ducts are varied and frequent. Those of the *gallbladder*
may be listed as follows: (1) *hypoplasia*—diminution in size or rudimentary,
(2) *hyperplasia*—increase in size, (3) *agenesis*—complete absence, (4)
variations in shape—fishhook, S-shaped, etc., (5) *duplication*—bifid dome,
septate, and complete duplication, (6) *variations in position*—subcutaneous,
intrahepatic, completely free, and left-sided instead of right with or without
situs inversus, and (7) *diverticula*. Developmental malformations of the
extrahepatic bile ducts consist of the following: (1) *variations* of the *points*
of *confluence* of the left and right hepatic ducts and the common hepatic
duct with the cystic duct, (2) *variations* in *lengths* of the ducts depending
upon the points of confluence, (3) *absence* of the *common bile duct*, (4) *variations* in *caliber* of the *lumen*—stenosis and atresia, (5) *variations* of *exit* of
common bile duct—into a diverticulum of the duodenum or into the stomach, (6) *duplication*—associated with duplication of the gallbladder, (7)
diverticula—terminal portion of the common bile duct, and (8) *cystic
dilatation* of the *common bile duct*. From a *clinical viewpoint* congenital
anomalies of the gallbladder are unimportant for the patient's health remains unimpeded regardless of the type or degree of the malformation.
Developmental abnormalities of the extrahepatic bile ducts, however, are
unimportant only as long as the continuity and caliber of the lumens are
not encroached upon. When these occur, the flow of bile is impeded and
jaundice and biliary cirrhosis develop. Of all the anomalies listed, diverticula of the gallbladder and cystic dilatation of the common bile duct only
are important enough to merit a few separate remarks.

Diverticula of the Gallbladder.—While a few diverticula of the gallbladder are *congenital*, most are acquired. The former consist of mural
outpocketings that are composed of all the layers of the gallbladder wall
while the latter consist of mucosal herniations that may extend all the way
to the serosa. *Acquired* diverticula have *also* been *called* Rokitansky-
Aschoff sinuses, Luschka's crypts or glands, false diverticula, mucosal
hernias, cholecystitis glandularis, adenomyosis, cholesterol cysts, etc.
(Robertson). The condition *occurs* infrequently in normal gallbladders and
frequently (in as high as 90%) in previously inflamed gallbladders with or
without stones. It predominates in females over males in the ratio of 2
to 1. The *pathogenesis* appears to depend upon two factors, namely: (1)
weakness of the wall caused by anatomic absence of the muscularis mucosa
and the presence of connective tissue between the muscle bundles of the
muscularis and (2) local increase of intraluminal pressure caused by hypertrophy of the muscle coat and/or unsynchronized contractions and relaxations of the gallbladder wall. As a result of these factors, the mucosa
herniates into and through the wall. *Grossly* the gallbladder may appear
normal or its wall may be thickened. Pinpoint or larger cystic spaces may
or may not be visible within the substance of the wall. *Histologically*

varisized crypts, glands, or cysts of mucosal epithelium may be found in the submucosa, between the muscle bundles, or beneath the serosa (Fig. 406). They may or may not be connected with the mucosal epithelium. The lumens of the structures may be empty or they may contain debris or calculi and the adjacent tissues may be permeated with leukocytes. The *clinical manifestations*, when present, are due to the associated inflammation. The condition should not be mistaken for carcinoma.

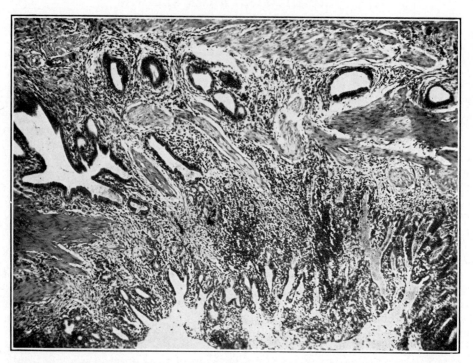

FIG. 406.—Diverticula of the gallbladder showing mucosal epithelium in glandular formation extending into the muscle coats. There is also an associated chronic inflammation. × 50.

Cystic Dilatation of the Common Bile Duct. —This condition, also known as *choledochus cyst*, is not too infrequent for 192 cases had been recorded in the literature by 1951 (Hertzler). The disorder is usually recognized before the age of twenty-five years and is three times as common in females as it is in males. The *cause* is probably an inequality of proliferation and subsequent canalization of the epithelial cells of the common bile duct (Shallow). Subsequently, torsion and angulation produce obstruction and increase dilatation. *Pathologically* the dilatation affects only that portion of the common bile duct that lies proximal to the wall of the duodenum. The cyst is spherical but eccentric and varies in capacity to as much as 8,000 cubic centimeters. The wall measures from 2 to 7.5 mm. in thickness. Histologically the normal components are usually replaced by collagenous connective tissue with only islands of mucosal epithelium and muscle remaining here and there. The contents of the cyst consist of viscid to watery fluid containing varying amounts of bile. The cystic and hepatic ducts are generally dilated. The chief *complications* are bile duct obstruction and infection. The cardinal *clinical manifestations* are tumor, jaundice, and pain. The *treatment* of choice consists of surgical excision. If this is impossible, anastomosis of the cyst to the duodenum or marsupialization may be carried out. The *prognosis* is fair to good with the current survival rate in surgically treated patients being about 50 per cent (Shallow).

DEGENERATIONS

Orientation. — Degenerative conditions of the extrahepatic biliary system are generally associated with other pathologic processes. Nevertheless, three disorders of the gallbladder that may be discussed under this heading are cholesterolosis, mucocele, and calcification.

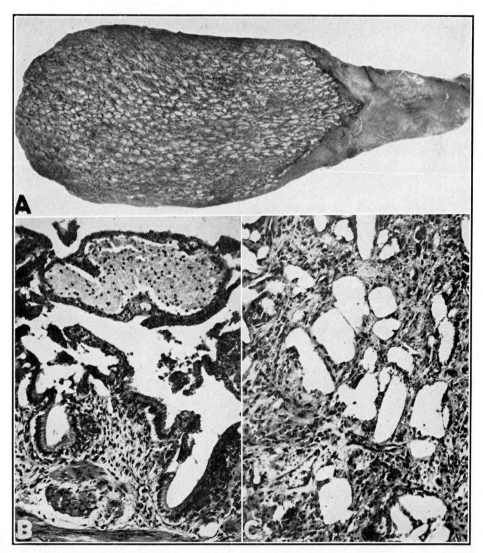

Fig. 407.—Cholesterolosis of the gallbladder illustrating *A*, the mucosa containing flecks of orange-yellow material, *B*, a typical bulbous villus filled with histiocytic foam cells. × 100, and *C*, a severe reaction consisting of a deposition of crystals and a permeation with foam cells, leukocytes, and fibroblasts. × 100.

Cholesterolosis of the Gallbladder.—Cholesterolosis of the gallbladder is also referred to as *strawberry gallbladder* (Womack). The condition is usually associated with cholesterol stones and is *due to* a deposition of cholesterol esters in the wall. *Grossly* the gallbladder wall is generally slightly thickened but may measure as much as 5 mm. across. The mucosa discloses innumerable, sharply demarcated, irregular, orange-yellow flecks that may measure as much as 0.2 cm. in greatest diameter (Fig. 407*A*). *Histologically* the villi are enlarged and club-shaped (Fig. 407*B*). Beneath the epithelial cells there are present collections of large polyhedral histiocytes with foamy cytoplasm and relatively small, round or oval, evenly staining nuclei. Usually the process ends here but sometimes, apparently in the presence of greater amounts of lipids and bile, a definite inflammatory reaction is set up. In such instances, crystals of cholesterol (and some-

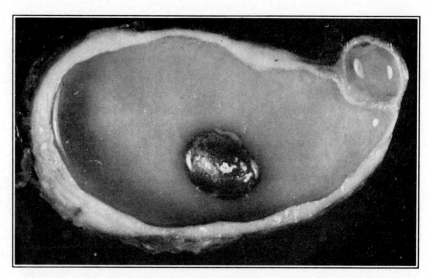

FIG. 408.—Mucocele of the gallbladder disclosing a thickened wall and a lumen filled with mucoid material and containing a solitary calculus.

times precipitates of bile itself) are deposited focally and are surrounded by giant cells, leukocytes, and fibroblasts (Fig. 407*C*). When the reaction is severe, actual necrosis and bacterial invasion may occur. The process heals by resolution and collagenous fibrous tissue replacement.

Mucocele of the Gallbladder.—Mucocele of the gallbladder, also known as *hydrops*, consists of a blockage of the cystic duct and a distention of the lumen of the gallbladder with viscid (but sometimes more watery) mucoid material (Fig. 408). The condition may occur in a previously normal or a previously diseased gallbladder. In the former the wall is thin, while in the latter it is usually thickened and fibrotic. The mucus forms as a result of excessive secretion by the mucosal epithelial cells. In the process, many of the cells become overdistended with secretion and undergo mucoid degeneration. Mucocele of the gallbladder is about four times as *frequent* in females as it is in males and usually occurs in the fifth decade of life (Blumberg). *Clinically* there may be no symptoms or the manifestations may consist of epigastric pain or discomfort, nausea, vomiting, slight fever, and (in about one-third of the cases) a palpable enlargement of the gallbladder.

The chief *complications* are inflammation and empyema. *Treatment* consists of cholecystectomy. The *prognosis* is good.

Calcification of the Gallbladder.—Calcification of the gallbladder has *also* been *called* petrified gallbladder, ossified gallbladder, porcelain gallbladder, china gallbladder, calcifying cholecystitis, cholecystopathia chronica calcarea, and simply calcified gallbladder (Jutras). The condition is rare, *occurring* about once in every 1,000 cholecystectomies. It is found chiefly in adults and affects females about three times as frequently as males. There are two theories to explain its *pathogenesis*: (1) mechanical — holding that the process is superimposed upon hydrops and that slowing of the circulation of the blood causes first degeneration of the wall of the organ and then calcification and (2) infectious — holding that calcification is the end result of a low-grade inflammation that first passes through a stage

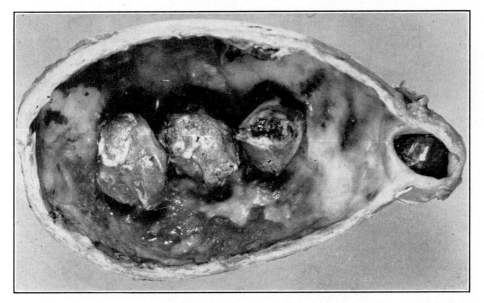

FIG. 409.—Calcification of the gallbladder disclosing thickening and streaking grayness of the wall. The wall was so firm that it had to be cut with a saw. The lumen of the organ contains four calculi.

of collagenous fibrosis. Of these, the latter is probably correct. *Pathologically* the gallbladder is usually large, rounded, hard or crackling to palpation, and reddish brown to gray in color. The wall is generally thickened and may not be cut with a knife (Fig. 409). The lumen, as a rule, is filled with mucus mixed with varying amounts of amorphous material and may contain stones. Histologically the normal layers of the wall are replaced with collagenous connective tissue and contain greater or lesser deposits of calcium. *Clinical manifestations* may be absent or are those of chronic cholecystitis. The organ may be palpated through the abdominal wall and is generally readily visualized roentgenographically. *Treatment* consists of surgical removal. The *prognosis* is good.

INFLAMMATIONS

Orientation.—Inflammation of the gallbladder is known as *cholecystitis* (Gr. = bile + bladder + inflammation) while inflammation of the bile ducts is referred to as *cholangitis* (Gr. = bile + vessel + inflammation). Inflammation of the extrahepatic bile ducts is virtually always associated with some obstructive phenomenon, is overshadowed by such a process, and by itself is thus of little or no significance.   Inflammation of the intrahepatic bile ducts has (directly or indirectly) already been referred to in connection with pylephlebitis (p. 379), infective biliary cirrhosis (p. 809), hepatic abscesses (p. 813), and viral hepatitis (p. 821).   In this section, therefore, inflammation of the gallbladder alone will be considered.

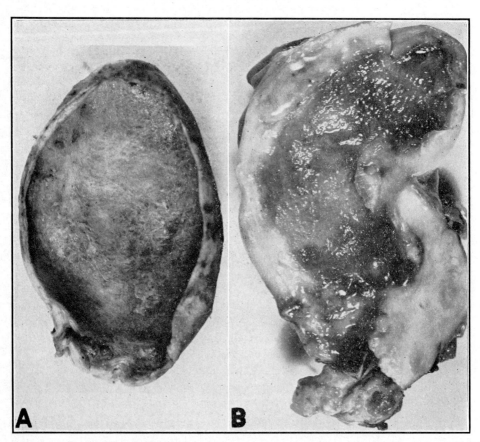

FIG. 410.—Cholecystitis disclosing *A*, an acute inflammation with hemorrhagic discoloration of the serosa, edema of the wall, and a fibrinous exudate covering the mucosa and *B*, a chronic inflammation in a typhoid carrier with marked fibrous thickening of the wall and considerable reduction in the size of the lumen.

Cholecystitis.—Inflammation of the gallbladder (recent or old) is a common disorder, especially in the United States where it has been estimated to occur in 2 out of every 3 autopsies on adults.   Its *incidence* among all patients with biliary tract disease is recorded as varying from 0.5 to 23.5 per cent of cases (Buxton).   It is most common between the ages of thirty and sixty years (DeCamp and Adams), but also occurs in the aged (Lyon) and even in children (Kahle).   It prevails in females over males in the ratio of 4 to 1.   *Experimentally*, many methods have been employed in producing cholecystitis in laboratory animals using especially chlorinated soda, bile, bile juice, amylase, and trypsin (Thomas and Womack).   One of

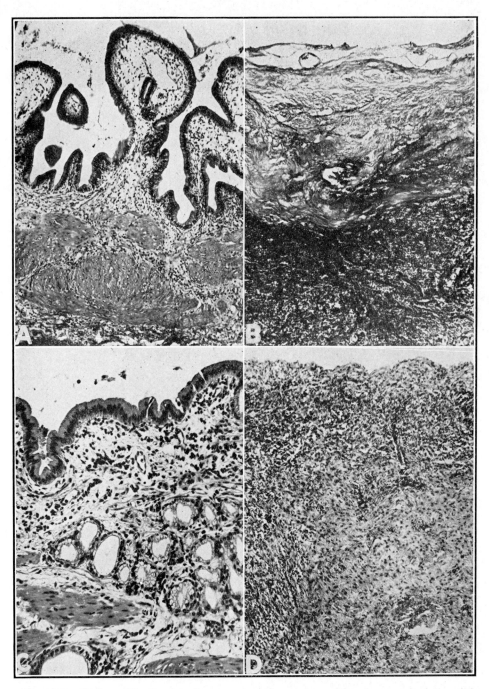

FIG. 411.—Cholecystitis showing *A*, an acute inflammation with enlargement of the villi, congestion and edema of the connective tissue of the villi and rest of the wall, and a diffuse infiltration with neutrophils. × 50, *B*, severe acute inflammation with gangrene of the mucosa and submucosa and marked neutrophilic infiltration of the rest of the wall. × 50, *C*, chronic inflammation with flattening of the villi, a moderate increase of connective tissue throughout the wall, and a diffuse infiltration with plasma cells and lymphocytes. × 100, and *D*, chronic inflammation with denudation of the mucosa, bile pigment in the tissue near the lumen, and an obscuring of the normal architecture by a deposition of collagenous connective tissue. × 50.

the most recent (and perhaps the most physiologic) is to withhold food from dogs for forty-eight hours (in order to concentrate the bile in the gall-bladder), obstruct the blood supply to the gallbladder, and ligate the cystic duct. An analogous situation apparently exists in *man*. Obstruction to the cystic duct is always present and is generally caused by a calculus. This initiates spasm of the gallbladder wall and the spasm, in turn, causes impairment of the blood flow (at least venous and lymphatic). Under such circumstances, the resistance of the gallbladder is lowered and the bile initiates a chemical inflammation. Once inflammation is underway, bacteria secondarily invade the organ. The most common organisms are colon bacilli, streptococci, and staphylococci (Twiss) but any pyogenic bacterium and even typhoid and tubercle bacilli may be found. Rarely, gas-producing (colon bacilli or *Clostridium welchii*) organisms invade the tissues producing a condition referred to as *emphysematous cholecystitis* (Retterbush).

Pathologically cholecystitis may be divided into two groups—acute and chronic (Figs. 410 and 411). As elsewhere in the body, *acute cholecystitis* is manifested by a rapidly developing procession of events resulting in (1) roughness, dullness, dryness, and pink, red, or blotchy purple and black discoloration of the serosa, (2) moderate to marked congestion, edema, and thickening of the wall, (3) roughening, ulceration, or fibrinous exudation of the mucosa, and (4) filling of the lumen with cloudy or frankly purulent material. As the inflammation advances, the wall of the gallbladder may be permeated with grossly apparent pus (suppurative cholecystitis) or may become completely necrotic (gangrenous cholecystitis) and the lumen may be filled with frankly purulent material (empyema). In acute cholecystitis the gallbladder is generally enlarged, sometimes to two or three times its normal size. An exception to this, however, occurs when the acute inflammation has been superimposed upon a previous chronic sclerosing process. Histologically the process is not specific. It consists essentially of congestion of the capillaries, edema of the connective tissue, and a diffuse permeation with neutrophils and varying numbers of other types of leuko-cytes. The degree of involvement of the various coats of the gallbladder wall varies from case to case but generally is more apparent in areas that contain a greater abundance of connective tissue. Thus the serosa, sub-mucosa, and muscle coats are generally affected in decreasing order of severity. Microscopically as grossly, when the process becomes more severe, the wall may be solidly infiltrated with neutrophils (suppurative cholecystitis) or it may become completely necrotic (gangrenous chole-cystitis). In *chronic cholecystitis* the organ may be larger than normal, of normal size, or smaller than normal. The serosa is usually pale, rough, and opaque. It may be covered with fibrous tags which form adhesions with adjacent organs. The wall is thickened, sometimes to as much as one or more centimeters. It is usually completely replaced with grayish-white, dense, sclerotic fibrous tissue. The mucosa may appear intact (but even in such cases is generally smooth) or it may appear roughened and ulcerated. The lumen may be enlarged, of normal caliber, or reduced in capacity and may be filled with bile or with clear watery fluid. Histologically the villi are usually flattened or completely erased and the mucosa may or may not be intact. Throughout the wall there are varying degrees of fibrous tissue deposition and plasma cell, lymphocytic, and monocytic infiltration. In less severe cases, the different coats of the vessel may be readily discerned while in more severe and older cases the layers are fused and may be completely replaced with the reparative process. In some instances, glands or cysts lined with cuboidal or columnar epithelium (cholecystitis glandularis) are present within the wall and either in these areas or between the connective tissue cells there may be deposits of bile or bile products. The incidence of *calculi* in cases of cholecystitis is high. Stones have been reported in the gallbladder and cystic duct in up to 98 per cent of all cases (Tunbridge and Clifford) and in the common bile duct in up to 11.5 per cent of all cases (DeCamp). As already stated, the calculi play a definite role in the pathogenesis of the disorder.

The *complications* of cholecystitis are many and, in the over-all, quite frequent (Freund, Lyon, DeCamp, and Johnstone). Since the recorded incidence of the complications varies greatly, specific figures will be omitted. The usual untoward effects are empyema, gangrene, jaundice (due to calculi in the common bile duct or to associated hepatitis), perforation, localized abscess formation, peritonitis, obstructive jaundice, biliary cirrhosis, and carcinoma. The last three complications listed are actually the effects of cholelithiasis but since stones are usually present in cholecystitis, they may also be listed as an accompaniment of inflammation. *Clinically, acute cholecystitis* is generally ushered in suddenly with abdominal pain (right upper abdominal quadrant or referred to the inferior angle of the right scapula or to the right shoulder), nausea, retching, vomiting, fever, leukocytosis to as high as 30,000, tenderness, rigidity, and a palpable mass in the region of the gallbladder (Tunbridge). *Chronic cholecystitis* is attended by variable manifestations. They consist of periodic attacks of abdominal discomfort and a sense of fullness, both being aggravated by cooked, greasy foods. In addition, there may be associated dull pain in the upper portion of the abdomen or in the region of the scapula, constipation, lethargy, belching and occasionally nausea. *Radiologic* studies (using radiopaque dye administered orally or intravenously) are great aids in studying patients with the chronic phase of the disease. Under such circumstances, gallstones and/or a nonfunctioning gallbladder are demonstrable in as high as 97.6 per cent of cases (Adams). The *diagnosis* of cholecystitis is usually made from a history of repeated attacks of the manifestations listed above and, in chronic cases, is generally verified by roentgenographic studies. A *differential diagnosis* should include peptic ulcer, appendicitis, acute pancreatitis, right-sided renal calculi, and myocardial infarction. In general, the *treatment* is operative. Although there is no unanimity of opinion, it is generally conceded that operation should be performed immediately on patients with acute cholecystitis with symptoms present for a shorter period than three to four days, or on patients exhibiting progression of the disease regardless of its duration (Lyon and DeCamp). If the disorder is of longer than three to four days' duration and the clinical manifestations are abating, treatment consists of supportive therapy and administration of antibiotics. In cases of chronic cholecystitis, especially with stone formation, cholecystectomy (in order to prevent obstructive jaundice, biliary cirrhosis, and carcinoma) is the treatment of choice (Adams). In general, the *prognosis* in cholecystitis is good. The over-all death rate in any large series of patients should not be greater than 6 to 9 per cent. The chief *causes* of *death* are peritonitis, pneumonia, and cardiac complications.

PHYSICAL DISTURBANCES

Orientation. — The more important Physical Disturbances of the Biliary System may be listed as follows: torsion of the gallbladder, calculi, trauma, obstruction of the bile ducts, and fistula.

Torsion of the Gallbladder.—Torsion or twisting of the gallbladder is an *unusual* condition, there having been only 77 cases recorded up to 1950 (Peck). Of these, 92 per cent occurred in females and the greatest incidence was in the seventh and eighth decades of life. The condition can occur only when the gallbladder is completely detached from the liver and lies freely suspended in the peritoneal cavity. The *pathogenesis* is unknown although peristalsis of the intestine is thought to initiate the process. Gallstones have been found in only a few of the recorded cases. *Pathologically* the torsion occurs in the region of the cystic duct and, depending upon its degree and tightness, the gallbladder is distended, acutely inflamed, or gangrenous. The *clinical manifestations* are like those in acute cholecystitis. *Treatment* consists of cholecystectomy. The recorded *mortality* has been 16 per cent.

Calculi.—Calculi of the biliary system are *also referred to* as gallstones, biliary concretions, and choleliths (Gr. = bile + stone). The term *cholelithiasis* indicates the presence or formation of gallstones. The recorded *incidence* of biliary calculi varies. In a study of 29,779 autopsies performed on patients over twenty years of age, Lieber noted the following occurrence: white females 21.7 per cent, white males 9.7 per cent, colored females 8.7 per cent, and colored males, 3.25 per cent. Other authors record a preponderance in females over males in ratios as high as 5 to 1 (Littler). They may be found at any age (Lawler), but the greatest incidence is in patients beyond the fourth decade. Although the *causes* of the formation of gallstones are unknown, heredity (by way of a fundamental disturbance of cholesterol metabolism), sedentary habits, infectious diseases, dietary indiscretions, and pregnancy are thought to be of etiologic significance. Despite the fact that the exact reason for their formation is unknown, it is known that the chief components of gallstones are cholesterol, bilirubin, biliverdin, and calcium salts. As a result of supersaturation or superconcentration of the bile these substances are precipitated out about a nucleus of mucin, dead epithelial cells, or bacteria and continued enlargement results from repeated precipitation of these substances layer upon layer.

Pathologically choleliths usually occur in the gallbladder but they are also found in the bile ducts. In the latter, the stones are generally located in the common bile duct where the average recorded incidence is around 11 per cent of all cases of biliary stones (Strohl). In general, three types of biliary calculi are usually recognized—cholesterol, pigment, and mixed (Walton). *Cholesterol* stones are always found in the gallbladder. They are single, oval, nodular, semitransparent, waxy, and light yellow (Plate II). They usually measure up to 2×4 cm. On section, they may disclose radiating crystals throughout or they may reveal radiating crystals centrally and amorphous material peripherally. Occasionally cholesterol stones are stained with bile and sometimes they may contain a slight amount of calcium. *Pigment* stones may be formed in the gallbladder or bile ducts. They are composed of biliverdin and bilirubin and, in the pure state, are soft, putty-like, easily crushed, and black. They are always multiple, are irregular in outline, and measure from a few millimeters to 1 cm. in diameter. *Mixed* stones are generally formed in the gallbladder and are usually found in the bile ducts only as the result of migration. They are composed of varying amounts of cholesterol, biliverdin, bilirubin, and calcium salts. They are multiple, mulberry-like or faceted, varicolored depending upon their composition, and measure from a few millimeters to 1 cm. in diameter. Occasionally mixed calculi are single and resemble cholesterol stones somewhat.

PLATE II

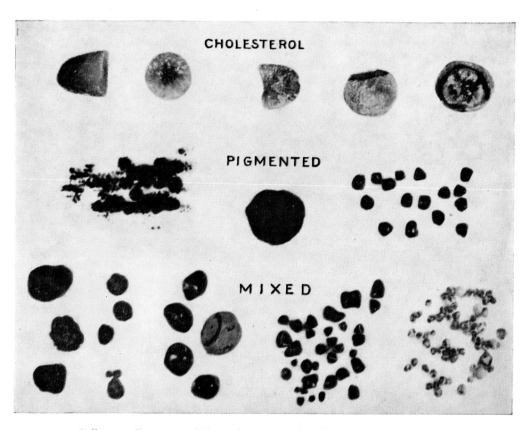

Gallstones illustrating cholesterol, pigmented, and mixed types of calculi.

The *complications* of gallstones are (1) cholecystitis, (2) pancreatitis, (3) cholangitis, (4) obstructive jaundice and cirrhosis (due to obstruction of the bile ducts), (5) biliary fistula, and (6) carcinoma of the gallbladder occurring in about 5 per cent of all cases (Love). The *clinical manifestations* may consist of biliary colic but are generally those of the complications with cholecystitis, obstructive jaundice, and biliary cirrhosis predominating. The *diagnosis* is made from the clinical manifestations and roentgenographic studies—ordinary studies in cases of stones that contain calcium and contrast medium studies in those that do not contain calcium. *Treatment* is surgical removal. This should be accomplished before complications develop. The *prognosis*, in general, is good but depends on the presence or absence of complications and upon the types of complications.

Trauma.—Trauma to the *gallbladder* as a result of penetrating abdominal wounds, blunt blows, or accidents is rare, there having been only 32 cases recorded up to 1946 (Norgore). The cases that are recognizable usually exist in the form of a rupture and the chief manifestations are those of bile peritonitis. In this connection, however, it should be pointed out that in most cases of abdominal trauma in which bile is found in the peritoneal cavity, the source of the bile is rupture of the liver itself rather than rupture of the gallbladder or bile ducts. Trauma to the *bile ducts* occurs most commonly as a result of operative procedures and consists of ligation, severance, or simple contusion that later may produce a stricture. Nonsurgical trauma to the bile ducts is rare but is more common than similar injury to the gallbladder. It consists of a contusion or tear (partial or complete tear). In any case, with the continuity of the biliary system disrupted, obstructive jaundice or bile peritonitis generally results.

Obstruction of the Bile Ducts.—The *causes* of obstruction of the extrahepatic bile ducts are protean (Cattell, Hsia, O'Malley, and Eisenstein). They may be listed as follows: (1) congenital anomalies—stenosis, atresia, or absence, (2) degenerations—mucous plug as a result of excessive secretion or degeneration of the epithelial cells, (3) inflammations—cholangitis, adhesions, duodenal ulcer, pancreatitis, and lymphadenitis, (4) physical disturbances—calculi, surgical trauma (benign stricture), nonsurgical trauma, and inspissated bile, and (5) tumors—benign and malignant primary tumors of the bile ducts and metastatic growths to the bile ducts or the liver lymph nodes. The *clinical manifestations* depend upon the location of the obstruction. If the cystic duct is affected, they will be primarily those of mucocele or cholecystitis whereas if the common duct or the hepatic ducts are involved they will be those of obstructive jaundice, cholangitis, or cirrhosis. *Treatment* consists of surgical re-establishment of the continuity of the lumen. The *prognosis* varies with the cause and duration of the obstruction.

Fistula.—Fistulas that connect the lumen of the biliary tree with the lumen of other organs or the outside of the body are referred to simply as *biliary fistulas* or are named after the *structures connected*. Some examples of the latter consist of cholecystocolic, cholecystoduodenal, cholecystogastric, cholecystopleural, cholecystobronchial, choledochoduodenal (common bile duct and duodenum), choledochocolic, choledochocutaneous, etc. While the *causes* of biliary fistulas are varied (trauma, tumors, etc.) the most common etiologic agents are gallstones and the most common associated condition is inflammation (Love, Calihan, Crenshaw, and Guy). The most common fistula is one that connects the gallbladder with the intestinal tract (usually the duodenum and less often the stomach, jejunum, ileum, and colon). When the opening in the gallbladder becomes large enough the stone (that is almost invariably present within its lumen) is discharged into the small intestine, stomach, or colon as the case may be (Fig. 412). Further, if the stone is large enough it may produce *intestinal obstruction* (small bowel, for the stone is discharged freely with the feces once it reaches the colon). Other *complications* of biliary fistulas may consist of abscess, peritonitis, pleuritis, pneumonia, etc., depending upon what structures are affected.

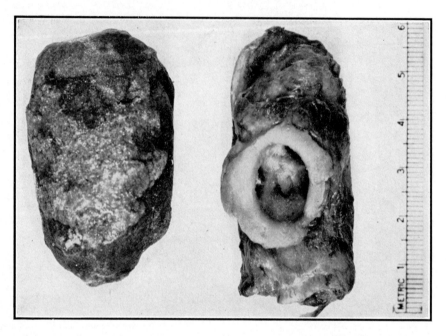

Fig. 412.—Cholecystoduodenal fistula with a discharged stone that produced intestinal obstruction. Specimen to the right is the gallbladder showing the ostium that connected with the duodenum.

TUMORS

Orientation.—Since the histologic composition of the gallbladder and extrahepatic bile ducts is similar, neoplasms that affect these portions of the biliary system are also similar. They may be listed as follows: papilloma, adenoma, carcinoid, carcinoma, fibroma, fibrosarcoma, myxoma, myxosarcoma, lipoma, myoma, myosarcoma, myoblastoma, neuroma, neurofibroma, neurofibrosarcoma, hemangioendothelioma, and secondary growths. Of these, the only lesions that need be considered further are papilloma of the gallbladder, carcinoma of the gallbladder, benign tumors of the hepatic ducts, and carcinoma of the hepatic ducts.

Papilloma of the Gallbladder.—Papilloma of the gallbladder is a rare lesion although the recorded incidence has varied from 0.4 to 8.5 per cent of all cholecystectomies (Kane). *Pathologically* the lesion is single or multiple, usually possesses a narrow pedicle, projects into the lumen in a funfating manner, is friable, and generally measures less than 1 cm. in diameter (Fig. 413). Histologically it is composed of thin stalks of connective tissue covered by relatively normal appearing columnar cells. Associated lesions, occurring in as high as 68 per cent of cases, consist of cholecystitis and cholelithiasis.   Papillomas are usually asymptomatic.   When *clinical manifestations* do occur they are due to the associated lesions.

Carcinoma of the Gallbladder. —Carcinoma of the gallbladder is the most common tumor of this organ.   The recorded *incidence* varies from 0.34 to 0.61 per cent of all autopsies and from 0.8 to 3.0 per cent of all operations on the biliary tract (Jones).   The condition is three to four times as common in females as it is in males and is usually seen after the age of fifty years.   As in other areas of the body the *cause* of the neoplasm is unknown.   Gallstones, however, are thought to play a predisposing role since they are present in from 86 to 100 per cent of cases (Russell).

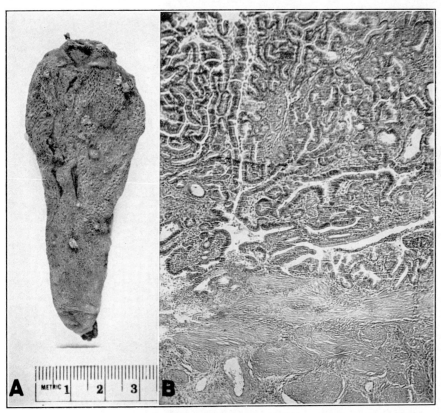

Fig. 413.—Papilloma of the gallbladder illustrating *A*, several mucosal growths and *B*, regular columnar epithelial cells forming well-defined glands that cover thin cores of connective tissue. × 50.

Pathologically the lesions are generally divided into two groups—infiltrating and fungating, with transitions from one to the other (Fig. 414). *Infiltrating* tumors are flat, penetrating, ill-defined, gray, firm growths that vary in size from one to several centimeters in greatest diameter.   Such tumors usually produce considerable distortion of the gallbladder as a whole or in focal areas.   The luminal portion has a tendency to ulcerate as the lesion penetrates, resulting ultimately in fistulous tract formation.   Fungating tumors grow into the lumen in a papillary fashion.   They are attached to the wall by a fairly broad pedicle and, at the point of attachment, the tumor is ill defined, permeating the tissues in an irregular fashion.   The portion protruding into the lumen is superficially serrated, usually reddish brown, and quite friable. Unlike in infiltrating tumors, the wall of the gallbladder is only focally affected and, therefore, permits considerable dilatation. *Histologically* carcinoma of the gallbladder is generally of the adenomatous variety with, in some instances, a tendency to papillary formation

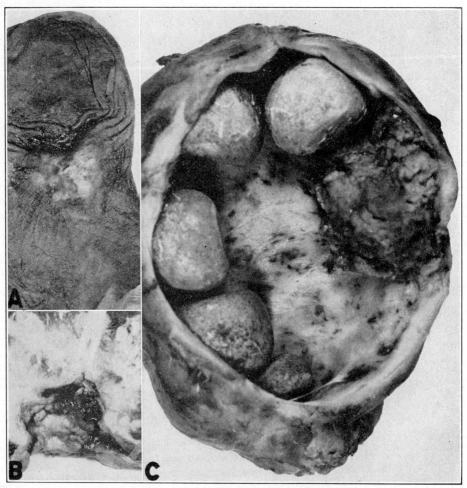

FIG. 414.—Carcinoma of the gallbladder showing *A* and *B*, infiltrating scirrhous growths and *C*, a fungating intraluminal tumor with the gallbladder containing five stones.

(Fig. 415). Actually the tumors are quite similar to those in the gastrointestinal tract. The better differentiated growths disclose rather regular appearing columnar or cuboidal epithelial cells in glandular formation. The cytoplasm is moderate in amount and may or may not disclose droplets of secretion. The nuclei are round or oval, hyperchromatic, and basally arranged. In the poorly differentiated growths the cells vary greatly in shape, size, and staining qualities and aimlessly infiltrate all the tissues they contact. Between the two extremes, there are all gradations. Occasionally the secretory activity of the cell is great enough to produce a typical mucinous appearance. Aside from the glandular types of tumors just men-

tioned the growth, on rare occasions, may be of a squamous variety.   Carcinoma of the gallbladder *spreads* by direct extension to the liver, stomach,
duodenum, and adjacent structures and by lymphatic channels and blood
vessels to liver hilar and other lymph nodes, lungs, pleura, adrenal glands,
pancreas, pertioneum, bones, etc.

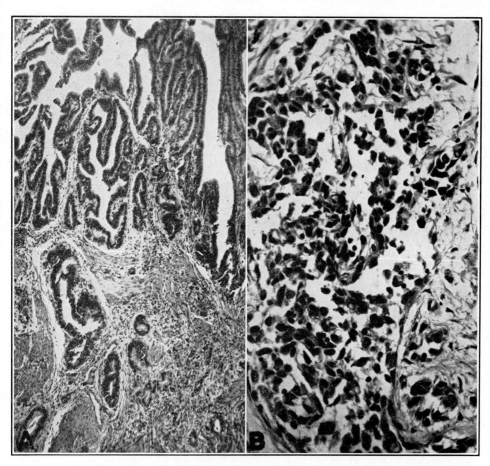

FIG. 415.—Carcinoma of the gallbladder illustrating *A*, a well-differentiated glandular tumor
penetrating the wall.   × 50 and *B*, a highly undifferentiated growth consisting of irregular cells
with no definite arrangement.   × 200.

The chief *complications*, aside from spread of the tumor to other tissues,
are jaundice (due to massive replacement of the liver by tumor or extension
of the process to obstruct the extrahepatic bile ducts) and fistulous tract
formation.   The *clinical manifestations* are nonspecific, being indistinguishable from those of cholecystitis or cholelithiasis.   The most common
symptoms and signs are jaundice, loss of weight, constant pain in the region
of the gallbladder, anorexia, vomiting, tenderness and a palpable mass in
the right upper quadrant, and ascites.   Roentgenograms generally show a
nonfunctioning gallbladder (Russell).   A clinical *diagnosis* of carcinoma of
the gallbladder is rarely made except at operation for, as already stated, the
symptoms and signs are not specific.   The only effective *treatment* is chole-

cystectomy. The *prognosis* is poor. The mortality rate is almost 100 per cent (Sainburt), although occasional five-year cures are reported (Booher).

Benign Tumors of the Extrahepatic Bile Ducts.—Although *rare*, benign tumors of the extrahepatic bile ducts are extremely important for because of their strategic locations they may cause death and yet, if properly diagnosed, the patient may be cured (Chu). They have been recorded in patients of all ages and have occurred twice as frequently in females as in

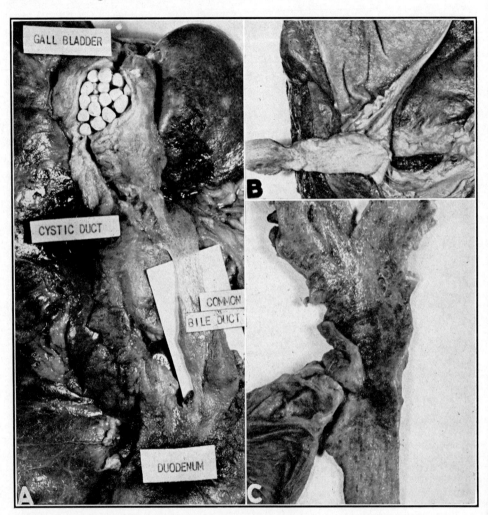

Fig. 416.—Carcinoma of the bile ducts demonstrating infiltrating tumors affecting *A*, the cystic duct, *B*, the common bile duct, and *C*, the confluence of the cystic and common bile ducts.

males. They may be *located* in any portion of the biliary tree but seldom measure more than 1 cm. in diameter. The most common *histologic types* of growths have been papilloma, adenoma, fibroma, and neuroma. *Clinically* they have a tendency to remain dormant for considerable periods of time. Gradually, however, they produce increasingly severe indigestion and then obstructive jaundice. The only effective *treatment* is surgical excision. The *prognosis* should be fair to good but in recorded cases it has been poor simply because of improper diagnoses.

Carcinoma of the Extrahepatic Bile Ducts. —Although statistics vary, carcinoma of the extrahepatic bile ducts has been recorded as constituting approximately 0.5 per cent of all operations on the biliary tract and 0.26 of all autopsies (Neibling). The condition *occurs* mostly in patients beyond fifty years of age and although some authors record an equal incidence in both sexes, others state that the disorder predominates slightly in males. The *cause* is unknown but, as in the gallbladder, gallstones may play a significant role since they are present in about two-thirds of all cases. *Pathologically* the lesions are usually single but may be multiple. The locations of the growths in approximately decreasing order of frequency are hepatic ducts, confluence of the cystic and common ducts, common duct, and cystic duct. Usually the tumors appear as firm, scirrhous, grayish-white infiltrations that affect varying lengths of the ducts and that cause narrowing and obstruction of the lumen (Fig. 416). Less frequently, the lesions are infiltrating but nodular and rarely they may be of a fungating variety (Martin). Histologically they are similar to carcinomas of the gall-bladder. The chief *complication* is biliary tract obstruction with subsequent jaundice, cholangitis, hepatic abscesses, and biliary cirrhosis. The chief clinical *symptoms* are jaundice, pain, and loss of weight (Neibling) while the chief physical findings are jaundice, palpably enlarged gallbladder, and tenderness in the right upper quadrant of the abdomen. The usual clinical *diagnosis* is obstructive jaundice but the cause of the obstruction (whether carcinoma of the pancreas, carcinoma of the bile ducts, or calculus) is generally not determined until the time of laparotomy. The only effective *treatment* is some type of surgical resection. The *prognosis* is poor, the average postoperative survival being only from three to four months.

REFERENCES

LIVER

Pathologic Physiology

BRACHET, J.: *Chemical Embryology* (translated by L. G. Barth), New York, Interscience, 1950 (Nuclear Function).

Henry Ford Hospital International Symposium, *Hepatitis Frontiers*, Boston, Little, Brown & Co., 1957 (Hepatitis).

MILLER, L. L., and BALE, W. F.: J. Exper. Med., *99*, 125, 1954 (Proteins).

POPPER, H., and SCHAFFNER, F.: *Liver; Structure and Function*, New York, The Blakiston Division, McGraw-Hill Book Co., Inc., 1957 (Physiology).

SHAY, H., *et al.*: Gastroenterology, *19*, 441, 1951 (Alkaline Phosphatase).

WATSON, C. J.: Ann. Int. Med., *45*, 351, 1956 (Bilirubin).

Congenital Anomalies

COMFORT, M. W., *et al.*: Gasteroenterology, *20*, 60, 1952 (Polycystic Disease).

KEREKES, E. S., and EWING, J.: Radiology, *55*, 861, 1950 (Traumatic Cyst).

MERRILL, G. G.: A. M. A. Arch. Path., *42*, 232, 1946 (Absence Left Lobe).

MILLER, S. E.: A. M. A. Arch. Path., *40*, 405, 1945 (Cruveilhier-Baumgarten Disease).

STOCK, F. E.: Brit. J. Surg., *39*, 530, 1952 (Cysts).

Degenerations

AHRENS, E. H., JR., *et al.*: Medicine, *29*, 299, 1950 (Primary Biliary Cirrhosis).

ARMAZ-CRUZ, R., *et al.*: Gastroenterology, *17*, 327, 1951 (208 Cases Portal Cirrhosis).

BEAN, W. B.: Am. Heart J., *25*, 463, 1943 (Palmer Erythema and Spider Nevi).

CAMPBELL, C. S.: J. Pediat., *41*, 582, 1952 (Juvenile Cirrhosis).

CORI, G. T., and CORI, C. F.: J. Biol. Chem. (Part II), *199*, 661, 1952 (Glucose-6-Phosphatase and Glycogen Storage Disease).

CRAIG, J. M.: A. M. A. Arch. Path., *49*, 665, 1950 (Cirrhosis and Erythroblastosis Fetalis).

CREVELD, S. V.: A. M. A. Arch. Dis. Child., *27*, 113, 1952, and Medicine, *18*, 1, 1939 (Glycogen Disease).

DOUGLASS, B. E., and SNELL, A. M.: Gastroenterology, *15*, 407, 1950 (444 Cases Portal Cirrhosis).

FRUMIN, A. M., *et al.:* Pediatrics, *9*, 290, 1952 (Exogenous Hemochromatosis).

GLASS, S. J.: Endocrinology, *27*, 749, 1940 (Sex Hormones and Liver Disease).

HERBUT, P. A., and TAMAKI, H. T.: Am. J. Clin. Path., *16*, 640, 1946 (Hemochromatosis).

HOMBERGER, F., and KOZOL, H. L.: J. A. M. A., *130*, 6, 1946 (Hepatolenticular Degeneration).

KOTIN, P., and HALL, E. M.: Am. J. Path., *27*, 561, 1951 (Cardiac Cirrhosis).

LUCKÉ, B.: Am. J. Path., *20*, 471, 1944 (Pathology Fatal Epidemic Hepatitis).

MARBLE, A., and BAILEY, C. C.: Am. J. Med., *11*, 590, 1951 (Hemochromatosis).

MILLER, W. R., and POLLARD, H. M.: Ann. Int. Med., *38*, 845, 1953 (Xanthomatous Biliary Cirrhosis).

MORRIONE, T. J.: A. M. A. Arch. Path., *37*, 39, 1944 (Testis in Hepatic Insufficiency).

MOSCHCOWITZ, E.: Ann. Int. Med., *36*, 933, 1952 (Cardiac Cirrhosis).

————: A. M. A. Arch. Path., *54*, 259, 1952 (Biliary Cirrhosis).

OLSEN, A. Y.: Am. J. M. Sci., *220*, 477, 1950 (Alcohol and Cirrhosis).

POPPER, H., *et al.:* Am. J. Clin. Path., *22*, 717, 1952 (Vascular Pattern in Cirrhosis).

PORTIS, S. A., and WEINBERG, S.: J. A. M. A., *149*, 1265, 1952 (Treatment Cirrhosis).

POST, J., and ROSE, J. V.: Am. J. Med., *8*, 300, 1950 (Portal Cirrhosis).

RICKETTS, W. E., *et al.:* Gastroenterology, *15*, 40, 1950 (Hepatic Function in Portal Cirrhosis).

RICKETTS, W. E., and KIRSNER, J. B.: Gastroenterology, *17*, 184, 1951 (Latent Portal Cirrhosis).

RICKETTS, W. E., and WISSLER, R. W.: Ann. Int. Med., *36*, 1241, 1952 (Cholangiolitic Biliary Cirrhosis).

SWEET, W. H., *et al.:* J. A. M. A., *117*, 1613, 1941 (Hepatolenticular Degeneration).

WARREN, S., and DRAKE, W. L., JR.: Am. J. Path., *27*, 573, 1951 (Hepatic Carcinoma in Hemochromatosis).

WARTHIN, T. A., *et al.:* Ann. Int. Med., *38*, 1066, 1953 (Idiopathic Hemochromatosis).

WATSON, C. J., and HOFFBAUER, F. W.: Ann. Int. Med., *25*, 195, 1946 (Cholangiolitic Cirrhosis).

YAZIGI, R., *et al.:* Gastroenterology, *18*, 587, 1951 (Postnecrotic Cirrhosis).

Inflammations

CHINN, A. B., *et al.:* Am. J. M. Sci., *222*, 530, 1951 (Hepatic Function in Weil's Disease).

CRAIG, C. F., and FAUST, E. C.: *Clinical Parasitology*, 5th Ed., Philadelphia, Lea & Febiger, 1951.

DRAKE, N. E., *et al.:* J. A. M. A., *152*, 690, 1953 (Gamma Globulin and Serum Hepatitis).

FARQUHAR, J. D., *et al.:* J. A. M. A., *149*, 991, 1952 (Viral Hepatitis).

FLYNN, J. E.: New England J. Med., *234*, 403, 1946 (Pyogenic Abscess).

GREENLEE, R. G., *et al.:* Texas State J. Med., *47*, 831, 1951 (Serum Hepatitis).

HAHN, R. D.: Am. J. Syph., *27*, 529, 1943 (Syphilis).

HALL, H. E., *et al.:* Ann. Int. Med., *35*, 981, 1951 (Leptospirosis).

HAVENS, W. P., JR.: Medicine, *27*, 279, 1948 (Infectious Hepatitis).

HAVENS, W. P., JR., *et al.:* Am. J. Med., *8*, 559, 1950 (Symposium on Viral Hepatitis).

KAUFMANN, G. G., *et al.:* J. A. M. A., *149*, 993, 1952 (Infectious Hepatitis).

KELLER, T. C., *et al.:* Military Surgeon, *109*, 425, 1951 (Nonfatal Hepatitis).

KINNEY, T. D., and FERREBEE, J. W.: A. M. A. Arch. Path., *45*, 41, 1948 (Abscess).

LEADER, S. A.: Ann. Int. Med., *37*, 594, 1952 (Tuberculosis).

LEIBOWITZ, S., *et al.:* Am. J. Med., *8*, 314, 1950 (Weil's Disease).

LESSES, M. F., and HAMOLSKY, M. W.: J. A. M. A., *147*, 727, 1951 (Serum Hepatitis).

LUCKÉ, B.: Am. J. Path., *20*, 471, 1944 (Fatal Epidemic Hepatitis).

MALLORY, G. K., and MALLORY, T. B.: McManus' *Progress in Fundamental Medicine* Philadelphia, Lea & Febiger, p. 102, 1952 (Viral Hepatitis).

MICHEL, M. L., and WIRTH, W. R.: J. A. M. A., *133*, 395, 1947 (Pyogenic Abscess).

OCHSNER, A., and DeBAKEY, M.: Surgery, *13*, 460, 1943 (Amebic Abscess).

REID, E. A. S., and REED, R. W.: Canad. M. A. J., *63*, 479, 1950 (Weil's Disease).

SAWITZ, W. G.: *Medical Parasitology*, New York, The Blakiston Co., 1950.

SBOROV, V. M., and KELLER, T. C.: Gastroenterology, *19*, 424, 1951 (Diagnosis Viral Hepatitis).

SHAPIRO, E., and WEINER, H.: Am. J. M. Sci., *222*, 494, 1951 (Tertiary Syphilis).

SHAY, H., *et al.*: Gasteroenterology, *19*, 441, 1951 (Sarcoidosis).
SOPER, F. L.: In *Clinical Tropical Medicine*, by Z. T. Bercovitz, New York, Paul B. Hoeber, Inc., p. 391, 1944 (Yellow Fever).
STEELE, H. H.: Gastroenterology, *15*, 59, 1950 (Serum Hepatitis).
SYMMERS, D., and SPAIN, D. M.: A. M. A. Arch. Path., *42*, 64, 1946 (Hepar Lobatum).
TRISMAN, A. S., *et al.*: J. Pediat., *37*, 174, 1950 (Viral Hepatitis in Infancy).

Physical Disturbances

ARMSTRONG, C. D., and CARNES, W. H.: Am. J. M. Sci., *208*, 470, 1944 (Chiari's Disease).
BLAKEMORE, A. H.: Surg., Gynec. & Obst., *94*, 443, 1952 (Portal Hypertension).
HERBUT, P. A., and SCARICACIOTTOLI, T. M.: A. M. A. Arch. Path., *40*, 94, 1945 (Sulfadiazine Necrosis).
LOSNER, S., *et al.*: A. M. A. Arch. Path., *49*, 461, 1950 (Infarction).
MALLORY, G. K., and MALLORY, T. B.: McManus' *Progress in Fundamental Medicine*, Philadelphia, Lea & Febiger, p. 117, 1952 (Chemical Necrosis).
MCCLOSKEY, J. F., and MCGEHEE, E. H.: A. M. A. Arch. Path., *49*, 200, 1950 (Carbon Tetrachloride Necrosis).
PAPEN, G. W., and MIKAL, S.: Rev. Gastroenterol., *17*, 633, 1950 (Trauma).
ROSENBAUM, D., and EGBERT, H. L.: J. A. M. A., *149*, 1210, 1952 (Infarction).
SAWYER, K. C., *et al.*: Am. Surg., *17*, 289, 1951 (Traumatic Rupture).
WELCH, C. T.: New England J. Med., *243*, 598, 1950 (Portal Hypertension).
WOOLLING, K. R., *et al.*: Gastroenterology, *17*, 479, 1951 (Infarction).
WRIGHT, L. T., *et al.*: A. M. A. Arch. Surg., *54*, 613, 1947 (Traumatic Rupture).

Tumors

BEAN, L. L.: Ann. West. M. & Surg., *3*, 391, 1949 (Primary Tumors).
BIGELOW, N. H., and WRIGHT, A. W.: Cancer, *6*, 170, 1953 (Primary Carcinoma in Children).
GALLUZZI, N. J., *et al.*: J. A. M. A., *152*, 15, 1953 (Primary Carcinoma).
LEVENSON, R. M., and MASON, D. G.: Ann. Int. Med., *38*, 156, 1953 (Hamartoma).
MCNAMARA, W. L., *et al.*: Am. J. Surg., *80*, 545, 1950 (Primary Carcinoma).
MILMAN, D. H., and GRAYZEL, D. M.: Am. J. Dis. Child., *81*, 408, 1951 (Mixed Tumor).
RIPSTEIN, C. B., and MILLER, G. G.: Canad. M. A. J., *64*, 240, 1951 (Primary Carcinoma).
SANFORD, C. H.: Ann. Int. Med., *37*, 304, 1952 (Primary Malignant Tumors).
SHALLOW, T. A., and WAGNER, F. B., JR.: Ann. Surg., *125*, 439, 1947 (Primary Fibrosarcoma).
STRONG, G. F., *et al.*: Ann. Int. Med., *30*, 791, 1949 (Primary Carcinoma).
WARVI, W. N.: A. M. A. Arch. Path., *37*, 367, 1944 (Primary Tumors).
WILSON, H., and TYSON, W. T., JR.: Ann. Surg., *135*, 765, 1952 (Hemangioma).

BILIARY SYSTEM

Pathologic Physiology

ARONSON, H.: A.M.A. Arch. Path., *34*, 843, 1942 (Experimental Gallstones).
BOYDEN, E. A., *et al.*: Anat. Rec., *88*, 423, 1944 (Functional Innervation).
GRAHAM, E. A.: Harvey Lectures, *29*, 176, 1933–34 (Applied Physiology).
IVY, A. C.: Am. J. Roentgenol., *57*, 1, 1947 (Biliary Dyskenesia).
ROUS, P. and MCMASTER, P. D.: J. Exper. Med., *34*, 47, 1921 (Gallbladder Absorption).
RYAN, J. D., *et al.*: Gastroenterol., *13*, 1, 1949 (Biliary-Pancreatic Dynamics).
SNAPE, W. J. and FRIEDMAN, M. H. F.: Gastroenterol., *10*, 496, 1948 (Choleystokinin Effectiveness).

Congenital Anomalies

BLEGEN, H. M., *et al.*: J. A. M. A., *148*, 196, 1952 (Entrance Common Bile Duct into Duodenal Diverticulum).
BLEICH, A. R., *et al.*: J. A. M. A., *147*, 849, 1951 (Left Upper Quadrant Gallbladder).
BULLARD, R. W., JR., *et al.*: J. A. M. A., *129*, 949, 1945 (Subcutaneous Gallbladder).
HERTZLER, J. H., and MAGUIRE, C. E.: A. M. A. Arch. Surg., *62*, 265, 1951 (Congenital Dilatation Common Bile Duct).
INGEGNO, A. P., and D'ALBORA, J. B.: Am. J. Roentgenol., *61*, 651, 1949 (Double Gallbladder).
LOCKWOOD, B. C.: J. A. M. A., *136*, 678, 1948 (Anomalies Gallbladder).

MOORE, T. C.: Surg., Gynec. & Obst., *96*, 215, 1953 (Atresia Extrahepatic Bile Ducts).
NELSON, W., *et al.:* Surgery, *25*, 916, 1949 (Absence Gallbladder).
OSLER, G. F., and DOW, R. S.: West. J. Surg., *53*, 316, 1945 (Anomalies Bile Ducts).
ROBERTSON, H. E., and FERGUSON, W. J.: A. M. A. Arch. Path., *40*, 312, 1945 (Diverticula Gallbladder).
SACHS, A. E.: J. A. M. A., *149*, 1462, 1952 (Absence Common Bile Duct).
SHALLOW, T. A., *et al.:* Ann. Surg., *117*, 355, 1943 (Cystic Dilatation Common Bile Duct).
SITES, E. C., and LAURIDSEN, J.: J. Internat. Coll. Surg., *14*, 420, 1950 (Opening Common Bile Duct into Stomach).
STERLING, J. A.: Am. J. Path., *25*, 325, 1949 (Diverticula Common Bile Duct).

Degenerations

BLUMBERG, G. N., and ZISSERMAN, L.: Rev. Gastroenterol., *13*, 97, 1946 (Hydrops of the Gallbladder).
JUTRAS, A., and LONGTIN, M.: Canad. M. A. J., *54*, 434, 1946 (Calcification Gallbladder).
WOMACK, N. A., and HAFFNER, H.: Ann. Surg., *119*, 391, 1944 (Cholesterolosis).

Inflammations

ADAMS, R., and STRANAHAN, A.: Surg., Gynec. & Obst., *85*, 776, 1947 (Cholecystitis, Cholelithiasis).
BUXTON, R. W., *et al.:* J. A. M. A., *146*, 301, 1951 (Acute Cholecystitis).
CLIFFORD, W. J.: New England J. Med., *241*, 640, 1949 (Gangrenous Cholecystitis).
DECAMP, P. T., *et al.:* Ann. Surg., *135*, 734, 1952 (Surgical Treatment Acute Cholecystitis).
FREUND, H. R.: Am. J. Surg., *82*, 703, 1951 (Acute Cholecystitis).
JOHNSTONE, G. A., and OSTNBORPH, J. E.: A. M. A. Arch. Surg., *53*, 1, 1946 (Cholecystitis with Perforation).
KAHLE, H. R., and JACKSON, J. T.: J. A. M. A., *151*, 1269, 1953 (Cholecystitis in Children).
LEADER, S. A.: Ann. Int. Med., *37*, 594, 1952 (Tuberculous Cholecystitis).
LYON, C. G.: West. J. Surg., *61*, 60, 1953 (Acute Cholecystitis in the Aged).
RETTERBUSH, W. C., *et al.:* Ann. Surg., *134*, 268, 1951 (Emphysematous Cholecystitis).
THOMAS, C. J., JR., and WOMACK, N. A.: A. M. A. Arch. Surg., *64*, 590, 1952 (Acute Cholecystitis).
TUNBRIDGE, R. E.: Practitioner, *170*, 33, 1953 (Gallbladder Dyspepsia).
TWISS, J. R., *et al.:* J. A. M. A., *147*, 1226, 1951 (Chronic Cholecystitis).

Physical Disturbances

CALIHAN, W. A., and HULBERT, H. F.: J. Internat. Coll. Surg., *16*, 325, 1951 (Intestinal Obstruction by Gallstones).
CATTELL, R. B.: J. A. M. A., *134*, 235, 1947 (Benign Biliary Stricture).
CRENSHAW, J. F.: South. M. J., *42*, 935, 1949 (Cholecystocolic Fistula).
EISENSTEIN, M. W., *et al.:* Surg., Gynec. & Obst., *95*, 93, 1952 (Obstruction Common Bile Duct).
GUY, C. C., and OLECK, H. T.: A. M. A. Arch. Surg., *55*, 316, 1947 (Biliary Bronchial Fistula).
HSIA, Z. Y., and GELLIS, S. S.: Am. J. Dis. Child., *85*, 13, 1953 (Biliary Obstruction in Infancy).
LAWLER, R. H., *et al.:* Am. J. Surg., *81*, 421, 1951 (Cholelithiasis in Children).
LIEBER, M. M.: Ann. Surg., *135*, 394, 1952 (Incidence Gallstones).
LITTLER, T. R., and ELLIS, G. R.: Brit. M. J., *1*, 842, 1952 (Gallstones).
LOVE, R. J. M.: Practitioner, *152*, 160, 1944 (Complications Gallstones).
NORGORE, M.: Ann. Surg., *123*, 127, 1946 (Rupture Gallbladder).
O'MALLEY, R. D., *et al.:* Ann. Surg., *134*, 797, 1951 (Biliary Tract Obstruction).
PECK, M. E., *et al.:* Surgery, *27*, 423, 1950 (Torsion Gallbladder).
STROHL, R. L., *et al.:* A. M. A. Arch. Surg., *64*, 788, 1952 (Common Duct Stones).
WALTON, J.: Brit. M. J., *2*, 593, 1945 (Etiology Gallstones).

Tumors

BOOHER, R. J., and PACK, G. T.: Am. J. Surg., *78*, 175, 1949 (Carcinoma Gallbladder).
CHU, P. T.: A. M. A. Arch. Path., *50*, 84, 1950 (Benign Tumors Extrahepatic Bile Ducts).
HERBUT, P. A., and WATSON, J. S.: Am. J. Clin. Path., *16*, 365, 1946 (Metastatic Tumors Extrahepatic Bile Ducts).

Jones, D. J.: Ann. Surg., *132*, 110, 1950 (Carcinoma Gallbladder).
Kane, C. F., *et al.*: Am. J. Surg., *83*, 161, 1952 (Papilloma Gallbladder).
Martin, W. F., and Page, G. D.: South. M. J., *44*, 109, 1951 (Carcinoma Extrahepatic Bile Duct).
Neibling, H. A., *et al.*: Surg., Gynec. & Obst., *89*, 429, 1949 (Carcinoma Extrahepatic Bile Ducts).
Russell, P. W., and Brown, C. H.: Ann. Surg., *132*, 121, 1950 (Primary Carcinoma Gallbladder).
Sainburg, F. E., and Garlock, J. H.: Surgery, *23*, 201, 1948 (Carcinoma Gallbladder).

Chapter

22

Pancreas

PATHOLOGIC PHYSIOLOGY

Franz Goldstein

The pancreas, *physiologically*, consists of two functionally separate units, an exocrine portion consisting of the pancreatic acini and ducts and an endocrine portion consisting of the islets of Langerhans. The *exocrine portion* of the pancreas produces a watery secretion rich in bicarbonate and containing the digestive enzymes trypsinogen and trypsin, chymotrypsinogen and chymotrypsin, amylase, lipase, and at least one peptidase, carboxypeptidase. There is evidence for a functional subdivision within the exocrine portion. The juice and bicarbonate appear to be elaborated by the lining cells of ducts, whereas the enzymes are produced by the acinar cells. The latter are stimulated by vagal and local reflex mechanisms, by chyme reaching the duodenum, and by a hormone, pancreozymin, manufactured by the duodenal mucosa. The ductal secretion is produced in response to hydrochloric acid reaching the duodenum and another hormone of small intestinal origin, secretin (Thomas).

The *beta cells* of the islets of Langerhans produce *insulin*, a hormone intimately associated with carbohydrate metabolism and indirectly also with the metabolism of lipids and proteins. Insulin increases the rate of glucose removal from body fluids and decreases the rate of addition of glucose to body fluids. These effects are accomplished (1) by increasing the rate of deposition of glycogen in the liver, muscle, and other tissues, (2) by increasing the rate of oxidation of glucose to carbon dioxide and water in the tissues, (3) by increasing the rate of conversion of glucose into fatty acids in the liver, (4) by depressing neoglucogenesis, and (5) by decreasing the rate of conversion of glycogen to glucose. The main chemical reaction catalyzed by insulin is the transformation of glucose to glucose-6-phosphate by means of the hexokinase reaction. Insulin appears to aid the formation of adenosine triphosphate and certain oxidative reactions of the Krebs cycle.

The *alpha cells* of the islet tissue produce *glucagon*, another hormone with effects on carbohydrate metabolism. Glucagon causes hepatic glycogenolysis and hyperglycemia and thus has actions antagonistic to insulin.

Another postulated hormone of pancreatic origin is *lipocaic* (Dragstedt). Its presumed action is the prevention of fatty liver but the existence of this hormone has been seriously questioned.

Abnormally, various *disease processes* may effect the pancreas. Disruption of the structural integrity of the gland may result in a variety of functional alterations of either the exocrine or the endocrine secretions or both.

Disease processes affecting the *exocrine secretion* may do so by means of two mechanisms working separately or together—obstruction to the out-

(864)

flow of pancreatic secretion into the duodenum and replacement of glandular by inflammatory or neoplastic tissue. Whenever *obstruction* is produced by blockage of the pancreatic ducts or the ampulla of Vater, and this occurs particularly in acute and chronic pancreatitis and in neoplasm, the exocrine sectetion will be prevented from reaching its destination in the duodenum. If the pancreas is at the same time stimulated to secrete, the blocked secretion may build up enough pressure to cause rupture of ductules and permit the enzyme containing secretion to enter the interstitial tissue of the pancreas. The proteolytic enzymes of the pancreatic juice, mainly activated trypsin, cause localized *autodigestion* and disruption of tissue, whereas the action of lipase contributes to the deposition of calcium soaps and so-called *fat necrosis*. Autodigestion may involve the walls of blood vessels with resulting hemorrhage into the gland. The state of the circulation is important in determining the extent and severity of the acute inflammatory process, a compromised vascular supply and ischemia adding to the primary insult and facilitating the occurrence of pancreatic necrosis. The enzyme containing secretions may find their way into the peritoneal cavity and cause local peritonitis manifested clinically by nausea, vomiting, local tenderness, and distention of small intestinal loops in the vicinity of the peritoneal inflammatory process. These processes are encountered most frequently in acute pancreatitis in which edema and obstruction occur suddenly and extend to the smaller ductules.

From the interstitial tissue, the juice and its enzymes will be gradually absorbed by regional lymphatic vessels and reach the blood stream. Elevations of *serum amylase* and *lipase* are easily detectable by means of laboratory tests and are of diagnostic importance. They signify pancreatic ductal obstruction in the presence of functioning pancreatic tissue. Efforts to measure blood *trypsin* levels have not been entirely satisfactory because of the presence of anti-trypsins in blood. However, the presence of excessive amounts of trypsin in blood has been incriminated in the production of shock frequently seen in acute pancreatitis.

If obstruction to the outflow of pancreatic juice is sufficiently complete and prolonged, significant interference with *digestion* and hence *absorption* of important *food stuffs* will occur. Actually, significant absorptive disturbances occur rarely in the absence of concomitant destruction of pancreatic parenchyma. The absence of sufficient quantities of amylase, lipase and trypsin in the small intestine will prevent adequate splitting of complex food stuffs, starches, fats, and proteins. Without this preliminary digestion these materials will be incompletely absorbed. Hence, varying amounts of undigested food material appear in the stools which may become bulky, greasy, and foul smelling. Because of the poor utilization of ingested food, patients may eat excessive amounts yet lose weight and become at times markedly malnourished. Along with *malabsorption* of fat, there is impaired absorption of fat-soluble vitamins which can result in clinical *vitamin deficiencies*. The prolonged excessive excretion of fats combined with calcium in the form of soaps may lead to marked lowering of serum calcium levels and clinical *tetany*. If pancreatic insufficiency develops early in life, as occurs especially in patients with *congenital fibrocystic disease*, physical growth may be stunted. When significant destruction of pancreatic tissue has occurred, the serum levels of amylase and lipase may be subnormal.

In borderline cases of pancreatic insufficiency, in which the digestive disturbances are not severe enough to give rise to clinical manifestations, *tests* designed to measure *pancreatic function* may disclose minimal or mild

55

abnormalities. The most accurate of these tests depends upon pancreatic stimulation by means of intravenously injected secretin and the subsequent measurement of the volume and bicarbonate concentration of pancreatic juice collected from the duodenum.

Disorders affecting the *endocrine portion* of the pancreas may result in excessive or deficient secretion of the hormones produced by pancreatic alpha and beta cells. Most commonly encountered is a deficiency, relative or absolute, in the production of *insulin*, resulting in the clinical syndrome of *diabetes mellitus*. Insulin production may be inadequate because of destruction of islet tissue by chronic inflammatory disease or neoplasm. More commonly, however, no such obvious lesions are present and the cause of the diabetes is "idiopathic." In these cases, there is poor correlation between the often insignificant, if at all demonstrable, degeneration of islet tissue and the metabolic defect resulting from an absolute or relative insulin deficit. Since idiopathic diabetes mellitus is found more commonly in over-eating, obese persons, the islets have been thought to become exhausted as the result of the overwork they are called upon to do. Experimentally, it has indeed been shown (Dohan and Lukens) that by placing an excessive load on the insulin-producing mechanism by means of intraperitoneal injections of glucose into laboratory animals, permanent diabetes may result. The same may be obtained from the prolonged action of insulin antagonists such as ACTH, pituitary growth hormone, adrenocortical steroids, and epinephrine. Conversely, diabetes may be ameliorated by extirpation of the anterior pituitary (Houssay phenomenon), that is, by removing the source of important insulin antagonists. The diabetes produced by pancreatic extirpation often requires less exogenous insulin for correction of the metabolic disturbance than do many cases of idiopathic diabetes mellitus, presumably because of the simultaneous elimination of the insulin antagonist glucagon.

Whatever its cause, a *deficient* supply of *insulin* will result in a train of *metabolic derangements*, the first of which is the inability to metabolize and utilize glucose. The resultant hyperglycemia leads to glycosuria when the renal threshold for glucose is exceeded. The body, not being able to satisfy its metabolic needs from metabolically unavailable glucose, draws upon protein and fat stores. The increased fat metabolism results in the appearance of excessive amounts of ketone bodies in the blood stream and urine. Both glucose and ketone bodies require water for excretion and therefore excessive water losses with resultant dehydration accompany the excessive solute losses. The anionic ketone bodies bind available cations and cause their excessive excretion with resultant acidosis and electrolyte depletion. The breakdown of depot fat and muscle protein for caloric purposes leads to weight loss and malnutrition. Cerebral metabolism dependent on glucose is also severely impaired. Such disturbances may become manifest as confusion deepening into coma and terminating in death. Although the above changes can be reversed and kept under control with a well-adjusted schedule of exogenous insulin, many diabetic patients eventually develop degenerative changes in the cardiovascular system, the kidneys, and retinas. Some of these changes have been attributed to disturbances in lipid metabolism which are an accompaniment of the altered carbohydrate metabolism. However, it is generally acknowledged that the full metabolic defect of diabetes mellitus has yet to be elucidated and that insulin alone may not correct all of the metabolic disturbances.

Overproduction of *insulin* is encountered in patients with benign or malignant *tumors* of beta cells. The insulin secretion in such patients is unchecked by low blood glucose levels. Especially after prolonged fasting or after exercise, the blood glucose may drop to dangerously low levels and result in symptoms. These may be caused by the compensatory release of epinephrine (tachycardia, diaphoresis, excitement), or by depression of cerebral metabolism (excitability followed by depression, convulsions, and coma), or both.

Oversecretion of pancreatic *alpha cells* may occur and recently a tumor composed of alpha cells has been recognized (Zollinger and Ellison). However, the oversecretion of these alpha cells does not result in excessive blood glucagon levels but in the excessive secretion of gastric acid and peptic ulcerations. A spontaneously occurring deficiency of alpha cell secretion has not been recognized, functionally or structurally.

Pain is a common accompaniment of pancreatic diseases, especially in association with inflammation and malignant tumors. Since the pancreas is located retroperitoneally, in close proximity to numerous nerve structures, the pain probably results from irritation of the many nerve plexuses around the pancreas by an edematous or enlarged gland or from exudation of inflammatory fluid and resulting peritoneal irritation. In some instances, however, the pain is out of proportion to the actual anatomic lesion and cannot be satisfactorily explained.

Marked *serum hyperlipemia* has been associated with some cases of pancreatic inflammation. The increase is predominantly in the neutral fat fraction. This interesting phenomenon has not been fully explained. Neither has it been established whether the hyperlipemia is the result of pancreatitis, whether hyperlipemia and fat emboli may cause pancreatitis, or whether either sequence may occur (Klatskin and Gordon).

An increased tendency for blood to coagulate and for the formation of *venous thrombosis* has been claimed in pancreatic disease, both neoplastic and inflammatory. Increased titers of anti-trypsins in blood could be responsible for this tendency.

CONGENITAL ANOMALIES

Orientation. — The chief developmental malformations of the pancreas consist of (1) *persistence* of *Santorini's* (dorsal) *duct* as the main duct and opening separately into the duodenum instead of the presence of the usual Wirsung's (ventral) duct uniting with the common bile duct, (2) *persistence* of the *dorsal* and *ventral pancreases* as separate structures, that is, failure of union of the two portions, (3) *agenesis* of the *dorsal pancreas*, (4) *hypoplasia* of the exocrine or the endocrine portion, (5) *aberrant pancreas*, (6) *annular pancreas*, (7) *solitary* and *multiple cysts*, and (8) *fibrocystic disease*. Of these, the five listed last may be considered further.

Aberrant Pancreas. — By aberrant pancreas is meant pancreatic tissue occurring outside its normal anatomic location (Pearson). The condition is also *referred to* as heterotopic or ectopic pancreas. The *incidence* is recorded as approximately 1 to 2 per cent of all autopsies. The *theories* of *origin* are many. Some may be listed as (1) incomplete regression of the left ventral anlage, (2) representation of an atavistic phenomenon, (3) isolation of pancreatic tissue during embryonic life by adhesions, (4) attachment of buds of pancreatic tissue to adjacent organs before relative changes in position of these organs occur, and (5) lateral buddings of rudimentary pancreatic ducts as they penetrate the intestinal wall. Of these, the last mentioned seems to be the most plausible. *Pathologically* accessory pancreatic tissue is found in the following locations: duodenum 30 per cent, stomach 25 per cent, jejunum 15 per cent, Meckel's diverticulum 6 per cent, ileum 3 per cent, and occasionally in the gallbladder, common bile duct, liver, spleen, and other sites of the abdominal cavity. In the gastrointestinal tract the tissue is located in the submucosa in one-half of the cases and in the muscle coats and serosa in the remaining cases. The deposits are single or multiple, appear yellowish gray to white, are lobulated, and measure from a few millimeters to 5 cm. across (Fig. 417). Histologically they consist of acini and islets of Langerhans. In some instances, there is accompanying proliferation of muscle tissue accounting for an appearance that has been called *adenomyoma* or myo-epithelial hamartoma. Physiologically, accessory pancreatic tissue may be as active as pancreatic tissue in the normal anatomic site. The *complications* consist of any of the disease processes (cysts, inflammation, tumors, etc.) that may affect the usual

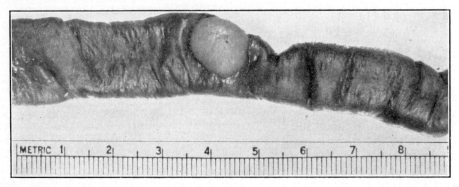

Fig. 417.—A mass of aberrant pancreatic tissue in the submucosa of the jejunum.

pancreas. *Clinically* most cases are asymptomatic but others are accompanied by manifestations that may mimic intestinal obstruction, peptic ulcer, gallbladder disease, common bile duct obstruction, intussusception, pancreatitis, and appendicitis. The *diagnosis* is usually made at operation or postmortem. *Treatment* is surgical excision. The *prognosis* is good.

Annular Pancreas.—An annular pancreas consists of a band or ring of pancreatic tissue arising from the head of the pancreas and encircling the second portion of the duodenum (Fig. 418). The amount of tissue forming the ring varies. The ring is usually complete but it may be incomplete, in which case the defect exists in the anterior portion. Histologically the tissue is normal in every respect. The chief *complication* is encroachment upon the lumen of the duodenum producing intestinal obstruction. Other complications consist of pancreatitis, peptic ulcer, and jaundice. Although there have been only 72 cases recorded in the literature up to 1953 (Castleton), the condition is doubtlessly more *common* than these reports would tend to indicate. It has been seen at all ages and in both sexes but, in surgically treated cases, it has been encountered two times as frequently in males as in females. The anomaly *arises* as a result of faulty fusion of the dorsal and ventral anlage of the developing pancreas in the presence of faulty rotation of the intestine. In symptomatic patients the usual *clinical manifestations* consist of epigastric pain, anorexia, nausea, and vomiting. The *diagnosis* is made from the clinical manifestations in the presence of a band-like constriction of the second portion of the duodenum demonstrated roentgen-ographically. *Treatment* consists of surgical removal of the obstruction by incision or excision of the constricting tissue. The *prognosis* is good.

Solitary and Multiple Cysts.—Cysts of the pancreas *occur* at all ages and affect both sexes. Some are *congenital* while others are *acquired*. They may be *classified* as follows: congenital, retention, pseudo, neoplastic, parasitic, and miscellaneous (Brilhart and Scott). The chief *complications* consist of pancreatic cachexia, diabetes, jaundice, rupture and peritonitis, secondary infection, and (in some cases) development of carcinoma. The *clinical manifestations* depend (among other things) upon (1) the number,

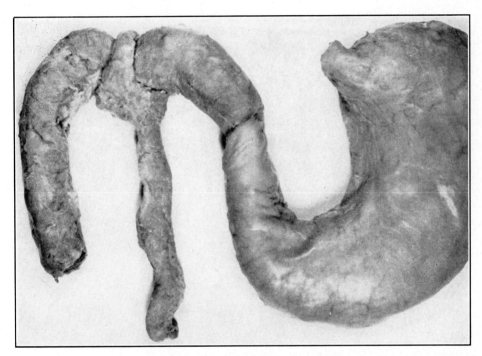

FIG. 418.—Annular pancreas, anterior view, showing a band encircling the second portion of the duodenum.

size, and exact anatomical location of the cysts, (2) the complications that arise, and (3) the amount of pancreatic tissue destroyed. They may consist of pain, dyspepsia, loss of weight, jaundice, and a palpable upper abdominal mass. *Roentgenographically* a tumor may or may not be demonstrated in the region of the pancreas. The *diagnosis* is usually made at operation or postmortem. *Treatment*, in general, consists of surgical excision. The *prognosis* varies but in the over-all is fair.

Congenital cysts of the pancreas arise as a result of segmentation, degenera-tion, and persistence (instead of disappearance) of portions of the ductal system of the developing organ (Norris). The portions of the system that persist then undergo progressive enlargement and cyst formation as a result of accumulation of intraluminal fluid secreted by the lining cells. The lesions are single or multiple (Nygaard). The former may measure as much as 20 cm. in diameter while the latter usually measure less than 1 cm. across (Fig. 419). The wall is thin; the inner surface is smooth, and the lumen (unless hemorrhage or infection occurs) is filled with clear, straw-colored fluid. The amount of remaining pancreatic tissue varies from almost normal to that which can scarcely be identified. Histologically the wall is composed of connective tissue lined with flattened cuboidal epithelial cells. The lesion is frequently accompanied by similar cysts in the kidneys and liver.

Retention cysts as such are of no clinical significance. They occur as a result of obstruction of the pancreatic duct by calculi, inflammations, or tumors. They consist of dilated ducts and acini and seldom measure more than 1 cm. across.

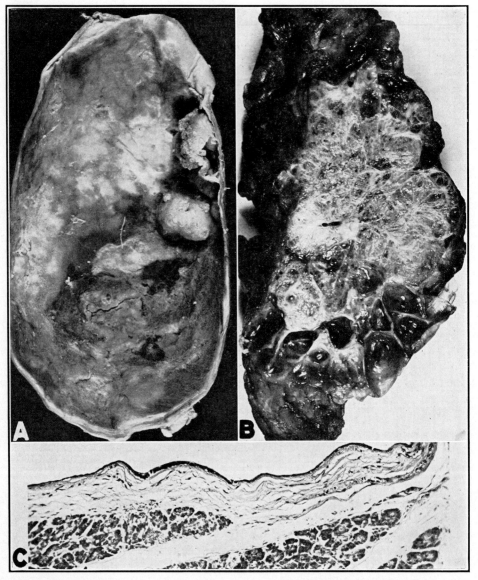

Fig. 419.—Congenital cysts of the pancreas illustrating *A*, a large unilocular cyst, *B*, multi-cystic disease, and *C*, a wall composed of fibrous tissue and lined with a single layer of cuboidal epithelial cells. × 100.

Pseudocysts are the most common (Brilhart and Collins). They arise as a result of trauma to, or inflammation of, the pancreas and consist essentially of an encapsulation of first hemorrhagic and later brownish, milky, or straw-colored fluid in the vicinity of the pancreas. Their most common location is the lesser peritoneal cavity. Grossly the cysts measure as much as 30 cm. in greatest diameter (Fig. 420). The wall is thick and fibrous and the inner surface may be rough and covered with fibrinous material. Histologically the wall is composed essentially of granulation or fibrous tissue and lacks an epithelial lining.

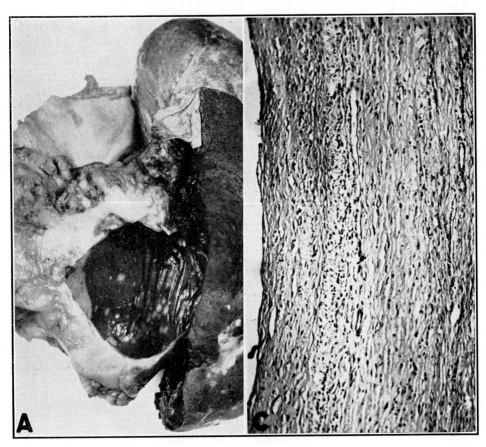

Fig. 420.—Pseudocyst of the pancreas disclosing *A*, a cystic space walled off by the pancreas, peritoneum, and spleen, and *C*, a wall composed of granulation and collagenous tissue and uncovered with epithelium. × 100.

Neoplastic cysts are progressively proliferative in nature and are thus true tumors. They are multiloculated, may be microscopic in size or measure many centimeters in diameter, and are composed of cuboidal or columnar epithelial cells in glandular formation (Fig. 421). The glands are located in the walls of the cysts and, beyond this, even in the pancreas proper. When the cells are irregular and/or invade the tissues the lesion is truly a cystadenocarcinoma.

Parasitic cysts are virtually limited to those found in echinococcus disease. The topic has been discussed in the Chapter on the Liver (p. 828).

Miscellaneous cysts include such conditions as cavernous hemangiomas, teratoid tumors, and cystic changes within otherwise solid tumors.

Fibrocystic Disease. — Fibrocystic disease of the pancreas, also known as cystic fibrosis, is a syndrome that has only recently been separated from the general category of celiac disease. Its exact *incidence* is difficult or impossible to establish but, from the recent upsurge of cases recorded in the literature, it may be stated that the condition is common. Changes in the pancreas similar to those in fibrocystic disease (but frequently unaccompanied by symptoms) have been noted, however, in as high as 3 per cent of all children coming to necropsy (Abbott). The disorder is most common

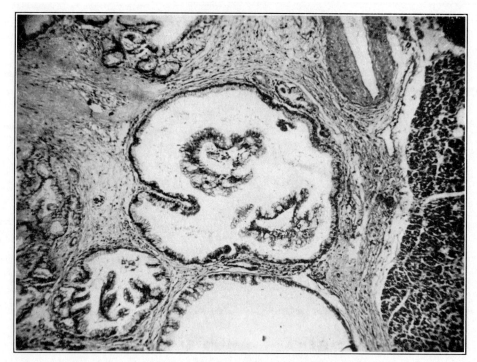

Fig. 421.—Neoplastic papillary cysts demonstrating spaces lined by a single layer of columnar epithelial cells. × 50.

during the first two years of life, but it may occur at any time during the first decade (Bostick). It does not have any predilection for either sex. Some of the many theories promulgated to explain the *cause* of the disorder are (1) heredity, (2) disturbance of parasympathetic innervation or autonomic imbalance in nervous control of secretions of the pancreas and mucous membranes of the respiratory tract resulting in inspissation of mucus and obstruction, (3) vitamin A deficiency producing metaplasia of the ductal epithelium with obstruction of the duct, and (4) congenital obstruction or stenosis of the pancreatic ductal system, especially in the region of the ampulla of Vater (Bostick and Baggenstoss). Needless to say, the exact causes and pathogenesis of the condition are still unknown.

Pathologically the *pancreas* grossly may appear relatively normal or it may be smaller than normal, fibrotic, and, upon close examination, permeated with tiny cysts (Fig. 422). Histologically it discloses the following: cystic dilatation of the duct, lining of the ducts with attenuated cuboidal or some-

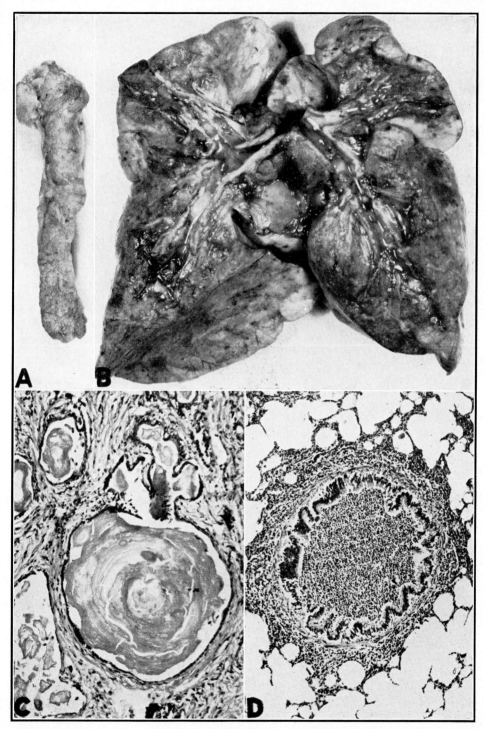

Fig. 422.—Fibrocystic disease of the pancreas showing *A*, a firm but otherwise relatively normal appearing pancreas, *B*, the bronchial tree filled with pus and the lungs distended with air (emphysema), *C*, pancreatic ducts filled with inspissated secretion and lined with attenuated cuboidal epithelial cells and the pancreatic acini replaced with fibrous tissue. × 100, and *D*, a bronchiole permeated with neutrophils and emphysema of the adjacent parenchyma. × 50.

times metaplastic (squamous) epithelium, filling of the ducts with pink-staining (granular or laminated) secretion, atrophy to complete disappearance of the exocrine portion of the gland, preservation of the islets of Langerhans, diffuse and extensive fibrosis, and varying degrees of leukocytic infiltration. If death occurs within a few days or weeks after birth, the *lungs* appear relatively normal. If death is delayed, however, they characteristically disclose the following changes: bronchitis, bronchiectasis, bronchopneumonia, and emphysema. *Other glands* of the body (such as Brunner's glands of the duodenum and the salivary glands) also disclose cystic changes in a high percentage of cases coming to autopsy.

Aside from the pulmonary changes which, in themselves, represent a part of the disease, the two *chief complications* occur *in utero* and consist of *meconium ileus* (obstruction of the ileum by inspissated meconium which, in turn, results from lack of pancreatic secretion) and *meconium peritonitis* (as a result of rupture of meconium ileus, see p. 898) (Montgomery and Forshall). In most instances, the onset of *clinical manifestations* is within the first few weeks of life (Abbott). In decreasing order of frequency the symptoms consist of (1) cough, (2) recurrent pneumonia, (3) abnormally loose, pale, bulky, foul stools, (4) vomiting, and (5) wheezing. *Physical examination* discloses malnutrition, abdominal distention, and pulmonary rales. Roentgen examination reveals pulmonary emphysema, increase in peribronchial markings, and pulmonary atelectasis. The *diagnosis* is readily made from the history, physical findings, and roentgen examination of the chest. *Treatment* is directed towards maintenance of nutrition by way of administration of pancreatic enzymes, high protein diet, vitamins, etc., and controlling the respiratory infection with antibiotics when necessary. The *prognosis*, as far as life is concerned, is fair to poor and the morbidity is high.

DEGENERATIONS

Orientation. —The pancreas is one of the most labile organs of the body as far as degenerative disturbances are concerned. It is, for example, one of the first organs to show postmortem autolytic and putrefactive changes — even when other tissues are still well preserved. As would be expected, therefore, most of the degenerative disorders commented upon in Chapter 4 (p. 29) may be represented in the pancreas. These include atrophy, parenchymatous degeneration, hydropic degeneration, hyaline degeneration, amyloidosis, mucoid degeneration, fatty infiltration, calcification, hemosiderosis, ordinary necrosis, fat necrosis, and avitaminosis A. Aside from their mention in Chapter 4, calcification of the pancreas is discussed in connection with pancreatic calculi (p. 883) and fat necrosis is referred to in connection with acute pancreatitis (p. 878). Since the above listed disturbances are fundamental pathologic processes, they may occur in conjunction with a variety of diseases. Conversely, purely degenerative diseases of the pancreas are few in number, with the only important condition being diabetes mellitus.

Diabetes Mellitus. —The caption diabetes mellitus (Gr. = through + to go + preparation made with honey) literally means a disease characterized by a discharge of excessive quantities of sweetened (glucose-containing) urine. It is a disorder of carbohydrate metabolism. While the *incidence* is difficult to determine, it is generally conceded that diabetes mellitus occurs in from 1 to 2 per cent of the total population (John). The disorder occurs at any age from birth on but with most of the cases occurring in the fifth decade and beyond. It is more common in females than in males in the approximate ratio of 3 to 2. The ultimate *cause* of diabetes mellitus is insulin deficiency (Warren). This may be (1) actual—due to decreased production, neutralization, or failure of transportation from the islets of Langerhans or (2) relative—due to increased demands or to insufficient facilities for the formation and storage of glycogen. In *man* three important general factors that appear to be concerned in the development of the disease are heredity, obesity, and infection (John). The role of *heredity* has been definitely established. It has been recorded in from 8.0 to 43.0 per cent of cases studied, but undoubtedly the incidence of heredity is even higher than these figures indicate. *Obesity* interferes with carbohydrate

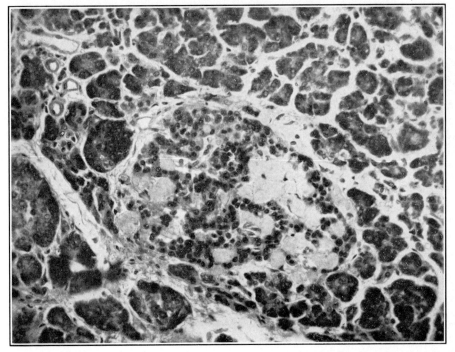

FIG. 423.—Hyalinization of an islet of Langerhans from a case of diabetes mellitus. × 200.

metabolism and is a definite factor. Any person who is excessively overweight for a prolonged period can expect to develop diabetes mellitus eventually. Conversely, it has been conclusively shown that a reduction in weight definitely improves carbohydrate tolerance. The question of *infection* is controversial. Diabetes mellitus, however, has been noted to develop following mumps, influenza, measles, pneumonia, and a host of other infections. Whether infection is just a trigger mechanism in a person already hereditarily predisposed to diabetes or whether infection, of itself, without the weak constitutional background is sufficient still remains unanswered. In a minority of cases, certain *anatomic* changes are noted to be responsible for the diabetic state. Some of these consist of (1) destruction of pancreatic tissue by inflammations, tumors, toxins, and surgical procedures, (2) selective destruction of insular tissue by hyalinization, fibrosis, toxins, and hydropic degeneration, (3) congenital deficiency in amount of insular tissue, and (4) inadequate blood supply to the pancreas as in cases of arteriosclerosis (Warren). *Experimentally* various laboratory animals have been used in the production of diabetes mellitus with the favorite ones being rabbits, rats, and dogs. The experimental aim has been to remove or to destroy (by direct chemical action or by exhaustion atrophy) the beta cells of the islets of Langerhans. The usual methods employed have been (1) total or subtotal pancreatectomy, (2) injection of alloxan or similar substances, (3) administration of anterior pituitary extract, (4) feeding thyroid in partially depancreatized animals, and (5) administration of excessive amounts of glucose over a prolonged period (Warren).

The *pathologic* changes may be outlined in connection with the various organs or systems affected. In most instances the *pancreas* is normal grossly. The most typical histologic change is hyalinization of the islets of Langerhans (Warren). The hyalin is deposited as homogeneous, eosinophilic, globular, or confluent material that partially or completely replaces islet cells (Fig. 423). It has no specific staining reaction but, on occasion, does take a positive amyloid stain. Hyalinization of the islets is seen in 6 per cent of diabetics up to forty years of age, in 45 per cent of diabetics over forty years of age, and in 50 per cent of diabetics who have had the disease ten years or more. The lesion, however, is not specific for diabetes mellitus, for it is occasionally seen in nondiabetic patients. Other islet changes that are occasionally seen are hydropic degeneration, pyknosis of the nuclei, necrosis, hypertrophy, and hemorrhage. In addition, the pancreas, as a whole, may disclose fibrosis and lymphocytic infiltration. The *kidneys* disclose two specific lesions—intercapillary or diabetic glomerulosclerosis (p. 1067) and (in uncontrolled diabetics) deposition of glycogen in the renal tubular cells (p. 49). Two important nonspecific lesions, occurring as complications, consist of pyelonephritis (p. 1087) and necrotizing renal papillitis (p. 1088). The most common and most important *vascular* change is arteriosclerosis (p. 359). In children the condition is encountered only after they have had diabetes for ten years or more; in adults it may precede or follow the development of diabetes, but in either case the process is accelerated by the diabetic condition. Although all tissues and organs of the body may be affected by the arteriosclerotic process, the more important changes produced by the vascular lesion consist of myocardial infarction, myocardial failure, encephalomalacia (degenerative ganglion changes leading to softening and necrosis), intracranial hemorrhage, gangrene of lower extremities, and intercapillary or diabetic glomerulosclerosis (Bell). The alterations in the *skin* may consist of the following: (1) changes due to secretion and excretion laden with excessive glucose—generalized pruritus and pruritus pudenda, (2) disorders due to increased susceptibility to bacterial and mycotic infection—furuncles, carbuncles, erysipelas, cutaneous gangrene, dermatophytosis, and moniliasis, and (3) disorders associated with abnormal metabolism of lipids—xanthelasma or xanthoma palpebrarum (round, oval, light yellow or orange, 1 to 4 mm., cutaneous deposits in the eyelids but seen also in nondiabetics), xanthoma diabeticorum (extensive papular, yellowish 2 to 10 mm. eruptions of the trunk, extremities, and especially soles and palms), and (4) necrobiosis lipoidica diabeticorum (pink or yellowish macules and plaques located on the lower extremity with healing occurring by central scar tissue formation) (Guy). The *ocular* changes that are characteristic (but not specific) for diabetes mellitus consist of (1) cataract formation, (2) vacuolization and glycogen deposition in the pigmented epithelium of the iris, (3) micro-aneurysms and capillary hemorrhages in the retina, (4) dilatation and sclerosis of the retinal vein, (5) protein-rich transudation in the retina, (6) proliferative retinitis, and (7) occlusion of central retinal vein with formation of a vascular connective tissue membrane on the anterior surface of the iris (Warren). Finally, *infants* born of *diabetic mothers* often disclose macrosomia (large body size), cardiac hypertrophy, excessive hematopoiesis in the liver, and hypertrophy of the islets of Langerhans (Miller).

Most of the *complications* have already been mentioned in connection with the description of the pathologic changes. For convenience, they may be listed as follows: (1) ketosis (p. 52) and diabetic coma, (2) renal failure, (3) myocardial infarction and cardiac failure, (4) visual disturbances, (5) gangrene of the extremities, and (6) susceptibility to infection. The *clinical manifestations* in diabetes mellitus are nonspecific. In uncomplicated cases, they may consist of the following: general weakness, loss of weight, excessive appetite and thirst, frequent passing of large quantities of urine, nocturia, generalized (and in females also vulvar) pruritus, backache, and impotency in the male (Duncan). When complications arise, the clinical manifestations are referable to the organs affected generally including the extremities, heart, eyes, brain, skin, kidneys, etc. The most important *laboratory findings* are elevation of blood sugar and glycosuria. A fasting blood sugar level above 120 mg. per cent is generally considered to indicate diabetes mellitus. In a normal person, the ingestion of 100 gm. of glucose causes a rise in the blood sugar to as much as 160 mg. per cent in the first hour and a return of the level to normal within the second hour. In a diabetic, the peak of the curve (over 160 mg. per cent) is not reached until the end of the second hour and the starting level may not be regained even at four hours. This test is referred to as the standard glucose tolerance test and the response, as outlined, is referred to as one of low tolerance. Ordinarily, glycosuria (sugar in the urine) occurs when the blood sugar level reaches 180 mg. per cent or more. Sometimes, however, the renal threshold may be higher or lower than 180 mg. per cent. Therefore, glycosuria of itself cannot be used as an absolute criterion for the diagnosis of diabetes mellitus and must be interpreted in conjunction with the blood sugar level (John). Aside from glycosuria, other urinary findings consist of an elevated specific gravity to 1.030 or over, increase in the twenty-four-hour volume of urine over 1500 cc. and, in cases of ketosis, the presence of ketone bodies. In addition to hyperglycemia, other corroboratory findings in the blood consist of increased cholesterol and fat values, accumulation of acetone bodies, and reduction of carbon dioxide combining power. The final *diagnosis* of diabetes mellitus is made on the basis of (1) glycosuria in the presence of hyperglycemia and (2) a typical glucose tolerance curve. *Treatment* consists of regulation of the diet and administration of insulin (Duncan). In the presence of infection and/or diabetic coma the insulin requirement is greatly increased over that of the daily need (Story). The objectives of treatment are (1) relief of symptoms, (2) maintenance of a normal nutrition, (3) preservation or minimization of complications (Ricketts). Since the insulin era, the *prognosis* in diabetes mellitus is good, for the mortality curve, with regard to age distribution, is the same in diabetics as it is in nondiabetics (John). With the exception of diabetic coma (which now is relatively rare) death in a diabetic is usually due to cardiac disease (failure or infarction), renal failure (intercapillary or diabetic glomerulosclerosis), postoperative state (including operation for gangrene), pneumonia, and a variety of other nondiabetic conditions. In other words, with proper treatment and care, the diabetic is assured of a relatively normal life.

INFLAMMATIONS

Orientation.—Inflammation of the pancreas is called *pancreatitis*. Although inflammations such as tuberculosis, Boeck's sarcoid, echinococcosis, etc., may rarely affect the pancreas, the only two conditions that occur frequently enough to warrant discussion are acute and chronic pancreatitis.

Acute Pancreatitis.—As the name suggests, acute pancreatitis is an acute inflammation of the pancreas. The caption includes such *designations* as acute pancreatic necrosis, acute interstitial pancreatitis, acute edematous pancreatitis, acute hemorrhagic pancreatitis, and acute hemorrhagic necrosis of the pancreas (Roberts and Pfeiffer). The condition has been recorded as *occurring* in about 0.2 per cent of all autopsies (Roberts) and 1 in 600 medical and surgical hospital admissions (Brobstein). It affects females with slightly greater frequency than males, is found in all decades of life with a preponderance in the sixth decade, and has no predilection for any race (Siler). The *causes* of the condition are doubtlessly many (Roberts and Morse). The disorder has been recorded as arising as a result of (1) bacterial invasion from adjacent structures, the bloodstream, the lymphatic vessels, and the duodenum and gallbladder (by way of the pancreatic ducts), (2) obstruction of the pancreatic ducts as a result of spasm of the sphincter of Oddi, biliary or pancreatic calculi, inspissated bile or pancreatic fluid, mucus, and metaplasia of the ductal epithelium, (3) reflux of bile by way of the common bile duct and pancreatic ducts, (4) reflux of duodenal contents by way of the ampulla of Vater and pancreatic ducts, (5) vascular occlusion by way of thrombi, emboli, or arteriosclerosis, and (6) trauma, either surgical or accidental. Whatever the initiating process, pancreatic enzymes are activated by bile, duodenal contents, degenerated ductal contents, or necrotic tissue products, releasing trypsin and lipase. Trypsin destroys all pancreatic (and other) tissue that it contacts, causing escape of lymph, blood, and bile while lipase attacks fat, producing fat necrosis (p. 87). The liberated tissue products are then absorbed into the bloodstream and produce a severe generalized toxic reaction. *Experimentally* (1) fat or hemorrhagic necrosis (without elevation of serum amylase and lipase) can be produced readily in dogs by oral administration of d, l-ethionine (an antagonist of the essential amino acid methionine) and (2) elevation of serum amylase and lipase (without fat or hemorrhagic necrosis) can be produced in dogs after (*a*) ligation of pancreatic ducts and stimulation of the gland by food or by food and intravenous injection of secretin and pancreozymin, or (*b*) ligation of pancreatic ducts and the injection of an oily emulsion into the arterial blood supply of the pancreas (Radakovich).

The *pathologic* changes vary with the severity of the process. In a minority of patients the peritoneal cavity appears relatively normal while in a majority it contains brownish or bloody fluid and occasionally even purulent fluid (Roberts). In *less severe cases*, the pancreas is slightly enlarged; its capsule is tense, and the parenchyma is swollen and firm. There is no evidence of softening, hemorrhage, or necrosis. Histologically the essential changes consist of congestion, edema, and a sparse to moderate interstitial permeation with neutrophils and other leukocytes. In *more severe cases* the pancreas is slightly, partially, or completely destroyed disclosing (1) small or large, sharply circumscribed, chalky areas of fat necrosis, (2) ordinary necrosis, and (3) hemorrhagic extravasation (Figs. 424 and 30, p. 88). Fat necrosis is found not only in the vicinity of the pancreas but also in the mesentery, omentum, retroperitoneum, peritoneum, pericardium, pleura, and mediastinum. Histologically a severely damaged organ reveals extensive, partial to complete destruction of tissue with varying degrees of erythrocytic and leukocytic extravasation. In areas of fat necrosis the necrotic cells are large and opaque. At their junction with

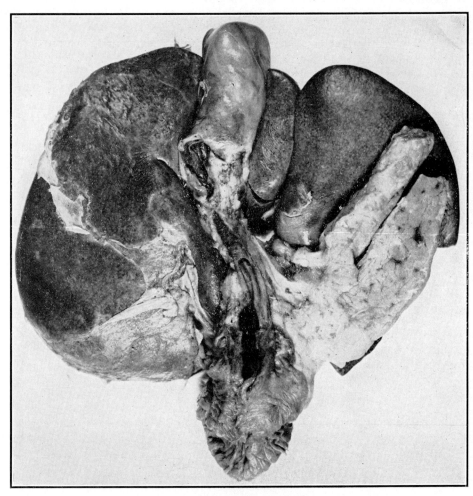

Fig. 424.—Acute pancreatitis disclosing chalky areas of fat necrosis in the pancreas and biliary calculi in the common bile duct.

normal tissue there is a zone of granular, bluish-staining material (calcium soap) and beyond this a zone of inflammation. Aside from the changes in the pancreas, associated biliary tract disease has been reported in as high as 94 per cent of all cases of acute pancreatitis and the presence of gall-stones has been recorded in as high as 80 per cent of cases.

The chief *complications* of acute pancreatitis are shock, peritonitis, localized suppuration, and pseudocyst formation. *Clinically* there is generally a history of recurrent or persistent indigestion (intolerance to certain foods, epigastric fullness, belching, pain, etc.) for months or years in almost one-half of the cases (Siler and Morse). The actual attack is ushered in by sudden, severe epigastric pain (due to stretching of the pancreatic capsule) followed by nausea, vomiting, occasionally hematemesis, constipation, slight fever, rapid pulse, at first elevated and then subnormal blood pressure, cyanosis, dyspnea, jaundice, abdominal tenderness and distention, rigidity of the abdominal muscles, and diminished peristalsis. The *laboratory* findings consist of anemia followed later by hemoconcentration (due to shock), leukocytosis, elevation of serum amylase and lipase, albuminuria,

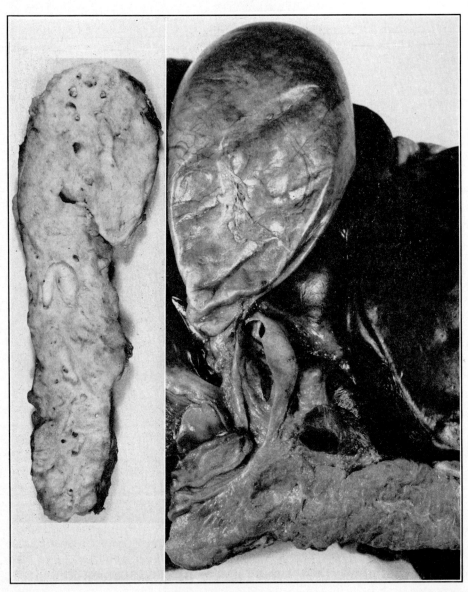

FIG. 425.—Chronic pancreatitis illustrating *A*, a diffuse perilobular and intralobular increase of fibrous tissue, dilatation of the pancreatic ducts, and a few calculi in the ducts in the head of the pancreas and *B*, obstruction of the common bile duct by the fibrotic pancreas. This lesion was mistaken at laparotomy for carcinoma of the head of the pancreas.

and glycosuria. *Roentgenographically* there is (1) an absence of air within the peritoneal cavity (distinguishing the disorder from ruptured peptic ulcer), (2) presence of calculi in the biliary system or pancreatic ducts in a high percent of cases, and (3) extrinsic pressure defect of a barium-filled stomach, later in the course of the disease. The *diagnosis* is made from the history, clinical findings, and the presence of an elevated serum amylase and lipase. A differential diagnosis should include ruptured peptic ulcer, cholecystitis and cholelithiasis, myocardial infarction, and renal colic. It is the concensus that conservative *treatment* should prevail. Among other things, it consists of (1) relief of pain, (2) abstinence from food, drink, etc.,

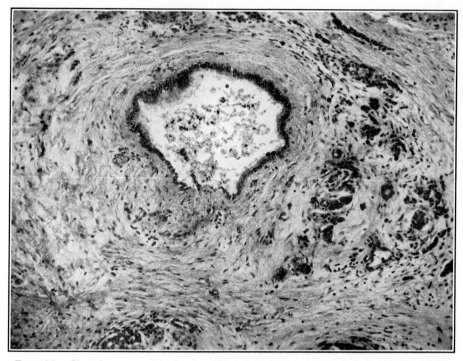

Fig. 426.—Chronic pancreatitis showing dilatation of a pancreatic duct and diffuse fibrous tissue and lymphocytic replacement of the rest of the tissue. × 100.

to minimize pancreatic secretion, and (3) combating infection by administration of antibiotics (Berk). Surgical interference should be delayed or withheld entirely (Morse). The operation consists essentially of draining the lesser peritoneal cavity. The *prognosis* is good in the less severe forms of the disease with the mortality being less than 4 per cent, but is fair to poor when necrosis and hemorrhage supervene with the mortality reaching as high as 85 per cent.

Chronic Pancreatitis.—Chronic pancreatitis, *also known* as chronic relapsing pancreatitis and chronic recurrent pancreatitis, represents a chronic protracted or recurrent inflammation and fibrosis of the pancreas. The disorder is *uncommon*, Edmondson recording 62 cases in 3,500 autopsies (1.18%). The condition may occur at any age beyond the third decade and is slightly more frequent in males than in females (Maimon). The precise *cause* is unknown. Some cases doubtlessly follow repeated attacks

56

of acute or subacute pancreatitis but others develop gradually with no evidence of any such antecedent disorder (Horton). Two other factors that are frequently stated as being of etiologic significance are cholelithiasis and chronic alcoholism.

Pathologically the appearance of the pancreas varies with the stage or severity of the process (Edmondson). In less severe or early stages the organ may actually be increased in size. Eventually, however, it becomes smaller than normal and presents a nodular distorted surface. It cuts with increased resistance. The cut surface discloses irregular patches of pancreatic tissue surrounded by depressed bands of fibrous tissue or a diffuse fibrous tissue replacement (Fig. 425). In either case, the pancreatic ducts are generally dilated, are filled with watery or more mucoid brownish fluid, or contain stones. *Histologically* there is a diffuse increase of fibrous tissue, more marked in the perilobular areas than within the lobules. Recently deposited connective tissue is more cellular while the older tissue is more collagenous and acellular. As the lesion advances, the fibrous tissue increases in amount, gradually producing atrophy and complete disappearance of the pancreatic acini (Fig. 426). Initially the islets of Langerhans and the ducts are fairly well preserved, but later even some of these become atrophic and replaced with fibrous tissue. The ducts that remain disclose dilatation, hyperplasia, and squamous cell metaplasia. Some of them are filled with pink-staining precipitate while others contain frank calculi. Erythrocytic and neutrophilic infiltration are present in the more acute cases, while lymphocytic and monocytic infiltration and hemosiderin deposition dominate the scene as the process ages.

The *complications* of chronic pancreatitis are calcification of the pancreas, pseudocyst formation of the pancreas, terminal acute pancreatitis, abscess formation in the pancreas, biliary cirrhosis (from calculi in or fibrosis about the common bile duct), and diabetes mellitus (in one-third of the cases). The most characteristic *clinical manifestation* is severe continuous or intermittent upper abdominal pain (Horton, Cattell, and Muether). The pain characteristically occurs in recurring attacks and is often associated with alcoholic excess. Other clinical manifestations consist of dyspepsia, loss of weight, nausea and vomiting, anorexia, weakness, jaundice, steatorrhea, and upper abdominal rigidity and tenderness. The important *laboratory* findings consist of (1) a glucose tolerance curve of the diabetic type, (2) elevation of serum diastase levels during exacerbations and low serum diastase levels in advanced pancreatic disease, and (3) demonstration of calcification of the pancreas roentgenographically. The *diagnosis* is arrived at from a consideration of the clinical manifestations and from the findings at laparotomy. A differential diagnosis should include cholecystitis, cholelithiasis, peptic ulcer, atypical appendicitis, and carcinoma of the head of the pancreas. The accepted *treatment* is conservative management. Unbearable pain, however, may be treated by sympathectomy, while jaundice may be treated by simple removal of stones or some short-circuiting operation on the biliary tract. The *prognosis* is only fair to poor. While the immediate death rate is low, the morbidity is extremely high.

PHYSICAL DISTURBANCES

Orientation. —Under the heading of Physical Disturbances may be included the following: obstruction of the pancreatic ducts, trauma, calcification and calculi, and fistulas.

Obstruction of the Pancreatic Ducts. —Sudden complete obstruction of the pancreatic ducts leads to dilatation of the ducts proximal to the occlusion (from accumulation of secretion), to atrophy and disappearance of the exocrine portion of the pancreas, and to moderate fibrosis. Gradual or partial obstruction brings about a slight dilatation of the ducts, gradual disappearance of the acinar tissue, lymphocytic and monocytic infiltration, and extensive fibrosis. In either case, the endocrine portion of the gland (islets of Langerhans) remains wholly or mostly unscathed. Some of the *causes* of obstruction of the pancreatic ducts are (1) congenital anomalies — stenosis and atresia, (2) degenerations — squamous metaplasia of the ductal epithelium and excessive secretion and inspissation of mucus, (3) inflammations — nonspecific inflammation in the region of the sphincter of Oddi, the terminal portion of the pancreatic duct, or the tributaries of the ducts, (4) physical disturbances — pancreatic or biliary calculi and spasm of the sphincter of Oddi, and (5) tumors — benign and malignant tumors of the pancreas or the terminal portion of the common bile duct.

Trauma. —Trauma to the pancreas may be *classified* as surgical or non-surgical (Shallow and Wright). The former *results* from various surgical procedures on the pancreas or in the vicinity of the pancreas while the latter follows penetrating wounds (resulting from blows sustained in fights, falls, or crushing accidents). Surgical trauma is generally limited to the pancreas. Nonsurgical trauma is usually associated with injury to other structures such as the spleen, liver, stomach, bowel, kidney, gallbladder, extrahepatic bile ducts, vena cava, diaphragm, and lungs. *Pathologically* the pancreatic lesion may consist of a puncture or cut wound, an irregular laceration, or a contusion. In the former two the capsule is penetrated and the injury (rupture) is said to be incomplete. In the latter, the capsule may or may not be interrupted and the injury (rupture) is accordingly complete or incomplete respectively. In any case, the trauma brings about rupture of vessels with hemorrhage and rupture of the pancreatic ducts with liberation of pancreatic enzymes. The latter, when activated, digest the contacting tissue and produce acute pancreatitis (p. 878).

Calcification and Calculi. —Under this heading may be included disorders of the pancreas that have been *termed* calcareous pancreatitis, disseminated calcification, pancreatitis petrificans, and diffuse parenchymatous calcification (Wirts). The condition is *rare*. It has been recorded as constituting 0.044 per cent of an aggregate total of 117,031 autopsies, although in individual series of carefully searched for cases the incidence has been as high as 5.3 per cent (Domzalski). The disorder is seen only in adults and is slightly more frequent in males than in females. The precise *cause* of calcification of the pancreas is unknown, although the condition is thought to arise as a result of repeated attacks of acute or subacute pancreatitis. The etiologic agents, therefore, are the same as those in acute pancreatitis (Wirts). As far as the calcification itself is concerned the factors involved appear to be obstruction of the pancreatic ducts, stasis of pancreatic secretion, supersaturation of the secretions with calcium carbonate and calcium phosphate, inflammation, and accumulation of protein debris (Edmondson). *Pathologically* three forms of the disorder are generally recognized — calculi, diffuse calcification, and mixture of both calculi and diffuse calcification (Domzalski). Pancreatic *calculi* are found to lie free in the ducts of Wirsung, Santorini, or their tributaries. The size varies from mere granules to structures that weigh as much as 60 gms. The stones are gray to brown and mulberry-like, elongated, or irregular. The external surface is smooth or sharp. Chemically the calculi consist mostly of calcium carbonate and calcium phosphate. *Diffuse calcification* consists of a permeation of most or all of the gland with minute or more plaque-like calcium deposits. Concomitantly there is extensive fibrosis and disappearance of most of the exocrine and even the endocrine portions of the gland. The third type of lesion consists of a *mixture* of calculi located within the pancreatic ducts and a dispersion of the calcific material throughout the gland proper.

The *complications* accompanying calcification and calculi of the pancreas are (1) diabetes mellitus occurring in approximately 50 per cent of cases, (2) erosion of the ducts and vessels of the pancreas by the stones resulting in hemorrhage and extravasation of pancreatic enzymes, and (3) biliary

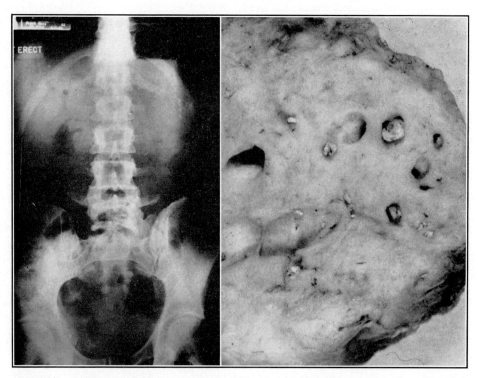

Fig. 427.—Pancreatic calcification and calculi illustrating multiple opacities in the region of the second and third lumbar vertebræ in the roentgenogram and ductal and interstitial calcific bodies in the gross specimen.

calculi. *Clinically* the condition is similar to chronic pancreatitis. The *diagnosis* is made from the clinical manifestations and the roentgen demonstration of calculi or calcific deposits in the region of the pancreas (Peters). *Treatment* is similar to that in chronic pancreatitis. Medical treatment, among other things, consists of combating the accompanying diabetes mellitus (by the use of insulin and appropriate diet) or steatorrhea (by use of the whole fat diet, high protein digest and amino acid preparations, pancreatin, vitamins, etc.). Surgical treatment is indicated in cases disclosing definite ductal stones or possessing intractable Pain. The *prognosis* is fair to poor.

Fistulas.—Fistulas of the pancreas usually *connect* the pancreatic ducts with (1) the lesser peritoneal cavity, forming an internal fistula or (2) the skin by way of the lesser peritoneal cavity, forming an external fistula (McCaughan). The former results in the formation of a cyst in the lesser peritoneal sac while the latter is accompanied by discharge of pancreatic juice onto the abdominal wall. Internal fistulas *result* from surgical procedures (partial pancreatectomy, biopsy, wedge resection, tumor enucleation, etc.) on the pancreas, penetrating injury, or nonpenetrating trauma. External fistulas eventuate from surgical procedures or penetrating injury. The two chief *complications* of pancreatic fistulas are (1) pancreatic cachexia (steatorrhea, loss of weight, etc.) and (2) secondary infection of the consequent cyst or fistulous tract.

TUMORS

Orientation. —Tumors of the pancreas may be primary or secondary. *Primary* growths may be listed as follows: cyst, adenoma, carcinoma, fibroma, fibrosarcoma, myxoma, lipoma, and lymphoblastoma. *Secondary* tumors may arise as a result of extension of neoplasms from the stomach, bile ducts, gallbladder, and transverse colon, or as a result of metastasis from distant areas. Of all the lesions listed, the only two groups that are significant enough to warrant separate consideration are carcinoma of the exocrine portion of the pancreas and islet cell tumors.

Carcinoma. —The caption "carcinoma of the pancreas" generally signifies carcinoma of the exocrine portion of the gland. While the *incidence* varies somewhat from group to group of cases analyzed, the tumor has been recorded as constitutng about 0.05 per cent of all hospital admissions, 0.61 per cent of all carcinomas (Broadbent), and 6 per cent of all carcinomas of the abdominal organs (Arkin). The disorder generally occurs in the sixth decade of life (Smith) and is from two to four times as common in males as it is in females. The *cause* of carcinoma of the pancreas, as in other tumors, is not known. Although inflammations, necrosis, etc., have been incriminated from time to time as predisposing factors, they are probably of little significance for, in most cases, the uninvolved portions of the pancreas do not show such lesions.

Pathologically carcinoma of the pancreas is about twice as common in the head of the organ as it is in the body and tail (Smith). Regardless of the location, most of the tumors grossly exist as sharply defined but not encapsulated, solid, grayish-white, extremely firm masses that may measure as much as 20 cm. in diameter but that, on an average, measure about 6 cm. across (Leach). The tumors cut with increased resistance and the cut surfaces generally disclose a rather sharp demarcation between neoplastic and normal tissue (Fig. 428). As a rule, the tumors are solid throughout but occasionally they may disclose small focal areas of necrosis, hemorrhage, liquefaction, and cyst formation. Careful inspection may reveal neoplastic tissue within vascular channels. Although most of the tumors are solid, occasionally the lesions are primarily cystic. The cysts may be large or small and unilocular or multilocular. In most instances the lesion is primarily a cyst (cystadenoma) which has secondarily undergone a malignant transformation. The cancerous change usually occurs in one area of the cyst and, as such, may be readily overlooked unless the specimen is carefully examined. The gross characteristics of the malignant area are the same as those in primarily solid tumors. Histologically carcinoma of the pancreas is primarily an adenocarcinoma (Fig. 429). As in other organs of the body harboring glandular tumors, the neoplastic cells are thus essentially cuboidal or columnar and are arranged in more or less typical acinar fashion. In some instances, the glandular formation is simple while in others it may disclose a tendency to papillary infoldings. As a rule, the cells are ill defined, possess a moderate amount of granular or vacuolated cytoplasm, and disclose round, oval, or irregular hyperchromatic basilar nuclei. Sometimes, secretion is abundant and not only the cells but the acinar lumens are filled

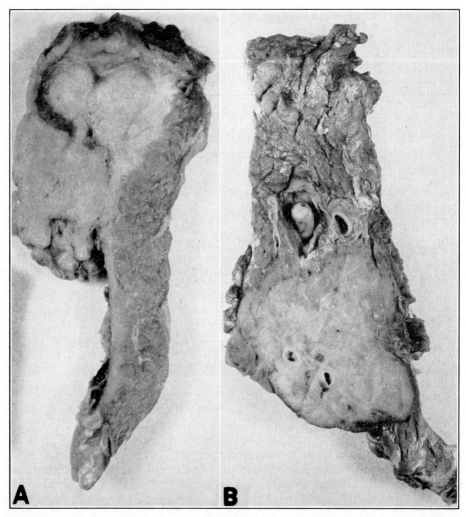

Fig. 428.—Carcinoma of the pancreas showing *A*, a tumor of the head of the pancreas and *B*, a tumor at the junction of the body and tail of the organ. Note the plug of neoplastic tissue within a large vein.

with mucoid material. As the tumors become more malignant, the glandular pattern becomes less and less distinct and the cells become more and more irregular. Ultimately they may exist as small, single, rounded, oval, or irregular cells composed of almost imperceptible cytoplasm and extremely hyperchromatic nuclei. The stroma varies from scanty to abundant in amount and from a loosely edematous to a densely collagenous variety. Leukocytic permeation varies in degree with the cells generally

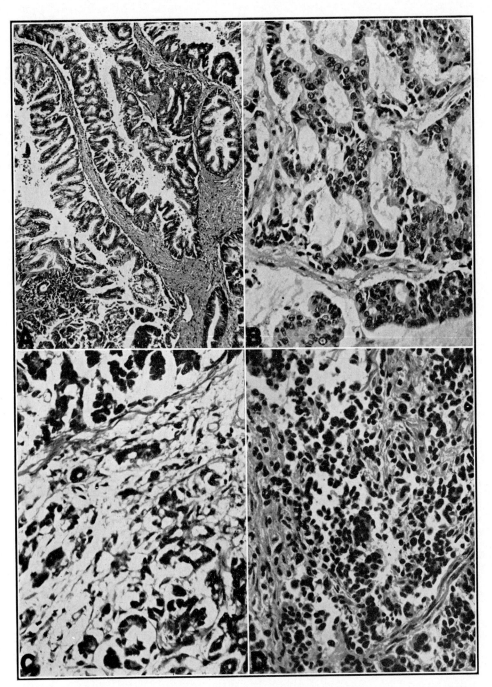

FIG. 429.—Carcinoma of the pancreas illustrating *A*, a low-grade adenomatous and papillary growth. × 50, *B*, a well-differentiated adenocarcinoma with abundant intraluminal secretion. × 100, *C*, a poorly differentiated tumor with still some attempt at glandular formation. × 200, and *D*, a poorly differentiated tumor with no attempt at glandular formation. × 200.

consisting of lymphocytes. Although, as already stated, most carcinomas of the pancreas are of a glandular variety, rarely squamous cell tumors are encountered. Carcinoma of the pancreas *spreads* by (1) direct extension to the duodenum, common bile duct, jejunum, colon, stomach, spleen, splenic and pancreatic arteries and veins, portal vein, and other adjacent structures, and (2) metastasis to the liver, abdominal and other lymph nodes, lungs, peritoneum, adrenals, mesentery, spleen, stomach, pleura, large intestine, omentum, gallbladder, heart, pericardium, small intestine, diaphragm, kidneys, bones, ovaries, etc. (Arkin). In general, metastasis occurs earlier, more widely, and more massively in carcinoma of the body and tail of the pancreas than in carcinoma of the head of the organ.

Aside from metastasis, the chief *complication* of carcinoma of the head of the pancreas is obstruction to the common bile duct with production of jaundice and even biliary cirrhosis, while the chief complication of carcinoma of the body and tail of the pancreas is widespread venous thrombosis (Smith and Mikal). Although the thrombosis is doubtlessly due to interference in the blood clotting mechanism, the reason for this disturbance is unknown. The thrombi may occur in any portion of the body but are particularly common in the veins of the lower extremities, portal vein, vena cava, and superior mesenteric vein. Such thrombi are noted in from 30 to 50 per cent of carcinomas of the body and tail of the pancreas but are infrequently seen or are altogether absent in cases of carcinoma of the head of the organ. The reason for this discrepancy is not known. The *clinical manifestations* in carcinoma of the body and tail of the pancreas (in decreasing order of frequency) may be listed as follows: deep gnawing pain, loss of weight, anemia, constipation, nausea and vomiting, anorexia, epigastric tenderness, ascites, weakness, venous thrombosis, jaundice, gas, epigastric mass, etc. (Smith). The clinical manifestations in carcinoma of the head of the pancreas are essentially similar except that jaundice moves from eleventh to fourth in frequency (Arkin). At this point, it should be stated that although jaundice is a frequent finding in carcinoma of the head of the pancreas it is by no means an early symptom and, therefore, should not be sought as a criterion for early diagnosis. In general, the *diagnosis* of carcinoma of the pancreas is made on the basis of clinical manifestations (especially abdominal pain in the presence of loss of weight), roentgenographic studies of the stomach and duodenum (noting mucosal changes, structural defects, and abnormalities of displacement), and exploratory laparotomy (Broadbent and Arkin). The only effective *treatment* of carcinoma of the pancreas is radical surgical resection. Even with this, however, the *prognosis* is poor. The average survival after the correct diagnosis is made is six months.

Islet Cell Tumors.—Under this heading may be included adenoma, carcinoma, and hyperplasia of the islets of Langerhans. Although not common, such lesions are by no means rare for over 400 cases had been recorded in the literature by 1952 (Whipple). They *occur* at all ages but predominate in the fourth and fifth decades and are somewhat more common in males than they are in females. The *causes* of the hyperplasia or tumor formation are not known although the action of the hypothalamus, anterior pituitary, or adrenal cortex has been thought to be of etiologic significance.

Pathologically, tumors (whether adenoma or carcinoma) are more or less evenly distributed throughout all portions of the pancreas (Howard). Occasionally, too, they are found in aberrant sites such as the wall of the duodenum, the hilum of the spleen, and posterior to the pancreas. As a rule, the tumors are single and measure 1.5 cm. or less in diameter. They appear to be well encapsulated, are moderately firm, and are homogeneously pink to tan in color. Histologically it may be extremely difficult to distinguish between an adenoma and a carcinoma for a rather bizarre looking tumor may remain entirely encapsulated and localized, while an innocuous appearing lesion may disclose widespread metastasis (Fig. 430). In general, the tumor exists in the form of rounded masses, cords, or glands. In tumors that grow in solid clusters, the cells resemble those of the normal islets of Langerhans. The cell borders are indistinct; the cytoplasm is moderate in amount and granular, and the nuclei are round or oval, centrally placed, and evenly stained. In tumors that form glands the cells are cuboidal or columnar. The borders are more distinct; the cytoplasm is somewhat more abundant and

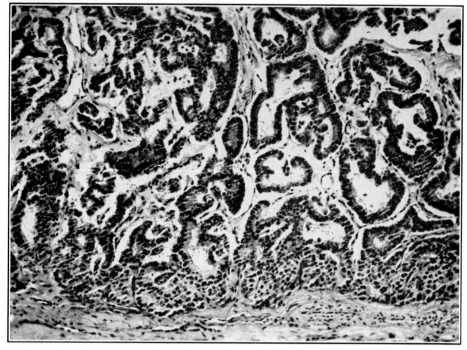

FIG. 430.—Adenoma of the islets of Langerhans showing, from below up, a capsule of collagenous fibrous tissue, several nests of relatively normal appearing islet cells, and glands composed of cuboidal epithelial cells. × 100.

occasionally vacuolated, and the nuclei are round or oval and basilar in position. Sometimes, however, the cellular patterns in either group are less regular with the cells showing considerable variation in shape, size, and staining qualities. Such bizarre appearances, however, need not necessarily indicate a carcinomatous transformation for, as already stated, many of these growths remain quite innocuous. The pancreas in cases of *hyperplasia* of the islets of Langerhans grossly appears normal. Histologically there is an increase in both the number of the islets and the size of the islets. The cells, however, remain relatively normal in appearance. As would be expected, the benign lesions remain localized while the carcinomas (37 cases recorded up to 1952—Howard) *spread* to extrapancreatic tissues. The most common sites of metastasis are the regional lymph nodes and the liver but in some instances tissues throughout the body are affected (Brearley).

The chief *complication* of islet cell tumors is hypoglycemia. In contrast to hypoglycemia of anterior pituitary (hypofunction), hypothalamic, and adrenocortical (hypofunction) origin, that present in connection with islet cell tumors is generally more severe with the level, as a rule, being lower than 50 mg. per cent. In connection with hypoglycemia, however, it should be pointed out that only about two-thirds of all islet cell tumors are functionally active. Other complications of islet cell tumors are neuromuscular disorders (Barris) and severe, more or less permanent, psychic disturbances (Pickard). Both of these are consequent to prolonged severe hypoglycemia. As would be expected, the *clinical manifestations* are those of hyperinsulinism or hypoglycemia coming on especially during the fasting period or after severe exertion (Whipple). They may be divided into (1) those due to disturbances of the vegetative nervous system—restlessness, pallor, sweating, nausea, and salivation, (2) those due to disturbances of the central nervous system—tonic and clonic spasms, uncontrolled motor activity, and opisthotonus, and (3) those due to disturbances of the higher psychic centers—confusion, anxiety, loss of consciousness, and coma. The *diagnosis* of islet cell tumors is made from the clinical manifestations, low blood sugar levels (below 50 mg. per cent), and rapid response to ingestion or parenteral administration of glucose. A differential diagnosis should include other causes of hypoglycemia (p. 50) (Whipple and Perkins). The only effective *treatment* is surgical removal of the tumor or, if a tumor is not found, subtotal pancreatectomy. The *prognosis* is good. In a collective review of 398 cases of islet cell tumors, Howard stated that 200 patients had undergone surgical treatment and that, of these, 79.5 per cent had been relieved of their hypoglycemia. Four patients in the group had a recurrence of symptoms after the original postoperative relief.

REFERENCES

Pathologic Physiology

DOHAN, F. C., and LUKENS, F. D. W.: Science, *105*, 183, 1947 (Diabetes mellitus).
DRAGSTEDT, L. R. *et al.*: Am. J. Physiol., *117*, 175, 1936 (Lipocaic).
DREILING, D. A., and JANOWITZ, H. J.: Advances Int. Med., *7*, 65, 1955 (Pathophysiology Pancreas).
KATSKIN, G., and GORDON, M.: Am. J. Med., *12*, 3, 1952 (Lipemia and Pancreatitis).
THOMAS, J. E.: The External Secretion of the Pancreas, Springfield, Ill., Charles C Thomas, 1950.
ZOLLINGER, R. M., and ELLISON, E. H.: Ann. Surg., *142*, 709, 1955 (Ulcerogenic Tumors Pancreas).

Congenital Anomalies

ABBOTT, V., *et al.*: Canad. M. A. J., *64*, 419, 1951 (Fibrocystic Disease).
BAGGENSTOSS, A. H., *et al.*: A. M. A. Arch. Path., *51*, 510, 1951 (Fibrocystic Disease).
BOSTICK, W. L., and RINEHART, J. F.: J. Pediat., *37*, 469, 1950 (Fibrocystic Disease).
BRILHART, K. B., and PRIESTLEY, J. T.: Am. J. Surg., *81*, 151, 1951 (Pseudocysts).
CASTLETON, K. B., *et al.*: Am. Surg., *19*, 38, 1953 (Annular Pancreas).
COLLINS, D. C.: A. M. A. Arch. Surg., *61*, 524, 1950 (Pseudocysts).
FORSHALL, I., *et al.*: Brit. J. Surg., *40*, 31, 1952 (Meconium Peritonitis).
MONTGOMERY, W. F.: J. A. M. A., *152*, 225, 1953 (Meconium Ileus).
NORRIS, R. F., and TYSON, R. M.: Am. J. Path., *23*, 485, 1947 (Polycystic Disease).
NYGAARD, K. K., and STACEY, L. J.: A. M. A. Arch. Surg., *45*, 206, 1942 (Solitary Cysts).
PEARSON, S.: A. M. A. Arch. Surg., *63*, 168, 1951 (Aberrant Pancreas).
SCOTT, J. V.: A. M. A. Arch. Surg., *59*, 1304, 1949 (Cysts).

Degenerations

BELL, E. T.: A. M. A. Arch. Path., *53*, 444, 1952 (Vascular Changes in Diabetes).
DUNCAN, G. G.: *Diseases of Metabolism*, 3rd Ed., Philadelphia, W. B. Saunders Co., p. 775, 1952.

Guy, W. B.: Pennsylvania M. J., *54*, 1052, 1951 (Cutaneous Lesions in Diabetes Mellitus).
Herbut, P. A., *et al.:* A. M. A. Arch. Path., *41*, 516, 1946 (Alloxan Diabetes in Rabbits).
————: A. M. A. Arch. Path., *42*, 214, 1946 (Alloxantin Diabetes in Rabbits).
John, H. J.: Ann. Int. Med., *33*, 925, 1950 (Diabetes Mellitus in Adults).
————: J. Pediat., *35*, 723, 1949 (Diabetes Mellitus in Children).
Miller, H. C., and Wilson, H. M.: J. Pediat., *23*, 251, 1943 (Infants of Diabetic Mothers).
Ricketts, H. T.: J. A. M. A., *150*, 959, 1952 (Treatment Diabetes Mellitus).
Story, R. D., and Root, H. F.: J. A. M. A., *144*, 86, 1950 (Diabetic Coma).
Warren, S., and LeCompte, P. M.: *Pathology of Diabetes Mellitus*, 3rd Ed., Philadelphia, Lea & Febiger, 1952.

Inflammations

Berk, J. E.: J. A. M. A., *152*, 1, 1953 (Acute Pancreatitis).
Brobstein, J. G., *et al.:* A. M. A. Arch. Surg., *59*, 189, 1949 (Acute Pancreatitis).
Cattell, R. B., and Warren, K. W.: Gastroenterology, *20*, 1, 1952 (Chronic Pancreatitis).
Edmondson, H. A., *et al.:* Am. J. Path., *25*, 1227, 1949 (Chronic Pancreatitis).
Horton, R. E.: Guy's Hospital Report, *96*, 226, 1947 (Chronic Pancreatitis).
Maiman, S. N., *et al.:* A. M. A. Arch. Int. Med., *81*, 56, 1948 (Chronic Pancreatitis).
Morse, L. J., and Achs, S.: Ann. Surg., *130*, 1044, 1949 (Acute Pancreatitis).
Muether, R. O., and Knight, W. A., Jr.: Gastroenterology, *12*, 24, 1949 (Chronic Pancreatitis).
Pfeiffer, D. B., and Miller, D. B.: Am. J. Surg., *80*, 18, 1950 (Acute Pancreatitis).
Radakovich, M., *et al.:* Surg., Gynec. & Obst., *94*, 749, 1952 (Acute Pancreatitis).
Roberts, N. J., *et al.:* Am. J. Clin. Path., *20*, 742, 1950 (Acute Pancreatitis).
Siler, V. E., and Wulsin, J. H.: J. A. M. A., *142*, 78, 1950 (Acute Pancreatitis).

Physical Disturbances

Domzalski, C. A.: Ann. Int. Med., *31*, 650, 1949 (Calcification).
Edmondson, H. A., *et al.:* Am. J. Path., *26*, 37, 1950 (Calculi).
McCaughan, J. M., and Werner, A. A.: Am. J. Surg., *35*, 595, 1937 (Fistulas).
Peters, B. J., *et al.:* A. M. A. Arch. Int. Med., *391*, 87, 1951 (Diffuse Calcification).
Shallow, T. A., and Wagner, F. B., Jr.: Ann. Surg., *125*, 66, 1947 (Trauma).
Wirts, C. W., Jr., and Snape, W. J.: Am. J. M. Sci., *213*, 290, 1947 (Diffuse Calcification).
Wright, L. T., *et al.:* Am. J. Surg., *80*, 170, 1950 (Trauma).

Tumors

Arkin, A., and Weisberg, S. W.: Gastroenterology, *13*, 118, 1949 (Carcinoma Pancreas).
Barris, R. W.: Ann. Int. Med., *38*, 124, 1953 (Islet Cell Tumor).
Brearley, B. F., and Laws, J. W.: Brit. M. J., *1*, 982, 1950 (Islet Cell Carcinoma).
Broadbent, T. R., and Kerman, H. D.: Gastroenterology, *17*, 163, 1951 (Carcinoma Pancreas).
Howard, J. M., *et al.:* Int. Abstracts of Surg., *90*, 417, 1950 (Islet Cell Tumors).
Leach, W. B.: Am. J. Path., *26*, 333, 1950 (Carcinoma Pancreas).
Mikal, S., and Campbell, A. J. A.: Surgery, *28*, 963, 1950 (Carcinoma Pancreas).
Perkins, H. A., *et al.:* New England J. Med., *243*, 281, 1950 (Islet Cell Tumors).
Pickard, K., *et al.:* Ann. Int. Med., *38*, 1306, 1953 (Islet Cell Tumor).
Smith, B. K., and Albright, E. C.: Ann. Int. Med., *36*, 90, 1952 (Carcinoma Pancreas).
Whipple, A. O.: Canad. M. A. J., *66*, 334, 1952 (Islet Cell Tumor).

23

Peritoneum

PATHOLOGIC PHYSIOLOGY

FREDERICK B. WAGNER, JR.

THE peritoneum is a serous membrane, *consisting of* loose connective tissue containing collagen and elastic fibers, fat cells, blood vessels, monocytes, and reticulum cells and covered by a single layer of mesothelial cells. It lines the inside of the abdominal wall and partially or almost wholly invests the abdominal organs. Except for an opening at the fimbriated end of each fallopian tube, it forms a closed cavity. There is much variation in the peritoneal reflections but the more extreme ones may produce pockets for internal hernias, or weak spots through which abdominal viscera may protrude as external hernias. Areas denuded of peritoneum by surgery may become points of adhesions for loops of bowel or other adjacent viscera.

The peritoneal cavity *normally* contains 75 to 100 cc. of clear, straw-colored *fluid* which is a transudate and has the function of lubricating the peritoneal surfaces. This fluid may be increased as much as 100 fold or more when ascites occurs. Other fluids may accumulate abnormally such as blood, chyle, pus, bile, pancreatic juice, or gastrointestinal contents as a result of rupture or inflammation of abdominal viscera. Irritation by these produces a chemical and/or bacterial peritonitis. The peritoneum has remarkable powers of absorption due to its rich supply of blood and lymph vessels, particularly in the upper part of the peritoneal cavity. This function has been utilized especially in children. Intact erythrocytes also are absorbed promptly.

The *removal* of bacterial and other *materials* from the peritoneal cavity is accomplished through the following mechanisms: (1) the bacteria penetrate the capillaires and lymphatics or are transported through by white cells which have phagocytosed them, (2) the endothelial cells of the blood and lymph capillaries selectively remove substances, (3) solutions are absorbed by osmosis, (4) respiratory movement increases the removal rate, and thus fixation of the diaphragm in the region of a subphrenic abscess is a protective mechanism, (5) the passage of bacteria is favored with increase of intra-peritoneal prressure and is decreased when the abdomen is opened during an operation. Factors which decrease the diffusion of infection in the peritoneal cavity are: (1) diminished intestinal activity and (2) the local reaction to the inflammatory process (fibrin network formation, agglutination of serous surfaces, enhanced phagocytosis, and peritoneal immunization).

The intraperitoneal *pressure* averages 8 cm. of water and breathing causes a fluctuation of 2 to 4 cm. Coughing, vomiting, and straining at stool elevate the pressure to levels as high as 150 cm. of water. The pressure rises in a variety of clinical conditions, as for example intestinal obstruction. A great increase produces (1) augmented thoracic respiratory activity, (2) upward displacement of the diaphragm, (3) venous stasis within the abdomen, (4) fall in arterial blood pressure and eventually a state of shock, (5) electrocardiographic changes, and (6) reduction of renal blood flow and renal oxygen consumption rate.

The *diagnosis* of peritoneal disorders depends first upon a careful history and physical examination. The differentiation of inflammatory and neoplastic lesions often requires special laboratory and operative aids. The study of aspirated fluid may yield information as to specific gravity, protein content, amylase concentration, bacterial growth and antibiotic sensitivity, neoplastic cells, and presence of blood. Plain *x*-ray examination may reveal the presence of fluid in ascites, air under the diaphragm in perforated viscus, elevation of the diaphragm in subphrenic abscess, the outline of soft tissue masses, and calcium flecks in meconium peritonitis. Peritoneoscopy permits direct visualization of the peritoneal cavity and the securing of biopsy specimens. In some instances, exploratory laparotomy must be the final resort.

CONGENITAL ANOMALIES

Orientation.—The only important developmental malformations of the peritoneum consist of (1) variations in size of the omentum—altogether absent, smaller than normal, or larger than normal, (2) greater or lesser degree of investment of the various organs—resulting respectively in retroperitonealization of organs that are normally completely or almost completely surrounded and pedunculation of organs that are normally more or less exteriorized, and (3) formation of potential weak spots or of actual defects through which abdominal viscera may protrude. Of these, the last mentioned is directly concerned with the formation of hernias and is thus of considerable importance.

Hernia.—Some of the general aspects regarding hernias have already been outlined in Chapter 6 (p. 225). Most hernias occur in connection with the peritoneal cavity. They are found at all ages, in both sexes, and in all races (Watson). The *fundamental cause* is a congenital or an acquired weakness or an actual defect in the peritoneum and supporting structures that permits a viscus or a portion of a viscus to escape from its normal location. Some of the *predisposing causes* of abdominal hernias are heredity, age, sex, obesity, disruption of tissues by trauma, and increase in bulk of abdominal viscera or contents (pregnancy, enlargement of the liver and spleen, neoplasms, excessive fat deposits in the omentum and mesentery, and ascites). The chief *exciting cause* is increase in intra-abdominal pressure occurring as a result of straining, coughing, lifting, or trauma.

Pathologically the viscus involved varies with the location and, to some extent, with the size of the hernial ring. Usually it is some portion of the gastrointestinal tract that escapes, but the female adnexa, urinary bladder, spleen, liver, and almost any other organ or tissue may be affected. Named according to the site of the hernial ring, the more important abdominal hernias may be listed as follows: (1) *inguinal*—constituting over 90 per cent of all hernias, more common in males than females, usually containing loops of small bowel with or without other organs, and being classified as indirect when the viscus leaves the abdomen by way of the internal inguinal ring, incomplete indirect when it remains in the inguinal canal, complete indirect when it emerges from the external inguinal canal, scrotal when it passes into the scrotum, and direct when it enters the inguinal canal directly through the abdominal wall medial to the internal inguinal ring, (2) *femoral* —constituting about 2.5 per cent of all hernias, also known as crural and pectineal hernias, consisting of a protrusion through the femoral ring into the femoral canal, usually containing omentum and less often small intestine and other organs, occurring mostly in women, and rarely found before the twentieth year, (3) *umbilical*—constituting about 2 per cent of all hernias, consisting of a protrusion through the umbilical ring, called omphalocele when it is found in the newborn with the contents never having entered the abdominal cavity, more common in infants than in adults, predominating in adult females (especially those who have borne children) over adult males in the ratio of 3 to 1, and generally containing omentum, transverse colon, and small intestine, (4) *incisional*—also known as postoperative, constituting about 1.5 per cent of all hernias, and occurring anywhere in the abdominal wall, (5) *ventral*—occurring anywhere in the anterior abdominal wall at points other than the inguinal, femoral, or umbilical openings or the linea alba, (6) *linea alba*—any protrusion through the linea alba and being epigastric or hypogastric in location, (7) *diaphragmatic*—protrusion through the diaphragm, also called phrenic, containing stomach and any of the other viscera, and including protrusions through the natural rings such as esophageal (esophageal hiatus hernia), aortic, vena caval, or through abnormal congenital (left diaphragmatic) or acquired (traumatic) rings, (8) *internal*—protrusions into one of the internal abdominal (paraduodenal, paracecal, intersigmoidal, and foramen of Winslow) fossas or postoperative apertures in the broad ligaments, (9) *lumbar*—protrusion through any portion of the lumbar region of the abdominal wall bounded by the twelfth rib above, crest of the ilium below, line drawn from the tip of the twelfth rib to the crest of the ilium in front, and vertebral column and erector spinæ muscles behind, (10) *obturator*—protrusion through the obturator foramen or canal in the innominate bone, (11) *sciatic*—protrusion through the greater or lesser sacrosciatic foramen, (12) *perineal*—protrusion through the muscles and fascias of the pelvic outlet and also known as ischiorectal pudendal, and subpubic, and (13) various *organs* such as bladder, ovaries, fallopian tubes, etc.

DEGENERATIONS

Degenerative disorders of the peritoneum are intimately bound with specific disease processes. While some authors consider pseudomyxoma of the peritoneum as a chemical reaction with an abundant secretion of mucoid material (hence also a degenerative disorder), the condition probably represents a true neoplasm and is, therefore, considered in connection with tumors.

INFLAMMATIONS

Orientation.—Inflammation of the peritoneum is known as *peritonitis*. Although the classifications are many, the more important lesions may be discussed under the following headings: nonspecific peritonitis, subphrenic abscess, benign paroxysmal peritonitis, meconium peritonitis, tuberculosis, and talcum powder granuloma.

Nonspecific Peritonitis.—Nonspecific peritonitis indicates inflammation of the peritoneum by the ordinary pyogenic organisms. The condition *occurs* at all ages, in both sexes, and in all races. Its incidence, in many instances, is inversely proportional to the promptness and adequateness of medical care. The precipitating *causes* are bacteria. Most commonly, they consist of colon bacilli, streptococci, and staphylococci but occasionally they include pneumococci, Friedländer's organisms, gonococci, etc. (Wright, Stanley, and Harvey). The *source* of the organisms is either (1) endogenous—from diseased or undiseased organs of the body or (2) exogenous—from without the body (Falk and Pedowitz). Some of the more common *conditions* that give rise to peritonitis are perforated appendicitis, perforated peptic ulcer, perforated cholecystitis, salpingitis, ruptured pyosalpinx, ruptured tubo-ovarian abscess, endometritis, abortion, ruptured diverticulitis, perforated enteritis or colitis, perforated carcinoma of the gastrointestinal tract, intestinal obstruction, gangrene of the bowel from whatever cause, traumatic rupture of abdominal organs, perforating (gunshot or stab) wounds of the abdomen, and surgical operations. In addition, it should be pointed out that peritonitis may occur as a result of metastasis from such distant infections as pneumonia or urethritis, and that in some instances (as in pneumococcic peritonitis of children) an antecedent infection cannot be found and the exact route of invasion is uncertain (Pahmer).

Pathologically peritonitis may be localized or generalized. *Localized* peritonitis usually results from nonperforating extension of an inflammation of an organ to the serosa. The adherence of the serosal surfaces to each other and the walling off of the infection by the omentum prevents the inflammation from spreading to distant portions of the peritoneum. *Generalized* peritonitis, as a rule, results from perforation of a viscus with continued spillage of infective material into the peritoneal cavity. In either case, the appearance of the inflammation is similar. The changes are those of any inflammatory reaction (Fig. 431). They consist of congestion of the serosal vessels, edema of the serosa, dulling of the surfaces, formation of an exudate, and adherence of apposing serosal surfaces to each other. The amount of exudate varies from scarcely perceptible to copious and the appearance of the exudate varies from serous to fibrinous, hemorrhagic, purulent, or combinations of these. *Histologically* the changes are similar to those in any inflammation consisting of congestion, edema, leukocytic (mostly neutrophilic) infiltration, complete breakdown (necrosis) of tissue, and later fibrosis. The termination in any case may be (1) death of the host at any stage of the infection, (2) complete resolution leaving no telltale evidence of infection, (3) extensive suppuration and necrosis with abscess formation, and (4) repair by fibrosis and adhesion formation (Boys).

The chief *complications* are paralytic ileus, toxemia, electrolytic imbalance, circulatory disturbance (shock), peritoneal abscess, and peritoneal adhesions with or without intestinal obstruction (Wright and Boys). *Clinically* the symptoms of the primary disease (if any) usually precede the peritonitis by varying intervals of time. The manifestations of the peritonitis itself are due to irritation of the peritoneum and absorption of toxic products both from the peritoneal cavity and obstructed (paralytic) bowel. They consist of abdominal pain (at first localized but then generalized), nausea, vomiting, clammy perspiration, diarrhea or constipation, rapid weak pulse, fever, low blood pressure, abdominal rigidity, abdominal tenderness, and leukocytosis. Roentgenograms of the abdomen reveal distention of loops of small intestine with air and fluid and, in cases of rupture of an air-containing viscus, air in the peritoneal cavity. The *diagnosis* is made from the history, symptoms, and signs. *Treatment* is primarily surgical whenever a viscus has been ruptured, perforated, or obstructed and the point of leakage has not been sealed off (Crile). Medical therapy, among other things, consists of administration of antibiotics (Wright). The *prognosis* is variable. Prior to the antibiotic and chemotherapeutic era the mortality rate, depending upon the cause, type of organism, delay in treatment, etc., was as high as 100 per cent. Today, in the presence of adequate and early treatment, most patients recover from the peritonitis and the ultimate prognosis depends, to a large extent, upon the associated condition.

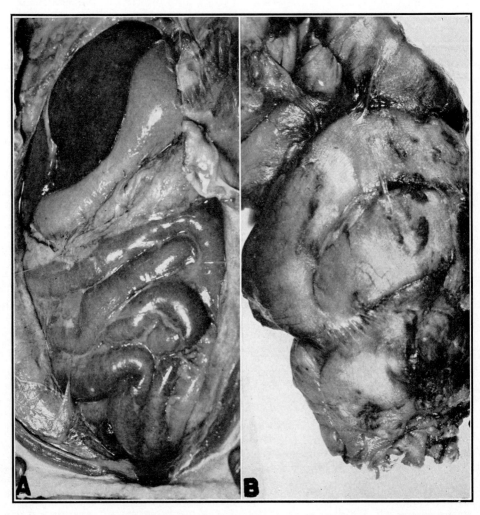

Fig. 431.—Nonspecific peritonitis showing *A*, an acute purulent exudate covering the serosal surfaces and *B*, fibrous adhesions binding together several loops of the small intestine.

Subphrenic Abscess.—*Subphrenic* or *subdiaphragmatic abscess*, as the name implies, is simply a collection of pus on the inferior surface of the diaphragm. The condition develops abruptly or insidiously and usually follows a previous abdominal operation, especially for perforated peptic ucler, appendicitis, or cholecystitis (Fraser). The *causative* organisms are *Staphylococcus aureus* (one third cases), *Streptococcus hemolyticus* (one third cases), and *Bacillus coli* combined with the two previously mentioned organisms (one third cases). *Pathologically* the right side is affected about ten times as frequently as the left. Superiorly the abscess is covered by diaphragm while inferiorly its wall is composed mostly of liver with, when the lesion is on the left, the addition of other organs of the upper abdominal cavity (Fig. 432). The size varies from a few millimeters in diameter to that covering virtually the entire under surface of the diaphragm. The central portion contains pus of varying quality while the periphery is composed of a wall that contains varying amounts of fibrous tissue. *Histologically* the wall, from within out, consists of debris, granulation tissue, and connective tissue. The *complications* consist of extension of the process to adjacent structures. These include the peritoneum, liver, pleura, and lungs. In addition, since most cases occur postoperatively, there may also be a breakdown of the surgical incision. The

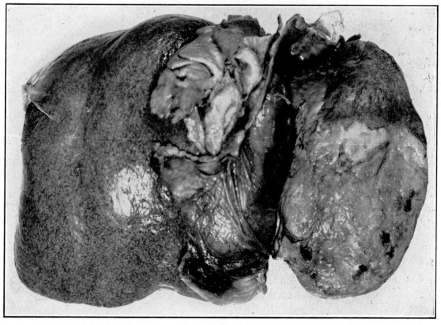

Fig. 432.—Subphrenic abscess showing a collection of pus over the superior surface of the left lobe of the liver. The diaphragm has been reflected toward the right lobe.

clinical manifestations may be masked by antibiotic therapy (Gerwig and Blades). They may consist of pain in the right or left lumbar area or hypochondrium, malaise, fever, increased respirations, cough, leukocytosis, tenderness over the twelfth rib, diminished movement of the chest, and dullness over the lower lung field on the side involved. Roentgenograms of the abdomen disclose elevation of the diaphragm, diminished diaphragmatic movements, trapped air bubble in the upper part of the abdomen, and, when the lesion is on the left side, depression of the stomach. The *diagnosis* is made from the history, clinical manifestations, and roentgenographic appearance. *Treatment* consists of surgical drainage. The *prognosis* is guarded for the death rate in surgically untreated cases is around 40 per cent and in surgically treated cases around 20 per cent.

Benign Paroxysmal Peritonitis.—This condition, also referred to as *periodic abdominalgia* of Reimann, is part of a little-understood syndrome that has been referred to as *"periodic disease."* There is no basis to consider the etiologic agents as infectious, allergic, endocrinologic, or neurologic and the group has been regarded as a "manifestation of a rhythm of life" (Brick). The disorder is *characterized* by recurrent bouts of abdominal pain and fever and may be attended by nausea, vomiting, malaise, abdominal muscle spasm, abdominal tenderness, and leukocytosis. The attacks usually start early in life, are of two to three days' duration, and continue at regular or irregular intervals for months or years. *Pathologically* the peritoneum may disclose widespread (1) edema, (2) fibrinous, purulent, or fibrinopurulent exudation, or (3) acute adhesions. Cultures are negative for ærobic and anærobic organsims. *Histologically* the reaction is nonspecific consisting of congestion, edema, and neutrophilic infiltration. Later, as healing occurs, fibrosis supervenes. There is no adequate *treatment* although the condition has been recorded as responding to para-amino-benzoic acid (Willis).

Meconium Peritonitis.—Meconium peritonitis is an inflammation of the peritoneum due to contamination with meconium (Olnick and Packard). The condition is *uncommon* although, by 1949, over 100 cases had been recorded in the literature. It may develop at any time from the second trimester of intra-uterine life to birth. The *cause* is perforation of the intestine and spilling of meconium into the peritoneal cavity. In 50 per cent of the cases the cause of the perforation is an organic obstruction of the intestine in the form of volvulus, intussusception, congenital bands, angulations, atresia, and stenosis. In the remaining 50 per cent of cases the cause is meconium ileus, congenital diverticula, ulcers, or indeterminable. *Meconium* consists of cast off epithelial cells, bile, fat, fatty acids, sebaceous material, mucin, and salts. When it reaches the peritoneal cavity it produces a severe *chemical irritation* which, in turn, evokes a leukocytic and later a fibroblastic response. Calcification occurs as the process ages and the ultimate picture, therefore, will depend upon the time of spillage. If the *infant* is *alive* at the time of birth it is acutely ill, exhibiting cyanosis, vomiting, absent or scanty stool, occasional blood in the vomitus and stool, and distention of the abdomen. *Roentgen* examination may disclose obstruction of the bowel, free air in the peritoneal cavity, and streaky, plaque-like peritoneal calcification. *Treatment* consists of surgical repair of the bowel, removal of the meconium, and release of the adhesions. The *prognosis* is poor, for even if the infant survives the operation it is likely to develop intestinal obstruction from adhesions which reform.

Tuberculosis.—Tuberculosis of the peritoneum is more common in females than in males and usually occurs between the ages of ten and forty years (Kahrs). The *cause* is, of course, *Mycobacterium tuberculosis.* The disease is always secondary to some other tuberculous infection elsewhere in the body. In females, the immediate *primary infection* is usually in the fallopian tubes but may be in the intestine or mesenteric lymph nodes while in males it is usually in the intestine or mesenteric lymph nodes. Less commonly, the immediate primary focus (in either sex) may be in the lungs, pleura, or pericardium and the route of spread is the vascular system. Both grossly and microscopically the basic *pathologic* lesion is the tubercle (Fig. 433). The tubercle may not, however, be always readily apparent to the naked eye for it is generally camouflaged by a serous, serofibrinous, fibrotic, caseous, or even purulent reaction. As a result of this response, the serosal surfaces of the abdominal structures are virtually always glued to each other in a hopelessly entangled mass. Between the adhesions there are pockets of encysted exudate.   Serous surfaces, other than those in the abdomen, are affected in almost one-half of the cases.   The *complications* are cachexia and occasionally intestinal obstruction.   The *clinical manifestations* ppear rapidly in two-thirds of the cases and in decreasing order of frequency consist of abdominal pain, fever, enlargement of the abdomen, anorexia, dizziness, diarrhea, emaciation, vomiting, meteorism (tympanitic distention of the abdomen), and indigestion.   The *diagnosis* may be readily established when the clinical manifestations listed are noted in a known tuberculous patient but in other instances it may be made only by exclusion.

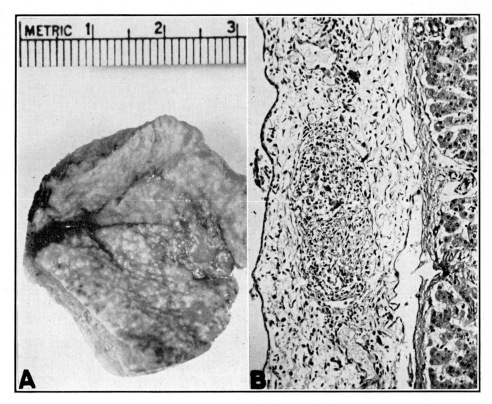

Fig. 433.—Tuberculous peritonitis illustrating *A*, numerous confluent and discrete tubercles covering a piece of parietal peritoneum and *B*, a well-defined tubercle in the submesothelial connective tissue.   × 100.

A differential diagnosis should include appendicitis, ascites, pleurisy, ileus, hernia, abdominal tumor, celiac disease, etc.   *Treatment* is generally medical with antibiotics assuming a prominent role.   Before the antibiotic era the *mortality* rate from the peritonitis was as high as 40 per cent with most of the deaths occurring within the first year.   Today the outlook is considerably better.

Talcum Powder Granuloma.—Talcum powder consists of 82.7 per cent magnesium silicate, 8.7 per cent calcium carbonate, 7.6 magnesium carbonate, and 1 per cent moisture (Ross).   When introduced parenterally it (crystals of magnesium silicate) evokes a severe chemical reaction that is characterized essentially by pseudotubercle formation (Fig. 434).   The tubercles are composed of collections of monocytes, epithelioid cells,

lymphocytes, fibroblasts, and foreign body giant cells. Both the monocytes and the giant cells contain talc crystals which may be readily visualized microscopically with polarized light but are also seen well with ordinary
subdued light. Grossly the lesion exists as disseminated tubercles, as
nodules, as larger conglomerate masses, or as dense fibrous adhesions.
Generally the talcum powder is deposited in the tissues from improperly
washed or finger-tip-perforated surgeon's gloves. The lesions have been
described in the following locations: peritoneal cavity, pleural cavity, skin,
vagina, rectum, brain, spinal canal, kidneys, breasts, ovaries, testes, penis,
and surgical wounds. Because of its proved irritating action, talcum
powder—as a dusting agent—should be replaced with a more innocuous
substance such as potassium bitartrate.

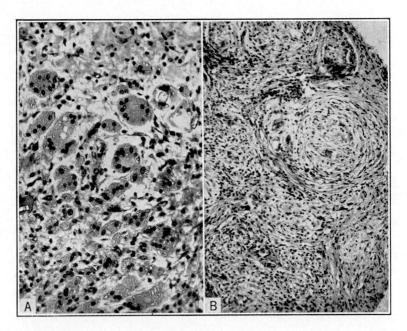

Fig. 434.—Talcum powder granuloma disclosing *A*, crystals of magnesium silicate within
monocytes and giant cells. × 200 and *B*, tubercles of epithelioid and giant cells surrounded and
permeated with fibroblasts. × 100. (Herbut's *Gynecological and Obstetrical Pathology*.)

PHYSICAL DISTURBANCES

Orientation.—Under this heading may be listed the following conditions: hernia (pp. 116 and 672), ascites, abdominal apoplexy, chylous effusion, pneumoperitoneum, trauma, foreign bodies, and omental infarction.

Ascites.—Ascites or hydroperitoneum is an accumulation of clear,
straw-colored fluid in the peritoneal cavity in amounts exceeding the usual
75 to 100 cc. The condition is intimately connected with obstructive
disorders of the lungs, heart, liver, and portal vein or with hypoproteinemic
(nephrotic or nutritional) states. Both of these have already been discussed
in connection with Chronic Passive Hyperemia (p. 193) and Edema (p.
203). The chief *complications* of the ascites as such consist of (1) pressure upon abdominal and thoracic organs from massive accumulation of
fluid, (2) anemia and nutritional deficiency from anorexia and loss of pro-

tein consequent to repeated abdominal paracentesis (withdrawal of fluid by abdominal tapping), and (3) infection (peritoneal or generalized) as a result of abdominal paracentesis or hypoproteinemia.

Abdominal Apoplexy.—Abdominal apoplexy connotes spontaneous non-traumatic intraperitoneal hemorrhage due to rupture of an intra-abdominal blood vessel (Saphir). Some of the causes of vascular disruption are (1) congenital anomalies—developmental defects in the media of small and medium-sized arteries at points of bifurcation leading to the formation of "berry" aneurysms, (2) degenerations—mucoid degeneration of the media

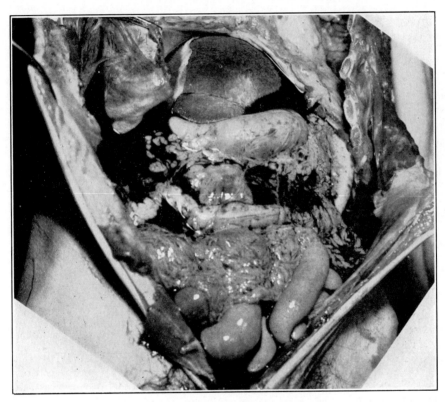

Fig. 435.—Abdominal apoplexy resulting from rupture of an arteriosclerotic aortic aneurysm. The peritoneal cavity contains a moderate amount of recently extravasated blood.

and arteriosclerosis, (3) inflammations—embolic (infective) emboli and local primary or secondary inflammation, (4) physical disturbances—ectopic gestation, infarcts, and varices of the diaphragm and broad ligaments, and (5) tumors—eroding vessels and consisting of primary or metastatic growths in any of the organs (Saphir, Shallow, and Reimann). Occasionally the hemorrhage is venous but usually it is arterial. Any *artery* in the abdomen may be affected with the most common being aorta, mesenteric, hepatic, splenic, renal, middle colic, celiac, and inferior pancreaticoduodenal. *Pathologically* the bleeding may be retroperitoneal, intraperitoneal, or in both locations (Fig. 435). It may be encapsulated (hematoma) or loosely extravasated. In recent hemorrhage the blood is dark red and both fluid and coagulated, while in older hemorrhage it discloses varying degrees of organization. Since extravasated blood acts as an irritant, it evokes a mild to moderate inflammatory reaction which, if the patient lives long enough, heals by resolution or fibrosis and adhesion formation. The chief *complications* are exsanguination and shock. The *clinical manifestations* consist of (1) sudden, severe, abdominal pain, (2) shock, and (3) signs of peritoneal irritation (rigidity and tenderness of the abdominal wall, mild leukocytosis, and low-grade fever). The *diagnosis* is made from the clinical manifestations and the appearance at the time of operation. *Treatment* consists of laparotomy and ligation of the vessel that has ruptured. The *prognosis* is poor. Most of the patients whose cases have been recorded in the literature have died.

Chylous Effusion.—Chylous effusion, also known as chylous ascites and chyloperitoneum, is the escape of chyle or lymph into the peritoneal cavity. The condition is analogous to the escape of chyle into the thoracic cavity (p. 392). *Clinically* it may be divided into three groups—(1) *acute chylous peritonitis*—rapid idiopathic escape of chyle into the peritoneal cavity producing acute peritonitis and responding promptly and adequately to simple drainage, (2) *true chylous ascites*—(*a*) producing abdominal distention, (*b*) occurring from traumatic rupture of cisterna chyli or its tributaries, rupture of chylous cysts, rupture of the thoracic duct, or obstruction of the thoracic duct as in filariasis or cervical venous thrombosis, and (*c*) responding poorly to treatment, and (3) *progressive chylous ascites* associated with palpable abdominal tumors—occurring as a result of obstruction of the cisterna chyli and its tributaries by tumor, tuberculous lymphadenitis, or mesenteric cysts and usually ending fatally (Karp and Thompson). The appearance of the fluid and the general clinical manifestations are similar to those in chylothorax (p. 393).

Pneumoperitoneum.—Pneumoperitoneum is the presence of air in the peritoneal cavity. It may *arise* as a result of (1) perforation of an abdominal viscus, (2) penetrating wounds from the outside, (3) retroperitoneal leakage of air from (*a*) an operation on the neck, (*b*) mediastinal emphysema, or (*c*) pneumothorax, (4) introduction of air during the performance of a peritoneoscopy (Jernstrom), (5) artificial introduction for treatment of tuberculosis and other pulmonary lesions (Banyai), and (6) idiopathic with the possibility of air arising on the basis of intestinal pneumatosis (Ayres). The *complications* are (1) air embolism to the heart and lungs as a result of massive entrance of air into a systemic vein, (2) pneumocele—herniation of an air-filled peritoneal sac (*a*) through the esophageal hiatus of the diaphragm, (*b*) into the scrotum, and (*c*) into the umbilicus, (3) pneumothorax, (4) mediastinal emphysema, (5) subcutaneous emphysema, (6) abdominal hernia, (7) peritoneal reaction in the form of inflammation and effusion, and (8) visceroptosis (Banyai, Hollander, Friedman, and Jernstrom).

Trauma.—Trauma to the abdomen (and hence peritoneum and abdominal viscera) occurs quite frequently in civilian life but reaches its zenith in military life (Metz, Bogle, and Gordon-Taylor). The general topic of trauma has been discussed in Chapter 6 (p. 222), while traumatic lesions of the stomach, small intestine, large intestine, liver, bile ducts, etc., have been referred to briefly in connection with Physical Disturbances under each of the organs concerned.

Foreign Bodies.—Foreign bodies usually gain entrance into the peritoneal cavity by the *external route* and occasionally by the internal route (Crossen). The former consists of entrance from the outside by way of the skin and occurs in connection with accidental penetrating injury (such as gunshot, stabbing, or lacerations) or in connection with operations. The objects deposited are quite diverse and include such articles as products of firearms, various types of metals, bits of clothing, splinters of wood, and surgical implements—most common among which are sponges (Fig. 436). Objects entering by the *internal route* usually do so by way of the gastro-intestinal, urinary, or genital tracts. While the objects vary considerably in nature they are, as a rule, pointed and include such articles as needles, pins, medicine droppers, etc. In general, foreign bodies in the peritoneal cavity

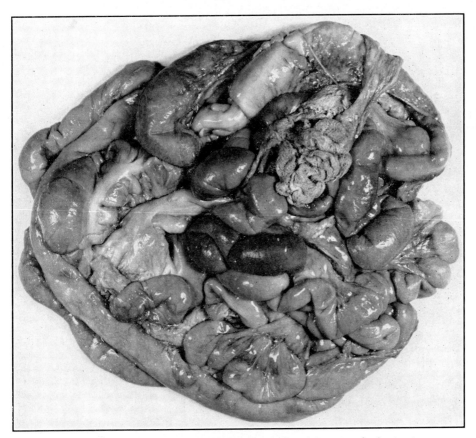

F<small>IG</small>. 436.—Sponge left in the peritoneal cavity during the course of a hysterotomy and appendectomy.

evoke three types of *reactions* (1) infective inflammation, (2) aseptic irrita-tion, and (3) tendency to extrusion in the direction of least resistance. Thus, they may bring about (1) peritonitis, (2) abscesses, (3) sinuses, or (4) fist-ulous tracts. They may be responsible for death of the patient in as high as 25 per cent of cases.

Omental Infarction.—Infarction of the omentum usually occurs in adults beyond forty years of age and is more common in males than in females (Cagney). The *causes* are trauma, thrombosis, embolism, torsion, and idiopathic. Torsion may result from (1) a primary (spontaneous) twist or (2) a secondary twist in connection with hernia or primary disease of an abdominal viscus (Sterling). The force causing the rotation is thought to come from (1) the movement of the intestines, (2) a deformity in anatomic configuration of, together with the flow of blood in, omental arteries and veins, or (3) external trauma. Of the causes listed, secondary torsion is by far the most common followed by primary torsion and then by the others named. *Pathologically* the initial changes consist of congestion, edema, and leukocytic infiltration. Later there is frank infarction and complete necrosis of tissue. The chief *complication* is toxemia from absorption of disintegration products. The *clinical manifestations* result from peritoneal irritation and absorption of the disintegration products referred to. They consist of pain, nausea, fever, rapid pulse, irregularity in function of the colon, and a palpable abdominal mass. The condition is generally *diagnosed* as acute appendicitis. *Treatment* consists of surgical excision. The *prognosis* is good.

TUMORS

Orientation.—Some tumors of the peritoneum are common while others are rare. They *occur* at all ages and in both sexes. While there is considerable difference of opinion regarding *classification* they may be divided into three main groups—primary, secondary, and retroperitoneal. Of these, the two mentioned last are most common. The chief *complications* are hemorrhagic ascites, neoplastic cachexia, and intestinal obstruction. The *clinical manifestations* accordingly consist of abdominal discomfort or pain, distention of the abdomen with blood-tinged fluid or by the tumor itself, indigestion, loss of weight, anorexia, weakness, nausea, vomiting, constipation, anemia, etc. The *diagnosis* is made from the history (especially in cases of secondary tumors), physical examination, finding of neoplastic cells in abdominal fluid obtained by paracentesis (Sattenspiel), peritoneoscopy, and laparotomy. *Treatment* in benign growths is surgical excision while that in malignant tumors is symptomatic. The *prognosis* in benign tumors is good whereas that in malignant tumors is poor.

Primary Tumors.—The confusion in nomenclature concerning primary tumors of the peritoneum is similar to that in connection with primary tumors of the pleura (p. 542). Since the peritoneum is a complex organ, each of its component cells (mesothelial, fibroblastic, fibrocytic, lipoblastic, lipocytic, reticulum, and vascular endothelial) should be capable of giving rise to a benign and a malignant growth. Further, the term *mesothelioma* should be reserved for tumors composed only of mesothelial cells. Actually, however, some authors prefer to speak of any primary tumor of the peritoneum as mesothelioma (Stout). Using the caption in the former sense, mesotheliomas of the peritoneum may be benign or malignant. *Benign mesotheliomas* have also been called adenomatoid tumors, adenomas, lymphangiomas, etc. (Wyatt, Rhind, and Horn). Among other places, they appear in the peritoneal covering of the epididymis, spermatic cord, uterus, fallopian tubes, ovaries, round ligaments, and canal of Nuck. They have not been described in the upper peritoneal cavity. They may be single or multiple, are sharply circumscribed, measure as much as 3 cm. in diameter, and present homogeneously gray or yellowish cut surfaces (Fig. 437*A*). Histologically they are characteristically composed of gland-like spaces lined with flattened to cuboidal epithelial cells (Fig. 437*B*). The stroma is of a connective tissue variety and usually discloses foci of lymphocytes. *Malignant mesotheliomas* are infrequent in comparison to benign mesotheliomas but are more common in the peritoneal cavity than in the pleura or pericardium (Stout and Rosenthal). Grossly they are nodular or diffusely spreading (Fig. 438). In the latter instance they encase the various structures with a thick sheet of neoplastic tissue. They do not, however, penetrate the underlying structures deeply nor do they metastasize widely. Histologically they are composed of sheets, cords, or glands of polyhedral, cuboidal, or columnar, often mucinous secreting cells embedded in a connective tissue stroma. In making a diagnosis of malignant mesothelioma, great care should be taken to exclude a secondary tumor, for the latter may grossly and microscopically be indistinguishable.

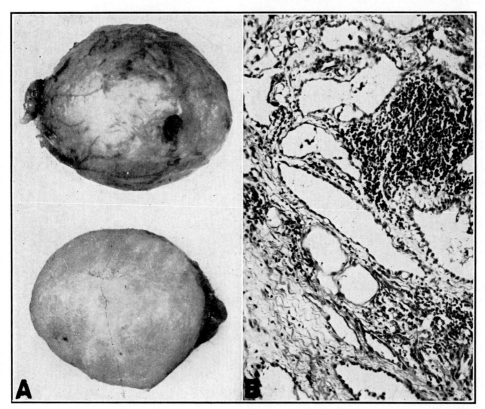

Fig. 437.—Benign mesothelioma (adenomatoid tumor) of the epididymis showing *A*, the external and cut surfaces and *B*, the microscopic appearance with gland-like spaces lined by low cuboidal cells and lymphocytic infiltration of the stroma. × 100.

Secondary Tumors.—Secondary neoplasms of the peritoneum are almost always malignant—the rare exception being a tumor such as a fibromyoma of the uterus that becomes attached to the peritoneum and then severs its connection with the parent organ. Further, a malignant tumor is most often a carcinoma. The most common primary sites are the abdominal organs, especially carcinoma of the female genital system (ovaries) and the gastrointestinal tract but, on occasion, any organ of the body may harbor the original growth. The neoplastic cells reach the peritoneum by direct extension (in cases of origin in an abdominal viscus) or by vascular metastasis (in cases of origin in an extra-abdominal viscus). Once in the peritoneal cavity the tumor spreads by direct permeation or by drop metastasis. Usually the serosal surfaces are studded with tiny or larger, grayish-white

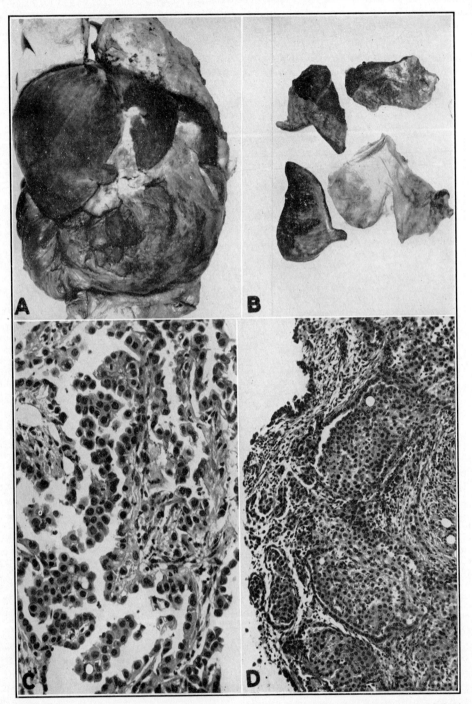

FIG. 438.—Malignant mesothelioma of the peritoneum showing A, the peritoneum and B, the pleural surfaces covered with neoplastic tissue, C, glandular arrangement of cuboidal cells. $\times$ 200, and D, more solid arrangement of both cuboidal and polyhedral cells. $\times$ 100.

foci or nodules that may resemble tubercles (Fig. 439), although sometimes
the tumor grows in plaques and sheets and may resemble a malignant
mesothelioma. The omentum is generally permeated with tumor and is
reduced to a small irregular mass or roll. Histologically the secondary
growths appear similar to the parent neoplasms.

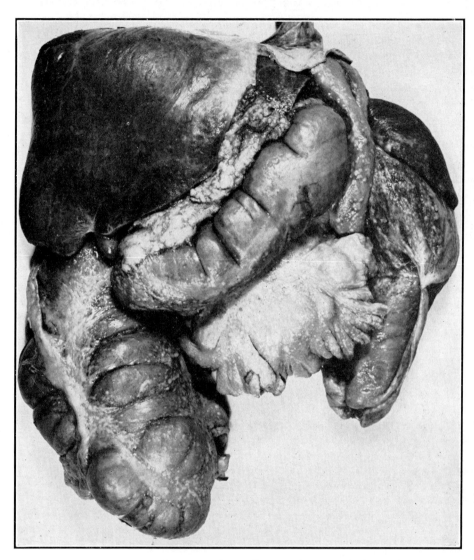

Fig. 439.—Metastatic peritoneal carcinoma from a primary tumor in the stomach.

A special type of secondary neoplasm of the peritoneum is what is referred to as *pseudomyxoma* of the *peritoneum* (Chaffee). The condition
occurs in both sexes but is much more common in females and usually develops after the age of thirty years. It is *caused* by rupture of (1) pseudomucinous cystadenoma of the ovary (p. 1186) or (2) a mucocele of the appendix (p. 742). The former thus represents a true tumor metastasis while
the latter is more in keeping with a chemical peritonitis. *Pathologically*

pseudomyxoma of the peritoneum exists as innumerable small or large, walled-off, mucin filled cysts distributed throughout the peritoneal cavity or as a more diffuse gelatinous and fibrous welding of the serosal surfaces of all the abdominal organs (Fig. 440). *Histologically* the lesion may consist of columnar, cuboidal, or flattened epithelial cells in more or less glandular formation or of structureless deposits of colloid. In either case, the support-

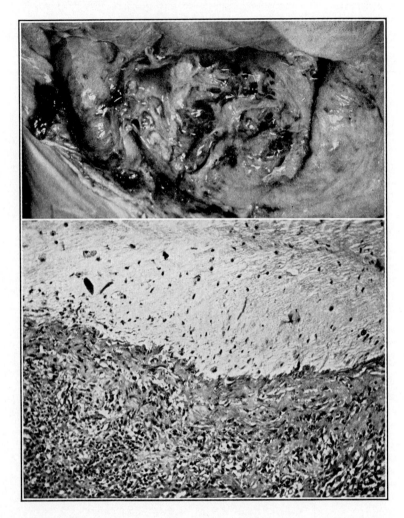

Fig. 440.—Pseudomyxoma of the peritoneum illustrating, above, a mottling of the serosal surfaces by gelatinous material and, below, mucinous material evoking a fibroblastic and leukocytic reaction. × 100.

ing tissue is fibrous and permeated with plasma cells, lymphocytes, neutrophils, and eosinophils. The *prognosis* is better in pseudomyxoma of the peritoneum in cases of appendiceal origin than it is in cases of ovarian origin. The usual *cause* of *death* is intestinal obstruction.

Retroperitoneal Tumors.—Since many of the abdominal organs are, strictly speaking, partially or wholly retroperitoneal in position, tumors that are generally classified as retroperitoneal are thus quite varied. Included in such classifications are (1) carcinoma and embryoma of the kidney, (2) carcinoma of the adrenal cortex, (3) neuroblastoma and other nerve tissue tumors of the adrenal medulla, sympathetic ganglion, and nerve trunks, (4) lymphoblastomas, (5) teratoid tumors, and (6) such soft tissue neoplasms as lipoma, liposarcoma, fibroma, fibrosarcoma, myxoma, myxosarcoma, myoma, rhabdomyosarcoma, embryoma, lymphangioma, and various mixtures of these (Snyder, Arnheim, Farbman, and Newman). Since most of the tumors are discussed in connection with the various organs mentioned and since soft tissue tumors are similar to corresponding growths of the subcutaneous tissues, further discussion at this time does not appear necessary.

REFERENCES

Pathologic Physiology

BOYD, WM.: *Pathology for the Surgeon*, 7th Ed., Philadelphia, W. B. Saunders Co., 1955, page 276.
COLE, W. H. and ELMAN, R.: *Textbook of General Surgery*, 6th Ed., New York, D. Appleton Century Co., 1952, page 768.
DAVIS, H. A.: *Principles of Surgical Physiology*, New York, Hoeber-Harper, 1957, Chapter 17

Congenital Anomalies

WATSON, L. F.: *Hernia*, 3rd Ed., St. Louis, C. V. Mosby Co., 1948.

Inflammations

BLADES, B.: Surg. Gynec. & Obst., *103*, 765, 1956 (Subphrenic Abscess).
BOYS, F.: Surgery, *11*, 118, 1942 (Peritoneal Adhesions).
BRICK, I. B., and CAGIGAS, M.: New England J. Med., *244*, 786, 1951 (Benign Paroxysmal Peritonitis).
CRILE, G., JR.: Am. J. Surg., *72*, 859, 1946 (Peritonitis).
————: Surg., Gynec. & Obst., *83*, 150, 1946 (Peritonitis Treated with Penicillin).
FALK, H. C., and BLINICK, G.: Am. J. Obst. & Gynec., *50*, 168, 1945 (Post-abortal Peritonitis).
FRASER, K.: J. Thor. Surg., *33*, 776, 1957 (Subphrenic abscess).
GERWIG, W. H. and BLADES, B.: Ann. Surg., *144*, 356, 1956 (Subdiaphragmatic Abscess)
HARVEY, H. D., and MELENEY, F. L.: Int. Abst. Surg., *67*, 339, 1938 (Peritonitis).
KAHRS, T.: Tubercle, *23*, 132, 1952 (Tuberculous Peritonitis—169 Cases).
OLNICK, H. M., and HATCHER, M. B.: J. A. M. A., *152*, 582, 1953 (Meconium Peritonitis).
PACKARD, G. B., and REYNOLDS, L. E.: Ann. Surg., *133*, 548, 1951 (Meconium Peritonitis).
PAHMER, M.: J. Pediat., *17*, 90, 1940 (Pneumococcic Peritonitis).
PEDOWITZ, P., and FELMUS, L. B.: Am. J. Surg., *83*, 507, 1952 (Adnexal Abscess and Peritonitis).
ROSS, W. B., and LUBITZ, J. M.: Ann. Surg., *130*, 100, 1949 (Talc Granuloma).
STANLEY, M. M.: A. M. A. Arch. Int. Med., *78*, 1, 1946 (Gonococcic Peritonitis).
WILLIS, W. H.: J. A. M. A., *147*, 654, 1951 (Benign Paroxysmal Peritonitis).
WRIGHT, L. T., *et al.*: Surg., Gynec. & Obst., *92*, 661, 1951 (Aureomycin in Peritonitis).

Physical Disturbances

AYRES, R. W., *et al.*: Am. J. Dig. Dis., *17*, 345, 1950 (Idiopathic Pneumoperitoneum).
BANYAI, A. L.: *Pneumoperitoneum Treatment*, St. Louis, C. V. Mosby Co., 1946.
BOGLE, J. H.: Am. J. Surg., *72*, 656, 1946 (War Wounds).
CAGNEY, M. S., and MILROY, G.: Brit. J. Surg., *35*, 95, 1947 (Omental Infarction).
CROSSEN, H. S., and CROSSEN, D. F.: *Foreign Bodies Left in the Abdomen*, St. Louis, C. V. Mosby Co., 1940.
FRIEDMAN, R. L.: J. A. M. A., *150*, 211, 1952 (Hiatus Pneumocele in Pneumoperitoneum).
GORDON-TAYLOR, G.: Brit. J. Surg., War Surgery Supplement III, p. 409 (War Wounds of the Abdomen).
HOLLANDER, A. G.: J. A. M. A., *147*, 568, 1951 (Air Embolism in Pneumoperitoneum).
JERNSTROM, P.: Am. J. Clin. Path., *21*, 573, 1951 (Air Embolism During Peritoneoscopy).

KARP, L. M., and HARRIS, F. I.: J. A. M. A., *147*, 656, 1951 (Chylous Peritonitis).

METZ, A. R., *et al.*: Am. J. Surg., *72*, 826, 1946 (Trauma with Ruptured Viscera).

REIMANN, D. L., and COWLEY, R. A.: Am. J. Surg., *71*, 328, 1946 (Intra-abdominal Hemorrhage).

SAPHIR, W.: Am. J. Dig. Dis., *15*, 408, 1948 (Abdominal Apoplexy).

SHALLOW, T. A., *et al.*: Surgery, *19*, 177, 1946 (Abdominal Apoplexy).

STERLING, J. A., and GOLDSMITH, G.: Rev. Gastroenterol., *18*, 106, 1951 (Torsion Omentum).

THOMPSON, M., and BUSCHEMEYER, W.: Ann. Surg., *135*, 615, 1952 (Chylous Peritonitis).

Tumors

ARNHEIM, E. E.: Pediatrics, *8*, 309, 1951 (Retroperitoneal Teratomas).

CHAFFEE, J. S., and LeGRAND, R. H.: A. M. A. Arch. Surg., *45*, 55, 1942 (Pseudomyxoma of the Peritoneum).

FARBMAN, A. A.: A. M. A. Arch. Surg., *60*, 343, 1950 (Retroperitoneal Fatty Tumors).

HORN, R. C., JR., and LEWIS, G. C., JR.: Am. J. Clin. Path., *21*, 251, 1951 (Mesothelioma Female Genital Tract).

NEWMAN, H. R., and PINCK, B. D.: A. M. A. Arch. Surg., *60*, 879, 1950 (Retroperitoneal Tumors).

RHIND, J. A., and WRIGHT, C. J. E.: Brit. J. Surg., *36*, 359, 1949 (Peritoneal Mesothelioma).

ROSENTHAL, J., and CONNOR, M.: New York State J. Med., *51*, 2507, 1951 (Peritoneal Mesothelioma).

SATTENSPIEL, E.: Surg., Gynec. & Obst., *89*, 478, 1949 (Cytologic Diagnosis of Cancer in Fluids).

SNYDER, W. H., JR.: A. M. A. Arch. Surg., *63*, 26, 1951 (Retroperitoneal Tumors).

STOUT, A. P.: Cancer, *3*, 820, 1950 (Mesothelioma).

WYATT, J. P., and KHOO, P. S. H.: Brit. J. Urol., *22*, 187, 1950 (Genital Adenomatoid Tumors)

Chapter

24

Reticulo-endothelial System

PATHOLOGIC PHYSIOLOGY

GORDON O. BAIN

IN 1881 Metchnikoff began the studies which lead to his theory of phago-cytosis in the defense of the organism against foreign invaders. He intro-duced the term *"macrophage"* for the large mononuclear phagocyte endowed with this function. Further studies of the phagocytic cells of the body by Marchand, Ranvier, Ribbert, Maximow and others culminated, in 1913, in Aschoff's concept of the *"Reticulo-endothelial System."* The reticulo-endo-thelial system was *defined* with the aid of vital dyes, the colloidal particles of which are phagocytosed and concentrated in the cytoplasm of reticulo-endothelial cells. Aptly termed the "macrophage system" by Maximow, the disseminated and morphologically variable reticulo-endothelial cells were identified as members of a functional system by the property of *phago-cytosis*. A great variety of body cells are capable of phagocytosis under certain conditions, but it is the intensity and frequency of phagocytosis which characterizes the cells of the macrophage system. It is possible, by the administration of a variety of colloidal substances, to saturate the reticulo-endothelial system and so to diminish temporarily its functional capacity. Such "blockade" has been used extensively in the experimental study of reticulo-endothelial function and also as a therapeutic measure in certain cases of hemolytic anemia.

The *cells* of the reticulo-endothelial system are derived from the *primitive embryonic mesenchyme*, an early function of which is the formation of blood vessels and blood cells. The mesenchyme invades developing organs and tissues, providing a vascularized supporting stroma which contains argyro-philic fibers. The ability to form argyrophilic reticulum is retained by cells of the reticulo-endothelial system. Furthermore, multipotent, primitive mesenchymal cells persist among the reticulo-endothelial cells of the adult and, under conditions of unusual need (*e.g.* myelophthisic anemia) or as a result of abnormal proliferative and differentiative activity (myeloprolifera-tive syndromes), may revert to embryological blood-forming activity (extra-medullary myeloid metaplasia). Cells of the reticulo-endothelial system are scattered diffusely throughout practically every organ and tissue but are concentrated particularly in the so-called "reticulo-endothelial" or "hemo-poietic" organs, namely, the spleen, hemopoietic bone marrow, liver, lymph nodes, and thymus.

The reticulo-endothelial cells (histiocytes, macrophages) are of two types, fixed and wandering. *Fixed histiocytes* (resting wandering cells of Maximow) may, under appropriate stimulation, become wandering macrophages, and vice versa. The fixed reticulo-endothelial cells include (1) *fixed histiocytes*

(911)

of the connective tissues—ovoid, fusiform, flat, or rhizopodal cells lying among the fibroblastic elements from which they may be distinguished by their ability to concentrate vital dyes. Many of these cells are perivascular, the "adventitial cells" of Marchand, (2) *reticulum cells* of the spleen, bone marrow, and lymphatic tissues—large cells with abundant syncytial cytoplasm which stains poorly with routine stains. They lie in the meshes of the argyrophilic reticulum fibers which they produce, (3) *littoral cells* of the sinusoids of the spleen, bone marrow, and lymph nodes, and endothelial-like cells lining the sinusoids of the liver (stellate cells of Kupffer), adrenal glands, and anterior hypophysis, and (4) *microglial phagocytes* of the central nervous system of pia-arachnoidal origin.

The *wandering cells* of *free histiocytes* of the reticulo-endothelial system include (1) wandering macrophages of the connective tissues (clasmatocytes of Ranvier), splenic pulp, lymphatic tissue, and bone marrow: the free microglia of the central nervous system (*e.g.* gitter-zellen, neuronophages), and the alveolar (septal) macrophages of the lungs (*e.g.* dust cells, heart failure cells), and (2) blood monocytes.

The *functions* of the reticulo-endothelial system are not well known, but in the light of present knowledge appear to be body defense (phaogcytosis and antibody production), blood cell metabolism (hemopoiesis, hemoclasis, bile pigment metabolism, and iron metabolism), and lipoid metabolism (lipoid formation and storage).

The reticulo-endothelial system is the body's main *organ* of *defense*. It functions principally against exogenous living and nonliving intruders, exogenous colloidal substances, endogenous debris, and metabolic products of particulate or colloidal nature. Pyogenic bacteria are attacked mainly by the *granulocytes* (microphages), the *macrophages* participating as scavengers in the later stages of the inflammatory reaction. Certain other infective agents, including acid-fast bacilli, rickettsiæ, fungi, and protozoal parasites, are dealt with primarily by reticulo-endothelial phagocytes. Stimulation of the macrophages results in proliferation to meet the demand. Locally, this may eventuate in the formation of a granuloma. Systemic stimulation of the reticulo-endothelial system results in widespread proliferation of reticulo-endothelial cells with enlargement of organs rich in such tissue. Thus, the reaction to a suture is a localized foreign body granuloma, while malaria and visceral leishmaniasis elicit a systemic response characterized by splenomegaly, hepatomegaly, *etc.* The mononuclear character of the *inflammatory exudate* in a variety of viral infections indicates that the reticulo-endothelial system is important in defense against viral invasion. Phagocytosis of viral elementary bodies is not readily observed because of their small size, but under direct observation phagocytosis of the large virus particles of psitticosis has occurred.

The phagocytic response is more intense in *animals* previously *sensitized* to the invading agent and it has long been suspected that the reticulo-endothelial system plays an important part in the elaboration of *immune antibodies* of antitoxic, complement-fixing, hemolytic, and agglutinating types. These are serum globulins found principally in the gamma and beta fractions. It is a logical assumption that the phagocytic cells within which particulate antigens such as bacteria have been observed to undergo dissolution, play a part in the elaboration of specific antibodies. There is experimental evidence in support of this assumption (Sabin). It has also been maintained, and denied, that the lymphocyte is the source of antibodies. There is considerable evidence that the plasma cell is an important source of antibody globulins. It has been suggested that reticulo-endothelial cells, in the process of antibody formation, assume the morphological characters of plasma cells (Fragraeus). As might be expected of an antibody-producing tissue, certain diseases (*e.g.* sarcoidosis, kala azar, *etc.*) in which the reticulo-endothelial system is strongly stimulated are characterized by hyperglobulinemia.

The reticulo-endothelial system plays a leading role in the *metabolism* of blood cells, bile pigment and iron, for it is both the cradle and the grave of the formed elements of the blood (p. 926).

The reticulo-endothelial system is implicated in *lipid metabolism*. In hyperlipemic states such as diabetes mellitus and familial hypercholesterolemia, reticulo-endothelial cells in certain sites (mainly skin and arterial intimas) may be laden with cholesterol. Reticulo-endothelial cells have the ability to form lipids, including cholesterol, and normally contain minute amounts of the glycolipid kerasin. In Gaucher's disease, kerasin accumulates in excessive amounts in reticulo-endothelial cells. In Niemann-Pick's disease the phospholipid sphingomyelin accumulates in the cells of the reticulo-endothelial system. Both kerasin and sphingomyelin are derived from lignoceryl sphingosine by enzyme action. Intracellular enzyme dysfunctions are thought to be the causes of these lipoid storage diseases. There is no evidence of disordered lipoid transport and the blood levels of glyco- and phospholipids are normal. In another group of reticulo-endothelial diseases, cholesterol accumulates in reticulo-endothelial cells as a secondary phenomenon. These disorders, comprising eosinophilic granuloma, Hand-Schüller-Christian's disease, and Letterer-Siwe's disease, are regarded as different manifestations of a fundamentally similar histiocytosis, possibly inflammatory in origin. According to Tannhauser, the excessive cholesterol originates in the foamy histiocytes within which it is found.

GENERAL CONSIDERATIONS

From a pathologic point of view, Congenital Anomalies and Physical Disturbances are unimportant as far as the reticulo-endothelial system is concerned, while Tumors fall in the category of lymphoblastoma and are discussed principally in the Chapters on the Blood (p. 953) and Lymph Nodes (p. 984). Thus only Degenerations and Inflammations are left to be considered forthwith.

DEGENERATIONS

Orientation.—Degenerative disorders of the reticulo-endothelial system resolve themselves into disturbances of lipoid metabolism, and together these conditions are referred to as *lipoid storage diseases* or *lipoidoses*. While the classifications of lipoid storage diseases are many and, in some instances, quite complicated the main disorders may be listed as follows: Gaucher's disease, Niemann-Pick's disease, Hand-Schüller-Christian's disease, eosinophilic granuloma of bone, and Letterer-Siwe's disease. Each of these may now be considered in the order mentioned.

Gaucher's Disease.—Gaucher's disease is a rare familial metabolic disorder characterized by a deposition of cerebrosides in the reticulo-endothelial cells of principally the spleen, bone marrow, and liver (Thannhauser). It has *also* been *called* primary idiopathic splenomegaly, Gaucher's large cell splenomegaly, lipoid cell splenohepatomegaly of the Gaucher's type, and

58

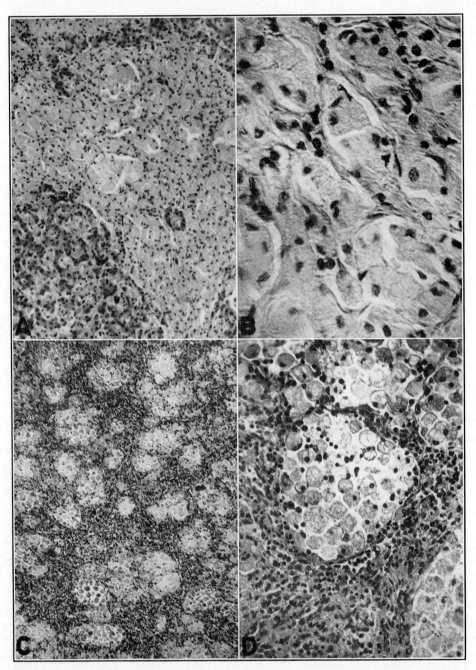

Fig. 441.—Gaucher's disease showing *A*, an infiltration of the liver by a sheet of Gaucher's cells. × 100, *B*, higher magnification of large polyhedral Gaucher's cells with abundant reticulated cytoplasm and rounded, relatively small, evenly stained nuclei. × 400, *C*, an infiltration of the spleen with collections of Gaucher's cells. × 40, and *D*, higher magnification of the splenic lesions. × 200.

cerebroside lipoidosis. The disorder may appear in two forms—adult and infantile. *Adult Gaucher's disease* is the chronic form of the disturbance and the commoner of the two, there having been about 200 cases recorded by 1949. It is apparently worldwide in *distribution* with most of the known cases occurring in Europe and America. It occurs among the white and colored population, is most frequent in Hebrews, predominates in females, and may appear at any time of life from childhood on. Aside from heredity, the *cause* is unknown but acute infection activates the disease and hastens its progress.

The important *pathologic changes* are found in the spleen, liver, lymph nodes, and skeletal system. The *spleen* may be enlarged to as much as 8,100 gm. in weight and 45 cm. in greatest diameter. The capsule is often fibrotic but the normal contour is maintained. The consistency is firm. Cut surfaces are deep brownish red and mottled and may show recent or old infarcts. The *liver* is enlarged but proportionately not as much as the spleen. The capsule may be thickened. The consistency is firm. Cut surfaces are brownish red and disclose ramifying gray streaks. The *lymph nodes*, both superficial and deep, are enlarged to as much as 2 cm. in greatest diameter, are soft, and appear brownish with grayish-white spots. The *skeletal system* is characteristically and sometimes primarily affected. All bones may be involved, especially the femur, sternum, and vertebræ. The marrow is soft and red and contains varisized nodules that measure as much as 2 cm. across. As the nodules enlarge, they encroach upon and erode the osseous tissue. The characteristic *histologic change* is the presence of Gaucher's cells (Fig. 441). The cells measure from 20 to 40 microns or more in diameter and are pale, round, oval, or polygonal. The cell borders are distinct; the cytoplasm is abundant, opaque, lightly basophilic, and reticulated, and the nuclei are single or multiple, round or oval, and regular.

The *complications* consist of (1) impairment of function of the lungs, heart, etc., due to the tremendous enlargement of the spleen, (2) anemia and thrombocytopenia due to replacement of the bone marrow by Gaucher's cells, and (3) superimposed secondary infection, especially tuberculosis. The *clinical manifestations* consist of massive splenomegaly, pains in the bones, osseous changes readily depicted roentgenographically, slight to moderate enlargement of the liver and lymph nodes, patchy melanin pigmentation of the skin, cuneiform thickening and brownish discoloration of the conjunctivæ, hemorrhagic tendency due to thrombocytopenia, microcytic anemia, leukopenia, fever, and emaciation. The *diagnosis* is made from (1) the clinical manifestations, (2) aspiration biopsy of the spleen, liver, or bone marrow, (3) the findings at autopsy, and (4) chemical analysis of affected tissue. There is no specific *treatment*. Splenectomy is advised in cases where the organ is tremendously enlarged. The *prognosis* is poor in cases in which the disease develops early in life and improves as the age of onset increases.

Infantile Gaucher's disease is the acute form of the disease. It starts during the first six months of age and results in death by the second year. Although splenomegaly is present, the manifestations are mostly neurological. They consist of lack of interest in the surroundings, rigidity of the neck, opisthotonus, increased muscular tone, laryngeal spasm, dysphagia, trismus, and strabismus.

Niemann-Pick's Disease.—Niemann-Pick's disease is a rare familial and congenital metabolic disorder characterized by a deposition of sphingomyelin in the reticulo-endothelial cells throughout the body (Thann-

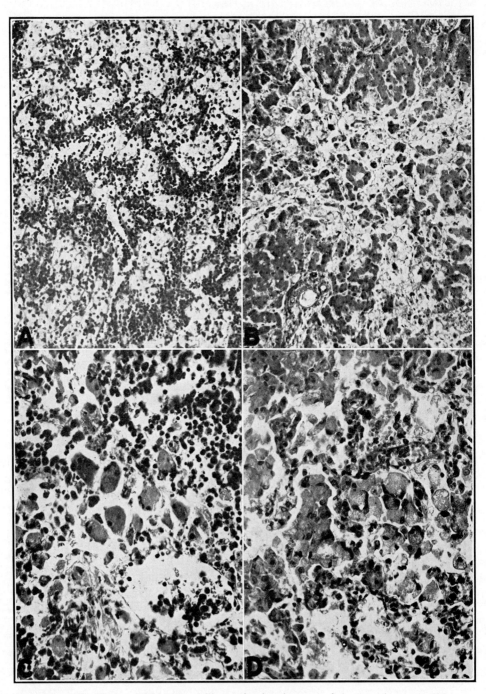

Fig. 442.—Nieman-Pick's disease illustrating involvement of *A*, the spleen. × 100, *B*, the liver. × 100, *C*, the bone marrow. × 200, and *D*, the lung. × 200.

hauser). It has *also* been *called* lipoid cell splenohepatomegaly of the Niemann-Pick's type, lipoid histiocytosis, essential lipoid histiocytosis, and phosphatide lipoidosis. While the disorder may rarely *occur* in adults (adult form) it is generally seen in infants (infantile form). It is more common in females than in males and predominates in Hebrews. The child appears normal at birth but within a few weeks or months it gradually stops eating, fails to gain, and loses weight. The remaining *clinical manifestations* consist of retardation of growth, enlargement of the abdomen, hepatomegaly, splenomegaly, yellowish-brown discoloration of the skin, apathy, open mouth, mongoloid expression, mental deterioration and blindness (amaurotic family idiocy), extreme emaciation, fever, and death

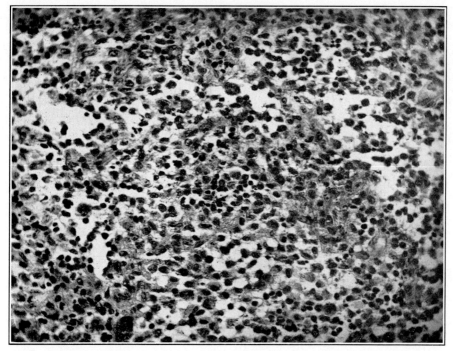

Fig. 443.—Hand-Schüller-Christian's disease demonstrating a granulomatous reaction composed of foam cells and leukocytes, with the latter consisting in part of eosinophils. × 200.

by the second year. The chief *gross pathologic changes* consist of splenomegaly, hepatomegaly, enlargement of the lymph nodes, yellowish mottling of the lungs, and a yellowish-gray appearance of the bone marrow. *Histologically* all of the organs of the body (including the eye and brain) contain Niemann-Pick cells to a greater or lesser degree (Fig. 442). The cells measure from 20 to 40 microns in diameter and are pale and ovoid or round. The cytoplasm is abundant, foamy, and finely vacuolated. The nuclei are single or, at most, double, round or oval, relatively small, and evenly stained. They usually do not evoke an accompanying inflammatory reaction.

Hand-Schüller-Christian's Disease.—This disease, *also known* as reticulo-endotheliosis, is a rare disorder of cholesterol and cholesterol ester metabolism (Horsfall and Wallace). It usually *starts* in childhood but is occasionally seen in young adults, and it affects males about three times as frequently as females. The disorder does not appear to be familial nor does it predominate in any particular race. *Pathologically* the disease is a granuloma that exists in three stages with transitions from one to another (Fig. 443). Initially it consists of focal collections of foam cells with sharply, defined borders, an abundant amount of foamy cytoplasm, and round, evenly stained, central or eccentric nuclei. The next stage is one of inflammatory reaction in which eosinophils are conspicuous. The third stage is one of fibrous tissue replacement and healing. While all organs of the

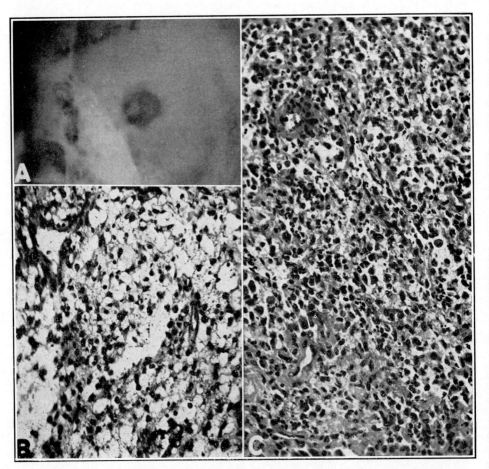

FIG. 444.—Eosinophilic granuloma of bone disclosing *A*, a punched-out defect in the skull, *B*, foam cells. × 200, and *C*, mostly leukocytes with numerous eosinophils. × 200.

body may be affected, the lesions characteristically appear in the bones, eye, and brain. The *bones* usually involved are skull, sella, pelvis, long bones, mandible, ribs, vertebræ, maxilla, and scapula. The process is destructive in nature and the defects are readily demonstrable roentgenographically. The *ocular* changes consist of an intra-orbital deposition of foam cells and granulations resulting in protrusion of the eye (exophthalmus). The deposits in the *brain* are in the region of the tuber cinereum and pituitary and, with the disruption of these structures, account for the development of diabetes insipidus. The usual *clinical manifestations* consist of bony defects, unilateral or bilateral exophthalmos, and diabetes insipidus.

In addition, there may be retardation of growth, gingivitis, dental caries, pains in the bones, slight lymphadenopathy, splenomegaly, cutaneous xanthomas, and hypogenitalism. The *diagnosis* is made from the clinical manifestations and is confirmed by biopsy. There is no special *treatment* although irradiation therapy has been effective. The *prognosis* is variable. Some cases progress slowly and terminate fatally while others remain more or less static for many years.

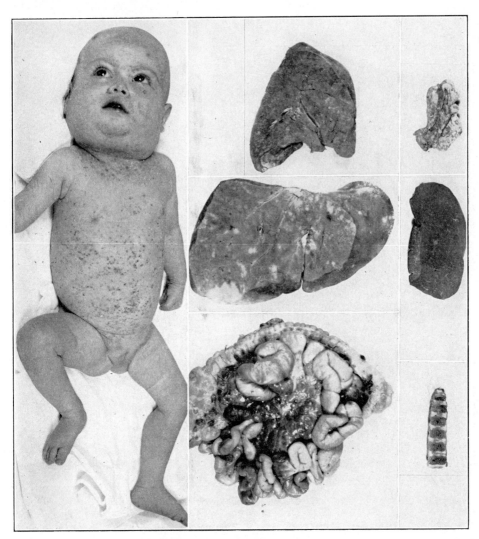

Fig. 445.—Letterer-Siwe's disease illustrating cutaneous petechiæ and enlargement of cervical lymph nodes as well as tumor nodules in the lung, thymus, liver, spleen, mesenteric lymph nodes and bone marrow in a six month old child.

Eosinophilic Granuloma of Bone.—It is generally considered that eosinophilic granuloma of the bone is closely related to or actually represents a benign form of Hand-Schüller-Christian's disease with the lesions limited to bone (Jaffe and Solomon). The condition is usually seen in children and young adults and predominates in males. *Pathologically* the osseous involvement may be single or multiple and, with the exception of the small bones of the hands and feet, any bones of the body may be affected. Those most often involved are cranium, ribs, vertebræ, humerus, and femur. The lesions are sharply circumscribed, measure as much as 2 cm. in diameter, and consist of cystic, hemorrhagic, and yellowish material when recent and more solid, gray, and fibrotic substance when older. They are readily demonstrable roentgenographically (Fig. 444*A*). *Histologically* they are similar to the lesions in the Hand-Schüller-Christian's disease (Fig. 444*B* and *C*). The usual *clinical manifestations* consist of osseous pain, swelling,

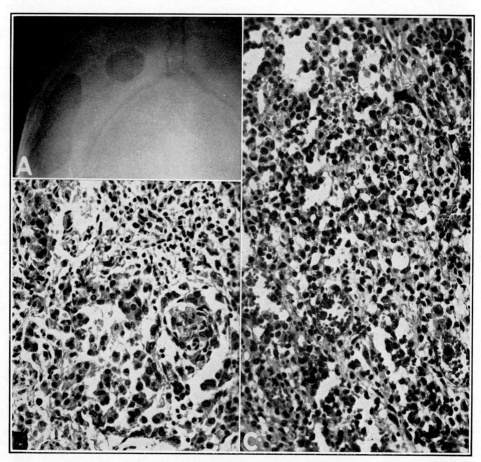

Fig. 446.—Letterer-Siwe's disease showing *A*, two punched-out defects in the skull, *B*, reticulum cells. × 200, and *C*, diffuse leukocytic reaction with numerous eosinophils. × 200.

and tenderness. The *diagnosis* is made from the clinical manifestations, the roentgenographic appearance, and biopsy. *Treatment* has consisted of curettage, irradiation, and watchful waiting. The *prognosis* is good for recovery has occurred in all recorded cases.

Letterer-Siwe's Disease.—It is generally believed that this disease is also closely related to or actually represents a malignant form of Hand-Schüller-Christian's disease (Claireaux and Havard). It has *also* been *called* aleukemic reticulosis and nonlipoid reticulo-endotheliosis. The disorder usually develops in patients between one and two years of age and is generally rapidly fatal. The *characteristics*, as listed by Siwe, are (1) hepatomegaly and splenomegaly, (2) hemorrhagic (petechiæ and purpura) diathesis (Fig. 445), (3) mild and generalized lymphadenopathy, (4) progressive anemia with a normal leukocytic count, (5) nonhereditary occurrence, (6) localized skeletal tumors readily demonstrable roentgenographically (Fig. 446*A*), and (7) generalized hyperplasia of the reticulo-endothelial cells with focal tumor proliferations in the spleen, liver, lymph nodes, thymus, skin, and bone marrow. The tumors possess a hemorrhagic tendency but no lipoid storage. Actually the histologic changes are similar to those in Hand-Schuller-Christain's disease and eosinophilic granuloma, with the exception that foam cells are not seen and that fibrosis is minimal or entirely absent (Fig. 446*B* and *C*).

INFLAMMATIONS

Orientation.—Because the reticulo-endothelial cells are so intimately connected with the various tissues and organs of the body, inflammation of the reticulo-endothelial system actually represents inflammation of the structures in which the cells happen to be located. Despite this, there are certain inflammatory diseases that have a preference for the system as such, thereby being of a widespread nature. Two such disorders, namely, Boeck's sarcoid and histoplasmosis, have already been discussed in Chapter 12 (pp. 501 and 513). Three others that may be considered in this section are brucellosis, leishmaniasis, and trypanosomiasis.

Brucellosis.—Brucellosis, also known as *undulant fever*, is primarily a disease of farm animals causing abortion in cattle, mares, sheep, rabbits, guinea pigs, and goats and occasionally transmitted to man by drinking unpasteurized milk or handling products of infected animals. The disease thus *prevails* among farmers and people handling farm products. It occurs at all ages but is from five to ten times as common in males as it is in females (Spink and Barrett). The *cause* is the *Brucella* group of organisms consisting of *Br. abortus* (cattle), *Br. suis* (swine), and *Br. melitensis* (goats). The organisms are small, gram-negative, nonmotile coccobacilli that are aerobic and micro-aerophilic and that grow best in 10 per cent carbon dioxide.

The *pathologic changes* are readily studied in the experimentally produced disease in guinea pigs and mice but are only infrequently seen in man due to the extremely low mortality. The lesions in experimental animals, however, are similar to those found in man (Spink and Barrett). Although the changes are widely distributed throughout the body, they are characteristically noted in the liver, spleen, lymph nodes, and bone marrow. The lesion is a granuloma (Fig. 447). The initial change consists of a focal collection of neutrophils containing ingested organisms. Within seventy-two hours the neutrophils are replaced by aggregations of epithelioid cells. The ultimate picture consists essentially of focal aggregations of epithelioid cells, occasional giant cells of the Langhans' type, scattered monocytes and lymphocytes, occasional neutrophils, and, in some instances, focal areas of acute necrosis. Caseation necrosis is not encountered. Occasionally the acute necrosis becomes more extensive with the formation of small abscesses. *Grossly* the liver, spleen, and lymph nodes are enlarged and these organs, along with the bone marrow, may be dotted with tiny grayish-white foci.

The *complications* of brucellosis consist of septicemia, bacterial endocarditis, neuritis and radiculitis, arthritis, and osteitis (Spink). *Clinically,* according to the time of affliction, the disease has been divided into three groups: (1) acute, lasting less than three months, (2) subacute, lasting from three to twelve months, and (3) chronic, lasting over twelve months. The *clinical manifestations* are nonspecific consisting of the following: intermittent fever, sweating, lassitude, chills or rigors, joint and other pains (diffuse rheumatism), gastrointestinal disturbances, and enlargement of the liver, lymph nodes, and spleen. Most ordinary *laboratory data* are of little aid in arriving at a correct diagnosis, although leukopenia and a relative lymphocytosis are important when they are present. More specific

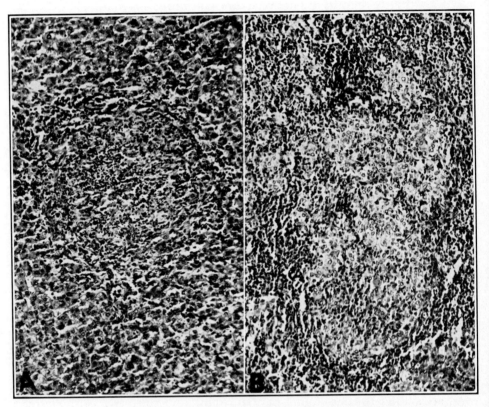

FIG. 447.—Brucellosis showing typical granulomas in *A*, the liver and *B*, the spleen. × 100. (Tissue submitted by Doctor E. Stubbs.)

laboratory procedures consist of agglutination tests, complement fixation tests, and culturing of the organisms from the blood (Barrett and Spink). The *diagnosis* is made from the clinical manifestations (especially when the patient is in an endemic area) together with the laboratory procedures outlined. *Treatment* is prevention. Once the disease is present, antibiotic and chemotherapeutic agents are administered. Currently, streptomycin and sulfadiazine, aureomycin, chloramphenicol, terramycin, dihydro-streptomycin, etc., are being employed (Spink and Simpson). The *prognosis* is good for, with proper treatment, there is an immediate response and a lasting clinical recovery without relapses in over 85 per cent of cases (Simpson).

Leishmaniasis.—Leishmaniasis connotes an infection with *Leishmania tropica*, *Leishmania brasiliensis*, or *Leishmania donovani*. Each of these is morphologically similar to the other and each passes through two stages in its life cycle—leishmania and leptomonas (Sawitz). The *leishmania stage* is the only stage found in man. The organisms live within the reticulo-endothelial cells, are oval, measure about 2 microns in diameter, lack a flagellum, and possess a nucleus, an axonema (rod-like body extending into the cytoplasm from the capsule) capped by a rounded blepharoplast and,

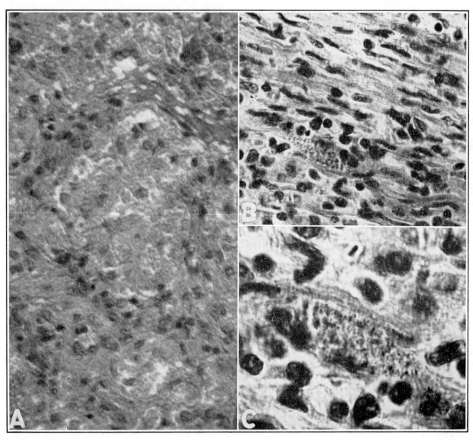

Fig. 448.—Parasitic infections of the reticulo-endothelial system illustrating *A, Leishmania donovani* within phagocytic cells of the spleen. × 400 and *B* and *C, Trypanosoma cruzi* within phagocytic cells of the heart. × 600 and 1380.

beyond this, by an elongated parabasal body (Fig. 448*A*). They multiply by fission, ultimately cause the cell to burst, are picked up by other cells, and repeat the cycle. When the resulting lesion becomes an open sore, the organisms are picked up by the *Phlebotomus* flies and in the flies they pass through the *leptomonas stage*. As such, the organisms are elongated, measure 15 microns in length, disclose an anterior flagellum, and possess a nucleus, an axonema, a blepharoplast, and a parabasal body. They multiply by fission and enter man at the time the flies are taking a blood meal.

Leishmania tropica causes cutaneous leishmaniasis or oriental sore which consists of a local inflammation of the skin that ultimately ulcerates and produces a crater that may measure as much as 3 cm. in diameter. Healing occurs by scar formation. The disorder prevails in the Orient. *Leishmania brasiliensis* causes mucocutaneous leishmaniasis, espundia, or American leishmaniasis. The lesions in the skin are similar to those in cutaneous leishmaniasis but, in addition, the disorder is characterized by inflammation and ulceration of the mucosa of the mouth, nose, and other mucocutaneous junctions. The disease occurs in Central and South America. *Leishmania donovani* causes visceral leishmaniasis or kala azar. The organisms are harbored in the liver, spleen, bone marrow, and lymph nodes. Because of interference in the function of these organs, the patient develops anemia and granulocytopenia and ultimately dies of secondary infection. The disorder occurs in the tropics. The *diagnosis* of leishmaniasis is made by isolating the organisms in smears or cultures of material aspirated from the lesions. Dogs serve as *reservoir hosts*.

Trypanosomiasis. —Trypanosomiasis signifies infection with *Trypanosoma gambiense*, *Trypanosoma rhodesiense*, and *Trypanosoma cruzi* (Sawitz). *Trypanosoma gambiense* and *Trypanosoma rhodesiense* occur in Central Africa where they cause African trypanosomiasis or sleeping sickness, are identical morphologically, and pass through two stages in their life cycles — crithidia and trypanosome. The *crithidia stage* occurs in the tsetse fly. The crithidiæ are spindle-shaped, measure 15 microns in length, multiply by fission, and possess an anterior flagellum and an undulating membrane that originates anterior to the nucleus. Crithidiæ are transformed into trypanosomes in the salivary glands of the fly, are transmitted to man when the fly is taking a blood meal, and circulate in the blood, lymph, and spinal fluid. *Trypanosomes* are similar to crithidiæ except that they are slightly longer and that the undulating membrane originates posterior to the nucleus. In man, fever occurs when the organisms circulate in the blood, and focal areas of the inflammation and cellular degeneration are present when organisms enter the tissues (especially the brain). The *diagnosis* is made by identifying the organisms in smears of blood, sternal marrow, spinal fluid, or aspiration of lymph nodes, or by experimentally reproducing the disease in dogs, guinea pigs, or rats by inoculating similar material. Pigs, cows, sheep, and wild animals such as antelopes serve as *reservoir hosts*.

Trypanosoma cruzi occurs in Central and South America where it causes American trypanosomiasis or Chagas' disease. The stages in its life cycle consist of (1) a trypanosome stage in man similar to that in other trypanosome infections, (2) a leishmania stage where leishmania-like organisms are found within the reticulo-endothelial cells of the body (Fig. 448*B*), and (3) a crithidia stage in transmitting insects similar to that in other trypanosome infections. The crithidiæ enter man by way of infected feces of an insect rubbed into the puncture wound made by the insect. Their sojourn in man is similar to the sojourn of *Leishmania donovani* in kala azar. The *diagnosis* is made by (1) isolating the organisms in smears or cultures of blood or splenic aspiration, (2) animal inoculation of similar material, or (3) complement fixation tests. The armadillo, opossum, and bat serve as *reservoir hosts*.

REFERENCES

Pathologic Physiology

Aschoff, L.: *Lectures on Pathology*, New York, Paul B. Hoeber, Inc., 1924, p. 1, (Reticulo-endothelial System).

Fagraeus, A.: Acta Med. Scand., Suppl. 204, Part III, 99, 1948 (Antibody Production and Plasma Cells).

Good, R. A.: J. Lab. Clin. Med., *46*, 167, 1955 (Agammaglobulinemia and Failure of Plasma Cell Formation).

Halpern, B. N., *et al.: Physiopathology of the Reticulo-endothelial System.* A Symposium, Springfield, Ill., Charles C Thomas, 1957.

Maximow, A. A.: *The Macrophages or Histiocytes in Cowdry's Special Cytology,* New York, Paul B. Hoeber, Inc., 1932, Vol. II, Section XIX, p. 711.

Sabin, F. R.: J. Exp. Med., *70*, 67, 1939 (Macrophages and Antibody Formation).

Tannhauser, S. J.: Lipoid Metabolism in Thompson and King's *Biochemical Disorders in Human Disease,* New York, Academic Press, Inc., 1957, Vol. VI, p. 697.

Wright, G. P.: The Reticulo-endothelial System in Hadfield's *Recent Advances in Pathology,* 6th Ed., London, J. A. Churchill, Ltd., 1953, p. 58.

General

Maximow, A. A., and Bloom, W.: *A Textbook of Histology,* 6th Ed., Philadelphia, W. B. Saunders Co., p. 63, 1952 (Reticulo-endothelial System).

Degenerations

Claireaux, A., and Lewis, I. C.: A. M. A. Arch. Dis. Child., *25*, 142, 1950 (Letterer-Siwe's Disease).

Havard, E., *et al.:* Pediatrics, *5*, 474, 1950 (Letterer-Siwe's Disease).

Horsfall, F. L., Jr., and Smith, W. R.: Quart. J. Med., *4*, 37, 1935 (Hand-Schüller-Christian's Disease).

Jaffe, H. L., and Lichtenstein, L.: A. M. A. Arch. Path., *37*, 99, 1944 (Eosinophilic Granuloma of Bone).

Solomon, H. A., and Schwartz, S.: J. A. M. A., *128*, 729, 1945 (Eosinophilic Granuloma of Bone).

Thannhauser, S. J.: *Oxford Medicine,* New York, Oxford University Press, Inc., Vol. IV, Part II, 1949 (p. 456—Gaucher's Disease and p. 531—Niemann-Pick's Disease).

Wallace, W. S.: Am. J. Roentgenol., *62*, 189, 1949 (Hand-Schüller-Christian's Disease).

Inflammations

Barrett, G. M., and Rickards, A. G.: Quart. J. Med., *22*, 23, 1953 (Brucellosis).

Sawitz, W. G.: *Medical Parasitology,* New York, The Blakiston Co., 1950.

Simpson, W. M.: U. S. Armed Forces M. J., *4*, 337, 1953 (Brucellosis).

Spink, W. W., *et al.:* J. Lab. & Clin. Med., *34*, 40, 1949; Am. J. Clin. Path., *22*, 201, 1952; A. M. A. Arch. Int. Med., *88*, 419, 1951 (Brucellosis).

Chapter

25

Blood

PATHOLOGIC PHYSIOLOGY

Robert T. Carroll

Blood is the principal fluid tissue of the body. It supplies other tissues with nutrients and oxygen and removes from them waste products of metabolic activity. It is composed of cellular elements—the erythrocytes, leukocytes and platelets, suspended in a protein liquid medium—the plasma. In healthy adults it makes up about 7 per cent of the total body weight.

Total blood volume may be determined by many procedures. The *dye dilution* method, using Evans blue dye, is a relatively simple technique. Several recent modifications have made it a fairly accurate procedure but the method is not sufficiently precise for measuring or following plasma volume. The use of *radioactive elements*, such as radioactive iron, radioactive phosphorus or radioactive chromium, while requiring special equipment, gives the worker a better means of evaluating the true red cell volume. The Ashby technique of *differential agglutination* of *red corpuscles* eliminates the necessity for special equipment and the potential hazards of radioactive element exposure. The *total blood volume* increases with increasing individual *height, weight,* and *surface area.* In terms of units of body weight, it is high in muscular or thin individuals and low in obese persons, while in terms of unit of surface area it is high in muscular and obese persons and low in thin individuals. Due to the higher red cell volume of the male, the total blood volume in terms of body weight is higher in the male (69.0 cc. per kg. body weight) than the female (64.4 cc. per kg. body weight). During life it tends to remain fairly stable although physiologic variations may occur. *Bed rest* has been reported to cause a reduction in blood volume, due primarily to a contraction of the plasma volume. In *pregnancy*, both blood and plasma volumes increase—the total blood volume amounting to 32 per cent or greater and returning to normal within one week following delivery. In abnormal states, such as following *acute hemorrhage*, there is a sharp decrease in total blood volume but the plasma volume is restored rapidly by the passage of fluid from the tissues. Following loss of blood, cells are liberated from the storage depots of the body and, to some degree, restore the corpuscular elements of the blood. Should the body not be able to compensate for the loss, and the volume not be restored by outside "artificial" means, shock will occur. When *blood* is *lost* over a *long period*, as in hemorrhoidal bleeding, the total blood volume is affected very slightly, an increase in plasma volume compensating for the loss of the cellular elements. In some of the chronic *leukemias*, particularly myeloid, increases in total blood volume have occurred, partly due to the increase in the cellular component and, to a lesser degree, to increases in plasma volume. In *polycythemia vera*, again primarily because of the increased cellular components, there is a marked increase in total blood volume.

Normal blood has a definite *specific gravity*, due primarily to its content of protein and cells. By means of the pycnometer method, it has been shown that the specific gravity of normal blood varies from 1.048 to 1.066, being higher for men (1.057) than for women (1.053). It is usually lower after meals and in the afternoon, rising after exercise and during the night. The specific gravity of serum varies from 1.026 to 1.031 and of cells from 1.092 to 1.095. Many of the blood donor centers throughout the country have found the specific gravity test a useful tool in determining the fitness of blood donors, as far as hemoglobin content of their blood is concerned. *Hemoglobin* is present in a concentration of 13.5 to 15.5 grams per cent in the adult male and of 12.5 to 14.5 grams per cent in the adult female. It is possible to prepare inert solutions of fixed specific gravity which may be used as "standards," the variable for practical purposes being the hemoglobin content in the drop of blood placed in the solution. For this purpose, it has been found that a copper sulfate solution offers many advantages, in that it is nontoxic, noninflammable, easily prepared, inexpensive, and therefore readily available to most laboratories. It has a temperature coefficient of expansion similar to that of blood. It has been calculated that this method indicates the protein content of blood within ±0.3 grams per 100 cc. blood. Routinely, copper sulfate solutions corresponding to a hemoglobin value of 12.5 grams per cent for females and 13.5 grams per cent for males are employed.

The determination of the *viscosity* of blood as an aid in differential diagnosis has now been almost abandoned. However, it is easily performed by the use of a viscometer and can be useful in determining if a circulatory impairment may be secondary to changes in the blood viscosity. Normally, in healthy adults it ranges from 3.5 to 5.4. The viscosity of the blood in men is 0.5 greater than it is in women. The primary cause of an *increase* in blood viscosity is an increase in the quantity of *erythrocytes*. Accordingly, polycythemia, whether primary or secondary, is the condition in which the greatest changes occur. Increases in *leukocytes* must be great, before they have any effect on blood viscosity. Changes in *plasma proteins*, particularly in multiple myeloma where one may find total plasma protein values as high as 16 or even 19 grams per cent, have a marked effect on the blood viscosity. An increase in the *carbon dioxide* content of the blood, by changing osmotic relationships, has been reported to increase the blood viscosity. Possibly because of this, venous blood has a higher viscosity than arterial blood.

The *sedimentation test*, because of its simplicity and in spite of its non-specificity, is still in wide use today. In this country, it probably finds its greatest field of usefulness as a crude screening test for following the progress of a chronic infectious process, such as *rheumatic fever*, or for determining the extent of the recovery phase of a *myocardial infarction*. Using the Wintrobe tube, the sedimentation rate of a normal adult male is 0 to 6 mm. in one hour, and that of a female 0 to 15 mm. The rate increases in *anemias* (except sickle cell anemia and when there is an increase in fibrinogen or globulin content), in *acute inflammatory states*, and in the normal *pregnancy*. A rapid sedimentation rate in the presence of other normal clinical and laboratory studies, should make one alert to the presence of occult organic disease. When the rate is rapid, it indicates an organic rather than a functional disorder. It is more often found in malignant rather than in benign tumors. In tuberculous patients, a rapid sedimentation rate has sometimes been found prior to the appearance of any new lesion of the chest film. It is of value in the "out-patient" management of patients with this condition, by demonstrating improvement, stability, or relapse of the infectious process. However, a normal sedimentation rate may occur in the presence of a fulminating infection, particularly in cachectic states, or if the infectious process is of viral origin.

The *erythrocytes*, or red blood cells, are manufactured in the bone marrow and, normally, mature there to the *reticulocyte* stage, after which they appear in the blood stream. Therefore, a measure of accelerated hematopoiesis in the blood is the number of reticulocytes present at any given time, the magnitude being influenced by, among other things, the extent of blood loss or destruction or the amount of stimulative material given. The normal red cell count in the blood of the adult male is 4,500,000 to 5,800,000 per c.mm. in the adult female 3,500,000 to 4,500,000. The life span of red cells is 100 to 130 days, as demonstrated by radiochromate survival studies. The primary function of the erythrocyte is the transport of oxygen, the amount of oxygen in combination with the hemoglobin molecule being determined by the partial pressure of this gas, more combining at higher pressures. Following release of the oxygen molecule to the tissues, the hemoglobin combines with and transports a molecule of carbon dioxide to the lungs, where it is released.

The *leukocytes*, or white blood cells, are manufactured in the bone marrow or in the lymphoid tissue. The normal white cell count is 5,000 to 10,000 per cu. mm. with no appreciable sex variation. These cells are divided into (a) the myeloid series, which in the blood stream is represented by the segmented neutrophil, eosinophil, and basophil, (b) the lymphocytic series, represented in the blood stream by the mature lymphocyte, and (c) the monocytic series, represented in the blood stream by the mature monocyte. The functions of leukocytes are discussed in the section on inflammation (p. 113). The segmented neutrophils and monocytes function primarily in phagocytosis, the neutrophils primarily against bacteria, the monocytes against protozoa and particulate matter. The lymphocytes appear to be most active probably in anitbody production. The eosinophils are thought to be important in detoxification and appear to have some obscure relationship to hypersensitive reactions. The basophils contain heparin and may function in delivering an anticoagulant to the site of inflammation. Neutrophils have a life span of 9 to 13 days; lymphocytes (short-lived) from 3 to 4 days, (long-lived) 100 to 200 days; and eosinophils and basophils from 8 to 12 days.

The third cellular elements of the blood, the *platelets*, are formed in the bone marrow as detached portions of the cytoplasm of megakaryocytes. They are normally present from 150,000 to 340,000 per cu. mm. of blood. It has been stated that 100,000 platelets are formed per cu. mm. of blood per day. Their average life span is 4 to 8 days. Platelets function to promote the coagulation of blood and aid in hemostasis. They are active in the first phase of coagulation and are believed to contain at least six factors which play separate roles in the early phase of blood coagulation.

GENERAL CONSIDERATIONS

ALTHOUGH the commonly used *blood values* in *normal* adults differ somewhat from author to author, the following may be considered as the figures generally accepted (Wintrobe): (1) *total blood volume*—7 per cent of body weight, 2,735 cc. per square meter of body surface, or 67 cc. per kg. of body weight, (2) *plasma volume*—45 cc. per kg. of body weight, (3) *red blood cell volume*—30 cc. per kg. of body weight, (4) *erythrocytic* (red blood cell) *count*—3.5 to 4.5 millions per c. mm. in females and 4.5 to 5.8 millions per c. mm. in males, (5) *hemoglobin*—12.5 to 14.5 gm. per 100 cc. in females and 13.5 to 15.5 gm. per 100 cc. in males, (6) *volume of packed erythrocytes* (hematocrit)—37 to 47 cc. per 100 cc. in females and 40 to 54 cc. per 100 cc. in males, (7) *mean corpuscular volume* or M.C.V. (hemotocrit per litter of blood divided by the number of erythrocytes in millions)—82 to 92 c. microns, (8) *mean corpuscular hemoglobin* or M.C.H. (hemoglobin in gm. per liter divided by the number of erythrocytes in millions)—27 to 31 micro-micrograms, (9) *mean corpuscular hemoglobin concentration* or M.C.H.C. hemoglobin in gm. per liter divided by the hematocrit per liter times one hundred) —32 to 36 per cent, (10) platelet count—250,000 per c. mm., (11) *leukocytic* (W.B.C.) *count*—5,000 to 10,000 per c. mm., (12) *differential leukocytic count*—neutrophils 55 to 75 per cent, eosinophils 2 per cent, baso-phils 0 to 1 per cent, monocytes 3 to 6 per cent, and lymphocytes 20 to 35 per cent, (13) *reticulocytes*—0.5 to 1.5 per cent of erythrocytes, and (14) *sedimentation rate*—0 to 6 mm. at the end of one hour in males and 0 to 15 mm. in females (Wintrobe method). Other values such as coagulation time, bleeding time, clot retraction time, prothrombin time, etc., vary so greatly with the methods used that over-all figures cannot be given. They may be found in any standard textbook on hematology.

Pathologically diseases of the blood are not readily classifiable into the five major categories of disease processes used in connection with other organs and systems of the body not only because the nature of many of the disorders is not understood, but also because diverse etiologic agents are responsible for similar conditions. Accordingly, the following disturbances may be considered in the order listed: anemia, polycythemia, purpura, hemophilia, malaria, granulocytopenia, infectious mononucleosis, infectious leukocytosis, and leukemia.

ANEMIA

Orientation.—As already stated or implied in Chapter 6 (p. 188), the term anemia (Gr. = negative + blood) literally means without blood and connotes a decrease in blood volume due to a reduction in the number of erythrocytes, the amount of hemoglobin, and the volume of packed erythro-cytes per 100 cc. of blood (Wintrobe). Thus, as usually used, the term indicates general rather than local changes in erythrocytes. Anemias *occur* at all ages, in both sexes, and in all races, with variations in each of these categories depending upon the type of anemia in question. The *causes* are also variable but, in general, may be listed as follows: (1) de-creased production of erythrocytes—consequent to (*a*) a deficiency of substances used in the manufacture of erythrocytes such as iron, protein, and vitamin B complex or (*b*) a fault in construction as in connection with infection, renal disease, poisons, etc., (2) increased destruction of erythro-cytes—consequent to hemolysis, (3) loss of erythrocytes from the body—consequent to acute or chronic hemorrhage, and (4) congenital dystrophies or inherited defects.

While the *classifications* of anemias are many, the simplest appears to be one that divides the disorders according to the morphologic appearance of the erythrocytes into (1) macrocytic, (2) normocytic, (3) microcytic normochromic, and (4) microcytic hypochromic. The characteristics of

59

each of these together with the specific causative factors and the respective clinical syndromes concerned are described briefly in the paragraphs that follow. Regardless of the type of anemia, the fundamental *pathologic changes* are similar. They are due to a decreased oxygen carrying capacity of erythrocytes (anoxia) and are mediated through the action of intra-cellular enzymes (p. 29). When the oxygen carrying capacity is reduced precipitously and severely (as in hemorrhage) toxic cellular metabolites flood the tissues and the patient develops shock (p. 205). When it is reduced gradually, even though severely (as in pernicious anemia), a variety of degenerative (especially atrophic and fatty) changes develop (pp. 29 and 51). More specifically, in any severe anemia the following organs may disclose the following alterations: (1) *skin*—jaundice, pallor, loss of elasticity, dermatitis, purpura, and ecchymosis, (2) *nails*—loss of luster, brittleness, and concavity instead of convexity, (3) *heart*—severe fatty change or frank infarction, (4) *lungs*—passive congestion, (5) *liver*—passive congestion and fatty change, (6) *gastrointestinal tract*—degenerations and inflammations, (7) *central nervous system*—degenerative and atrophic changes in the brain and spinal cord, and (8) *bone marrow*—replacement of hematopoiesis by fat and/or fibrous tissue.

The *clinical manifestations* are extremely variable and, in addition to those listed above, may consist of combinations of the following: dyspnea, shallow breathing, cardiac murmurs, headache, vertigo, faintness, tinnitus, irritability, paresthesis, anorexia, nausea, flatulence, abdominal discomfort, constipation, diarrhea, vomiting, dysphagia, menorrhagia, amenorrhea, albuminuria, edema, fever, etc. The *diagnosis* is made from a consideration of the clinical manifestations, hematologic (peripheral and bone marrow) studies, and, in some instances, roentgenographic findings. *Treatment* consists of ridding the body of the cause or of replacing the element or elements that are deficient. As an adjunct, or if this approach is impossible, blood transfusions are used rather freely. The *prognosis* depends upon the type of anemia present and upon the promptness and adequacy of the treatment.

Macrocytic Anemia.—In this type of anemia there is a decrease in the number of circulating erythrocytes, increase in size of erythrocytes, increase in amount of hemoglobin carried by the erythrocytes, increase in mean corpuscular volume, increase in mean corpuscular hemoglobin, and a normal or slightly reduced mean corpuscular hemoglobin concentration (Wintrobe). The more common anemias in this group are known as (1) *pernicious anemia,* (2) *macrocytic anemia associated* with *sprue* and *celiac disease* (pp. 698 and 699), (3) *nutritional macrocytic anemia*—occurring in tropical and (to a lesser extent) temperate zones, being similar to pernicious anemia, and apparently arising from a diet high in carbohydrate, low in protein and fat, and deficient in vitamins (Wills and Rubie), (4) *macrocytic anemia of pregnancy*—accounting for a minority of anemias of pregnancy, usually seen in women of the poorer class, affecting multiparas more often than primiparas, generally occurring in the third trimester of pregnancy, probably dietary in origin, and consisting of anemia similar to that in pernicious anemia with prominence of vomiting, diarrhea, sore tongue, edema, and even hypertension and albuminuria (Callender and Scott), (5) *macrocytic anemia associated* with *organic lesions* of the *gastrointestinal tract*—uncommon or rare and seen in connection with gastric carcinoma, gastric syphilis, gastric polyposis, destruction of gastric mucosa by acid, gastrectomy, gastro-enterostomy, intestinal strictures, chronic dysentery, regional enteritis, chronic pancreatic disease, resection of the small intestine, and diseases of the liver (Wintrobe), (6) *macrocytic anemia* accompanying infection with *Diphyllobothrium latum* (p. 722), (7) *macrocytic anemia* in *hypothyroidism*—due to defective gastric secretion and lack of appetite leading to a deficiency of the anti-anemic substance of the liver or of iron respectively (Lerman and Stern), and (8) *achrestic anemia*—an anemia of unknown cause that morphologically resembles pernicious anemia but that does not respond to liver therapy, that steadily progresses, and that is usually fatal (Israels and Davidson). Of all the macrocytic anemias mentioned above, pernicious anemia may be taken as the prototype and thus merits separate discussion.

Pernicious Anemia.—Pernicious anemia may be defined as a hereditary chronic disorder that develops insidiously and that is characterized by the presence of macrocytic anemia, achylia gastrica, and certain gastrointestinal and neurologic disturbances (Wintrobe). It is *also known* as primary anemia and Addison's anemia. The disease *occurs* chiefly in temperate zones, predominates in the white race, is uncommon in Hebrews and Orientals, and is rare in Negroes. It usually appears after forty years of age and affects males more frequently than females in England and the United States, but females more frequently than males in Sweden. The fundamental *cause* of pernicious anemia is faulty blood construction—a deficiency of a hematopoietic principle or substance without which normal maturation of erythrocytes cannot occur. Normally the hematopoietic principle or substance is apparently produced in the stomach during digestion by a reaction between an intrinsic and an extrinsic factor. The *intrinsic factor* is an enzyme present in gastric juice while the *extrinsic factor* consists of folic acid and vitamin B_{12} and is derived from the diet (beef muscle and other foods). In pernicious anemia there is a decreased secretion of gastric juice and thus a decreased production of the intrinsic factor. This, often coupled with a deficiency of the extrinsic factor (due to an inadequate diet), results in a deficiency of the hematopoietic principle or substance which, in turn, causes an arrest of maturation of erythrocytes and produces the anemia. The cause of decreased secretion of gastric juice, except for heredity, is unknown.

Pathologically, as a result of modern therapy, the typical changes are only rarely encountered at autopsy (Fig. 449). They consist of (1) yellowish appearance of the skin in the presence of lack of wasting, (2) fatty changes in the heart, liver, kidneys, and other organs, (3) hemosiderosis of the liver, spleen, lymph nodes, and other tissues abounding in reticuloendothelial cells, (4) megaloblastic (primitive type of nucleated red blood cell) hyperplasia of the bone marrow rendering the marrow deep red and jelly-like grossly, (5) extramedullary hematopoiesis in the spleen and liver, (6) atrophic glossitis, (7) atrophic gastritis, and (8) myelin degeneration and loss of nerve fibers in the dorsal and lateral column of the spinal cord and degeneration of the peripheral nerves.

The *complications* of pernicious anemia are (1) cardiac failure, (2) renal insufficiency, (3) decubitus ulcers and cystitis (from central nervous system changes), (4) gastric carcinoma (higher incidence than in normal people), and (5) variety of other associated (but not necessarily related) diseases. The *clinical manifestations* are explainable on the basis of the pathologic changes listed and vary with the severity of the disease. The onset is insidious with the complaints consisting of fatigability, weakness, faintness, numbness and tingling of the extremities, headache, nausea, anorexia, vomiting, dizziness, dyspnea, palpitation, diarrhea, loss of weight,

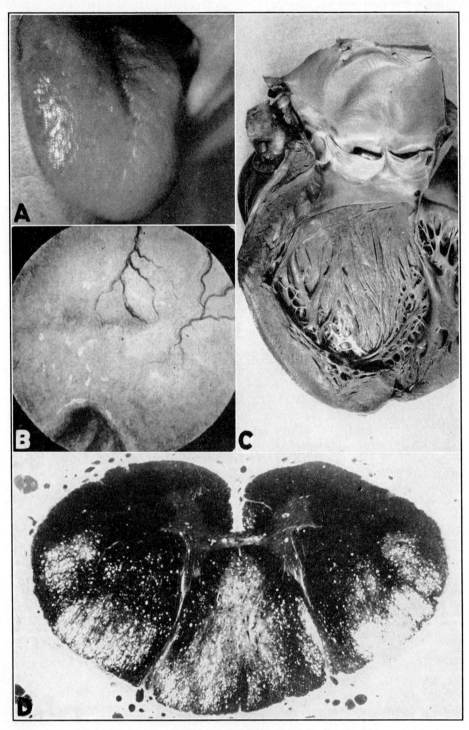

Fig. 449.—Pernicious anemia showing *A*, atrophic glossitis, *B*, atrophic gastritis (gastroscopically), *C*, fatty change in the heart (stippling), and *D*, degeneration (light areas) of the posterior and lateral columns of the spinal cord.

pallor, abdominal pain, and sore tongue. The skin is lemon yellow in appearance; there is no wasting; the tongue is wholly or partially beefy red in color; the lower extremities disclose a loss of vibratory sense and in-co-ordination; the marrow reveals megaloblastic proliferation (Fig. 450); the blood shows macrocytosis, poikilocytosis (variation in shape), increase in mean corpuscular volume, increase in mean corpuscular hemoglobin, and a normal or slightly reduced mean corpuscular hemoglobin concentration; the gastric juice reveals achlorhydria, and gastroscopic examination discloses atrophic gastritis. The *diagnosis* is made from a consideration of the clinical manifestations as listed, especially in the presence of sore tongue

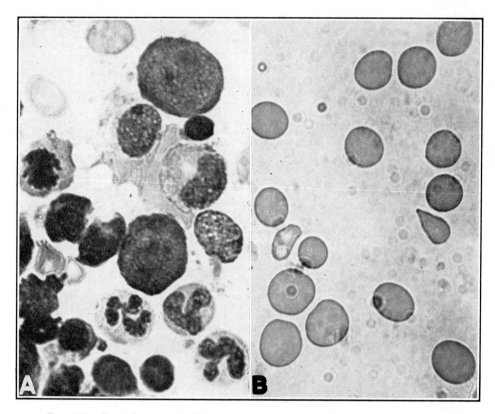

Fig. 450.—Pernicious anemia illustrating *A*, megaloblastic hyperplasia of the bone marrow and *B*, macrocytes in the peripheral blood. × 1380.

numbness and tingling, weakness, macrocytic anemia, and achlorhydria. Specific *therapy* consists of administration of folic acid (which controls the blood picture) and/or vitamin B_{12} (which controls both the blood picture and the neurologic manifestations). The *prognosis* is good for, with adequate therapy, most patients can be maintained in normal health.

Normocytic Anemia.—In this type of anemia there is a decrease in number of circulating erythrocytes, a normal size and normal hemoglobin content of the erythrocytes, no change or only a slight increase in mean corpuscular volume and mean corpuscular hemoglobin, and a normal mean corpuscular hemoglobin concentration (Wintrobe). Normocytic anemias are due to (1) loss of blood, (2) lack of blood formation, and (3) destruction of blood. They include such conditions as (1) *acute posthemorrhagic anemia* —any sudden and excessive loss of blood from whatever cause, (2) *primary refractory anemia*—also known as aplastic or hypoplastic anemia, caused by a disappearance of hematopoiesis in the bone marrow and its replacement with fatty or fibrous tissue, associated with granulocytopenia (lack of formation of leukocytes) and the thrombocytopenia (lack of formation of platelets), and occasionally occurring hereditarily (Fanconi syndrome) but more commonly and more specifically brought about by the administration of or accidental exposure to chemicals and physical agents such as benzol, arsenicals, gold compounds, nitrogen mustards, bismuth, mercury, silver colloids, dinitrophenol, trinitrotoluene, hair dye, volatile insecticides, antibiotics, sulfonamides, ionizing irradiation, etc. (Hunter and Jacobson),

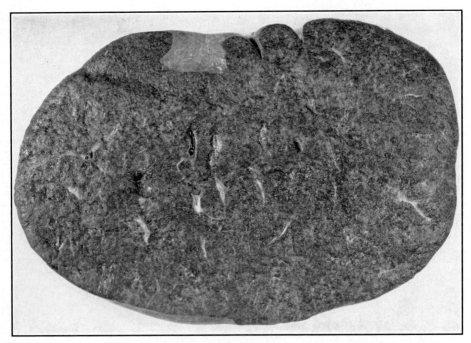

FIG. 451.—Congenital hemolytic anemia showing marked enlargement of the spleen.

(3) *simple chronic anemia*—the most common of all anemias, usually mild in degree, and seen in connection with a variety of inflammatory disorders (rheumatic fever, tuberculosis, syphilis, bacterial endocarditis, arthritis, osteomyelitis, bronchiectasis, dysentery, parasitic infections, etc.), renal diseases, malignant tumors, chronic pancreatic disease, chronic hepatic disorders, endocrine imbalances, vitamin deficiencies, and most pregnancies (Hubbard, Braverman, Middleton, Callen, Wintrobe, Daughaday, and Adair), (4) *myelophthisic anemia*—associated with space taking diseases of the marrow, also called leuko-erythroblastic anemia and leuko-erythroblastosis (because it is accompanied by the presence of erythroblasts and immature leukocytes in the blood), and seen in connection with metastatic tumors, multiple myeloma, myelofibrosis (replacement of the marrow with fibrous tissue), osteosclerosis (replacement of the marrow with osseous tissue), Hodgkin's disease, leukemia, lipoid storage diseases, etc. (Erf and

Herbut), and (5) *hemolytic anemia*—being acute to chronic in nature, resulting from destruction or hemolysis of erythrocytes, accompanied by a variety of clinical manifestations (varying degrees of jaundice, sudden or gradually developing weakness, malaise, headache, restlessness, irritability, pain in the extremities, nausea, vomiting, diarrhea, hemoglobinuria, hemorrhages, etc.), and occurring in conjunction with infections (malaria, septicemia, etc.), chemical agents (phenylhydrazine, benzene, aniline, acetanilid, sulfonamide, etc.), physical agents (burns), vegetable and animal poisons (fava bean, snake venom, etc.), immune body reactions (isoagglutinins, cold hemolysins, and cold, warm, and blocking antibodies), other diseases (as Hodgkin's disease, leukemia, lymphosarcoma, liver disorders, etc.), and intracorpuscular defects (as congenital hemolytic jaundice, sickle cell anemia, hemoglobinuria, and thalassemia) (Wintrobe). Of all the normocytic anemias listed above, the hemolytic anemias associated with intracorpuscular defects merit short separate discussions.

Congenital Hemolytic Anemia or Jaundice.—This condition is *also known* as chronic familial jaundice or icterus, hemolytic splenomegaly, chronic acholuric jaundice, hereditary spherocytosis, and spherocytic anemia (Wintrobe). The condition is a chronic form of jaundice that *occurs* in both sexes with equal frequency, is rare in Negroes, is hereditary, is associated with abnormally large amounts of hemoglobin F, and is transmitted as a mendelian dominant. The *cause* of excessive hemolysis is an abnormal fragility of erythrocytes but the reason for the abnormal fragility is unknown. The *pathologic changes* are disappointing. The spleen is enlarged to as much as 1,500 gm., discloses a smooth surface and a dark, purplish-red, homogeneous parenchyma, and histologically reveals small malpighian bodies widely separated by dilated sinusoids and a pulp packed with erythrocytes (Fig. 451). The bone marrow shows erythropoietic hyperplasia of the normoblastic type. Mild hemosiderosis may be present in the liver, lymph nodes, spleen, kidney, and other organs (Fig. 452). The *complications* are associated congenital anomalies of other portions of the body, impairment of body and mental development, biliary tract disease, and ulceration of the lower extremities. The *clinical manifestations* develop at any time during infancy, childhood, or adulthood and the symptoms and signs may be slight and barely noticeable or severe and readily apparent. Jaundice, varying in degree from presenting a sallow complexion to a true lemon color, is the most constant manifestation. Other than this, the condition is characterized by crises and remissions. A crisis develops suddenly and is due to a rapid increase in blood destruction. It is accompanied by chills, fever, lassitude, dyspnea, abdominal pain, vomiting, and anorexia. Otherwise, congenital hemolytic jaundice is characterized by splenomegaly, sometimes hepatomegaly, anemia to as low as 1,000,000 erythrocytes, spherocytosis (rounded erythrocytes), increased numbers of reticulocytes, increased fragmentation of erythrocytes in hypotonic saline solutions, leukocytosis after a crisis, normal or increased number of platelets, high icterus index, increased urobilinogen in the urine, normoblastic hyperplasia of the bone marrow, and roentgen changes in the bones similar to, but less severe than, those in sickle cell anemia. The *diagnosis* is made from the history, clinical manifestations, and hematologic studies. *Treatment* of choice is splenectomy. The prognosis following splenectomy is good. If this is not performed, the complications listed above may develop, or death may occur during a crisis.

Sickle Cell Anemia.—This is a form of hereditary, hemolytic anemia peculiar to Negroes and characterized by elongated, sickle-shaped distortions of erythrocytes (Wintrobe). The *sickling trait* occurs in about 10 per cent of the Negro population as a whole, but sickle cell anemia occurs only in 1 out of every 40 people with the trait. Sickle cell anemia almost always *occurs* before the age of thirty years and is as common in males as in females. Although the condition is hereditary, and associated with pathologic hemoglobins S, D, and G, the precise *cause* for the sickling remains unknown. *Pathologically* fatty changes are found in the heart and

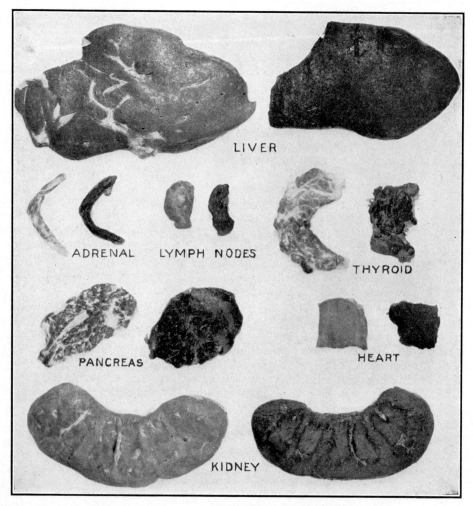

Fig. 452.—Hemosiderosis in severe normocytic anemia. The organs are labeled. One-half of each organ as it appeared in its natural state is on the left while the other half subjected to the Prussian blue reaction and staining dark is on the right.

liver; hemosiderin is noted in the liver, spleen, kidneys, lymph nodes, and bone marrow, and thrombosis with resulting necrosis and hemorrhages may occur in any of the organs (Fig. 453). Early in the course of the disease the spleen is enlarged and shows congestion of the sinusoids with sickled erythrocytes. Later, as a result of repeated infarctions and fibrosis, it diminishes in size and may weigh as little as 16 gm. The marrow of the bones of the calvarium, trunk, and extremities is grossly hyperplastic, jelly-like, and dark

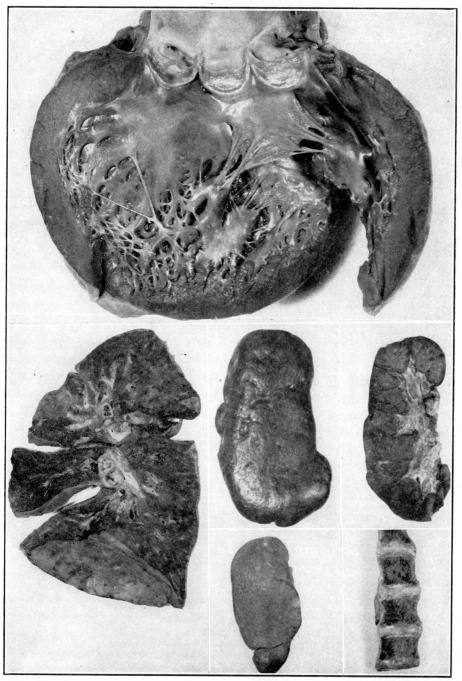

FIG. 453.—Sickle cell anemia illustrating enlargement of the heart, thrombi in the pulmonary vessels, scars in the kidneys resulting from previous infarcts, a small spleen with two scars and several recent infarcts, and hyperplasia of the marrow.

red and microscopically discloses hyperplasia of nucleated red blood cells.
The *complications* consist of (1) intercurrent (often tuberculous) infection,
(2) cardiac failure, (3) thrombosis and hemorrhage, (4) renal failure, and
(5) gallstones. The *clinical manifestations* consist of pale mucous membranes,
jaundice, fatigue, episodes of pains in the joints and bones, pain and tenderness in the abdomen, hepatomegaly, rarely palpable enlargement of the
spleen, cardiac abnormalities (enlargement, changes in rhythm, murmurs,
etc.), dyspnea, leg ulcers, bone deformities (kyphosis, scoliosis, and saber
shins), roentgenographic changes in the bones (especially thickening, ground
glass appearance, and radial striations—the so-called "hair-on-end" appearance of the skull), neurologic disturbances (consisting of drowsiness, stupor,

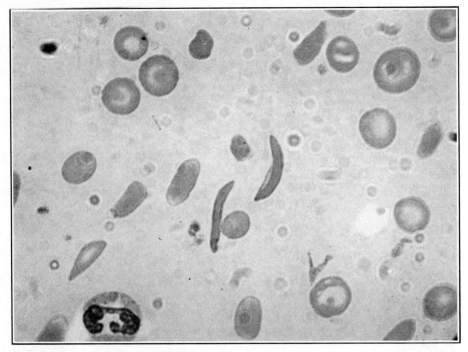

FIG. 454.—Sickle cell anemia disclosing distorted, elongated, and sickle cells. × 1380.

hemiplegia, aphasia, blindness, convulsions, etc.), anemia to 1,000,000,
sickling of erythrocytes (due to decreased oxygen tension and seen particularly well when blood is sealed under a cover slip and incubated) (Fig. 454),
presence of normoblasts (nucleated red blood cells) to as high as 40 per cent,
increase in reticulocytes to as high as 25 per cent, luekocytosis to as high as
30,000, increase in platelets to as high as 500,000, increased resistance of
erythrocytes to hypotonic saline solutions, slow sedimentation of erythrocytes, and changes in the bone marrow as indicated. The *diagnosis* is
achieved finally upon demonstrating sickling in properly prepared blood
smears. The differential diagnosis includes appendicitis, rheumatic fever,
osteomyelitis, and a variety of neurologic disorders. *Treatment* is unsatisfactory, consisting principally of administering blood transfusions. The *prognosis* is poor with most patients dying in the first and second decades of life.
   Hemoglobinuria.—Hemoglobinuria (Gr. = hemoglobin + urine) con-

notes the presence of hemoglobin in the urine. It results from a rapid destruction of erythrocytes in the bloodstream rather than in the reticulo-endothelial cells, with a consequent high concentration of free hemoglobin in the circulating blood. There are at least four entities in which hemoglobinuria occurs (Wintrobe)—(1) *blackwater* or *hemoglobinuric fever*—an acute hemolytic anemia with hemoglobinuria occurring in malaria and considered to represent a hypersensitivity to malarial proteins from previous infections (Blackie and Fernán-Nunez), (2) *paroxysmal* or *cold hemoglobinuria*—passage of hemoglobin in the urine after exposure (local or general) to cold, explainable on the basis of an autohemolysin uniting with erythrocytes in the presence of complement at low temperatures and causing

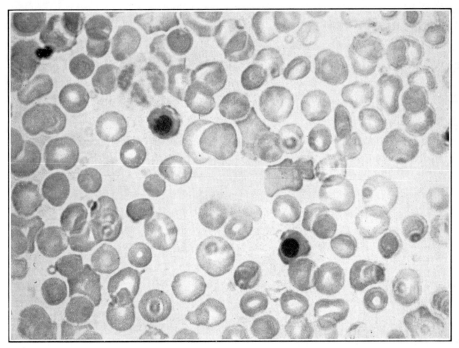

FIG. 455.—Thalassemia major showing poikilocytosis, a few target cells, and two nucleated red blood cells. × 1380.

hemolysis when the blood is again warmed, and characterized by generalized pain (in the back, legs, and/or abdomen), headache, malaise, vomiting, and diarrhea followed by a shaky chill, fever, and passage of dark brown or black urine (Jordan and Mackenzie), (3) *march hemoglobinuria*—presence of hemoglobin in the urine after marches (soldiers) or runners (marathon) with the cause unknown (Gilligan and Hobbs), and (4) *paroxysmal nocturnal hemoglobinuria*—chronic hemolytic anemia punctuated by attacks of hemoglobinuria developing essentially at night, occurring more often in males than in females, prevailing in the third decade of life, and characterized by slight jaundice and passage of dark red urine upon rising in the morning (Crosby). Two factors involved in the pathogenesis of the disorder are defective erythrocytes and the properdin system (Pillemer). That the properdin system is implicated is demonstrated by the following *in vitro* observations: (1) serum deprived of properdin only, fails to produce hemolysis of erythrocytes from a patient with the disorder, (2) the addition of properdin to such serum restores its hemolytic activity, (3) serum deficient in complement or magnesium ions (the necessary components of the properdin system) fails to produce hemolysis and the addition of properdin to such serum does not restore its hemolytic property, and (4) the higher the properdin titer of serum used in the *in vitro* experiment the greater is the hemolytic activity of that serum.

Thalassemia. — Thalassemia (Gr. = sea + blood) is an anemia that occurs in people originating around the Mediterranean sea. It is *also known* as Mediterranean anemia, Cooley's anemia, von Jaksch's anemia, and erythroblastic anemia (Wintrobe). The condition is hereditary, occurs in several members of a single family, is found in both males and females, and is associated with pathologic hemoglobins C, D, E, and G and abnormally large amounts of hemoglobin F. When the anomaly is *inherited* from both parents, the offspring develops a severe form of the disease known as thalassemia major, but when it is inherited from only one parent the offspring develops a mild form of the disease known as thalassemia minor. In *thalassemia major* the following are noted: insidious onset, pallor within the first two years of life, intercurrent infections, splenomegaly, hepatomegaly, stunting of stature, large head, mongoloid facies, slight jaundice, moderate lymphadenopathy, cardiac enlargement and failure, roentgen changes in the bones ("hair-on-end" appearance of the skull and medullary widening and thinning of the cortex in the long bones), elevated icterus index, leukocytosis, anemia to as low as 1,000,000 and, in smears of peripheral blood, poikilocytosis, presence of target cells (erythrocytes appearing as a peripheral rim with a dark circular area in the center) and nucleated red blood cells (Fig. 455). In *thalassemia minor* clinical manifestations are entirely lacking or consist only of fatigability and the diagnosis is made upon careful examination of the peripheral blood.

Microcytic Normochromic Anemia. — In this type of anemia there is a reduction in the number and size of circulating erythrocytes, a normal hemoglobin content of erythrocytes, a normal or decreased mean corpuscular volume, a normal or decreased mean corpuscular hemoglobin, and a normal or slightly decreased mean corpuscular hemoglobin concentration (Wintrobe). The entire group is associated with subacute or chronic inflammation and is poorly defined etiologically, clinically, and morphologically.

Microcytic Hypochromic Anemia. — In this type of anemia there is a reduction in the number and size of circulating erythrocytes, a below normal hemoglobin content of erythrocytes, a decrease in the mean corpuscular volume, a decrease in the mean corpuscular hemoglobin, and a decrease in the mean corpuscular hemoglobin concentration. Some of the many *synonyms* and subgroups are iron deficiency anemia, nutritional hypochromic anemia, chronic hypochromic anemia, idiopathic hypochromic anemia, chloranemia, chlorosis, chloritic anemia, asiderotic anemia, hypochromic anemia of pregnancy, hypochromic anemia of prematurity, and hypochromic anemia of infancy and childhood (Wintrobe). As some of these names indicate, it *occurs* at all ages and, although it is present in both sexes, it is more common in females than in males. The fundamental *cause* is a deficiency in iron. This may come about as a result of (1) chronic blood loss as from menorrhagia, metrorrhagia, bleeding peptic ulcer, bleeding hemorrhoids, ulcerating carcinoma, hookworm infection, etc., (2) disorders of the gastrointestinal tract in which digestion is impaired as in dysentery, sprue, postgastrectomy, postgastroenterostomy, etc., (3) deficiency of iron in the diet, that is, a diet lacking in meat, liver, vegetables, and fruit, and (4) excessive physiologic demand as in pregnancy. There are no specific or characteristic *pathologic* changes. The *clinical manifestations* may consist of the following: insidious onset, gradual progress, weakness, fatigability, pallor, edema of the extremities, hepatomegaly, splenomegaly, flatulence, heartburn, constipation or diarrhea, sore tongue, dysphagia, palpitation, cardiac failure, neurologic pains, etc. The hematological findings are those outlined at the beginning of this section. In addition, there may be poikilocytosis, increase in reticulocytes, normal or increased resistance of erythrocytes to hypotonic saline solutions, normal leukocytic and platelet counts, and normoblastic hyperplasia of the bone marrow. The *diagnosis* is made from the history, the clinical manifestations, and a careful hematologic examination. *Treatment* consists of correcting the primary condition and of administering iron. The *prognosis* is good.

POLYCYTHEMIA

As indicated in Chapter 6 (p. 188) *polycythemia* indicates an above normal increase in number of circulating erythrocytes. It is dividable into two groups — primary and secondary.

Primary Polycythemia. — Primary polycythemia is also known as polycythemia vera, polycythemia rubra, erythrocythemia, and erythremia. The condition *occurs* in all races but is rare in Negroes, affects males two to three times as frequently as females, and generally appears in middle or late life (Wintrobe). Although the disorder is distinctly familial in a certain proportion of cases, the *cause* is unknown. Among other things, the disease has been thought to develop as a result of oxygen want, simple hyperactivity of the blood-forming organs, excessive formation of the intrinsic gastric hematopoietic factor, abnormalities of endocrine secretion, and an unknown stimulus but analogous to that causing leukemia. The chief *pathologic* findings consist of (1) extreme vascular engorgement of all the organs imparting a deep red to cyanotic color, (2) thrombosis of arteries and veins with consequent hemorrhages, infarcts, and gangrene of the various organs affected, (3) enlargement of the spleen and liver, (4) hyperplasia of all the marrow elements causing the medullary cavities of the bones to be filled with dark red cellular material, and (5) extramedullary hematopoiesis in the spleen and liver (Fig. 456). Some of the many *complications* consist of vascular thromboses (various organs and so common that they are considered as part of the disease), intercurrent infection, duodenal ulcer, cirrhosis, hypertension and renal disease, bone marrow exhaustion with myelofibrosis, and (especially after the use of radioactive phosphorus) acute leukemia (Wiseman). The *clinical manifestations* are due principally to (1) the excessive amount of circulating blood, (2) vascular thromboses, and (3) the other complications enumerated. They may be listed as follows: headache, lassitude, dizziness, syncope, weakness, visual disturbances, mental changes, numbness and tingling in the extremities, deep red to cyanotic discoloration of the face and distal portions of the extremities, hypertension, gastrointestinal disturbances, splenomegaly, and hemorrhages. The *blood* discloses a count over 7,000,000 relatively normal appearing erythrocytes, increase in hemoglobin to as high as 40 gm., normal reticulocyte count, leukocytosis to as high as 50,000, increase in platelets to as high as 6,000,000, increased resistance of erythrocytes to hypotonic

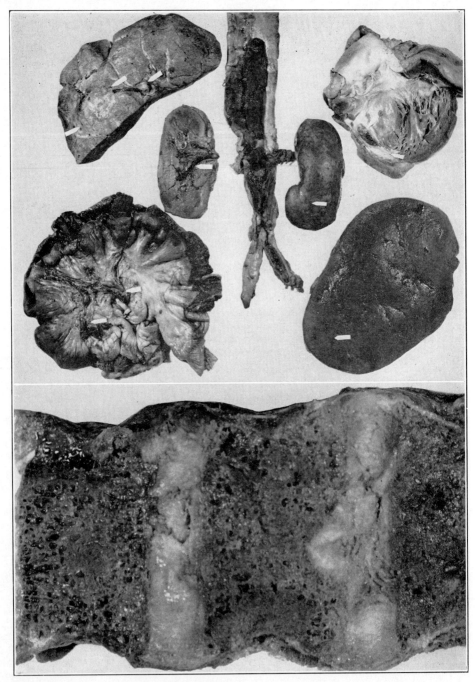

FIG. 456.—Primary polycythemia illustrating, above, deep red color to all the organs along with thrombi in the liver, aorta, kidneys, endocardium, and mesenteric vessels and, below, hyperplasia of the bone marrow.

saline solutions, increased viscosity and specific gravity of the blood as a whole, and delayed sedimentation rate. The *diagnosis* is made from the clinical manifestations and hematologic studies just listed, especially ruddy cyanosis, splenomegaly, and polycythemia. *Treatment* consists of phlebotomy and administration of phenylhydrazine, Fowler's solution, nitrogen mustards, and irradiation (Wiseman). Of these, the use of radioactive phosphorus (P^{32}) appears to be the most popular (Lawrence). The *prognosis* is fair with the course protracted to from ten to twenty years. The usual causes of death are vascular thrombosis, myelofibrosis, or acute leukemia (Dameshek).

Secondary Polycythemia.—Secondary polycythemia, also known as erythrocytosis, is a physiologic increase of circulating erythrocytes consequent to deficiency in oxygenation. Among other conditions it is seen in connection with newborn infants, congenital or acquired heart diseases, pulmonary diseases (emphysema, interstitial fibrosis, arteriovenous fistulas, arteriosclerosis, anthracosilicosis, etc.), and sojourns at high altitudes (Wintrobe).

PURPURA

Purpura (L. = purple) signifies the presence of deep red hemorrhagic extravasations in the skin, mucous membranes, and other organs of the body. It represents a heterogeneous collection of unrelated disorders that have bleeding as a common denominator (Wintrobe). The *classifications* are numerous and not entirely satisfactory. A workable division is based upon whether the platelets are numerically deficient—thrombocytopenic or normal—nonthrombocytopenic. *Thrombocytopenic purpura* may be divided into two groups—*purpura hemorrhagica* and *symptomatic*. *Symptomatic thrombocytopenic purpura* may be caused by (1) chemicals such as arsenicals, gold salts, benzol, dinitrophenol, quinine, ergot, organic hair dyes, antibiotics, etc., (2) vegetable products such as orris root, (3) animal products such as snake venoms, vaccines, and protein disintegration products (burns), (4) physical agents such as heat and ionizing irradiation, and (5) disease processes such as leukemia, anemia, splenic disorders, septicemia, bacterial endocarditis, typhus, etc. *Nonthrombocytopenic purpura* may also be divided into two groups—*allergic* and *symptomatic*. *Symptomatic nonthrombocytopenic purpura* may be caused by (1) chemicals such as iodides, copaiba, belladonna, atropine, bismuth, mercury, phenacetin, salicylic acid, chlorohydrate, etc., (2) animal products such as snake venoms, and (3) disease processes such as nephritis, chronic cardiac and hepatic disorders, avitaminosis C, bacterial endocarditis, septicemia (meningococcic), typhoid, influenza, scarlet fever, etc. Of the disorders mentioned, only two—purpura hemorrhagica and allergic purpura may be pursued further.

Purpura Hemorrhagica.—This type of purpura is *also known* as essential purpura, primary purpura, Werlhof's disease, thrombocytolytic purpura, and hemogenic syndrome (Wintrobe). Most cases *occur* within the first two decades of life; males are affected twice as frequently as females, and the disorder is uncommon in Negroes. The *cause* is unknown. *Clinically* there is usually a history of nosebleed or bruising readily. The disorder itself may appear suddenly with the usual manifestations consisting of pinpoint, larger, or ecchymotic areas of hemorrhage appearing in the skin and mucous membranes of the mouth and nose. This is followed by bleeding into the gastrointestinal, genitourinary, central nervous, and other systems. Accordingly, the symptoms may consist of epistaxis, hemoptysis, hematemesis, melena, hematuria, menometrorrhagia, and a variety of manifestations caused by bleeding into (rather than from) the various organs. *Hematologic* examination discloses reduction in or total absence of platelets, prolongation of the bleeding time, lack of clot retraction, positive tourniquet test (petechiæ or larger cutaneous hemorrhages of an extremity distal to an applied tourniquet), normal coagulation time, little or no anemia, and no change in leukocytes. The *bone marrow* reveals increased or normal numbers of megakaryocytes with only minor changes (lack of granules, vacuolization, etc.) in the cytoplasm. The *pathologic* changes (aside from the alterations in the blood and bone marrow already mentioned) consist only of varisized hemorrhages in the skin, mucous membranes, and other organs of the body (Fig. 457). The *diagnosis* is made from the

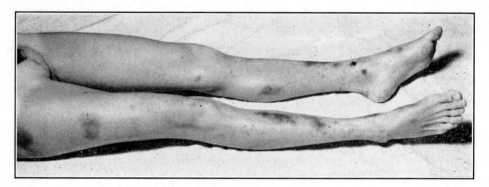

FIG. 457.—Purpura hemorrhagica illustrating numerous pinpoint to ecchymotic hemorrhages in the skin.

history, appearance of the lesions, and hematologic studies. There is no specific *treatment*. The *prognosis* is variable. In most cases, the disorder is marked by prolonged remissions; in some it disappears spontaneously, while in a few it is fulminating and rapidly fatal.

Allergic Purpura.—This caption encompasses the nonthrombocytopenic purpuras that are associated with allergic manifestations such as erythema, urticaria, angioneurotic anemia, etc. (Wintrobe). The disorders are due to increased capillary permeability rather than to any changes in the hemato-poietic system (blood studies are normal) and may occur in connection with hypersensitivity to bacteria, cold, or foods such as milk, eggs, potatoes, wheat, beans, meats, etc. Included in the group are (1) *Henoch's purpura*—purpura associated with a serohemorrhagic effusion into the gastrointestinal tract, attended by colic and other abdominal manifestations, and occurring most frequently in children and adolescents, and (2) *Schonlein's purpura*—purpura associated with hemorrhages into the periarticular tissues and seen most frequently in young adults.

HEMOPHILIA

Hemophilia (Gr. = blood + to love) is an inherited "bleeder's" disease transmitted as a sex-linked recessive from an affected father to a grandson by way of an outwardly normal daughter (Wintrobe). The sons of an affected male are normal and incapable of transmitting the disease, while the daughters are capable of transmitting the disease as an apparent defect to one-half of their sons and as a hidden defect to one-half of their daughters. The condition *represents* some defect in thrombin formation and is manifested by a greatly delayed coagulation time. The chief *clinical manifestation* is repeated, prolonged, persistent, slow, oozing of blood from various parts of the body, occurring spontaneously or after slight trauma, and being out of all proportion to the severity of the injury. The regions of the body commonly affected are skin, subcutaneous tissues, muscles, joints, gastrointestinal tract, urinary tract, lungs, and mesothelial-lined cavities (Fig. 458). Aside from the bleeding, the symptoms and signs will vary with the organ affected. Examination of the *blood* reveals only prolongation of coagulation time and reduced prothrombin consumption with a normal (except during or shortly after bleeding) erythrocytic count, leukocytic

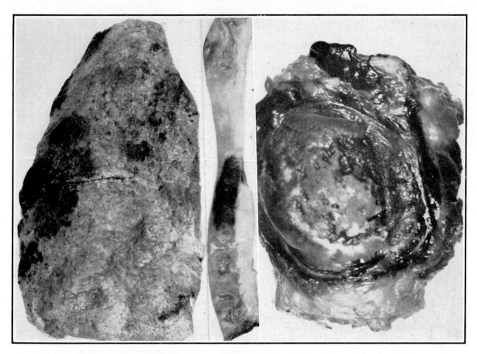

Fig. 458.—Hemophilia demonstrating, from left to right, hemorrhages into the lung, bowel, and joint of the upper end of the humerus.

count, platelet count, bleeding time, and clot retraction time. The *diagnosis* is made from the history, physical findings, and hematologic examination. *Treatment* is nonspecific and consists principally of transfusion of whole blood or plasma. Locally, application of (1) a pseudo-globulin fraction from rabbit or other plasma, (2) coagulating snake venoms, and (3) thromboplastic substances is carried out with success. The *prognosis* is guarded for over one-half of the patients die during the first five years of life. The most common *cause* of *death* is exsanguination.

Pseudohemophilia is a designation reserved for a hereditary disorder (transmitted by either sex and in direct line from one generation to the next) characterized by an excessive tendency to bleed in the presence of normal platelets, normal coagulation time, normal serum fibrinogen, normal prothrombin time, and prolonged bleeding time (Estren).

60

MALARIA

Malaria (It. = bad air) is an acute to chronic protozoan disease caused by organisms of the genus *Plasmodium* and, in nature, transmitted to man by the bite of an infected *Anopheles* mosquito (Craig and Faust). Artificially, transfusion of infected blood may also transmit the disease. There are four species of *Plasmodium* that are infective for man: (1) *P. vivax*—causing vivax or tertian malaria, (2) *P. ovale*—causing ovale or tertian malaria, (3) *P. malariæ*—causing malariæ or quartan malaria, and (4) *P. falciparum*—causing falciparum, malignant tertian, or estivo-autumnal malaria (Sawitz).

There are two stages in the *life cycle* of plasmodia—sexual and asexual. The *sexual stage* (sporogony) occurs in the female of an appropriate species of the *Anopheles* mosquito (Plate III). The blood-sucking female mosquito

---

EXPLANATION OF PLATE III.

Partly schematic. Drawn and rearranged by Williams, partly from Muir and Ritchie, partly from Kolle and Hetsch and partly original. Giemsa's stain.

The asexual forms show cycle of the organism in the red blood cells of the human host. They show schematically the time of fever and the day of segmentation.

A. *Plasmodium vivax (Benign tertian malaria)*.
　First day:
　　1. Segmented organism.
　　2. Young ring form in cell and a young form on surface.
　　3. Growing schizont; irregular form due to great motility; beginning pigment formation; red blood cell becoming paler and slightly enlarged.
　Second day:
　　4. Larger schizont with dividing nucleus. Red blood cells pale, stippled (Schüffner's dots), and enlarged.
　　5. Nucleus divided into four clumps.
　　6. Further division of chromatin and formation of irregular rosette. Pigment finely granular in center.
　Third day:
　　7. Segmentation. Note eighteen merozoites (usually sixteen).
　　8. Red blood corpuscle infested by merozoite from 7.—same as 2.—Cycle started again.
　　9. Same stage as 3.
B. *Plasmodium malariæ (Quartan)*.
　　Red blood corpuscles not enlarged. Rings are coarse. All developmental stages occur in peripheral circulation. Tendency to band forms. Segmentation every seventy-two hours. Merozoites are fewer, larger, usually 8. Pigment coarse.
C. *Plasmodium falciparum (Aestivo-autumnal, Malignant tertian malaria)*.
　First day:
　　1. Merozoites numerous, usually 32 in number.
　　2. Red blood corpuscle infested with delicate hair-like rings with chromatin dot. Frequently more than one parasite attacks corpuscle.
　Second day:
　　3, 4, 5, developmental stages occur in internal organs not found in the peripheral circulation. Parasites are sticky, adhere to themselves and intimal lining of capillaries.
　Third day:
　　6 and 7, completion of developmental cycle in internal organs.
　　8 amd 9, red corpuscles reinfected. Same as 2.
D. *Sexual forms.* Show cycle of development in mosquito.
　Fig. 1—(A to E)—Male (♂) and female (♀) forms of tertian type formed in human blood; F, flagellation of male type in stomach of mosquito; G, H, changes in female type and fertilization in stomach of mosquito.
　Fig. 2—Development of sporocyst within mosquito. Liberation of sporozoites which find their way to the salivary gland.
E. Sexual forms of *Plasmodium falciparum* found in human blood, showing development of sickle-shaped bodies.

PLATE III

A. PLASMODIUM VIVAX

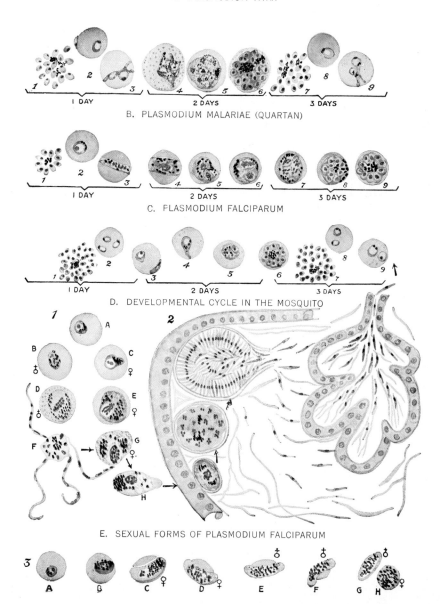

I DAY　　2 DAYS　　3 DAYS

B. PLASMODIUM MALARIAE (QUARTAN)

I DAY　　2 DAYS　　3 DAYS

C. PLASMODIUM FALCIPARUM

I DAY　　2 DAYS　　3 DAYS

D. DEVELOPMENTAL CYCLE IN THE MOSQUITO

E. SEXUAL FORMS OF PLASMODIUM FALCIPARUM

becomes infected by ingesting male and female gametocytes—sexually differentiated but immature organisms with the female being called a macrogametocyte and the male a microgametocyte. In the mosquito, the macrogametocyte loses part of its chromatin and develops into a female gamete (mature sexual cell) while the microgamete (by nuclear and cytoplastic division) develops into from six to eight flagellum-like motile male gametes. Union of a male and female gamete forms a zygote which becomes motile and is then known as an oökinete. The oökinete migrates through the stomach wall and, upon encysting, becomes the oöcyst. As a result of nuclear division, innumerable sporozoites are formed in the oöcyst and the latter is thus transformed into a sporocyst. Upon rupturing, sporozoites are liberated into the body cavity of the mosquito and those that reach the salivary glands are transmitted to man during the bite of the mosquito. The sojourn in the mosquito varies with the species but, in the over-all, lasts from eight to ten days.

The *asexual stage* (schizogomy) takes place in man. Upon being inoculated into the skin of man the sporozoites enter the bloodstream and, within thirty minutes, are deposited in the hepatic cells. By nuclear division, sporozoites develop into cryptozoites; the latter, in turn, develop into merozoites (measuiring 0.7 to 1.5 microns in diameter), and the merozoites are liberated into the bloodstream. Here they invade erythrocytes and are transformed into trophozoites—organisms consisting of a nucleus and a vacuole in the cytoplasm rendering it a signet-ring-like appearance. Obtaining nutrition from the erythrocytes, the organisms grow and in the process produce dark brown, finely granular, malarial pigment. Further multiplication results in the formation of a mature schizont—a spherical body containing varying numbers of nuclei (depending upon the species) that surround a collection of pigment granules. Rupture of the schizont and erythrocyte liberates the pigment and the daughter organisms or merozoites. The pigment is picked up by the reticulo-endothelial cells of the body while the merozoites repeat the erythrocytic cycle. Finally, the merozoites of the fifth generation develop into macrogametocytes and microgametocytes and these must be ingested by the mosquito for the cycle to be repeated.

Geographically malaria is worldwide in distribution, occurring in practically all localities where the warmest part of the year has a mean temperature of more than 72° F. (Craig and Faust). Of the four species, *P. vivax* is the most widely distributed. *Clinically* (after an incubation period of about fourteen days) the usual manifestations consist of paroxysms of chills, fever, and sweating, occurring every three days in connection with *P. vivax* and *P. ovale*, every fourth day in connection with *P. malariæ*, and every thirty-six to forty-eight hours in connection with *P. falciparum*. In addition, combinations of the following may be noted: (1) pains in the head, back, neck, muscles, etc., (2) gastrointestinal disturbances consisting of vomiting, pain, and diarrhea or constipation, (3) respiratory embarrassment, (4) jaundice, (5) cerebral manifestations consisting of convulsions, mental confusion, and coma, and (6) blackwater fever (p. 707). *Hematologically* the following changes are often noted: macrocytic anemia, poikilocytosis, leukopenia, relative monocytic leukocytosis, and the presence of the parasite and malarial pigment within erythrocytes.

Pathologically in fatal cases (1) the brain discloses congestion, edema, and focal hemorrhages, (2) the liver and spleen are enlarged, (3) the kidneys reveal congestion, edema, and hemorrhages, (4) the gastrointestinal tract

TABLE 5.—THE DIFFERENTIAL DIAGNOSIS OF THE MALARIA PARASITES OF MAN. (WRIGHT'S STAIN.)

	Plasmodium vivax	Plasmodium malariae	Plasmodium falciparum	Plasmodium ovale
Duration of schizogony	48 hours	72 hours	36 to 48 hours	48 hours
Motility	Active ameboid until about half-grown	Slightly ameboid during trophozoite stage	Seldom ameboid during trophozoite stage	Slightly ameboid during trophozoite stage
Pigment (Hematin)	Yellowish-brown, in fine grains and minute rodlets	Dark brown or almost black in coarse grains, rods, or irregular small clumps	Very dark brown or black in coarse granules or small masses	Dark brown in coarse granules or irregular masses
Infected red blood corpuscle	Much enlarged, pale with eosinophilic stippling (Schüffner's dots)	Not enlarged. Normal color. No granular stippling	Not enlarged or smaller than normal. Darker green (brassy). Basophilic dots and brick-red clefts in cytoplasm (Maurer's clefts or dots)	Somewhat enlarged, oval or irregular in shape, with eosinophilic stippling (Schüffner's dots)
Stages of development seen in peripheral blood	Trophozoites, schizonts and gametocytes	Trophozoites, schizonts and gametocytes	Usually only trophozoites and gametocytes. In pernicious infections rarely schizonts may be seen	Trophozoites, schizonts and gametocytes
Multiple infection of red blood corpuscle	Quite common	Very rare	Very common	Rare

Area of red blood corpuscle occupied by fully developed schizont	Entire red blood corpuscle which is enlarged	Almost entire red blood corpuscle which is not enlarged	From two-thirds to three-quarters of red blood corpuscle which is not enlarged	About three-quarters of red blood corpuscle which is enlarged
Trophozoites (ring-forms)	Small and large rings with vacuole and usually one chromatin dot. Ameboid	Small and large rings with vacuole and usually one chromatin dot; or early "band" forms	Very small and larger rings with vacuole and frequently with 2 chromatin dots. Peripheral forms common. (Forms appliqué)	Small and large rings with vacuole
Segmenting schizonts	Irregular, bizarre forms. Vacuole present in early stage. Chromatin in fine grains or small irregular clumps	Oval or round, with vacuole in early stage. Chromatin in coarse granules or irregular clumps. Band forms often seen	Not usually seen in peripheral blood. Oval or round with chromatin in large granules and in small clumps	Round and oval with vacuole in early stage. Chromatin in irregular clumps or filamentous masses
Segmented schizonts	Fill greatly enlarged red blood corpuscle. 12 to 24 merozoites (usually 18 to 20) irregularly arranged about a mass of pigment	Almost fill a normal sized red blood corpuscle. 6 to 12 merozoites (usually 8 to 10) arranged like the petals of a flower surrounding a central pigment mass	Not usually seen in peripheral blood. Fill two-thirds to three-quarters of red blood corpuscle. 8 to 36 merozoites (usually 18 to 24) arranged about a central pigment mass	Fill about three-quarters of red blood corpuscle. 6 to 12 merozoites arranged about a central or eccentric pigment mass
Gametocytes	Round and fill the enlarged red blood corpuscle. Chromatin undistributed in cytoplasm	Round and fill the normal sized red blood corpuscle. Chromatin undistributed in cytoplasm	Crescentic or kidney-bean in shape. Usually appear free in blood. Chromatin undistributed in cytoplasm	Round and fill about three-quarters of the enlarged red blood corpuscle. Chromatin undistributed in cytoplasm

(CRAIG and FAUST, *Clinical Parasitology*, Lea & Febiger, 5th Edition, 1951, pages 246 and 247).

shows congestion, focal hemorrhages, and mucosal ulcerations, (5) the heart discloses a fatty change and sometimes infarction, and (6) all the organs reveal a slate gray discoloration (due to the presence of malarial pigment). The *histologic* changes consist of (1) plugging of the capillaries with malaria-filled erythrocytes, (2) capillary thrombi, (3) focal hemorrhages, and (4) ingestion of malarial pigment by reticulo-endothelial cells, especially in the liver, spleen, and bone marrow (Plate IC, facing p. 66).

The *diagnosis* is made by identifying the malarial parasite in thick or thin smears of peripheral or sternal (marrow) blood stained by Wright's or Giemsa's method. In such preparation the cytoplasm of the organism stains light blue, the nucleus red, and the malarial pigment remains dark brown. In any infection, not only should the organisms be identified as malarial but the precise type of organism should be noted. The appearance of the organisms and the details of differentiation are given in Plate III and Table 5. *Treatment* is (1) preventive by eliminating breeding places of and destroying gametocytes through early treatment and (2) actual by administering antimalarial preparations such as chloroquine, pentequine, and quinine (Sawitz). The *prognosis* regarding life is excellent in cases of infection with *P. vivax*, *P. ovale*, and *P. malariæ* but is guarded in cases of infection with *P. falciparum*. The response even of this infection, however, to early and adequate treatment is good.

GRANULOCYTOPENIA

Granulocytopenia (Gr. = granulocytes + poverty) connotes a reduction in the number of granulocytes (myeloid cells) in the circulating blood. Some of the many *synonyms* are agranulocytosis, agranulocytic angina, agranulosis, granulopenia, agranulocythemia, hypogranulocytosis, granulocytic hypoplasia, and idiopathic malignant or pernicious leukopenia (Wintrobe). The condition is worldwide in distribution, *occurs* about two to three times as frequently in females as in males, and is usually seen in adults beyond the age of forty years. Although infection has been recorded as a *cause* most, if not all, cases are due to drugs such as benzene, organic arsenicals, gold salts, amidopyrine, dinitrophenol, sulfonamides, barbiturates, thiouracil, antibiotics, etc. While the exact mechanism involved is not understood, the condition may be brought about by an abnormal destruction of granulocytes in the peripheral blood as well as an arrest of their maturation in the bone marrow. The *clinical manifestations* develop suddenly and consist primarily of chills, fever, sore throat, and prostration. These are followed rapidly by necrotic pseudomembranous ulcers of the mucosal surface of the oropharynx, nose, vagina, anus, etc., and by a variety of gastrointestinal and central nervous system symptoms and signs. Jaundice is frequently present. The *hematologic changes* consist of leukopenia to as low as 1,000 or less, depletion of granulocytes to as low as 0, and a relative lymphocytosis and monocytosis. The *bone marrow* discloses (1) normal erythropoiesis, (2) agranulocytosis, and (3) relative increase in plasma cells, lymphocytes, and reticulum cells. *Pathologically* the most striking changes consist of (1) absence of granulocytes within blood vessels, (2) hemorrhages, and (3) multiple foci of necrosis in the lungs, liver, spleen, and other organs and ulcers of mucosal-lined surfaces all flooded with bacteria and devoid of leukocytic reaction. The chief *complications* are toxemia and secondary bacterial infection. The *diagnosis* is made from the history, symptoms and signs, and hematologic studies. *Treatment* has been varied with administration of antibiotics, transfusions, and nucleic acid derivatives favored. The *prognosis* is guarded although, with early and adequate antibiotic therapy, the outlook is considerably improved.

INFECTIOUS MONONUCLEOSIS

Infectious mononucleosis may be *defined* as an acute infectious, febrile and self-limited disease affecting primarily the hematopoietic system and related organs. It *occurs* at any age but is most common in the third decade of life, affects males more frequently than females, and is rare in Negroes (Schultz, Stevens, and Bernstein). The *cause* is unknown. Although the disorder is probably due to a virus, attempts to isolate the organism or to transmit the disease to laboratory animals have failed.

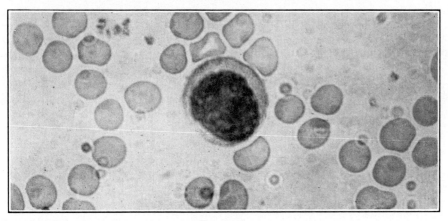

Fig. 459.—Infectious mononucleosis showing a large atypical lymphocyte with scanty reticulated or vacuolated cytoplasm and a large rounded nucleus filled with chromatin arranged in blurred coarse strands. × 1380.

The most outstanding *pathologic* change is the atypical lymphocyte or the infectious mononucleosis cell. In *smears* of *peripheral blood* the cell is variable in size but is at least as large as a normal lymphocyte. The cytoplasm is moderate in amount, light blue, and vacuolated or foamy (Fig. 459). The nucleus is large, and ovoid, rounded, kidney-shaped, or lobulated. The chromatin is distributed in coarse blurred or clumped strands. In *histologic sections* the infectious mononucleosis cell measures from 12 to 15 microns in diameter and is rounded. The cytoplasm is homogeneously and faintly acidophilic. The nucleus is central or slightly eccentric in position and is sharply delineated. The nuclear membrane is thin and occasionally indented or folded and the chromatin is irregularly distributed and mottled (Smith). While most of the organs of the body may be affected, the more important changes have been described in the spleen, lymph nodes, liver, and nervous system. The *spleen* is three to four times the normal size. Histologically the architectural pattern is blurred, the follicles are poorly defined and are devoid of germinal centers, and infectious mononucleosis cells infiltrate the capsule, trabeculæ, adventitia of arteries, and intima of the veins. The *lymph nodes* disclose a preservation of the architectural pattern, maintenance of the follicles with blending of the borders of the follicles with the adjacent pulp, proliferative activity of the pulp, and a diffuse infiltration of the pulp and periphery of the follicles with infectious mononucleosis cells (Gall). Biopsy of the *liver* discloses changes similar to those seen in nonfatal epidemic hepatitis (p. 824) (Wadsworth). The most commonly recorded changes in the *nervous system* consist of serous meningitis and meningo-encephalitis while the rarely recorded changes encompass neuritis and polyneuritis (Garvin). More specifically, the changes consist of congestion, edema, and hemorrhages of the leptomeninges and brain proper, focal collections of mononuclear cells in the same areas, and degeneration of ganglion cells. The nerves reveal degeneration of the myelin sheets and disruption of the axis cylinders (Bernstein).

The recorded *complications* of infectious mononucleosis are pneumonia, myocarditis, thrombophlebitis, hepatitis, edema of the glottis, hemorrhage from deep tonsillar ulcers, splenic rupture, serous meningitis and meningo-encephalitis, and peripheral neuritis (Shultz, Smith, and Garvin). The *clinical manifestations* usually consist of fever, malaise, sore throat, headache, weakness, anorexia, nausea, chilliness, chills, cough, abdominal pain, vomiting, diarrhea, stiff neck, general lymphadenopathy, splenomegaly, hepatomegaly, skin eruptions, jaundice, abdominal tenderness, and gingivitis. The pertinent *laboratory findings* consist of leukopenia followed by leukocytosis, lymphocytosis over 50 per cent, presence of atypical lymphocytes or infectious mononucleosis cells, occasionally anemia, demonstration of heterophile antibodies (by agglutination of sheep cells) in dilutions over one to fifty-six, hyperplastic (simple) or normal bone marrow, abnormal liver function tests, and frequently a false positive serologic test for syphilis. The *diagnosis* is made from (1) the clinical findings (especially pharyngitis, splenomegaly, and generalized lymphadenopathy), (2) lymphocytosis over 50 per cent, (3) presence of infectious mononucleosis cells in the peripheral blood, and (4) positive heterophile antibiotic reaction in titers over one to fifty-six (Schultz and Bender). The *treatment* generally is symptomatic only. Attempts to modify the course of the disease with antibiotics and chemotherapeutic agents have failed, but ACTH in seriously ill patients does have a salutary effect (Doran). The *prognosis* is good. As already stated, the disease is generally self-limited but relapses may occur within the first four months (Stevens). *Deaths* occasionally result from pneumonia, edema of the glottis, hemorrhage from tonsillar ulcers, or splenic rupture (Smith).

INFECTIOUS LYMPHOCYTOSIS

Infectious lymphocytosis is a benign, self-limited disease characterized by the presence of an increased number of small mature lymphocytes in the peripheral blood and bone marrow (Riley). The condition *occurs* primarily in children but may be found in young adults, is infectious and contagious, and has an incubation period of from twelve to twenty-one days (Lemon). The *cause* is unknown. *Pathologic* changes have been described only in lymph nodes. They are inconsequential, consisting essentially of degeneration of the follicles and proliferation of the reticulo-endothelial cells. There are no *complications*. *Clinically* the condition may be asymptomatic or it may be accompanied by infection of the upper respiratory tract, abdominal disturbances that simulate appendicitis, or manifestations that resemble early poliomyelitis. The only *hematologic* finding of note is a leukocytosis of from 20,000 to 140,000 with practically all of the cells (97%) being small mature lymphocytes. The *bone marrow* discloses an increase of mature lymphocytes. The *heterophile antibody* agglutination is negative. The *diagnosis* is made from the positive clinical findings, the normal appearance of the lymphocytes, and the negative heterophile antibody reaction. A differential diagnosis should include (among other things) infectious mononucleosis and leukemia. *Treatment* is symptomatic. The *prognosis* is excellent, for complete recovery is the rule.

LEUKEMIA

Leukemia (Gr. = white + blood) signifies an increase of normal and immature leukocytes in the peripheral blood and the hematopoietic organs. The terms *aleukemic* or *subleukemic* leukemia are reserved for the form of the disease in which the number of leukocytes in the circulating blood is normal or subnormal. Leukemia is a disease that is *widespread* throughout the animal kingdom, being found in man, dogs, mice, other mammals, and fowl (Wintrobe). In man it is a common disorder that appears to be on the increase for in the United States the recorded death rate was 1.9 per 100,000 in 1920 and 3.7 per 100,000 in 1940 (Sacks). Similar increases have been noted in other countries. The disease is worldwide in distribution, affects people of all strata of life, is uncommon in Negroes, occurs at all ages, and is about three times as frequent in males as in females. The *cause* is unknown. By most observers, leukemia is looked upon as cancer of the white blood cells of the body. If this is so, then the condition must be hereditarily predisposed. In fact, there are a number of reports recording its occurrence in several members of the same family (Ardashnikov and Anderson). Since, however, all members of the same family do not develop the disorder, there must be additional predisposing factors. Some of these are infection, ionizing irradiation, toxins, chemicals (arsenicals, benzol, aniline dyes, sulfonamides, etc.), hormones, and trauma (physical or mental). From a *metabolic* point of view, F. R. Miller has isolated two closely related and interconvertible acids—myelokentric and lymphokentric. Myelokentric (noncarbinol) acid occurs in urine of patients with chronic myeloid leukemia, chronic lymphoid leukemia, monocytoid leukemia, and Hodgkin's disease, and in normal livers while lymphokentric (hydroxy) acid occurs in urine of patients with acute or chronic lymphoid leukemia, lymphosarcoma, chronic myeloid leukemia, monocytoid leukemia, and Hodgkin's disease, and in normal livers. Myelokentric acid stimulates myelopoiesis and matures lymphoid cells while lymphokentric acid stimulates lymphopoiesis and matures myeloid cells. It is Miller's contention that leukemia results from an upset of the balance between these two acids. Myeloid leukemia is due to an excess of myelokentric acid and a depletion or withdrawal of lymphokentric acid; lymphoid leukemia is due to an excess of lymphokentric acid and a depletion or withdrawal of myelokentric acid, and monocytoid leukemia is due to an excess of both of these acids attended by pleomorphism and varying degrees of maturation of the cells.

The best *pathologic classification* is based on the types of cells affected. The most common and well-established groups are myeloid, lymphoid, and monocytoid. Each of these may be divided into (1) acute—lasting several weeks and attended by the presence of a high per cent of immature leukocytic cells in the circulating blood and hematopoietic organs and (2) chronic —lasting longer than a year (chronic monocytoid leukemia is extremely rare) and attended by the presence of a high per cent of mature leukocytic cells in the circulating blood and hematopoietic organs. In addition, some authors speak of a subacute form that is put between the acute and chronic forms of the disease. Other rare and less well-established forms of leukemia that need only be listed are eosinophilic, basophilic, plasma cell, and megakaryocytic. In *acute leukemia* the most outstanding grossly detectable change is hemorrhage. Bleeding may be in the form of petechiæ, purpuric spots, or hematomas. It may occur in any of the tissues of the body but is particularly prone to develop in the skin, mucous membranes of the

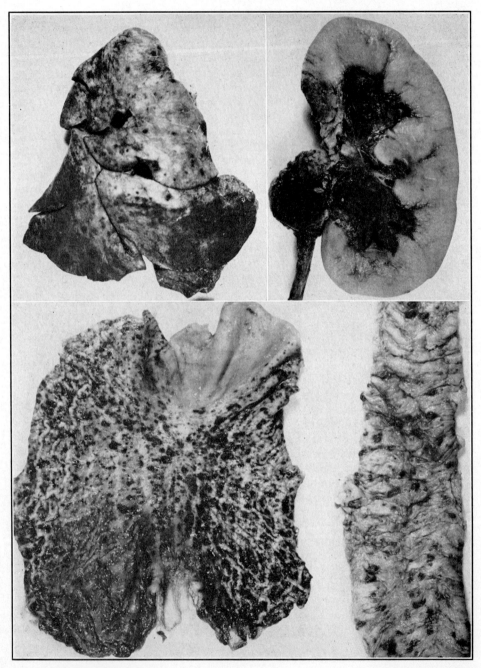

FIG. 460.—Acute leukemia illustrating hemorrhages in the lung, kidney, stomach, and intestine.

mouth and other portions of the gastrointestinal tract, urinary tract, lungs, and central nervous system (Fig. 460). The hemorrhagic extravasation resolves, progresses to form large masses, or, when near the surface, breaks through and produces an ulcer. The lymph nodes, spleen, and liver are generally only moderately increased in size. Indistinct, irregular, streaky

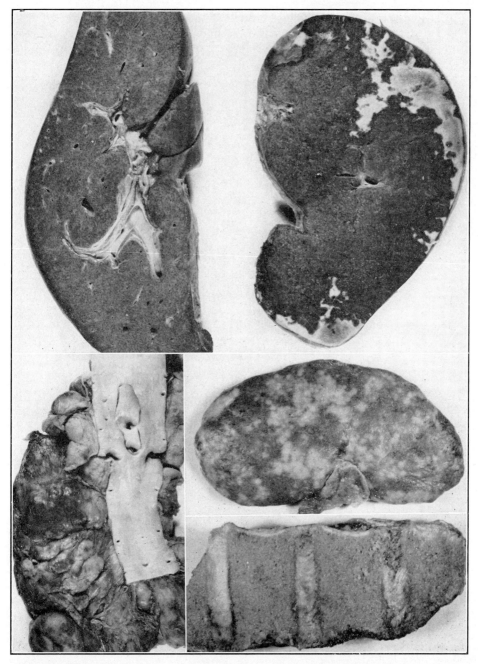

FIG. 461.—Chronic leukemia showing hepatomegaly, splenomegaly with infarcts, enlarged para-aortic lymph nodes, nodular leukemic infiltrations of the kidney, and diffuse replacement of the marrow by gray leukemic tissue.

infiltrations with grayish-white tissue may be noted in each of these organs and, in addition, may be seen in the kidneys, adrenals, heart, submucosa of the gastrointestinal tract, bone marrow, and subperiosteum. The subperiosteal changes (readily demonstrable roentgenographically) are limited to children and young adults. In *chronic leukemia* hemorrhages occur only terminally at a time when the disease has been transformed into an acute form. The lymph nodes, spleen, and liver are almost always diffusely enlarged but the increase in size varies somewhat with the type of leukemia (Fig. 461). Thus, the enlargement of the lymph nodes is greatest in lymph-

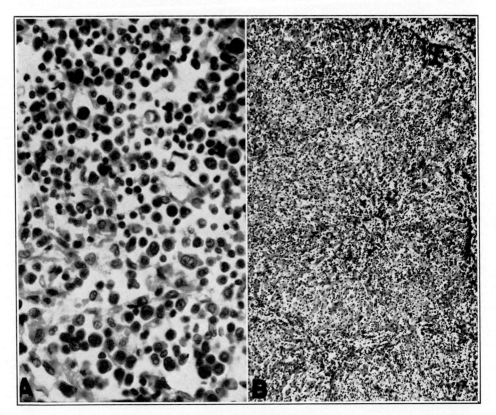

FIG. 462.—Myeloid leukemia showing *A*, myeloid cells in a lymph node. × 400 and *B*, myeloid cells diffusely permeating hepatic lobules. × 50.

oid leukemia and that of the spleen and liver reaches its zenith in myeloid leukemia. In addition, diffuse or nodular infiltrations of grossly identifiable, grayish-white (sometimes slightly greenish) tissue are found in virtually all organs of the body including the skin (leukemids), wall of the gastrointestinal tract, genitourinary tract, liver, spleen, lymph nodes, bone marrow, pancreas, adrenals, heart, lungs, and brain.

Microscopically the characteristic findings consist of the presence of increased numbers of mature and immature leukocytic cells in the bloodstream and the tissues throughout the body, especially bone marrow, liver, spleen, and lymph nodes. In acute leukemia the *peripheral leukocytic count* may at first be normal or subnormal but as the disease progresses it gradually increases and terminally may reach as high as 100,000. In chronic

PLATE IV

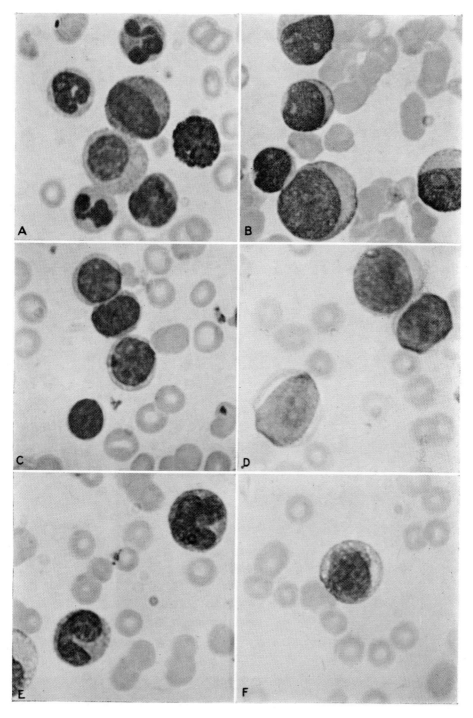

Leukemia illustrating *A*, mature and immature myeloid cells, *B*, myeloblasts, *C*, lymphocytes, *D*, lymphoblasts, *E*, monocytes, and *F*, a monoblast.   × 1350.

leukemia, counts as high as 800,000 in myeloid leukemia and 250,000 in lymphoid leukemia are not infrequent. The types of leukocytic cells vary with the types of leukemia (Plate IV). In acute leukemia, as high as 90 per cent of the cells may be of the blastic type and cannot be differentiated with any degree of certainty as to myeloid, lymphoid, or monocytoid. They are large, disclose scanty, basophilic, agranular cytoplasm, and reveal large, rounded nuclei with reticulated or condensed chromatin and one or more nucleoli. In addition to the undifferentiated cells, however, there are almost always present other more mature cells of the myeloid, lymphoid, or monocytoid series, thus allowing a precise diagnosis to be made. In chronic

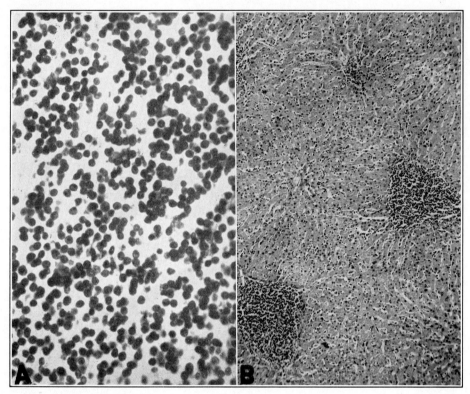

Fig. 463.—Lymphoid leukemia disclosing *A*, lymphoid cells in a lymph node. $\times$ 400 and *B*, lymphoid cells collected in clusters in the portal radicles of the liver. $\times$ 50.

leukemia, the majority of the cells are sufficiently differentiated to readily permit an exact classification. In *tissues* the microscopic changes consist of infiltrations with similar leukemic cells (Figs. 462, 463 and 464). The infiltrations may occur in any or all of the organs but are most prevalent in areas where reticulo-endothelial cells predominate. Generally the cellular permeations are diffuse and irregularly distributed but, in the liver, they tend to predominate between the hepatic cords in myeloid leukemia, in the portal areas in lymphoid leukemia, and in either or both sites in monocytoid leukemia. When the leukemia is acute the cells are immature and may be unclassifiable but when the leukemia is chronic they are generally differentiated enough to permit identification readily.

The usual *complications* of leukemia are hemorrhage, ulceration, infarction, anemia, intercurrent infection, and a physiologic failure of any of the organs (heart, kidneys, etc.) that may be affected. Regardless of the morphologic type of leukemia, the *clinical manifestations* are essentially similar and may be divided into two groups—acute and chronic (Wintrobe). In *acute leukemia* the following may be noted: sudden onset, weakness, general malaise, headache, sore throat, fever, constipation, pallor, hemorrhages (especially in the skin and mucous membranes of the mouth and throat), pains in the bones (especially children), a variety of

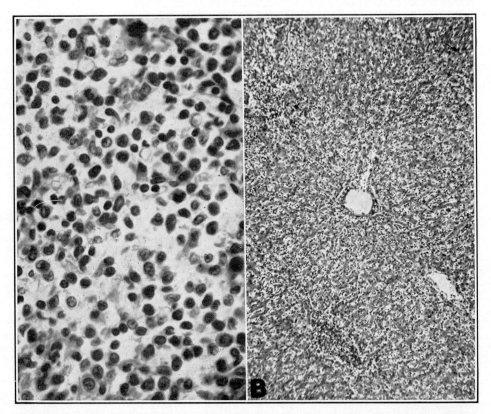

Fig. 464.—Monocytoid leukemia illustrating *A*, monocytic cells in a lymph node. × 400 and *B*, monocytic cells permeating hepatic lobules and, in one area, collected in a small clump in a portal radicle. × 50.

central nervous system symptoms and signs, and slight to moderate enlargement of the lymph nodes, liver, and spleen. In *chronic leukemia* the onset is insidious, ultimately culminating in symptoms and signs referable to (1) anemia, (2) pressure from enlarged lymph nodes, liver, and spleen or from leukemic infiltrations of other organs, or (3) systemic disturbances as a whole, including loss of weight, nervousness, weakness, and fever. From the *laboratory standpoint*, the chief findings occur in the peripheral blood. In acute leukemia there are severe anemia, thrombocytopenia, and leukocytosis or leukopenia with immature cells composing a large proportion of the entire leukocytic cells. Chronic leukemia may exhibit an unexplained, ordinary leukocytosis for months before the true picture of leukemia develops. When this occurs, examination of the peripheral blood reveals an increase in leukocytic cells with only a relatively small proportion being immature, varying degrees of anemia, and generally a normal platelet count until the terminal stages of the disease. Whether the leukemia is acute or chronic, the bone marrow discloses an abnormal proliferation of both mature and immature leukocytic cells and a decrease in erythropoiesis. The *diagnosis* of leukemia is made from the clinical manifestations together with hematologic (peripheral blood and bone marrow) studies. *Treatment* has been most varied and quite unsatisfactory. Among other things, it has consisted of administration of the following: transfusions, irradiation, and chemicals such as arsenic, benzol, urethane, nitrogen mustards, folic acid antagonists, hormones, etc. The *prognosis* is poor with death eventually occurring in all cases. Most patients with acute leukemia die within a few weeks or, at most, within six months. Patients with chronic leukemia, however, are more fortunate for the average duration of life is about four years and, in individual instances, may reach as high as twenty years or more.

REFERENCES

Pathologic Physiology

KRACKE, R. R.: *Diseases of the Blood*, 2nd Ed., Philadelphia, J. B. Lippincott Co., 1941.
TOCANTINS, L. M.: *Progress in Hematology*, New York, Grune & Stratton, 1956.
WINTROBE, M. M.: *Clinical Hematology*, 4th Ed., Philadelphia, Lea & Febiger, 1956.

General

WINTROBE, M. M.: *Clinical Hematology*, 3rd Ed., Philadelphia, Lea & Febiger, 1951.

Anemia

ADAIR, F. L., et al.: Am. J. Obst. & Gynec., *32*, 560, 1936 (Anemia in Pregnancy).
BLACKIE, W. K.: Clin. Proc. Cape Town, *3*, 272, 1944 (Blackwater Fever).
BRAVERMAN, M. M.: Am. Rev. Tuberc., *46*, 27, 1942 (Anemia in Tuberculosis).
BUTTERWORTH, C. E., JR., et al.: Blood, *5*, 793, 1950 (Spherocytic Anemia in the Negro).
CALLEN, I. R., and LIMARZI, L. R.: Am. J. Clin. Path., *20*, 3, 1950 (Anemia in Renal Disease).
CALLENDER, S. T. E.: Quart. J. Med., *13*, 75, 1944 (Pernicious Anemia of Pregnancy).
CARROLL, D. S., and EVANS, J. W.: Radiology, *53*, 834, 1949 (Roentgen Findings in Sickle Cell Anemia).
CHINI, V., and MALAGUZZI VALERI, C.: Blood, *4*, 989, 1949 (Mediterranean Anemia).
COFFEY, J.: Am. J. Roentgenol., *37*, 293, 1937 (Skeletal Changes in Hemolytic Anemias).
CROSBY, W. H.: Blood, *6*, 270, 1951 (Paroxysmal Nocturnal Hemoglobinuria).
CUMMER, C. L., and LaROCCO, C. G.: Arch. Dermat. & Syph., *42*, 1015, 1940 (Leg Ulcers in Sickle Cell Anemia).
DARBY, W. J.: J. A. M. A., *130*, 830, 1946 (Iron Deficiency Anemia and Oral Lesions).
DAUGHADAY, W. H., et al.: Blood, *3*, 1342, 1948 (Anemias in Endocrinopathies).
DAVIDSON, L. S. P.: Blood, *3*, 107, 1948 (Refractory Megaloblastic Anemia).
DAVIDSON, L. S. P., et al.: Brit. M. J., *2*, 95, 1943 (Nutritional Anemia).
DEBRÉ, R., et al.: Am. J. Dis. Child., *56*, 1189, 1938 (Congenital Hemolytic Jaundice).
DIGGS, L. W., and BIBB, J.: J. A. M. A., *112*, 695, 1939 (Erythrocyte in Sickle Cell Anemia).
DIGGS, L. W., et al.: Ann. Int. Med., *7*, 769, 1933 (Sickle Cell Trait).
DOAN, C. A.: J. A. M. A., *105*, 1567, 1935 (Splenectomy and the Hemolytic Equilibrium).
ERF, L. A., and HERBUT, P. A.: Ann. Int. Med., *21*, 863, 1944 (Myelofibrosis and Osteosclerosis).
FERNAN-NUNEZ, M.: Am. J. Trop. Med., *16*, 563, 1936 (Hemoglobinuric Fever).
GILLIGAN, D. R., and ALTSCHULE, M. D.: New England J. Med., *243*, 944, 1950 (March Hemoglobinuria).
GRAY, L. A., and WINTROBE, M. M.: Am. J. Obst. & Gynec., *31*, 3, 1936 (Hypochromic Anemia in Women).
HEATH, C. W., and PATEK, A. J., JR.: Medicine, *16*, 267, 1937 (Iron Deficiency Anemia).
HOBBS, R. E.: Am. J. Clin. Path., *14*, 485, 1944 (March Hemoglobinuria).
HUBBARD, J. P., and McKEE, M. H.: J. Pediat., *14*, 66, 1939 (Anemia in Rheumatic Fever).

HUGHES, J. G., et al.: J. Pediat., 17, 166, 1940 (Nervous System in Sickle Cell Anemia).
HUNTER, D.: Quart. J. Med., 12, 185, 1943 (Anemias and Industrial Poisons).
ISRAELS, M. C. G., and WILKINSON, J. F.: Quart. J. Med., 9, 163, 1940 (Achrestic Anemia).
JACOBSON, L. O., et al.: Radiology, 52, 371, 1949 (Ionizing Irradiation).
JORDAN, W. S., JR., et al.: J. Clin. Invest., 30, 11 and 22, 1951 (Cold Hemoglobinuria).
KLINEFELTER, H. F.: Am. J. M. Sci., 203, 34, 1942 (Heart in Sickle Cell Anemia).
LERMAN, J., and MEANS, J. H.: Endocrinology, 16, 533, 1932 (Anemia in Myxedema).
MACKENZIE, G. M.: Medicine, 8, 159, 1929 (Paroxysmal Hemoglobinuria).
MIDDLETON, W. S., and BURKE, M.: Am. J. M. Sci., 198, 301, 1939 (Anemia in Bacterial Endocarditis).
OGDEN, M. A.: A. M. A. Arch. Int. Med., 71, 164, 1943 (Sickle Cell Anemia in Whites).
PEMBERTON, J. DEJ.: Ann. Surg., 94, 755, 1931 (Splenectomy in Hemolytic Jaundice).
PILLEMER, LOUIS: Trans. N. Y. Acad. Med., 17, 526, 1955 (Paroxysmal Nocturnal Hemoglobinuria).
RUBIE, J., and CALNAN, C. D.: Brit. M. J., 1, 1079, 1949 (Nutritional Macrocytic Anemia in Temporate Zones).
SCOTT, J. M., and GOVAN, A. D. T.: J. Obst. & Gynaec. Brit. Emp., 56, 28, 1949 (Anemia of Pregnancy).
SMITH, C. H.: Am. J. Dis. Child., 75, 505, 1948 (Cooley's Anemia).
STERN, B., and ALTSCHULE, M. D.: J. Clin. Invest., 15, 633, 1936 (Blood in Hypothyroidism).
TAYLOR, E. S.: J. A. M. A., 112, 1574, 1939 (Leg Ulcers in Hemolytic Jaundice).
TOMLINSON, W. J.: Am. J. M. Sci., 209, 722, 1945 (Abdominal Crisis in Sickle Cell Anemia).
WHIPPLE, G. H., and BRADFORD, W. L.: J. Pediat., 9, 279, 1936 (Mediterranean Disease).
WILLS, L.: Blood, 3, 36, 1948 (Tropical Macrocytic Anemia).
WINSOR, T., and BURCH, G. E.: A. M. A. Arch. Int. Med., 76, 47, 1945 (Habitus in Sickle Cell Anemia).
WINTROBE, M. M.: A. M. A. Arch. Int. Med., 57, 289, 1936 (Anemia in Liver Disease).

Polycythemia

DAMESHEK, W.: J. A. M. A., 142, 790, 1950 (Course).
LAWRENCE, J. H.: J. A. M. A., 141, 13, 1949 (Treatment with Radioactive Phosphorus).
WISEMAN, B. K., et al.: Ann. Int. Med., 311, 1951 (Treatment).

Purpura

ALEXANDER, H. L., and EYERMANN, C. H.: J. A. M. A., 92, 2092, 1929 (Allergic Purpura).
BARTHELME, F. L.: J. Allergy, 1, 170, 1930 (Allergic Purpura).
DAMESHEK, W., and MILLER, E. B.: Blood, 1, 27, 1946 (Megakaryocytes in Idiopathic Thrombocytopenic Purpura).
GAIRDNER, D.: Quart. J. Med., 17, 95, 1948 (Schönlein-Henoch Syndrome).
HERTZOG, A. J.: J. Lab. & Clin. Med., 32, 618, 1947 (Autopsy Findings in Essential Thrombocytopenic Purpura).
JONES, H. W., and TOCANTINS, L. M.: Ann. Med. Hist., 5, 349, 1933 (History of Purpura Hemorrhagica).
PETERS, G. A., and HORTON, B. T.: Proc. Staff Meetings, Mayo Clin., 16, 631, 1941 (Allergic Purpura Due to Cold).
ROBERTS, M. H., and SMITH, M. H.: Am. J. Dis. Child., 79, 820, 1950 (Thrombopenic Purpura).
WINTROBE, M. M., et al.: J. A. M. A., 109, 1170, 1937 (Purpura Hemorrhagica).
WISEMAN, B. K., et al.: J. A. M. A., 115, 8, 1940 (Thrombocytopenic Purpura).

Hemophilia

ADAMS, M. A., and TAYLOR, F. H. L.: Am. J. M. Sci., 205, 538, 1943 (Use of Rabbit Thrombin in Hemophilia).
DAVIDSON, C. S., et al.: Blood, 4, 97, 1949 (Forty Cases Hemophilia).
ESTREN, S.: Blood, 1, 504, 1946 (Pseudohemophilia).
LOZNER, E. L., and TAYLOR, F. H. L.: J. Clin. Invest., 18, 821, 1939 (Coagulation Defect in Hemophilia).
MACKLIN, M. T.: Am. J. M. Sci., 175, 218, 1928 (Heredity in Hemophilia).
QUICK, A. J., and HUSSEY, C. V.: Am. J. M. Sci., 223, 401, 1952 (Diagnosis and Inheritance Hemophilia).
WRIGHT, C., et al.: J. Lab. & Clin. Med., 33, 708, 1948 (Theories in and Management of Hemophilia).

Malaria

CRAIG, C. F., and FAUST, E. C.: *Clinical Parasitology*, 5th Ed., Philadelphia, Lea & Febiger, 1951.
SAWITZ, W. G.: *Medical Parasitology*, New York, The Blakiston Co., 1950.

Granulocytopenia

FISHER, S., *et al.*: Arch. Dermat. & Syph., *55*, 57, 1947 (Agranulocytosis).
GOLDMAN, A., and HABER, M.: J. A. M. A., *107*, 2115, 1936 (Granulopenia Due to Dinitrophenol).
KATO, K., *et al.*: J. Pediat., *22*, 432, 1943 (Agranulocytosis Due to Sulfathiazole).
KRACKE, R. R.: Am. J. Clin. Path., *1*, 385, 1931 (Recurrent Agranulocytosis).
LOVEMAN, A. B.: Ann. Int. Med., *5*, 1238, 1932 (Granulocytopenia after Arsphenamines).
MOORE, F. D.: J. A. M. A., *130*, 315, 1946 (Toxic Manifestations of Thiouracil Therapy).
PLUM, P.: *Clinical and Experimental Investigations in Agranulocytosis*, London, H. K. Lewis & Co., Ltd., p. 410, 1937.
ROSENTHAL, N., and VOGEL, P.: J. A. M. A., *113*, 584, 1939 (Granulocytopenia Due to Sulfapyridine).

Infectious Mononucleosis

BENDER, C. E.: J. A. M. A., *149*, 7, 1952 (Diagnosis).
BERNSTEIN, T. C., and WOLFF, H. G.: Ann. Int. Med., *33*, 1120, 1950 (Central Nervous System Involvement).
DORAN, J. K., and WISEBERGER, A. S.: Ann. Int. Med., *38*, 1058, 1953 (Treatment with ACTH).
GALL, E. A., and STOUT, H. A.: Am. J. Path., *16*, 433, 1940 (Lesion in Lymph Nodes).
GARVIN, J. S.: J. A. M. A., *151*, 293, 1953 (Involvement of Nervous System).
SCHULTZ, A. L., and HALL, W. H.: Ann. Int. Med., *36*, 1498, 1952 (100 Cases).
SMITH, E. B., and CUSTER, R. P.: Blood, *1*, 317, 1946 (Rupture of Spleen).
STEVENS, J. E., *et al.*: Am. J. Med., *11*, 202, 1951 (210 Cases).
WADSWORTH, R. C., and KEIL, P. G.: Am. J. Path., *28*, 1003, 1952 (Hepatic Changes).

Infectious Lymphocytosis

LEMON, B. K., and KAUMP, D. H.: J. Pediat., *36*, 61, 1950.
RILEY, H. D., JR.: New England J. Med., *248*, 92, 1953.

Leukemia

ANDERSON, R. C.: Am. J. Dis. Child., *81*, 313, 1951 (Familial).
ARDASHNIKOV, S. N.: Brit. M. J., *2*, 955, 1947 (Genetics).
BETHELL, F. H.: Ann. Int. Med., *18*, 757, 1943 (Radiation Therapy).
BOWDITCH, M., and ELKINS, H. B.: J. Indust. Hyg. & Toxicol., *21*, 321, 1939 (Benzol as Cause).
BURCHENAL, W. P., *et al.*: Cancer, *2*, 1, 1949 (Nitrogen Mustard Treatment).
COOKE, J. V.: J. A. M. A., *101*, 432, 1933 (Acute in Children).
CROSS, F. S.: J. Pediat., *24*, 191, 1944 (Congenital).
DAMESHEK, W., *et al.*: Blood, 5, 890, 1950 (Treatment with Folic Acid Antagonists).
FISHER, J. H., *et al.*: New England J. Med., *246*, 477, 1952 (Splenectomy).
GELLHORN, A., and JONES, L. O.: Am. J. Med., *6*, 188, 1949 (Chemotherapy).
GOLDBLUM, F. C., *et al.*: J. Invest. Dermat., *20*, 1, 1953 (Leukemids).
HERBUT, P. A., and MILLER, F. R.: Am. J. Path., *23*, 93, 1947 (Histopathology Monocytic Leukemia).
KALAYJIAN, B. S., HERBUT, P. A., and ERF, L. A.: Radiology, *47*, 223, 1946 (Bone Changes in Children).
MARCH, H. C.: Am. J. M. Sci., *220*, 282, 1950 (In Radiologists).
MARLOW, A. A., and BARTLETT, G. A.: J. A. M. A., *152*, 1033, 1953 (Survival in Chronic Lymphoid).
MICHAEL, B., *et al.*: Ann. Int. Med., *35*, 194, 1951 (Myeloid).
MILLER, F. R., HERBUT, P. A., and JONES, H. W.: J. Hematol., *2*, 15, 1947 (Lymphoblastic Treated with Myelokentric Acid).
MOFFITT, H. C., JR., and LAWRENCE, J. H.: Ann. Int. Med., *30*, 778, 1949 (Longevity Chronic Leukemia).

Osgood, E. E., and Seaman, A. J.: J. A. M. A., *150*, 1372, 1952 (Irradiation Therapy in Chronic).

Reinhard, E. H., *et al.:* J. Lab. & Clin. Med., *31*, 107, 1946 (Treatment with Radioactive Phosphorus).

Sacks, M. S., and Seeman, I.: Blood, *2*, 1, 1947 (Mortality).

Silverman, F. N.: Radiology, *54*, 665, 1950 (Treatment with Folic Acid Antagonists).

Southam, C. M., *et al.:* Cancer, *4*, 39, 1951 (Natural History Acute Leukemia).

Wilson, S. J.: Blood, *6*, 1002, 1951 (Treatment with Folic Acid Antagonists).

Wintrobe, M. M., and Hasenbush, L. L.: A. M. A. Arch. Int. Med., *64*, 701, 1939 (Chronic).

Yaguda, A., and Rosenthal, N.: Am. J. Clin. Path., *9*, 311, 1939 (Relation Trauma to Leukemia).

Chapter

26

Spleen

PATHOLOGIC PHYSIOLOGY

GORDON O. BAIN

The spleen in the *normal* adult of average size weighs 150 to 200 grams. It is covered by peritoneum and is unattached except at the pedicle. The resulting mobility permits exercise of the splenic capacity for contraction and massive expansion. These properties are attributed to the presence of smooth muscle and elastic tissue in the fibrous capsule and trabeculæ and to the sponge-like character of the splenic pulp. Splenic contraction occurs in response to epinephrine but, in man, no significant change in blood volume results.

For descriptive purposes the splenic parenchyma is divisible into white and red pulp. The *white pulp* comprises the malpighian corpuscles. The *red pulp* consists of a reticulo-endothelial meshwork, the littoral cells of which form the walls of the pulp sinuses. The meshes of the pulp contain red and white blood cells in transit between the terminal arteries and the venous sinuses, as well as varying numbers of lymphocytes and plasma cells and large numbers of reticulo-endothelial phagocytes, some of which contain granular debris.

The spleen contains the greatest concentration of *reticulo-endothelial tissue* of any body organ. Since lymphatic vessels are confined to the capsule and trabeculæ, the splenic pulp is located exclusively within the blood vascular system. The spleen derives its blood supply from the splenic artery which is the largest branch of the celiac artery. After a serpentine course retroperitoneally along the upper border of the pancreas, this vessel passes through the lieno-renal ligament to enter the hilus of the spleen as several branches. Within the spleen, the splenic arterial branches, accompanied by veins, are located within the trabecular processes of the capsule. When about 0.2 mm. in diameter, they leave the trabeculæ to enter the pulp where, at intervals, they are ensheathed in nodules of lymphatic tissue, the malpighian corpuscles. The splenic arterioles terminate in brush-like tufts of penicilliary branches. Whether the capillary branches of the latter join the venous sinuses or empty into the tissue spaces of the pulp is disputed, but the latter seems probable. The pulp sinuses, which have perforated walls, are lined by the littoral cells of the reticulo-endothelial framework of the pulp. The sinuses unite to form pulp veins, trabecular veins, and ultimately the splenic vein which, after traversing the splenic pedicle, joins the inferior and superior mesenteric veins behind the neck and head of the pancreas to form the portal vein. Thus, the spleen is located in the venous system which serves the pancreas, the gastrointestinal tract from lower esophagus to the anal columns, and forms an important part of the blood supply to the liver.

The blood vascular relationships of the spleen are of great importance, for all known splenic functions, whether normal or pathological, appear to depend upon them.

Splenic *functions* relate principally to blood formation and blood destruction. During intra-uterine life the spleen is an active *hemopoietic* organ between the third and seventh months. In postnatal life, under conditions of unusual need such as myelophthisis or severe hemolysis, the spleen may again become the site of extramedullary hemopoiesis as a compensatory phenomenon. In addition, the spleen may exhibit extramedullary myeloid metaplasia apart from compensation for bone marrow or blood destruction in such myeloproliferative syndromes as agnogenic myeloid metaplasia, polycythemia vera, and chronic myelocytic leukemia.

Under physiologic conditions the spleen is the principal site of *destruction* of erythrocytes, leukocytes, and thrombocytes. At the end of their normal life spans, the formed elements of the blood are removed from the circulation by the scavenger cells of the reticulo-endothelial system, located largely in the splenic pulp. Under pathological conditions the hemoclastic function of the spleen may become exaggerated, with the production of *hemocytopenias*. This is thought to be one of the mechanisms involved in the abnormal functional state termed hyperpslenism.

The concept of *hypersplenism* (p. 971) presupposes an influence of the normal spleen on bone marrow function, either directly by a hormonal mechanism governing formation and release of blood cells, or indirectly through an effect upon the blood. Evidence that the spleen does exert some such regulatory function is derived from abnormalities present in the peripheral blood in splenic agenesis, consisting of target cells, Howell-Jolly bodies, occasional nucleated red blood cells, siderocytosis, leukocytosis, and thrombocytosis. Similar alterations in the blood follow splenectomy. In any of a great variety of conditions characterized by splenomegaly, there may develop changes in the peripheral blood which suggest overactivity of the regulatory functions of the spleen. The hypersplenic activity may be directed against any or all of the formed elements of the blood resulting in anemia, leukopenia, thrombocytopenia, or pancytopenia. Anemia of hypersplenic type may be accompanied by jaundice, hyperbilirubinemia, reticulocytosis, and excessive bile pigment excretion, or may show no such evidence of hemolytic activity. In the former cases it is thought that hypersplenic acitivity has taken the form of abnormal destruction of erythrocytes within the spleen. In cases of the latter type, it is presumed that inhibition of release of blood cells from the bone marrow is the mechanism of the anemia. Some cases of hypersplenism are complicated by the development of auto-hemagglutinins, and the separation of these cases from so-called acquired auto-immune hemolytic anemia is often difficult.

Some cases of hypersplenism are *"idiopathic"* and the pathologic alterations in the enlarged spleen are nonspecific in nature. In other instances, hypersplenism *complicates* some *other disease* characterized by splenomegaly (*e.g.* malignant lymphoma, leukemia, sarcoidosis, disseminated lupus erythematosus, hyperthyroidism). In all instances, the underlying *pathogenetic mechanism* appears to be a stimulation of the reticulo-endothelial elements of the spleen to increased activity. There appear to be three principal ways in which this may influence the formed elements of the blood, namely, (1) by increased phagocytic activity in the splenic pulp, (2) by depression of bone marrow release of blood cells, and (3) by the elaboration of auto-immune antibodies against erythrocytes, luekocytes, and/or thrombocytes.

The relative importance of these mechanisms is disputed but, under various circumstances, all three probably occur. The results of *splenectomy* are variable, being best in cases without evidence of abnormal blood cell destruction, that is, in cases in which the mechanism appears to be one of inhibition of release of blood cells from the bone marrow. The frequent failures in cases of hemoclastic type are commonly attributed to implication of reticuloendothelial elements in other organs and tissues in the pathologic process. Included in the latter group is a considerable proportion of cases which manifest auto-immune phenomena, including acquired hemolytic anemia of auto-immune type, in which postsplenectomy remission is often incomplete.

It is implicit in the designation "hypersplenism" that the *pathologic process* in the *spleen* is the primary process, antedating alterations in the blood cells. Such may not necessarily be the case. Congestion in the spleen is a finding common to many of the conditions associated with hypersplenism. In some instances, as in hypersplenism associated with hepatic cirrhosis, the congestion is clearly a passive process, but this is not necessarily the case in other instances. It is one of the functions of the spleen to sequester damaged or altered erythrocytes. Thus blood cells, the integrity of which has been challenged by such agents as viruses, toxins, or antibodies, may accumulate within the spleen as the result of an active, selective process. As a result, the splenic reticulo-endothelial tissue may be stimulated to increased activity. In this way, hypersplenic activity may, in some instances, be secondary to acquired alterations in blood cells, with the establishment of a vicious cycle which may have phagocytic, immunologic, and/or marrow depressing facets.

The relationship of the spleen to the occurrence of *anemia* in *hereditary spherocytosis* is better known. In this disease the hemoclastic activities of the spleen are clearly secondary to an hereditary, intrinsic, metabolic defect in the erythrocytes characterized by enzymatic defects in glycolytic metabolism which render the erythrocytes highly vulnerable to the effects of stasis. A concomitant of the enzymatic defect is the property of increased erythrocyte thickness, an abnormality which increases in degree as the cell ages. The spleen, indeed any spleen, selectively retains spherocytes in the pulp. Congestion of an actively selective type occurs in the splenic pulp subjecting the red cells to conditions of stasis to which they are highly susceptible. Under stasis, the thick erythrocytes become progressively more spherocytic and increasingly fragile. Many are destroyed in the splenic pulp. Others are released in fragile spherocytic form to breakdown elsewhere in the circulation. In hereditray spherocytosis *splenectomy* is curative of the anemia although the erythrocyte defect persists. This is because splenectomy removes an organ which selectively sequesters spherocytes and subjects them to stasis resulting in increased spheroidicity, increased mechanical fragility, and destruction. Since, in hereditary spherocytosis, the fundamental defect is known to be in the erythrocyte rather than in the spleen, it does not seem advisable to classify this disorder as a form of hypersplenism.

A special relationship between the *spleen* and *bone marrow* was suggested by the experiments of Jacobson demonstrating that animals could survive lethal total body *irradiation* providing the spleen were shielded. It appeared that the spleen elaborated a humoral factor which promoted recovery of the bone marrow from the effects of irradiation. While there are still many unanswered problems in this field, recent evidence suggests that protection may have been due in part to repopulation of the irradiated marrow spaces by hemopoietic cells from the shielded spleen.

Because of the special anatomic relationships of the venous drainage of the spleen, this organ undergoes certain structural and concomitant functional alterations in the presence of pathologic lesions of the portal venous system which cause *portal hypertension*. The pathologic lesions which may produce portal hypertension are numerous, but by far the most common is cirrhosis of the liver. Increased portal venous pressure is transmitted by way of the splenic vein to the spleen which, because of the discontinuous nature of its arteriovenous circulation, takes up the pressure in the sinusoids and pulp spaces. As a result of the sustained high venous pressure, the sinusoids increase in prominence and number ("sinus hyperplasia") and the pulp exhibits fibrosis and areas of hemorrhage. Because of its sponge-like structure, the spleen is capable of considerable enlargement under these conditions. Secondary to the splenic alterations there arises in many cases a *hypersplenic syndrome* characterized by anemia and leukopenia. In some instances, thrombocytopenia is also present. The association of chronic congestive splenomegaly, anemia, leukopenia, and hemorrhage from esophageal varices is referred to as *Banti's syndrome*. Banti's original concept of a primary disorder in the spleen, with the elaboration therein of a toxin producing the hepatic and other alterations, has been discarded in most quarters. The syndrome of chronic congestive splenomegaly with hypersplenism does not occur in chronic generalized systemic venous congestion, because portal venous pressure in this condition does not approach the sustained high levels seen in portal hypertension due to obstructive lesions located in the portal venous system.

Being in free and intimate contact with the blood, the reticulo-endothelial phagocytes of the splenic pulp are ideally situated for the removal of particulate *infectious agents*. Since it is a reticulo-endothelial organ, the spleen is capable of elaborating *antibodies* in response to antigenic stimulation. Thus, the spleen plays a dual role in defense against infection—phagocytosis and antibody production. Under a variety of septicemic states of bacterial, viral, protozoal, or mycotic types, splenomegaly is a frequent finding. Secondary hyperslpenism may complicate some of these conditions. In addition, splenomegaly and secondary hypersplenism may occur in certain reactive states such as rheumatoid arthritis, disseminated lupus erythematosus, and Boeck's sarcoid.

The spleen, being a reticulo-endothelial organ, is implicated in *lipid metabolism* (p. 51) and in the metabolism of *iron* and *bile pigments*. Since it is a principal site of red cell destruction, the reticulo-endothelial cells of the spleen are of major importance as elaborators of bilirubin. Iron released in the breakdown of hemoglobin is stored in the reticulo-endothelial cells as ferritin (an iron hydroxide—protein complex) and, when present in larger quantities, as hemosiderin. In many disorders, characterized by increased red cell destruction, hemosiderin is found in the spleen in increased quantities. Splenic *hemosiderosis* is also seen in states characterized by decreased blood formation as a result of depressed bone marrow function (such as pernicious anemia, hypoplastic anemia), especially following repeated blood transfusions. Iron stored in the reticulo-endothelial system is available for hemopoiesis upon demand, being transported to sites of erythropoiesis in combination with the plasma iron-binding protein transferrin (siderophilin). Thus, stainable iron is not demonstrable in reticulo-endothelial organs in iron deficiency anemia.

Finally, the spleen is an important *source* of blood *lymphocytes* and probably *monocytes*.

CONGENITAL ANOMALIES

Developmental malformations of the spleen consist of *changes* in *shape, fissuring, accessory spleen,* and *right-sided spleen* (in cases of *situs inversus*). The chief importance of *accessory spleen* lies in the fact that, if overlooked

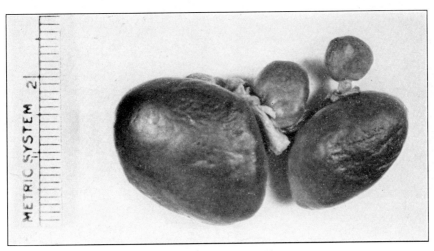

FIG. 465.—Accessory spleens showing four well-encapsulated and separated structures.

at the time of splenectomy, it may hypertrophy and cause a recurrence of the malady for which the operation was originally performed (Curtis). In most instances, accessory spleen results from a congenital segregation of splenic tissue but sometimes it occurs as a result of autotransplantation following rupture (p. 972). The incidence is recorded as high as 44.4 per cent in cases of splenectomy and as high as 35 per cent in cases at necropsy. While it occurs at all ages it is most frequent in the first two decades of life. The usual location is near the hilum of the spleen, but other sites include retroperitoneum, pancreas, omentum, mesentery of the large and small intestines, left adnexa in the female, and left spermatic cord, epididymis, and testis in the male (Bennett-Jones). *Grossly* an accessory spleen is rounded, encapsulated, and of varying sizes (Fig. 465). *Histologically* it resembles a normal organ.

DEGENERATIONS

Although degenerative or retrogressive changes occur in the spleen in conjunction with other disease processes, a few disorders that may be mentioned separately are (1) *atrophy*—small organ, wrinkled capsule, firm consistency, light reddish-brown parenchyma, and due chiefly to contraction of the organ following acute blood loss, (2) *hyaline degeneration*— affecting especially the capsule, producing what has been termed hyaline perisplenitis or "sugar-coated" spleen, seen in connection with polyserositis (Pick's disease) and other low-grade or organizing inflammatory processes, and characterized by an irregular or diffuse, gray to almost bluish, hyaline fibrosis of a part or of the entire capsule of the organ (Fig. 466), (3) *amyloid-*

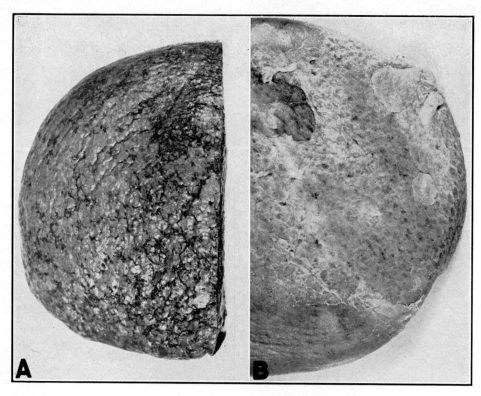

FIG. 466.—Hyaline degeneration of the splenic capsule illustrating
A, an irregular and *B*, a more diffuse thickening.

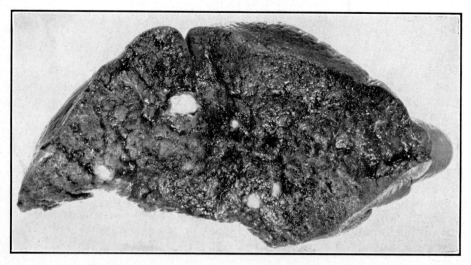

FIG. 467.—Multiple calcific foci in the spleen representing healed tubercles.

osis (p. 39), (4) *disturbances* of *lipid metabolism*—lipoid storage diseases
(p. 913), (5) *calcification*—found in connection with phlebitis, arteriosclerotic
splenic artery, aneurysm of the splenic artery, infarcts, hemorrhage in the
capsule, perisplenitis, parasitic or other cysts, and tumors, but most commonly encountered in healed tuberculosis and consisting of multiple,
varisized (to 1 cm.), sharply circumscribed, grayish-white, firm nodules
scattered throughout the parenchyma (Fig. 467) (Gray), and (6) *pigmentation*—seen especially in connection with hemosiderosis (p. 804) and malaria
(pp. 74 and 946).

INFLAMMATIONS

Orientation.—Inflammation of the spleen is called *splenitis.* The more
important inflammatory disorders of the organ may be listed as follows:
acute splenitis, abscess, tuberculosis, Boeck's sarcoid, syphilis, brucellosis
(p. 921), histoplasmosis (p. 513), and parasitic infection including echinococcosis (p. 828), visceral leishmaniasis (p. 923), and malaria (p. 946). Of
these, all but brucellosis and parasitic infections merit a few separate
remarks.

Acute Splenitis.—This condition, *also known* as acute splenic tumor and
acute hyperplastic splenitis, is seen in a host of acute systemic infections
including septicemia, pyemia, typhoid fever, acute tuberculosis, bubonic
plague, generalized anthrax, etc. (Symmers and Rich). The spleen is enlarged to as much as 500 grams and discloses the following changes: tense
capsule, rounded edges, soft consistency, mushy parenchyma, intense congestion, and a diffuse infiltration with neutrophils and their precursors.

Abscess.—Abscess of the spleen has been recorded as occurring in from
0.4 to 0.7 per cent of autopsies (Andrus). The condition has no predilection
for either sex, any age, or any race. The *cause* is any pyogenic organism
and the infection eventuates as a result of (1) trauma with local hemorrhage, (2) extension from an adjacent infection, and (3) metastasis from a
distant focus of infection. *Pathologically* the abscesses are usually multiple
and present the gross and microscopic appearance of any localized suppurative process (p. 135). The chief *complication* is the presence of abscesses
in other organs. The *clinical manifestations* consist of pain in the left upper
quadrant of the abdomen, fever, chills, leukocytosis, palpable spleen, abdominal muscle spasm, and elevation of the left leaf of the diaphragm as
demonstrated roentgenographically. The *diagnosis* is made from the
clinical manifestations, especially in the presence of a history of trauma.
Treatment consists of splenotomy or splenectomy. The *prognosis* in surgically treated cases with the lesion confined to the spleen is good.

Tuberculosis.—Tuberculosis of the spleen is always secondary to tuberculosis of other tissues or organs of the body, notably the lungs (Symmers,
Coffee, and Englebreth-Holm). By *primary* tuberculosis of the spleen is
meant those infections in which the spleen is noticeably affected but in
which infection of other organs is minimal or not readily apparent. *Pathologically* the disturbance in the spleen is of two types, namely, (1) acute
splenitis—seen in cases of acute tuberculosis with the reaction being entirely nonspecific and (2) actual tuberculous infection of the spleen. In
the latter, the involvement is usually of a miliary or disseminated (active
or calcified) type and, less commonly, of a caseating variety (Fig. 468). The
general *clinical manifestations* are those of tuberculosis while the local manifestations consist of splenomegaly (pathologically to as much as 3,780 gm.).
When the disease is to all intents and purposes limited to the spleen, splen-

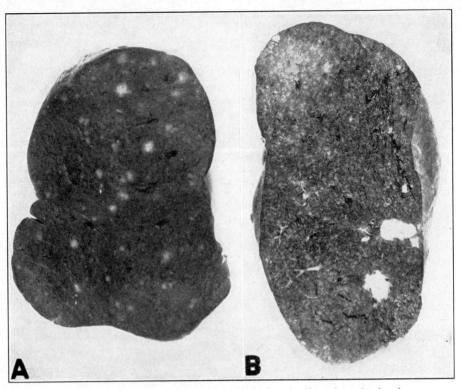

Fig. 468.—Tuberculosis of the spleen disclosing *A*, disseminated tubercles and *B*, miliary tubercles with two larger caseous foci.

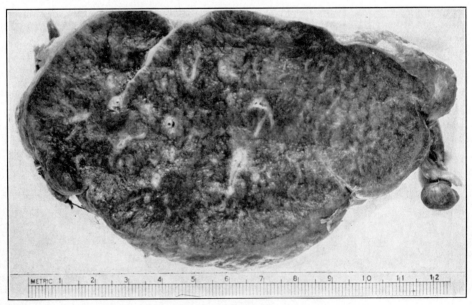

Fig. 469.—Boeck's sarcoid of the spleen showing nodulations that resemble those in cirrhosis of the liver.

ectomy has been advocated by some authors in order to remove an active focus of infection. This form of *treatment* has not, however, been universally accepted.

Boeck's Sarcoid. — In Boeck's sarcoid the spleen usually attains a weight of from 700 to 1,000 gm. but weights reaching as much as 4,800 gm. have been recorded (Symmers and Kay). *Grossly* the organ is diffusely enlarged showing a tense capsule and rounded edges. Both external and cut surfaces disclose either minute nodules that resemble miliary tubercles or larger confluent masses that bear a striking resemblance to the nodulations in portal cirrhosis of the liver (Fig. 469). *Histologically* the changes are similar to those in other organs with the characteristic unit being the hard tubercle (p. 501). The disease is always part of a general infection, but *clinically* splenomegaly may be the most outstanding manifestation.

Syphilis. — In *congenital syphilis* the spleen is increased in size to as much as twice normal. The pathologic changes are nonspecific consisting of dilatation of the sinusoids, lining of the sinusoids with prominent endothelial cells, some fibrosis of the pulp, and the presence of hematopoietic foci. In *acquired syphilis* the involvement may consist of the following: (1) diffuse splenomegaly in about one-third of all cases with the early form of the disease due to either a diffuse hyperplasia of the lymph follicles or an acute splenitis, (2) nonspecific congestion, fibrosis, and foci of iron-calcium incrustation (focal hemosiderosis, fibrous tissue reaction, and calcium deposition) seen in conjunction with advanced hepar lobatum, and (3) rarely single or multiple circumscribed gummas (Symmers and Harmos).

PHYSICAL DISTURBANCES

Orientation. — Under this heading may be listed the following disorders of the spleen: (1) *simple passive hyperemia* — seen in conjunction with hyperemia due to disturbances in the heart and lungs (p. 193), (2) *congestive splenomegaly* — seen in conjunction with portal hypertension (p. 831), (3) *infarction* — seen as a result of simple vascular occlusion (p. 190) but occasionally also as a result of torsion of the organ about a long pedicle (Adkins), (4) *hypersplenism*, (5) *Felty's syndrome*, (6) *rupture*, and (7) *indications* for *splenectomy*. Of these, the four mentioned last merit brief separate consideration.

Hypersplenism. — This condition, also *referred to* as splenic neutropenia and splenic panhematopenia, is a syndrome characterized by splenomegaly, decrease in some or all of the circulating elements (leukocytes, platelets, and erythrocytes) of the blood, hyperplasia of the bone marrow, and demonstration of splenic overactivity by the epinephrine test (shrinkage of the spleen after injection of epinephrine) (Schatken). *Clinically* the condition has been divided into two groups — primary and secondary (Zollinger). *Primary hypersplenism* encompasses those conditions attended by a primary reduction of platelets (purpura hemorrhagica), of erythrocytes (congenital hemolytic jaundice), of neutrophils (primary splenic neutropenia), or of combinations of these (primary pancytopenia). *Secondary hypersplenism* produces a picture similar to that in primary hypersplenism but occurs as a complication of chronic leukemia, portal hypertension, Boeck's sarcoid, Hodgkin's disease, acquired hemolytic anemia, Felty's syndrome, etc. The *pathologic* changes in the spleen vary with the type of hypersplenism. In the primary form, prominent ring-like cuffing zones about malpighian follicles have been described as characteristic (Leffler).   In the secondary form, the alterations are those of the predisposing condition (p. 964).

Felty's Syndrome.—Felty's syndrome consists of polyarthritis, fever, secondary anemia, leukopenia, and splenomegaly (Rogers and Kanar). The cause of the syndrome is unknown.   In fact, some authors do not accept it as an entity, looking upon the disorder as rheumatoid arthritis with associated complications or, conversely, as primary splenic neutropenia in which arthritis develops.   At any rate, splenectomy ameliorates the symptoms and signs.

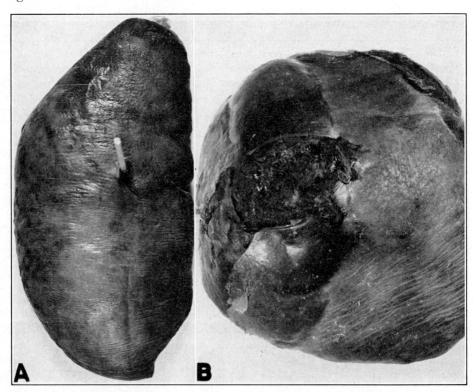

FIG. 470.—Rupture of the spleen illustrating *A*, a stab wound and *B*, irregular tear with a sugcapsular hematoma.

Rupture.—Rupture of the spleen may be spontaneous or traumatic. *Spontaneous rupture* usually occurs in connection with a previously diseased organ (malaria, infectious mononucleosis, leukemia, typhoid fever, infarction, systemic infections, etc.) or, rarely, in connection with a previously healthy organ (Brines). It must hastily be added, however, that some authors doubt the latter possibility.   In support of this, they state that a slight unnoticed or forgotten trauma or that the possibility of an infarct or other focus can never be ruled out entirely. *Traumatic rupture* of the spleen is relatively common (Byrne). It occurs at any age and results from direct, indirect, penetrating, or nonpenetrating injury (automobile or bicycle accident, fall, gunshot wound, stab wound, etc.). *Pathologically* any portion of the spleen may be affected. The organ is generally enlarged; the capsule is intact, penetrated, or irregularly torn; the parenchyma is irregularly lacerated or punctured, and bleeding occurs into the spleen, beneath the splenic capsule, or into the perisplenic tissues (Fig. 470). The types, shapes, sizes, and number of the defects depend, to a considerable extent, upon the types of injuries sustained. The chief *complications* consist of (1) hemorrhage—immediate (within twenty-four hours) or delayed (beyond twenty-four hours), (2) secondary infection, and (3) peritoneal autotransplantation of splenic tissue (Waugh). The *clinical manifestations* consist of (1) pain in the abdomen, shoulder, or chest, (2) abdominal tenderness and rigidity, (3) dullness in the flanks, and (4) acute anemia. The picture is modified somewhat in cases of severe trauma or severe bleeding in which shock is superimposed. *Treatment* consists of blood transfusions and surgical excision of the organ (Larghero). The *prognosis* is fair to good, with mortality rates as high as 15 to 20 per cent being recorded.

Indications for Splenectomy.—The more important indications for surgical removal of the spleen may be listed as follows: portal hypertension, Felty's syndrome, hemolytic jaundice, purpura hemorrhagica, primary splenic neutropenia, primary pancytopenia, rupture, primary tumors, abscesses, certain cases of Gaucher's disease, certain cases of malaria, and ptosis (Welch and Bate). The usual *contraindications* for splenectomy are acute splenitis, Hodgkin's disease, leukemia, metastatic tumor, most parasitic infections, pernicious anemia, polycythemia, and sickle cell anemia. Some of the *complications* of splenectomy are as follows: (1) venous thrombosis—portal, pulmonary, cerebral, etc., (2) hemorrhage—massive or oozing and coming from the splenic pedicle, pancreas, or injured adjacent structures, (3) infection—subdiaphragmatic abscess, peritonitis, or wound infection, and (4) miscellaneous—peritoneal transplantation of splenic tissue, failure to remove all splenic (accessory) tissue, fever, and hemolytic crisis (Martin).

TUMORS

Orientation.—Tumors of the spleen are not nearly as common as tumors of other organs of comparable size. They *occur* at all ages, in all races, and in both sexes. Some are congenital while others are acquired but, in either case, the *causes* remain unknown. *Pathologically* they are characterized by diffuse or focal enlargements (sometimes to enormous proportions) of the spleen with or without the presence of grossly detectable masses (Fig. 471). *Histologically* they vary with the type of growth and are classified as primary or secondary. Primary tumors are further dividable into the following: hamartoma, hemangioma, hemangio-endothelioma (hemangiosarcoma), lymphoblastoma, cyst, fibroma, fibrosarcoma, leiomyoma, leiomyosarcoma, neuroma, and neurosarcoma (Bostick and Lazarus). The chief *complication* is in connection with malignant tumors in which metastases to other (usually liver, lungs, lymph nodes, pancreas, and bones) organs of the body occur. In primary splenic growths, metastases occur after the local origin of the tumor while in secondary splenic growths they may occur before, at the same time, or after the tumor appears in the spleen. *Clinically* benign tumors may be entirely asymptomatic or may be associated only with splenomegaly. Malignant tumors, on the other hand, are accompanied by a rapidly growing mass in the region of the spleen, pain in the same area, loss of weight, downward displacement of the left kidney (visualized roentgenographically), anemia, and often thrombocytopenia (Wachstein). The *diagnosis* of splenomegaly is readily made, but the nature of the splenic enlargement is more difficult to ascertain. Aspiration biopsy of the spleen has been both advocated and condemned. *Treatment* consists of splenectomy. The *prognosis* in benign tumors is good while that in malignant tumors is poor. Aside from the general comments just concluded, a few separate words may be said about the more common growths.

Cysts.—Cysts of the spleen are uncommon for, by 1948, there were only 168 cases recorded in the literature (Tamaki). While classifications are many, the lesions may be divided into parasitic and nonparasitic. The latter, in turn, may be considered as primary and secondary. *Primary nonparasitic cysts* are about one-fourth as frequent as secondary nonparasitic cysts. They may be lymphangiomatous or epidermoid in nature (Fischl and Bean). Lymphangiomatous cysts are usually multiple, vary in size, are filled with clear fluid, and are lined with endothelial cells (Fig.

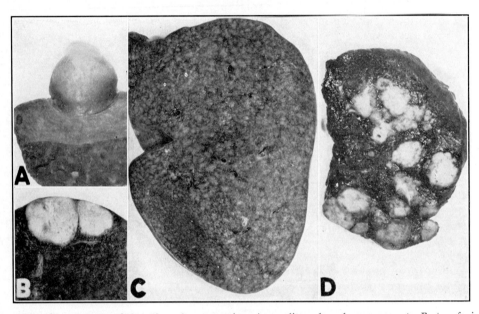

Fig. 471.—Tumors of the spleen demonstrating *A*, a solitary lymphogenous cyst, *B*, two foci of metastatic carcinoma from the urinary bladder, *C*, lymphosarcoma with diffusely distributed, ill-defined foci, and *D*, Hodgkin's disease with many rather sharply defined tumor masses.

471*A*). Epidermoid cysts are usually single but may be multiple, are filled with clear, greenish or blood-tinged fluid, and are lined by squamous epithelial cells. *Secondary nonparasitic cysts* almost always occur as a result of trauma and are thus, in reality, hematomas that have become cystic. They may be single or multiple and vary in size from a few millimeters to many centimeters (Fig. 472). The wall is composed essentially of dense or cellular fibrous tissue and may or may not be calcified. The inner surface usually lacks a lining of endothelial or epithelial cells. The lumen contains fluid or coagulated blood, or clear fluid filled with shimmering cholesterol crystals.

Hamartoma.—Benign splenic tumors composed of mixtures of normal splenic elements abnormally arranged are uncommon for, by 1952, there were only 23 cases recorded (Coe). The growths are spherical, possess a pseudocapsule that demarcates them from the adjacent parenchyma, measure from 0.8 to 23 cm. in diameter, are generally solitary and solid, and histologically consist principally of varying combinations of lymphoid and sinusoidal tissue.

Hemangioma.—Hemangioma of the spleen is rare, there having been a total of 31 cases reported on by 1947 (Hodge). The tumors vary in size, sometimes reaching large proportions. Grossly they appear as a sponge-like network of trabeculæ filled with blood and may or may not disclose larger cystic spaces. Histologically they are generally of the cavernous variety. The chief complication is rupture with serious intraperitoneal hemorrhage.

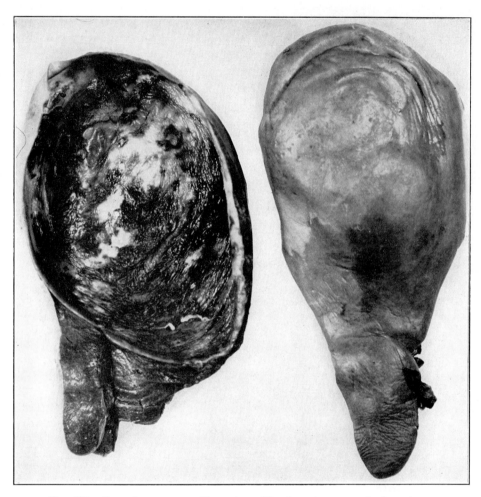

FIG. 472.—Secondary nonparasitic cyst resulting from trauma and a hematoma.

Lymphoblastoma.—Lymphoblastomas of the spleen are similar to lymph-oblastomas of lymph nodes and other organs (p. 984). This group is the most common of all primary tumors of the spleen. In leukemia, the organ is diffusely and homogeneously enlarged and, in the chronic forms of the disease, may attain a weight of as much as 5,000 gm. (Krumbhaar). In other types of lymphoblastoma (Hodgkin's disease, lymphosarcoma, etc.) the enlargement is usually less and the distribution may be diffuse and homogeneous, finely nodular, or massive (Fig. 471C and D). Histologically the lesions are similar to those in the lymph nodes.

Secondary Tumors. — Secondary tumors of the spleen are uncommon in comparison with secondary tumors of other organs, for they constitute only from 0.3 to 4.8 per cent of all cases coming to necropsy (Herbut and Hirst). As far as malignant tumors of the spleen are concerned, however, they are more common than primary growths. Almost every organ of the body has served as the initial site of the neoplasm with the most common being carcinoma of the stomach, lung, pancreas, and breast. The lesions affect the spleen by metastasis, direct extension, or peritoneal implantation. Grossly the spleen may be diffusely enlarged, may disclose innumerable foci of tumor, or may reveal one or more large circumscribed masses (Fig. 471*B*). Histologically the growths appear similar to the parent neoplasms.

REFERENCES

Pathologic Physiology

CHERTKOW, G., and DACIE, J. V.: Brit. J. Haematol., *2*, 237, 1956 (Auto-immune Hemolytic Anemia).

DAMESHEK, W.: Bull. N. Y. Acad. Med., *31*, 113, 1955 (Hypersplenism).

DOAN, C. A.: Sodeman's *Pathologic Physiology*, 2nd Ed., Philadelphia, W. B. Saunders Co., 1956, p. 852 (Spleen and Reticulo-Endothelial System).

DOAN, C. A.: Halpern's *Physiopathology of the Reticulo-Endothelial System*, Springfield, Ill., Charles C Thomas, 1957, p. 290, (Hypersplenism).

EMERSON, C. P., et al.: A.M.A. Arch. Int. Med., *97*, 1, 1956 (Hereditary Spherocytosis and Spleen).

MAINGOT, R.: Lancet, *262*, 625, 1952 (Splenectomy, General Review).

General

WINTROBE, M. M.: *Clinical Hematology*, 3rd Ed., Philadelphia, Lea & Febiger, 1951.

Congenital Anomalies

BENNETT-JONES, M. J., HILL, C. A., and HILL, S. T.: Brit. J. Surg., *40*, 259, 1952 (Accessory Spleen in Scrotum).

CURTIS, G. M., and MOVITZ, E.: Ann. Surg., *123*, 276, 1946 (Accessory Spleen).

Inflammations

GRAY, E. F.: Am. J. Roentgenol., *51*, 336, 1944 (Calcification).

Degenerations

ANDRUS, D. L., et al.: U. S. Armed Forces M. J., *2*, 233, 1951 (Abscess).

COFFEE, H. D., and LIPTON, S.: A. M. A. Arch. Surg., *47*, 478, 1943 (Primary Tuberculosis).

ENGELBRETH-HOLM, J.: Am. J. M. Sci., *195*, 32, 1938 (Tuberculosis).

HARMOS, O., and MYERS, M. E.: Am. J. Clin. Path., *21*, 737, 1951 (Gummas).

KAY, S.: Am. J. Path., *26*, 427, 1950 (Boeck's Sarcoid).

RICH, A. R., et al.: Bull. Johns Hopkins Hosp., *65*, 311, 1939 (Acute Splenitis).

SYMMERS, D.: A. M. A. Arch. Path., *45*, 385, 1948 (Splenomegaly).

Physical Disturbances

ADKINS, E. H.: Ann. Surg., *107*, 832, 1938 (Torsion of Pedicle).

BATE, T. N.: J. Internat. Coll. Surg., *15*, 531, 1951 (Surgical Diseases).

BRINES, O. A.: A. M. A. Arch. Path., *36*, 163, 1943 (Spontaneous Rupture).

BYRNE, R. V.: A. M. A. Arch. Surg., *61*, 273, 1950 (Traumatic Rupture).

KANAR, E. A., et al.: West. J. Surg., *58*, 670, 1950 (Felty's Syndrome).

LARGHERO, P., and GIURRA, F.: Surg., Gynec. & Obst., *92*, 385, 1951 (Traumatic Rupture).

LEFFLER, R. J.: Am. J. Path., *28*, 303, 1952 (Hypersplenism).

MARTIN, J. D., JR., and COOPER, M. N.: South. Surgeon, *16*, 1047, 1950 (Complications of Splenectomy).

Rogers, H. M., and Langley, F. H.: Ann. Int. Med., *32*, 745, 1950 (Felty's Syndrome).
Schatken, R. V.: Ann. Surg., *135*, 536, 1952 (Hypersplenism).
Waugh, R. L.: New England J. Med., *234*, 621, 1946 (Peritoneal Autotransplantation Splenic Tissue after Rupture).
Welch, C. S., and Dameshek, W.: New England J. Med., *242*, 601, 1950 (Splenectomy in Blood Dyscrasias).
Zollinger, R. M.: J. A. M. A., *149*, 24, 1952 (Hypersplenism).

Tumors

Bean, L., and Stahlgren, L. H.: U. S. Armed Forces M. J., *4*, 305, 1953 (Epidermoid Cyst).
Bostick, W. L.: Am. J. Path., *21*, 1143, 1945 (Primary Tumors).
Coe, J. I., and von Drashek, S. C.: Am. J. Path., *28*, 663, 1952 (Hamartoma).
Fischl, A. A., and Papps, J.: Ann. Int. Med., *31*, 1105, 1949 (Cysts).
Herbut, P. A., and Gabriel, F. R.: A. M. A. Arch. Path., *33*, 917, 1942 (Secondary Tumors).
Hirst, A. E., Jr., and Bullock, W. K.: Am. J. M. Sci., *223*, 413, 1952 (Secondary Tumors).
Hodge, G. B., and Wilson, D. A.: Surgery, *21*, 343, 1947 (Cavernous Hemangioma).
Krumbhaar, E. B., and Stengel, A.: A. M. A. Arch. Path., *34*, 117, 1942 (Leukemia).
Lazarus, J. A., and Marks, M. S.: Am. J. Surg., *71*, 479, 1946 (Malignant Tumors).
Tamaki, H. T.: A. M. A. Arch. Path., *46*, 550, 1948 (Cyst).
Wachstein, M.: J. A. M. A., *152*, 237, 1953 (Hemangiosarcoma).

27

Lymph Nodes

PATHOLOGIC PHYSIOLOGY

Gordon O. Bain

THE *functions* of lymphatic tissue may be regarded as activities of its two principal structural components, the reticulo-endothelial cells and the lymphatic cells proper. Situated strategically in the lymphatic vascular system, the lymph nodes form an extended line of defense against invasion of the body by bacteria or other noxious agents in lymph drained from distal tissues. Afferent lymphatics penetrate the capsule, delivering lymph into the peripheral lymph sinus. Radial sinuses conduct the lymph stream to the medullary sinuses which converge at the hilus to form one or more efferent vessels. The sinus lining cells differ from the common endothelium of lymphatic vessels, for they are phagocytic littoral cells of the reticulo-endothelial framework of the lymph node (p. 912). The sinus walls are incomplete, permitting iteinrant lymph to bathe the interior of the node, in intimate contact with its cells.

Thus, the lymph node has the structure of an effective *filter*. Large particles, such as tumor cells, may be arrested in the sinuses and, in metastatic carcinoma, groups of tumor cells are often seen in the peripheral sinus in stages preceding destruction of the node by the tumor. Smaller particles such as bacteria, viruses, and colloidal particles are engulfed by reticulo-endothelial pahgocytes in the sinuses and pulp. Hypertrophy and hyperplasia of these cells is a common feature of chronic nonspecific lymphadenitis. This reaction is sometimes pronounced, as in tuberculous lymphadenitis, with the formation of nodular collections of macrophages.

In addition to serving as reticulo-endothelial filters, lymph nodes are an important *source* of *blood lymphocytes* (p. 119). Whether lymphocytopoiesis occurs in the cortex or in the medulla is disputed. The primary follicles of the cortex commonly exhibit pale central areas called secondary follicles. Some authorities regard these as germinal centers for lymphocyte production but their absence during intra-uterine life and in experimental animals reared in germ-free environments, suggests that they may represent a reaction to antigenic stimulation. Necrobiotic changes occur in the secondary follicles (reaction centers) in a variety of toxic and infective states.

Lymph nodes are important sites of *antibody formation* but precisely which cells are responsible is controversial. Recent studies indicate that plasma cells found among the lymphocytes are an important source of antibody globulin (p. 121). Plasma cells are absent in utero and in agammaglobulinemia, gradually appear after birth, and are particularly abundant following antigenic stimulation. The origin of plasma cells is disputed. According to different theories they arise by morhpological alteration of reticulo-endothelial cells, or of lymphocytes, or by differentiation of a lymphocyte precursor cell. Cells morphologically intermediate between lymphocytes and plasma cells are seen in certain viral diseases (*e.g.* infectious mononucleosis, rubella, and hepatitis) and in Waldenstrom's macroglobulinemia. It has been suggested that lymphocytes may serve as stores of nucleic acids to guide the synthesis of protein antibodies (Hamilton).

Lymphatic tissue is subject to *endocrine influences.* Adrenocorticotropic hormone (ACTH), adrenal steroids, androgens, and estrogens are capable of causing involution of lymphatic tissue. Such stresses as extremes of temperature, burns, trauma, and toxic states cause involution of lymphatic tissue by release of pituitary ACTH. The plasma cells are unaffected. Administration of adrenal cortical steroids causes dissolution of lymphocytes, an increase in immature plasma cells and, in the immunized animal, a rise in the serum levels of specific antibodies (Dolowitz, Dougherty, *et al.*). Modest lymphoid hyperplasia may follow gonadectomy, adrenalectomy, administration of desoxycorticosterone acetate (DOCA), progesterone, thyroid extract, or thyroid stimulating hormone (TSH).

Factors responsible for the occurrence of *lymphoblastoma* are largely unknown. In experimental animals the thymus contains a factor favoring tumor induction, while bone marrow contains an inhibitory factor. Estrogen has a leukomogenic effect in mice. The effects of other hromones parallel their effect on thymic growth and involution. The relationship of these findings to human lymphoid tumors is not clear. *X*-radiation has a leukemogenic effect in experimental animals and there is considerable evidence that this is also true in man. Lymphatic tissue is highly susceptible to ionizing radiation, the most mature cells being most susceptible. The reticuloendothelial cells and plasma cells are highly resistant. Following sublethal irradiation the lymphatic cells are reconstituted by multiplication and differentiation of primitive reticular cells.

GENERAL CONSIDERATIONS

Of the different pathologic processes affecting lymph nodes, *Congenital Anomalies* are unimportant for the slight variations in locations and the differences in the numbers of lymph nodes are of no consequence. *Degenerations* exist chiefly in the form of (1) *atrophy*—the normal physiologic process occurring with advancing age, (2) *hyalinization*—occurring primarily as the end stage of inflammation, (3) *amyloidosis*—seen in connection with amyloidosis of other organs, (4) *fibrinoid necrosis*—encountered as part of a group of disorders referred to collectively as "collagen diseases," (5) *disturbances* of *lipoid metabolism*—giving rise to lipoid storage diseases, and (6) *pigmentation* —occurring especially in conjunction with pneumoconioses. *Physical Disturbances*, like developmental malformations, are of no significance. This leaves *Inflammations* and *Tumors* only to be considered.

INFLAMMATIONS

Orientation.—Inflammation of lymph nodes is known as *lymphadenitis.* The *causes* of lymphadenitis are virtually the causes of diseases in general and include such agents as bacteria, spirochetes, rickettsia, viruses, fungi, parasites, chemicals, physical agents, foreign bodies, and trauma. Some of the more important lesions may be listed as follows: acute nonspecific lymphadenitis, chronic nonspecific lymphadenitis, dermatopathic lymphadenitis, tuberculosis, Boeck's sarcoid (p. 501), syphilis, tularemia (p. 491), brucellosis (p. 921), typhoid and paratyphoid fever (p. 707), filariasis (p. 379), leishmaniasis (p. 923), granuloma inguinale (p. 1112), lymphogran-uloma venereum (p. 1112), infectious mononucleosis (p. 951), cat scratch fever, berylliosis (p. 468), and anthracosilicosis (p. 462). Some of these lesions (except as indicated) may now be considered in the order mentioned.

Acute Nonspecific Lymphadenitis.—As the name suggests, this type of inflammation occurs as a result of infection with ordinary pyogenic organisms. It is by far the most common type of lymphadenitis. *Clinically* it is most noticeable in conjunction with *peripheral* lymph nodes that can be both seen and felt. It is encountered in lymph nodes that drain any cutaneous abrasion or infection, in submental lymph nodes in cases of injuries or inflammations of the gums or mucosa of the mouth, and in cervical lymph nodes in conjunction with tonsillitis and pharyngitis. The condition, however, is also encountered *internally*—notably in the mediastinum in conjunction with acute pneumonia and in the mesentery in a condition generally known as *acute mesenteric lymphadenitis* (Postlethwait). Regardless of the localization of the process, the lymph nodes are enlarged, painful, and tender. *Pathologically* they usually remain discrete although in severe infections with breakdown of tissue they may become confluent. They are firm, reddened, and may or may not disclose suppuration. *Histologically* they reveal congestion and edema of the sinusoidal spaces, diminution or increase in the size of the lymph follicles, and a diffuse sinusoidal infiltration with neutrophils. In cases of suppuration there is complete breakdown of tissue. The process heals by resolution when the damage has not been too great, and by granulation tissue formation and fibrosis when necrosis of tissue has occurred.

Chronic Nonspecific Lymphadenitis.—This type of inflammation occurs as a sequel of acute nonsuppurative lymphadenitis or appears as a low-grade chronic process from the start. Depending upon the site of the primary inflammation, any lymph node of the body may be affected. The nodes are enlarged but generally not tender or painful. They are less sharply circumscribed than in acute nonspecific lymphadenitis, more matted together, and firmer. Histologically they disclose varying degrees of plasma cell and monocytic infiltration, sinusoidal reticulum cell hyperplasia, and fibrosis. Some, in addition, reveal hyperplasia of the follicles.

Dermatopathic Lymphadenitis.—This condition, also known as lipomelanotic reticulosis, is a lymph nodal reaction to a variety of chronic nonspecific dermatologic conditions including exfoliative dermatitis, neurodermatitis, parapsoriasis, eczema, pityriasis, seborrheic dermatitis, lichen planus, etc. (Hurwitt and Obermayer). Grossly there is usually generalized lymphadenopathy of a minor degree. Microscopically the following changes are present: (1) moderate to marked sinusoidal reticulum cell hyperplasia, (2) varying degrees of fibrosis, (3) scanty to abundant deposition of melanin and, to a lesser extent, hemosiderin within and adjacent to the proliferated reticulum cells, and (4) fair preservation of the follicular architecture (Fig. 473). The condition as such is quite innocuous. The chief importance lies in its recognition and its differentiation from Hodgkin's disease and mycosis fungoides.

Tuberculosis.—Tuberculous lymphadenitis is always secondary to tuberculosis of the tissues or organs that are drained by the lymph nodes in question. While such an infection may involve any of the lymph nodes in the body (and sometimes may mimic lymphoblastoma in distribution) the

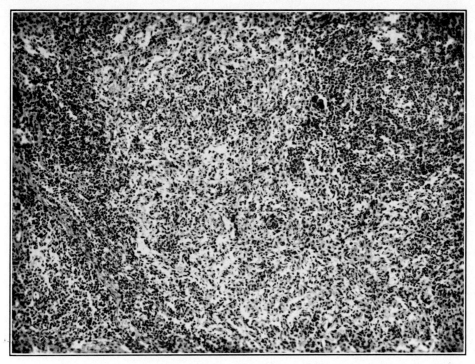

FIG. 473.—Dermatopathic lymphadenitis showing sinusoidal reticulum cell hyperplasia and deposition of brown pigment. × 100.

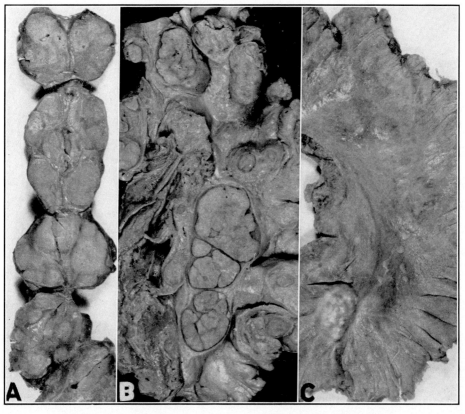

FIG. 474.—Tuberculosis demonstrating *A*, a chain of affected cervical lymph nodes, *B*, caseating mesenteric lymph nodes, and *C*, calcified mesenteric lymph nodes.

three most common *sites* are (1) mediastinal lymph nodes from tuberculosis of the lungs, (2) mesenteric lymph nodes from tuberculosis of the ileocecal region, and (3) cervical lymph nodes from tuberculosis of the tonsils. Of these sites, the cervical area appears to be the most important for, being superficial, it is the most apparent (Davies and Lester). Cervical and mesenteric lymphadenitis are most often bovine in type while mediastinal lymphadenitis is most often human in type. Since the *incidence* of the disorder parallels the incidence of tuberculosis in general, its frequency has been steadily on the decline in the United States. Regardless of the location of the infection, the pathologic picture is the same. *Grossly* the lymph

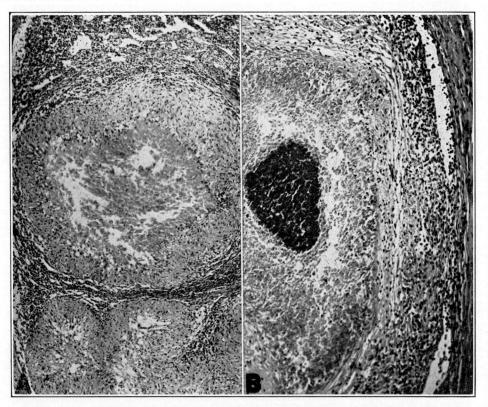

Fig. 475.—Tuberculosis illustrating *A*, several large tubercles, one with a caseating center and a periphery of epithelioid cells. × 50 and *B*, a larger mass with a caseating and calcific center and a periphery of fibroblasts, lymphocytes, and fewer epithelioid cells. × 100.

nodes are enlarged, firm, and matted. Cut surfaces vary with the type of tuberculous process. In miliary tuberculosis they are dotted with tiny gray foci; in fibrocaseous tuberculosis they contain large or small irregular areas of caseation necrosis surrounded peripherally by varying amounts of fibrous tissue; in tuberculoma they consist of a single homogeneous mass of necrotic or more elastic tissue, while in calcifying tuberculosis they are partially or completely replaced with calcium salts (Fig. 474). *Histologically* they are composed of soft or hard tubercles, of larger tubercles with caseous centers and peripheral epithelioid cells arranged at right angles to the main mass, or of large caseous masses with or without calcification and surrounded by fibroblasts and tuberculous granulation tissue (Fig. 475). The process *heals* by resolution, fibrosis, or calcification. The chief *complications* are (1) extension to adjacent structures with fistulous tract formation and (2) remaining as a focus of infection for dissemination to other parts of the body. *Clinically* the nodes are enlarged, may be putty-like in consistency, and are not attended by pain or tenderness. Calcification is readily demonstrable roentgenographically. The *diagnosis* is made from the clinical manifestations, roentgen appearance, and, inadvertently, biopsy. *Treatment* is that of tuberculosis in general together with surgical excision if the nodes are located in the neck. The *prognosis* is fair to good.

Syphilis.—Syphilitic lymphadenitis may occur in conjunction with any of the stages of syphilis. In keeping with the clinical picture, the pathologic changes may be divided into those associated with early (first and

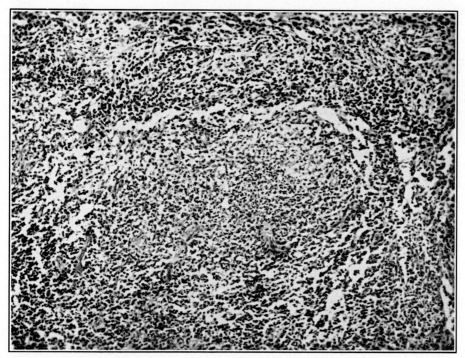

Fig. 476.—Cat-scratch fever showing an area of beginning necrosis surrounded at the periphery by plasma cells, lymphocytes, neutrophils, and eosinophils. × 100.

second stages) and late (third stage) syphilis (Evans). In *early syphilis*, the lymph nodes draining the chancre and those found throughout the body when mucous patches and syphilids occur are similar. They are moderately enlarged, discrete, soft to firm, and do not suppurate. Histologically they disclose marked enlargement of the lymph follicles and an increase in reticulum cells, plasma cells, and lymphocytes in the interfollicular sinusoidal areas. *Late* (tertiary) *syphilis* is usually localized to a node or group of nodes and is often located in the neck (Cummer). The nodes are enlarged and hard and may be homogeneously gray and firm or may contain one or more large or small, circumscribed, rubbery areas of necrosis. Histologically they consist of either a diffuse infiltration with principally plasma cells and lymphocytes or of typical gummas.

Cat Scratch Fever.—This condition, also known as benign inoculation reticulo-endotheliosis and nonbacterial regional lymphadenitis, characteristically *consists of* a cutaneous cat scratch followed in about three weeks by enlargement and perhaps tenderness and redness of regional lymph nodes, and by fever and other systemic manifestations such as malaise, anorexia, lassitude, chills, headache, etc. (Daniel and Campbell). Subsequently the nodes may gradually recede spontaneously or may proceed to suppuration. The disorder is presumably *caused* by a virus. Recorded methods of transmission other than cat scratch have been cat lick, insect bite, cat urine, prick with porcupine quill, scratch on meat crate, handling wild rabbits, and unknown. *Pathologically* the *skin* lesion usually occurs on exposed portions of the body, is generally single but may be multiple, and consists of a scratch, papule, pustule, ulcer, scab, or prick. The *lymph nodes* most commonly affected are axillary, cervical, and epitrochlear. They may measure as much as 5 cm. in diameter and, as already stated, may or may not suppurate. Histologically the first change in the lymph nodes consists of reticulo-endothelial hyperplasia. It is followed by focal areas of necrosis and nuclear fragmentation surrounded by infiltrations with neutrophils, eosinophils, plasma cells, and monocytes (Fig. 476). The lesion should not be confused with Hodgkin's disease, lymphogranuloma venereum, brucellosis, or tularemia. The *diagnosis* is made from the history, clinical manifestations, and histologic examination of a removed lymph node. In addition, a positive skin test using antigen prepared from a suppurating lymph node is of value. Active *treatment* in the form of surgical excision of the affected nodes is indicated only in cases of suppuration to forestall sinus tract formation. The *prognosis* is good.

TUMORS

Orientation.—Tumors and tumor-like conditions of lymph nodes may be *classified* as *primary* and *secondary.* Most primary tumors are generally grouped collectively under the heading *lymphoblastoma.* Ordinarily, however, this caption does not include two closely related conditions that also merit consideration, mainly, *mycosis fungoides* and *extramedullary plasmocytoma.*

Lymphoblastoma.—The term lymphoblastoma (or simply lymphoma) is used to encompass most primary tumors or tumor-like conditions not only of lymph nodes but of other organs of the reticulo-endothelial system that are composed of reticulum, lymphoid, myeloid, and monocytoid cells. While the disorders are variously *classified* (Wetherley-Mein, Hellwig, and Berman), your author has found the following division to be quite satisfactory: leukemia, leukosarcoma, reticulum cell sarcoma, Hodgkin's disease, lymphosarcoma, and giant follicular lymphoblastoma (giant follicular hyperplasia, follicular lymphoblastoma, follicular lymphoma, Brill's disease, etc.). That all these conditions are closely *related* has been amply demonstrated by (1) the fact that all cells listed above ultimately originate from a common stem cell that is known as the reticulum or primitive mesenchymal cell, (2) morphologic mixtures of the various cells in different lymph nodes from the same patient or even different portions of the same lymph node (Herbut), (3) the fact that the condition may (*a*) start as a lymphosarcoma, pass through a stage of Hodgkin's disease, and terminate as reticulum cell sarcoma, (*b*) start as giant follicular lymphoblastoma and terminate as lymphosarcoma, lymphatic leukemia, Hodgkin's disease, or reticulum cell sarcoma, or (c) start as lymphosarcoma and terminate as lymphatic leukemia, etc. (Herbut and Custer), (4) tissue cultures from one part of a node resembling Hodgkin's disease and from another part of the same node resembling lymphosarcoma, and (5) the finding of both myelo-kentric and lymphokentric acids in a patient with any one of the conditions mentioned (p. 953). Since the disorders are closely related, they have many features in common and, except for leukemia which has already been discussed (p. 953), may be considered together. As a group, the *incidence* of lymphoblastoma appears to be on the increase. It is said to constitute about 5 per cent of all malignant tumors. While there are variations in each of the categories listed, the condition has been described at all ages from birth on and is from two to four times as common in males as it is in females (Wintrobe). It is worldwide in distribution and affects all races. The *cause* remains undetermined and, in fact, even the nature of the disorder is not agreed upon. Many authors accept all the conditions listed as true tumors (with which your author agrees), but others do not include Hodgkin's disease in this category. They look upon Hodgkin's disease as a granuloma with the etiologic agent unknown despite the incrimination by some of tubercle bacilli, diphtheroids, amebæ, viruses, etc. (Hoster and Bostick).

Pathologically lymphoblastoma, as already stated, is a disturbance of the reticulo-endothelial system with the lymph nodes generally disclosing the characteristic changes. As a rule, the deep lymph nodes, especially those of the retroperitoneum, are more extensively affected than the superficial nodes. Terminally the lesions are always multiple although they may start with involvement of a single node or group of nodes. Initially the enlargement is only slight and the nodes are discrete. Ultimately, however, the individual nodes may measure 6 cm. or more in diameter and since they have a tendency to coalesce as they enlarge, they may form conglomerate masses that measure as much as 30 cm. across (Fig. 477). In most instances, the enlargement is due to infiltration with diffusely grayish-white moderately firm tissue. In Hodgkin's disease, however, there is a tendency to spontaneous necrosis and fibrosis, while in giant follicular lymphoblastoma the large follicles may actually be visualized with the naked eye as circumscribed mottlings. Aside from the lymph nodes, some of the *other organs* that show focal or tumorous (and less commonly diffuse) permeations with neoplastic tissue are spleen, liver, bone marrow, submucosa of the gastrointestinal tract, kidneys, lungs, and heart.

Histologically, as already stated, the patterns are generally quite distinct but, on occasion, may be mixed. From the onset it should be recorded that the most important single change is an obliteration of the normal architecture. The term *leukosarcoma* is used in retrospect. It connotes a tumefaction that is composed of mature or immature lymphoid cells (lymphoid leukosarcoma), myeloid cells (myeloid leukosarcoma), or monocytoid cells (monocytoid leukosarcoma) and that after months, weeks, or even years terminates respectively as a lymphoid, myeloid, or monocytoid leukemia. *Reticulum cell sarcoma* consists of a diffuse permeation with primitive reticulum cells (Fig. 478A). The cells are large and disclose the following: rounded or polyhedral-shaped with long processes (demonstrated by reticulum stains) continuous with the supporting reticulum, abundant eosinophilic but sometimes lightly basophilic cytoplasm, and large, round, hyperchromatic nuclei. In *Hodgkin's disease* the picture is characterized by pleomorphism (Fig. 479). Generally (in the granulomatous variety) there is a diffuse permeation with neutrophils, eosinophils, plasma cells, lymphocytes, monocytes, and reticulum cells. Characteristically, too, there are present varying numbers of Sternberg-Reed cells. These are single or multinucleated giant cells and possess a scanty amount of cytoplasm and large, round or oval, deeply stained and (when multiple) piled-up nuclei. In addition, there are often foci or larger areas of necrosis and increases in cellular or collagenous connective tissue. Less commonly (in the sar-

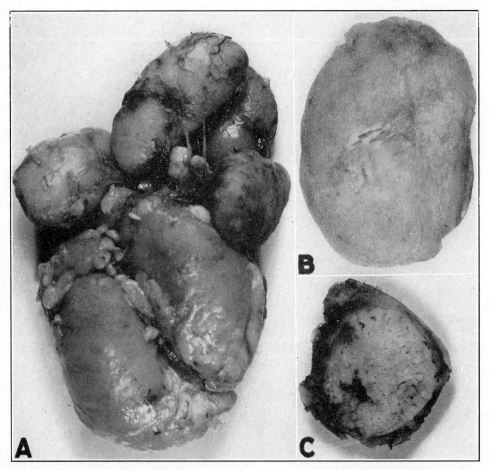

FIG. 477.—Lymphoblastoma illustrating *A*, a conglomerate mass of enlarged nodes in a case of Hodgkin's disease, *B*, cut surface with diffuse involvement in a case of lymphosarcoma, and *C*, cut surface with prominent follicular markings in a case of giant follicular lymphoblastoma.

comatous variety) Hodgkin's disease consists predominantly of primitive reticulum cells that resemble reticulum cell sarcoma. *Lymphosarcoma* consists of diffuse permeation with rather normal appearing lymphocytes or lymphoblasts (Fig. 478*B*). The characteristic change in *giant follicular lymphoblastoma* is the presence of increased numbers of enlarged follicles (Figs. 478*C* and *D*). Because of the large size of the follicles, the interfollicular sinusoidal structure is compressed and erased.

The *complications* of lymphoblastoma are (1) neoplastic cachexia and (2) impairment of function of the organs affected. The *clinical manifestations*

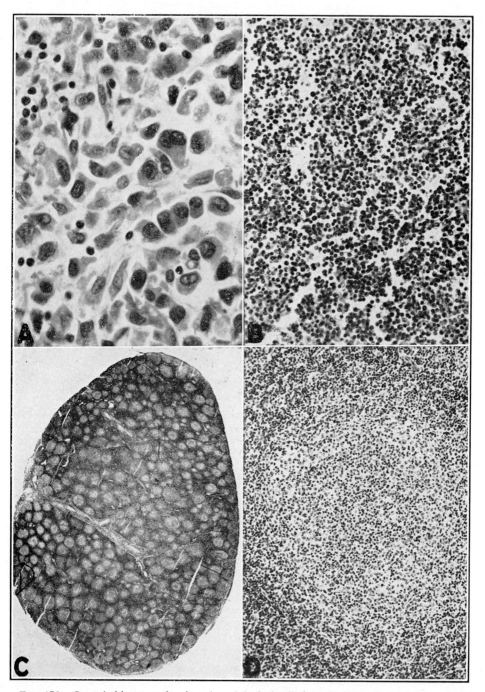

FIG. 478.—Lymphoblastoma showing *A*, polyhedral cells in reticulum cell sarcoma. × 400 *B*, lymphocytes in lymphosarcoma. × 200, *C*, hypertrophy and hyperplasia in giant follicular ymphoblastoma. × 4, and *D*, a large follicle in giant follicular lymphoblastoma. × 100.

vary somewhat with the type of lymphoblastoma and, of course, with the system most severely affected but, in general, the following may be noted at one time or another: painless lymphadenopathy, splenomegaly, hepatomegaly, anorexia, loss of weight, fever, weakness, sweating, cough, expectoration, dyspnea, hemoptysis, indigestion, hematemesis, melena, jaundice, pains in the abdomen and other sites, hematuria, paresthesias, pruritus (Hodgkin's disease), cutaneous eruptions (especially in Hodgkin's disease), anemia, occasionally leukocytosis, and normal, hypoplastic, or specifically affected bone marrow. The *diagnosis* is made from the history, careful hematologic examination (including bone marrow studies) and

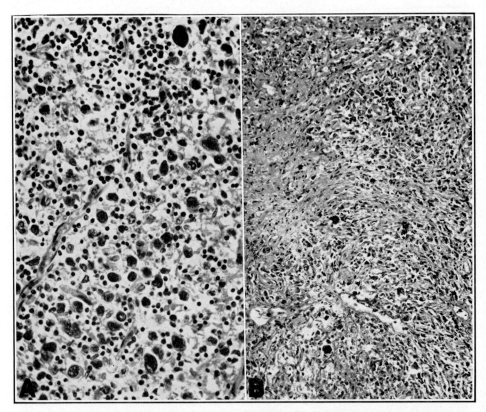

Fig. 479.—Hodgkin's disease illustrating *A*, a pleomorphism of cells with numerous Sternberg-Reed cells. × 200 and *B*, a later phase with abundant fibrosis. × 100.

biopsy of an affected lymph node. The differential diagnosis includes any inflammation (tuberculosis, infectious mononucleosis, brucellosis, histoplasmosis, etc.), degeneration (lipoid storage diseases), or other enlargement of lymph nodes. *Treatment* has been most varied with chemotherapeutic (especially nitrogen mustard and related compounds) agents and some type of irradiation therapy being most popular. Surgical interference is advocated only when the disorder is localized to an accessible area. The *prognosis* depends essentially upon the type of lymphoblastoma with recorded survivals reaching twenty years or more in giant follicular lymphoblastoma and lasting only a few weeks in cases of reticulum cell sarcoma. In general, the comparative malignancy (from least to most) may be listed

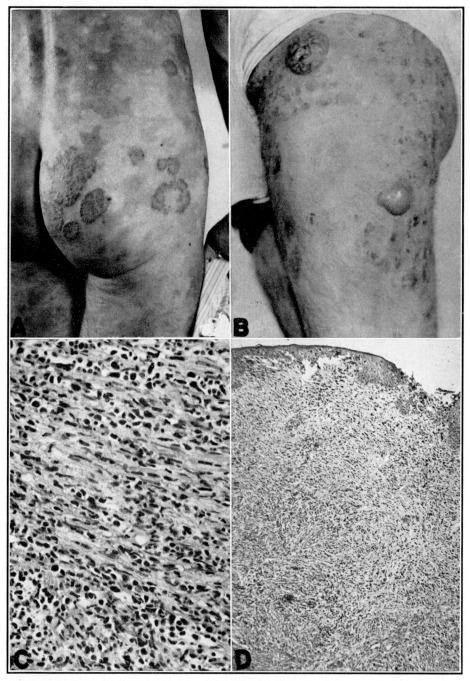

FIG. 480.—Mycosis fungoides showing *A*, plaque-like lesions of the second stage, *B*, fungating lesions of the third stage, *C*, a variety of leukocytes permeating the corium. × 200, and *D*, diffuse permeation of the entire dermis by leukocytes. × 50.

as follows: giant follicular lymphoblastoma, Hodgkin's disease, lymphosarcoma, leukosarcoma, and reticulum cell sarcoma.

Mycosis Fungoides.—Mycosis fungoides is considered by some as a separate disease but by most observers is looked upon as a cutaneous manifestation of a lymphoblastoma, especially Hodgkin's disease, lymphosarcoma, or reticulum cell sarcoma (Cawley). The disorder thus is a clinical rather than a pathologic entity. The *cutaneous lesions* are generally divided into three stages: (1) red, scaly, indefinite eruptions, (2) few or many round, oval, horseshoe-shaped, angular, linear, or serpiginous infiltrated plaques that vary in color from red to purple (Fig. 480*A*), and (3) fungating and ulcerating, mushroom-like, reddish-purple tumors predominating on the trunk and measuring up to 5 cm. or more in diameter (Fig. 480*B*). The clinical manifestations consist chiefly of the cutaneous eruptions but in the first two stages there may be, in addition, severe pruritus. *Pathologically* the epidermis discloses hypertrophy of the prickle cell layer (acanthosis), micro-abscesses, intercellular edema, dissolution of the basal layer of cells, and atrophy in areas overlying tumors. Early in the course of the disease the outer third of the dermis discloses infiltration with reticulum cells, fibroblasts, lymphocytes, basophils, neutrophils, eosinophils, monocytes, plasma cells, and occasional giant cells of the Sternberg-Reed type (Fig. 480*C*). Later the infiltration occupies the entire thickness of the dermis and is composed mostly of reticulum cells (Fig. 480*D*). Sooner or later the disease affects most of the *other organs*, notably lymph nodes, bone marrow, spleen, liver, heart, lungs, and kidneys. The *diagnosis* is made from the clinical manifestations and biopsy of the skin. The *course* of the disease is protracted, with death occurring on an average of about five years after the diagnosis is established. The causes of death are cachexia, lymphoblastomatous involvement of other organs, and intercurrent infection.

Extramedullary Plasmocytoma.—Ordinarily plasmocytoma (plasma cell myeloma) is a tumor of bone marrow (p. 1264), but occasionally tumors of plasma cells also originate in extramedullary sites. Some of these areas consist of upper respiratory tract, larynx, tonsils, floor of the mouth, conjunctivæ, lymph nodes, pleura, thyroid, lacrimal glands, ovaries, fallopian tubes, intestines, kidneys, spermatic cord, skin, etc. (Hellwig). The tumors may be single or multiple and are composed of adult, normal appearing plasma cells. They are more common in males than in females and usually appear in the fifth and sixth decades of life. Some of the growths remain localized for years but sooner or later most of them become malignant and metastasize to lymph nodes, bones, and other organs.

Secondary Tumors.—Secondary tumors of lymph nodes are far more frequent than primary neoplasms. Most commonly, they consist of carcinomas and only infrequently are they sarcomas. At first the lesions usually affect the lymph nodes that drain the primary neoplastic site but sometimes skip metastases (that is, distant lymph nodes) only occur and at other times most of the lymph nodes of the body may be uniformly affected. It is also most important to be aware of the fact that although the primary site is usually apparent, not infrequently (especially in connection with carcinoma of the nasopharynx, carcinoma of the tail of the pancreas, or carcinoma of the prostate) it is so small that it must be searched for with meticulous care before it is discovered. *Grossly* the affected lymph nodes are, as a rule, enlarged, may be matted together, are firm, and are partially or wholly replaced with tumor. The neoplastic tissue is usually gray and it may or may not show areas of necrosis. The nodes thus may be readily mistaken for lymphoblastoma or tuberculosis. *Histologically* the tumors generally mimic the parent growths. They are readily identified as metastatic when the neoplasms are well differentiated but they are easily mistaken for lymphosarcoma or reticulum cell sarcoma when they are highly anaplastic. The *prognosis* depends upon the nature of the primary growth and upon the localization of the metastases. In general, the outlook is usually better in well-differentiated growths than it is in poorly differentiated tumors and it is also better in cases of regional as compared with more widespread metastases.

REFERENCES

Pathologic Physiology

BURNET, F. M.: *The Production of Antibodies*, Melbourne, Macmillan & Co., Ltd., 1941.
DOLOWITZ, D. A., *et al.*: A.M.A. Arch. Otolaryng., *66*, 245, 1957 (Adrenal Influence on Lymphatic Tissue).
GOOD, R. A.: J. Lab. Clin. Med., *46*, 167, 1955 (Agammaglobulinemia).
HAMILTON, L. D.: Function of the Lymphocyte in Rebuck's *The Leukemias*, New York, Academic Press, Inc., 1957, p. 381.
KAPLAN, H. S.: Cancer Res., *14*, 535, 1954 (Etiology and Pathogenesis of Leukemias).
MARSHALL, A. H. E.: *An Outline of the Cytology and Pathology of the Reticular Tissue*, Springfield, Ill., Charles C Thomas Co., 1956.
MAXIMOW, A. A.: The Lymphocytes and Plasma Cells in Cowdry's *Special Cytology*, New York, Paul B. Hoeber, Inc., 1932, Vol. II, p. 601.

Inflammations

BAILEY, H.: Lancet, *1*, 313, 1948 (Tuberculosis).
CAMPBELL, W. N., and ANDERSON, T. G.: Pennsylvania M. J., *56*, 188, 1953 (Cat Scratch Disease).
CUMMER, C. L.: Am. J. Syph., *12*, 13, 1928 (Tertiary Syphilis).
DANIELS, W. B., and McMURRAY, F. G.: Ann. Int. Med., *37*, 697, 1952 (Cat Scratch Disease).
EVANS, N.: A. M. A. Arch. Path., *37*, 175, 1944 (Secondary Syphilis).
HURWITT, E.: J. Invest. Dermat., *5*, 197, 1942 (Dermatopathic Lymphadenitis).
LESTER, C. W.: Surg., Gynec. & Obst., *87*, 719, 1948 (Tuberculosis).
OBERMAYER, M. E., and FOX, E. T.: A. M. A. Arch. Dermat. & Syph., *60*, 609, 1949 (Lipomelanotic Reticulosis).
POSTLETHWAIT, R. W., and CAMPBELL, F. H.: A. M. A. Arch. Surg., *59*, 92, 1949 (Acute Mesenteric Lymphadenitis).

Tumors

BERMAN, L.: Blood, *3*, 195, 1953 (Classification Lymphomas).
BOSTICK, W. L.: California Med., *70*, 87, 1949 (Hodgkin's Disease).
————: California Med., *74*, 111, 1951 (Etiology Hodgkin's Disease).
CAWLEY, E. P., *et al.*: A. M. A. Arch. Dermat. & Syph., *64*, 255, 1951 (Mycosis Fungoides).
CUSTER, R. P., and BERNHARD, W. G.: Am. J. M. Sci., *216*, 625, 1948 (Interrelationship of Lymphblastomas).
HELLWIG, C. A.: Am. J. Clin. Path., *16*, 564, 1946 (Malignant Lymphoma).
————: A. M. A. Arch. Path., *36*, 95, 1943 (Extramedullary Plasmocytoma).
HERBUT, P. A., *et al.*: Am. J. Path., *21*, 233, 1945 (Relationship of Lymphblastomas).
HOSTER, H. A., *et al.*: Cancer Research, *8*, 1 and 49, 1948 (Hodgkin's Disease).
REIMANN, H. A., HAVENS, W. P., and HERBUT, P. A.: A. M. A. Arch. Int. Med., *70*, 434, 1942 (Hodgkin's Disease with Primary Cutaneous Lesions).
SYMMERS, D.: A. M. A. Arch. Path., *45*, 73, 1948 (Lymphoid Diseases).
WEATHERLEY-MEIN, G.: St. Thomas' Reports, *7*, 5, 1951 (Malignant Lymphoma).
WETHERLEY-MEIN, G., *et al.*: Quart. J. Med., *21*, 327, 1952 (Follicular Lymphoma).
WINTROBE, M. M.: *Clinical Hematology*, 3rd Ed., Philadelphia, Lea & Febiger, 1951.

Thymus

PATHOLOGIC PHYSIOLOGY

JOSEPH J. RUPP

There is no acceptable data which indicate that the thymus secretes a *hormone* or alters the internal secretions of other glands. The frequent association of *myasthenia gravis* and thymic tumors, and the observation that thymectomy even in the absence of thymic tumors often decreases the severity of the myasthenia, would seem to indicate that the thymus may play a role in acetylcholine-cholinesterase metabolism.

Although the thymus has no known endocrine function, its bulk can be *altered by hormones*. In experimental animals, for example, the size of the thymus is increased following adrenalectomy and decreased by treatment with glucocorticoids but not mineralocorticoids. In some patients with myasthenia gravis and thymic tumors ACTH will decrease the size of the thymus. Often the symptoms of myasthenia in patients with or without thymic enlargement will be temporarily ameliorated by a short course of treatment with ACTH. Initially, this treatment may increase the muscle weakness by alterations in potassium levels.

Thymic *enlargement* is an occasional finding at necropsy in patients with untreated thyrotoxicosis. This finding is probably a result of increased thymic lymphoid tissue and is only a reflection of the general lymphoid hyperplasia which occurs in thyrotoxicosis.

The high incidence of *thyroid carcinoma* which is noted in children exposed to irradiation of the thymus in infancy is probably the result of irradiation of the thyroid gland at a critical period in its development, rather than an effect of thymic irradiation as such.

GENERAL CONSIDERATIONS

THE thymus makes its appearance about the fifth week of embryonic life as a paired structure that arises from the third pharyngeal pouches. At first, it is hollow but soon it is transformed into solid bars of epithelial tissue. Then the lower ends of the bars unite and descend with the pericardium into the mediastinum as the definitive organ. Meanwhile, the upper portions have severed their connections with the pharynx. By the third month, the original pharyngeal epithelium, remaining as Hassell's or thymic corpuscles, becomes surrounded with an appreciable amount of lymphoid tissue and the latter ultimately constitutes the bulk of the organ. Normally the thymus weighs about 15 gm. at birth, between 20 and 35 gm. around puberty, and gradually decreases in weight thereafter. As already stated in the section on Pathologic Physiology, the physiologic functions of the thymus are not definitely known. Whatever may be its endocrinologic connections, the organ is usually enlarged in hyperthyroidism, Addison's disease, acromegaly, status thymicolymphaticus, congenital hypoplasia of the adrenals, and anencephaly and is sometimes enlarged in myasthenia gravis, ricketts, after hypophysectomy and after adrenalectomy (Carr). It is persistent in eunuchs and cases of early castration and is small in marasmus and wasting diseases.

CONGENITAL ANOMALIES

Orientation.—There are three noteworthy developmental malformations of the thymus—aberrant thymic tissue, cysts, and status thymicolymphaticus.

Aberrant Thymic Tissue.—Aberrant thymic tissue may occur at any point along the path of descent of the normal organ from the level of the third pharyngeal pouches to its ultimate position behind the sternum. The anomaly generally consists of failure of descent of the entire thymic tissue on the affected side—there being no corresponding thymic tissue in the usual position (Gilmour). Sometimes the aberrant thymic tissue is located in the thyroid and at other times it surrounds the inferior parathyroids (which also develop from the third pharyngeal pouches).

Cysts.—Cysts of the thymus are uncommon (Crellin and Weller). They probably arise as a result of inclusion of branchial cleft remnants, persistence of the tubular lumen of the original thymus, or distention of Hassell's corpuscles. The cysts may be single and measure as much as 11 cm. in diameter or multiple and measure up to 1 or 2 cm. across. They may be located in the region of the normal thymus or they may be found at any point along the line of descent of the thymic tissue. Grossly they disclose a thin wall, a smooth inner surface, and a lumen filled with clear amber or hemorrhagic watery fluid. Histologically the wall is composed of connective tissue containing thymic remnants and is lined by flat or squamous cells or is devoid of an epithelial covering.

Status Thymicolymphaticus.—This caption connotes the association of sudden death from trivial injury (such as pinprick, sudden immersion in cold water, induction anesthesia, etc.) with enlargement of the thymus and other lymphoid tissues throughout the body and hypoplasia of the heart, aorta, and adrenal glands (Carr). Two explanations advanced for the participation of the thymus in such deaths are mechanical and hormonal. The *mechanical theory* (now discarded by most observers) holds that the enlarged thymus presses upon the trachea thereby causing suffocation, that it compresses the great vessels in the mediastinum producing cerebral anemia and syncope, or that it produces irritation of the recurrent pharyngeal nerves causing laryngeal spasm. The *hormonal theory* includes (1) the presence of a thymic lymph toxin, (2) the sudden liberation of nuclear proteins from foci of necrosis in the thymus and lymphoid tissue with the production of an anaphylactic reaction, and (3) adrenal insufficiency (due to hypoplasia) similar to that seen in Addison's disease. Thus the mechanism of death in the syndrome is not well understood. Not only is this so but the very existence of the condition as an entity is doubted by many observers. Such an attitude doubtlessly stems from the fact that in the past the caption has been used as a catchall—whenever another diagnosis was wanting. Despite the protests, however, the diagnosis of status

63

thymicolymphaticus is valid, in your author's opinion, in properly selected cases.

DEGENERATIONS

Degenerations of the thymus occur (1) as a natural physiologic phenomenon after the organ has reached its maximum size at puberty, (2) in connection with inflammations, and (3) in connection with tumors. Of themselves, they are of no clinical significance.

INFLAMMATIONS

Inflammation of the thymus is known as *thymitis*. The condition is uncommon and is generally of little clinical significance. It may occur in conjunction with (1) *pyemia*, (2) *extension of a suppurative process in the mediastinum*, (3) mediastinal, pulmonary, or miliary *tuberculosis*, and (4) congenital *syphilis*. Syphilitic thymitis usually consists of a diffuse fibrosis of the organ but, on occasion, may disclose multiple gummas and, rarely, may reveal small abscesses (Dubois abscesses) originating within Hassell's corpuscles.

TUMORS

Thymic tumors may be primary or secondary. *Secondary growths* occur as a result of extension from primary tumors in the mediastinum or lung or from metastasis from the lung or other organs of the body. They may mimic primary growths both clinically and pathologically.

Primary tumors of the thymus are often collectively referred to as *thymomas*. The term was coined as a result of the confusion which had existed with regard to classification and for practical purpose has been quite satisfactory. Thymomas may *occur* at any age from birth on, but are most common in the second and third decades of life (Lowenhaupt). They occur in all races and affect males as frequently as they do females. In comparison with other tumors of the body they are uncommon for the literature up to 1949 contained approximately 300 recorded cases (Reid). The *causes* of the tumors are unknown.

Pathologically thymomas are almost always located in the normal position of the thymus, that is, in the anterior mediastinum beneath the sternum. At first they maintain the normal shape of the thymus, but as they increase in size, they become more globular and more irregular. They are almost always well encapsulated until late in the course of the disease when the capsule is broken and the tumor extends in an irregular fashion to adjacent structures. As a rule, the external surface is irregularly bossed and the consistency is firm. Cut surfaces usually disclose homogeneous, gray, firm, lobulated masses separated by depressed grayish-white bands of fibrous tissue that appear to be connected with the capsule of the tumor (Fig. 481). Less frequently they are variegated, being composed in part of solid gray tumor, in part of yellowish or hemorrhagic neoplastic tissue, and in part of cystic spaces filled with necrotic material or fluid. In tumors in which cysts develop, foci or large plaques of calcification are common within the walls of the cystic structures. As the tumor becomes larger and more malignant, the capsule is broken in one or more areas and the neoplastic tissue invades the pericardium, heart, blood vessels, trachea, bronchi, sternum, lungs, and any of the tissues which it contacts. Following the confusion that has existed regarding the types of cells that normally compose the thymus, thymomas have been variously classified microscopically. Since, however, as already stated it is convenient to look upon the normal cells as epithelial and lymphoid, the tumors may accordingly be classified histologically as *carcinoma* and *lymphoblastoma*. Since the epithelial cells arise from the pharynx the tumor which they give rise to may be a *squamous cell carcinoma* or a lympho-epithelioma (Figs. 482 and 483*A*). The former is composed of polyhedral or less well-defined cells that resemble those arising in other epithelial structures. The cell borders are usually indistinct but the cells are distinctly polyhedral. The cytoplasm is abundant and diffusely lightly eosinophilic. The nuclei are round or oval, central in

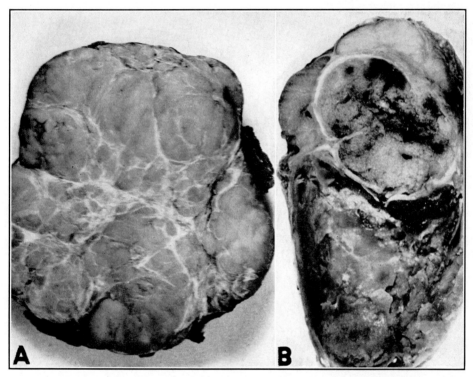

Fig. 481.—Thymoma showing *A*, a solid lobulated tumor and *B*, a variegated solid and cystic growth. Each tumor is well encapsulated and each was removed surgically.

position, and evenly stained. As a rule, despite the definite squamous cell overgrowth there remains a sprinkling of lymphocytes throughout the tissue. *Lympho-epithelioma* is similar to lympho-epithelioma in the naso-pharynx (p. 431). The tumor is composed of ill-defined nests of epithelial cells intermingled at the periphery with varying numbers of lymphocytes. As in lymph nodes (p. 984), *lymphoblastoma* may exist as leukemia, leuko-sarcoma, reticulum cell sarcoma, Hodgkin's disease, lymphosarcoma, and giant follicular lymphoblastoma. Of these, leukemia and giant follicular lymphoblastoma are usually part of a systemic process but the other types of lymphoblastoma may be present, originally at least, as primary thymic neoplasms. In any case, the lymphoblastomas are identical morphologi-cally with similar tumors in lymph nodes and other lymphoid structures (Fig. 483*B*, *C* and D). Thymomas generally remain localized for considerable periods of time but ultimately they *spread* to adjacent structures (as already indicated) and, less commonly, they metastasize to (1) mediastinal, cervical, and retroperitoneal lymph nodes and (2) to distant areas such as pleura, lungs, and even abdominal organs.

The *complications* of thymoma are (1) compression of the great vessels, nerves, trachea, and bronchi on the mediastinum, (2) erosion of the sternum, (3) metastasis to distant organs, and (4) myasthenia gravis (p. 1307). Myasthenia gravis is said to occur in as high as 75 per cent of all thymomas and, conversely, it is said to be attended by a thymoma or a persistent thymus in 15 per cent of cases (Seybold). *Clinically* thymomas are usually asympto-

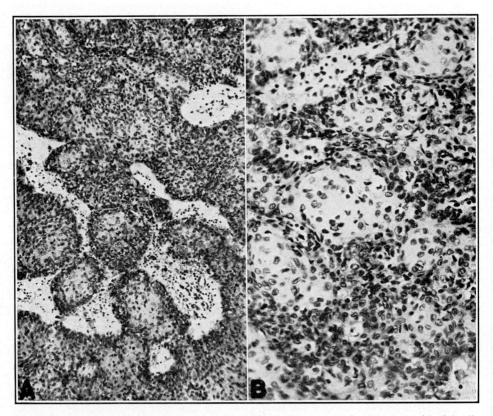

Fig. 482.—Thymoma of a carcinomatous variety illustrating groups of polyhedral epithelial cells surrounded by varying numbers of lymphocytes. *A*, × 100 and *B*, × 200.

matic for considerable periods of time. Sooner or later, however, they are attended by pain in the chest or beneath the sternum and compression symptoms referable to the structures already listed. The more important of these manifestations include dyspnea, couge, hoarseness, and (from compression of the superior vena cava) swelling of the upper portion of the chest, neck, and upper extremities and serous effusions into the pleural cavities. *Roentgenographically* a calcifying or noncalcifying tumor mass in the anterior mediastinum beneath the sternum is generally readily demonstrable. The appearance, however, is not distinctive enough to differentiate the growth from other mediastinal neoplasms. The *diagnosis* may be suspected when pain and compression symptoms develop but generally it is arrived

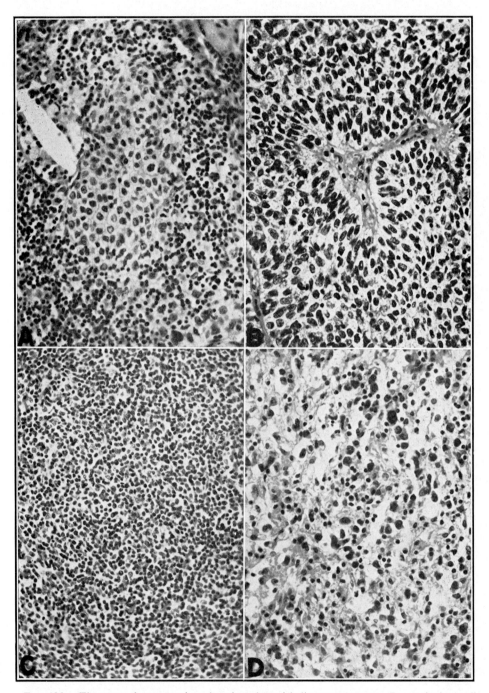

FIG. 483.—Thymoma demonstrating *A*, a lympho-epitheliomatous tumor, *B*, a reticulum cell type of growth, *C*, a lymphocytic variety of neoplasm, and *D*, a Hodgkin's type of tumor. × 200.

at from the roentgenographic changes. A differential diagnosis should, of course, encompass all other tumors of the mediastinum including benign cysts. The *treatment* of choice is complete surgical excision. This should be accomplished as soon as the tumor is discovered for when symptoms and signs of compression develop it is probably too late. Failing surgical extirpation, irradiation therapy is accompanied by good palliative results in cases of thymic lymphoblastoma but is ineffective in cases of thymic carcinoma. The *prognosis* is good in instances in which the tumor has remained localized and is completely removed surgically. Otherwise it is poor.

REFERENCES

Pathologic Physiology

SEGALOFF, A.: *Glandular Physiology and Therapy*, 5th Ed., Philadelphia, J. B. Lippincott Co., 1954, p. 417.

Congenital Anomalies

CARR, J. L.: J. Pediat., *27*, 1, 1945 (Status Thymicolymphaticus).
CRELLIN, J. A., *et al.:* Dis. Chest., *18*, 154, 1950 (Benign Thymic Cyst).
GILMOUR, J. R.: J. Path. & Bact., *52*, 213, 1941 (Aberrant Thymus).
WELLER, R. W., *et al.:* A. M. A. Arch. Path., *52*, 569, 1951 (Cyst).

Tumors

BIGELOW, N. H., and EHLERS, A. A.: J. Thoracic Surg., *23*, 528, 1952 (Lipothymoma).
HUBBELL, D. S., and LIEBOW, A. A.: Am. J. Path., *28*, 321, 1952 (Lymphangioendothelial Tumors).
LOWENHAUPT, E.: Cancer, *1*, 547, 1948 (Classifications of Tumors).
LOWENHAUPT, E., and BROWN, R.: Cancer, *4*, 1193, 1951 (Carcinoma).
MARGOLIS, H. M.: Am. J. Cancer, *15*, 2106, 1931 (Classification of Tumors).
POPE, R. H., and OSGOOD, R.: Am. J. Path., *29*, 85, 1953 (Reticular Perithelioma).
REID, H., and MARCUS, R.: Brit. J. Surg., *36*, 271, 1949 (Thymoma).
SEYBOLD, W. D., *et al.:* J. Thoracic Surg., *20*, 195, 1950 (General Discussion on Tumors).
SYMMERS, D.: Ann. Surg., *95*, 544, 1932 (Tumors).
WILSON, F. N., and PRITCHARD, J. E.: Canad. M. A. J., *53*, 444, 1945 (Malignant Thymoma).

29

Adrenal Glands

PATHOLOGIC PHYSIOLOGY

Joseph J. Rupp

EACH adrenal gland consists actually of two glands in one—a medulla developing from primitive ganglia of the celiac plexus and a cortex arising from peritoneal epithelium.

ADRENAL MEDULLA

The adrenal medulla secretes two *hormones*, epinephrine (adrenalin) and norepinephrine (noradrenalin). These sympathetic amines are adrenergic and have actions similar to those produced by activity of the sympathetic nervous system. *Epinephrine* causes contraction of some vessels and dilatation of others, the sum effect being a decrease in peripheral resistance and tachycardia. *Norepinephrine* constricts vessels, increases peripheral resistance, and decreases or has no effect on the heart rate. Both hormones are also calorogenic and glycogenolytic, although the activities of epinephrine are greater in these respects than are those of norepinephrine.

Although *functional tumors* of the adrenal medulla or of the extra adrenal chromaffin tissue secrete large amounts of epinephrine and norepinephrine, the ratio of the one to the other is not constant in any given tumor. The clinical manifestations of such tumors are persistent or paroxysmal hypertension, tremor, headache, flushing, nausea, and vomiting.

ADRENAL CORTEX

The adrenal cortex secretes *four groups* of *hormones*, designated according to their major physiological activities as glucocorticoids, adrenal androgens, adrenal estrogens, and mineralocorticoids.

The most potent naturally occurring *glucocorticoid* is *17 hydroxycorticosterone* (cortisol or compound F). Its rate of production is regulated by ACTH—the pituitary adrenocorticotrophic hormone. The rate of formation and release of ACTH in turn is regulated by neurohormones of the hypothalmus. Once secreted, the adrenal steroid exerts an inhibitory influence on the pituitary release of ACTH. Similarly, exogenous cortisol suppresses ACTH production. This results in atrophy of the adrenal cortex. Conversely, when the adrenal is destroyed or removed, ACTH production is increased above normal.

17 hydroxycorticosterone is both protein catabolic and diabetogenic with the resulting hyperglycemia representing the sequel of gluconeogenesis from protein. The hormone is anti-inflammatory, antifibroblastic, lympholytic, and eosinophilopenic. It also causes plethora and a tendency to polycythemia. It (1) helps regulate the renal clearance of water, (2) plays a part in the renal tubular regulation of sodium, potassium, hydrogen, and bicarbonate, and (3) in excessive amounts, may cause metabolic alkalosis. Because of changes in the protein matrix of bone and loss of calcium in the excreta, this steroid may ultimately produce osteoporosis. In excessive amounts, from either exogenous or endogenous sources, it may also result in *Cushing's syndrome* (hyperadrenocorticalism). In this disorder, the clinical manifestations result from excessive amounts of 17 hydroxycorticosterone and are the same regardless of whether the basic lesion is a hyperplasia or a tumor. The patients usually have hypertension, impaired carbohydrate metabolism, metabolic alkalosis, plethora, moon fact, truncal obesity, and purplish abdominal striae. Amenorrhea and varying degrees of hirsutism are usually present in the female. Osteoporosis, bone pain, and pathological fractures occur. In cases due to adrenal hyperplasia, treatment with ACTH for a few days results in a greater than normal increase in the plasma and urinary levels of 17 hydroxycorticosterone and its metabolites. When tumor is the cause, the changes following ACTH therapy are less marked and not as consistent. This failure of response to ACTH by a tumor, however, is not an invariable finding for some cases of tumor and even carcinoma, which responded to ACTH with a marked increase in cortisol production, have been reported. One explanation for this difference may be that a pituitary factor is necessary for adrenal hyperplasia whereas it is not necessary for adrenal tumors which are usually autonomous.

Adrenal androgens are excreted in the urine as 17 ketosteroids and, as such, account for about two thirds of the total urinary 17 ketosteroids. The adrenal production of androgens is regulated by ACTH and excessive secretion of these hormones may be brought about by adrenal cortical tumors. In overabundance they cause *virilization* in the *female*. Such patients disclose acne, hirsutism, a large clitoris, amenorrhea, and increased urinary levels of 17 ketosteroids.

Excessive production of adrenal androgens, as in congenital adrenal hyperplasia, may also result in *female pseudohermaphroditism* or *male pseudoprecocious puberty*. In these conditions, a congenital defect with respect to a hydroxylating enzyme in the adrenal gland limits the rate of synthesis of 17 hydroxycorticosterone. The most common abnormality is at the level of 17 hydroxyprogesterone which normally is completely transformed to compound S and this, in turn, is converted into 17 hydroxycorticosterone. When the defect is present, 17 hydroxyprogesterone is converted to compound S at a slower than normal rate, its level increases, and it is changed to pregnandiol which is excreted in the urine. Since the production of ACTH is increased because of the lowered levels of cortisol, the adrenal glands become hyperplastic and the production of adrenal androgens is increased. The androgenic steroids cause either pseudoprecocious puberty or pseudohermaphroditism. These conditions can be treated by use of a natural or synthetic steroid which has glucocorticoid activity. The steroid supplies the body's need and suppresses ACTH production. As a result, the adrenal glands decrease in size, their function decreases, and androgen production drops. On the other hand, adrenal stimulation with ACTH results in a greater than normal increase in secretion of androgens. Congenital adrenal hyperplasia must be differentiated from ovarian tumors in females and testicular tumors or idiopathic precocious puberty in males.

Estrogen producing tumors of the adrenal cause feminization in males and are accompanied by gynecomastia and decreased libido and potentia.

The most potent *mineralocorticoid* produced by the adrenal is *aldosterone*. For the most part, the adrenal production of this steroid is not regulated by the pituitary but is probably regulated by changes in the serum sodium or potassium or perhaps by changes in serum volume. Aldosterone (1) is excreted by the kidneys, with the urinary levels being increased by salt restriction and decreased by salt feeding and (2) acts on the kidney tubules to enhance the resorption of sodium and bicarbonate and to increase the excretion of potassium and hydrogen ions. Excessive amounts of aldosterone cause hypernatremia, hypokalemia, and alkalosis. Polyuria, polydypsia, and inability to produce a concentrated urine even in response to pitressin are present when continuous overproduction of aldosterone occurs. Such manifestations, along with hypertension, fatigue, muscle weakness, and muscle cramps, may be seen in connection with adrenal cortical tumors or hyperplasia in which case the disorder is referred to as *primary aldosteronism*. Despite the defect in serum potassium its correction by use of exogenous potassium is difficult. Indeed, some patients initially thought to have a potassium losing nephritis have been proved later to have primary aldosteronism. *Secondary aldosteronism* occurs in nephrosis, congestive heart failure with edema, cirrhosis with ascites, and during toxemia of pregnancy. In both primary and secondary aldosteronism, aldosterone is excreted in excessive amounts in the urine. In toxemia of pregnancy, however, the interpretation of high levels of the hormone in the urine must be interpreted with caution for they are elevated in normal pregnancy.

Hypoadrenalism, as seen in *Addison's disease* and referred to as *primary adrenal insufficiency*, develops when the production of adrenal steroids is inadequate for maintenance of normal homeostasis. This condition may be idiopathic or may result from adrenal surgery, infections, amyloid infiltration, or tumor metastases. In such instances, the glucocorticoids, mineralocorticoids, androgens, and estrogens are decreased or absent. This differs from the *adrenal insufficiency secondary* to *pituitary failure* in which aldosterone production, not under ACTH control, continues. For this reason, the electrolyte disturbances are less marked in secondary adrenal failure than they are in primary adrenal failure. The absence of cortisol production permits continuous ACTH production and this pituitary hormone, or a closely related pituitary factor, is responsible for the development of the hyperpigmentation which is characteristic of the patient with Addison's disease. The insulin sensitivity, tendency to hypoglycemia with fasting, and inability to excrete a water load found in patients with adrenal failure are reflections of the need for 17 hydroxycorticosterone. The absence of adrenal androgens is reflected by the low levels of 17 ketosteroids excreted in the urine. Hypotension, hyponatremia, and hyperkalemia are manifestations of lack of aldosterone action. Since patients with adrenal failure cannot increase their production of steroids as normally occurs in response to stressful situations, they are prone to develop adrenal crises when exposed to even minor injuries or illnesses. The shock which develops is rapidly fatal unless adequate treatment is instituted.

CONGENITAL ANOMALIES

Developmental malformations of the adrenal glands may consist of the following: (1) *absence*—of importance only when both glands are lacking, in which case the condition is incompatible with life, (2) *hypoplasia*— usually occurring as a result of hypoplasia of the pituitary gland, consisting of diminution in size of the cortex, and seen in conjunction with anencephalia or other malformations of the brain (Hartman), and (3) *aberrant adrenal tissue*—generally consisting of cortical tissue only, occurring in as high as 32 per cent of cases, and located in the area of the celiac plexus, beneath the renal capsule, beneath the hepatic capsule, in the pancreas, in the mesentery, and along the course of descent of the ovaries or testes (Gualtieri and Graham).

DEGENERATIONS

Orientation.—The adrenal glands are sensitive to virtually all of the ordinary degenerative disorders that affect the tissues of the body (p. 29). Specific references have already been made to amyloidosis and atrophy (p. 41) and to parenchymatous degeneration and focal necrosis (p. 209). Of particular interest, perhaps, are calcification, myeloid formation, and atrophy of sufficient degree to produce Addison's disease.

Calcification.—Calcification of the adrenal glands is the end stage of a variety of conditions, especially (1) hemorrhage, (2) tuberculosis, (3) other infections that may or may not be associated with hemorrhage, and (4) benign or malignant primary tumors (Snelling and Boyce). Pathologically the calcific deposits vary in size and location. Those resulting from hemorrhage are generally found in the medulla, those from inflammation in the cortex, and those associated with tumor within the neoplastic tissue. Histologically telltale evidence of the causative process is usually found.

Myeloid Formation.—Myeloid formation indicates simply the presence of bone marrow within the adrenal gland. The condition has *also* been *called* myeloid metaplasia, bone marrow heterotopia, and myelolipoma. Although the lesion probably arises as a metaplastic response to irritation, inflammation, or fibrosis it has been considered to represent misplaced marrow, embolism of marrow cells, and reactivation of hematopoiesis (Giffen) and it has been produced in female rats by treatment with testosterone and crude anterior pituitary preparations (Selye). *Pathologically* the lesion exists as a circumscribed encapsulated mass of orange-yellow tissue of an over-all diameter of as much as 8 cm. Histologically it is composed of normal appearing marrow that rarely contains bony trabeculæ.

Addison's Disease.—Addison's disease is a chronic type of adrenal cortical insufficiency characterized by asthenia, pigmentation of the skin and mucous membranes, hypotension, and gastrointestinal disturbances. Although the disorder is *uncommon* it is estimated that the death rate is approximately 4 per 1,000,000 people (Hartman). The condition is most common in the third and fourth decades of life, affects males about twice as frequently as females, and is as common in Negroes as it is in the white population (Tucker). The most common *causes* of the disappearance of adrenal cortical tissue to a degree sufficient to produce hypofunction are tuberculosis and idiopathic atrophy (Duffin). The precise reasons for the atrophy have not been determined although mythical toxic agents, decrease in vascular bed, arteriolar occlusion, etc., have been incriminated. Other uncommon or rare causes of disappearance of cortical tissue are fibrosis and calcification from previous septicemia (Tucker), amyloidosis (Heller), blastomycosis (Torres), metastatic (bronchial) carcinoma (Wallach and Butterly), trauma, amebiasis, fungous and yeast-like infections, avitaminosis, adrenal denervation, pituitary failure, etc. (Hartman).

Pathologically both adrenals are always affected. In cases of idiopathic atrophy, the amount of adrenal tissue present may be so small that it is scarcely identifiable or it may not be found at all. In the latter instance, histologic sections made of the areolar tissue in areas where the adrenal normally is located usually discloses remnants of the adrenal. In either case, the cortex is completely or almost completely absent and all that remains is the medulla (Fig. 484). Generally, the amount of medullary tissue and the appearance of medullary cells are within normal limits. Throughout the medulla, however, and throughout the cortical area, there are usually varying degrees of lymphocytic infiltration. The vessels may appear relatively normal or they may show varying degrees of arterio-

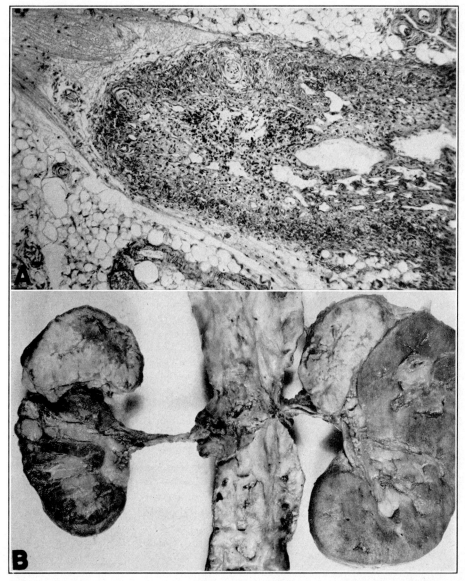

FIG. 484.—Addison's disease showing A, idiopathic atrophy of the adrenal with complete loss of cortical tissue and a permeation of the medulla with lymphocytes. × 100 and B, tuberculosis with diffuse enlargement and destruction of the adrenals by caseous tissue.

sclerosis. In cases of tuberculosis, the adrenals are always enlarged although they retain their normal shape (Fig. 484). The capsules are relatively intact but virtually all of the adrenal tissue is replaced with caseous, fibrocaseous, or fibrotic and calcified material. Histologically normal cortical cells are scarcely identifiable and even the medullary tissue is destroyed. The appearances of the adrenals in cases caused by other than atrophy or tuberculosis vary according to the etiologic agents and need not be discussed here. *Associated lesions* in Addison's disease are melanin pigmentation of the basal layer of the skin and mucous membranes, small heart, lymphoid hyperplasia or infiltration (especially of organs of the reticulo-endothelial system), atrophy and fibrosis of the thyroid gland, and increase in connective tissue and decrease of basophil cells of the anterior lobe of the pituitary gland (Duffin).

Aside from the manifestations that are part of the syndrome itself, the chief *complications* of Addison's disease are (1) intercurrent infection as a result of decrease in general resistance and (2) the effects of the disorder (such as tuberculosis, carcinoma, etc.) that originally causes the disappearance of adrenal cortical tissue. The *clinical manifestations* consist of the following (Duffin and Hartman): (1) gradually developing and slowly progressing physical and mental asthenia, (2) hypotension with palpitation, dyspnea, dizziness, faintness, etc., (3) gastrointestinal disturbances in the form of anorexia, loss of weight, hiccough, gaseous distention, nausea, vomiting, diarrhea, or constipation, (4) brown to black melanin pigmentation of the skin, mucous membranes, and occasionally hair, and (5) addisonian crisis characterized by an intensification of the above mentioned symptoms and signs with development of a shock-like picture (p. 209). The crisis may be precipitated by withholding sodium chloride from the diet. The *laboratory* findings consist of low basal metabolic rate, low blood sugar, low adrenalin hyperglycemia (due to low storage of glycogen in the liver), low creatinine and uric acid outputs, reduced excretion of ascorbic acid in the urine, relative neutropenia and lymphocytosis, normal erythrocytic count, impaired renal function, low plasma sodium, and decreased excretion of 17-ketosteroids. The *diagnosis* is generally made from a combination of the clinical manifestations and laboratory findings listed above. Of importance, is the combination of asthenia, pigmentation of the skin, hypotension, and gastrointestinal disturbances. *Treatment* is threefold. In essence it consists of (1) replacement of adrenocortical hormones, (2) administration of sodium salts and fluids to replace the loss due to the missing sodium factor and administration of glucose, especially in crisis, and (3) prevention of unnecessary stresses that call for increased production of hormones (Hartman). The *prognosis*, prior to hormonal therapy, was poor for the course was progressively downhill and invariably terminated fatally. Today, with the availability of adequate adrenocortical hormones, life can be prolonged indefinitely.

INFLAMMATIONS

Orientation. — Inflammation of the adrenal gland is known as *adrenalitis* or *adrenitis*. The more important inflammations consist of (1) *nonspecific adrenalitis* — caused by the ordinary pyogenic organisms and occurring as a result of direct extension from adjacent structures (such as the peritoneum), septicemia or pyemia, and rarely from the outside in conjunction with penetrating injuries or operation, (2) *tuberculosis* — always occurring as a result of bloodstream infection from another focus within the body, being found as a miliary or a fibrocaseous process, and, when extensive, producing Addison's disease, and (3) *fungous* and *yeast-like adrenalitis* — particularly blastomycosis and histoplasmosis and always occurring as a result of hematogenous spread in systemic disease.   In addition to the above listed conditions, a few words should be said about the Waterhouse-Friderichsen syndrome.

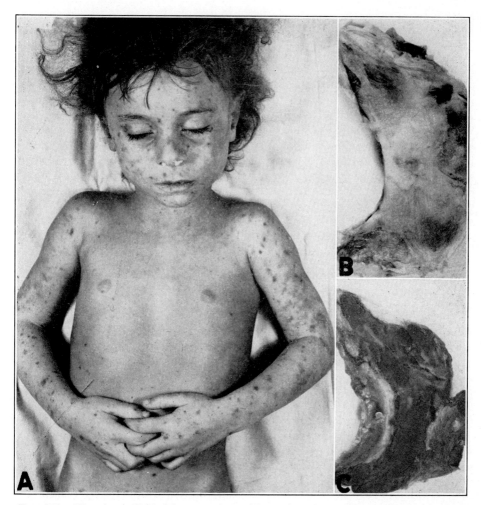

Fig. 485.—Waterhouse-Friderichsen syndrome illustrating *A*, numerous petechiæ, especially over the face and extremities, *B*, external, and *C*, cut surfaces of an adrenal destroyed by hemorrhage.

Waterhouse-Friderichsen Syndrome. —This syndrome may be *defined* as a fulminating septicemia attended by massive bilateral adrenal hemorrhages, acute adrenal insufficiency, profound shock, and frequently death. The condition is *uncommon*, but over 125 cases had been recorded in the literature up to 1943 (Herbut) and many others have been reported on since (Nelson and Walker).   While the syndrome may occur at any age, it usually affects children in the first decade of life and has no predilection for either sex. Most cases are *caused* by meningococci and, conversely, from 2 to 4 per cent of meningococcic infections develop the syndrome (Nelson). Other infrequent causes are staphylococci, streptococci, and pneumococci. *Clinically* there is a rapid onset of fever, headache, malaise, and chills. This is followed by widespread petechiæ and larger hemorrhages (Fig. 485*A*), unobtainable pulse, cyanosis, coma, and usually death—all within a matter of six to twelve hours. The causative organisms may be recovered from the blood, spinal fluid, or cutaneous hemorrhages. *Pathologically* the general findings are those of *septicemia* and include acute splenitis, generalized hyperemia, petechiæ or larger hemorrhages throughout all the organs (especially the lungs), and sometimes acute meningitis. Sections through the hemorrhagic areas of the skin disclose the causative organisms within thrombotic vessels and among extravasated erythrocytes. The most striking change, however, is in the adrenal gland (Fig. 485 *B* and *C*). Each organ discloses a massive hemorrhage that starts within the medulla, gradually permeates and destroys the cortex, and ultimately distends the adrenal capsule. The shape of the organ is maintained but the size is two or more times that of normal. The *complications* consist of death (septicemia and acute adrenal insufficiency), renal failure, and, rarely, (in some of the survivors) Addison's disease. The *clinical diagnosis* is made from the manifestations as outlined together with the demonstration of causative organisms in smears of blood from the cutaneous hemorrhages. *Treatment* consists of combating septicemia and shock and restoring the adrenocortical hormones. The *prognosis* is grave, although more and more cases of recovery are constantly being recorded following heroic treatment.

PHYSICAL DISTURBANCES

The only important disorder in this category is *hemorrhage* or *apoplexy*. Massive bilateral adrenal hemorrhage occurring in connection with fulminating septicemia has already been considered in connection with the Waterhouse-Friderichsen syndrome. Other possible *causes* of bleeding into the adrenal gland are birth and other trauma, neonatal involution, pregnancy, venous thrombosis, hemorrhagic diathesis, heparin therapy, tumors, burns, hypertension, arteritis, and idiopathic (Emery, Berte, and Greene). It may *occur* at all ages from birth on. *Pathologically* the process may be unilateral or bilateral and may consist of (1) massive hemorrhage replacing the entire parenchyma of the gland, (2) central hemorrhage replacing the medulla only and leaving the cortex relatively intact, or (3) multiple small foci of bleeding scattered throughout both the cortex and the medulla. The *clinical manifestations* result from the causative condition, irritation of the nerves by the extravasated blood, absorption of protein products, and adrenocortical insufficiency. A *newborn* infant with adrenal hemorrhage discloses the following: lack of desire to eat, paleness, pyrexia, restlessness, weakness, coma, and perhaps a palpable mass in the region of the adrenal. An *adult* may reveal pain (epigastrium, upper quadrant, or simply abdomen), abdominal tenderness, localized abdominal hyperesthesia, pallor, prostration, hypotension, cyanosis, nausea, vomiting, shock, fever, and leukocytosis. The *diagnosis* may be suspected from the clinical manifestations as outlined. *Treatment* is directed toward the primary condition and combating shock. The *prognosis* depends upon the causative factor and upon the distribution and extent of the bleeding.

TUMORS

Orientation.—Since the adrenal gland is composed of connective tissue, fat, nerves, blood vessels, and parenchyma, the organ is capable of giving rise to a variety of neoplasms. Also, because the blood supply is abundant, metastatic tumors (particularly bronchogenic carcinoma) are quite com-

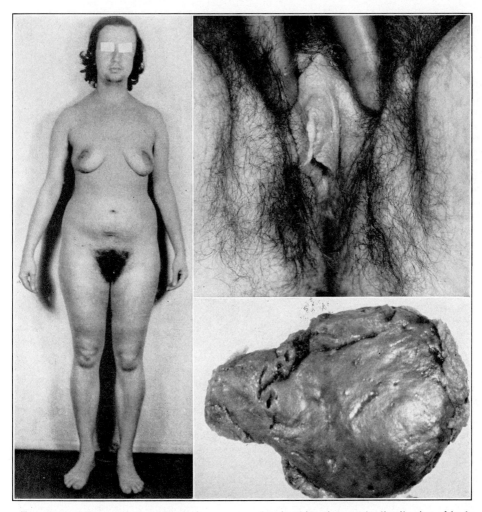

FIG. 486.—Adrenogenital syndrome in a woman showing hirsutism, male distribution of body hair, some atrophy of the breasts, hypertrophy of the clitoris, and the causative circumscribed adenoma. (Photographs of the patient by courtesy of Dr. A. E. Rakoff.)

mon. Of all the growths, however, those arising in the parenchyma proper are the most important. They are readily dividable into tumors originating in the cortex and those originating in the medulla.

Cortical Tumors.—Tumors or tumor-like conditions of the adrenal cortex may be *classified pathologically* into the following three groups: hyperplasia, adenoma, and carcinoma. Each of these may or may not be associated with increased hormonal excretion and, accordingly, may be further divided *clinically* into functional and nonfunctional. Morphologically, however, functional tumors cannot be differentiated from nonfunctional growths and, clinically, any of the various syndromes may be produced by any of the morphologic type of neoplasms. Thus, the discussion of the topic may be simplified by first outlining the clinical syndromes and then describing briefly each of the tumors or tumor-like conditions.

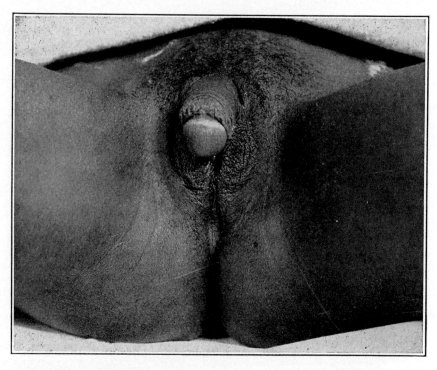

FIG. 487.—Adrenogenital syndrome in a nine year old Negro girl illustrating marked enlargement of the clitoris. (Herbut's *Urological Pathology*.)

Functional Tumors.—Functional adrenocortical growths produce combinations of clinical manifestations that have been variously classified (Cahill, Kepler, Wilkins, and Walters). One of the simplest perhaps is that of Kenyon. It consists of the following five categories: (1) *adrenogenital syndrome*—seen most commonly in girls but occurring occasionally in women and even in boys and characterized by masculinization which includes the following: precocious or heterosexual growth of phallus, deepening of the voice, male distribution of body hair, enhancement of somatic growth in children, failure of normal development of the breasts in female children, and amenorrhea in women (Figs. 486 and 487), (2) *Cushing's syndrome*—occurring mostly in women and less often in children and characterized by hirsutism, adiposity of the "buffalo" type, moon-shaped facies, acne, purple cutaneous striæ, ecchymoses, hypertension, osteoporosis, diabetes mellitus, and amenorrhea (Fig. 488 and 489), (3) *combinations* of *adrenogenital* and *Cushing's syndromes*, (4) *isolated expressions* of the *above*—diabetes or amenorrhea alone, and (5) *feminization*—in girls characterized by precosity and in men (seen rarely) characterized by atrophy of the testes, loss of body hair, and overdevelopment of the breasts.

Cortical Hyperplasia.—Hyperplasia of the adrenal cortex signifies an increase in the size and number of cortical cells. It may occur at any age and is usually bilateral. *Grossly* the normal shape of the gland is more or less maintained but the over-all size may be many times that of normal (Fig. 490). *Histologically* the normal architecture of the cortex is not disturbed but the different zones are larger and more prominent than normal and the component cells are likewise more conspicuous. The supporting connective tissue is scanty and well vascularized and the medulla remains relatively normal. While it is not known for certain, the *cause* of adrenocortical hyperplasia may be overstimulation by adrenocortical hormone

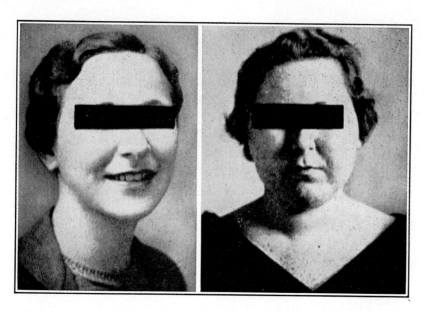

FIG. 488.—Cushing's syndrome due to adrenal cortical hyperplasia showing the patient before and after the illness developed. The latter photograph illustrates a moon-shaped facies, acne, and hirsutism. (Herbut's *Urological Pathology*.)

(ACTH) of the pituitary gland. Excessive production of ACTH may result from lesions in the pituitary (for Cushing's syndrome is often associated with basophilic adenoma or hyalinization of the basophil cells of the pituitary) or from external stimuli of the pituitary such as occurs after adrenalectomy, after estrogenic therapy, or during absolute increase in cortical hormone requirement (Tepperman and Paschkis). Hyperplasia of the adrenal cortex is recognized clinically only when it is hormonally overactive.

Cortical Adenoma.—Adenoma of the adrenal cortex may appear at any age and is unilateral or bilateral. It occurs in two forms—the presence of one or several circumscribed small nodules often referred to as *adenomatous hyperplasia* and the presence of a *solitary nodule* that may measure 3 cm. or more in diameter (Fig. 491). In either case, the adenoma is sharply circumscribed and even encapsulated, light yellowish orange, and of the consistency of the normal cortex. When larger, it may disclose focal areas of necrosis and hemorrhage. Histologically it is usually composed of relatively normal appearing cortical cells that are distributed irregularly rather than in radiating parallel columns. The supporting stroma is

64

generally scanty and well vascularized. Adenoma of the adrenal cortex is benign and, therefore, does not metastasize. Aside from its sporadic connection in cases of adrenogenital and Cushing's syndromes, some authors have tried to incriminate adenomatous hyperplasia of the adrenal cortex as a cause of essential hypertension (Reinhart and Russi). Other authors, however, have shown that such changes occur in both hypertensive and nonhypertensive patients and that they are not necessarily concerned with the production of high blood pressure (Dempsey and Commons). Adenoma of the adrenal is asymptomatic unless it is hormonally overactive.

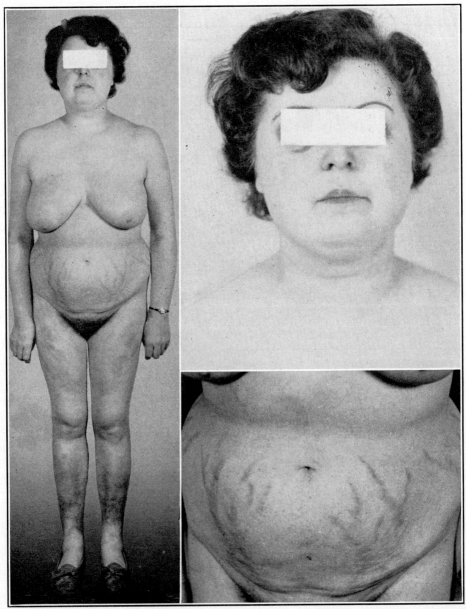

FIG. 489.—Cushing's syndrome illustrating adiposity of the "buffalo" type, moon-shaped face, acne about the face, and abdominal striæ.

Cortical Carcinoma.—Carcinoma of the adrenal cortex may occur at any age and is approximately as frequent in males as it is in females (Cleveland and Anderson). The *tumor* is unilateral in about 90 per cent of cases and bilateral in 10 per cent of cases. In unilateral cases it is about twice as frequent on the left side as on the right. It may arise in any part of the

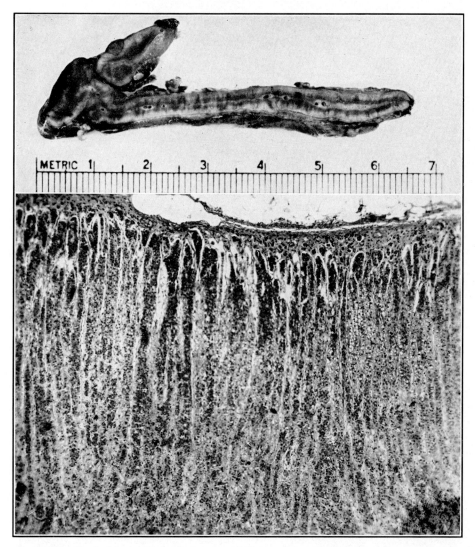

Fig. 490.—Cortical hyperplasia of the adrenal illustrating moderate enlargement of the gland due to increase in size of the cortex and hypertrophy and hyperplasia of the cortical cells with prominence of cords. × 50.

cortex, may partially or completely replace the homolateral gland, and, at the time of discovery, may measure as much as 25 cm. in diameter. As a rule, the growth is encapsulated, moderately firm, friable, and yellowish orange to tan (Fig. 492). As it enlarges, it generally discloses foci of necrosis, hemorrhage, and cyst formation. The *histologic* picture varies greatly from case to case. At one extreme, the cells may resemble those seen in an

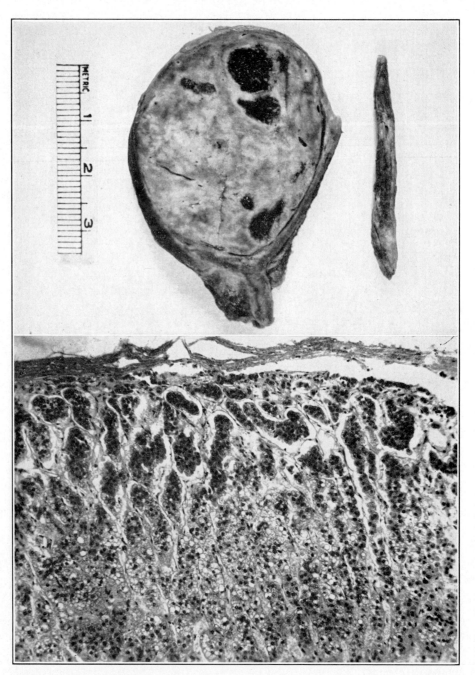

Fig. 491.—Cortical adenoma of the adrenal showing a well-encapsulated tumor with foci of necrosis and hemorrhage (compared with the remaining adrenal gland) and regular appearing cortical cells irregularly arranged. × 100.

adenoma while at the other extreme the cells (1) are large, rounded, or polyhedral, (2) possess an abundant amount of granular, reticulated, or vacuolated eosinophilic cytoplasm, and (3) disclose round, oval, or irregular, varisized, hyperchromatic nuclei. When the capsule is invaded and neo-plastic cells are found within vascular channels, a diagnosis of carcinoma is warranted regardless of how innocent the tumor appears. Carcinoma of the adrenal *spreads* by (1) direct extension to adjacent structures and (2)

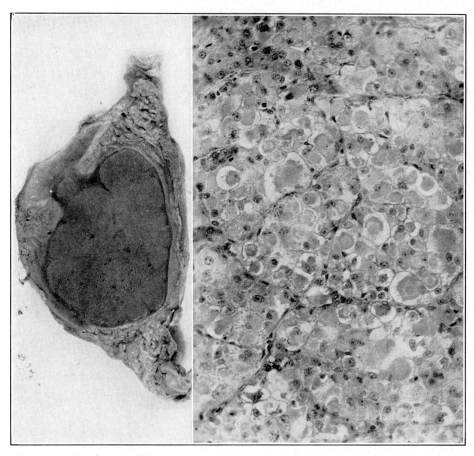

Fig. 492.—Carcinoma of the adrenal cortex demonstrating grossly a well-encapsulated, deep brown tumor and microscopically large polyhedral cells with granular and vacuolated cytoplasm and rounded nuclei. × 200.

vascular channels to the lymph nodes, liver, lungs, and other tissues of the body. *Clinically* hormonally overactive tumors may be readily recognized. Functionless tumors are symptomless in the early stages. In time, however, they are attended by pain, malaise, loss of weight, and a palpable ab-dominal mass (Griffiths). Pressure upon adjacent organs may, in addition, produce symptoms referable to the gastrointestinal tract, kidneys, etc. *Treatment* consists of surgical excision of the tumor. The *prognosis* is poor for the neoplasm grows rapidly and metastasizes early.

Medullary Tumors.—The important neoplasms of the adrenal medulla are of nerve tissue origin and are similar to those that arise in sympathetic ganglia and, in some instances (pheochromocytoma), paraganglia cells. In order to appreciate the various types or mixtures of tumors, one should remember the *histogenesis* of the cells in the areas concerned. Embryologically, neural crests give rise to primitive cells called medullary epithelial cells and these differentiate into mother or sympathogonia cells. The latter, in turn, differentiate into (1) neurilemma or Schwann cells of the nerve fibers, (2) neuroblasts (sympathoblasts), and (3) pheochromoblasts. The neuroblasts differentiate further into ganglion cells and the pheochromoblasts differentiate into pheochromocytes. Each of the cells listed is capable of giving rise to (or at least constituting) a tumor. Thus the following four

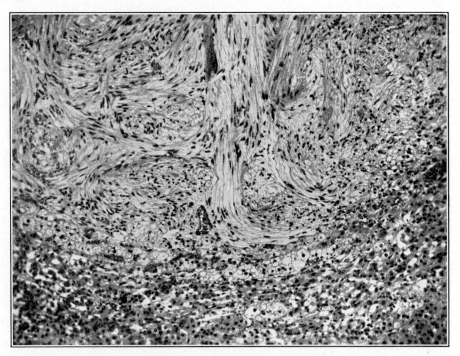

Fig. 493.—Neurilemmoma of the adrenal medulla showing interlacing bundles of fibrous tissue-like cells. × 100.

groups of tumors are generally recognized: (1) neurilemmoma or schwannoma, (2) neuroblastoma or sympathoblastoma (including also tumors of the more primitive medullary epithelial or sympathogonia cells), (3) ganglioneuroma, and (4) pheochromocytoma (including pheochromoblastoma).

Neurilemmoma.—Neurilemmoma or schwannoma is a benign tumor of the supporting structure of the nerve fibers, and in your author's opinion, is indistinguishable from neurofibroma. As far as the adrenal gland is concerned, the growth is rare and unimportant. It occurs alone or in conjunction with similar tumors of nerve trunks, may be microscopic or several centimeters in size, and is composed of elongated, fibrous tissue-like cells in interlacing bundle formation (Fig. 493). Nerve fibers may or may not be readily recognizable.

Neuroblastoma.—Neuroblastoma has also been called sympathoblastoma, sympathicoblastoma, sympathogonioma, neurocytoma, and medullary epithelioma (Beck). The tumor is as frequent in males as it is in females and is usually seen in children within the first five years of life. Occasionally, however, it does occur in older children and in adults. The *cause* of the tumor is unknown. *Pathologically* the neoplasm is most common in the adrenal glands but it may also occur in any of the vertebral sympathetic ganglia as well as the celiac plexus and organ of Zuckerkandl near the bifurcation of the aorta (Beck). Regardless of its precise location, the tumor is generally of unicentric origin and is thus, of course, unilateral. It varies greatly in size from a few to many centimeters in diameter, is at first well encapsulated but later breaks through the capsule, appears gray to hemorrhagic, usually discloses large areas of necrosis, and may reveal foci of calcification (Fig. 494). *Histologically* it is composed of round cells with scanty cytoplasm and relatively large, round, evenly but deeply staining nuclei. Some of the cells resemble lymphocytes while others resemble lymphoblasts. Usually the cells are diffusely arranged but when enough sections are made and studied carefully rosette formation is generally apparent. Neuroblastoma *spreads* by direct extension to the spinal canal, inferior vena cava, and other structures and by vascular channels to distant organs. In the past, neuroblastoma of the right adrenal was thought to metastasize characteristically to the liver and the tumor was referred to as one of the Pepper type. Neuroblastoma of the left adrenal, on the other hand, was thought to metastasize characteristically to the skull and retro-orbital tissue and was referred to as one of the Hutchinson type. In recent years, however, it has been shown that such precise metastases are not constant enough to warrant the use of the eponyms listed. Aside from the liver, skull, and retro-orbital tissues, metastasis may occur to any of the organs of the body. The chief *complication* of neuroblastoma is metastasis. There are no endocrinologic disturbances from the tumor as such. The *clinical manifestations* are extremely variable (Boyd). The most common local manifestation is enlargement of the abdomen but frequently metastases to the skull or retro-orbital tissues may constitute the first sign of the disorder. In addition, patients usually exhibit pain, pallor, wasting, fatigue, listlessness, loss of weight, anorexia, fever, hepatomegaly, headache, and vomiting. *Roentgenographic* examination of the abdomen may disclose a tumor mass with foci of calcification and roentgenograms of the skull and other bones may reveal destructive lesions together with spicules of new bone formation at right angles to the surface. The *diagnosis* of neuroblastoma is made from the clinical manifestations, from the roentgen appearance, and by exclusion. A differential diagnosis should include, among other things, Wilms' tumor of the kidney and lymphoblastoma. *Treatment* consists of surgical excision when the tumor is excisable and of irradiation therapy when local extension or metastasis has occurred. The *prognosis* is fair. In general, about 10 per cent of reported cases are recorded as cures (Beck), although Wittenborg listed a cure rate of about 30 per cent in a series of 73 cases studied. The best outlook is in those patients in whom the disease is confined to the abdomen. Conversely patients with metastasis to the chest or bones have thus far not been salvagable.

Ganglioneuroma.—A ganglioneuroma may arise in the adrenal medulla or any of the sympathetic ganglia (McFarland, Willis, and Lewis). *Grossly* the tumor may measure as much as 15 to 20 cm. in diameter (Fig. 495). It is sharply circumscribed, smooth or bossed, well encapsulated, and diffusely grayish white. Some tumors may, in addition, show areas of necrosis, calcification, hemorrhage, or cyst formation. *Histologically* they consist of mixtures of nerve bundles, ganglion cells, and edematous stroma. Ganglio-

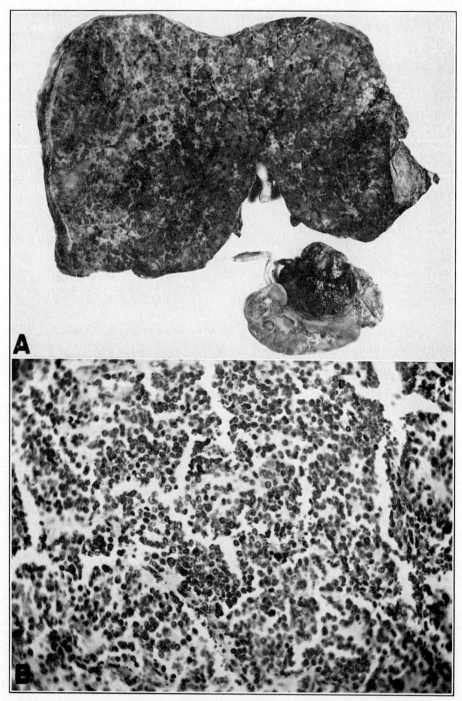

Fig. 494.—Neuroblastoma illustrating A, a primary tumor of the right adrenal compressing the kidney and metastasizing to the liver and B, the microscopic appearance with a diffuse infiltration of lymphoid-like cells. × 200.

neuroma is ordinarily *benign* but, in a certain proportion of cases, it may become *malignant*. When such a change occurs the affected tissue reverts to a more primitive form, constituting in fact a *neuroblastoma*. The *clinical manifestations* of a ganglioneuroma are those referable to a slowly growing, space taking lesion and thus vary with the location of the neoplasm. *Treatment* consists of surgical excision. The *prognosis* is good.

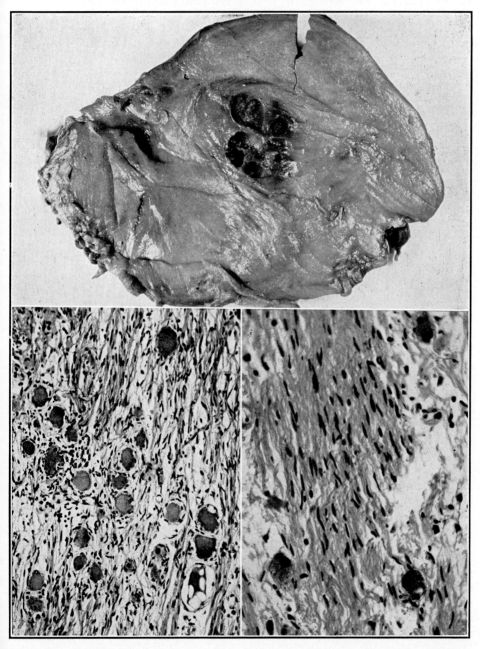

FIG. 495.—Ganglioneuroma showing grossly a large tumor with a neuroblastomatous transformation in its central portion and microscopically mixtures of ganglion cells, nerve fibers, and edematous stroma. × 100 and 200.

Pheochromocytoma. — Because it is often impossible to differentiate between a benign tumor of pheochromocytes (pheochromocytoma) and a
malignant tumor of pheochromoblasts (pheochromoblastoma or malignant
pheochromocytoma) the two are generally discussed together under the
heading of pheochromocytoma. The tumor, *also called* chromaffinoma and
paraganglioma, is more common than generally supposed. It *occurs* at all
ages but is relatively infrequent in children (Snyder and Hubble).

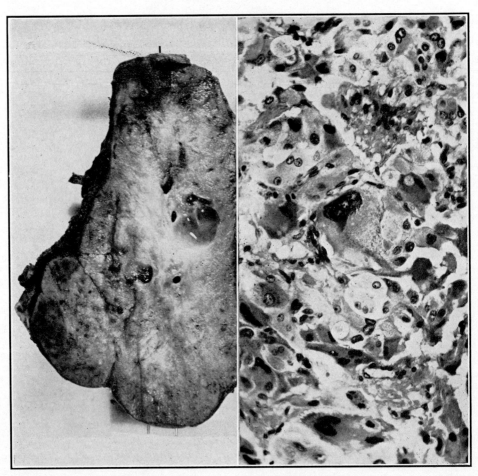

Fig. 496.—Pheochromocytoma demonstrating a mottled light and dark brown cut surface containing several small cysts and irregular large cells containing fine brown granules. × 200.

Pathologically it usually arises in the adrenal but it may also occur in
other sites such as the carotid body, organ of Zuckerkandl, retroperitoneal
tissues, intestinal wall, and thorax (Walton and Ortega). In the adrenal,
the growth is usually unilateral and may measure as much as 12 cm. in
diameter. It starts in the medulla and gradually destroys the adrenal as
it enlarges. The tumor is usually well encapsulated, rounded, and moderately firm. Cut surfaces are homogeneously reddish brown and may
reveal areas of necrosis, hemorrhage, and cyst formation (Fig. 496). Biochemical assays on the tumor disclose large amounts of adrenalin and
noradrenalin (Hatch). *Histologically* remnants of adrenal cortex may be

found peripherally. The tumor varies greatly in its microscopic composition. The cells are diffusely arranged. In the better differentiated growths, they resemble those of a normal adrenal medulla. In the more poorly differentiated tumors, the cells may be extremely large and irregular possessing an abundant amount of granular or vacuolated cytoplasm and irregular hyperchromatic nuclei. When fixed in chrome salts, the cytoplasm discloses fine brown granules. In either case, the stroma is usually scanty and inconspicuous. As already stated, it is virtually impossible to predict the benignity or malignancy of the growth from the microscopic appearance of the cells. As a rule, the growth remains *localized*, but when it becomes definitely malignant it *metastasizes* to the regional and distant lymph nodes, liver, bones, lungs, pleura, skin, intestines, and kidney (Brines).

The chief *complications* are a malignant transformation and development of shock after adrenalectomy from withdrawal of adrenalin. The most characteristic *clinical manifestation* consists of *paroxysmal hypertension* (Howard, Calkins, and Snyder). An attack usually lasts one to two hours and may be repeated at intervals ranging up to six years. It consists of hypertension to as high as 300 mm. of mercury together with headache, palpitation, perspiration, nausea, and occasionally vomiting (deVries). In addition, the following are of importance: hyperglycemia accompanying the hypertension, low glucose tolerance test, increased metabolic rate, precipitation of an attack by administration of histamine or mecholyl, demonstration of increased amounts of adrenalin in the blood during an attack, and reduction of blood pressure by an adrenalin antagonist such as benzodioxane (Cahill). *Roentgenography* (plain films, pyelograms, or peri-adrenal air insufflation) is often useful in outlining the tumor. The *diagnosis* is made from the clinical manifestations as listed. *Treatment* consists of surgical removal of the tumor. The *prognosis* is good in surgically treated cases but is poor in patients in whom the tumor is not removed.

REFERENCES

General

HARTMAN, F. A., and BROWNELL, K. A.: *The Adrenal Gland*, Philadelphia, Lea & Febiger 1949.

HERBUT, P. A.: *Urological Pathology*, Philadelphia, Lea & Febiger, p. 695, 1952.

Pathologic Physiology

COOK, J. R., and SCHNEIDER, R. W.: *Glandular Physiology and Therapy*, 5th Ed., Philadelphia, J. B. Lippincott Co., 1954, p. 132 (Adrenal Medulla).

PINCUS, G., and THIMAN, K. V.: *The Hormones*, New York, Academic Press, Vol. 3, 1955.

THORN, G. W.: *The Diagnosis and Treatment of Adrenal Insufficiency*, 2nd Ed., Springfield, Charles C Thomas, 1951.

VENNING, E. H., *et al.*: *Glandular Physiology and Therapy*, 5th Ed., Philadelphia, J. B. Lippincott Co., 1954, p. 99 (Adrenal Cortex).

Congenital Anomalies

GRAHAM, L. S.: Cancer, *6*, 149, 1953 (Celiac Accessory Adrenals).

GUALTIERE, T., and SEGAL, A. D.: J. Urol., *61*, 949, 1949 (Aberrant Adrenal Tissues).

Degenerations

BOYCE, C. L., and SEARS, W. N.: Radiology, *56*, 731, 1951 (Calcification in Adrenal Neoplasms).

BUTTERLY, J. M., *et al.:* Ann. Int. Med., *37*, 930, 1952 (Addison's Disease Due to Metastatic Carcinoma).
DUFFIN, J. D.: A. M. A. Arch. Path., *35*, 649, 1943 (Addison's Disease from Cortical Necrosis).
GIFFEN, H. K.: Am. J. Path., *23*, 613, 1947 (Myeloid Formation).
HELLER, E. L., and CAMARATA, S. J.: A. M. A. Arch. Path., *49*, 601, 1950 (Addison's Disease from Amyloidosis).
SELYE, H., and STONE, H.: Am. J. Path., *26*, 211, 1950 (Experimental Myeloid Formation).
SNELLING, C. E., and ERB, I. H.: J. Pediat., *6*, 22, 1935 (Calcification Following Hemorrhage).
TORRES, C. M., *et al.:* Am. J. Path., *28*, 145, 1952 (Destruction of Adrenals in Blastomycosis).
TUCKER, H. ST. G., JR., *et al.:* Am. J. M. Sci., *223*, 479, 1952 (Addison's Disease in the Negro).
WALLACH, J. B., and SCHARFMAN, W. B.: J. A. M. A., *148*, 729, 1952 (Addison's Disease from Bronchogenic Carcinoma).

Inflammations

HERBUT, P. A., and MANGES, W. E., A. M. A. Arch. Path., *36*, 413, 1943 (Waterhouse-Friderichsen Syndrome).
NELSON, J., and GOLDSTEIN, N.: J. A. M. A., *146*, 1193, 1951 (Waterhouse-Friderichsen Syndrome).
WALKER, S. H., *et al.:* Ann. Int. Med., *38*, 610, 1953 (Waterhouse-Friderichsen Syndrome and Renal Failure).

Physical Disturbances

BERTE, S. J.: Ann. Int. Med., *38*, 28, 1953 (Spontaneous Adrenal Hemorrhage in Adults).
EMERY, J. L., and ZACKARY, R. B.: Brit. M. J., *2*, 857, 1952 (Adrenal Hematoma in Newborn).
GREENE, R. C.: J. A. M. A., *152*, 133, 1953 (Idiopathic Adrenal Apoplexy).

Tumors

ANDERSON, A. F., *et al.:* J. Path. & Bact., *55*, 341, 1943 (Adrenal Carcinoma).
BECK, S. M., JR., and HOWARD, P. J.: Am. J. Dis. Child., *82*, 325, 1951 (Neuroblastoma).
BOYD, R. W.: Canad. M. A. J., *63*, 153, 1950 (Neuroblastoma).
BRINES, O. A., and JENNINGS, E.: Am. J. Path., *24*, 1167, 1948 (Paraganglioma).
CAHILL, G. F.: Surgery, *16*, 233, 1944 (Hormonal Tumors of Adrenal Gland).
CAHILL, G. F., and ARANOW, H., JR.: Ann. Int. Med., *31*, 389, 1949 (Pheochromocytoma).
CALKINS, E., and HOWARD, J. E.: J. Clin. Endocrinol., *7*, 475, 1947 (Bilateral Pheochromocytoma).
CLEVELAND, M., and KNOX, L. C.: A. M. A. Arch. Surg., *47*, 192, 1943 (Bilateral Carcinoma of Adrenal Cortex).
COMMONS, R. R., and CALLAWAY, C. P.: A. M. A. Arch. Int. Med., *81*, 37, 1948 (Adenomas of Adrenal Cortex).
DEMPSEY, W. S.: A. M. A. Arch. Path., *34*, 1031, 1942 (Adrenal Cortex in Hypertension).
DEVRIES, A., *et al.:* Am. J. Med., *6*, 51, 1949 (Pheochromocytoma).
GRIFFITHS, E.: Brit. J. Surg., *37*, 311, 1950 (Carcinoma Adrenal Cortex).
HATCH, F. N., *et al.:* Am. J. Med., *6*, 633, 1949 (Pheochromocytoma).
HOWARD, J. E., and BARKER, W. H.: Bull. Johns Hopkins Hosp., *61*, 371, 1937 (Pheochromocytoma).
HUBBLE, D.: A. M. A. Arch. Dis. Child., *26*, 340, 1951 (Pheochromocytoma in Children).
KENYON, A. T.: Surgery, *16*, 194, 1944 (Adrenocortical Tumors).
KEPLER, E. J., *et al.: Pathologic Physiology of Adrenocortical Tumors and Cushing's Syndrome,* Recent Progress in Hormonal Research, Proc. Laurentian Hormone Conference, Vol. II, New York, Academic Press, Inc., pp. 345–389, 1948.
LEWIS, D., and GESCHICKTER, C. F.: A. M. A. Arch. Surg., *28*, 16, 1934 (Tumors Sympathetic Nervous System).
McFARLAND, J.: A. M. A. Arch. Path., *11*, 118, 1931 (Ganglioneuroma).
ORTEGA, P., JR.: A. M. A. Arch. Path., *53*, 78, 1952 (Paraganglioma Arising from the Organ of Zuckerkandl).
PASCHKIS, K. E., *et al.:* J. Clin. Endocrinol., *3*, 212, 1943 (Cushing's Syndrome).
RINEHART, J. F., *et al.:* A. M. A. Arch. Path., *32*, 169, 1941 (Adenomatous Hyperplasia of Adrenal Cortex).
RUSSI, S., *et al.:* A. M. A. Arch. Int. Med., *76*, 284, 1945 (Adenomas of the Adrenal Cortex).
SNYDER, C. H., and VICK, E. H.: Am. J. Dis. Child., *73*, 581, 1947 (Pheochromocytoma in Children).

TEPPERMAN, J., *et al.:* Endocrinology, *32*, 373, 1943 (Adrenocortical Hypertrophy).

WALTERS, W., and SPRAGUE, R. G.: J. A. M. A., *141*, 653, 1949 (Functioning Adrenocortical Tumors).

WALTON, J. N.: Lancet, *1*, 438, 1950 (Pheochromocytoma).

WILKINS, L.: J. Clin. Endocrinol., *8*, 111, 1948 (Feminizing Adrenal Tumor in a Boy and Virilizing Tumor in a Girl).

WILLIS, R. A.: *Pathology of Tumors*, St. Louis, C. V. Mosby Co., p. 843, 1948.

WITTENBORG, M. H.: Radiology, *54*, 679, 1950 (Roentgen Therapy in Neuroblastoma).

Chapter

30

Lower Urinary System

PATHOLOGIC PHYSIOLOGY

WILLARD M. DRAKE, JR.

THE *function* of the *lower urinary system* which begins with the collecting tubules, is to collect, store, and transport the urine formed by the kidney, until it has been expelled from the body. The pelvis collects urine from the collecting ducts and funnels it into the ureter. Intrapelvic pressures range from 4 to 13 cm. of water. The ureter transports urine from the pelvis to the bladder and is capable of exerting pressures up to 80 mm. Hg. The bladder both stores and expels urine and exerts pressures up to 150 mm. Hg. Some (Narath) believe that the calyces undergo active effective peristalsis coordinated with the pelvis. Others (Kiil) have recently challenged such a contention. All workers, however, concede that urine is normally transported by peristalsis of the pelvis and ureter, although the mechanism of peristaltic conduction is not clear. In this connection, no effect on ureteral activity was demonstrated by Kiil by using adrenalin, ephedrine, atropine, prostigmin, urocholine chloride, banthine, probanthine, narcotics such as morphine hydrochloride, or general or spinal anesthesia. Similarly, Butcher, in studying action potentials of ureteral peristaltic waves, found no change from nicotine, curare, hexamethonium, xylocaine, prostigmin, and acetylcholine with or without eserine, atropine, epinephrine, and regitine. Adaptation of resting pressure and volume allow for storage in the bladder of urine in volumes from 500 to 750 cc. Although the bladder is composed principally of smooth muscle, initiation and inhibition of expulsive contractions are under voluntary control. Contractions producing pressures ranging from 18 to 42 cm. of water are necessary to overcome urethral resistance. Opening of the external urethral sphincter is reflex but active voluntary closure is possible. The bulbocavernosus muscles aid in expulsion of the final drops of urine in the male. The normal bladder is capable of emptying itself completely in a single sustained contraction usually producing pressures in the range of 50 to 60 mm. Hg., and producing a urine flow of more than 20 cc. per second, provided the void is 200 cc. or more.

Obstruction anywhere in the tract is the chief cause of *abnormal function*. This may be the result of (1) congenital malformation as ureteropelvic vessels, bands or narrowing, concentric contracture of the vesical orifice, or urethral meatal stenosis, (2) scars or strictures secondary to truama, or infections such as tuberculosis or gonorrhea, (3) stone formation due either to metabolic disease or associated with obstruction and infection, or (4) tumors either intrinsic or extrinsic which distort, compress, or invade the organs. The response of the lower urinary system to obstruction is twofold.

Early, there is hypertrophy of the muscles above the site of obstruction. This hypertrophy may be quite marked as in the heavily trabeculated and thick-walled bladder sometimes seen in benign hypertrophy of the prostate. Later, as the obstruction continues or becomes more severe, there follows decompensation, dilatation, atony, and atrophy. The effects of obstruction are related to structures more proximal. In far advanced and prolonged obstruction of the urethra with bladder decompensation, hydroureter and hydronephrosis with impaired renal function may develop, again following the pattern of hypertrophy early and decompensation with dilatation later.

Neurogenic dysfunctions of both the ureter and bladder have been described. Dysfunction of the ureter on a neurogenic basis, however, has been challenged by some who believe that proof of such is still lacking (Swenson, Lewis, and Kiil). Neurogenic dysfunctions of the bladder, on the other hand, are well documented with the bladder response depending on the location and magnitude of the neurologic defect. That this is so, is demonstrated by the fact that the tabetic bladder is atonic with large capacity, while the autonomous bladder, due to a lesion in the sacral chord, is usually of small capacity and thick walled (Bors). A peculiar bladder dysfunction without apparent neurogenic or obstructive cause occurs with interstitial cystitis. This bladder is of small capacity because of intrinsic fibrosis.

Obstruction of the *urethra* causes a decrease in the size and force of the stream. It results in a low uroflometric reading and is often associated with frequency, urgency, double voiding, enuresis, dribbling, and even episodes of complete retention. Residual urine indicates bladder decompensation. As to diagnosis—strictures may be demonstrated by exploration of the urethra with bulbs or bougies and urethral lesions and bladder neck obstructions are determinable by panendoscopy. Urethrograms are helpful in demonstrating some urethral lesions, particularly diverticula. The type of *bladder* response is elicited by cystometry while lesions of the bladder are visually demonstrated by cystoscopy and by cystograms. Cystograms also demonstrate adequacy of the ureterovesical junction. Renal function tests, such as the determination of blood urea nitrogen, or PSP excretion, are helpful in evaluating obstructions of the lower urinary tract but must be considered in conjunction with other findings for they may also be abnormal in nonobstructive diseases.

Obstruction of the *ureter* or *pelvis* may produce pain in the involved side varying from mild discomfort to the severe pain of renal colic. Related gastrointestinal symptoms, including nausea, vomiting, and meteorism, are common. Hydronephrosis may produce tenderness in the flank and a palpable mass. Smear and culture of the freshly voided urine of the male or of a catheterized specimen in the female reveal the presence or absence of infection. In the presence of stones, microscopic examination will usually show hematuria and/or pyuria. In the presence of cancer, properly stained smears of urinary sediment may be of value.

The *diagnosis* of a *stone* in the pelvis or ureter can often be made by a plain roentgenogram of the abdomen, but more exact information about size, shape, and emptying ability of the urinary tract is desirable and is obtained by intravenous urography or retrograde pyeloureterography. Finally, Kiil's method of urometry combined with cinepyelography (making of moving roentgenographic pictures) may prove of value in studying ureteral dysfunctions such as dilatations of pregnancy and meaglo-ureter, which at present are not well understood.

GENERAL CONSIDERATIONS

In keeping with the organization in other Chapters, the Lower Urinary System will be discussed briefly under the headings of Urethra, Bladder, and Ureters and Pelves. Also, in each the disorders will be considered under the usual major divisions of disease processes.

URETHRA

CONGENITAL ANOMALIES

Developmental malformations of the urethra are common, often complicated, and so trivial that they go unnoticed for years or so grave that they are incompatible with life. In general, they produce symptoms and signs because of obvious deformity, deviation of the urinary stream, obstruction of the urinary stream, or secondary infection. They may be grouped as follows: (1) *persistent cloaca*—occurring as a result of failure of the urorectal septum (Baker) and dividable into (*a*) persistent cloacal duct with failure of formation of the anus and communication of the rectum with the urethra or bladder, (*b*) persistent cloacal duct with failure of formation of the urethra and communication of the bladder with the rectum, (*c*) true cloaca with the intestines, ureters, and genital system opening into a common receptacle, and (*d*) absence of anterior abdominal wall leaving the cloaca exposed to the exterior, (2) *ectopic ureteral openings*—associated with a double ureter, usually draining the upper pelvis, and located near the external urethral orifice in the female and the prostatic urethra in the male (Herbst), (3) *hypospadias*—occurring in both males and females and consisting of an abnormal opening in the ventral portion of the urethra at any point between the external urethral meatus and the perineum (Creevy), (4) *epispadias*—abnormal opening of the urethra on the dorsal surface of the penis or clitoris or an absence of the anterior wall of the urethra (Dees), (5) *accessory urethra*—partial or complete duplication of the urethra with the former (*a*) opening exteriorly and ending blindly or connecting with the urethra at a more proximal level or (*b*) opening into the urethra and ending blindly (Gross), (6) *stenosis*—occurring more frequently in males than in females, located at the external meatus, and consisting of partial occlusion of the lumen (Boyd and Campbell), (7) *atresia*—consisting of a lack of any opening, predominating in males, and affecting any portion of or the entire urethra (Dourmashkin), (8) *diverticulum*—consisting of an outpocketing of the urethra, seen more commonly in females than in males, located in the floor of the urethra, and possessing a wide or narrow ostium that opens at any point along the course of the canal (Bergman and Dees), (9) *cysts*—rare, originating in any of the glands that drain into the urethra, and usually attaining a size less than 1.5 cm. in diameter (Wesson), (10) *hypertrophy of the verumontanum*—consisting of enlargement of the urethral crest and occurring only in males (Pilcher), and (11) *congenital valves*—found mostly in males, located in the prostatic urethra, and consisting of ridges or folds that project into the lumen in the vicinity of the verumontanum (Landes).

INFLAMMATIONS

Inflammation of the urethra is known as *urethritis*. The condition occurs at all ages and affects both sexes. The *causes* are varied and include bacteria, spirochetes, viruses, fungi, parasites, chemicals, foreign bodies, and trauma. The *clinical manifestations* consist of (1) urethral discharge—from local destruction of tissue and exudation, (2) urgency, frequency, and nocturia—from irritation of the vesical orifice and internal sphincter, and (3) pain—from spasm and flow of urine over the sensitized mucosa. In general, the more important disorders may be classified as follows: (1) *nonspecific urethritis*—due to a variety of predisposing factors and non-specific precipitating agents including the ordinary pyogenic organisms, occurring more commonly in females than in males, being acute or chronic in its course, characterized by a nonspecific inflammatory reaction, and sometimes complicated by periurethral abscess, prostatitis, cystitis, and stricture of the urethra, (2) *gonorrheal urethritis*—due to *Neisseria gonor-rhœæ*, occurring more often in males than in females, predominating in the lower strata of society and between the ages of twenty and fifty years, transmitted by sexual intercourse, characterized clinically by exquisite tenderness of the urethra with discharge of yellowish pus, diagnosed by finding gonococci within neutrophils, treated effectively by antibiotics and chemotherapeutic agents, and occasionally complicated by balanitis, epididymitis, prostatitis, abscess of Cowper's glands, seminal vesiculitis, urethral abscess, urethral stricture, skenitis, bartholinitis, vaginitis, cervicitis, salpingitis, tubo-ovarian abscess, arthritis, proctitis, septicemia, endocarditis, meningitis, dermatitis, ophthalmitis, and myositis, (3) *Reiter's disease*—of unknown cause but thought to be due to a virus, almost confined to men between the ages of fifteen and forty-five years, usually self-limited in its course (lasting about one month), and characterized by mucopurulent urethritis, mucopurulent conjunctivitis, and migratory arthritis affecting especially the larger joints such as the ankle and knee (Creecy and Hall), (4) *cowperitis*—inflammation of Cowper's glands, generally part of nonspecific or gonorrheal urethritis, and sometimes complicated by the production of recurrent posterior urethritis, abscess, or fistula leading to the perineum, urethra, or rectum (Firestone and Harkness), (5) *verumontinitis*—inflammation of the verumontanum and occurring in conjunction with posterior urethritis (Helvestine), (6) *abscess*—usually a sequel of gonorrhea and classified as periurethral (around the urethra), para-urethral (near the urethra), parafrenal (to one side of the frenum), and suburethral (along the inferior surface of the urethra), (7) *tuberculosis*—rare, almost always a complication of tuberculosis of the urogenital system, located in the posterior urethra, consisting first of tiny tubercles and later of caseation necrosis and ulceration, and occasionally complicated by hemorrhage, fistula, or stricture (Kilburn and Pelouze), (8) *syphilis*—occurring essentially in the form of a chancre and only rarely as secondary or tertiary lesions (Loveman), and (9) *trichomonal urethritis*—caused by *Trichomonas vaginalis*, usually seen in women but occasionally found in men, characterized by a frothy exudation and marked redness and edema of the mucosa, and usually complicated by extension of the process into the trigone of the bladder (Glen and Heckel).

PHYSICAL DISTURBANCES

The more important Physical Disturbances of the urethra consist of the following: (1) *foreign bodies*—rather common, occurring mostly in males (because of the length of the urethra), generally inserted from below accidentally or purposefully, consisting of a great variety of objects from a pencil to a decapitated snake, and complicated by inflammation, fistulous tract formation, stricture, and urinary obstruction (Gutierrez), (2) *calculi*— arising locally as a result of stagnation or urine and infection or migrating from the more proximal portion of the urinary tract, sometimes formed about a foreign body, generally single and measuring less than 2 cm. in diameter, of varied composition (but consisting mostly of phosphates, uric acid, and calcium oxalate), and attended by complications similar to those caused by foreign bodies (Beilan), (3) *rupture*—loss of continuity of the urethra, occurring in a normal or previously diseased urethra, caused by trauma (falls, blows, instrumentation, coitus, etc.), usually seen in males and most commonly affecting the bulbous urethra, attended by a variety of clinical manifestations (but usually shock, bleeding, disturbances in urination, and swelling along the fascial planes of the penis, scrotum, lower abdominal wall, etc.), and complicated by stricture or infection from extravasation of urine (Simpson-Smith and Mulholland), (4) *fistula*—resulting from virtually any disorder of the urethra (congenital anomalies, inflammations, physical disturbances, or tumors) and directly or indirectly connecting the urethra with the skin, scrotum, perineum, rectum, vagina, and vas deferens, (5) *stricture*—being congenital or acquired, when acquired generally resulting from inflammation (gonorrhea) or trauma, located most commonly in the posterior portion of the urethra in the male and in the distal portion of the urethra in the female, and complicated by urinary retention, infection of the proximal portion of the urinary tract, periurethral abscess, urethral fistula, and urinary extravasation (Attwater, Bottsford, Wynne, and Dourmashkin), (6) *prolapse*—protrusion of the urethral mucosa through the external meatus, confined to females (children or adults), often caused by straining in the presence of undue mobility of the mucosa and enlarged meatus, characterized by the presence of a painful, red, urethral tumor, and sometimes complicated by infection and acute urinary retention (Zeigerman, Kloman, and Moffett), and (7) *obstruction*— caused by most of the congenital anomalies, inflammations, and physical disturbances already listed, and by primary or secondary tumors.

TUMORS

Orientation.—Tumors of the urethra are uncommon. They affect both sexes and, while they may *occur* at any age, they are more frequent in adults than they are in children. *Pathologically* the tumors may be classified as primary or secondary. *Secondary* growths arise as a result of direct extension from the bladder, prostate, penis, vagina, vulva, etc., or as a result of metastasis from a distant focus. *Primary* growths may originate from any of the tissues that compose the normal urethra. The more important lesions may be listed as cysts, papilloma, carcinoma, adenoma, fibroma, leiomyoma, fibromyoma, hemangioma, caruncle, carcinoma of Cowper's glands, sarcoma, and melanoblastoma. Regardless of the type of growth, they produce *clinical manifestations* as a result of obstruction (difficulty in urination, slow stream, straining, etc.), ulceration (bleeding and fistulous tracts), infection (pain and frequency), and the tumor itself (palpable mass). The *diagnosis* is made from the clinical manifestations, urethroscopy, and biopsy. *Treatment* of choice is surgical excision. The *prognosis* varies with the type of tumor. In general, the outlook in benign growths is good while that in malignant tumors is poor. Aside from the general considerations outlined above, a few separate words should be said concerning caruncle, papilloma, and carcinoma.

Caruncle.—A urethral caruncle consists of an exquisitely painful and tender mass of tissue protruding from the terminal portion of the urethra. It is confined to adult females and reaches a peak incidence in the sixth decade of life (Palmer). The protrusion is generally single, soft, and deep red, and seldom measures more than 2 cm. in greatest diameter. Histologically it may be composed predominantly of epithelium (squamous, transitional, or glandular), of thin-walled blood capillaries or sinuses, or of granulation tissue.

Papilloma.—Papillomas of the *anterior portion* of the *urethra* generally originate in response to local irritation such as gonorrhea, balanitis, vaginitis, cervicitis, etc. They are often associated with venereal warts (condyloma acuminata), usually arise just within the meatus, are cauliflower-like, measure up to 2 cm. in diameter, and are composed mostly of squamous epithelium in finger-like projections. They rarely if ever become malignant. Papillomas of the *posterior portion* of the *urethra* are similar to papillomas of the urinary bladder. They are usually located in the vicinity of the verumontanum, are frequently multiple, may measure as much as 5 cm. across, are pinkish gray and friable, and consist of stalks of well-vascularized connective tissue covered with relatively regular or more bizarre transitional epithelium. These growths have a propensity to become cancerous. In fact, the change is usually so subtle that a morphologic interpretation as to whether a certain lesion is benign or malignant is often hazardous. For this reason, some pathologists call all papillary tumors in this area carcinoma adding the caption "low grade" for the more innocent appearing growths.

Carcinoma.—Carcinoma of the urethra is uncommon. It *occurs* in adults, is about as frequent in males as it is in females, and has no racial immunity or susceptibility. The *cause* is unknown but papilloma and leukoplakia are often precursors and infection and trauma are thought to act as predisposing factors. *Pathologically* the growth may originate in any portion of the urethra, although in females the immediate suprameatal portion is involved more often than the more proximal segments. Growths that extrude into the exterior are generally large, fungating, sessile, granular, superficially ulcerated, gray to reddish brown, and friable. Those that are located within the urethral canal are infiltrating, sharply defined but not encapsulated, constricting, and superficially ulcerated (Figs. 497 and 498). *Histologically* the tumors may be of a squamous cell, transitional cell, or adenomatous type, each showing varying degrees of differentiation. Usually, squamous cell carcinomas are well differentiated. They exist as sheets and masses of sharply defined polyhedral cells with moderate amounts of eosinophilic cytoplasm and round or oval, centrally placed, hyperchromatic nuclei. Pearl formation is, as a rule, not abundant. Transitional cell carcinomas exist as infiltrating masses or as finger-like projections of rounded or polyhedral, moderately well-defined, evenly staining cells with moderate amounts of cytoplasm and round, centrally placed, evenly staining nuclei. Adenocarcinomas consist of acini of cuboidal or columnar cells disclosing reticulated or secretory cytoplasm and round, hyperchromatic nuclei. Carcinoma of the urethra *spreads* (1) by direct extension in all directions, (2) by lymphatics to the inguinal, external iliac, and hypogastric lymph nodes, and (3) rarely by the blood vessels to the scrotum, epididymis, liver, and lungs. The *prognosis* is at best only fair. In general, the outlook is better in males than in females and is also better the more distally the tumor is located.

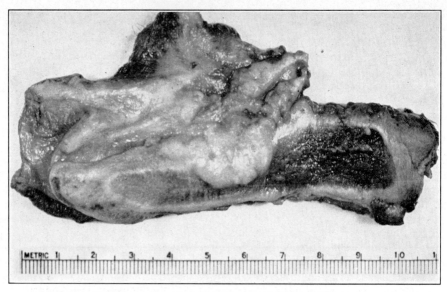

FIG. 497.—Carcinoma of the male urethra showing an ill-defined, grayish white infiltrating tumor starting just within the external meatus.

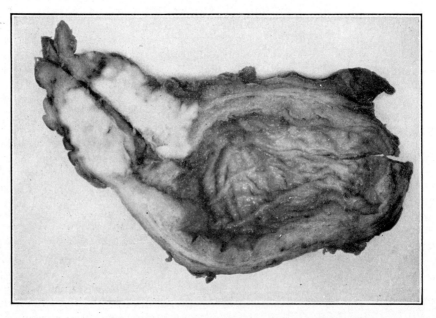

FIG. 498.—Carcinoma of the female urethra disclosing a sharply-circumscribed, grayish white tumor surrounding the entire canal (courtesy Dr. George Shoup and Dr. George H. Strong).

BLADDER

CONGENITAL ANOMALIES

Developmental malformations of the urinary bladder are often associated with malformations of other portions of the urinary and genital tracts. They may be listed as follows: (1) *fistulas*—rare, associated with cloacal anomalies, and consisting of vesicorectal, vesicovaginal, and vesico-enteric communications, (2) *absence*—extremely rare with ureters opening into the urethra or onto the anterior abdominal wall, (3) *hypoplasia*—also rare and associated with other urinary tract anomalies, (4) *hyperplasia*—enlargement to a degree filling most of the abdomen and generally associated with some obstruction at the urethral orifice but occasionally being free of such an impediment (Steinhardt), (5) *hour glass deformity*—incomplete transverse

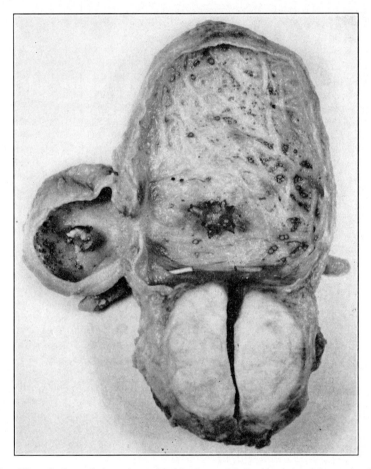

<small>Fig. 499.—Diverticulum of the urinary bladder located just above the right ureteral orifice. It discloses a wide ostium and both it and the bladder contain calculi.</small>

constriction dividing the bladder into an upper and a lower compartment (Zellermayer), (6) *duplication*—consisting of two or more compartments separated by complete or incomplete, usually longitudinal but occasionally transverse, septa with the ureters opening into a single chamber or into two compartments (Burns), (7) *diverticulum*—occasionally arising on a congenital basis as a result of growths of accessory urethral buds or coalescence of ridge-like elevations of mucosa, more commonly arising on an acquired obstructive (urethra) basis, being single or multiple, generally located near the ureteral orifices (Fig. 499), measuring from a few millimeters to many centimeters in diameter, connected with the bladder by a wide or constricted ostium, composed of a wall similar to that of the urinary bladder with greater or lesser amounts of smooth muscle, and complicated by infection, calculi, tumor, or perforation (Kimbrough and Kretschmer), (8) *contracture vesical orifice* —also called hypertrophy of the vesical neck, occurring as a stenosis of the vesical ostium of the urethra, and consisting of hypertrophy of peri-urethral glands, connective tissue, and muscle fibers (Campbell), (9)

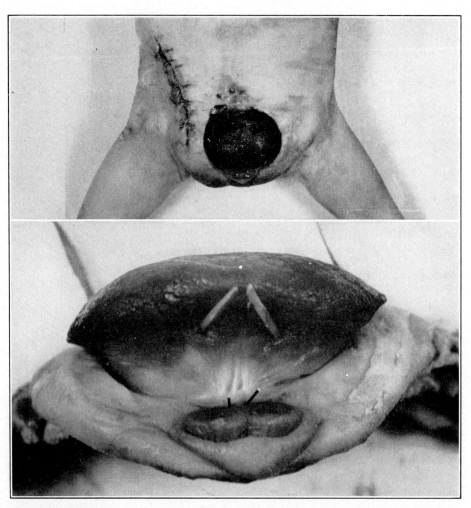

Fig. 500.—Exstrophy of the urinary bladder showing (above) the reddened mucosa of the posterior bladder wall *in situ* and (below) the postmortem specimen with the ureters and ureteral (with applicators) openings, ejaculatory duct openings (pins), and epispadias.

exstrophy —defined (Gr. = out + to turn) as an absence of the anterior wall of the urinary bladder and corresponding portion of the anterior abdominal wall, occurring once in every 30,000 births, affecting males more often than females, complicated by infection (local and upper urinary tract) and occasionally carcinoma, and consisting of (*a*) a bright red circumscribed area of exposed posterior bladder wall containing the openings of the ureters and ejaculatory ducts (Fig. 500), (*b*) epispadias, (*c*) absence of the symphysis pubis, and (*d*) other local or distant anomalies (Gross and Higgins), and (10) *urachal abnormalities*—malformations of the canal that connects the bladder with the allantois in the fetus, consisting of (*a*) a complete patency (vesico-umbilical fistula), (*b*) patency at the umbilical end only (urachal sinus), (*c*) patency at the vesical end only, and (*d*) patency at some point between the umbilical and vesical ends (urachal cyst), and complicated by (*a*) associated anomalies (urethral stricture, umbilical hernia, etc.), (*b*) infection (with drainage of pus or abscess formation), (*c*) calculi, and (*d*) tumors (fibroma, sarcoma, and mucinous carcinoma) (Brodie, Lloyd and Wessell).

DEGENERATIONS

The only important, albeit rare, specific retrogressive process of the bladder is *amyloid degeneration.* The condition may be *secondary* to a debilitating (usually suppurative) process or it may be *primary.* The latter is often referred to as *amyloid tumor* (Senger and Roen). It consists of an ill-defined, irregular, plaque-like thickening or more protruding tumor mass that may measure as much as 8 cm. in diameter. Histologically it is composed of a diffuse infiltration of homogeneously eosinophilic material that discloses the usual properties of amyloid (p. 39).

INFLAMMATIONS

Inflammation of the urinary bladder is called *cystitis.* Some types of cystitis are common; others are rare. The condition occurs in both sexes, at all ages, and in all races. The *precipitating causes* include bacteria, spirochetes, viruses, fungi and yeast-like organisms, parasites, chemicals, foreign bodies, trauma, tumors, etc., and the most important *predisposing cause* is obstruction at the vesical orifice or at any point along the course of the urethra (Mathé). The chief *clinical manifestations* consist of (1) frequency of urination—due to decreased capacity of the bladder as a result of contraction and to the irritative effect of the infection on the vesical orifice and internal sphincter, (2) pain—located in the perineal or suprapubic region, most severe during the termination of micturition, and due to irritation of the sensitive trigone, (3) pyuria—grossly seen as cloudy urine, microscopically characterized by pus cells in the urine, and due to exudation from the vesical wall, (4) hematuria—occurring as a result of diapedesis, ulceration of the vesical wall, and rupture of the blood vessels, and (5) general—consisting of fever, chills, loss of appetite, nausea, and vomiting and due to absorption of toxic material and tissue products and resulting more from associated renal infection than from the cystitis as such. The chief *complications* are infection and dilatation of the upper urinary tract eventually culminating in renal insufficiency. *Treatment* consists of removal of the cause and administration of antibiotics and chemotherapeutic agents. The *prognosis* varies with the cause.

Pathologically cystitis may be classified as follows: (1) *nonspecific cystitis*—dividable into acute and chronic, usually caused by colon bacilli and staphylococci, being localized to the base of the bladder or general in distribution, characterized in the acute stage by congestion edema, and exudation (Fig. 501) and in the chronic stage by reduction in capacity, fibrosis and ulceration, and microscopically attended by congestion, edema, ulceration, and nonspecific infiltration with neutrophils, plasma cells, lymphocytes, and other leukocytes (Berry, Higgins, and Kretschmer), (2) *gangrenous cystitis*—

inflammation of the bladder attended by massive necrosis and sloughing of the mucosal surface, caused by (*a*) interference with the circulation of the bladder, (*b*) debilitating conditions such as uncontrolled diabetes mellitus, typhoid fever, and diphtheria, (*c*) chemicals—consisting of strong alkaloids or acids instilled into the bladder, and often attended by overwhelming toxemia (Cristol), (3) *trigonitis*—inflammation of the trigone of the bladder, occurring often in women, and similar to nonspecific cystitis except that the process is localized (Bassow), (4) *interstitial cystitis*—chronic inflammation

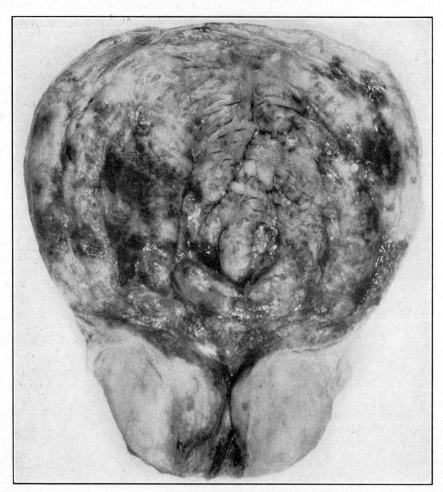

Fig. 501.—Acute cystitis illustrating marked congestion
and edema and irregular superficial ulceration.

of the interstitial tissue of the bladder, also known as Hunner's ulcer, often seen following some type of pelvic operation, of unknown cause but probably arising as a result of stasis of lymph, and characterized pathologically by (*a*) reduction in capacity of the bladder, (*b*) single or multiple lesions most often affecting the dome and always sparing the trigone, (*c*) irregular, ill-defined, salmon colored, or ulcerating ulcers that have a tendency to crack and bleed, and (*d*) nonspecific congestion, edema, leukocytic infiltration, and fibrous tissue proliferation of the interstitial connective tissue of the bladder (Seaman), (5) *malakoplakia*—of unknown cause, and characterized pathologically by the presence of (*a*) several to numerous, smooth, centrally umbilicated, yellowish-gray to brown, mucosal plaques that may measure as much as 8 cm. across, (*b*) central ulceration of the larger parts, (*c*) the presence of malakoplakic cells—large, single or multinucleated, giant cells, and (*d*) Michaelis-Gutmann bodies—round or irregular, granular or centrally laminated bodies that have a strong affinity for hemotoxylin (Boonstra and French), (6) *incrusted cystitis*—the deposition of phosphatic crust upon a vesical mucosa that has been previously demaged by inflammation, tumor, chemicals, or trauma (Hager), (7) *proliferative cystitis*—associated with similar lesions in the ureters (proliferative ureteritis) and renal pelves (proliferative pyelitis), occurring as a result of any low-grade chronic inflammatory process and classified pathologically into (*a*) *cystitis* (ureteritis or pyelitis) *follicularis*—presence of innumerable 1 to 2 mm. mucosal nodules composed of lymph follicles, (*b*) *cystitis* (ureteritis or pyelitis) *granulosa*—presence of cluster-like projections of granulation tissue, (*c*) *cystitis* (ureteritis or pyelitis) *glandularis*—presence of clusters of epithelial cells in glandular formation, and (*d*) *cystitis* (ureteritis or pyelitis) *cystica*—presence of small, bead-like mucosal cysts lined with epithelium (Patch and Warrick), (8) *cystitis emphysematosa*—inflammation of the bladder associated with the presence of gas-filled cysts, often seen in conjunction with diabetes mellitus, and caused by organisms (colon bacilli and *Cl. welchii*) that are capable of producing gas (Milner), (9) *tuberculous cystitis*—always seen as a complication of tuberculosis of the kidneys, usually encountered in early adult life, prevailing in females, consisting microscopically of tubercles or tuberculous granulation tissue, and characterized grossly by reduction in capacity of the bladder together with the following lesions in the trigonal area: intense hyperemia, edema, mulberry-like mucosal protrusions, tubercles, excrescences or larger accumulations of granulation tissue, or sharply defined, undermined ulcers (Lazarus and Greenberger), (10) *leukoplakia*—of unknown cause, more common in males than in females, usually seen in patients beyond the third decade of life, occasionally complicated by carcinoma, consisting microscopically of squamous metaplasia with hyperkeratosis of the epithelium, and characterized grossly by the presence of sharply defined, elevated, grayish-white, irregular mucosal patches usually located near the trigone (Thompson), (12) *syphilis*—caused by *Treponema pallidum*, usually occurring in adults in the third to the fifth decades of life, affecting both sexes with equal frequency, and consisting of macules and superficial mucosal ulcerations in the secondary stage of the disease and of gummas and papillomas in the tertiary stage (Finestone), (13) *fungous* and *yeast-like cystitis*—rare and encompassing mostly actinomycosis and moniliasis (Hatch and Moulder), and (14) *parasitic cystitis*—encompassing trichomoniasis (p. 1154), schistosomiasis (p. 775), echinococcosis (p. 828), and amebiasis (p. 770).

PHYSICAL DISTURBANCES

The more important Physical Disturbances of the bladder consist of the following: (1) *trauma*—consisting of contusion (bruise) or actual rupture (break in the wall), occurring as a result of (*a*) penetrating wounds (gunshot, stab, fractured pelvic bones, instrumentations, foreign bodies, etc.), (*b*) concussion (crush, blast, blow, fall, kick, etc.), and (*c*) physiologic increase of interabdominal pressure (as during lifting, micturition, etc.)

acting upon a diseased bladder wall, and complicated by (*a*) hemorrhage, (*b*) extravasation of urine, (*c*) extravesical abscess or peritonitis, (*d*) fistulas, and (*e*) associated trauma to other viscera (Michels, Feigal, and Crastnopol), (2) *fistulas*—occurring as a result of congenital, inflammatory, physical, or neoplastic disturbances and consisting of the following: vesicocutaneous, vesicotubo-ovarian, tubovesical, uterovesical, cervicovesical, vesicovaginal, uterovesicovaginal, urethrovesicovaginal, vesico-intestinal, vesico-enteric, vesico-appendiceal, vesicocecal, vesicosigmoidal, vesicorectal, etc., (3) *neurogenic bladder*—also called cord bladder, resulting from a disturbance of the normal physiologic function of the bladder consequent to a disruption of the nerve pathways between the bladder and the spinal cord and brain, caused by a variety of nerve tissue lesions (myelomeningocele, spina bifida, spinal cord abscess, penetrating trauma or fracture of the cord, brain tumors or injuries, degenerative changes in the cord and brain, etc.), complicated principally by infection of the urinary tract and calculous formation, and characterized clinically by lack of sensation to void, overdistention of the bladder, and incontinence (Nesbit), (4) *irradiation changes*—resulting from roentgen or radium therapy applied to the bladder or to adjacent structures, dividable into an acute stage occurring up to six weeks after treatment and a chronic stage occurring after a lapse of a year or more following treatment, being extremely refractive to any type of therapy, and characterized pathologically by congestion, edema, superficial ulceration, and nonspecific leukocytic infiltration in the acute stage and by reduction in capacity, fibrosis, indolent ulceration, and vascular occlusion by endothelial proliferation in the chronic stage (Dean and Watson), (5) *obstruction*—caused by any lesion of the urethra (p. 1024) or prostate that encroaches upon the urethral lumen and, in addition, by the following lesions at the vesical orifice: congenital contracture of the vesical outlet (Howard), nonspecific cystitis, trigonitis, proliferative cystitis, tuberculosis, syphilis, schistosomiasis, echinococcosis, benign and malignant tumors, neurogenic bladder, calculus, and foreign bodies, (6) *urinary incontinence*—lack of voluntary control of urination, known also as enuresis (nocturnal when occurring at night and diurnal when occurring during the day), and caused by (*a*) the following functional disorders: improper training, emotional instability, or ingestion of too large quantities of fluid before going to bed, and (*b*) the following organic lesions: exstrophy of the bladder, patent urachus, hypoplasia of the bladder, epispadias, phimosis, preputial adhesions, contracture of the vesical orifice, hypertrophy of the verumontanum, underdevelopment of the internal sphincter, ectopic urethral orifices, inflammation of the bladder or urethra, tumors of the urethra or vesical orifice of the bladder, neurogenic bladder, urethral stricture, vesical fistulas, relaxation of the vesical sphincter in women who have borne children, after perineal prostatectomy, etc. (Forsythe and Stewart), (7) *hernia*—usually a protrusion of the bladder through the inguinal ring in males and the femoral ring in females and rarely a protrusion through the obturator foramen, linea alba, rectus abdominus muscle, and ischiorectal fossa (Iason), (8) *calculi*—migrating from the upper urinary tract or formed locally as a result of urinary obstruction (causing concentration of urine) and infection, frequently precipitated about a foreign body (such as a nail, pencil, rubber drain, etc.), varying in size from barely perceptible to 32 cm. in diameter, being single or multiple (Figs. 499 and 502), composed mostly of calcium, ammonium, and magnesium phosphate but also containing carbonate, oxalate, urate, uric acid, and attended by vesical irritation and inflammation (Twinem, Cristol, Prentiss, Wilson, and Vermeulen), and (9) *foreign bodies*—occasionally gaining entrance from within the body as a result of migration from adjacent structures but more commonly inserted from below, consisting of a varied assortment of objects (nails, pencils, pins, needles, tacks, wire, teeth, hairs, matches, fountain pens, etc.), and attended by trauma, infection, and urinary obstruction (Nitschke and Vors).

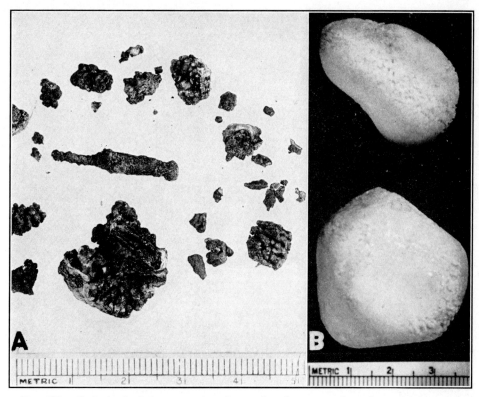

FIG. 502.—Vesical calculi demonstrating *A*, a nail and numerous irregular varisized stones and *B*, two large smooth stones unassociated with a foreign body.

TUMORS

Orientation.—Some tumors of the urinary bladder are common while others are extremely rare. They *occur* at all ages, in both sexes, and in all races. The *causes* are unknown although many authors point to trauma and chronic irritation and some incriminate endogenous (hormones) or exogenous (chemicals such as aniline dyes) carcinogens excreted in the urine as of etiologic significance (Kirwin). *Pathologically* the tumors may be classified as primary or secondary. *Primary* tumors may originate in any of the tissues that normally compose the bladder with, however, epithelial neoplasms constituting about 95 per cent of all growths. They may be listed as follows: adenoma, papilloma, carcinoma, fibroma, myxoma, fibromyxoma, fibrosarcoma, myxosarcoma, neurofibroma, neurogenic sarcoma, hemangioma, hemangio-endothelioma, lipoma, liposarcoma, leiomyoma, leiomyosarcoma, rhabdomyoma, rhabdomyosarcoma, myoblastoma, lymphoblastoma, teratoid tumors, osteoma, chondroma, osteosarcoma, chondrosarcoma, and urachal tumors. *Secondary* tumors are mostly carcinomas that reach the bladder as a result of (1) direct extension from the cervix, prostate, seminal vesicles, rectum, or sigmoid colon, (2) implantation from the ureter or renal pelvis, or (3) metastasis from a distant focus in the stomach, gallbladder, etc. In addition, endometriosis may also be added as a tumor arising from tissue that is not native to the bladder. The *complications* of tumors of the bladder are cystitis, ureteral or urethral obstruction, torsion of the tumor with gangrene, ulceration with hemor-

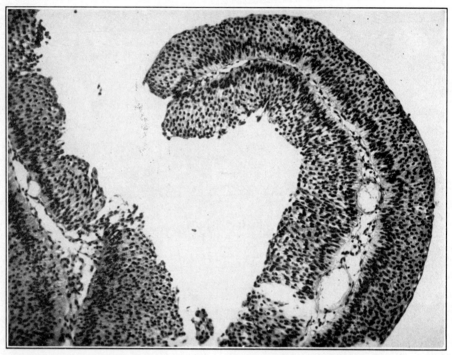

FIG. 503.—Papilloma of the bladder showing two slender villi composed of a thin stalk of connective tissue covered with hyperplastic but regular transitional epithelium. × 100.

rhage, and, in cases of malignant tumors, extension to adjacent structures, fistulous tract formation, and metastasis. The *clinical manifestations* result from irritation of the vesical mucosa by the tumor causing contraction of the bladder and from the complications listed. The more important symptoms and signs may be enumerated as follows: frequency, nocturia, dysuria, hematuria, increasing slowness in starting the stream, weakness of the stream, terminal dribbling, palpable mass in the region of the bladder, cloudy or hemorrhagic urine (containing albumin, pus cells, and erythrocytes), and visualization of the tumor roentgenographically (by use of contrast medium) or cystoscopically. The *diagnosis* is made from the clinical manifestations together with cystoscopy and biopsy. *Treatment* is surgical (incisional or electrical) excision and, less often, cystectomy. The *prognosis* varies with the location, type, and size of the tumor and the age of the patient. In general, the outlook in strictly benign tumors is good while that in malignant tumors is at most only fair. It is poor in children as compared with adults. Aside from the general remarks just concluded, a few separate words should be said in connection with papilloma, carcinoma, and sarcoma.

Papilloma.—Papillomas of the urinary bladder are similar in behavior and pathologic appearance to papillomas of the posterior portion of the urethra (p. 1027). The condition usually occurs in patients beyond thirty years of age, reaches a maximum in the sixth and seventh decades, and is three times as common in males as it is in females (Deming and Winsbury-White). The lesion is single about as often as it is multiple and it is *located* in the vicinity of the trigone in one-half the cases, in the posterior wall in the majority of the remaining cases, and in the anterior wall relatively infrequently. *Grossly* a papilloma appears as a delicate, thinly pedunculated, multiply branched, pink, villous outgrowth that floats gracefully in a bladder filled with urine or saline. It is friable and bleeds easily upon manipulation. *Histologically* it is composed of a thin stalk of well-vascularized connective tissue, covered with hyperplastic but otherwise regular transitional epithelium (Fig. 503). As in the urethra, great care must be taken not to underdiagnose an epithelial tumor of the bladder. In general, the following characteristics indicate a papillary carcinoma rather than a papilloma: (1) broad base, (2) fixation of the base to the submucosal tissues, (3) coalescence of the peripheral portions of the villi, (4) variations in shape, size, and staining qualities of the cells, and (5) invasion of the base by epithelial cells. The earliest *clinical manifestation* is hematuria. *Treatment* consists of excision with fulguration of the base. The *prognosis* is variable. Some authors have found that less than 10 per cent of originally benign papillary tumors become malignant (Deming) while others report a malignant transformation in almost 50 per cent of cases (Winsbury-White). The difference in these statistics doubtlessly lies in the criteria used in making the original diagnosis.

Carcinoma.—Carcinoma of the urinary bladder is said to account for approximately 4 per cent of all cancers. Like papilloma, it affects men about three times as frequently as women, is uncommon before the age of thirty years, and is most prevalent in the seventh decade of life. *Pathologically* from one-half to two-thirds of the lesions are located in the vicinity of the trigone and most of the others are situated in the posterior wall. Tumors located in the summit of the bladder are generally of urachal origin. In the over-all, about 90 per cent of the growths are of a papillary nature (Fig. 504). In any given case, the tumors are single or multiple, usually sessile, and occasionally pedunculated. The surface is covered with villi that are often adherent to each other, frequently ulcerated and, on a whole, less graceful than those of papilloma. The base is, as a rule, indurated with the infiltration affecting not only the mucosa but, as the tumor ages, penetrating all the way through the wall. In the minority of cases (about (10%) the tumor is *nonpapillary* appearing as a flat, penetrating, and usually centrally ulcerated mass. In either instance, the neoplastic tissue is, as a rule, white, firm, friable, and fairly sharply demarcated from the normal tissues of the wall but not encapsulated. *Histologically* carcinoma of the bladder is most often of a transitional cell type, occasionally of a squamous cell variety, and rarely of an adenomatous nature. Each, in turn, may be well differentiated to highly anaplastic in appearance. Well-differentiated *transitional cell carcinoma* approaches the appearance of a papilloma. It is composed of thin cores of well-vascularized connective tissue with hyperplastic but somewhat irregular transitional epithelial cells. As the lesion becomes more malignant, the adjacent villi become fused and the cells become more and more irregular (Fig. 505). At the base they infiltrate the submucosal tissues in irregular clumps, masses, or individually. In highly malignant growths the cells become so irregular that it is virtually impossible to identify them as transitional in origin. *Squamous cell carcinoma* is similar to squamous cell carcinoma in other organs. It usually exists as nests of well-defined, polyhedral, prickle cells possessing irregular hyperchromatic nuclei and exhibiting a marked tendency to pearl formation. *Adenocarcinoma* is composed of irregular cuboidal

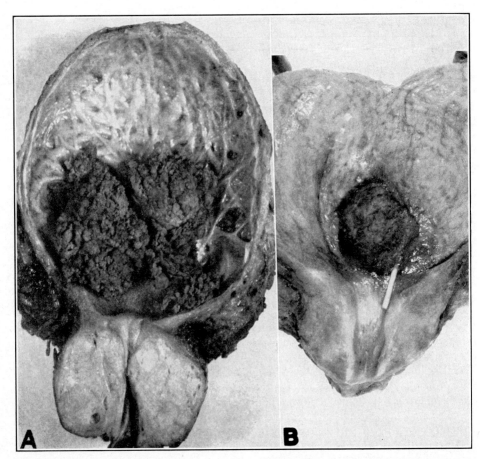

Fig. 504.—Papillary carcinoma of the bladder illustrating *A*, numerous papillary tumors covering the entire posterior surface of the bladder and *B*, a sessile tumor located medial to the left ureteral orifice.

or columnar cells in glandular formation and is generally located in the region of the urachus. Carcinoma of the bladder *spreads* by (1) implantation to involve the mucosa of the rest of the bladder or that of the urethra, (2) continuity to involve the entire thickness of the bladder wall and beyond this the perivesical tissues and organs, and (3) metastasis to the draining lymph nodes, kidneys, adrenals, colon, lungs, pleura, skin, etc. The final *diagnosis* of vesical carcinoma is made by cystoscopy and biopsy, with examination of urinary sediment for neoplastic cells as a good adjunct.

Treatment depends upon the size and extent of the growth. It consists of (1) local destruction with a cautery, (2) local surgical excision, (3) partial cystectomy, (4) total cystectomy, or (5) some form of irradiation therapy. The most recent of these procedures, namely, total cystectomy with transplantation of the ureters into the colon is not as ideal as originally thought for it is attended (1) by hyperchloremia and acidosis (from absorption of urinary chloride by the colonic mucosa) and (2) by ascending pyelonephritis and hydronephrosis (Creevy). If uncorrected, either of these untoward effects may cause death of the patient. The *prognosis* is variable. In small superficial growths, the five-year survival rate should be from 60 to 80 per cent but in large penetrating tumors it is less than 3 per cent.

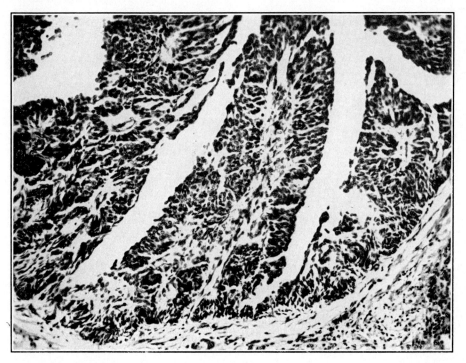

Fig. 505.—Papillary carcinoma of the bladder showing a rather broad core of connective tissue covered with irregular transitional epithelium.   × 100.

Sarcoma.—Sarcoma of the urinary bladder is rare. It occurs at all ages but is the most common type of malignant tumor of the bladder in children (Way, Henry, and Crane). Most of the growths are located in the vicinity of the trigone. They *start* within the wall and protrude intravesically, extravesically, or in both directions. Generally they are composed of moderately firm, grayish-white, brain-like tissue with varying degrees of necrosis and hemorrhage. They vary in size but usually measure about 10 cm. in diameter at the time of discovery. *Histologically* any of the mesodermal tissues may be represented with fibrosarcoma, myxosarcoma, leiomyosarcoma, and rhabdomyosarcoma being the most common. The method of spread is similar to that in carcinoma. The *prognosis* is poor for the mortality rate is between 90 and 100 per cent.

URETERS AND PELVES

CONGENITAL ANOMALIES

Developmental abnormalities of the ureters and renal pelves are said to occur in about 3 per cent of the population. They consist of the following: (1) *variations* in *number*—occurring in as high as 10 per cent of urologic patients studied, affecting the right ureter more often than the left, being twice as frequent in males as in females, generally discovered in the third and fourth decades of life, arising on the basis of premature or increased number of cleavages of the ureteral bud, usually consisting of one (but

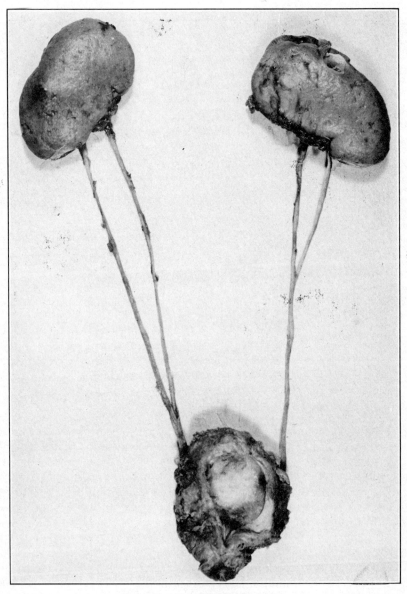

FIG. 506.—Duplication of ureters.

sometimes two or even more) accessory ureter that (*a*) joins the main ureter before it empties into the bladder, (*b*) ends blindly, or (*c*) empties ectopically into the vestibule, vagina, urethra, bladder, cervix, uterine cavity, or Gartner's duct in the female and the posterior urethra, seminal vesicles, vermontanum, ejaculatory duct, and vas deferens in the male (Fig. 506), generally associated with duplication (united or completely separated) of the corresponding kidney and renal pelvis, and complicated by hydronephrosis, pyonephrosis, pylonephritis, and associated genito-urinary and distant abnormalities (Nation, Smith, and Eisendrath), (2) *hypoplasia*—diminution in size, usually terminating blindly (cranially), and associated with agenesis of the corresponding kidney (Hamilton), (3) *kinks*—resulting from failure

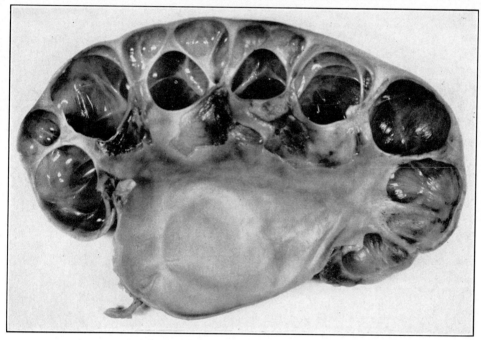

Fig. 507.—Congenital stenosis at the ureteropelvic junction with severe hydronephrosis.

of the kidney to ascend, elongation of the ureter, and external pressure, (4) *twists*—due to failure of the ureter to rotate with the kidney, (5) *agenesis*—consisting of complete failure of formation, being unilateral or bilateral, and associated with agenesis of the corresponding kidney (Grim), (6) *megalo-ureters*—enlargement of the ureters, usually occurring bilaterally, and resulting from neurogenic dysfunction of the lower ends of the ureters, obstruction of the intravascular portion of the ureters, developmental arrest, or abnormal function of the bladder consequent to a defect in the parasympathetic ganglion cells (Campbell and Swenson), (7) *stenosis*—being unilateral or bilateral, usually occurring at the ureteropelvic junction and, less often, at the ureterovesical junction, and complicated by hydronephrosis (Fig. 507) (Soley and Henline), (8) *retrocaval ureter*—resulting from faulty development of the inferior vena cava, consisting of the right ureter passing behind, medial, and then anterior to the venous trunk, and complicated by hydronephrosis, pyonephrosis, and calculous formation (Parks), (9) *diverticulum*—consisting of a true outpocketing of the entire

66

wall (true diverticulum) or of a herniation of the mucosa (false diverticulum) and occurring most commonly at the ureteropelvic junction or less commonly at the sacro-iliac level and the ureterovesical junction (McGraw), (10) *valves*—extremely rare, consisting of a mucosal fold that occurs with decreasing frequency in the juxtavesical area, iliac region, and lumbar region (MacLean), (11) *ureterocele*—occurring as a sacculation of the lower end of the ureter that bulges into the bladder and caused by stenosis of the ureteral ostium together with weakness of the wall of the luminal portion of the ureter (Campbell), (12) *aberrant renal vessels*—accounting for almost one-half of all cases of obstruction at the ureteropelvic junction, usually being unilateral, disclosing no preference for either side, affecting renal arteries much more frequently than renal veins, and consisting of an origin from the renal arteries, aorta, suprarenal arteries, or iliac arteries, and of a termination in either the upper or the lower pole of the kidney (Aaron, Henline, and Soley), (13) *variations* in *number* of *renal pelves* and *calyces*, (14) *variations* in *position* of *renal pelvis*—within or outside the renal parenchyma and displaced anteriorly or posteriorly (Herbst), and (15) *calyceal diverticulum*—rare and consisting of a cavity within the renal parenchyma lying distal to and connected with a minor calyx (Prather).

INFLAMMATIONS

Inflammation of the ureter is known as *ureteritis* and inflammation of the renal pelvis is called *pyelitis*. The two usually occur concomitantly and, in addition, the kidney is also generally affected. The latter, however, is considered in the succeeding Chapter. The more important inflammatory conditions may be listed as follows: (1) *nonspecific ureteritis* and *pyelitis*— usually associated with inflammation of the kidney and, therefore, better termed pyelo-ureteronephritis, seen frequently in children and pregnant women, predisposed by any obstructive lesion of the lower urinary tract, precipitated by bacteria (usually colon bacilli, staphylococci, and streptococci) that gain entrance from the bloodstream, by way of the lymphatics, ascension along the lumen, or extension from adjacent structures, attended by a variety of local and general clinical manifestations (chills, fever, pain in the back, hematuria, polyuria, frequency, dysuria, enuresis, etc.), and characterized pathologically by (a) congestion, edema, thickening, fibrosis, mucosal ulceration, and dilatation of the ureter and pelvis, (b) elongation, tortuosity, and kinking of the ureter, (c) hydronephrosis (p. 1095), and pyelonephritis (p. 1087), and (d) nonspecific leukocytic infiltration followed by fibrosis (Riches, Kobak, and Heaney), (2) *gangrenous ureteritis*—inflammation of the ureter associated with gangrene and caused by (a) nonspecific ureteritis of severe intensity, (b) injection of strong chemicals, and (c) pelvic operations (especially for carcinoma of the cervix) where the ureter is both stripped of its blood supply and directly traumatized (Hepburn and Michaels), (3) *spastic ureteritis*—consisting primarily of spasm of the ureter, occurring as a result of hyperirritability, characterized clinically by intense pain, and responding temporarily to ureteral dilatation and permanently to ureteral denervation (Wharton), (4) *proliferative ureteritis* and *pyelitis*—similar to proliferative cystitis (p. 1033), (5) *tuberculous ureteritis* and *pyelitis*—always secondary to renal tuberculosis where the process is usually of the ulcerocavernous type (Fig. 508), characterized pathologically by (a) congestion, roughening, and dulling of the mucosa initially, (b) the development of large granulations, ulcerations, fibrosis, distortion, and calcification as the lesion advances, and (*c*) the formaton of tubercles or tuberculous granulation tissue microscopically, and complicated by hydronephrosis and pyonephrosis (Gorro and Rinker), (6) *leukoplakia*—rare, affecting either the ureter or pelvis, and appearing similar to that in the bladder (Laughlin), (7) *parasitic ureteritis* and *pyelitis*—usually consisting of schistosomiasis and being similar to that in the bladder (p. 775) (Makar), and (8) *empyema*—consisting of a collection of pus in the stump of the ureter after an incomplete ureterectomy (Senger).

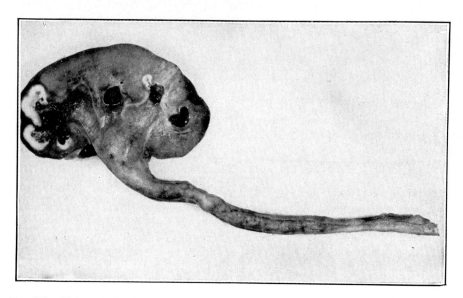

FIG. 508.—Tuberculosis of the kidney, pelvis, and ureter showing caseation necrosis and cavitation in the kidney and granularity, ulceration, and fibrosis in the pelvis and ureter. (Herbut's *Urological Pathology*.)

PHYSICAL DISTURBANCES

Orientation.—In this section, the following disturbances may be included: (1) *calculi*, (2) *trauma*—caused by (*a*) surgical injury during operation on the female pelvic organs, large intestine, appendix, hernia, kidney, ureter, and bladder, (*b*) cystoscopic maneuvers including ureteral catheterization and ureterography, (*c*) external trauma such as gunshot and stab wounds, and (*d*) foreign bodies such as filiform, catheter, stone extractor, pipe stem, straws, pins, wires, etc., predisposed by congenital or acquired lesions of the ureters (previous operations, anomalous position of the ureter, adnexal adhesions, carcinoma of the fundus of the uterus, intraligamentous tumors, etc.), consisting of a variety of lesions (contusions, cuts, tears, punctures, clamp wounds, ligations, cauterization, pulverization, etc.), and complicated by urinary extravasation, infection, fistulas, calculi, and ureteral stricture (Rusche and Novak), (3) *irradiation changes*—caused by roentgen or radium irradiation for pelvic conditions, characterized by changes similar to those seen in the bladder, and complicated by fistulas and ureteral strictures (Diehl), (4) *fistulas*—being (*a*) congenital, (*b*) inflammatory, (*c*) traumatic, or (*d*) neoplastic and connecting the ureter with the urethra, bladder, vagina, uterus, seminal vesicles, verumontanum, ejaculatory ducts, vas deferens, peritoneum, bowel, skin, and even vessels, and (5) *obstruction*—encompassing (*a*) congenital anomalies—duplication, hypoplasia, stenosis, kinks, twists, retrocaval ureter, diverticulum, cysts, valves, ureterocele, and aberrant vessels, (*b*) inflammation—nonspecific ureteritis, irradiation ureteritis, spastic ureteritis, proliferative ureteritis, tuberculosis, leukoplakia, schistosomiasis, and periureteritis, (*c*) physical disturbances—calculi, trauma, fistulas, intussusception, hernias, and (*d*) tumors.

Calculi.—Calculi of the urinary tract are called uroliths and the process of their formation or the state of their presence is known as *urolithiasis*. The condition *occurs* at all ages but is most frequent in patients between twenty and fifty years of age and is about three times as common in men as it is in women (Higgins).

The *causes* of urinary calculi may be discussed briefly under two headings—extrinsic factors and intrinsic factors. *Extrinsic factors* are those conditions outside of the urinary tract that have a bearing on calculous formation (Doherty). They consist of (*a*) geographic zones such as along the Volga, Northern and Eastern India, Africa, etc., and probably operating as a result of increased calcium in drinking water, hot and dry climate with concentration of urine, avitaminosis A, improper balance of acid and alkaline ash foods, and heredity, (*b*) increased excretion of calcium as seen in cases of prolonged recumbent position (Kimbrough) and in cases of hyperparathyroidism (Keating), (*c*) distant foci of infection causing initial changes in the renal papillæ (Randall), and (*d*) metabolic disorders such as gout. *Intrinsic factors* encompass the conditions present in the urinary tract itself. They include stasis and infection. *Stasis* of urine occurs simply as stagnation when a patient lies on his back for prolonged periods of time or as a result of any of the many causes of urinary tract obstruction. It operates by allowing urine to concentrate, thereby facilitating precipitation of its salts. *Infection* operates by changing the pH of the urine and thus also favoring precipitation of its salts. Given some of the suitable conditions listed above, the first step in the development of a calculus is the formation of the *nucleus*. In noninfected urine the nucleus develops as a result of precipitation and later crystallization of colloidal particles of the salts or chemicals concerned. In infected urine, collections of dead epithelial cells, blood clots, and bacteria act as nuclei upon which urinary salts are gradually deposited.

Experimentally, urinary calculi have been produced in (*a*) dogs by feeding oxamide, by avitaminosis A, and by injecting streptococci derived from human stones into devitalized teeth of dogs, (*b*) rats by avitaminosis A, by traumatizing the bladder and producing carbon monoxide poisoning, by changing the mineral salts in the diet, and by administering large doses of estradiol diproprionate, (*c*) mice by avitaminosis A, and by prolonged administration of estrogens, (*d*) chickens by avitaminosis A, and (*e*) rabbits by producing a chemical cystitis and injecting proteus organisms into the bladder (Wilson).

Chemically urinary calculi are composed of the following: calcium carbonate, calcium phosphate, urates, and mixtures of calcium carbonate, calcium phosphate, urates, and oxalates (McKay).

Pathologically most urinary tract calculi originate in the renal pelvis, calyces, or papillæ. They are unilateral in from 80 to 90 per cent of cases and bilateral in from 10 to 20 per cent of cases. In unilateral stones there is no predilection for either side. In the renal pelvis, the most common locations of the stones are ureteropelvic junction, lower calyx, filling the entire

PLATE V

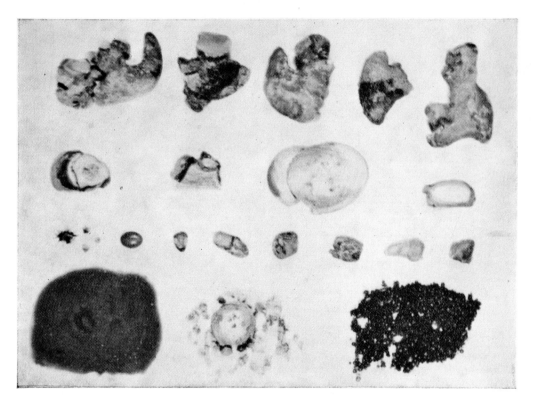

Uroliths showing the following from above down: Row 1, "staghorn" calculi; Row 2, cross sections of stones with and without lamellation; Row 3, varishaped stones from pelves and ureters; and Row 4, brown sand (left) calculus with crystalline deposits (center), and numerous brown, small faceted stones (right).

pelvis and calyces, and attached to a papilla. In the ureters, the most common location is the pelvic portion. The number of stones varies from one to thousands. The size of the calculus varies from that approaching a grain of sand to that measuring 10 cm. or more in greatest diameter and weighing as much as 567 gm. (Landes). The shape depends upon the size (Plate V). When the stones are small they are rounded but as they enlarge they tend to conform to and produce casts of the cavities in which they lie. Thus, when they fill the entire pelvis and calyces they produce a replica of the structures and since they contain many points they are often referred to as "staghorn calculi" (Fig. 509). Externally the stones may be smooth,

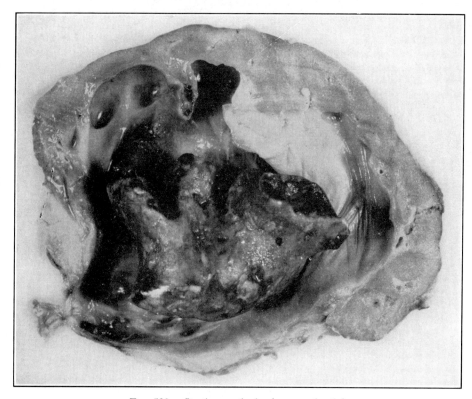

Fig. 509.—Staghorn calculus in a renal pelvis.

pebbled, or actually spinous. The color varies with the chemical composition from white to black. Cut surfaces often disclose a central nucleus surrounded by concentrically arranged amorphous or crystalline lamellæ.

The most common *complications* of urinary calculi are obstruction, hydronephrosis, pyonephrosis, pyelonephritis, septicemia, and perforation of the pelvis, ureter, etc., with infection of adjacent structures. The *clinical manifestations* consist of (*a*) renal colic resulting from muscular contraction of the ureter in an attempt to get rid of the stone, (*b*) renal pain due to ureteral contraction and hydronephrosis, (*c*) frequency and urgency caused by secondary infection of the urinary bladder, (*d*) digestive disturbances (nausea and vomiting) resulting from reflex impulses from the urinary tract to the digestive tract, and (*e*) general symptoms (fever, chills, leukocytosis, etc.) consequent to absorption of toxic material from the urinary tract. *Urinalysis* discloses erythrocytes, albumin, leukocytes, and casts and cultures of the urine usually reveal colon bacilli and staphylococci. The *diagnosis* of uroliths is made from the history, clinical manifestations, urinalysis, and demonstration of the stones roentgenographically (in plain films or using a contrast medium). *Treatment* consists of eliminating the factors that cause the stones and, once the stones have formed, of cystoscopic or incisional removal. The *prognosis* depends to a large extent upon the cause, the presence or absence of complications, the unilateral or bilateral nature, etc. Recurrences are common.

TUMORS

Orientation.—Tumors of the ureters and pelves are similar to tumors of the urinary bladder although they are much less frequent. They *occur* at all ages but are much more common in adults than in children and affect both sexes. Pathologically they may be classified as follows: adenoma,

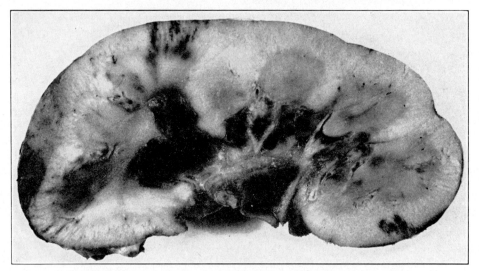

FIG. 510.—Hemangioma of the kidney showing several deeply hemorrhagic areas encroaching upon the renal pelvis.

papilloma, carcinoma, fibroma, myxoma, myoma, myosarcoma, leiomyosarcoma, fibromyoma, fibrolipoma, hemangioma, neurofibroma, sarcoma, mixed tumor, lymphoblastoma, and secondary tumors. The chief *complications* are hydronephrosis, pyonephrosis, pyelonephritis, and calculous formation in both benign and malignant tumors, and metastasis in malignant tumors. The most common *clinical manifestations* are hematuria (due to ulceration and secondary infection), pain (due to attempts at expulsion of the tumor and blood and hydronephrosis), bladder symptoms of dysuria, urgency, etc. (due to cystitis), and palpable tumor in the lumbar region (due to hydronephrosis). The *diagnosis* is made from the clinical manifestations, the demonstration of filling defects roentgenographically, and, in carcinoma, the finding of neoplastic cells in the urine. *Treatment* consists of surgical excision—usually by nephro-ureterectomy. The *prognosis* depends upon the type of tumor. In general, it is good in benign growths and at most only fair in malignant growths. Of all the tumors listed, only four need be dwelt upon further—hemangioma, papilloma, carcinoma, and secondary tumors.

Hemangioma.—Hemangioma of the upper part of the urinary tract is virtually confined to the kidney (Rives and Rappaport). It is usually located beneath the mucosa of the pelvis, calyx, or tip of a papilla, is single or multiple, measures as much as 3 to 4 cm. across, and is composed of sponge-like spaces filled with blood (Fig. 510). *Histologically* it is generally composed of cavernous spaces lined by endothelial cells and filled with erythrocytes.

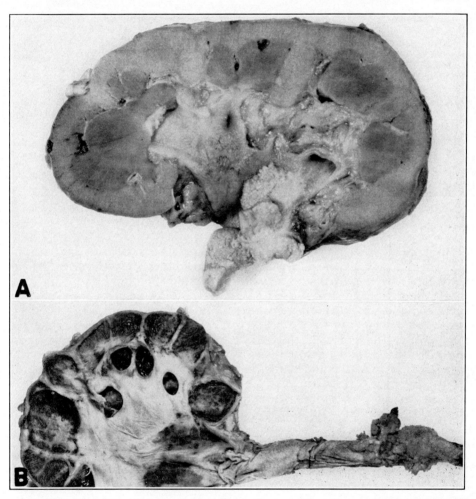

Fig. 511.—Carcinoma of *A*, renal pelvis illustrating a papillary tumor near the ureteropelvic junction and *B*, ureter showing multiple papillary tumors. The ureteral growths are associated with marked hydronephrosis.

Papilloma.—Papilloma of the ureter and renal pelvis is similar to papilloma of the urethra and bladder (Moore, Barnes, and Vest). The tumor is usually unilateral and is either single or multiple. When many tumors are present the condition is referred to as *papillomatosis*. *Grossly* the neoplasms exist as pedunculated and, less often, sessile, brown to pink, villous growths that are freely movable at their bases. *Histologically* they are composed of thin stalks of connective tissue covered with transitional epithelium. Although they are irregular in distribution, tumors of the pelvis are most often *located* at the ureteropelvic junction while those in the ureters are generally found in the distal portion. Papillomas of the pelvis and ureter are associated with similar tumors in the bladder in about one-third of the cases (Smith).

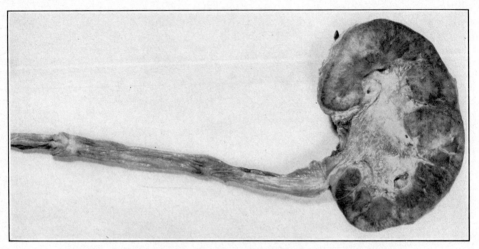

FIG. 512.—Metastatic carcinoma of the ureter from the colon demonstrating an infiltrating scirrhous growth.

Carcinoma.—Carcinoma of the ureter and pelvis is similar in distribution to papilloma and *pathologically* the lesion resembles that of carcinoma of the bladder. The growths are usually single and unilateral and, as a rule, are of a fungating, cauliflower-like variety (Fig. 511). The external surface is serrated and often superficially ulcerated; the base is infiltrated, and the growth, as a whole, is friable. Flat infiltrating tumors do occur but are rare. *Histologically* most of the lesions are of a transitional cell variety and only rarely are they of a squamous or adenomatous nature. The growths *spread* by (1) implantation onto the mucosa of the more distal portion of the urinary tract, (2) continuity to other portions of the urinary tract and adjacent tissues, and (3) metastasis to the lymph nodes, liver, bones, lungs, kidneys, bladder, adrenals, etc. (Scott).

Secondary Tumors.—Secondary tumors of the ureters and renal pelvis arise as a result of direct extension from adjacent structures or metastasis from distant organs (Presman, Moore, and Lazarus). The usual primary sites are uterus, prostate, bladder, kidney, stomach, lymph nodes, breast, lung, bowel, ovary, ureter, vagina, and pancreas. *Grossly* the growths are generally infiltrating but may be papillary (Fig. 512). *Histologically* they resemble the primary neoplasms.

REFERENCES

General

Herbut, P. A.: *Urological Pathology*, Philadelphia, Lea & Febiger, 1952.

Pathologic Physiology

Bors, E.: Urol. Survey, 7, 201, 1957 (Neurogenic Bladder).
Butcher, H. R., Jr. *et al.*: J. Urol., 78, 221, 1957 (Peristaltic Conduction Mechanism in Canine Ureter).

References

KIIL, F.: *The Function of the Ureter and Renal Pelvis*, Philadelphia, W. B. Saunders Co., 1957.

LEWIS, E. L., and KIMBROUGH, J. C.: South. Med. J., *45*, 171, 1952 (Concept Megaloureter).

NARATH, P. A.: The Physiology of the Renal Pelvis and Ureter. In Campbell's *Urology*, Philadelphia, W. B. Saunders Co., 1954, p. 64.

SWENSON, O., *et al.*: N. England J. Med., *246*, 41, 1952 (Etiology of Megaloureter).

URETHRA

Congenital Anomalies

BAKER, W. J., and WILKEY, J. L.: J. Urol., *59*, 642, 1948 (Persistent Cloaca).

BERGMAN, R. K.: Urol. & Cutan. Rev., *53*, 590, 1949 (Diverticulum Female Urethra).

BOYD, M. L.: J. A. M. A., *92*, 2154, 1929 (Stricture Female Urethra).

CAMPBELL, M. F.: Tr. Am. A. Genito-urin. Surgeons, *36*, 183, 1943 (Stenosis External Urethral Meatus).

CREEVY, C. D.: Surgery, *3*, 719, 1938 (Hypospadias).

DEES, J. E.: Surgery, *12*, 621, 1942 (Epispadias).

————: Urol. & Cutan. Rev., *54*, 480, 1950 (Diverticulum Anterior Male Urethra).

DOURMASHKIN, R. L.: J. Urol., *50*, 747, 1943 (Complete Urethral Occlusion).

GROSS, R. E., and MOORE, T. C.: A. M. A. Arch. Surg., *60*, 749, 1950 (Duplication of Urethra)

HERBST, R. H., and POLKEY, H. J.: J. Urol., *17*, 61, 1927 (Ectopic Urethral Openings).

LANDES, H. E., and RALL, R.: J. Urol., *34*, 254, 1935 (Valves Posterior Urethra).

PILCHER, F., JR., and PRICE, H. W.: J. A. M. A., *115*, 2072, 1940 (Hypertrophy Verumontanum).

WESSON, M. B.: J. Urol., *13*, 605, 1925 (Cyst of Prostate and Urethra).

Inflammations

CARSON, R. B.: Urol. & Cutan. Rev., *51*, 23, 1947 (Urethritis in Female).

COHN, A., and GRUNSTEIN, I.: Am. J. Obst. & Gynec., *48*, 339, 1944 (Gonorrhea in the Female).

CREECY, A. A., and BEAZLIE, F. S., JR.: J. Urol., *59*, 234, 1948 (Reiter's Syndrome).

FIRESTONE, A.: Urol. & Cutan. Rev., *41*, 590, 1937 (Cowper's Glands).

GLEN, J. E., JR., and BAILEY, R. S.: J. Urol., *66*, 294, 1951 (Trichomoniasis in the Male).

HALL, W. H., and FINEGOLD, S.: Ann. Int. Med., *38*, 533, 1953 (Reiter's Syndrome).

HARKNESS, A. H.: Brit. J. Venereal Dis., *13*, 119, 1937 (Cowper's Glands).

HECKEL, N. J.: J. Urol., *35*, 520, 1936 (Trichomonal Urethritis and Cystitis).

HELVESTINE, F., JR.: Virginia M. Monthly, *68*, 407, 1941 (Verumontanitis).

HODGES, C. V.: J. A. M. A., *149*, 753, 1952 (Chronic Urethritis).

JACOBY, A., and KRAFF, H.: Am. J. Syph., *27*, 415, 1943 (Gonorrhea in Women).

KILBURN, I. N.: New England J. Med., *215*, 112, 1936 (Tuberculous Urethritis).

LOVEMAN, A. B., and MORROW, R. P., JR.: Am. J. Syph., *28*, 79, 1944 (Intraurethral Chancres).

PELOUZE, P. S.: *Gonorrhea in the Male and Female*, 3rd Ed., W. B. Saunders Co. 1939.

————: Tr. Am. Urol. Assoc., *11*, 59, 1917 (Tuberculosis Urethra).

STONE, E.: A. M. A. Arch. Surg., *18*, 1315, 1929 (Gonorrheal Posterior Urethritis).

VOSE, S. N.: New England J. Med., *229*, 610, 1943 (Gonorrhea).

Physical Disturbances

ATTWATER, H. L.: Brit. J. Urol., *15*, 39, 1943 (Urethral Stricture).

BEILIN, L. M., and GRUENEBERG, J.: J. Urol., *52*, 596, 1944 (Calculus).

BOTSFORD, T. W., *et al.*: Am. J. Surg., *70*, 153, 1945 (Stricture Male Urethra).

DOURMASHKIN, R. L.: J. Urol., *68*, 496, 1952 (Stricture).

GUTIERREZ, R.: J. Urol., *49*, 865, 1943 (Foreign Bodies).

KLOMAN, E. H., *et al.*: South. M. J., *42*, 929, 1949 (Prolapse in Females).

MOFFETT, J. D., and BANKS, R., JR.: J. A. M. A., *146*, 1288, 1951 (Prolapse in Girls).

MULHOLLAND, S. W., and MADONNA, H. M.: J. Urol., *68*, 489, 1952 (Rupture).

SIMPSON-SMITH, A.: Brit. J. Surg., *24*, 309, 1936 (Rupture).

WYNNE, H. M. N.: Am. J. Obst. & Gynec., *27*, 373, 1934 (Stricture Female Urethra).

ZEIGERMAN, J. H.: Urol. & Cutan. Rev., *49*, 403, 1945 (Prolapse Female Urethra).

Tumors

BRACK, C. D., and FARBER, G. J.: J. Urol., *64*, 710, 1950 (Carcinoma Female Urethra).

EISENSTADT, J. S.: Am. J. Surg., *81*, 612, 1951 (Carcinoma Female Urethra).

HAHN, G. A.: J. Urol., *67*, 319, 1953 (Carcinoma Female Urethra).
KIRKMAN, N. F.: Brit. J. Surg., *37*, 162, 1950 (Carcinoma Penile Urethra).
NANSON, E. M.: Brit. J. Urol., *23*, 222, 1951 (Carcinoma Male Urethra).
PALMER, J. K., *et al.:* Surg., Gynec. & Obst., *87*, 611, 1948 (Caruncle).
RICHES, E. W.: Brit. J. Urol., *16*, 12, 1944 (Papilloma).
RICHES, E. W., and CULLEN, T. H.: Brit. J. Urol., *23*, 209, 1951 (Carcinoma Urethra).
ZASLOW, J., and PRIESTLEY, J. T.: J. Urol., *58*, 207, 1947 (Carcinoma Male Urethra).

BLADDER

Congenital Anomalies

BRODIE, N.: Am. J. Surg., *69*, 243, 1945 (Urachal Cysts).
BURNS, E., *et al.:* J. Urol., *57*, 257, 1947 (Duplication).
CAMPBELL, M. F.: South. M. J., *41*, 99, 1948 (Congenital Bladder Neck Obstruction).
GROSS, R. E., and CRESSON, S. L.: J. A. M. A., *149*, 1640, 1952 (Exstrophy).
HIGGINS, C. S.: J. Urol., *63*, 852, 1950 (Exstrophy).
KIMBROUGH, J. C.: J. Urol., *45*, 368, 1941 (Diverticulum).
KRETSCHMER, H. L.: Surg., Gynec. & Obst., *71*, 491, 1940 (Diverticulum).
LLOYD, F. A., and PRANKE, D.: Urol. & Cutan. Rev., *55*, 734, 1951 (Patent Urachus).
STEINHARDT, B.: Urol. & Cutan. Rev., *48*, 261, 1944 (Hypertrophy).
WESSEL, M. S., *et al.:* J. Urol., *67*, 523, 1952 (Urachal Carcinoma).
ZELLERMAYER, J., and CARLSON, H.: J. Urol., *51*, 24, 1944 (Hour Glass Deformity).

Degenerations

ROEN, P. R., and WIENER, J.: J. Urol., *66*, 119, 1951 (Primary Amyloid Tumor).
SENGER, F. L., *et al.:* J. Urol., *63*, 790, 1950 (Amyloidosis).

Inflammations

BASSOW, S. H.: Urol. & Cutan. Rev., *51*, 559, 1947 (Trigonitis).
BERRY, J. V., and BERRY, N. E.: J. Urol., *58*, 260, 1947 (Acute Cystitis).
BOONSTRA, C. E., and BATES, P. L.: U. S. Armed Forces M. J., *1*, 1029, 1950 (Malakoplakia).
CRISTOL, D. S., and GREENE, L. F.: Surgery, *18*, 343, 1945 (Gangrenous Cystitis).
DEAN, A. L., and SLAUGHTER, D. P.: J. Urol., *46*, 917, 1941 (Irradiation Cystitis).
FINESTONE, E. O.: Surg., Gynec. & Obst., *62*, 93, 1936 (Syphilis).
FRENCH, A. J., and MASON, J. T.: J. Urol., *66*, 229, 1951 (Malakoplakia).
GREENBERGER, A. J., and GREENBERGER, M. E.: J. Urol., *67*, 222, 1952 (Tuberculosis).
HAGER, B. H.: J. Urol., *16*, 447, 1926 (Incrusted Cystitis).
HATCH, W. E., and WELLS, A. H.: J. Urol., *52*, 149, 1944 (Actinomycosis).
HIGGINS, C. C.: M. Clin. North America, *19*, 1959, 1936 (Cystitis).
KRETSCHMER, H. L.: New England J. Med., *233*, 339, 1945 (Cystitis).
LAZARUS, J. A.: J. Urol., *55*, 160, 1946 (Tuberculosis).
MATHÉ, C. P.: J. Urol., *62*, 308, 1949 (Cystitis).
MILNER, W. A., *et al.:* New England J. Med., *246*, 902, 1952 (Cystitis Emphysematosa).
MOULDER, M. K.: J. Urol., *56*, 420, 1946 (Thrush).
PATCH, F. S.: New England J. Med., *220*, 979, 1939 (Proliferative Cystitis).
ROEN, P. R., and WIENER, J.: J. Urol., *66*, 119, 1951 (Amyloid Tumor).
SEAMAN, J. A.: J. Urol., *63*, 105, 1950 (Interstitial Cystitis).
THOMPSON, G. J., and STEIN, J. J.: J. Urol., *44*, 639, 1940 (Leukoplakia).
WARRICK, W. D.: J. Urol., *45*, 835, 1941 (Cystitis Cystica).
WATSON, E. M., *et al.:* J. Urol., *57*, 1038, 1947 (Irradiation Cystitis).

Physical Disturbances

BORS, E., and BOWIE, C. F.: J. Urol., *55*, 358, 1946 (Foreign Bodies).
CRASTNOPOL, P., *et al.:* A. M. A. Arch. Surg., *60*, 1093, 1950 (Spontaneous Rupture).
CRISTOL, D. S., and GREENE, L. F.: Surg. Clin. N. America, p. 987, 1945, (Vesical Calculi in Women).
FEIGAL, W. M., and POLZAK, J. A.: J. Urol., *56*, 196, 1946 (Spontaneous Rupture).
FORSYTHE, W. E., JR., and KARLAN, S. C.: J. Urol., *54*, 22, 1945 (Enuresis).
HOWARD, T. L., and BUCHTEL, H. A.: J. A. M. A., *146*, 1202, 1951 (Vesical Neck Obstruction in Children).
IASON, A. H.: Am. J. Surg., *63*, 69, 1944 (Hernia).

MICHELS, L. M.: Ann. Surg., *123*, 999, 1946 (Wounds).
NESBIT, R. M., and GORDON, W. G.: Pennsylvania M. J., *43*, 1261, 1940 (Neurogenic Bladder).
NITSCHKE, P. H.: Am. J. Surg., *40*, 560, 1938 (Foreign Bodies).
STEWART, C. B.: Canad. M. A. J., *55*, 370, 1946 (Enuresis).
TWINEM, F. P., and LANGDON, B. B.: J. Urol., *66*, 201, 1951 (Bladder Stones).
VERMEULEN, C. W., *et al.:* J. Urol., *64*, 541, 1950 (Experimental Uroliths).

Tumors

BARSOTTI, M., and VIGLIANI, E. C.: Arch. Indust. Hyg. & Occupat. Med., *5*, 234, 1952 (Bladder Lesions and Aromatic Amines).
CRANE, A. R., and TREMBLAY, R. G.: Ann. Surg., *118*, 887, 1943 (Sarcoma).
CREEVY, C. D., and REISER, M. P.: Surg., Gynec. & Obst., *95*, 589, 1952 (Renal Effects of Cholecystectomy).
DEMING, C. L.: J. Urol., *63*, 815, 1950 (Papilloma).
DUKES, C. E., and MASINA, F.: J. Urol., *21*, 173, 1949 (Epithelial Tumors).
FLOCKS, R. H.: J. A. M. A., *145*, 295, 1951 (Treatment Carcinoma).
GRAVES, R. C., *et al.:* J. Urol., *63*, 821, 1950 (Cystectomy for Carcinoma).
HENRY, G. W.: Am. J. Roentgenol., *62*, 843, 1949 (Sarcoma).
JEWETT, H. J.: J. A. M. A., *148*, 187, 1952 (Infiltrating Carcinoma).
KERR, W. S., JR., and COLBY, F. H.: J. Urol., *63*, 842, 1950 (Treatment Carcinoma).
————: J. Urol., *65*, 841, 1951 (Correlation Pathology, Treatment, and Prognosis in Carcinoma).
KIRWIN, T. J.: J. Internat. Coll. Surgeons, *13*, 1, 1950 (Tumors).
MARSHALL, V. F., and WHITMORE, W. F., JR.: J. Urol., *63*, 232, 1950 (Cystectomy for Carcinoma).
ROYCE, R. K., and ACKERMAN, L. V.: J. Urol., *65*, 66, 1951 (Clinical and Pathologic Aspects Carcinoma).
WAY, R. A.: J. Urol., *67*, 688, 1952 (Sarcoma).
WINSBURY-WHITE, H. B., *et al.:* Lancet, *2*, 797, 1950 (Papilloma).

URETER AND PELVIS

Congenital Anomalies

CAMPBELL, E. W.: J. Urol., *60*, 31, 1948 (Megalo-ureter).
CAMPBELL, M.: Surg., Gynec. & Obst., *93*, 705, 1951 (Ureterocele).
EISENDRATH, D. N.: Urol. & Cutan. Rev., *42*, 404, 1938 (Ending Ectopic Ureter).
GRIM, K. B.: J. Urol., *44*, 397, 1940 (Ureteral Agenesis).
HAMILTON, J. L.: J. Urol., *56*, 530, 1946 (Hypoplasia Ureter).
HENLINE, R. B., and HAWES, C. J.: J. A. M. A., *137*, 777, 1948 (Ureteropelvic Obstruction).
HERBST, W. P.: J. A. M. A., *137*, 775, 1948 (Posterior Renal Pelvis).
MacLEAN, J. T.: J. Urol., *54*, 374, 1945 (Ureteral Valve).
McGRAW, A. B., and CULP, O. S.: J. Urol., *67*, 262, 1952 (Diverticulum Ureter).
NATION, E. F.: J. Urol., *51*, 456, 1944 (Duplication Kidney and Ureter).
PARKS, R. E., and CHASE, W. E.: Am. J. Dis. Child., *82*, 442, 1951 (Retrocaval Ureter).
SMITH, I.: Brit. J. Surg., *34*, 182, 1946 (Triplicate Ureter).
SOLEY, P. J.: J. Urol., *55*, 46, 1946 (Ureteropelvic Obstruction).
SWENSON, O., *et al.:* New England J. Med., *246*, 41, 1952 (Megalo-ureters).

Inflammations

GORRO, A. P., *et al.:* Urol. & Cutan. Rev., *51*, 209, 1947 (Tuberculosis).
HEANEY, N. S., and KRETSCHMER, H. L.: J. A. M. A., *128*, 407, 1945 (Pyelitis in Pregnancy).
HEPBURN, T. N.: Ann. Surg., *93*, 1114, 1931 (Gangrene Ureter from Silver Nitrate).
KOBAK, A. J., and SCHIRMER, E. H.: Urol. & Cutan. Rev., *47*, 659, 1943 (Pyelitis in Pregnancy).
LAUGHLIN, V. C., and BILOTTA, J. F. L.: J. Urol., *44*, 358, 1940 (Leukoplakia).
MAKAR, N.: Brit. J. Surg., *36*, 148, 1948 (Schistosomiasis).
MICHAELS, J. P.: Surg., Gynec. & Obst., *86*, 36, 1948 (Necrosis Ureter Following Operation).
RICHES, E. W., *et al.:* Proc. Roy. Soc. Med., *38*, 188, 1944 (Pyelitis).
RINKER, J. R.: J. A. M. A., *142*, 87, 1950 (Tuberculosis).
SENGER, F. L., *et al.:* Am. J. Surg., *73*, 69, 1947 (Empyema).
WHARTON, L. R.: South. M. J., *26*, 677, 1933 (Denervation Ureter).

Physical Disturbances

DIEHL, W. K., and HUNDLEY, J. M.: Surg., Gynec. & Obst., *87*, 705, 1948 (Irradiation Ureteritis).

DOHERTY, W. E.: Practitioner, *151*, 341, 1943 (Urinary Calculi).

HIGGINS, C. C.: J. Urol., *62*, 403, 1949 (Renal Lithiasis).

KEATING, F. R., and COOK, E. N.: J. A. M. A., *129*, 994, 1945 (Lithiasis in Hyperparathyroidism).

KIMBROUGH, J. C., and DENSLOW, J. C.: J. Urol., *61*, 837, 1949 (Urinary Calculi in Recumbent Patients).

LANDES, R. R.: J. A. M. A., *152*, 514, 1953 (Giant Calculus).

McKAY, H. W., *et al.*: J. A. M. A., *137*, 225, 1948 (Urinary Calculi).

NOVAK, J.: Urol. & Cutan. Rev., *48*, 321, 1944 (Ureteral Injuries in Gynecological Operations).

RANDALL, A.: Internat. Abstracts of Surgery, *71*, 209, 1940 (Etiology Renal Calculus).

RUSCHE, C. F.: J. Urol., *60*, 63, 1948 (Gunshot Wound Ureter).

RUSCHE, C. F., and BACON, S. K.: J. A. M. A., *114*, 201, 1940 (Injury Ureter).

WILSON, J. G., *et al.*: J. Urol., *54*, 503, 1945 (Experimental Calculi).

Tumors

BARNES, R. W., and KAWAICHI, G. K.: Urol. & Cutan. Rev., *48*, 430, 1944 (Tumors of Ureter).

GAHAGEN, H. Q., and REED, W. K.: J. Urol., *62*, 139, 1949 (Squamous Cell Carcinoma Pelvis).

GUALTIERI, T., *et al.*: J. Urol., *59*, 1083, 1948 (Carcinoma Ureter).

LAZARUS, J. A.: J. Urol., *45*, 527, 1941 (Metastatic Carcinoma Ureter).

LAZARUS, J. A., and MARKS, M. S.: J. Urol., *54*, 140, 1945 (Primary Carcinoma Ureter).

McDONALD, J. R., and PRIESTLEY, J. T.: J. Urol., *51*, 245, 1944 (Carcinoma Renal Pelvis).

MOORE, T.: Brit. J. Surg., *29*, 371, 1942 (Tumors of Ureter).

PRESMAN, D., and EHRLICH, L.: J. Urol., *59*, 312, 1948 (Metastatic Tumor Ureter).

RAPPAPORT, A. E.: A. M. A. Arch. Path., *40*, 84, 1945 (Hemangioma).

RIVES, H. F., and POOL, T. L.: J. A. M. A., *125*, 1187, 1944 (Hemangioma).

SCOTT, W. W.: J. Urol., *50*, 45, 1943 (Carcinoma Ureter).

SMITH, G. G.: Am. J. Surg., *30*, 130, 1935 (Tumors of Kidney and Ureter).

VEST, S. A.: J. Urol., *53*, 97, 1945 (Benign Tumors of Ureter).

Chapter

31

Kidneys

PATHOLOGIC PHYSIOLOGY
WILLIAM V. McDONNELL

THE vital responsibility of maintaining the body's internal environment falls mainly on the kidneys. Although other organs partake to some extent, the kidneys play the *main role* in maintaining the chemical balance in tissues and body fluids. They are the organs responsible for the regulation of fluid, electrolyte, osmotic, and acid-base balance. In the performance of this regulatory mechanism the ultimate end product is urine. A second aspect of renal function is concerned with the regulation of arterial blood pressure. Although variously interpreted, the latter is generally considered to be controlled by an endocrine mechanism. It will be discussed in a later section of this chapter (Hypertension).

It is not in the province of this text to discuss in detail the many intricacies of normal and abnormal renal function. Only a consideration of those factors which form the basis for an understanding of the effects of morphologic change will be attempted. For elaboration on this subject a textbook on physiology is recommended.

If the kidneys are responsible for regulating the composition of blood, the entire *blood volume* must pass through them at frequent intervals. This is indeed the case. It is estimated that 20 per cent of the cardiac output at rest goes to the kidneys despite the fact that these organs comprise less than 0.5 per cent of the total body weight. To accomplish this the *vascular structure* of the kidneys is unique in many respects. The organs lie close to the aorta where they receive blood from the short, wide renal arteries. Upon entering the kidney, the renal artery promptly divides into from seven to nine interlobar arteries which in turn divide to form the looped arcuate arteries. These give rise to the interlobular arteries which terminate as afferent arterioles. Each afferent arteriole divides into approximately 50 convoluted capillaries to form the tuft of the glomerulus. The tuft invaginates into a proximal sac-like dilatation of a renal tubule to form Bowman's space. Each capillary loop is, therefore, ensheathed in a reflected layer of epithelium continuous with that lining Bowman's space and the corresponding tubule. The convoluted capillaries of the tuft reunite to form the efferent arteriole which emerges from Bowman's space and subsequently empties into a capillary bed. This serves as the source of blood for the corresponding renal tubule (peritubular capillaries). Close to the efferent arteriole, and bearing a relation also to the distal convoluted tubule, is a collection of cells probably derived from the arteriole and possibly having a humoral effect on glomerular blood flow. This is called the *juxta-glomerular apparatus*.

The *renal tubule* is usually described as having four anatomic divisions. The *proximal convoluted tubule* begins at the glomerulus. It is a coiled segment located entirely in the cortex and lined by a single layer of rather high cuboidal epithelium. This segment enters the column of Bertini and becomes first the *descending limb of Henle's loop* and then, the *ascending limb of Henle's loop*. In these two portions of the tubule the epithelium becomes gradually flatter with a noticeable clearing of the cytoplasm. The ascending limb ends at the level of the cortex where the tubule again assumes a tortuous course forming the *distal convoluted tubule*. In this portion, the lining epithelial cells again become higher but their cytoplasm remains somewhat clearer than those of the proximal segment. The distal convoluted tubule drains into a collecting tubule which in turn empties into one of the calyces.

This arrangement of glomerulus and tubule forms the *functioning* unit of the kidney and is referred to as the *nephron*. Renal function is the summation of the activity of the more than one million nephrons present in each kidney. The activity of a nephron, culminating in the formation of urine, encompasses filtration, reabsorption, and secretion.

Filtration of blood occurs in the glomerulus. The unusual vascular system of the kidney, referred to previously, provides for the delivery of a massive amount of blood (1700 cc. per day) to the glomeruli at an unusually high pressure (75 mm. Hg.). The rate at which plasma is filtered into Bowman's space is determined by a simple interplay of *three forces*. Capillary blood pressure (75 mm. Hg.) tends to force fluid into the capsular space while the colloidal osmotic pressure of the blood (25 mm. Hg.) and the pressure in the capsular space (10 mm. Hg.) oppose filtration. The effective filtration pressure is, therefore, equal to the capillary blood pressure minus the two opposing pressures or $EFP = 75 - (25 + 10) = 40$ mm. Hg. Under normal conditions, this allows filtrate to be formed by the total glomerular membrane at a rate of approximately 120 cc. per minute or about 170 liters per day.

From the foregoing, it is readily evident that the *quantity* of *filtrate* formed is affected by any alteration in the pressure relationships of the three forces concerned. Accordingly, a fall in the systemic blood pressure (shock) to a level that allows the capillary blood pressure to be equal or less than the combined capsular and osmotic pressures causes a complete cessation of filtration and anuria results. Conversely, an elevation in systemic blood pressure (hypertension) increases filtration rate but usually only to a slight degree. Lowering of the osmotic pressure of the blood (hypoproteinemia) increases filtration rate and a sudden obstruction of the flow of urine (ligation of ureter) raises the capsular pressure to a level exceeding capillary blood pressure and filtration ceases. Another factor having a quantitative effect on filtration is the patency of the glomerular capillaries. Narrowing of their lumens due to swelling or proliferation of the lining cells (acute diffuse glomerulonephritis) decreases filtration often to a marked degree.

Since filtration is purely a mechanical process, the quality of the resultant filtrate is determined solely by particulate size. Substances of a smaller *molecular size* pass the glomerular membrane and appear in the filtrate while particles of larger size will not. The critical threshold is apparently between the molecular size of albumin (70,000) and hemoglobin (68,000). Albumin will not pass through an intact glomerular membrane while hemoglobin, if present free in the blood, passes easily. Alterations in the *glomerular membrane* which increase its permeability (nephrotic syndrome) or disrupt its continuity (diffuse glomerulonephritis) will cause the appearance in the urine of protein and other substances of a molecular size too large to pass the normal filtering membrane. Of the several protein fractions of the blood, albumin has the smallest molecular size and, therefore, under conditions of abnormal glomerular permeability constitutes the bulk of the protein in the urine thus accounting for the commonly used term *albuminuria* rather than *proteinuria*, which actually is more accurate.

It is obvious that if the massive volume of glomerular filtrate formed were allowed to be lost in the urine fatal dehydration would ensue in minutes. Reduction of the approximately 170 liters filtered in 24 hours to a liter or so of urine that is normally passed within this period takes place in the renal tubules. This process is essentially one of *reabsorption*. That this reabsorption is selective is evidenced by the fact that substances in the filtrate that are needed by the body are reabsorbed while substances that are the end products of metabolism, and which are not needed by the body, are allowed to pass on into the urine. Substances which are needed include water, glucose, sodium, potassium, calcium, chloride, vitamin C, and amino acids. All of these are normally reabsorbed to such a degree that they are either absent from urine or present in extremely low concentrations. Excessive amounts of these substances in the urine may indicate either defective tubular absorption, such as loss of sodium in Addison's disease, or a concentration in the blood that is too great for normal tubular activity, such as glycosuria in diabetes mellitus. Other substances are normally reabsorbed in relatively small amounts and, therefore, are highly concentrated in the urine. These include urea, uric acid, phosphates, and sulfates. Creatinine is concentrated to a greater degree than any other consitutent of urine since, under normal conditions, it is not reabsorbed at all.

Reabsorption by the renal tubules is a relatively complex phenomenon involving many physical, chemical, and humoral processes. A few of these, because they are readily evident in renal and systemic disease, may be briefly mentioned. The *adrenal cortex* (aldosterone) acts to increase the excretion of potassium and decrease the excretion of sodium and water. In adrenal insufficiency (Addison's disease), loss of sodium and water occurs and excess potassium is retained. The *posterior lobe* of the *pituitary gland* plays a role in the reabsorption of water by the distal renal tubules through its antidiuretic hormone. When this activity of the pituitary is obliterated a large volume of urine is excreted, as is the case in diabetes insipidus. A third important factor concerned with reabsorption, and important for an understanding of chronic renal disease, is the *rate* of *flow* of fluid along the tubules. As the rate of flow increases the time for reabsorption decreases and the output of urine therefore has a tendency to increase.

Although *secretion* by the tubular epithelium of creatinine, H-ions, potassium, and certain foreign substances occurs, this phenomenon of tubular activity appears to be of little importance in man under ordinary conditions of health.

Renal insufficiency or failure is the inability of the kidneys to adequately carry out their functions. It may develop slowly or rapidly as the result of a wide variety of disease processes and leads eventually to a complex syndrome called *uremia* (see later section in this chapter). The loss of ability to function adequately may develop suddenly in a kidney which has previously been morphologically and physiologically normal or it may develop gradually and relentlessly over a long period of time. It is valid, therefore, to speak of acute renal failure and chronic renal failure.

Acute renal failure is also referred to as *kidney shutdown*. It occurs when the great majority of nephrons in both kidneys are suddenly rendered non-functional. Although it is seen in association with many pathologic processes, the effect produced is similar, namely, a decrease in the formation of urine (oliguria) which in many cases progresses to complete cessation (anuria) leading to uremia. The anuria of acute renal failure may occur as the result of decreased glomerular filtration, excessive and indiscriminate tubular reabsorption, or a combination of both. Some of the causes of decreased glomerular filtration have been previously enumerated. In the presence of normally functioning tubules reabsorption will continue despite the greatly decreased filtrate, and *retention of water, electrolytes* and *nitrogenous wastes* will occur rapidly. Urine, therefore, will be decreased in amount and heavily concentrated (*hypersthenuria*). Necrosis of tubular epithelium (acute toxic nephrosis) removes the physiologic barrier between the filtrate and the concentrated blood in the peritubular capillaries. There is loss of the selective power of the tubular cells to absorb or reject the various components of the filtrate. As a result, there is indiscriminate and massive reabsorption of the filtrate across the naked basement membrane into the peitubular capillaries which, added to the usually coexisting impairment of filtration, leads to anuria.

Chronic renal failure occurs when there has been gradual destruction of at least 75 per cent of functioning nephrons. The chronicity of the process is emphasized by the realization that destruction is brought about essentially by scarring, and therefore does not occur suddenly. The most typical examples are the atrophic scarred kidneys of chronic diffuse glomerulonephritis, bilateral chronic pyelonephritis and, less commonly, benign nephrosclerosis. As more and more nephrons are destroyed certain changes occur in those that remain. Due to an increase in extracellular fluid and the increased blood pressure which accompanies chronic renal disease, glomerular blood flow, glomerular blood pressure, and consequently filtration increase per glomerulus even though the total filtrate is probably reduced. The rate of tubular flow increases and, as has already been mentioned, this decreases tubular reabsorption primarily of water but also to some extent of solutes. The urine from such a kidney, therefore, often increases in quantity (*polyuria*) but the impairment of the reabsorptive and concentrating ability of the tubules causes it to be of a low fixed specific gravity (*hyposthenuria*). This lack of ability to concentrate or dilute urine as needed is an indication of severe renal destruction no matter what the cause. Inevitably there is a progressive loss of tubular activity, both regarding water and solutes, until the urine passed is essentially unchanged as far as content and specific gravity is concerned from that of glomerular filtrate (isothenuria). There thus exists failure of renal function with all that it implies in the presence of continued and often excessive urine formation. It is important to note that renal failure thus produced is inexorable in its progression toward uremia and death. Acute renal failure, on the other hand, need not be premanent. Whether due to decreased filtration or necrosis of tubular epithelium, if the patient can be supported through his uremia for approximately 14 days, the kidneys will again begin to function usually with no clinical evidence of residual damage. It is, therefore, evident that acute renal failure offers best use of such a device as an artificial kidney.

An important aspect of altered renal physiology is *edema*. In acute diffuse glomerulonephritis the moderate edema that occurs in other than dependent sites in the absence of lowered plasma protein is thought to be due to a general increase in capillary permeability caused by the same toxic agent that is responsible for the renal changes. The most important factor in the production of renal edema is damage to the glomerular filter with consequent loss of large amounts of protein in the urine. Albumin, because it has a smaller molecular size than globulin or fibrinogen, makes up the bulk of the lost protein. When the amount of proteinuria is sufficient to lower the plasma proteins below 5 grams per 100 cc., edema ensues. The complex of proteinuria, hypoproteinemia, edema and, for reasons unknown, hypercholesterolemia is referred to as the *nephrotic syndrome*. It is a common feature of subacute diffuse glomerulonephritis, diabetic glomerulosclerosis, and renal amyloidosis.

Numerous *renal function tests* are available to help detect clinically the presence and also the severity of damage to the kidneys. In addition to urinalysis and determination of nitrogenous constituents of the blood, procedures are available to evaluate tubular excretion (phenolsulfonphthalein test), tubular reabsorption (concentration and dilution tests), and glomerular filtration (urea clearance test). For details of technique and interpretation of these and other renal function tests, a textbook of clinical pathology is recommended.

Uremia.—*Uremia* (Gr. = urine + blood) may be *defined* as a complex clinical syndrome associated with renal failure. In general, it may be said that uremia occurs as a result of failure of the kidneys to excrete waste products and to retain substances essential for the proper maintenance of the internal environment. As has already been pointed out, renal failure may occur on an extrarenal basis due to low blood pressure and low blood volume. The state thus produced is frequently referred to as "*prerenal*" or "*extrarenal*" uremia.

Uremia is the *common ground* upon which all severe damaging renal diseases meet. Some of the more common of these *conditions* are polycystic disease, nephrosclerosis, acute toxic nephrosis, amyloidosis, myeloma kidney, diffuse glomerulonephritis, periarteritis nodosa, pyelonephritis, bilateral cortical necrosis, hydronephrosis, and pyonephrosis. The specific *biochemical alterations* that occur in uremia are variable depending to some extent on the rapidity of onset of renal insufficiency, the underlying renal disease, and also for reasons which are not clear. Within the scope of this text, however, only certain basic alterations need be mentioned. The levels of urea, creatinine, uric acid, ammonia, amino acids, and other nonprotein nitrogeneous substances in the blood increase. In addition, there is usually loss of chloride and sodium and retention of potassium, phosphates, and sulfates. On the basis of these biochemical alterations, and also for reasons which are obscure, certain clinical and pathologic alterations in various systems occur with sufficient regularity to warrant special consideration.

Cardiovascular System.—*Hypertension* is commonly associated with uremia, but this association is seen only when the underlying renal failure is chronic. Renal failure developing rapidly (acute toxic nephrosis) is not regularly associated with an increase in blood pressure. A sterile, serofibrinous *pericarditis* is present in about one third of the cases of uremia. The precise etiologic factor of the pericarditis is not known but it has been suggested that it is due to the accumulation of one or more waste products. It is now believed that the precipitating cause of death in many cases of uremia is myocardial failure brought about by an increase in the blood level of potassium.

Central Nervous System.—Most cases of uremia show profound central nervous system disturbances. These include headache, vertigo, convulsions, twitching, muscular weakness, apathy, coma, and delirium. Most of these are attributable to the lowered calcium level in the blood which, in turn, is the result of phosphate retention. Pathologically, there are no constant or pathognomonic central nervous system findings other than edema of the brain proper and the meninges.

Gastrointestinal System.—Nausea, vomiting, and either diarrhea or constipation are seen commonly in uremic patients. These symptoms are associated with a variety of pathologic lesions occurring anywhere in the gastrointestinal tract, from the esophagus to the rectum, and consisting of discrete ulcers or diffuse areas of acute inflammation. The reason for the association of this involvement with the uremic state has not been clearly established.

Respiratory System.—Patients in uremia commonly have dyspnea or marked deep sighing respiration (*Kussmaul breathing*). There is a typical ammoniacal odor to the breath which is thought to be due to the production of ammonia from the decomposition of the abnormally large amount of urea in the saliva. Pathologically a mild interstitial pneumonitis and intra-alveolar deposition of fibrin are often found.

Skin.—The skin in uremia is often dry, yellow brown, and pruritic. In advanced cases, crystals of grayish-white urea are deposited on the integument especially of the face, neck, and chest producing what has been referred to as "uremic frost" (Fig. 513).

Blood.—Some of the many chemical alterations in the blood have already been mentioned. In addition, there is almost always an anemia of varying severity. The basis for the anemia is not known with certainty. Both bone marrow depression and hemolysis have been cited, with most workers favoring the former.

Parathyroid Glands.—In certain cases of prolonged renal insufficiency, another facet of the uremic picture is provided by *parathyroid hyperplasia*. Retention of phosphates by the kidneys, with a consequent excessive excretion by the intestinal tract removing at the same time unabsorbed calcium, and increased levels of blood phosphorus contribute to the increase in parathyroid activity. The severest manifestations of this aspect of chronic renal insufficiency are seen in *children*. Before the age of puberty the mobilization of calcium from the bones by the increased activity of the parathyroids leads to the changes of *osteitis fibrosa cystica*. The occurrence of osseous deformities in association with chronic renal insufficiency is referred to as *renal rickets*.

The *importance* of recognizing *uremia* in clinical practice is not lessened by the fact that in the majority of (but definitely not all)cases it is caused by destructive renal disease of a progressive irreversible nature. It has been mentioned previously that uremia associated with acute kidney shutdown (acute toxic nephrosis) may be temporary and, therefore, early recognition and the institution of proper supportive measures are of the utmost importance.

Hypertension.—The term *hypertension* (Gr. = over + tension) signifies a persistent increase in both the systolic and particularly the diastolic blood pressure. Opinion differs as to what constitutes a hypertensive blood pressure level but generally an elevation of the systolic beyond 140 and diastolic beyond 90 extending over a period of months and years is thought to be significant. Although all cases of hypertension are not of renal origin, the frequent association of the kidney and the hypertensive state prompts a consideration of the subject at this time. The condition is *common*. It is estimated that approximately 12 per cent of all persons die of hypertension and that 20 per cent of the population can expect to have high blood pressure at some time during life. While it may occur at all ages, the majority of patients are beyond the fourth decade. It is found more commonly in Negroes than in whites.

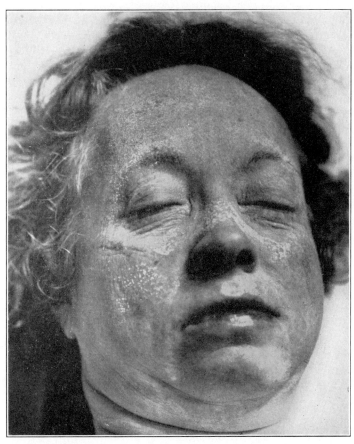

Fig. 513.—Uremic frost distributed about the face and forehead.

The *causes* of hypertension may be enumerated as follows: (1) *Neurogenic*. This occurs on the basis of vasoconstriction from stimulation of the sympathetic ganglia or the vasomotor centers in the brain. In man, hypertension may be seen in bulbar poliomyelitis, tabes dorsalis, sclerosis of the carotid sinus, increased intracranial pressure (as from tumor or hemorrhage), psychic disturbance, and resection of the glossopharyngeal nerve. In animals, it has been produced by sectioning the carotid sinus and the aortic depressor nerve, cerebral ischemia, diathermy stimulation of the medulla in dogs, and subjecting rats to the sound of an air blast over 167 times daily. (2) *Cardiovascular*. Experimentally, cardiovascular hypertension is produced by clamping the aorta above the renal vessels while in man hypertension on a cardiovascular basis is seen in coarctation of the aorta, arteriovenous fistula, arteriosclerosis, and occasionally heart failure. (3) *Endocinogenic.* Experimental evidence of endocrinogenic participation consists of the following: diminution in blood pressure after removal of the anterior lobe of the pituitary or both adrenals, and increase of blood pressure upon administration of adrenalin or (under certain circumstances) desoxycorticosterone acetate. In man, hypertension is seen in cases of basophilic adenoma of the pituitary, pheochromocytoma of the adrenal, hyperplasia or tumor of the adrenal cortex, and toxemia of pregnancy. (4) *Renal Humoral.* It seems evident that a renal humoral mechanism for the production of hypertension has been clearly established and that the mechanism works through the medium of renal ischemia. Experimentally, hypertension has been produced by constriction of renal arteries, compression of ureters, and wrapping of the kidney with silk or cellophane (perinephritis). In man, it is seen in association with acute and chronic glomerulonephritis, obstruction to the main renal vessels, nephrosclerosis, diabetic glomerulosclerosis, pyelonephritis, hydronephrosis, and polycystic kidney. The mechanism of renal hypertension apparently involves the formation by the renal tubules of a proteolytic enzyme renin which is released into the blood stream in increased amounts when renal circulation is disturbed. In the blood renin acts upon a globulin, hypertensinogen, also called renin substrate, which is produced in the liver and which is normally in the blood. The result of this interaction is a polypeptide called hypertensin or angiotonin. Hypertensin acts directly on the cardiovascular system causing vasoconstriction, increased peripheral resistance, and hypertension. (5) *Unknown.* It is an unfortunate fact that approximately 90 per cent of hypertensive people cannot be placed in any of the above mentioned etiologic categories. Hypertension of this nature is referred to as *primary* or *essential.* When essential hypertension is characterized by a moderate blood pressure elevation extending over relatively long periods of time it is referred to as *benign* hypertension. When the elevation of blood pressure is severe, the onset sudden and progression to death rapid, the condition is referred to as *malignant* or accelerated hypertension. At autopsy the kidneys of patients with essential hypertension, usually reveal extensive arteriolarsclerosis with consequent ischemic atrophy and scarring of renal tissue (*benign nephrosclerosis*). The kidneys of patients dying with malignant hypertension reveal extensive necrosis as well as sclerosis of arterioles and other findings which will be described later in this chapter (*malignant nephrosclerosis*).

Despite extensive research over the past 25 years the exact *pathogenesis* of essential hypertension remains obscure. Neurogenic, endocrine, and renal factors have received greatest attention. The common association of essential hypertension with an ischemic scarred kidney would suggest that the renal humoral theory referred to above is the mechanism of action. It is the general opinion today that renal change may accentuate the hypertensive state but not initiate it. The not infrequent absence of renal change in patients dying early in the course of essential hypertension tends to substantiate this belief. Although lacking in proof, it might be possible that a person of susceptible constitutional, psychological, and hereditary makeup possesses alterations in the vasomotor or endocrine system or both which produce peripheral vasoconstriction with consequent increase in peripheral resistance and elevated blood pressure. As outlined in Chapter 9, page 359. prolonged vasospasm and elevated intravascular pressure lead to arteriolarsclerosis. The effect of arteriolarsclerosis on the kidney is ischemia thus initiating the humoral maintenance and accentuation of the hypertensive state.

The *pathologic* changes in hypertension consist of (1) a great variety of renal lesions (described in subsequent sections of this Chapter), (2) arteriosclerosis and arteriolarsclerosis (page 359), and (3) the complications that arise as a result of the renal and arterial changes. The chief *complications* consist of uremia, myocardial failure (from simple decompensation or infarction), and cerebral hemorrhage. The *manifestations* consist of restlessness, asthenia, loss of accustomed zest for living, headache, vertigo, epistaxis, insomnia, syncope, aphasia, paresthesia, monoplegia, hemiplegia, coma, heart consciousness, palpitation, cardiac decompensation, symptoms of coronary artery occlusion, nocturia, polyuria, elevation of blood pressure (beyond 140 systolic and 90 diastolic), full pulse, cardiac enlargement, eye ground changes (tortuosity and narrowing of the vessels, nicking of the veins at points crossed by arteries, edema, hemorrhages, and exudates), and often albumin, hyaline and granular casts, and erythrocytes in the urine. The *diagnosis* of hypertension is based upon the clinical manifestations, especially the sustained, elevated blood pressure. *Treatment* is directed toward elimination of the cause whenever possible. Failing this, it consists of allaying anxiety, dietary measures, hypotensive drug therapy, and sympathectomy. The *prognosis* depends upon the age of the patient at the time of onset, the rapidity of development, the elevation of (especially the diastolic) pressure, and the complications that arise. Of particular prognostic significance are the changes in the eye grounds—the outlook being favorable when the changes are minimal and poor when they are maximal. In general, about 75 per cent of the patients with benign essential hypertension may be expected to live fifteen years or longer while few patients with malignant hypertension survive more than one or two years.

CONGENITAL ANOMALIES

Developmental malformations of the kidneys are varied, frequent, and often associated with malformations of the remaining portions of the urinary tract. They may be outlined as follows: (1) *aplasia* or *agenesis*—rare, occurring unilaterally or bilaterally, and consisting of the presence of a small mass of embryonic tissue instead of the normal kidney or of a complete absence of renal substance (Nation, Levin, and Leffler), (2) *hypoplasia*—normal in structure but diminutive in size, said to constitute about 4 per cent of all renal anomalies, being unilateral or bilateral, and complicated by infection, obstruction, calculous formation, and uremia (Graham), (3) *hypertrophy*—normal in structure but increased in size, usually occurring on a compensatory basis, and being congenital or acquired (Welsh), (4) *inclusions*—consisting most commonly of adrenocortical tissue located beneath the renal capsule (Mitchell) and rarely of islands of cartilage (Bigler), (5) *abnormalities* of *shape*—including short, long, L-shaped, globular poles, square poles, and fetal lobulations, (6) *horseshoe kidney*—consisting of fusion of the lower poles of the kidneys resulting in a horseshoe-shaped structure (Fig. 514), occurring in from 1 in 600 to 1 in 800 autopsies, located inferiorly with the isthmus crossing the spine at the level of the fourth lumbar vertebra or lower, rotated so that the pelves and ureters arise anteriorly or even laterally, crossed by the ureters anteriorly, possessing a vascular supply from any of the adjacent arteries (aorta, inferior mesentery, iliac, or internal or external iliac), and subjected to inflammatory and

obstructive disorders more commonly than normal kidneys (Lowsley),
(7) *simple ectopia*—congenital downward displacement, arising as a result
of an arrest of ascension and failure of rotation, usually occurring unilaterally, located at any point between the normal position of the kidney
and the bony pelvis, and disclosing an anterior or extrarenal pelvis, short
ureter descending anterior to the kidney, and vessels arising from neighboring arteries (Culp, Nation, and Fetter), (8) *crossed ectopia*—congenital
medial displacement of one kidney to the opposite side, known also as
crossed ectopia with or without fusion and as unilateral fused kidney,
frequently subjected to infection and obstruction, and consisting of separate

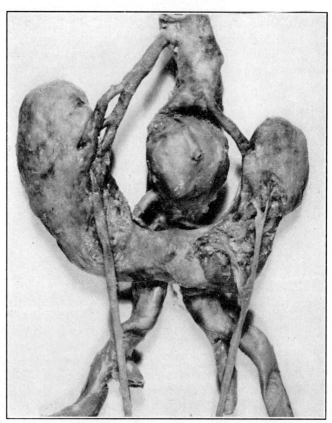

FIG. 514.—Horseshoe kidney showing union of the lower poles at the level of the bifurcation of
the aorta, vascular supply from the aorta, and ureters crossing anterior to the renal substance.

kidneys or of fusion with the following deformities: simple end to end, S-
shaped, lobular (lumped kidney) mass, discoid-shaped, and L-shaped
(Abeshouse), (9) *abnormalities of rotation*—actually brought about by
irregular proliferation of metanephrogenic tissue or by late insertion of
the ureter and characterized by the following anomalous positions of the
pelvis: ventral, ventromedial, lateral, or dorsal (Weyrauch), (10) *duplication*—consisting of two or more pelves on one side associated with two or
more ureters and two or more masses of renal substance and each exhibiting
fusion or complete separation (supernumerary kidney) of the renal substance (Carlson), and (11) *cystic disease*—resulting from failure of union

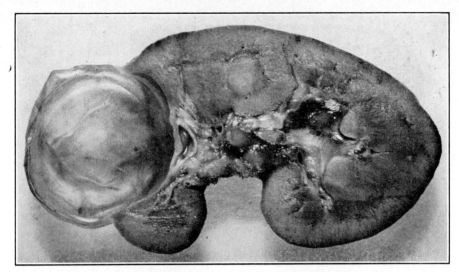

FIG. 515.—Solitary simple cyst at one pole of a kidney.

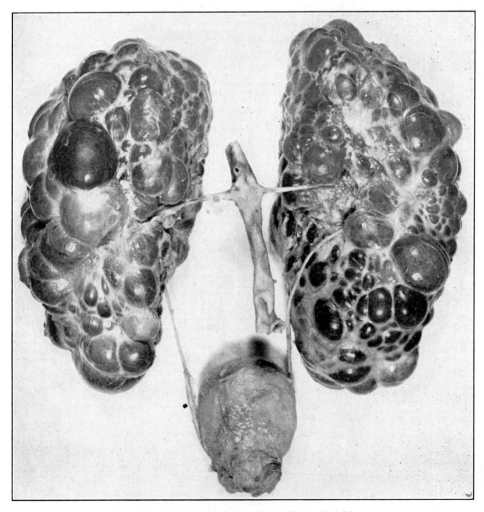

FIG. 516.—Polycystic disease illustrating both kidneys
completely replaced with varisized cysts.

of the nephron with the collective tubules or from the failure of absorption of the second to the fourth generations of uriniferous tubules and consisting of (*a*) solitary or multiple varisized (usually 2 to 8 cm. in diameter) cysts filled with clear fluid (Fig. 515), generally lined by attenuated epithelium, and sometimes complicated by calcification, infection, hemorrhage, tumor, calculi, hydronephrosis, and pyelonephritis (Powell, Ravitch, Glaser, and Lowsley) and (*b*) polycystic disease where the kidney is completely replaced with innumerable cysts measuring up to 1 or 2 cm. in diameter (Fig. 516), usually occurring bilaterally, affecting both sexes with equal frequency, generally discovered after the age of thirty years, attended by complications similar to those in solitary cysts, and usually terminating in hypertension and uremia (Ochsner and Newman).

DEGENERATIONS

Orientation. — The renal tubular and, to a lesser extent, glomerular cells are quite sensitive to retrogressive changes. Consequently virtually all of the degenerative alterations (atrophic, parenchymatous, hydropic, hyaline, amyloid, carbohydrate, fatty, etc.) described in Chapter 4 are represented at one time or another. Although most of these changes are not specific by themselves, they may nevertheless, singly or in combinations, be associated with well-defined renal disease processes. Accordingly, the following degenerative disturbances may be considered: acute toxic nephrosis, lipoid nephrosis, kidney in lupus erythematosus, kidney in scleroderma, kidney in eclampsia, amyloid kidney, myeloma kidney, diabetic glomerulosclerosis, nephrocalcinosis, benign nephrosclerosis, malignant nephrosclerosis, senile arteriosclerotic kidney, and Goldblatt kidney.

Acute Toxic Nephrosis. — Acute toxic nephrosis may be defined as a clinicopathologic *syndrome* that includes conditions called toxic nephritis, hepatorenal syndrome, nephrosis, clinically acute nephritis, acute hematogenous interstitial nephritis, extrarenal azotemia, acute interstitial nephritis, crush syndrome, renal changes in secondary shock, acute tubular nephrosis, lower nephron nephrosis, acute renal failure associated with injury, glomerulonephrosis, etc. (Herbut, French, Oliver, Lucké, and Moon). A few of the protean *causes* of the syndrome are (1) infection such as peritonitis, septicemia, abscess, pneumonia, etc., (2) blood transfusion reactions, (3) prolonged operations, (4) intestinal obstruction, (5) crushing injuries, (6) cutaneous burns, (7) hepatic disorders associated or unassociated with jaundice, and (8) chemicals such as sulfonamides, bichloride of mercury, carbon tetrachloride, iodides, quinine, cantharidin, etc. Regardless of the precise cause, the *mechanism* involved appears to be simple cortical ischemia resulting from vasoconstriction and shunting of the blood from the cortex through the medulla (Trueta).

Pathologically both kidneys are affected with equal severity. They are enlarged to as much as twice the normal size and are firm and edematous. The capsules strip with ease; the capsular surface is generally smooth; the cortex is broadened; the cortico-medullary demarcations are often distinct; the cortex is pale, and the medulla is congested (Fig. 517). *Histologically* the fundamental process consists of degeneration to complete necrosis of the tubular epithelial cells with the alterations being most severe in the proximal convoluted tubules and less severe as the lower portion of the nephron is approached (Fig. 518). In addition, the tubules show varying degrees of dilatation and the tubular lumens contain pigment, granular, or cellular

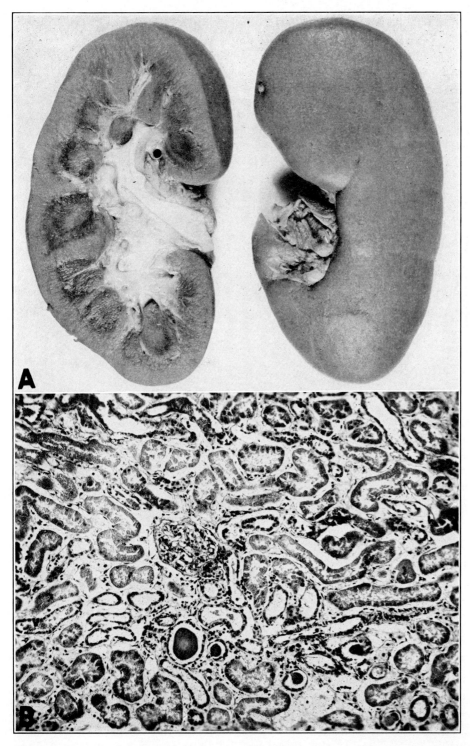

FIG. 517.—Acute toxic nephrosis showing A, a large kidney with a swollen pale cortex and a dark medulla and B, tubular degeneration and dilatation, tubular casts, and edema and leukocytic infiltration of the interstitial tissue. × 100.

casts. The interstitial tissue discloses congestion, edema, and leukocytic (plasma cell, lymphocytic, monocytic, and neutrophilic) infiltration and the glomeruli may be ischemic or congested.

The chief *complication* is death from uremia. The *clinical manifestations* are those of rapidly developing or incipient shock and renal failure. They consist of pale ashen face, cold extremities, low blood pressure, rapid pulse, hiccoughs, vomiting, dryness of the tongue, nausea, hallucinations, restlessness, edema, increasing oliguria ending in anuria, hemoconcentration, nitrogen retention in the blood, and urinalysis disclosing a specific gravity between 1.014 and 1.018, albumin, casts, erythrocytes, and pus cells. The *diagnosis* is made from the history, the symptoms and signs, and the

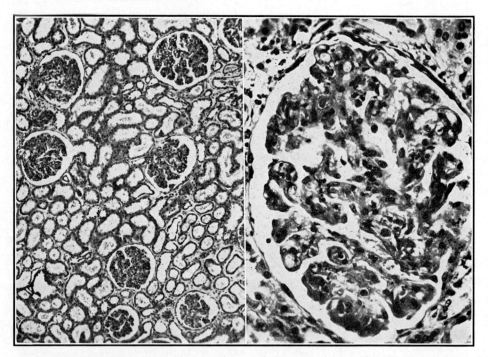

FIG. 518.—Eclampsia illustrating prominence of glomeruli and considerable thickening of the capillary basement membrane. × 50 and 200.

laboratory findings. *Treatment* is directed toward combating the cause, preventing shock (which is the common denominator in the pathogenesis), maintaining the fluid and electrolytic balance, and attempting to restore renal function. The *prognosis* is guarded for once the syndrome is fully developed a mortality rate as high as 90 per cent has been recorded.

Lipoid Nephrosis.—The term lipoid nephrosis of Epstein or genuine lipoid nephrosis has been used to indicate a renal disorder characterized by albuminuria, hypoproteinemia, hypercholesterolemia, doubly refractile lipoid droplets in the urine, secondary anemia, anasarca with low protein content in the fluid, normal renal function, normal blood pressure, low basal metabolic rate, fatty change in the renal tubular epithelial cells, and normal appearance of the rest of the parenchyma (Moschowitz). Actually the term is no longer tenable for, as the years advanced, it has become apparent that the condition is not a disease but a *nephrotic syndrome* due to

hypoproteinemia and most often encountered in subacute glomerulonephritis (albuminuria) but also seen in cases of deficient intake of protien
(famine), failure of absorption of protein from the intestine (sprue), or
failure of utilization of protein by the liver (cirrhosis).

Kidney in Lupus Erythematosus.—In lupus erythematosus (atypical
verrucal endocarditis or Libman-Sacks disease) the kidneys reveal a
hyaline thickening (wire looping) of the basement membrane of the glomre-
ular capillaries and occasionally intracapillary hyaline bodies (p. 309). In
some instances, albuminuria is present and occasionally uremia develops,
but generally the urine is normal and renal insufficiency does not exist
(Bell).

Kidney in Scleroderma.—In scleroderma some of the patients develop
oliguria, progressive renal failure, and die within a few weeks of uremia
(Moore). The kidneys disclose elongation and intimal mucoid degeneration
of the intralobular arteries, fibrinoid necrosis of the media and intima of
the distal portions of the intralobular arteries and of the afferent arterioles,
ischemic atrophy or necrosis of the renal parenchyma supplied by these
vessels, and occasionally wire looping of the glomerular capillaries.

Kidney in Eclampsia.—Eclampsia (Gr. = out + to flash) may be defined
as an acute toxic condition in a pregnant, parturient, or puerperal woman
usually accompanied by tonic and clonic convulsions and coma (Greenhill). The *cause* is probably an estrogen-progesterone-chorionicgonado-
tropin imbalance with a marked decrease in estrogen (Smith). This
decrease liberates a necrotizing toxin which is destructive to tissues in
general and vessels in particular and which is responsible for the condition.
The *pathologic* changes in eclampsia consist of the following: (1) *liver*—
periportal degeneration, necrosis, and hemorrhages, (2) *kidney*—(*a*) pre-
existing lesion of glomerulonephritis, pyelonephritis, etc., (*b*) glomeruli—
prominent, large, bloodless, and showing a diffuse increase of endothelial
cells, thickening of the capillary basement membrane, fibrinoid necrosis of
the glomerular tufts, adhesions of the glomerular tufts to the capsules, and
later fibrosis, (*c*) afferent arterioles—swelling and necrosis of the walls and
thrombosis of the lumens, (*d*) tubules—parenchymatous, hydropic, hyaline
droplet, and fatty degeneration, and (*e*) interstitial tissue—varying degrees
of congestion, edema, and leukocytic infiltration (Way), (3) *adrenals*—
lipoid depletion, foci of degeneration to necrosis, and varying degrees of
erythrocytic extravasation, and (4) *brain*—congestion, edema, ischemic
degeneration of the ganglion cells, vascular necrosis, and hemorrhages.

Amyloid Kidney.—The specific changes in the kidney in amyloidosis
have already been listed (p. 41). In addition, the tubular epithelial cells
may show degeneration and the tubular lumens usually contain casts.
Clinically, amyloidosis of the kidneys generally produces a rather typical
nephrotic syndrome (p. 1066).

Myeloma Kidney.—In advanced cases of multiple myeloma the tubules
disclose hyaline casts and peripheral foreign body giant cells (Fig. 519),
degeneration of the adjacent tubular epithelium, and dilatation of the tubules proximally. In addition, the stroma reveals fibrosis and infiltration
with chronic inflammatory cells and the cortex shows focal or more diffuse
areas of atrophy. Clinically the patient reveals Bence-Jones proteinuria
and terminally (because of obstruction of the tubules by casts) renal insufficiency and uremia (Armstrong).

Diabetic Glomerulosclerosis.—In 1936, Kimmelstiel and Wilson described a *syndrome* (which they called intercapillary glomerulosclerosis)

characterized clinically by mild diabetes, hypertension, retinal arteriosclerosis, albuminuria, and edema and pathologically by hyaline sclerosis of
the intercapillary connective tissue of the renal glomeruli (Kimmelstiel
and Herbut). Since then the disorder has been more commonly called
diabetic glomerulosclerosis and Kimmelstiel-Wilson syndrome. It usually
occurs in patients beyond the age of forty years, but has been recorded in
patients in the third and even the second decade of life and is about twice
as common in males as it is in females (Wilson and Mann). *Clinically*,
aside from the features already mentioned, the serum discloses an elevation
of cholesterol, phospholipids, total lipids, lipoproteins, and alpha-2 globulin
(Engelberg and Rifkin). *Grossly* the kidneys may appear normal or may
be indistinguishable from those of benign nephrosclerosis (Fig. 520).

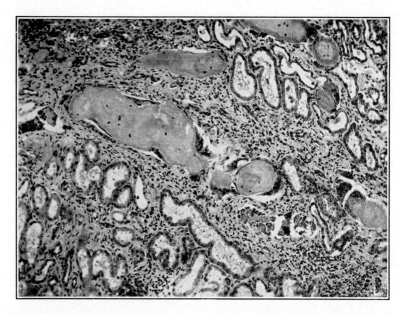

Fig. 519.—Myeloma kidney disclosing hyaline casts with peripheral foreign body giant cells,
destruction of tubular epithelium, dilatation of the more proximal tubules, and interstitial fibrosis
and leukocytic infiltration. ×100. (Herbut, *Urological Pathology.*)

Histologically the characteristic lesion consists of a deposition of hyaline
material between the capillaries of the glomerular tufts. The deposition
may affect only a portion of the tuft or it may involve the entire tuft and
it may be uniformly distributed or it may be deposited in the form of
nodules. In addition to the glomerular changes, the arterioles usually
reveal sclerosis, the tubules show varying degrees and types of degenerations,
and the interstitial tissue may disclose fibrosis and leukocytic infiltration.
The *causes* of *death* in the syndrome are cardiac failure, diabetes with its
complications, and uremia.

Nephrocalcinosis.—Nephrocalcinosis denotes deposition of calcium salts
in the renal parenchyma in sufficient amounts to be demonstrable roentgenographically (Ostry and Engel). When the condition occurs in children
it is generally associated with osteoporosis, bony deformity, and dwarfism
and is referred to as *renal rickets* and when it occurs in adults it may be
associated with bony changes consistent with *osteitis fibrosia cystica* (p. 1251)

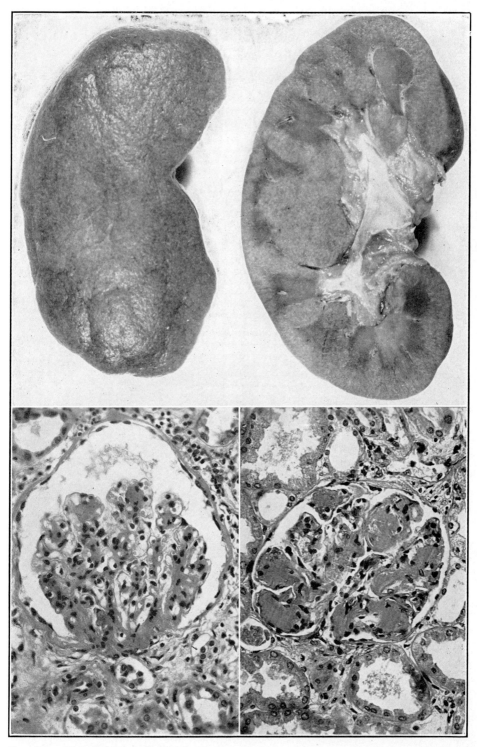

Fig. 520.—Diabetic glomerulosclerosis showing relatively normal appearing kidneys grossly and moderate and massive deposition of hyaline material in the glomeruli. × 200.

(Albright). Some of the many *causes* of nephrocalcinosis are (1) systemic conditions such as hyperparathyroidism, hypervitaminosis D, certain chemical poisonings, and high intestinal obstruction and (2) local renal lesions such as pyelonephritis, glomerulonephritis, hydronephrosis, and pyonephrosis.

Pathologically the kidneys may appear normal grossly or may disclose the lesions already listed. In addition, they may reveal calcific deposits scattered irregularly throughout the parenchyma. *Histologically* calcium salts are seen as granular precipitates or as more homogeneous collections in the tubular lumens, in the epithelial cells and basement membrane of the tubules, in the basement membrane of the glomeruli, and in the stroma. The renal changes produce secondary hyperplasia of the parathyroid glands (p. 592) and the hyperplasia, in turn, mobilizes calcium from the bones accounting for the osseous lesions already referred to.

The chief renal *complications* are urolithiasis and uremia. The *clinical manifestations* are referable to the skeletal system and to the kidneys (Rule). The latter consist of nocturia, polyuria, polydypsia, signs of acidosis, and those consequent to uremia. Urinalysis discloses a fixed low specific gravity, albumin, erythrocytes, leukocytes, and casts and the blood reveals normal serum calcium, elevated phosphates, elevated nonprotein nitrogen, and a normal or slightly reduced carbon dioxide combining power. The *diagnosis* is based upon (1) roentgenographic changes in the bones, (2) demonstration of renal dysfunction, and (3) alterations in blood chemistry. *Treatment* depends upon the cause. The *prognosis* varies with the degree of functional renal impairment and, of course, with the causative factors.

Familial Idiopathic Oxalate Nephrocalcinosis.—As indicated by the caption, this condition is a type of nephrocalcinosis characterized by a familial occurrence, an unknown cause, the persistent finding of almost pure calcium oxalate crystals in the urine, the presence of renal calculi, and frequently an elevation of the serum uric acid level (Aponte). The disorder usually becomes apparent around the age of 10 years by the presence of renal colic and the passage of urinary calculi. Despite surgical and dietary treatment, the urinary tract episodes not only continue but worsen progressively and death ensues in from 3 to 6 years from renal failure. Pathologically the kidneys are slightly enlarged (Fig. 521*A*). Roentgenograms reveal diffusely scattered, cortical and medullary opacities. Cutting through the parenchyma is accompanied by a gritty sensation. Cut surfaces disclose obscuring of the cortico-medullary demarcations, calcific deposits in the cortex and medulla, and calculi in the calyces and pelves. Chemical analysis of these deposits reveals them to be composed almost entirely of calcium oxalate. Histologic sections disclose the deposition of the crystals within the tubular lumens as well as in the interstitial tissue. In the latter area they are accompanied by mononuclear cell infiltration and fibroblastic proliferation. The latter ultimately leads to extensive destruction of the renal parenchyma. The only other finding of note is the presence of calcium oxalate crystals in the bone marrow.

Benign Nephrosclerosis.—Benign or arteriolar nephrosclerosis represents the renal lesion in benign (essential) hypertension (Allen). The disorder is usually *encountered* in patients in the fifth to seventh decades of life and is more frequent in males than in females. The *cause* of most of the renal changes is attributable to arteriolar sclerosis and the causes of these have already been discussed in connection with arteriosclerosis (Chapter 9, p. 359). The *pathologic* changes in the kidneys vary with the severity and

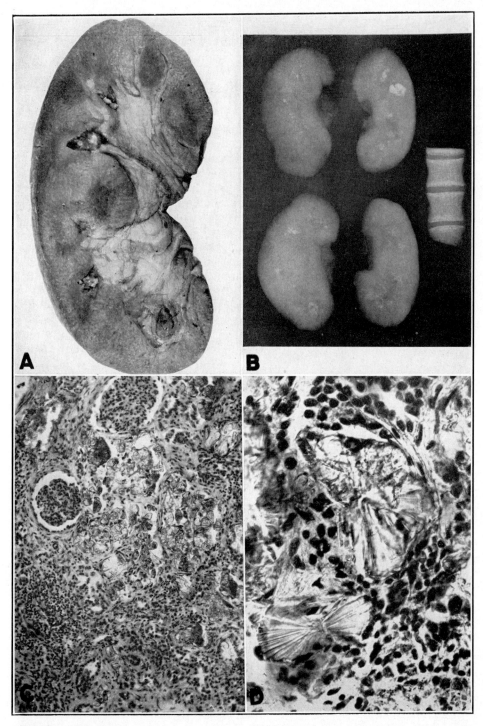

FIG. 521.—Familial idiopathic oxalate nephrocalcinosis illustrating *A*, obscuring of the cortico-medullary demarcations, calcific deposits in the parenchyma, and calculi in the calyces, *B*, opacities in the kidneys roentgenographically, and *C* and *D*, calcium oxalate crystals, inflammation, and fibrosis of the renal parenchyma.   × 100 and 400 respectively.

duration of the disease. The disorder is always bilateral; each kidney is equally affected, and the process is uniform in each organ. In a typical case the kidneys are reduced in size to about one-half normal; the capsules are slightly thickened and moderately adherent; the external surface is light brown and finely pebbled; the cortex is irregularly atrophied and its demarcation from the medulla is obscured; the cortex often reveals scattered, 1 to 3 mm. cysts; the interlobular arteries are prominently sclerotic; the medulla is normal or reduced in width, and the peripelvic fat tissue is increased in amount (Fig. 522A). *Histologically*, although the entire kidney is affected, the initial lesions are spotty and only in advanced stages is all of the parenchyma involved (Fig. 522B). The chief vascular change consists of hyaline sclerosis of the arcuate and interlobular arteries and especially the afferent arterioles (p. 365) (Jones). The remaining alterations result from the gradual ischemia produced by the arterial and arteriolar occlusion. The glomeruli show progressive deposition of collagen between the capillary loops of the tufts and within the basement membrane of Bowman's capsule. As a result of this the glomerular capillaries become encroached upon and obliterated, Bowman's space becomes smaller and smaller, and ultimately the entire glomerulus becomes replaced with a hyaline mass. The tubules likewise disclose degenerative and atrophic changes and finally completely disappear. Concomitantly, as the glomeruli and tubules disappear, the interstitial tissue shows leukocytic infiltration and fibroblastic proliferation. Also, as the glomeruli in corresponding tubules are lost, the remaining glomeruli and tubules become more prominent and hyperplastic—undergoing work hypertrophy as it were. These tubules are dilated, often show papillary infoldings, and frequently contain hyaline or other casts. The *complications* of benign nephrosclerosis are those of benign hypertension (p. 1061). In advanced cases, the renal lesions as such produce uremia.

The *clinical manifestations* are likewise those of benign hypertension together with those of uremia when renal failure has developed. The changes in the urine consist of increased volume, fixed low specific gravity, presence of albumin, and a few granular casts, leukocytes, and erythrocytes in the sediment. The *diagnosis* of nephrosclerosis is based on the clinical findings of hypertension together with the urinary changes listed. *Treatment* is primarily that of the accompanying hypertension. The *prognosis* depends upon the age of onset, the rapidity of development, and the severity of the process. In general, it parallels that of benign hypertension.

Malignant Nephrosclerosis.—Malignant nephrosclerosis represents the renal lesion in malignant hypertension (Allen). The condition generally *occurs* about a decade earlier than does benign nephrosclerosis. When it is seen in young patients it always starts as malignant nephrosclerosis, but when it is seen in older patients it is usually superimposed terminally upon a previously benign nephrosclerosis. The *pathologic* picture will thus vary accordingly. In a typical case occurring as a rapidly progressive disease in a patient in the fourth decade of life, the kidneys are enlarged to about 200 or 250 gm. each. The capsules are slightly thickened and adherent and the external surface is dull but smooth. It is light to dark brown and characteristically discloses scattered, pinpoint hemorrhages (Fig. 523A). The cortex is somewhat thickened and its demarcation from the medulla is generally sharp. The vessels are not prominent and the peripelvic fat tissue is not increased. *Histologically* the lesions are spotty, involving from 10 to 40 per cent of the parenchyma (Fig. 523B). The smaller arteries,

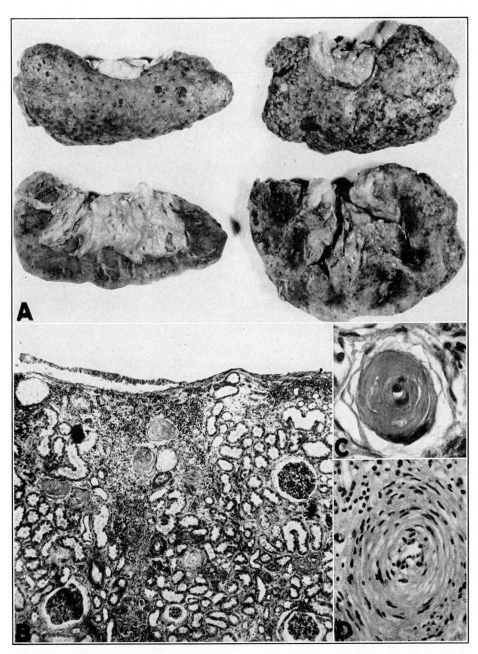

FIG. 522.—Benign nephrosclerosis disclosing *A*, external and cut surfaces of two kidneys with marked reduction in size, granularity and cyst formation of the external surface, cortical atrophy, obscuring of the cortico-medullary demarcations, prominence of the smaller arteries, and increase in peripelvic fat tissue, *B*, spotty involvement of the parenchyma with arteriosclerosis, glomerulosclerosis, tubular dilatation, and interstitial fibrosis and leukocytic infiltration. × 5, *C*, hyaline arteriolar sclerosis. × 400, and *D*, proliferative arteriolar sclerosis. × 200.

especially the afferent arterioles, disclose necrotizing and proliferative arteriolar necrosis (p. 365) (Fig. 524*A*, *B* and *C*). Because of the necrotizing changes, the vessels not only look smudgy but are also permeated with extravasated erythrocytes and may even be thrombotic (Jones). The glomeruli reveal focal areas of fibrinoid necrosis similar to those seen in the

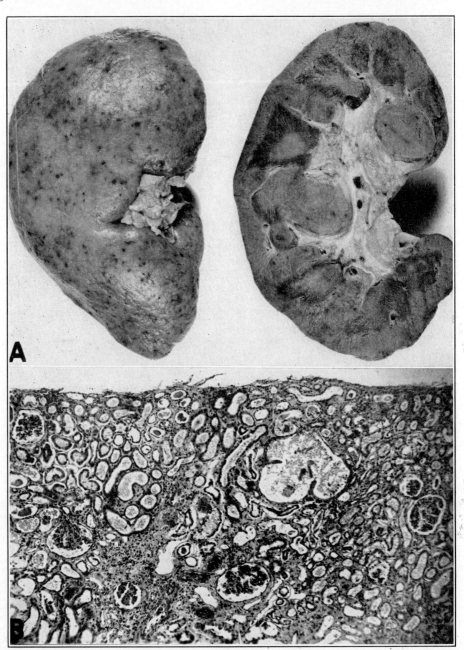

Fig. 523.—Malignant nephrosclerosis illustrating *A*, enlarged kidneys with numerous petechiæ scattered throughout the cortex and *B*, spotty involvement of the parenchyma with arteriolar necrosis, necrosis of one of the glomeruli, tubular dilatation, and some interstitial edema and leukocytic infiltration. × 50.

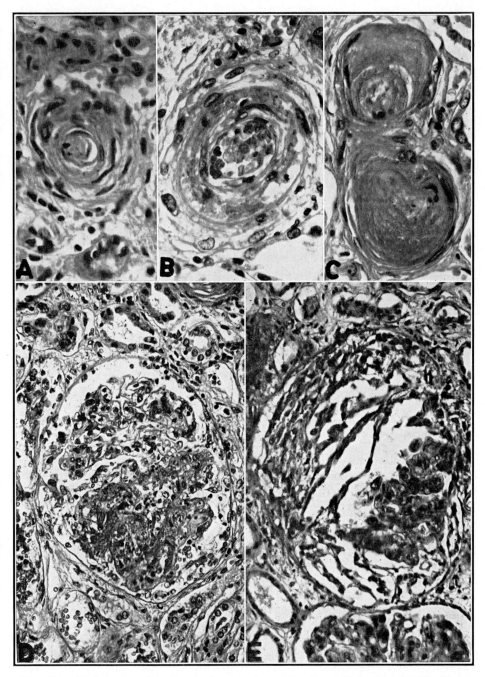

Fig. 524.—Malignant nephrosclerosis showing *A*, proliferative endarteritis. × 400, *B*, proliferative endarteritis with necrosis and erythrocytic extravasation. × 400, *C*, hyaline arteriolar sclerosis with superimposed necrosis. × 400, *D*, fibrinoid necrosis of one-half of a glomerulus with erythrocytic extravasation in the necrotic area and in Bowman's space. × 200, and *E*, glomerular crescent. × 200.

arterioles, leukocytic and erythrocytic extravasation in the areas of necrosis, and fibroblastic proliferation with frequent formation of adhesions between the tufts and Bowman's capsule and occasional formation of glomerular crescents (crescent-shaped proliferations of epithelium covering Bowman's capsule (Fig. 524*D* and *E*). The renal tubules disclose degeneration of their epithelial cells and erythrocytes and casts within their lumens. The interstitial connective tissue reveals congestion, edema, and varying degrees of leukocytic infiltration. Thus, the chief renal findings in malignant nephrosclerosis are endarteritis obliterans, arteriolar necrosis, glomerular necrosis, and occasional glomerular crescent formation. The *complications* are those of malignant hypertension with uremia assuming a prominent position. The *clinical manifestations* are also those of rapidly progressing and severe hypertension (p. 1061). In addition to casts and leukocytes, the urine discloses numerous erythrocytes, frequently to a degree producing gross hematuria. The *diagnosis* is made from the clinical manifestations (especially the young age of the patient in the presence of rapidly progressive and severe hypertension) together with the urinary findings. *Treatment* is directed toward the hypertension. The *prognosis* is poor with death usually occurring in about six months.

Senile Arteriosclerotic Kidney.—In cases of advanced arteriosclerosis, as generally exhibited in old age, the larger branches of the renal arteries are affected by the same sclerotic changes that affect other vessels of the body (p. 359). When the lumens of these vessels become sufficiently occluded, the peripheral parenchyma becomes atrophied and fibrotic, leaving wedge-shaped or irregular areas of cortical scarring. Such a kidney is referred to as a senile arteriosclerotic kidney. The changes are seldom accompanied by renal insufficiency.

Goldblatt Kidney.—Starting in 1928, Goldblatt performed a series of *experiments* in an attempt to elucidate the causes of essential hypertension. Using the dog, sheep, goat, rat, and other animals, his method, in essence, consisted of partial constriction (by means of a clamp) of one or both renal arteries or of the aorta just about the exit of the renal arteries, thus producing renal ischemia. His findings may be briefly summarized as follows: (1) constriction of one renal artery results in hypertension that may be sustained several months, but removal of the clamped vessel and kidney allows the blood pressure to return to normal, (2) constriction of both renal arteries produces permanent hypertension, (3) constriction of one renal artery and nephrectomy on the opposite side produces permanent hypertension and if the constriction is great enough the animal dies in uremia, (4) constriction of the aorta above the renal vessel produces hypertension, (5) the pathologic changes in the kidney with the constricted vessel vary from necrosis to ischemia and fibrosis depending upon the rapidity and severity of the vascular occlusion, but they do not correspond to those in benign nephrosclerosis in man, and (6) malignant hypertension produced by constriction of one renal artery and ligation of the ureter to the opposite kidney. There are no specific findings in the kidney with the constricted artery (the protected kidney) but the kidney with the occluded ureter (the unprotected kidney) discloses changes identical with those seen in malignant nephrosclerosis. Other workers, however, have shown (1) that simple constriction of the renal artery to one kidney may result in infarction, atrophy, or fibrosis of the corresponding kidney depending upon the degree and rapidity of the vascular occlusion, (2) that lesions corresponding to those of malignant nephrosclerosis do not develop in the corresponding

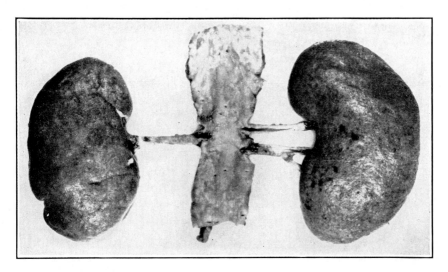

Fig. 525.—Goldblatt kidney showing arteriosclerotic occlusion of the orifices of both main renal arteries but with a widely patent accessory artery to the left kidney, ischemic atrophy of the protected right kidney, and enlargement of the unprotected left kidney with scattered petechiæ. (Herbut's *Urological Pathology*.)

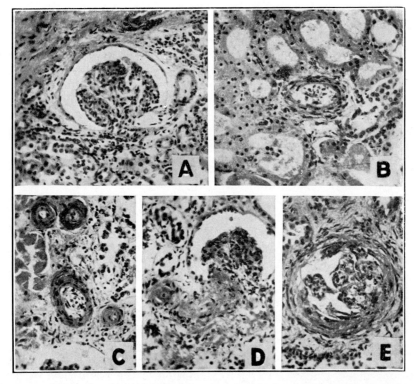

Fig. 526.—Goldblatt kidney from the same case illustrated in Figure 431 illustrating *A*, a normal glomerulus, *B*, a normal arteriole from the protected right kidney, *C*, endarteritis obliterans, *D*, afferent arteriolar and glomerular necrosis, and *E*, glomerular crescent from the unprotected left kidney. × 200. (Herbut's *Urological Pathology*.)

(protected) kidney, but (3) that such lesions do develop in the opposite (unprotected) kidney. The *human* counterpart to the experimentally produced lesions just referred to is known as the Goldblatt kidney. Ideally, the lesion results from occlusion of one renal artery. Some of the many *causes* of arterial occlusion are arteriosclerosis, embolism, thrombosis, pressure from an extrarenal (neoplastic or inflammatory) mass, kinking from nephroptosis, and aneurysm (Yuile, Herbut, and Laforet). In addition, however, a variety of unilateral renal diseases have been recorded as causing hypertension. Some of them are developmental abnormalities of the pelvis, hypoplasia, pyelonephritis, perinephritis, tuberculosis, neoplasms, nephroptosis, hydronephrosis, calculus, and trauma (Smith).

Pathologically the changes vary with the initial process. In cases caused by arterial occlusion the alterations correspond to those seen in experimental animals (Figs. 525 and 526). The protected kidney discloses only ischemia while the unprotected kidney reveals lesions that are typical of those seen in malignant nephrosclerosis. The chief *complication* is uremia. The *clinical manifestations* are those of the primary disease and hypertension. The *diagnosis* is made from the history, clinical manifestations, and urologic studies. *Treatment* is directed towards eradication of the causative factor, with the performance of nephrectomy when necessary. The *prognosis* varies with the causative factor and the severity of the hypertension.

INFLAMMATIONS

Orientation.—Inflammation of the kidney is known as *nephritis*. The term as such, however, is seldom used alone for it is usually embellished by adjectives and prefixes in order to make the connotations more precise. Thus, *glomerulonephritis* indicates primarily an inflammation of the glomeruli, *pyelonephritis* an inflammation of the pelvis, peripelvic tissues, and renal parenchyma, *embolic glomerulonephritis* an inflammation affecting the glomeruli and occurring as a result of emboli, etc. Formerly the eponym *Bright's disease* was quite popular but, since it encompasses any chronic renal disorder (usually glomerulonephritis, nephrosclerosis, and pyelonephritis) that is accompanied by albuminuria and edema, it is gradually being dropped from the usual nomenclature in favor of more precise terms. Although renal inflammations are varied, the following may be enumerated as the more common disorders: diffuse glomerulonephritis, embolic glomerulonephritis, pyelonephritis, acute necrotizing papillitis, abscess, perinephritis and perinephric abscess, periarteritis nodosa, tuberculosis, syphilis, actinomycosis (p. 515) and echinococcosis (p. 828).

Diffuse Glomerulonephritis.—Diffuse glomerulonephritis may be *defined* as a nonsuppurative renal inflammation affecting primarily the glomeruli and being uniformly distributed throughout all parts of both kidneys. The disorder is relatively uncommon, being exceeded in frequency by both pyelonephritis and nephrosclerosis. While the condition may *occur* at any age, its onset is usually in the first three decades of life. It has no predilection for either sex or any race. The *cause* is doubtlessly a hypersensitivity to a foreign protein—most commonly the bacterial protein of streptococci. The most convincing evidence of this association is the frequency with which diffuse glomerulonephritis follows (by two to three weeks) streptococcic sore throat, rheumatic fever, and scarlet fever (Brod and Robertson). Other evidence in man consists of (1) the type of renal reaction, (2) failure to recover organisms from the affected kidneys, (3) frequent association of

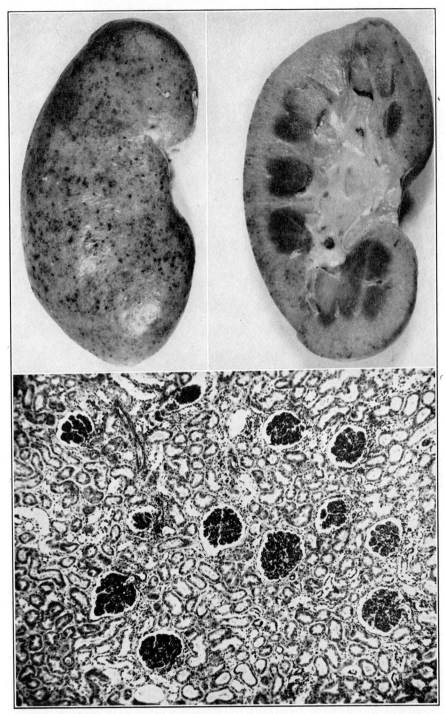

FIG. 527.—Acute diffuse glomerulonephritis showing enlargement of the kidneys, petechiæ of the cortex, and sharp corticomedullary demarcations grossly and diffuse glomerular involvement with interstitial congestion and edema microscopically. × 50.

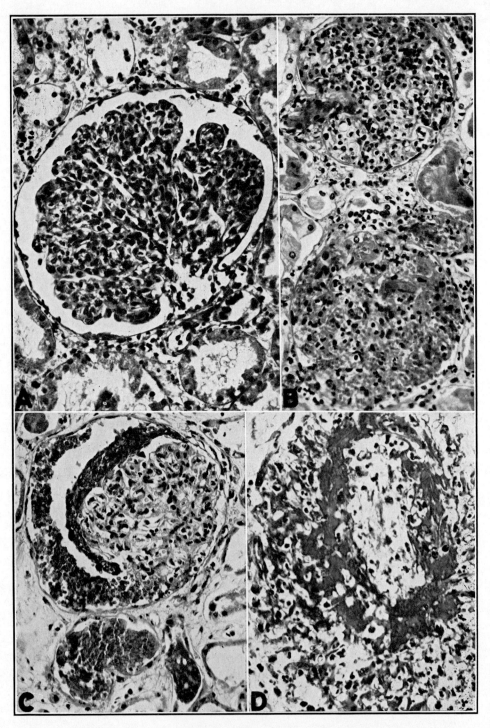

Fig. 528.—Acute diffuse glomerulonephritis illustrating *A*, proliferation of glomerular epithelium and endothelium. × 200, *B*, glomerular exudation above and hemorrhagic extravasation below. × 200, *C*, fibrinoid necrosis of a glomerular tuft, erythrocytic extravasation into Bowman's space, and exudate within a proximal convoluted tubule. × 200, and *D*, acute necrotizing arteriolitis. × 400.

the disease with outright manifestations of serum sickness or other allergic disorders, (4) development of high antistreptolysin titers and cutaneous sensitivity to streptococci in patients with glomerulonephritis, and (5) demonstration of a nephrotoxic substance and of auto antibodies to human kidney tissue in the serum of patients with glomerulonephritis (Herbut, Lippman, and Allen).

Experimentally diffuse glomerulonephritis may be readily produced in rabbits by (1) repeated small or (2) one or several large intravenous injections of bovine gamma globulin or horse serum (McLean and More). It may also be produced in rabbits, rats, or dogs by intravenous injection of specific nephrotoxic serum obtained by the injection of macerated kidney from these animals into ducks, rats (rabbit or dog kidney), and rabbits (dog or rat kidney) (Lippman). Even more specifically it has been determined by ultracentrifugalization and sonic vibration that the nephrotoxic antigen is located in the basement membrane of the glomerulus (Krakower).

Pathologically diffuse glomerulonephritis is dividable into three stages—acute (first), subacute (second), and chronic (third), with transitions from one to the other (Bell, Allen, and Jones). In each of these stages, the kidneys are bilaterally, diffusely, and uniformly affected. In *acute diffuse glomerulonephritis* the kidneys may be enlarged to twice the normal size. The capsules are slightly thickened and slightly adherent. The external surface is reddish brown, for the most part smooth, and covered with petechiæ (Fig. 527). Cut surfaces reveal some swelling of the cortex, petechial hemorrhages in the cortex, a sharp demarcation between the cortex and medulla, congested medulla, normal peripelvic fat tissue, and normal or congested calyces and pelvis.

Histologically virtually all of the glomeruli are affected and the lesions may be proliferative, exudative, or combinations of the two (Fig. 528). *Proliferative* lesions consist principally of diffuse hypertrophy and hyperplasia of the epithelial and endothelial cells of the glomerular tuft. The glomerulus thus appears more cellular than normal and is quite conspicuous. In addition, the capillary basement membrane may become swollen, somewhat hyalinized, and prominent. As a consequence of both of these changes, the glomerulus becomes bloodless and the vascular supply to the remaining portion of the nephron is impeded. *Exudative* lesions consist of varying degrees of congestion, hemorrhagic extravasation, neutrophilic infiltration, and fibrinoid necrosis of the glomerulus. In either case (but especially in the exudative lesions) Bowman's space contains some protein precipitates, erythrocytes, and leukocytes. Similar material is also found in the tubules where it either lies freely or forms casts. The tubules in acute diffuse glomerulonephritis show varying degrees of degeneration but such changes do not reach their acme until the subacute stage is approached. The interstitial tissue discloses congestion, edema, and varying degrees of leukocytic infiltration. The arterioles may be normal or may disclose acute necrotizing arteriolitis similar to that seen in periarteritis nodosa (p. 370).

In *subacute diffuse glomerulonephritis* the kidneys retain many of the changes seen in the acute stage but also show some of the alterations seen in the chronic stage. Grossly they are generally large (Fig. 529). The capsule is slightly thickened and may be adherent or, due to edema, loosely attached. The external surface is pale, grayish white, and may or may not disclose petechiæ. Cut surfaces reveal a swollen, pale cortex, a darker medulla, fairly sharp demarcations between the cortex and medulla, some edema of the peripelvic fat tissue, and normal or congested calyces and pelvis. *Histologically* the proliferative and/or exudative changes seen in the acute stage persists, but in addition, the glomeruli disclose adhesions between the loops of the tuft and Bowman's capsule, moon-shaped proliferation of capsular epithelium with formation of glomerular crescents, (in some cases) marked hyaline accentuation of the basement membrane, and

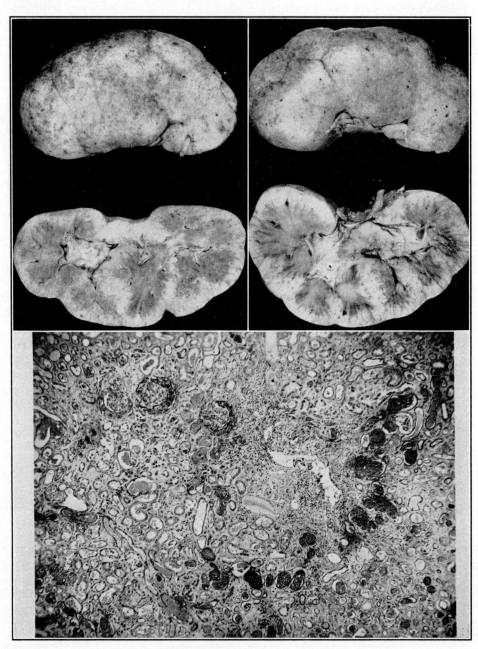

Fig. 529.—Subacute diffuse glomerulonephritis demonstrating large pale kidneys with scattered petechiæ grossly and diffuse glomerular, tubular, and interstitial involvement microscopically. × 50.

abundant edema fluid in Bowman's space (Fig. 530). The tubular epithelium characteristically discloses parenchymatous, hydropic, hyaline droplet, and fatty degeneration (Figs. 5, 6, and 18, p. 33) and tubula lumens show protein precipitate, cellular exudate, or casts. The interstitial tissue and vessels are similar to those seen in the acute stage or show the beginning fibrosis and sclerosis of the chronic stage.

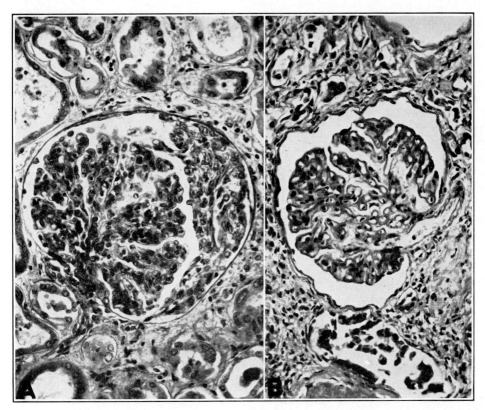

Fig. 530.—Subacute diffuse glomerulonephritis showing *A*, glomerular crescent formation and *B*, hyaline thickening of the capillary basement membrane. $\times$ 200.

In *chronic diffuse glomerulonephritis* the emphasis is on healing and fibrosis. Grossly the kidneys are small and contracted and resemble those seen in advanced benign nephrosclerosis (Fig. 531). The capsule is thick, fibrotic, and adherent to the underlying cortex. The external surface is diffusely finely granular and may disclose tiny retention cysts. Cut surfaces reveal extreme atrophy of the cortex, obscuring of the corticomedullary demarcations, decreased amount of medulla, occasional prominence of the arcuate and interlobular arteries, increase in peripelvic fat tissue, and relative increase in size of the calyces and pelvis. *Histologically* most of the glomeruli disclose varying degrees of fibrosis to complete obliteration but occasional glomeruli are only moderately or slightly affected and even hypertrophied. Also, the tubules corresponding to glomeruli are respectively either completely atrophic or hyperplastic with the latter showing dilatation of the lumens, papillary infoldings of the lining epithelium, and cellular or hyaline casts (Fig. 532). The interstitial tissue shows extensive

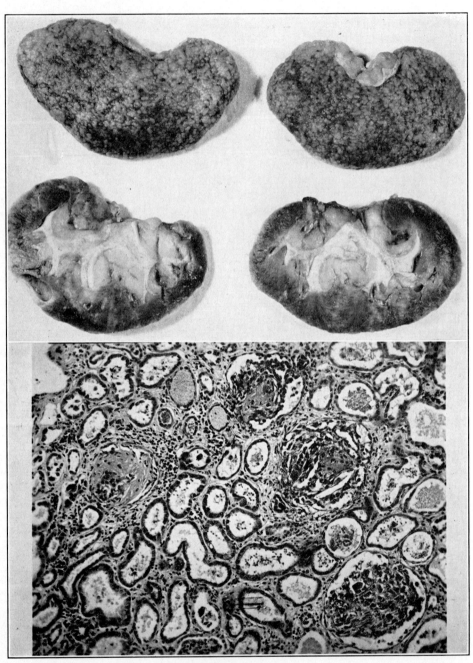

Fig. 531.—Chronic diffuse glomerulonephritis illustrating contracted granular kidneys with increase in peripelvic fat tissue grossly and varying degrees of glomerular and interstitial fibrosis together with leukocytic infiltration and tubular dilatation microscopically. × 100.

fibrosis and fusion with the atrophic glomeruli and tubules. The smaller arteries and arterioles reveal secondary sclerotic changes that are indistinguishable from those encountered in benign nephrosclerosis.

The chief *complications* in diffuse glomerulonephritis are (1) acute renal failure in the acute stage, (2) hypoproteinemia and secondary infection in the subacute stage, and (3) hypertension and renal insufficiency with uremia in the chronic stage. The *clinical manifestations* vary with the stage of the disease. In acute diffuse glomerulonephritis the following may be encountered: edema (especially about the eyes and ankles), dyspnea, headache, hematuria, backache, lassitude, exaggerated thirst, fever, frequency

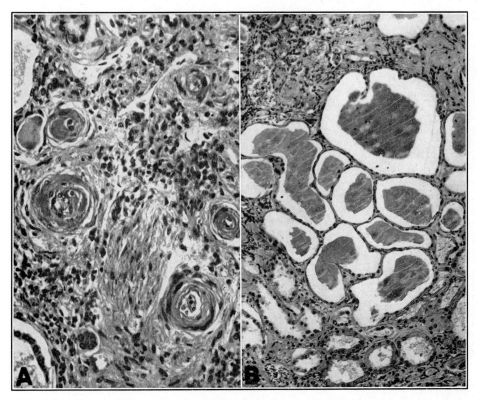

Fig. 532.—Chronic diffuse glomerulonephritis disclosing *A*, marked arteriolar sclerosis together with interstitial fibrosis and leukocytic (mostly lymphocytic and plasma cell) infiltration. × 200 and *B*, marked tubular dilatation with hyaline casts in the tubular lumens. × 100.

of urination, vomiting, dysuria, epistaxis, oliguria, anuria, albuminuria, casts and erythrocytes in the urine, occasional effusion into serosal cavities, mild to moderate hypertension, pulmonary edema, hypertensive encephalopathy, hypertensive retinal changes, diminished renal function tests, and nitrogen retention in the blood (Brod). *Subacute diffuse glomerulonephritis* is characterized clinically by the *nephrotic syndrome* which consists of massive albuminuria, hypoproteinemia, anasarca, hypercholesterolemia, anemia, normal blood pressure or slight hypertension, and sometimes oliguria and terminal uremia. *Chronic diffuse glomerulonephritis* is characterized by hypertension and progressive renal failure ending in uremia (pp. 1058 and 1057).

The *diagnosis* of diffuse glomerulonephritis is made from the history, the symptoms and signs as indicated, urinalysis, and chemical determinations on the blood. *Treatment* is more or less symptomatic. In essence it consists of bed rest, dietary restriction of sodium chloride, and prevention of attacks of pharyngitis or other infection. The *course* and *prognosis* are variable. The first indication of the disease may consist of symptoms referable to the acute, subacute, or chronic stage. Also, the disorder may first appear in the acute or subacute stage and then progress to the chronic stage or it may be arrested in any of the stages. Although the course is unpredictable, in general, the outlook in acute and subacute diffuse glomerulonephritis is good (for death occurs in less than 5% of cases) while it is poor in chronic glomerulonephritis with evidence of nitrogen retention in the blood.

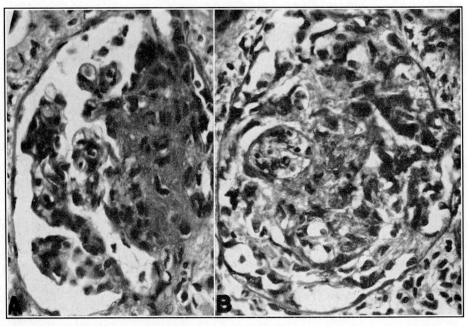

Fig. 533.—Embolic glomerulonephritis showing *A*, part of a glomerulus and *B*, an entire glomerulus affected by fibrinoid necrosis, erythrocytic extravasation, and cellular proliferation with adhesions. × 400.

Embolic Glomerulonephritis.—In some cases of bacterial endocarditis, and rarely of rheumatic fever, small emboli from the cardiac vegetations or verrucæ lodge in the capillaries of the glomerular tufts and, as a result of liberation of toxic products, produce thrombosis and necrosis (Bell). Such a lesion is called embolic glomerulonephritis. Grossly the only typical change is scattered petechiæ throughout the cortex producing what has been referred to as the "flea-bitten kidney." Histologically the lesions are found in scattered glomeruli and a portion or the entire glomerulus may be affected (Fig. 533). In the acute stage the changes consist of hyaline thrombosis, fibrinoid necrosis, erythrocytic extravasation, and epithelial proliferation. As the lesion ages it either resolves or is replaced with fibrous tissue. The only noteworthy sign is the escape of erythrocytes in the urine. Renal insufficiency seldom if ever occurs.

Pyelonephritis.—Pyelonephritis may be defined as a bacterial inflammation of the kidneys, usually affecting the ureter, pelvis, and renal parenchyma. The condition has already been referred to briefly in connection with nonspecific ureteritis and pyelitis (p. 1042). It is the most common inflammatory and degenerative disease of the kidneys, *occurring* to a greater

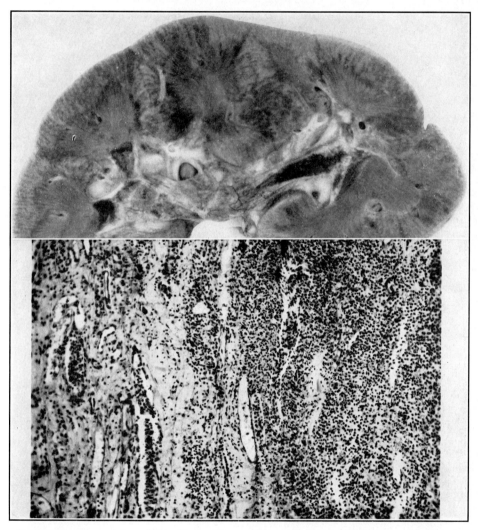

Fig. 534.—Acute pyelonephritis illustrating swelling of the kidney, obscuring of the cortico-medullary demarcations, radial streaking and congestion of the pelvis grossly and severe interstitial infiltration with neutrophils microscopically. × 100.

or lesser degree in about 50 per cent of all autopsies and outnumbering by far both nephrosclerosis and diffuse glomerulonephritis (Birchall and Saphir). It is found at all ages but is most frequent in children, pregnant women, and elderly men. The *causes* are predisposing and precipitating. The former consist of obstructive lesions of the pelvis, ureter, bladder, or urethra, while the latter consist of bacteria—usually of the colon group but including also proteus and pyocyaneus bacilli and streptococci and staphylococci. The routes of bacterial invasion are bloodstream, peri-ureteral lymphatic channels, ureteral lumen, or adjacent structures.

Pathologically the lesions may be divided into acute and chronic with transitions from one to the other. In either case, the inflammation may be unilateral or bilateral but, even when bilateral, the degree of involvement is not uniform. In *acute pyelonephritis* the kidney is enlarged; the capsule is thickened and adherent; the external surface is smooth or finely granular and may disclose irregular varisized but usually small abscesses; the cortex is thick and edematous; the demarcations between the cortex and medulla are obscure; the cortex and medulla disclose considerable radial streaking; peripelvic fat tissue is edematous and firm, and the calyces, pelvis, and ureter are usually reddened but may or may not be dilated (Figs. 534 and 536*A*). *Histologically* the lesion is characterized by a nonspecific inflammatory reaction consisting mostly of neutrophils. It is patchy in distribution, is located primarily in the stroma, and while it affects both the cortex and medulla it generally predominates in the latter. In *chronic pyelonephritis* the emphasis is on atrophy of the parenchyma and fibrosis (Fig. 535). The affected kidney is reduced in size, sometimes to about one-quarter that of normal. The capsule is fibrotic and adherent; the external surface is coarsely and finely scarred; the cortex is irregularly reduced in volume; the corticomedullary demarcations are obscured; the arcuate and interlobular arteries are often sclerotic; the peripelvic fat tissue is increased in amount, and the calyces and pelvis are thickened and fibrotic. *Histologically* the interstitial tissue discloses extensive fibrosis and infiltration with plasma cells, lymphocytes, and monocytes. The tubules and glomeruli in the affected areas are atrophic or completely replaced with scar tissue. The remaining glomeruli and tubules are hypertrophic and the tubular lumens are not only dilated but often contain hyaline casts. In advanced lesions the arteries and arterioles disclose marked sclerosis.

The chief *complications* are uremia and hypertension. The *clinical manifestations* vary with the type of renal involvement. In *acute pyelonephritis* they consist of (1) fever, chills, pallor, anemia, and leukocytosis — due to systemic absorption of products of inflammation, (2) renal pain and tenderness — due to inflammation in the kidney and adjacent tissues, and (3) dysuria, frequency, pyuria, and hematuria — due to concomitant inflammation of the bladder. In *chronic pyelonephritis* the manifestations may be similar with, in addition, superimposed symptoms and signs of hypertension and uremia. The *diagnosis* of pyelonephritis is made from the history (children, pregnant women, or older men), clinical manifestations as outlined, and urologic studies (often demonstrating an obstruction). *Treatment* consists of relieving the urinary tract obstruction when such a lesion is found and of administering antibiotics and chemotherapeutic agents. The *prognosis* depends upon the cause, the amenability of the obstructive lesion to therapy, and the degree of renal damage.

Acute Necrotizing Papillitis. — This condition, also known as renal papillary necrosis, is a severe form of pyelonephritis attended by necrosis of the renal papillæ (Silberstein and Knutsen). It is usually (but not always) seen in diabetics and generally *occurs* in the sixth and seventh decades of life (Tamaki). The *causes* are the same as those in pyelonephritis with obstruction of the urinary tract, infection with colon bacilli or staphylococci, and diabetes playing dominant roles. *Pathologically* the condition may be unilateral or bilateral. The affected kidney discloses the usual picture of acute pyelonephritis with or without abscess formation (Fig.

536). In addition, the tips or the greater portions of the pyramids reveal characteristic red to gray necrosis with a prominent hemorrhagic line of demarcation separating the necrotic from the viable tissue. *Histologically* the involved papillæ show simple coagulation necrosis; the line of demarcation reveals a nonspecific inflammatory reaction, and the rest of the kidney discloses typical pyelonephritis. The *complications* are toxemia and uremia. The *clinical manifestations* are those of severe pyelonephritis. The *diagnosis*

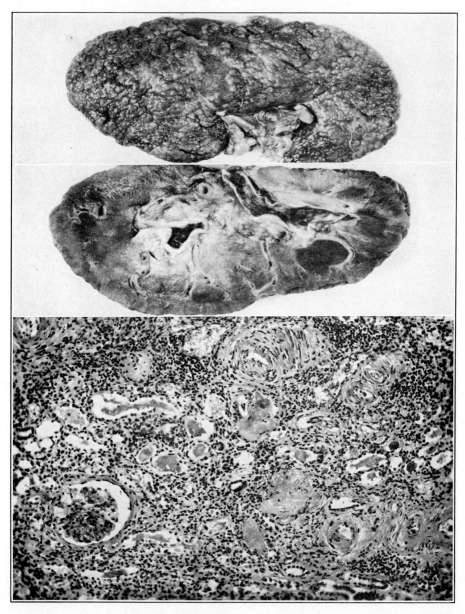

Fig. 535.—Chronic pyelonephritis showing irregular granularity of the external surface, thinning of the cortex, and obscuring of the corticomedullary demarcations grossly and interstitial fibrosis and leukocytic infiltration, hyalinization of the glomeruli, tubular dilatation, tubular casts, and sclerosis of the arteries microscopically. × 100.

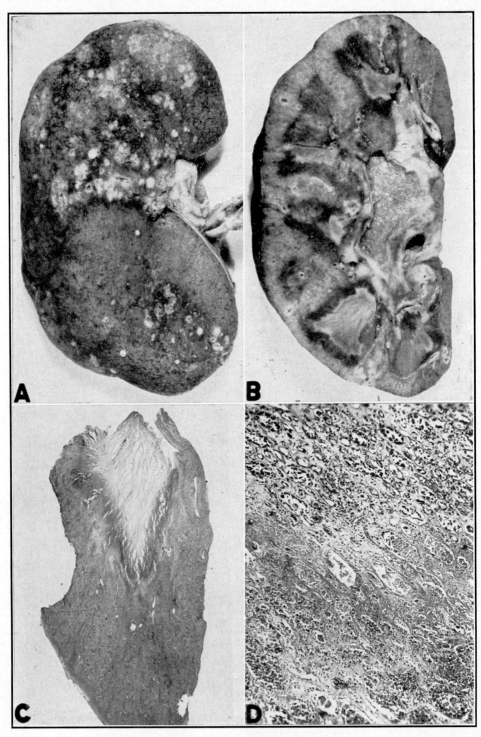

FIG. 536.—Acute necrotizing papillitis demonstrating *A*, multiple small cortical abscesses, *B*, massive necrosis of virtually all of the papillæ, *C*, necrosis of a papilla. × semigross, and *D*, zone of junction of necrotic with viable tissue. × 50.

can be suspected in any patient beyond the fifth decade of life having both diabetes and manifestations of renal infection. *Treatment* consists of controlling diabetes (when present), of relieving the urinary tract obstruction, and of administering antibiotics and chemotherapeutic agents. The *prognosis* is grave for the mortality rate is high.

Abscess.—Abscesses of the kidney occur in conjunction with pyelonephritis, pyemia, and such distant suppurative foci as boils, carbuncles, abscesses, felons, etc. (Welch). An abscess in the last mentioned category is often called *renal carbuncle*. The renal *infection* is unilateral, solitary, and cortical in location. It consists of an ordinary, nonspecific, pyogenic abscess. The *cause* is usually *Staphylococcus aureus*. The condition *occurs* at all ages but is most common in the third decade of life and it affects males two times as frequently as females. The chief *clinical manifestations* consist of renal pain and tenderness, fever, chills, sweating, weakness, malaise, loss of weight, and leukocytosis. The lesion may encroach upon a calyx and be demonstrable roentgenographically. The *diagnosis* is made from a history of a boil, etc., followed by the clinical manifestations listed. *Treatment* consists primarily of administration of antibiotics and chemotherapeutic agents and, only if these fail, of nephrectomy. The *prognosis* is good.

Perinephritis and Perinephric Abscess.—Perinephritis connotes inflammation of the fibrous and fatty tissues surrounding the kidney and confined by the renal fascia. A perinephric (perinephritic) abscess is local suppuration in the same area. The condition *occurs* in both sexes and at all ages (Parks). The *causes* are usually colon bacilli, staphylococci, and streptococci and the routes of infection are kidney, adjacent tissues, or bloodstream. *Pathologically* the process is generally unilateral and more common on the right side. It consists simply of diffuse thickening, induration, and permeation with purulent material of all tissues surrounding the kidney. As the disease advances the pus may collect into one or more abscesses. The *clinical manifestations* are similar to those in renal abscess with the exception that a mass is generally palpable and that roentgenograms disclose (among other things) obscuring of the lateral border of the psoas muscle and curvature of the spine. *Treatment* consists of incision and drainage and administration of antibiotics and chemotherapeutic agents. The *prognosis* is good.

Periarteritis Nodosa.—Periarteritis nodosa as a disease has been discussed in Chapter 9 (p. 230). Renal involvement is said to occur in from 73 to 87 per cent of all cases (Davson and Wold). It consists of infarcts or diffuse parenchymatous lesions. The *infarcts* are similar grossly and microscopically to any other infarcts of the kidney. They are due to specific involvement and thrombosis of the arteries and their shape and distribution depend upon the vessels affected. *Diffuse parenchymatous* lesions may be accompanied by no gross abnormality or they may disclose changes similar to those seen in malignant nephrosclerosis (p. 1072). Histologically the vessels show changes typical of periarteritis nodosa (p. 370); the glomeruli disclose focal areas of fibrinoid necrosis and later fibrosis; the periglomerular tissue reveals nonspecific inflammation; the tubules exhibit perenchymatous degeneration, and the interstitial tissue shows congestion, edema, and varying degrees of leukocytic infiltration.

Tuberculosis.—Tuberculosis of the kidney is always *secondary* to tuberculosis of some other organ of the body and the organisms almost always arrive on the scene by the hematogenous route (Sporer and Auerbach). The condition usually *occurs* between twenty and forty years of age and has no predilection for either sex (Plummer). *Pathologically* both kidneys are generally affected although the process is, as a rule, more severe in one organ than in the other. Grossly the lesions may be (1) *miliary* — generally part of widespread miliary tuberculosis and consisting of tiny varisized gray nodules scattered throughout the parenchyma, (2) *coalescing nodular* — composed of one or more, conglomerate but irregular, grayish-white, solid or necrotic areas arising in the cortex and extending to the medulla, (3)

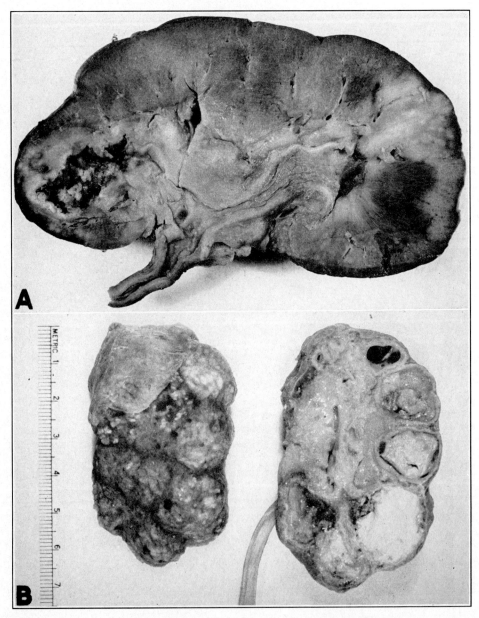

FIG. 537.—Renal tuberculosis showing *A*, coalescing nodular and ulcerocavernous lesions of the parenchyma and nodular lesions of the pelvic mucosa and *B*, irregular nodular lesions externally and ulcerating caseous lesions on cut surface.

ulcerocavernous—similar to the nodular type with the exception that the masses, upon reaching the pelvis, discharge their caseous material into the urinary tract and leave irregular, intercommunicating, cavernous spaces, (4) *hydronephrotic*—resulting from stricture at the ureteropelvic junction (or ureter) and consisting of a hydronephrotic kidney filled with caseous material and of ulcerating, tuberculous lesions of the parenchyma, (5) *contracted scarred calcified kidney*—representing the healed end stage, and (6) *tuberculoma* (Fig. 537). *Histologically* the lesions consist of miliary tubercles, of larger caseating or more solid tubercles, or of tuberculous granulation tissue. The chief *complications* are (1) spread of the infection to the lower urinary tract and to the genital tract and (2) uremia.

The *clinical manifestations* are (1) constitutional—due to the general effects of tuberculosis on the body and (2) local urinary—due to involvement of the kidney and bladder and consisting of frequency, dysuria, and hematuria, and occasionally of pain in the back and renal colic. The *diagnosis* is made from a history of tuberculosis elsewhere with current manifestations focused on the urinary tract. Tubercle bacilli should be isolated from the urine in over 80 per cent of cases. *Treatment* consists of administration of antibiotics and chemotherapeutic agents, often supplemented by nephrectomy (Ljunggren and Oppenheimer). The *prognosis* depends essentially upon the extent of the extrarenal tuberculosis and the presence and extent of tuberculosis of the rest of the urinary tract. In general, it is fair to good.

Syphilis.—Syphilis of the kidney is uncommon. The condition has been described in three forms (1) *nephrosis*—occurring in conjunction with secondary syphilis, clinically similar to subacute diffuse glomerulonephritis, and accompanied by complete recovery (Thomas), (2) *syphilitic nephritis*—seen in conjunction with secondary or tertiary syphilis and consisting of interstitial infiltration with mononuclear cells (Rich), and (3) *gumma* (Hunter).

PHYSICAL DISTURBANCES

Orientation.—In this section the following unrelated disorders may be briefly considered: aneurysm of the renal artery, trauma, movable kidney, infarction, hydronephrosis and pyonephrosis, hematuria, chyluria, and benign albuminuria.

Aneurysm of the Renal Artery.—Aneurysm of the renal artery is uncommon. The *causes* are (1) congenital—on the basis of developmental defect in the elastic and muscle tissue, (2) degenerative—arteriosclerosis, (3) inflammatory—syphilis, tuberculosis, and periarteritis nodosa and inflammations associated with pneumonia, pleurisy, endocarditis, malaria, dysentery, rheumatic fever, nephritis, and embolism, and (4) traumatic—falls, blows, stab or gunshot wounds, and operative (Mathé, Lazarus, and Herbut). *Pathologically* the aneurysm may be (1) true—consisting of all the coats, measuring up to 6 cm. in diameter, located in the main artery or any of its branches, and being saccular, fusiform, or pyriform, or (2) false—consisting of rupture of the vessel with hemorrhage into the coats of the vessel and adjacent tissues and measuring up to 15 cm. in diameter. Two important *complications* are (1) rupture with fatal hemorrhage and (2) occlusion of the vascular lumen producing renal ischemia and hypertension. The *clinical manifestations* are (1) pain from pressure on adjacent structures, (2) tumefaction due to the aneurysm itself and to the extravasation of blood, (3) hematuria occurring when the escaping blood finds its way into the calyces and pelvis, and (4) symptoms and signs referable to the hemorrhage and hypertension. The *diagnosis* is made from the clinical manifestations, roentgenograms (plain and angiographic films), and the findings at operation. *Treatment* consists of nephrectomy. The *prognosis* is good in patients treated surgically but is poor in those not operated upon.

Trauma. —Disturbances of the kidney in this category may consist of spontaneous rupture and traumatic injury. *Spontaneous rupture* follows such minor injuries as muscle effort or turning in bed. It occurs in such renal conditions as hydronephrosis, pyonephrosis, calculus, pyelonephritis, abscess, infarct, tuberculosis, aneurysm of the renal artery, and stricture of the ureter. The rupture may occur in the renal substance but is more common in the pelvic area (Councill). It varies in extent and is attended by little or no bleeding. *Traumatic injury* may occur in a previously diseased or a previously healthy kidney. The injury may be (1) closed— from a direct blow or indirect force such as muscular exertion, (2) open— from penetrating injury as by knife, sword, bullet, etc., or (3) instrumentation—from the use of a catheter, bougie, forceps, etc. (Cheetham). The localization, size, and type of wound varies with the type of injury. It may consist of a puncture or of an irregular laceration and it may involve the renal capsule, the renal parenchyma, and/or the calyces and pelvis. The injury is *attended by* varying degrees of hemorrhage, urinary extravasation, infection, and later ureteral obstruction and calculous formation (Hodges). The *clinical manifestations* consist of hematuria, pyuria, pains, tenderness, renal mass, abdominal rigidity, shock, and later symptoms and signs of infection (Sargent). Pyelography may disclose extravasation of the dye beyond the pelvis and calyces. The *diagnosis* is made from a history of trauma in association with the clinical manifestations listed. *Treatment* consists of watchful waiting, surgical exploration and drainage, or nephrectomy (McCague). The *prognosis* is generally good.

Movable Kidney. —A movable kidney is one that has a greater than normal range of mobility and, because of this mobility, produces clinical manifestations. The condition is *also known* as nephroptosis, ptosis, ptotic kidney, and mobile kidney. It usually *occurs* between the ages of twenty and forty years and is much more common in females than it is in males (Deming and Bandler). The *predisposing causes* are shallow renal fossa, long renal pedicle, separation of the anterior and posterior layers of the perirenal fascia, depletion of perirenal fat, long lumbar segment, and poor muscular development. *Precipitating causes* are sudden jar, fall, blow, or contraction of muscles. *Pathologically* the condition is usually unilateral and is about ten to twelve times as frequent on the right side as it is on the left (Livermore). The only changes occurring as a result of *complications* consist of hydronephrosis, infection, and calculous formation. The *clinical manifestations* consist of (1) pain—from pull on the pedicle and kinking of the vessels and ureter, (2) gastrointestinal disturbances comprising nausea, vomiting, abdominal distention, etc.—from reflex nervous stimuli, and (3) general symptoms of fever, leukocytosis, etc., and local urinary symptoms of urgency, dysuria, pyuria, hematuria, etc.—from inflammation in the kidney and lower urinary tract. Roentgenograms disclose altered position of the kidney upon lying down and standing up. The *diagnosis* is made from the clinical manifestations and roentgenographic appearance. *Treatment* consists of conservative measures such as application of a belt and, if this fails, of nephropexy. The *prognosis* is good.

Infarction. —Infarctions of the kidney may be divided into three groups — uric acid infarcts, simple infarcts, and diffuse cortical necrosis.

Uric acid infarcts are usually deposits of urates in the medullary pyramids rather than true infarcts (Bell). They are usually seen in newborn infants and arise as a precipitation of excessive uric acid which comes from disintegration of nuclei of erythroblasts. Grossly they appear as streaks of yellow material covering the pyramids, while microscopically urate crystals are seen in the collecting tubules.

Simple infarcts arise on the basis of (1) arterial occlusion—rheumatic fever, bacterial endocarditis, embolism, thrombosis, or arterial occlusion, (2) venous occlusion—primary or in association with sepsis such as pneumonia, enteritis, puerperal sepsis, pyelonephritis, pyemia, or thrombophlebitis of the leg veins, or (3) trauma (Regan, Warren, and Kobernick). The *pathologic* appearance has already been described (p. 190). The condition may be unilateral or bilateral and the area of involvement may be small or massive. When the infarcts are small they are asymptomatic but when they are large the *clinical manifestations* consist of pain in the flank, palpable mass, hematuria, albuminuria, pyuria, anorexia, leukocytosis, and fever. The *diagnosis* is made from a history of a predisposing condition coupled with the clinical manifestations listed. *Treatment* in massive unilateral infarcts has been nephrectomy. The *prognosis* depends upon the causative factor and extent of the lesion. It is poor in bilateral massive infarcts.

Diffuse cortical necrosis consists of massive necrosis of the cortex of both kidneys. The condition usually occurs in connection with pregnancy but is also seen in nonpregnant patients. The latter group includes males and is not limited to any age group. The specific *causes* are generally unknown although the condition has been thought to arise on the basis of (1) toxic agents (chemical, bacterial, tissue, etc.) in hypersensitive patients and (2) ischemia resulting from actual emboli, thrombi, or spasm (Smith, Haft, and Campbell). *Pathologically* the kidneys are enlarged; the capsule is thickened and slightly adherent, and the external and cut surfaces present a characteristic mosaic pattern of light areas alternating with dark areas (Fig. 538). The infarcts are usually limited to the cortex but when they are extensive, the medulla too may be affected. *Histologically* the affected tissue shows the usual loss of architectural pattern seen in any infarct with an inflammatory zone of reaction seen at the junction of the dead and living tissue. The chief *complication* is renal insufficiency ending in uremia. The *clinical manifestations* consist of oliguria, anuria, hematuria, albuminuria, pyuria, epigastric or renal pain, leukocytosis, edema, and symptoms and signs of uremia. The clinical *diagnosis* of diffuse cortical necrosis is seldom possible. *Treatment* is symptomatic and unsatisfactory. The *prognosis is* poor.

Hydronephrosis and Pyonephrosis.—*Hydronephrosis* (Gr. = water + kidney) may be defined as a collection of watery fluid in the renal pelvis attended by progressive (1) dilatation of the pelvis and calyces and (2) atrophy of the renal parenchyma. *Pyonephrosis* (Gr. = pus + kidney) connotes pus in the kidney. It actually means an infected hydronephrosis and is thus a complication of hydronephrosis. Hydronephrosis (or its sequel pyonephrosis) *occurs* at all ages and in both sexes. The *cause* is partial or intermittent obstruction to the urinary tract at or below the ureteropelvic junction and the renal changes are brought about not only by direct pressure on the renal parenchyma from a dilated pelvis, but also by vascular occlusion and renal ischemia (Hinman). The obstructive lesions may be congenital or acquired and may be due to any of the many developmental, degenerative, inflammatory, mechanical, or neoplastic conditions considered in the various sections on the urinary system (Davis and Campbell). The organisms producing the infection in pyonephrosis are similar to those in pyelonephritis (p. 1087).

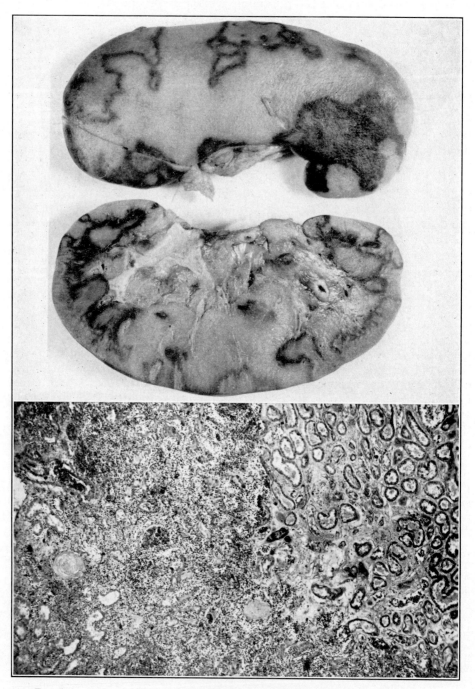

FIG. 538.—Diffuse cortical necrosis showing massive infarction of the cortex grossly and necrosis with leukocytic infiltration microscopically.   × 50.

Pathologically the process may be unilateral or bilateral, depending upon whether the obstruction occurs above or below the level of the entrance of the ureter into the bladder. The degree of dilatation of the pelvis and calyces varies from that which is scarcely perceptible to that occupying a capacity of 7,000 cc. or more. Initially the fluid is urine but gradually it becomes more watery and when infection supervenes it becomes distinctly purulent. As the process advances the renal parenchyma gradually becomes more and more atrophic, the corticomedullary demarcations become more and more obscured, and the entire renal substance is reduced to a mere shell of tissue (Fig. 539). When infection supervenes, the parenchyma

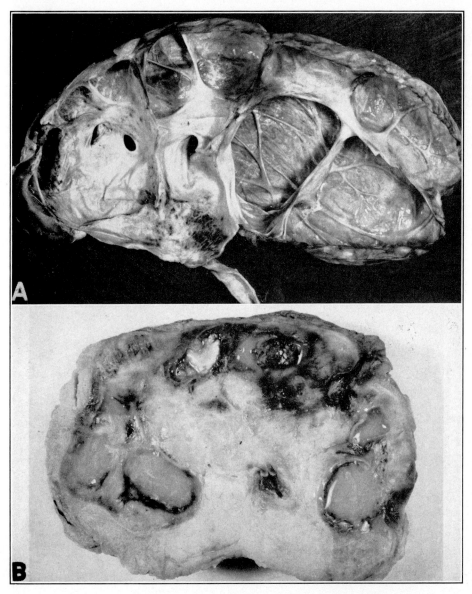

Fig. 539.—Effects of ureteral obstruction on the kidney showing *A*, severe hydronephrosis due to ureteropelvic occlusion and *B*, pyonephrosis from calculi in the renal pelvis.

becomes streaked with pus and ultimately undergoes fibrosis. *Histologically* the changes are those of ischemic atrophy with gradual disappearance of the renal parenchyma and replacement with fibrous tissue (Fig. 540). Superimposed infection is indicated by leukocytic permeation.

The chief *complication* of hydronephrosis is disturbance of sufficient amount of renal parenchyma to produce renal insufficiency and uremia. The *clinical manifestations* consist of a tumor mass in the renal area, frequency, pyuria, chills, fever, anorexia, loss of weight, malaise, backache, nausea, etc. Retrograde and intravenous pyelography disclose dilatation of the renal pelvis and calyces and/or a nonfunctioning kidney. The *diagnosis* is made from the clinical manifestations and complete urologic (including cystoscopic) studies. *Treatment* consists essentially of relieving the ob-

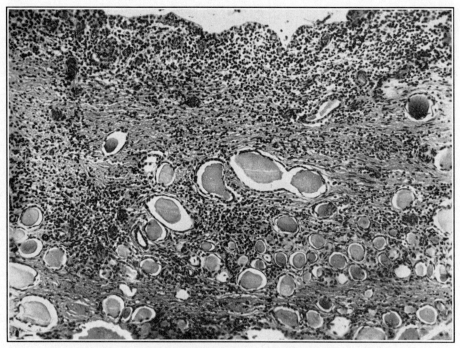

FIG. 540.—Hydronephrosis illustrating marked atrophy of the renal parenchyma, extensive fibrosis, and diffuse permeation with plasma cells and lymphocytes. × 100.

struction and combating the infection with antibiotic and chemotherapeutic agents. Nephrectomy is performed only when all other measures fail. The *prognosis* depends upon the cause and the extent of the renal damage.

Hematuria.—Hematuria (Gr. = blood + urine) is the passage of blood in the urine. It is a symptom and not a disease. It may be caused by (1) virtually any disease in any portion of the urinary tract—with inflammations and tumors heading the list, (2) diseases of adjacent organs invading the urinary tract—including appendicitis, salpingitis, diverticulitis, and tumors, or (3) systemic diseases—encompassing purpura, hemophilia, inflammations (septicemia, typhoid fever, endocarditis, etc.), lymphoblastoma, avitaminosis C and K, etc. (Cahill). Of the various parts of the urinary tract affected, the bladder and kidneys are most commonly involved.

Chyluria.—Chyluria (Gr. = chyle + urine) means the presence of lymph (chyle) in the urine. It occurs as a result of obstruction of the lymphatic channels and their subsequent communication with the urinary tract, usually at the pelvic level. Some of the many causes of obstruction are *Wuchereria bancrofti*, posterior mediastinal tumors or inflammations, perirenal abscess, pregnancy, syphilis, tuberculosis, etc. (Logan). The urine is milky but does not clear on centrifugalization and it may contain clots of coagulated chyle. Retrograde pyelography may disclose extravasation of contrast medium into the communicating lymphatic channels.

Benign Albuminuria.—Benign albuminuria may be defined as albumin in the urine unassociated with serious or progressive renal disease (King). It is said to occur in from 11.6 to 16 per cent of college students and military inductees. It may be divided into transitory and postural. *Transitory albuminuria* accounts for about 75 per cent of all cases and consists of albumin in the urine without regular duplication of its presence. It may be caused by contamination with seminal or prostatic fluid, infection of the bladder or urethra, toxic systemic conditions, severe emotional strain, injury to the brain, encephalography, etc. *Postural albuminuria* (also called orthostatic, lordotic, variable, and juvenile albuminuria) is that form of albuminuria that can be produced regularly by the lordotic (erect or recumbent) position. The assumption is that the position interferes with the renal circulation and that this produces the albumin in the urine. The importance of benign albuminuria lies in its recognition as an innocuous condition and its differentiation from pathologic albuminuria caused by organic renal disease.

TUMORS

Orientation.—Tumors of the kidneys are as varied as the tissues that compose these organs. They may be listed as follows: adenoma, carcinoma, hemangioma, hemangio-endothelioma, lipomatosis, xanthomatosis, lipoma, liposarcoma, fibroma, fibrosarcoma, myoblastoma, leiomyoma, leiomyosarcoma, rhabdomyoma, rhabdomyosarcoma, dermoid cysts, Wilms' tumor, osteoblastoma, lymphoblastoma, neurofibroma, neurocytoma, and secondary tumors. Most of the benign growths are small, asymptomatic, and discovered as incidental findings at autopsy while the more important malignant neoplasms are carcinoma and Wilms' tumor.

Carcinoma.—Carcinoma of the kidney, also called Grawitz tumor and hypernephroma, is one of the more common malignant growths of the body, constituting about 1 per cent of all cancers. It usually *occurs* after the age of forty years and is from two to three times as common in males as it is in females (Fryfogle, Griffiths, and Herger). The *cause* of the neoplasm is unknown and, although there is still some debate as to whether the growth arises from renal parenchyma or adrenal rests, it is the concensus that the tubular epithelial cells are the progenitors (O'Crowley).

Pathologically the neoplasm is generally single and unilateral although, on rare occasions, simultaneous bilateral growths have been recorded. In unilateral tumors, the right kidney is favored somewhat over the left. Although any part of the kidney may serve as the starting point, the most common site of origin is the upper pole (Fig. 541). The size is variable but by the time the neoplasm is discovered it generally measures from 3 to 10 cm. in diameter. As a rule, the tumor is well delineated from the kidney substance and adjacent tissues. It is firm, usually solid but occasionally cystic in part, and variegated gray to yellow to deep red in appearance. As it grows it bulges in all directions and finally affects the perirenal tissue, calyces and pelvis, and lumens of the renal veins and vena cava (Ney). *Histologically* the tumors are fundamentally of two types—clear cell and granular cell with transitions from one to the other. *Clear cell carcinoma* is composed of large, polyhedral, sharply defined cells consisting of an abundant amount of watery or clear cytoplasm and round or, at most, oval, centrally placed, evenly stained nuclei (Fig. 542*A*). The cells are arranged in cords, nests, glands, or papillæ. *Granular cell carcinoma* is composed of

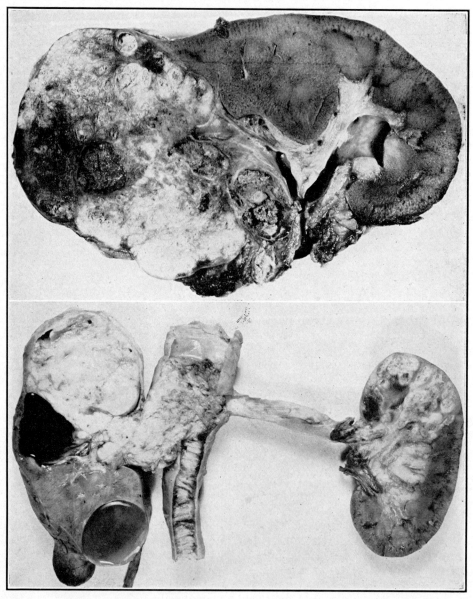

FIG. 541.—Carcinoma of the kidney showing *A*, a large variegated tumor destroying the upper pole of the kidney and growing into the pelvis and *B*, a tumor that has replaced the upper half of the right kidney, extended into the renal vein and inferior vena cava, and metastasized to the left kidney.

smaller, rounded or polyhedral, sharply defined cells with a moderate amount of granular cytoplasm and relatively larger, round or oval, hyperchromatic, centrally placed nuclei (Fig. 542*B*). In either case, the cells become more irregular as the lesions increase in degree of malignancy. The *stroma* is generally scanty, of a loose connective tissue variety, and well vascularized. Calcification is occasionally present. Carcinoma of the kidney *spreads* by (1) direct extension to adjacent structures, renal pelvis, and blood vessels (especially renal vein and inferior vena cava), (2) lymphatics to the lymph nodes, and (3) bloodstream to the lungs, liver, bones, and virtually every organ and tissue of the body.

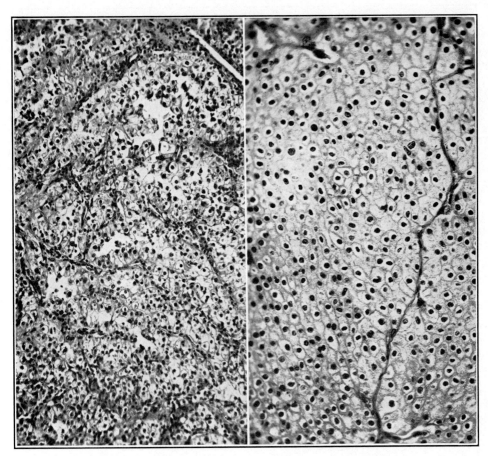

Fig. 542.—Carcinoma of the kidney demonstrating *A*, a clear cell tumor. × 100 and *B*, a granular cell tumor. × 200.

The most important *complication* is metastasis. Clinically it is not unusual to find metastasis to such areas as the skin, thyroid, tongue, parotid gland, bones, etc., months or even years before manifestations of the primary growth become apparent. When symptoms and signs do appear they consist characteristically of the triad of (1) hematuria—due to invasion of the calyces and pelvis by the tumor, (2) pain—due to stretching of the renal capsule, transitory urostasis, and passage of blood clots by the ureter, and (3) tumor mass—due to the growth itself. In addition, there may be (1) constitutional symptoms such as anorexia, fever, loss of weight, etc.—from absorption of pyrogenic substances from the tumor, (2) varicocele—from occlusion of the spermatic vein, and (3) edema of the legs—from occlusion of the inferior vena cava. The *diagnosis* is made from the clinical manifestations and urologic and roentgenographic findings. Neoplastic cells can be demonstrated in the urine so infrequently that this procedure is of little practical value. The only effective *treatment* is nephrectomy. Unlike most other malignant tumors, a solitary metastasis is not a contraindication for nephrectomy because the neoplasm grows slowly and removal of both

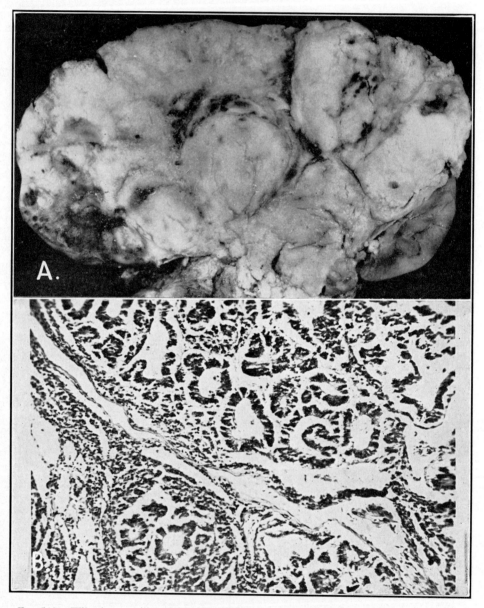

FIG. 543.—Wilms' tumor illustrating *A*, a fleshy mass replacing most of the renal substance and *B*, embryonal cells attempting to form tubules. × 100.

the primary growth and the metastatic focus may be consistent with years of survival. The *prognosis* is variable but the over-all results are good. A five-year survival rate of approximately 40 per cent can be expected.

Wilms' Tumor.—This tumor is also known as embryoma, malignant embryoma, embryonal mixed tumor, mesoblastic nephroma, and carcino-sarcoma (Culp). Although it may *occur* in adults (Eskersky) it is usually found in children under three years of age (Ladd, Eisel, Nesbit, and Dickey) and is somewhat more common in females than in males. The *cause* is unknown. *Histogenetically* the growth is thought to arise from wolffian remnants, pluripotent mesonephric elements, displaced myotomes, or renal blastema.

Pathologically the tumor is usually unilateral, having no predilection for either side. It appears fairly well encapsulated, is irregularly rounded, generally measures 15 to 20 cm. in diameter, replaces most of the kidney substance as it gets larger, is soft to firm in consistency, and, on cut surface, is homogeneously grayish white and brain-like (Fig. 543*A*). In larger masses, however, necrosis, hemorrhage, and liquefaction may be noted. *Histologically* most of the tumor is composed of small, ill-defined, rounded or elongated, mesoblastic cells with from scanty to imperceptible, lightly basophilic cytoplasm and rounded or elongated, deeply staining nuclei (Fig. 543*B*). The cells are arranged in sheets or cords or they attempt to form tubules and glomeruli. In addition, most tumors contain varying amounts of striated and smooth muscle, myxomatous tissue, nerve fibers, fat, cartilage, calcium, and even bone. Wilms' tumor usually remains localized for long periods of time. As it grows, it *spreads* locally to involve the vessels, diaphragm, spleen, liver, and any of the tissues it contacts and infrequently by way of the lymphatics and blood vessels to the lymph nodes, liver, lungs, brain, and other tissues.

The most important *complication* is spread to adjacent tissues and distant organs. The only important *clinical manifestations* are abdominal mass (due to the tumor itself) and abdominal pain (due to distention of the renal capsule and pressure upon the adjacent structures). Hematuria is present infrequently and other manifestations such as loss of weight, nausea, vomiting, etc., occur only in advanced stages of the disease. The precise clinical *diagnosis* is readily made when a child three years of age or younger develops an expanding mass in the region of the kidney. It is more difficult to arrive at in an older child or in an adult where other lesions such as hydronephrosis, renal carcinoma, splenic enlargement, etc., have to be taken into consideration. *Treatment* of choice is complete surgical removal of the tumor and kidney followed by irradiation therapy. The *prognosis* is fair to good with the cure rate being around 50 per cent (Gross and Gahagan).

REFERENCES

Pathologic Physiology

ALLEN, A. C.: *The Kidney, Medical and Surgical Diseases*, New York, Grune & Stratton, 1951.

BELL, E. T.: *Renal Diseases*, 2nd Ed., Philadelphia, Lea & Febiger, 1950.

BEST, C. H., and TAYLOR, N. B.: *The Physiological Basis of Medical Practice*, 5th Ed., Baltimore, Williams & Wilkins Co., 1950.

BULL, G. M.: Lancet, *1*, 731, 1955 (Uremia).

CASTLEMAN, B., and SMITHWICK, R. H.: N. England J. Med., *239*, 729, 1948 (Kidney in Essential Hypertension).

DEXTER, L.: Am. J. Med., *4*, 279, 1948 (Pathogenesis of Hypertension).

Editorial: Circulation, *15*, 1, 1957 (Pathogenesis of Hypertension).

GOLDBLATT, H.: *The Renal Origin of Hypertension*, Springfield, Charles C Thomas, 1948.

GUYTON, A. C.: *Textbook of Medical Physiology*, Philadelphia, W. B. Saunders Co., 1956.
HERBUT, P. A.: *Urological Pathology*, Philadelphia, Lea & Febiger, 1952.
MILLER, S. E.: *A Textbook of Clinical Pathology*, 4th Ed., Baltimore, Williams & Wilkins Co., 1952.
MORITZ, A. R., and OLDT, M. R.: Am. J. Path., *13*, 679, 1937 (Kidney in Hypertension).
PAGE, I. H.: J.A.M.A., *140*, 451, 1949 (Hypertension).
PAGE, I. H., and HELMER, O. M.: J. Exp. Med., *71*, 29, 1940 (Renin in Hypertension).
PLENTL, A. A., PAGE, I. H., and DAVIS, W. W.: J. Biol. Chem., *147*, 143, 1943 (Renin in Hypertension).
ROBBINS, S. L.: *Textbook of Pathology*, Philadelphia, W. B. Saunders Co., 1957.
SODEMAN, W. A.: *Pathologic Physiology*, Philadelphia, W. B. Saunders Co., 1956.
STEAD, E. A., WARREN, J. V., and BRANNEN, E. S.: Am. Heart J., *35*, 529, 1958 (Renal Physiology).
WAKERLIN, G. E.: Arch. Int. Med., *92*, 889, 1953 (Pathogenesis of Hypertension).
WAKIM, K. G.: Proceedings of the Staff Meetings of the Mayo Clinic, *29*, 65, 1954 (Renal Physiology).

Congenital Anomalies

ABESHOUSE, B. S.: Am. J. Surg., *73*, 658, 1947 (Crossed Ectopia).
BIGLER, J. A., and KILLINGSWORTH, W. P.: A. M. A. Arch. Path., *47*, 487, 1949 (Cartilaginous Inclusion).
CARLSON, H. E.: J. Urol., *64*, 224, 1950 (Supernumary Kidney).
CULP, O. S.: J. Urol., *52*, 420, 1944 (Renal Ectopia).
FETTER, T. R., and SMITH, B.: J. Urol., *63*, 403, 1950 (Renal Ectopia).
GLASER, S.: Brit. J. Surg., *40*, 74, 1952 (Simple Cysts).
GRAHAM, A. P.: J. Urol., *60*, 581, 1948 (Bilateral Hypoplasia).
LEFFLER, R. J.: Am. J. Clin. Path., *21*, 752, 1951 (Renal Agenesis).
LEVIN, H.: J. Urol., *67*, 86, 1952 (Bilateral Renal Agenesis).
LOWSLEY, O. S.: J. Urol., *67*, 565, 1952 (Horseshoe Kidney).
LOWSLEY, O. S., and CURTIS, M. S.: J. A. M. A., *127*, 1112, 1945 (Cystic Disease).
MITCHELL, N., and ANGRIST, A.: A. M. A. Arch. Path., *35*, 46, 1943 (Adrenal Rests).
NATION, E. F.: Am. J. Surg., *68*, 67, 1945 (Renal Ectopia).
————: Surg., Gynec. & Obst., *79*, 175, 1944 (Renal Agenesis).
NEWMAN, H. R.: Am. J. Surg., *80*, 410, 1950 (Polycystic Disease).
OCHSNER, H. C.: Am. J. Roentgenol., *65*, 185, 1951 (Cysts).
POWELL, T., *et al.*: Brit. J. Urol., *23*, 142, 1951 (Multilocular Cysts).
RAVITCH, M. M.: Pediatrics, *4*, 769, 1949 (Unilateral Multicystic Disease).
WELSH, C. A., *et al.*: J. Clin. Invest., *23*, 750, 1944 (Hypertrophy).

Degenerations

ALBRIGHT, F., *et al.*: Bull. Johns Hopkins Hosp., *60*, 377, 1937 (Renal Osteitis Fibrosis Cystica).
APONTE, G. E., and FETTER, T. R.: Am. J. Cl. Path., *24*. 1363, 1954 (Onalate Nephrocalcinosis)
ARMSTRONG, J. B.: Am. J. M. Sci., *219*, 488, 1950 (Myeloma Kidney).
ENGEL, W. J.: J. A. M. A., *145*, 288, 1951 (Nephrocalcinosis).
ENGELBERG, H., *et al.*: Diabetes, *1*, 425, 1952 (Diabetic Glomerulosclerosis).
FRENCH, A. J.: A. M. A. Arch. Path., *49*, 43, 1950 (Glomerulonephrosis).
GOLDBLATT, H.: Am. J. Med., *4*, 100, 1948 (Experimental Renal Hypertension).
————: Physiol. Rev., *27*, 120, 1947 (Renal Origin of Hypertension).
GREENHILL, J. P.: *Principles and Practice of Obstetrics*, 10th Ed., Philadelphia, W. B. Saunders Co., 1951.
HERBUT, P. A.: Ann. Int. Med., *25*, 648, 1946 (Renal Changes in Secondary Shock).
————: A. M. A. Arch. Path., *31*, 501, 1941 (Diabetic Glomerulosclerosis).
HERBUT, P. A., and PRICE, A. H.: A. M. A. Arch. Path., *39*, 274, 1945 (Aneurysm Renal Artery and Hypertension).
JONES, D. B.: Am. J. Path., *29*, 619, 1953 (Nephrosclerosis).
KIMMELSTIEL, P., and PORTER, W. B.: New England J. Med., *238*, 876, 1948 (Intercapillary Glomerulosclerosis).
LAFORET, E. G.: Ann. Int. Med., *38*, 667, 1953 (Renal Artery Occlusion and Hypertension).
LUCKÉ, B.: Military Surgeon, *99*, 371, 1946 (Lower Nephron Nephrosis).
MANN, G. V., *et al.*: Am. J. Med., *7*, 3, 1949 (Diabetic Glomerulosclerosis).
MOON, V. H.: Ann. Int. Med., *39*, 51, 1953 (Acute Tubular Nephrosis).
MOORE, H. C., and SHEEHAN, H. L.: Lancet, *1*, 68, 1952 (Kidney in Scleroderma).

Moschcowitz, E.: Am. J. M. Sci., *216*, 146, 1948 (Lipoid Nephrosis).
Oliver, J., *et al.*: J. Clin. Invest., *30*, 1307, 1951 (Acute Renal Failure from Injury).
Ostry, H.: Canad. M. A. J., *65*, 465, 1951 (Nephrocalcinosis).
Rifkin, H., and Petermann, M. L.: Diabetes, *1*, 28, 1952 (Diabetic Glomerulosclerosis).
Rule, C., and Grollman, A.: Ann. Int. Med., *20*, 63, 1944 (Nephrocalcinosis).
Smith, G. van S., and Smith, O. W.: Physiol. Rev., *28*, 1, 1948 (Eclampsia).
Smith, H. W.: Am. J. Med., *4*, 724, 1948 (Hypertension and Urologic Disease).
Trueta, J., *et al.*: *Renal Circulation*, Springfield, Ill., Charles C Thomas, 1947.
Way, G. T. C.: Am. J. Obst. & Gynec., *54*, 928, 1947 (Eclampsia).
Wilson, J. L., *et al.*: New England J. Med., *245*, 513, 1951 (Diabetic Nephropathy).
Yuile, C. L.: Am. J. M. Sci., *207*, 394, 1944 (Renal Arterial Occlusion and Hypertension).

Inflammations

Auerbach, O.: The New Internat. Clinics, *3*, 21, 1940 (Tuberculosis).
Birchall, R., and Alexander, J. E.: Medicine, *29*, 1, 1950 (Pyelonephritis).
Brod, J.: Am. J. Med., *7*, 317, 1949 (Acute Diffuse Glomerulonephritis).
Davson, J., *et al.*: Quart. J. Med., *17*, 175, 1948 (Periarteritis Nodosa).
Herbut, P. A.: Am. J. Path., *20*, 1011, 1944 (Diffuse Glomerulonephritis Following Vaccination).
Hunter, A. W.: J. Urol., *42*, 1176, 1939 (Gumma).
Jones, D. B.: Am. J. Path., *29*, 33, 1953 (Glomerulonephritis).
Knutsen, A., *et al.*: Am. J. Clin. Path., *22*, 327, 1952 (Papillary Necrosis).
Krakower, C. A., and Greensbon, S. A.: A. M. A. Arch. Path., *51*, 629, 1951 (Experimental Nephrotoxic Glomerulonephritis).
Lippman, R. W., *et al.*: A. M. A. Arch. Path., *53*, 1, 1952 (Nephrotoxic Globulin Nephritis).
Ljunggren, E.: J. Urol., *67*, 129, 1952 (Tuberculosis).
McLean, C. R., *et al.*: A. M. A. Arch. Path., *51*, 1, 1951 (Horse Serum Glomerulonephritis in Rabbits).
More, R. H., and Kobernick, S. D.: A. M. A. Arch. Path., *51*, 361, 1951 (Globulin Glomerulonephritis in Rabbits).
Oppenheimer, G. D., and Narins, L.: J. Urol., *62*, 804, 1949 (Tuberculosis).
Parks, R. E.: J. Urol., *64*, 555, 1950 (Perinephric Abscess).
Rich, A. R.: Bull. Johns Hopkins Hosp., *50*, 357, 1932 (Syphilis).
Robertson, H. F., and Schlamowitz, S. T.: Ann. Int. Med., *33*, 708, 1950 (Rheumatic Nephritis).
Saphir, O., and Taylor, B.: Ann. Int. Med., *36*, 1017, 1952 (Pyelonephritis).
Silberstein, J. S., and Paugh, J. T.: Ann. Int. Med., *38*, 689, 1953 (Necrotizing Papillitis).
Sporer, A.: Quart. Bull. Sea View Hosp., *8*, 120, 1946 (Tuberculosis).
Tamaki, H. T., and Whitman, M. A.: J. A. M. A., *150*, 1304, 1952 (Papillary Necrosis).
Thomas, E. W., and Schur, M.: A. M. A. Arch. Int. Med., *78*, 679, 1946 (Syphilis).
Welch, N. M., and Prather, G. C.: J. Urol., *62*, 646, 1949 (Renal Carbuncle).
Wold, L. E., and Barker, N. W.: Minnesota Med., *32*, 715, 1949 (Periarteritis Nodosa).

Physical Disturbances

Bandler, C. G., *et al.*: New York State J. Med., *44*, 1541, 1944 (Movable Kidney).
Cahill, G. F.: J. Urol., *47*, 224, 1942 (Hematuria).
Campbell, A. C. P., and Henderson, J. L.: A. M. A. Arch. Dis. Childhood, *24*, 269, 1949 (Cortical Necrosis).
Campbell, M.: J. Urol., *65*, 734, 1951 (Hydronephrosis in Children).
Cheetham, J. G.: Internat. Abst. Surg., *72*, 573, 1941 (Renal Trauma).
Councill, W. A., and Councill, W. A., Jr.: J. Urol., *63*, 441, 1950 (Spontaneous Rupture).
Davis, D. M.: M. Ann. District of Columbia, *22*, 73, 1953 (Hydronephrosis).
Deming, C. L.: Pennsylvania M. J., *48*, 207, 1944 (Movable Kidney).
Haft, D. E., and Prior, J. T.: Ann. Int. Med., *34*, 1483, 1951 (Diffuse Cortical Necrosis).
Herbut, P. A., and Price, A. H.: A. M. A. Arch. Path., *39*, 274, 1945 (Aneurysm Renal Artery).
Hodges, C. V., *et al.*: J. Urol., *66*, 627, 1951 (Renal Trauma).
King, E. S., and Gronbeck, C., Jr.: Ann. Int. Med., *36*, 765, 1952 (Benign Albuminuria).
Kobernick, S. D., *et al.*: Am. J. Path., *27*, 435, 1951 (Thrombosis Renal Veins).
Lazarus, J. A., and Marks, M. S.: J. Urol., *52*, 115, 1944 (Aneurysm Renal Artery).
Livermore, G. R.: J. Urol., *65*, 964, 1951 (Movable Kidney).
Logan, A. H., Jr., *et al.*: Am. J. M. Sci., *216*, 389, 1948 (Chyluria).
Mathé, C. P.: J. Urol., *60*, 543, 1948 (Aneurysm Renal Artery).

McCague, E. J.: J. Urol., *63*, 773, 1950 (Renal Trauma).

Regan, F. C., and Crabtree, E. G.: J. Urol., *59*, 981, 1948 (Renal Infarction).

Sargent, J. C., and Marquardt, C. R.: J. Urol., *63*, 1, 1950 (Renal Injuries).

Smith, A., and Muirhead, E. E.: Texas State J. Med., *47*, 88, 1951 (Bilateral Cortical Necrosis).

Warren, H., *et al.:* J. A. M. A., *152*, 700, 1953 (Thrombosis Renal Veins).

Tumors

Culp, O. S., and Hartman, F. W.: J. Urol., *60*, 552, 1948 (Mesoblastic Nephroma).

Dickey, L. B., and Chandler, L. R.: Pediatrics, *4*, 197, 1949 (Embryoma).

Esersky, G. L., *et al.:* J. Urol., *58*, 397, 1947 (Wilms' Tumor in Adults).

Fryfogle, J. D., *et al.:* J. Urol., *60*, 221, 1948 (Carcinoma).

Gahagan, H. Q., and Yearwood, H. M.: J. Urol., *62*, 295, 1949 (Wilms' Tumor).

Griffiths, I. H., and Thackray, A. C.: Brit. J. Urol., *21*, 128, 1949 (Carcinoma).

Gross, R. E., and Neuhauser, E. B. D.: Pediatrics, *6*, 843, 1950 (Mixed Tumor).

Herger, C. C., and Sauer, H. R.: Surg., Gynec. & Obst., *78*, 584, 1944 (Carcinoma).

Ladd, W. E., and White, R. R.: J. A. M. A., *117*, 1858, 1941 (Wilms' Tumor).

Nesbit, R. M., and Adams, F. M.: J. Pediat., *29*, 295, 1946 (Wilms' Tumor).

Ney, C.: J. Urol., *55*, 583, 1946 (Malignant Tumors).

O'Crowley, C. R., and Martland, H. S.: J. Urol., *50*, 756, 1943 (Carcinoma).

Weisel, W., *et al.:* J. Urol., *50*, 399, 1943 (Wilms' Tumor).

32

Male Generative System

PATHOLOGIC PHYSIOLOGY

A. E. Rakoff

THE *testes* are the center of functional activity in the male reproductive system. As in the case of the ovaries, the function of the male gonads is stimulated by the gonadotropic hormones of the anterior pituitary. The *gonadotropic hormones* secreted by the *male pituitary* are identical qualitatively with those secreted by the female, namely FSH (follicle-stimulating hormone), LH (luteinizing hormone), and LTH (luteotropic hormone or prolactin), but there are quantitative differences in that in the male the proportion of FSH appears to be higher, and there is no regular cycling of the various gonadotropins as occurs in the female in conjunction with the menstrual cycle. *FSH* stimulates growth of the speramtic tubules and spermatogenesis. Whether it also stimulates the secretion of a hormone by the tubules is still a controversial subject. The secretion of such a hormone has been suspected on the basis of analogy to the secretion of estrogen by the growing ovarian follicles under FSH stimulation, and also because of the presence of high FSH in some conditions associated with hyalinization of the tubules but intact Leydig cells. It has been suggested that *estrogen*, secreted by the *Sertoli cells*, may be the tubular hormone. *LH* stimulates the *interstitial cells* of *Leydig* and the secretion by these cells of the *male sex hormone;* for this reason LH is sometimes also termed *ICSH* (interstitial-cell-stimulating hormone). The function of LTH in the male is not known, although it may act as a synergist with LH.

The male sex hormone secreted by the testis is *testosterone*—a steroid hormone with high androgenic activity. A number of steroids with less marked *androgenic activity* are also secreted by the adrenal cortex and indeed the latter accounts, by weight, for two thirds of the androgens excreted in the urine. Like estrogens, the androgens are metabolized and conjugated chiefly in the liver and excreted in the urine as a variety of steroids, the most important of which are androsterone, isoandrosterone, dehydroisoandrosterone, and etiocholanolone. Chemically, the *urinary* androgens are characterized by being neutral (nonphenolic) *ketosteroids* with a ketone group on the 17th carbon atom, and can be detected by a somewhat specific colorimetric reaction with metadinitrobenzene (Zimmerman reaction). Therefore, chemical determination of the neutral 17-ketosteroids serves as a measure of the urinary androgens, which in the male is an index of combined testicular and adrenal cortical activity, but only of the latter in the female.

The *biologic actions* of the *androgens* in the male include growth of the penis, prostate, and seminal vesicles. The stimulation of the epithelium and secretory functions of the accessory glands also are particularly influenced by androgens. Both alkaline and acid phosphatase activity are stimulated, along with an increase in the fructose content of the semen. Androgens are responsible for the secondary male sex characteristics such as growth of the beard and pubic and axillary hair as well as deepening of the voice. Closure of the epiphyses is also fostered by androgens. In addition, they exert many other metabolic effects including protein anabolism and favoring positive calcium balance and salt and water retention. Androgens also exert a back action on the pituitary and inhibit gonadotropin release.

There is good evidence to indicate that the testis also produces some *estrogen*, although there is a difference of opinion as to whether this arises from the Sertoli cells or the Leydig cells, or perhaps both. Small amounts of estrogen are also secreted by the adrenal cortex.

Most *disturbances* of *function* of the *male generative organs* arise from (1) genetic or acquired conditions affecting the testes or systemic, or (2) metabolic and extragonadal endocrine disturbances which may indirectly alter testicular function. Less commonly, functional genital tract disorders result from congenital abnormalities or acquired lesions of the prostate, seminal vesicles, epididymis, spermatic cord, or penis.

Hypofunction of the *testes* is more common than excessive activity. Although *congenital absence* of the testes is rare, the discovery that many of the apparent "females" with Turner's syndrome (p. 1145) are actually chromosomal males, increases the incidence of *anorchia* and also clarifies our understanding of some of the findings in *pseudohermaphroditism*. Absence of functioning testicular tissue in embryonic development leads to failure of development of the Wolffian system and permits development of the Müllerian derivatives. If the testes have been partially damaged during intra-uterine life, varying degrees and types of male pseudohermaphroditism may result depending upon the period of fetal development in which the defect occurred. Conversely, the secretion of excessive amounts of angdroen during fetal life in a female child with congenital adrenal hyperplasia will cause the appearance of a phallus (enlarged clitoris) and other evidences of female pseudohermaphroditism, often including a urogenital sinus.

Acquired deficiencies of the *testes* may involve both spermatogenic (tubular) and hormonal (Leydig cell) function, or either of these separately. If there is *failure* of *Leydig cell function* prior to puberty, the syndrome of *eunuchoidism* develops, which is characterized by rudimentary or absent testes, small penis, and lack of development of the accessory structures and secondary male sex characteristics. The epiphyses are late in closing so that the limbs become disproportionately long, causing "eunuchoid" skeletal proportions. This syndrome can result from castration, physical injuries to the testes (p. 1130), irradiation damage, inflammatory lesions (p. 1130) and (in some cases) cryptorchidism (p. 1128), although spermatogenesis is more often impaired than Leydig cell function in the latter condition. In these examples of *primary testicular failure* there is a high FSH excretion in the urine, diminished urinary 17-ketosteroids, and aspermia or marked oligospermia. *Prepubertal hypogonadism* may also result from a lesion in or near the pituitary or from a chronic systemic or metabolic disease such as celiac disease or ulcerative colitis, affecting the ability of the pituitary to secrete gonadotropic hormones. In such instances, FSH levels in the urine are low or absent and there may also be laboratory and clinical evidence of a deficiency in other tropic hormones of the pituitary . Occasionally, there may be a functional deficiency in the secretion of gonadotropic hormone alone without any apparent cause, producing the syndrome of pituitary eunuchoidism.

An *increase* in the *estrogen level*, either exogenously or endogenously produced, also causes testicular atrophy, primarily by inhibiting the gonadotropins and possibly also by a direct action on the testes. This may occur in cirrhosis of the liver in which the endogenous estrogen can not be properly inactivated by the damaged liver so that there is a high free estrogen level favoring gynecomastia and testicular atrophy. Estrogen-producing tumors of the testis may also produce *feminization* (see below). Similarly, a physiologic castration may be produced by the exogenous administration of estrogens. This principle is made use of in the treatment of metastatic carcinoma of the prostate, since this tumor is favored by the presence of androgen.

Leydig cell failure, resulting from these same etiologic factors after puberty, causes some decrease in the size of the penis and accessory organs, and also some regression of secondary sex characteristics but not their complete disappearance. Libido and potency diminish but in some instances may persist, since sexual patterns are partially controlled by endocrine factors and partially by acquired nervous system reflexes.

Testicular deficiency, in which there is seminal failure but normal or nearly normal Leydig cell function, is seen clinically in men with *sterility* but no clinical or laboratory evidence of male sex hormone deficiency. Among the *causes* for this state are (1) congenital defects affecting the seminiferous tubules but not the Leydig cells, (2) arrest in the maturation of the sperm beyond the stage of the primary spermatocytes or other defects in the process of spermatogenesis, and (3) progressive fibrosis of the tubules. Among the etiologic factors, other than genetic causes, that have been suspected for seminal failures of these types are systemic diseases, acute and chronic infections, malnutrition, vitamin deficienceis, diabetes, and hypothryoidism. Frequently, no etiologic factor can be found and attempts at treatment usually are discouraging. In men with aspermia, but normal Leydig cell function, *testicular biopsy* is helpful in determining whether the sterility is caused by an obstructive lesion in the vas or a spermatogenic defect. *Gonadotropin assays* are valuable in determining if a spermatogenic deficiency is caused by a primary testicular factor or secondary to pituitary hypofunction, while assays for *17-ketosteroids* help in deciding whether there is concomitant Leydig cell failure.

The *Klinefelter syndrome* is characterized not only by spermatogenic failure and normal or moderately diminished Leydig cell function, but also by the presence of gynecomastia and high urinary FSH. The testes are small and exhibit extensive pericanalicular fibrosis. The probability of a genetic defect is suggested by the finding of a "female" sex chromatin pattern in some cases of this syndrome.

In rare instances, *spermatogenesis* has been observed in *eunuchoid* men with clinical and laboratory evidence of poor Leydig cell function. However, the amount of ejaculate is small or absent.

The occurrence of a *climacteric* or *"menopausal" syndrome* in the male is much less frequent than in the female. Indeed, gonadal function and fertility may continue well into old age, and does not cease abruptly as it does in the female. In occasional instances, however, the male climacteric syndrome may occur in men in their fifties or sixties, characterized by vasomotor symptoms, nervous system disturbances, and loss of libido and potency, with associated high gonadotropin excretion in the urine. The differentiation from psychoneurosis is often difficult. The male climacteric syndrome responds promptly to testosterone therapy.

Hyperfunction of the testes occurs in association with certain tumors of the testis. Some growths, such as chorionepithelioma (p. 1133), secrete chorionic gonadotropic hormone, so that a positive pregnancy test may be obtained on examining of the urine or even serum. Gynecomastia usually is present in men with testicular chorionepitheliomas. In some instances, a moderate increase in the urinary estrogen level is obtained and the presence of pregnandiol has also occasionally been noted. In patients with *seminoma* (p. 1132) or nonfunctioning tumors of the testis, increased titers of gonadotropin of pituitary origin, usually FSH, is noted. Unless present in quite large amounts, however, this gonadotropin will not give a positive pregnancy test reaction but can be detected by other appropriate bio-assay methods. Occasionally, chorionic gonadotropin has been reported in cases of seminoma, but in these it is probable that teratoid tissue was present and overlooked. It is to be emphasized that not all teratoid tumors or seminomas of the testis are associated with increased excretion of gonadotropins and that the tests may be negative even in a widely metastasizing testicular tumor.

Interstitial cell (Leydig) tumors of the testes (p. 1132) secrete androgens, sometimes in enormously high amounts as indicated by 17-ketosteroid levels ranging, in one case, to more than 1000 mg. per 24 hours. If such a tumor occurs in childhood it causes masculinizing precocious pseudopuberty. In the adult, the endocrine effect is not really noticeable. Gynecomastia may occur in both adults and children. The explanation for this is not entirely clear. Atrophy of the nontumor bearing testicle is generally the rule.

Estrogen producing tumors of the testis are generally thought to be of *Sertoli cell* origin, although it has been suggested that some of these may be atypical Leydig cell tumors. Sertoli cell tumors are rare in humans but are found rather frequently in dogs. These tumors produce a syndrome of feminization and are attended by an increased excretion of estrogens in the urine.

The frequently discussed question of an *endocrine disturbance* as the *cause* for *testicular tumors* has been reviewed by Twombly. Although there appears to be a higher incidence of tumors of the cryptorchid testis, the role of cryptorchidism in tumorgenesis is still undecided. The higher incidence of testicular cancer in the years of active sexual life also suggests the possibility of a hormonal factor. In addition, testicular tumors including teratomas and Leydig cell tumors can be produced in various laboratory animals by altering the hromonal status of the animal.

GENERAL CONSIDERATIONS

In keeping with the descriptions in other portions of the text, the diseases of the Male Generative System will be considered from a regional rather than from a systemic point of view. Accordingly, they will be discussed under the headings of Penis, Prostate, Seminal Vesicles, Spermatic Cord, Epididymides, Testes, and Scrotum.

PENIS

CONGENITAL ANOMALIES

Developmental malformations of the penis may be listed as follows: (1) *hypoplasia*—small penis, (2) *hyperplasia*—large penis, (3) *curvature*—consisting of twisting with the frenum directed upward or of ventral or dorsal curvature usually associated with hypospadias and epispadias respectively, (4) *concealed*—location beneath the skin of the lower abdomen, scrotum, perineum, or thigh, (5) *adherent*—attachment of the under surface to the scrotum, (6) *absence*—rare, consisting of complete lack of penile tissue in the normal position, occasionally accompanied by nubbins of erectile tissue in the perineum or within the anus, and attended by a urethral opening anterior to the scrotum or uncommonly in the perineum, rectum, or anus (McCrae), (7) *duplication*—consisting of the presence of one or more penes in addition to the regular organ, varying in degree from duplication of the glans to complete duplication of the entire organ, and usually attended by duplication of the urethra corresponding in degree to that of the penis (Blanco and Davis), (8) *abnormalities* of the *genitoperineal raphe*—comprising squamous epithelial-lined canals and cysts that are located along the raphe of the penis, scrotum, or perineum and that are frequently complicated by secondary inflammation (Neff), (9) *bone formation*—most infrequent, rarely congenital, usually acquired, and consisting of osseous tissue or calcium deposition in the outer border of the erectile tissue just beneath the capsule or within the erectile tissue proper (Hirsch), (10) *short frenum*—causing curvature of the penis ventrally, (11) *absence* of *prepuce*, (12) *redundance* of *prepuce*, (13) *adherent prepuce* to *glans*—seen as a congenital lesion in association with phimosis and as an acquired lesion after inflammation, (14) *phimosis*—signifying (Gr. = closure) an opening of the prepuce small enough to prevent the foreskin from being drawn over the glans and often attended by inflammation and obstruction to the flow of urine, and (14) *paraphimosis*—connoting (Gr. = amiss + closure) retraction of a narrow preputial orifice over the glans with constriction and swelling of the penis.

DEGENERATIONS AND INFLAMMATIONS

Since the penis is covered with integument it is subjected to a variety of degenerations and inflammations similar to those affecting the skin of other portions of the body. Because these two broad groups of disease processes are usually intimately interwoven, they may be considered under one heading. Inflammation of the penis is known as *penitis*, of the glans penis as *balanitis*, of the prepuce as *posthitis*, of the glans and prepuce as *balanoposthitis*, and of the cavernous bodies as *cavernitis* or *cavernositis*. The more important lesions may be enumerated as follows: (1) *acute balanoposthitis*—common in persons with a redundant or phimotic prepuce, caused by the usual pyogenic organisms including gonococci, and attended by local itching, burning, pain, swelling, redness, and purulent discharge, (2) *diphtheria*—usually seen in newborn infants and grafted upon a recent circumcision (Borovsky), (3) *caruncle*—(p. 1027), (4) *erysipelas*—(p. 1330), (5) *cellulitis*—(p. 135), (6) *acute cavernositis*—caused by the usual pyogenic organisms, secondary to a local urethral or systemic infection, characterized by suppuration and destruction of the cavernous bodies, (7) *gangrene*—caused by (*a*) physical agents (such as trauma, chemicals, heat, or cold) alone, or (*b*) physical agents contaminated by virulent organisms (streptococci, staphylococci, colon bacilli, and *B. gangrenous cutis*) and characterized by an explosive inflammation with death and sloughing of the integument and immediately underlying tissues (McCrea), (8) *genital fusospirochætosis*—progressive and destructive ulceration starting in the vicinity of the cor-

onal sulcus and extending proximally and distally, caused by a fusiform
bacillus and spirochete both resembling those found in Vincent's angina
(p. 603), and complicated by mutilation of the penis or acquired phimosis
(von Hamm and Lev), (9) *chemical penitis*—consisting of a variety of
eczematoid lesions caused by sensitivity to rubber condoms, ephedrine,
sulphonamides, etc., (10) *metabolic balanoposthitis*—inflammatory fissures
and ulcers of the glans caused by irritation of urine in patients with diabetes
or other metabolic disorders (Madden), (11) *herpes progenitalis*—(p. 607),
(12) *plastic induration*—known also as *Peyronie's disease*, consisting of
collagenous fibrosis of the tunics surrounding the corpora cavernosa penis
or the separating septum, of unknown cause but thought to be part of a
fibrous diathesis, attended by curvature of the penis and pain upon erection,
variously treated (surgical excision, irradiation, diathermy, administration
of tocopherol, etc.), and resulting in a good prognosis in from 50 to 75 per
cent of cases (Calloman and Scott), (13) *tuberculosis*—rare, usually primary, contracted as a result of (*a*) ritual circumcision, (*b*) using sputum as
a penile lubricant, or (*c*) coitus from vaginal infection, generally involving
the glans penis, and characterized pathologically by an undermined ulcer
showing the typical histologic changes of tuberculosis (Lewis), (14) *syphilis*
—constituting the most common portal of entrance of *Treponema pallidum*
in males, virtually always acquired by sexual intercourse, and characterized
by (*a*) a *chancre*—appearing up to forty days after exposure as an elevated,
indurated, painless, 1 cm., superficial ulcer located on the mucosa of the
prepuce or glans penis (Fig. 544), possessing sloping edges and a clean floor
covered with serum, disclosing endothelial proliferation of the vessels and
perivascular infiltration with plasma cells and lymphocytes, attended by
painless enlargement of the draining lymph nodes, and disappearing with
or without treatment in from three to eight weeks, (*b*) *syphilids*—affecting
the skin of the shaft and appearing similar to those in the skin elsewhere
(p. 180), and (*c*) *condyloma latum*—located in moist areas such as around the
anus and in the folds between the perineum and scrotum, and composed of
elevated, macerated, cauliflower-like excrescences of loose connective
tissue covered with hyperplastic epithelium (Ormsby and Montgomery),
(15) *chancroid*—a genital lesion that looks like a chancre, caused by the
Hemophilus ducreyi which is harbored by prostitutes and transmitted by
sexual intercourse, consisting of a primary 1 to 2 cm. ulcer that, in males, is
located about the glans but spreads to the adjacent skin and, in females, is
located about the vulva and anus, and complicated by inflammation of
lymph nodes in the groin (bubos) in 50 per cent of cases (Sullivan and
Satulsky), (16) *lymphogranuloma venereum*—also called lymphopathia
venereum, caused by a virus, transmitted by sexual intercourse, consisting
of (*a*) an acute stage that is characterized by a primary evanescent papule,
vesicle, or erosion located on the glans penis in the male and on the vulva,
cervix, or vaginal mucosa in the female, (*b*) involvement, usually in males,
of inguinal lymph nodes (bubos) in from two to eight weeks after the appearance of the primary sore, and (*c*) chronic phase of the disease, usually
in females, characterized by stricture at the anorectal junction and elephantiasis (edema, ulceration, and fibrosis) of the vulva, composed histologically
of a central collection of neutrophils and nuclear fragments surrounded
peripherally by epithelioid cells (Fig. 545), diagnosed not only by the clinical appearance and biopsy but also by the Frei test, treated effectively by
sulfonamides, and attended by a good prognosis when treated early (Pund,
Koteen, and Smith), (17) *granuloma inguinale*—genital and extragenital

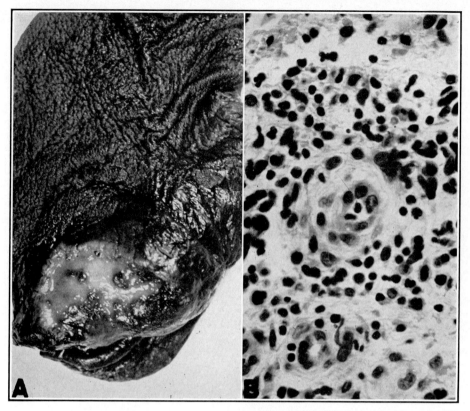

Fig. 544.—Chancre of the penis showing *A*, a rather large ulcer on the prepuce and *B*, characteristic endothelial proliferation and perivascular infiltration with plasma cells and lymphocytes. × 400.

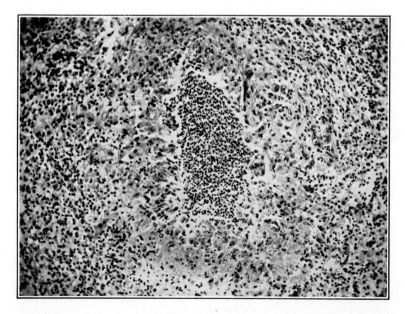

Fig. 545.—Lymphogranuloma venereum illustrating a typical stellate abscess composed centrally of neutrophils and peripherally of epithelioid cells. × 100. (Herbut's *Urological Pathology*.)

disease, occurring in both females and males, prevailing in Negroes over white people in the ratio of 10 to 1, caused by the *Donovania granulomatis* (encapsulated organism found within mononuclear cells in smears from the lesion and in histologic sections) (Fig. 546), initially showing a subcutaneous nodule measuring 1 to 4 cm. in diameter but later disclosing ulceration, cicatrization, and distortion, histologically consisting of a diffuse infiltration that is rich in neutrophils, plasma cells, and monocytes (containing *Donovania granulomatis*) but poor in lymphocytes, occasionally complicated by

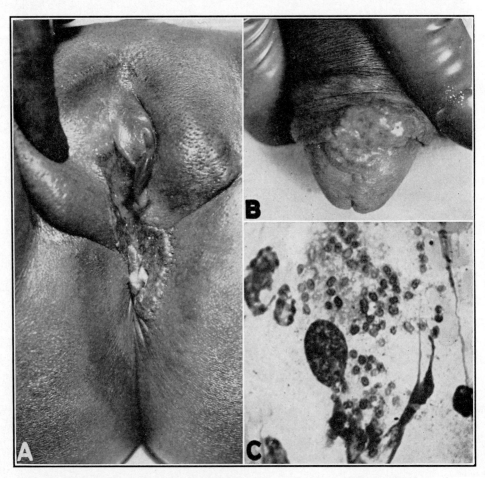

FIG. 546.—Granuloma inguinale demonstrating *A*, a relatively small ulcer of the perineum, vulva, and vagina, *B*, granular and ulcerating lesion of the glans and prepuce, and *C*, *Donovania granulomatis* within a monocyte in a smear of the pus. × 1350.

systemic dissemination, treated effectively by antimony compounds and antibiotics, and attended by a fair to good prognosis (D'Aunoy, Chen, Marshak, and Pund), (18) *balanitis xerotica obliterans*—an atrophic shrinking process affecting the glans penis and prepuce, associated with stenosis of the urethra, of unknown cause, characterized grossly by parchment-like ivory plaques and histologically by atrophy of the epidermis, disappearance of the rete pegs and hyalinization of the dermis, complicated occasionally by carcinoma, and responding poorly to treatment (Freeman and Farrington), and (19) *erythroplasia* of *Queyrat*—occurring principally on the glans penis, consisting grossly of an erythematous plaque and histologically of irregular hyperplasia of the epidermis, and sometimes complicated by a carcinomatous transformation (Klinger).

PHYSICAL DISTURBANCES

The important Physical Disturbances of the penis consist of the following: (1) *preputial calculi*—stones located in the space between the prepuce and glans penis, always associated with phimosis, originating in the upper urinary tract or locally, being single or multiple, measuring up to 8 cm. in diameter, and weighing as much as 224 gm. (Ingraham), (2) *incarceration*—rare, seen at all ages, caused by constriction of the penis by a variety of objects (strings, hairs, bushings, nuts, bottles, rings, etc.) and, depending upon the tightness of the constriction, disclosing redness, edema, ulceration, gangrene, and secondary infection (Hoffman), (3) *avulsion* of the *skin*—rare, consisting of denudation of a part or most of the skin of the penis and scrotum, and generally caused by catching a redundant prepuce in a revolving wheel of some type (Judd and Davis), (4) *contusion*—caused by direct trauma, characterized by the formation of a hematoma, and occasionally complicated by infection, (5) *fracture*—connoting rupture of the corpora cavernosa, usually occurring as a result of trauma to the erected but sometimes to the flaccid penis, and attended by urethral obstruction, loss of power of erection, and penile deformity (Fetter and O'Connor), (6) *dislocation*—rare, consisting of a traumatic displacement of the organ from its integument into the adjacent subcutaneous tissue, and complicated by urinary extravasation and infection (Curr), and (7) *priapism*—uncommon, defined as a persistent and painful erection unaccompanied by sexual desire, and caused by urethritis, carcinoma of the penis or urethra, vesical calculus, leukemia, metastatic tumors of the cavernous bodies, sickle cell anemia, and central nervous system lesions such as multiple sclerosis, syphilis, cord injury, and cerebral hemorrhage (Cave and Blazier).

TUMORS

Orientation.—Histogenetically tumors of the penis may be classified as follows: sebaceous cyst, Paget's disease, papilloma, carcinoma, fibroma, fibrosarcoma, glomus tumor, angioma, endothelioma, Kaposi's sarcoma, myoma, lipoma, melanoblastoma, lymphoblastoma, sarcoma, teratoma, and secondary tumors. Of these, only papilloma and carcinoma are frequent enough to warrant separate discussion.

Papilloma.—Papillomas of the penis are of two types—penile horn and condyloma acuminatum. The *penile horn* is a papilloma disclosing masses of proliferated prickle cells covered with an overabundance of keratin (Winterkoff). The base is broad while the free end is tapering and the structure may measure as much as 9 cm. in length and 4 cm. in diameter. The condition usually occurs as the result of prolonged irritation by a long prepuce and it may be complicated by carcinoma. *Condyloma acuminatum*, also known as venereal wart, connotes a tapering wart. The condition is most frequent in early adult life and is caused by a virus. In males, the lesions are located on the inner surface of the prepuce, coronal sulcus, glans, or body of the penis while in females, they are usually present about the labia and vagina.　In both sexes they may occur around the anus umbilicus, axillæ, face, and even within the mouth (Gersh and Culp). *Grossly* the disorder usually consists of multiple, sessile to pedunculated, pink to gray, wart-like elevations measuring not more than 1 cm. in diameter.　*Histologically* the nodules are composed of finger-like papillary projections of well-vascularized connective tissue covered with hyperplastic nonkeratinizing epithelium.　The condition is usually accompanied by a discharge and foul odor due to secondary infection.　The lesions *respond* readily to treatment with podophyllin.

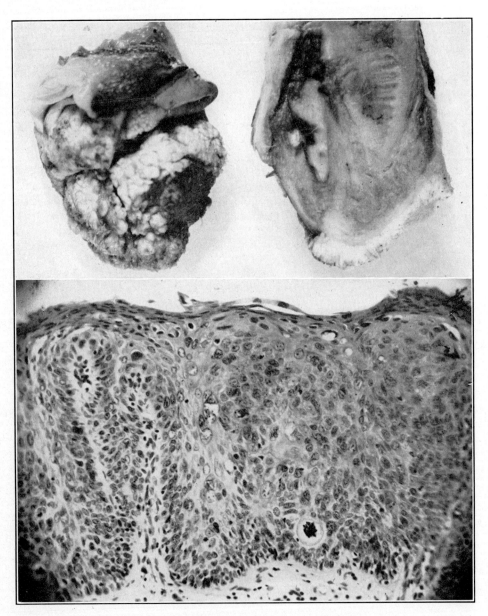

Fig. 547.—Carcinoma of the penis showing a fungating tumor affecting most of the glans grossly and a squamous cell growth still limited by the basement membrane microscopically.　× 200.

Carcinoma.—Carcinoma is the most important malignant tumor of the penis and is said to constitute from 1 to 3 per cent of all cancers in males (Colon). It usually *occurs* between the ages of forty and seventy years, and although it affects most races it is practically nonexistent in Jews and Mohammedans—those races who practice circumcision at birth (Harlin). Thus, it follows that a long prepuce complicated by phimosis, accumulation of smegma, and secondary infection acts as a predisposing *cause*.

Pathologically the more common sites of origin are frenum, inner surface of the prepuce, surface of the glans, and junction of the meatus with the glans while the less common sites are external surface of the prepuce and skin of the shaft (Lenowitz). The lesion may start as an eczematous patch, papule, nodule, ulcer, or leukoplakia. As it increases in size it assumes one of two forms—papillary or infiltrating. A *papillary* tumor exfoliates on the surface as a fungating, cauliflower-like growth with a rough, serrated, or superficially ulcerated surface and a broad base that is firmly united with the underlying structures (Fig. 547). In the early stages it is localized to a small area but in later stages it may measure several centimeters in diameter and may cover the entire glans or most of the inner surface of the prepuce. Cut surfaces disclose grayish-white tissue that penetrates only superficially. An *infiltrating* tumor grows beneath the surface. As it penetrates the underlying tissues it usually ulcerates, producing a crater 3 or more cm. in diameter. It thus mutilates the penis more than does the papillary growth. *Histologically* carcinoma of the penis is of a squamous nature and is generally fairly well differentiated. Initially, it is confined by the basement membrane and exists as irregular polyhedral prickle cells disclosing varying amounts of cytoplasm and varisized, relatively large, hyperchromatic nuclei (Fig. 547). Mitoses are often abundant. As the growth penetrates the basement membrane, it exists as masses and nests of keratinizing epithelial cells permeating first the connective tissue and then even the cavernous bodies. The tumor *spreads* by (1) direct extension to involve and destroy most of the penis, (2) lymphatics to the inguinal and less often deep femoral and perirectal lymph nodes, and (3) blood vessels (rarely) to the lungs, liver, and other organs (Dean and Hudson). Aside from extension and metastasis, the *complications* consist of fistulous tract formation with the urethra and skin, obstruction of the urethra, infection, and hemorrhage. The *clinical manifestations* consist of tumor and, as a result of infection, itching, burning, pain, purulent discharge, and painful urination. The final *diagnosis* is made by biopsy. *Treatment* consists of prophylaxis by way of circumcision at birth (Bleich) and of amputation of the penis or irradiation therapy once the lesion has developed (Dean and Lenowitz). The *prognosis* is fair to good, with an expected five-year survival of about 50 per cent.

PROSTATE

CONGENITAL ANOMALIES

Developmental abnormalities of the prostate are few and generally not too important. They may be listed as follows: (1) *hypoplasia*, (2) *aplasia*, (3) *median bar*—proliferation of prostatic tissue spanning the vesical exit of the urethra and either of congenital or acquired origin, (4) *fistulas*—connecting the prostate with the rectum in cases of persistent cloaca and the prostate with the kidney in cases of ectopic ureteral opening, (5) *cysts*—being (*a*) congenital—arising in the prostate proper, wolffian bodies, or

mullerian ducts, and being single, large, and located in the midline and
superior portion of the prostate or (*b*) acquired—arising as a result of retention of secretions or breakdown of septa in adenomatous hyperplasia
and being multiple, small, and located in any portion of the prostate
(Emmett, Lazarus, and Dees), and (6) *diverticula*—cavities communicating
with the urethra and being (*a*) congenital—due to malformations of the
prostatic acini and generally consisting of a single outpocketing measuring
4 to 5 cm. in diameter or (*b*) acquired—due to rupture of prostatic abscesses
and consisting of small, intercommunicating, branched outpocketings
(Senger and Hock).

DEGENERATIONS

Degenerative disorders of the prostate always accompany the various
disease processes. In addition, however, an important lesion from a differential histologic point of view that may be put in this category is *squamous
metaplasia* of the prostatic acini. The specific *cause* of the condition is

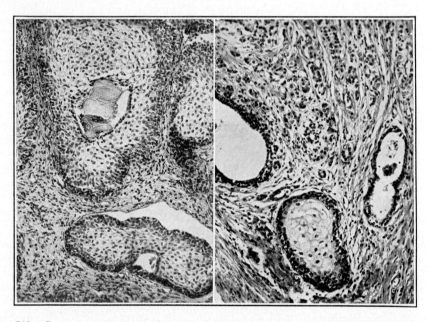

F ig. 548.—Squamous metaplasia of the prostate occurring (on the left) in connection with
hypertrophy and (on the right) in connection with carcinoma. × 100. (Herbut's *Urological
Pathology*).

unknown but the lesion has been noted to occur in connection with prostatic trauma (transurethral resection), infarction, inflammation, hypertrophy, and carcinoma and in connection with estrogenic therapy and
avitaminosis A (Baird, Mostofi, and Nanson). If *gross* changes are present
in the prostate they are those of the primary condition. *Histologically* the
acini are filled with polyhedral, squamous-like cells showing an abundant
amount of cytoplasm and round or oval, small, centrally placed nuclei
(Fig. 548). Intercellular bridges, however, are usually not seen. As far
as is known, the condition does not become malignant and its greatest
importance is its differentiation from occult squamous cell carcinoma.

INFLAMMATIONS

Inflammation of the prostate gland is known as *prostatitis*. The more important lesions may be listed as follows: (1) *nonspecific prostatitis*—predisposed by prostatic trauma (masturbation, prolonged sexual excitement, alcoholism, instrumentation, etc.), caused by any of the pyogenic organisms (colon bacilli, staphylococci, streptococci, and gonococci) that usually gain entrance from the posterior urethra but occasionally come by way of the bloodstream, consisting (*a*) grossly of enlargement of the gland with or without permeation with pus and of fibrosis, and (*b*) microscopically of neutrophilic infiltration in the acini and stroma in the acute stage and of plasma cell, lymphocytic, and monocytic infiltration and fibrosis in the chronic stage, readily mistaken for carcinoma in the chronic stage, complicated by urethral obstruction and occasionally by systemic spread of the infection, attended clinically by local pain, frequency, urinary disturbances, and erythrocytes and leukocytes in the urine, treated primarily by antibiotics and chemotherapeutic agents and secondarily (chronic cases) by prostatic massage, electrocoagulation, etc., and responding satisfactorily to treatment in from two-thirds to three-quarters of all cases (Buchert, Fetter, Peterson, and Cumming), (2) *abscess*—consisting of one or more focal collections of pus, generally occurring as a progression of nonspecific prostatitis, and frequently secondary to distant foci of infection such as pneumonia, furuncle, carbuncle, abscessed teeth, etc. (Schwartz and Forsythe), (3) *granulomatous prostatitis*—occurring as a foreign body reaction to retained secretions in nonspecific prostatitis, found at all ages frequently mistaken for tuberculosis, and consisting of complete replacement of the acini by focal collections of neutrophils, plasma cells, lymphocytes, normal and reticulated monocytes, and occasionally foreign body giant cells (Tanner and Baker), (4) *tuberculosis*—almost always secondary to tuberculosis of other portions of the genito-urinary tract and (less commonly) distant foci, occurring as a result of entrance of the organisms by way of the prostatic ducts or (less frequently) hematogeneously, occasionally consisting of miliary tubercles but more often being of a fibrocaseous nature, complicated by extension along the paravertebral veins to the meninges and directly to adjacent structures, manifested by local obstructive symptoms and general manifestations of tuberculosis, treated by the usual antituberculosis measures and by local removal (transurethral resection or prostatectomy) when obstruction arises, and attended by a guarded prognosis (Baker, Auerbach, Nesbit, and de la Pena), (5) *syphilis*—rare and consisting either of gummas or of a diffuse type of chronic inflammatory response (Crowley), (6) *fungous* and *yeast-like prostatitis*—rare and consisting principally of coccidioidomycosis and blastomycosis and generally occurring as part of a systemic infection, and (7) *parasitic prostatitis*—rare and consisting of trichomoniasis, schistosomiasis, and echinococcosis.

PHYSICAL DISTURBANCES

The more important Physical Disturbances of the prostate consist of (1) *infarction*—occurring most often as a result of trauma (instrumentation, catheters, physical examination, constipation, etc.) or of relative ischemia secondary to irregular growth, producing no characteristic clinical manifestations, always accompanied by benign hypertrophy of the prostate, appearing grossly as a sharply circumscribed area of hemorrhagic discoloration that measures as much as 3 to 4 cm. in diameter, consisting histologically of varying degrees of tissue necrosis and, at the periphery, of squamous metaplasia, and rarely complicated by infection and abscess formation (Rogers, Baird, and Mostofi), (2) *calculi*—occurring after the age of forty years, arising on the basis of obstruction of prostatic acini, complicated by infection, formed around corpora amylacea, located in any portion

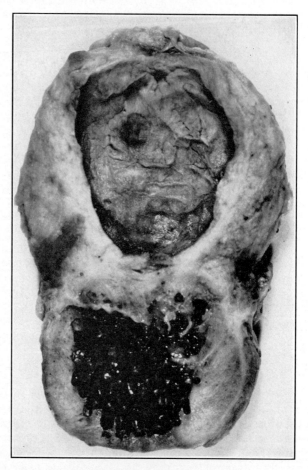

FIG. 549.—Prostatic calculi illustrating innumerable black stones
within the right lobe of the organ.

of the prostate, generally being multiple and measuring 3 to 4 mm. in diameter (Fig. 549), varying in color from gray to black, and complicated by infection and rarely carcinoma (Ward, Henline, and Gentile), (3) *complications following prostatectomy*—consisting of hemorrhage (primary or secondary), incontinence (from disturbance of sphincters), infection, osteitis pubis, pulmonary embolism, coronary artery occlusion, oliguria and uremia, cerebral hemorrhage, impotency, subsequent benign prostatic hypertrophy, subsequent carcinoma, calcification in cystotomy wound, and fibrous occlusion of the vesicourethral orifice (Jacobs).

TUMORS

Orientation.—Histogenetically tumors of the prostate may be classified as follows: benign hypertrophy, adenoma, carcinoma, fibroma, fibrosarcoma, myxoma, myxosarcoma, leiomyoma, leiomyosarcoma, rhabdomyosarcoma, angioma, hemangioendothelioma, lymphoblastoma, neurofibroma, neurofibrosarcoma, chondroma, chondrosarcoma, and secondary growths. Of these, only benign hypertrophy and carcinoma are common enough to warrant further consideration.

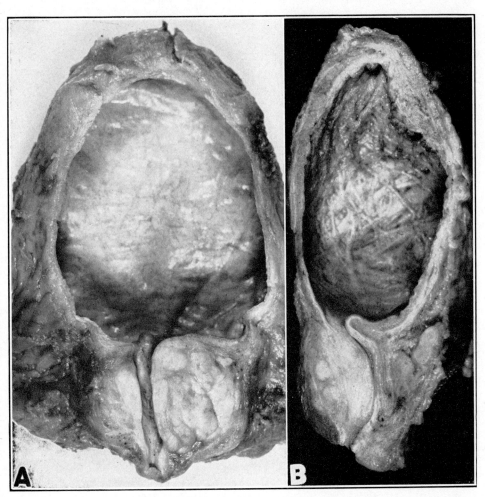

Fig. 550.—Benign hypertrophy of the prostate demonstrating *A*, enlargement of lateral lobes and *B*, enlargement of the anterior lobe with dislocation of the urethra.

Benign Hypertrophy.—Benign hypertrophy of the prostate is *also known* as hyperplasia, fibroglandular hyperplasia, benign prostatic hypertrophy, adenomatous hypertrophy, nodular hyperplasia, and benign enlargement. The condition usually *occurs* in patients beyond the age of forty-five years and increases in incidence until about 80 per cent of men beyond eighty years of age are affected (Moore). Although the *cause* of the enlargement in man is not definitely known, it is thought that it arises on the basis of a stimulant originating in the testes and acting over a prolonged period (Huggins). It is further thought that this stimulant is androgenic because prostatic hypertrophy is not seen in feminized dogs and castration (in dogs and man) brings about decrease in height of acinar cells and shrinkage of the gland. *Experimentally* prostatic hypertrophy may be produced in Macacus monkeys, mice, rats, and guinea pigs by administration of estrogens (Lipschutz).

Pathologically the enlargement may start either in the periurethral glands in the vicinity of the prostate or in the prostate proper. In the prostate, any part of the gland may serve as the point of origin but most often it is the middle and lateral lobes that are involved (Fig. 550). The enlargement starts as multiple, circumscribed nodules that steadily increase in size to ultimately produce a gland that may weigh as much as 820 gm. (Ockerblad). As the nodules coalesce and enlarge they gradually push aside the original prostatic tissue until it forms a peripheral capsule. Simultaneously they encroach upon the urethra causing X-shaped, Y-shaped, and other distortions. Regardless of their location, the nodules are moderately firm, fairly sharply circumscribed, and pinkish gray. They bulge on cut surface and are bathed in a milky fluid. *Histologically* they are composed of varying degrees of proliferation of fibrous tissue, muscle tissue, and glands. Sometimes one of these elements proliferates almost exclusively at the expense of the other two but generally all three are intermixed. The glands may be small, may disclose papillary projections into the lumen, and may be lined with tall columnar cells or they may be large, cystic, and lined with low cuboidal cells (Fig. 551). In either case, they contain corpora amylacea, fluid, and degenerated epithelial cells and phagocytes. The prostatic tissue adjacent to the nodules is usually compressed and atrophic.

The more common *complications* consist of (1) urethral obstruction, (2) infection of and stone formation in the more proximal portion of the urinary tract, (3) prostatic hemorrhage (from infection and ulceration), (4) prostatic carcinoma (as an associated lesion rather than a result), and (5) systemic (cardiovascular, etc.) disorders commensurate with the age of the patient (Higgins). The *clinical manifestations* are due to urethral obstruction, infection, and encroachment upon the vesical sphincters. They consist of frequency, difficulty in starting the stream, diminished force of stream, nocturia, dysuria, dribbling, hematuria, and urinary retention. Rectal examination discloses symmetrical enlargement of the prostate; a cystourethrogram reveals distortion of the urethra (Colby), and urinalysis usually shows leukocytes, erythrocytes, and albumin. The *diagnosis* is made from the history, clinical manifestations, rectal examination, and cystoscopic appearance of the enlargement. *Treatment* is indicated when obstruction occurs and consists of transurethral resection or prostatectomy (suprapubic or perineal). The *prognosis* in nonobstructive cases and in obstructive cases treated surgically is good, while that in obstructive cases not treated surgically is poor.

Carcinoma.—Carcinoma of the prostate is one of the more *common* tumors of the body. It is rare before the age of forty-five years but increases steadily thereafter. As a whole, it is said to constitute about 10 per cent of all cancers in males (Dixon and Moore), to occur in an occult form in from 14 to 46 per cent of all prostates in men over the age of fifty years (Rich and Baron), and to account for over 8,000 deaths in the United States each year. The *cause* of prostatic carcinoma is unknown but its origin is thought to be related to sex hormones. This contention is supported *clinically* by the following: (1) stimulation of growth by injection of androgens, (2) inhibition of growth by castration or injection of estrogens, and (3) increase of appetite, relief of pain, gain in weight, and improvement in anemia after castration (Huggins). *Experimentally*, growth of carcinoma of the prostate can be initiated in the anterior chamber of the eye of the guinea pig in males and pregnant females but not in castrated males or nonpregnant females, indicating that androgens are necessary for its establishment (Deming).

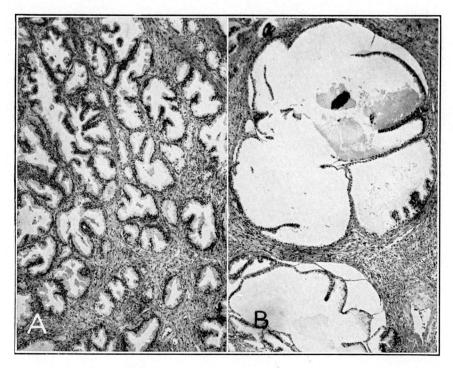

Fig. 551.—Benign hypertrophy showing *A*, numerous glands with papillary infoldings lined by tall columnar epithelial cells and *B*, cystically dilated glands lined by low cuboidal epithelium. × 50.

Pathologically the growth may arise in any part of the gland but most commonly it starts in the posterior lobe near the outer border (Rich, Moore, and Kahler). The initial lesion is better felt than seen. It exists as a single nodule or as multiple nodules that protrude beneath the prostatic fascia toward the rectum. As the growth expands, it gradually involves more and more of the prostate until a large portion or the entire organ is affected (Fig. 552). The tumor is generally ill defined, grayish white to yellowish, and extremely firm. *Histologically* the lesion is, in most instances, an adenocarcinoma showing varying degrees of differentiation (Fig. 553). Most commonly the tumor forms small, well-defined glands composed of relatively regular appearing cuboidal or columnar cells with regular basal nuclei. In fact, so innocuous may the lesion appear that it can be distinguished from a benign hyperplasia only by (1) diffuse permeation of the glands rather than their usual lobular formation, (2) penetration of the capsule of the prostate, or (3) the presence of the glands or cells in blood vessels or perineural lymphatic channels. As the tumor becomes more malignant, however, it generally discloses a greater variation in appearance of the cells and its differentiation from benign hyperplasia becomes easier. Aside from adenocarcinoma, carcinoma of the prostate may also be of a squamous cell nature. The term *occult carcinoma* is reserved for lesions that

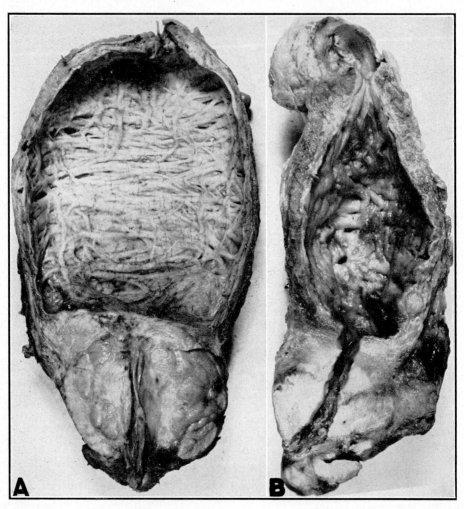

Fig. 552.—Carcinoma of the prostate illustrating *A*, a gray tumor affecting the lateral sub-capsular portion of the right lateral lobe and *B*, a grayish-white tumor involving most of the prostate and encroaching upon the urethra.

are so small that they are undetected clinically. Carcinoma of the prostate *spreads* by (1) local extension to the urethra, vesical orifice of the bladder, seminal vesicles, vasa deferentia, perineum, ureters, and pelvic tissues, (2) lymphatics to the pelvic, lumbar, thoracic, and supraclavicular lymph nodes, and (3) blood vessels to the lower vertebræ, pelvis, liver, lungs, and other tissues. Of all sites of metastasis, bones deserve special mention. They are often involved early—even before the primary lesion is detected, and the metastasis elicits an osteoblastic reaction that is readily demonstrable roentgenographically as an increase in osseous density. Along with metastasis to the bones, the serum acid phosphatase level is increased (due to the action of the neoplastic cells themselves) above the normal ten unit level in over 85 per cent of cases (Huggins and Creevy).

Aside from metastasis, the chief *complication* of carcinoma of the prostate is obstruction of the urinary tract. The *clinical manifestations* consist of (1) frequency, dysuria, nocturia, decrease in force of the urinary stream, and later urinary retention—due to obstruction of the urethra and infection of the posterior urethra and trigone of the urinary gladder, (2) pain in the

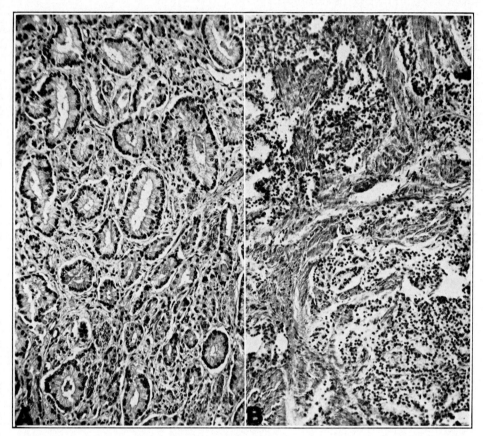

Fig. 553.—Carcinoma of the prostate demonstrating *A*, the usual well-defined adenomatous type of growth composed of columnar and cuboidal cells and *B*, a more irregular and anaplastic type of lesion. × 100.

pelvis, bones, etc.—due to involvement of nerves and bones by tumor, and (3) late systemic manifestations of anemia, weakness, loss of weight, loss of strength, etc.—due to tumor cachexia, metastasis, and replacement of bone marrow by neoplastic, osteoblastic, and fibrous tissue cells. Rectal examination discloses irregular nodularity of the prostate. Cystoscopy reveals encroachment of the tumor on the urethra or bladder. Cysto-urethrograms also show the encroachment of the tumor on the urinary tract and roentgenograms of the bones reveal osteoblastic changes in cases of metastasis. The *diagnosis* is made from the history, rectal examination, roentgenograms, serum acid phosphatase elevation, and biopsy. Cytologic examination of prostatic secretions may be of value in doubtful cases (Herbut). By way of differential diagnosis, the osseous changes may be confused with Paget's disease. *Treatment* consists of total prostatectomy when the lesion is small and of palliative transurethral resection, orchiectomy, estrogenic therapy, or bilateral adrenalectomy when the local tumor is not removable (Hudson and Harrison). The final *prognosis* of carcinoma of the prostate is poor with most patients ultimately dying of the disease. The chief reason for the poor outcome is late diagnosis. With modern methods of hormonal therapy, however, satisfactory palliation is often achievable for years.

SEMINAL VESICLES

Diseases of the seminal vesicles are intimately associated with diseases of the prostate. The more important lesions may be listed as follows: (1) *Congenital Anomalies*—consisting of absence, hypoplasia, duplication, stricture, entrance of ectopic ureter, and cysts, (2) *Degenerations*—consisting of calcification and being either on a postinflammatory or purely degenerative basis, (3) *Inflammations*—consisting of nonspecific seminal vesiculitis (caused by the usual pyogenic organisms and generally associated with prostatitis), abscess (sequel to nonspecific inflammation), and tuberculosis (almost always secondary to tuberculosis of other portions of the genitourinary tract), (4) *Physical Disturbances*—consisting of calculi, hemorrhage (generally traumatic, inflammatory, or idiopathic and constituting one cause of hemospermia), and fistula (being congenital and disclosing a connection with an ectopic ureter or acquired traumatic, inflammatory, or neoplastic and disclosing a connection with the urethra, prostate, or rectum), and (5) *Tumors*—consisting more commonly of secondary tumors (extension from the prostate, rectum, etc.) and rarely of primary tumors chief among which are leiomyoma, carcinoma, and sarcoma.

SPERMATIC CORD

The spermatic cord (also called funiculus spermaticus) connects each epididymis with the corresponding seminal vesicle and consists of the vas deferens, arteries, lymphatics, nerves, and stroma of fat and connective tissue. The more common disorders may be listed as follows: (1) *Congenital Anomalies*—consisting of absence, atresia, or duplication of the vas deferens and shortening, elongation, or displacement of the cord as a whole (Nelson, Coe, and Mathé), (2) *Degenerations*—consisting essentially of calcification of the vas deferens, (3) *Inflammations*—called *funiculitis* when the entire cord is affected and *deferentitis* when the vas deferens alone is involved and generally consisting of (*a*) *nonspecific funiculitis* and *deferentitis*—caused by the ordinary pyogenic organisms (including gonococci), occurring (1) as a complication of posterior urethritis, (2) as a result of metastasis from a distant focus, or (3) as a result of extension from adjacent structures, accompanied by pain, swelling, and tenderness along the course of the spermatic cord, and responding well to antibiotic and chemotherapy (Ibrahim, Power, and Oeconomos), (*b*) *thromboangiitis obliterans* (p. 374), (*c*) *tuberculosis*—secondary to tuberculosis of the epididymis or seminal vesicle and consisting of small nodular lesions or of a tuberculoma (Heckel), (*d*) *syphilis*—extremely rare, (*e*) *lymphogranuloma venereum* (p. 1112), and (*f*) *filiariasis* (p. 379), (4) *Physical Disturbances*—consisting of (*a*) *torsion*—precipitated by strong contraction of the cremasteric muscle and predisposed by hypermobility of the testis, tumor of the testis, long or absent mesorchium, abnormalities of the gubernaculum testis, and long spermatic cord, occurring at all ages but more common in children, complicated by gangrene of the epididymis and testis, and accompanied clinically by sudden excruciating pain, nausea, and vomiting (Campbell and Peck), (*b*) *varicocele*—consisting of dilatation and tortuosity of the veins of the pampiniform plexus, occurring at all ages, located mostly on the left side, and being idiopathic or secondary to occlusion of the spermatic vein or its tributaries by renal tumors, hydronephrosis, hepatic congestion, constipation, muscular strain, etc. (Campbell, Palomo, and Skinner), (*c*) *severance* of *vas deferens*—accidental or purposeful to prevent ascending infection or to produce sterility (O'Conor), (*d*) *hematoma*, and (*e*) *fistula*, and (5) *Tumors*—consisting of benign and malignant tumors of virtually all the tissues that compose the spermatic cord but more commonly being of a fatty nature (lipoma and liposarcoma) and corresponding both pathologically and clinically to similar tumor in other portions of the body (Thompson, Schulte, and Strong).

EPIDIDYMIDES

CONGENITAL ANOMALIES

Developmental malformations of the epididymides consist of the following: (1) *absence*, (2) *duplication*, (3) *failure* to *descend*—situated at any point along its normal descent from the abdomen and associated with failure of descent of the testes (Lazarus), (4) *anomalous position*—generally located anterior to the testis (Waddy), (5) *failure* of *fusion* with the *testis*, (6) *adrenal inclusions* (Freeman), (7) *Walthard cell rests*—rare and located on the serosa, and (8) *cysts*—consisting of dilatations of the epididymis proper, appendix of the testis (hydatid of Morgagni), appendix of the epididymis, paradidymis, and cysts of the vas aberrans, being unilocular or multilocular, and generally measuring less than 1 cm. in diameter but occasionally (as in cysts of the epididymis proper) containing a liter or more of fluid, lined by attenuated epithelial cells, and usually filled with clear or opalescent fluid that may or may not contain spermatozoa (Campbell, McCrae, and Wakeley).

INFLAMMATIONS

Inflammation of the epididymis is known as *epididymitis*. The lesions may be classified as follows: (1) *nonspecific epididymitis*—caused by the usual pyogenic organisms (gonococci, staphylococci, streptococci, colon bacilli, etc.), occurring as a result of extension from the posterior urethra and, less commonly, as metastasis from distant areas, seen at all ages but predominating in the third decade of life, generally affecting only one side, consisting of nonspecific permeation with neutrophils, complicated by abscess and hydrocele, attended clinically by local pain and tenderness and by chills, fever, nausea, vomiting, etc., and responding well to supportive measures and antibiotic and chemotherapy (Robertson, Tunbridge, and Handley), (2) *tuberculosis*—of common occurrence, generally seen in younger adults, usually secondary to tuberculosis of the genitourinary tract, often unaccompanied by symptoms unless the bladder is also affected, as a rule consisting of a fibrocaseous lesion, and complicated by secondary infection with abscess formation, scrotal fistula, and hydrocele (Auerbach and Borthwick), (3) *syphilis*—rare, unilateral in 90 per cent of cases, and consisting of a diffuse or gummatous type of infection (Cokely), (4) *blastomycosis*—extremely rare and always part of a disseminated process (Jacobson), (5) *filariasis* (p. 379), and (6) *mumps epididymitis*—associated with a similar lesion in the testis.

PHYSICAL DISTURBANCES

In this section the following disorders may be listed: (1) *wounds*, (2) *contusions*—usually resulting from a kick or fall (Halpert), (3) *traumatic epididymo-orchitis*—caused by trauma, consisting of massive swelling and edema, and attended by considerable pain (Henline and Mason), (4) *foreign bodies*—extremely rare and consisting of objects brought in from the outside, (5) *infarction*—resulting from torsion of the spermatic cord, and (6) *torsion* of the *appendix testis* and *appendix epididymis* (Seidel).

TUMORS

As in the spermatic cord, benign and malignant tumors of the epididymis may arise from virtually all other tissues that normally compose this structure. The more common benign growths consist of benign mesothelioma or adenomatoid tumor (p. 904), cholesteatoma, lipoma, and leiomyoma while the more common malignant tumors consist of carcinoma, fibrosarcoma, and secondary growths (Longo, Gibson, Falk, and Glaser). The only clinical manifestation is a mass in the region of the epididymis and the only way a definitive diagnosis can be made is by pathologic examination of the removed mass. The prognosis depends upon the type of neoplasm.

TESTES

CONGENITAL ANOMALIES

Developmental malformations of the testes may be outlined as follows: (1) *anorchidism*—complete absence of testes, rare, accompanied by a feminine habitus and lack of sexual desire, and associated with anomalies of the epididymides and spermatic cord (Hepburn), (2) *monorchidism*—absence of one testis only, exhibiting no physical changes, and associated with anomalies of the epididymis and spermatic cord on the homolateral side (Kawaichi), (3) *polyorchidism*—more than two testes, present in the scrotum or more superiorly, and serviced by a separate or a common vas deferens (Handley), (4) *synorchidism*—fusion of the two testes, located in the abdomen or the scrotum, and being extremely rare, (5) *cryptorchidism*—failure of complete descent of the testis from its abdominal position, also known as undescended testis or testicond, occurring in approximately 1 per cent of the population, thought to result from (*a*) a hereditary defect, (*b*) hormonal imbalances, or (*c*) some mechanical obstruction, being unilateral or bilateral and (when unilateral) more common on the right than on the left side, disclosing no pathologic change until after puberty when it reveals distinct tubular atrophy, characterized clinically by absence of the testis in the scrotum, and complicated by (*a*) hernia, (*b*) sterility (when bilateral), and (*c*) cancerous transformation (probably not more often than in a normal testis), and treated by (*a*) watchful waiting, (*b*) hormones, or (*c*) orchio-pexy (Lewis), (6) *ectopia*—displacement outside of its normal position and normal line of descent, occurring about once in every 25,000 males, and being interstitial (superficial inguinal), puboperineal, femoral, transverse (both testes in the same scrotal sac arriving by way of the same inguinal canal), perineal, or pelvic in position (Hunt), (7) *hyperplasia*—of unknown cause and rare, (8) *hermaphroditism*—(p. 1182), (9) *pseudohermaphroditism*—(p. 1182), (10) *rests*—adrenal or splenic, and (11) *abnormalities* of the *processus vaginalis*—consisting of a distinct band, partial or complete patency, or cysts.

DEGENERATIONS

The only important degenerative change as such in the testis is *atrophy*. Although this is an acquired lesion it differs from a congenital process known as *hypoplasia* and the two may therefore be considered together.

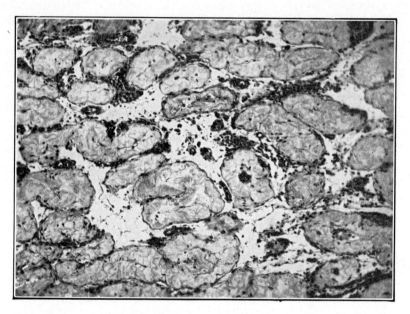

FIG. 554.—Atrophy of the testes showing complete replacement of the tubular cells with hyaline substance.

The *causes* of *atrophy* are arteriosclerosis, syphilis, tuberculosis, leprosy, mumps, hypothyroidism, hyperthyroidism, anterior pituitary deficiency, diabetes mellitus, adrenocortical disturbance, hepatic insufficiency (due to failure of inactivation of estrogens), malnutrition, avitaminosis A and B, fever, alcoholism, tumors, trauma, circulatory disturbances, obstruction of the genital ducts, irradiation, and androgenic or estrogenic therapy. The causes of *hypoplasia* are cryptorchidism, defective germ plasm, congenital obstruction of the genital duct system, congenital endocrine deficiency, and idiopathic (Rather, Werner, Engle, and Pollak).

Pathologically the process may be unilateral or bilateral. The organ is generally of normal shape but reduced in size. The tunica vaginalis is thickened; the cut surface presents a homogeneously gray appearance, and the tubules do not pull away in a string-like fashion. *Histologically* there is a gradual disappearance of the testicular cells starting with spermatozoa and affecting, in turn, spermatids, spermatocytes, spermatogonia, and finally Sertoli cells. As the cells disappear, the basement membrane becomes progressively hyalinized and finally the entire tubule is replaced with a hyaline mass (Fig. 554). The interstitial tissue may show fibrosis and the interstitial cells of Leydig may reveal focal hyperplasia. The most important *complication* is sterility. It occurs only when both testes are involved.

INFLAMMATIONS

Inflammation of the testis (orchis) is known as *orchitis* or *orchiditis*, of the tissues around the testis as *periorchitis*, and of the tunica vaginalis as *vaginalitis*. The more important inflammations may be listed as follows: (1) *nonspecific orchitis*—simple inflammation caused by the usual pyogenic (including gonococci) organisms, rather uncommon, almost always representing a progression of epididymitis, attended by the same clinical manifestations as epididymitis, usually unilateral, disclosing nonspecific congestion, edema, and leukocytic (mostly neutrophilic) infiltration, and complicated by abscess formation, hydrocele, fibrosis, and sterility (Campbell and Clem), (2) *abscess*—nonspecific orchitis with suppuration, (3) *vaginalitis* —caused by bacteria, chemicals, or trauma and usually associated with hydrocele (p. 1130), (4) *brucellosis*—part of a systemic infection (Sanborn), (5) *mumps orchitis*—occurring in from one-quarter to one-third of all cases of mumps developing in adult males, usually unilateral, consisting essentially of interstitial congestion and edema and secondarily of atrophy of tubular cells, occurring clinically as a painful testicular swelling just before the parotid swelling subsides, and complicated by extension of the inflammation to adjacent tissues, testicular atrophy but (since the process is unilateral) rarely sterility, and hydrocele (Werner, Charny, and Gall), (6) *tuberculosis*—almost always seen as an extension of tuberculous epididymitis and being similar to the latter clinically and pathologically (Thomas and Auerbach), (7) *syphilis*—rather common, of diminished incidence in recent years, occurring in the congenital or acquired form of the disease, being unilateral or bilateral, consisting of diffuse fibrosis with testicular atrophy or of gummatous formation, characterized clinically by swelling of the testis and only slight pain and tenderness, and complicated by sterility when the process is bilateral and of a diffuse inflammatory type (Menninger and London), (8) *leprosy*—described as occurring in up to 97 per cent of leprous patients, usually being bilateral, consisting essentially of obliterative vasculitis followed by interstitial fibrosis and tubular atrophy, and attended by gynecomastia in up to 90 per cent of cases (Grabstald), (9) *fungous* and *yeast-like orchitis*—consisting of blastomycosis and actinomycosis and generally being part of a systemic disease, and (10) *parasitic orchitis*— consisting of filariasis and echinococcosis.

PHYSICAL DISTURBANCES

The more important lesions in this category may be outlined as follows: (1) *hydrocele*—collection of serous fluid in the sac of the tunica vaginalis, occurring as a result of excessive production of fluid rather than as a result of defective absorption, arising on the basis of (*a*) a congenital anomaly (found at birth and often associated with hernia), (*b*) inflammation of any type, (*c*) tumors of the testis, epididymis, or tunica vaginalis, (*d*) trauma

such as that caused by a truss, (*e*) systemic conditions such as cardiovascular and renal diseases, and (*f*) idiopathic, clinically consisting of a
rapid or gradual enlargement of the scrotum to as much as 15 cm. in diameter, generally transmitting light, usually confined to the scrotum but occasionally extending into the abdomen, as a rule consisting of a thin, smooth-
walled sac filled with clear, straw-colored fluid (Fig. 555) but composed of

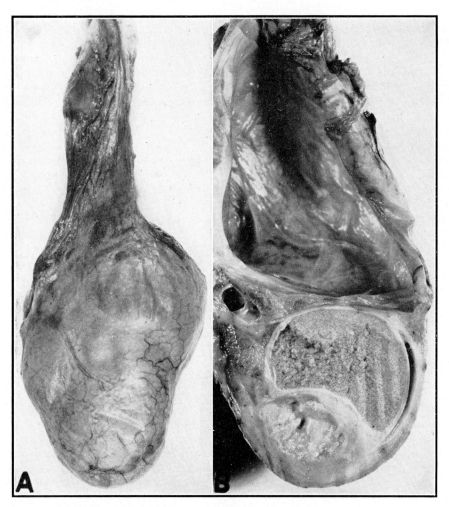

FIG. 555.—Hydrocele illustrating *A*, an intact and *B*, an opened sac.

a thick fibrous wall filled with pus or inspissated material once it becomes
infected, often disappearing spontaneously when it occurs in newborn
infants, and treated by injection of a sclerosing fluid or by open operation
(with incision and eversion of the sac) in lesions that do not disappear or
that recur (Wilson, Bruskewitz, and Prather), (2) *hematocele*—blood within
the cavity of the tunica vaginalis, resulting from (*a*) trauma, (*b*) puncturing
a vessel when tapping a hydrocele, or (*c*) irritation by a malignant tumor,
but occasionally being idiopathic (Neligan), (3) *lymphocele*—chylous effusion into the tunica vaginalis generally seen in filariasis, (4) *traumatic*

rupture—rare (Senger), (5) *luxation*—displacement of the testis from the scrotal cavity into the inguinal canal, subcutaneous tissues, or through the scrotum, occurring as a result of trauma, and usually being unilateral (Ockuly), (6) *calculi*—occurring in connection with inflammation of the tunica vaginalis, and (7) *infarction*—seen in conjunction with torsion of the spermatic cord.

TUMORS

Orientation.—Tumors of the testes may arise from the tunics of the testes or from the testes proper. They may be either benign or malignant and include such lesions as mesothelioma, lipoma, leiomyoma, leiomyosarcoma, rhabdomyosarcoma, fibroma, hemangioma, hemangio-endothelioma, neurofibroma, lymphoblastoma, Sertoli cell tumors, Leydig cell tumors, malignant epithelial tumors, and secondary growths. Of these, only Leydig cell tumors and malignant epithelial tumors need be discussed further.

Leydig Cell Tumors.—These tumors, known also as interstitial cell tumors, are *rare*, there having been only thirty-seven cases described up to 1952 (Christeson). *Pathologically* the growths are usually unilateral, diffusely yellowish or dark brown, and may measure up to 10 cm. in diameter. *Histologically* they are composed of fairly sharply defined polyhedral cells that may resemble normal Leydig cells or that are similar to those of the adrenal cortex. Generally they are quite regular but pleomorphism has been described. The cellular arrangement is usually diffuse. While most of the neoplasms remain localized, a few have been known to metastasize to the regional lymph nodes, lungs, and femur. The chief *clinical manifestations* are precocity in boys and gynecomastia in adults. *Treatment* consists of surgical removal. The *prognosis* is good.

Malignant Epithelial Tumors.—In this category may be included primary epithelial tumors of the testes excluding Leydig cell and Sertoli cell tumors. The *incidence* is difficult to determine but it may be said with assurance that the lesion represents one of the more common tumors in the male. In World War II the incidence in the United States Army population was 2.8 per 100,000 (Dixon). The majority of patients are in the third and fourth decades of life and Negroes appear to be relatively immune (Kaplan and Jensen). The *cause* of the tumors is unknown but, because of the age incidence, hormonal activity has been incriminated. While there is still some difference of opinion, the growths are considered to arise, by most authors, from totipotent germ cells (Melicow and Milton Friedman).

Pathologically the tumors are usually unilateral and have no predilection for either side. They vary in size from microscopic to 20 cm. in diameter. They may start in any part of the testis and as they enlarge they replace more and more of the testicular tissue until the entire organ is absorbed. Externally the neoplasms, even when large, are well encapsulated, smooth, and glistening. Their consistency is moderately firm. Cut surfaces disclose tissue that is (1) uniformly gray, (2) necrotic and hemorrhagic, (3) cystic, or (4) combinations of these (Fig. 556). Rarely bone, cartilage, hair, and sebaceous material may be encountered. While the *histologic* classifications of the tumors have been many (Gray, Dean, Sauer, O'Connell, etc.), the one first proposed by Friedman and Moore appears to be quite satisfactory. Accordingly, the tumors may be divided into (1) *seminoma*—being most common and consisting of diffusely arranged, uniform, large, rounded, or polyhedral cells with abundant, light staining, clear cytoplasm and round or oval, uniformly staining, centrally placed nuclei (Fig. 557), (2) *embryonal carcinoma* (trophocarcinoma)—composed of cuboidal, columnar, or irregular cells arranged in glands, papillæ, diffusely, or in structures that resemble chorionic villi and including the group composed of irregular Langhans' and syncytial cells (chorionepithelioma or choriocarcinoma), (3) *teratoma*—composed of adult appearing (adult type) or embryonal appearing (immature type) bone, cartilage, epithelium, muscle, lymphoid tissue, and occasionally fat, either irregularly arranged or

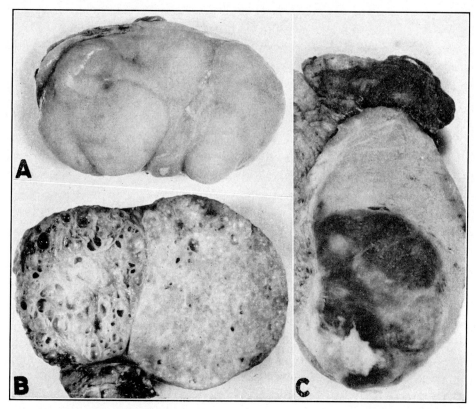

Fig. 556.—Malignant epithelial tumors of the testes showing *A*, a solid homogeneously gray growth, *B*, a cystic mass, and *C*, a solid gray mass with areas of necrosis and hemorrhage.

in organoid formation, and (4) *teratocarcinoma*—consisting of combinations of teratoid and carcinomatous elements. In general, the most benign growths are pure adult teratomas and pure seminomas. When these tumors are mixed with more primitive elements the growths as a whole are then as malignant as these elements indicate and the neoplasms should be so labeled. The tumors *spread* by lymphatics to the internal iliac, common iliac, periaortic, and later mediastinal lymph nodes and by blood vessels to the lungs, liver, and other tissues of the body.

Aside from metastasis the *complications* consist of hydrocele and, in hormone-producing tumors such as embryonal carcinoma, chorionepithelioma, and teratocarcinoma, of gynecomastia. The *clinical manifestations* consist of tumor of the testis later associated with testicular pain and, when metastases occur, with loss of weight, anorexia, cough, indigestion, back-

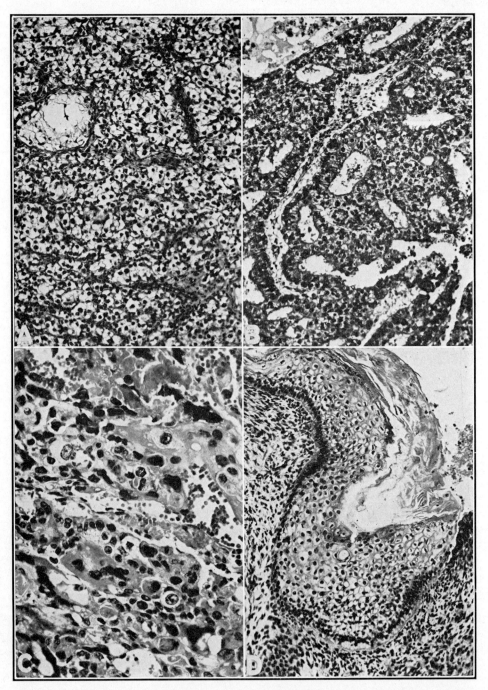

Fig. 557.—Malignant epithelial tumors of the testes disclosing *A*, seminoma. × 100, *B*, glandular embryonal carcinoma. × 100, *C*, embryonal carcinoma (chorionepithelioma). × 200, and *D*, teratoma with a focus of keratinizing squamous epithelium. × 100.

ache, etc. The *diagnosis* is made by careful palpation of the testis. Hormonal assays (chorionic gonadotropins) are of confirmatory rather than of diagnostic value. *Treatment* consists of surgical extirpation, irradiation, or a combination of the two. The *prognosis* depends upon the type of growth. It is excellent in pure adult teratoma, good in pure seminoma, and fair to poor in other tumors.

SCROTUM

CONGENITAL ANOMALIES

Developmental malformations of the scrotum may be listed as follows: (1) *hypoplasia*—seen in connection with undescended testes, (2) *hyperplasia*, (3) bifid scrotum—relatively common and seen in connection with duplication of the penis, exstrophy of the bladder, and perineal hypospadias (Mackenzie), and (4) *splenic inclusions*—rare (Andrews).

DEGENERATIONS AND INFLAMMATIONS

Being composed mostly of integument, the scrotum is subjected to most of the degenerative and inflammatory disorders that affect the skin of the penis (p. 1111) and other portions of the body. The more common disturbances may be listed as follows: furuncle, abscess, erysipelas, cellulitis, gangrene, scabies, psoriasis, syphilis, chancroid, lymphogranuloma venereum, granuloma inguinale, filariasis, erythroplasia of Queyrat, actinomycosis, and paraffinoma. A *paraffinoma* of the scrotum is similar to a paraffinoma (lipid pneumonia) of the lungs (p. 312). It is, in reality, a foreign body reaction to prolonged exposure to paraffin and other oils. In the case of the scrotum it has resulted from injection of material for devious reasons (Brown).

PHYSICAL DISTURBANCES

The more important lesions in this category may be listed as follows: (1) *elephantiasis* (p. 381), (2) *injury*—including contusion, hematoma, wounds, and traumatic avulsion (p. 1115) (Vernon), (3) *fat necrosis*—rare and usually resulting from trauma (Hinman), (4) *air* in the *scrotum*—known as *pneumocele* when it is within the tunica vaginalis and *aerocele* or *emphysema* when it is outside of the tunica vaginalis, indicated by crepitant or noncrepitant swelling of the scrotum, and caused by pneumoperitoneum, pneumoradiographic studies on the genitournary tract, gas bacillus infection, ulcers of the penis and scrotum, urethral stricture, operations on the prostate, and trauma (Wynn–Williams and Speed), (4) *calculi*—rare and usually occurring within the tunica vaginalis rather than in the scrotum proper, (6) *fistula*—connecting (*a*) the scrotum with the posterior urethra and found in connection with hypospadias, urethral abscess, urethral carcinoma, and urethral stricture or (*b*) the scrotum with the vas deferans and seen in connection with urethral stricture, obstruction of the opening of the ejaculatory ducts, operative removal of the verumontanum, and operative removal of the seminal vesicles (Bessesen).

TUMORS

Orientation.—Tumors of the scrotum are as varied as the normal tissues that compose this organ. They may be enumerated as follows: cutaneous horn, epithelial cyst, carcinoma, sebaceous cyst, Paget's disease, fibroma, myxoma, myxofibroma, lipoma, leiomyoma, angiokeratoma, hemangioma, lymphangioma, neurofibrosarcoma, melanoblastoma, chondroma, osteoma, and sarcoma. Of these, the most important is carcinoma.

Carcinoma.—Carcinoma of the scrotum is infrequent. It usually occurs in the sixth decade of life and has no racial predilection (Dean and Higgins). In most instances the *cause* is unknown but occupational exposure to chimney soot, mineral oil, or petroleum and its products acts as a definite precipitating cause (Henry, Brockbank, and Kennaway).

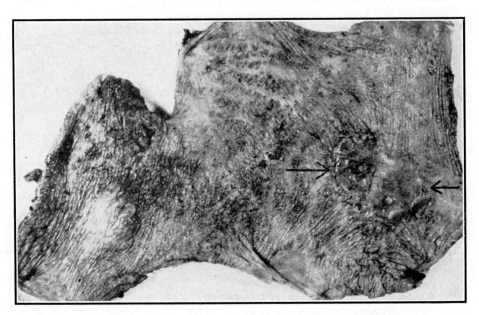

FIG. 558.—Carcinoma of the scrotum illustrating two ill-defined superficially ulcerating lesions.

Pathologically any part of the scrotum may be affected and the lesion may be single or multiple. It starts as a papule, roughened area, or ulcer and as it grows it forms a papillary tumor or an excavating indurated mass (Fig. 558). *Histologically* the growth is always of a stratified squamous cell type of low or intermediate grade malignancy. It usually *spreads* by extension to adjacent structures and by lymphatics to the inguinal and femoral lymph nodes. Hematogenous metastasis is rare and occurs only in the terminal stages of the disease. Aside from extension of the growth, the *complications* consist of infection and hemorrhage. The chief *clinical manifestation* consists of a scrotal sore. The final *diagnosis* is made by biopsy. *Treatment* consists of prophylaxis (in industry) and of irradiation, surgical excision, or combinations of these. The *prognosis* is poor for most of the patients die within two years after they first seek aid.

REFERENCES

General

HERBUT, P. A.: *Urological Pathology*, Philadelphia, Lea & Febiger, 1952.

Pathologic Physiology

CHARNEY, C. W., and WOLGIN, W.: *Cryptorchism*, New York, Hoeber-Harper, 1958.

DORFMAN, R. I., and SHIPLEY, R. A.: *Androgens. Biochemistry, Physiology and Clinical Significance*, New York, John Wiley & Sons, Inc., 1956.

NELSON, W. O.: Mammalian Spermatogenesis. In *Recent Progress in Hormone Research*, New York, Academic Press, Inc., 1951, Vol. VI.

PASCHKIS, K. E., RAKOFF, A. E., and CANTAROW, A.: *Clinical Endocrinology*, 2nd Ed., New York, Hoeber-Harper, 1958.

SOHVAL, A. R.: *Soffer's Diseases of the Endocrine Glands*, 2nd Ed., Philadelphia, Lea & Febiger, 1956 (Diseases of the Testis).

TWOMBLY, G. H.: *Soskin's Progress in Clinical Endocrinology*, New York, Grune & Stratton, 1950, (Hormonally Active Testicular Tumors).

PENIS

Congenital Anomalies

BLANCO, S.: J. Urol., *53*, 786, 1945 (Duplication).

DAVIS, D. M.: J. Urol., *61*, 111, 1949 (Duplication).

HIRSCH, E. W.: Urol. & Cutan. Rev., *34*, 453, 1930 (Ossification).

McCREA, L. E.: J. Urol., *47*, 818, 1942 (Absence).

NEFF, J. H.: Am. J. Surg., *31*, 308, 1936 (Canals and Cysts of Raphe).

Degenerations and Inflammations

BOROVSKY, M. E.: J. A. M. A., *104*, 1399, 1935 (Diphtheria).

CALLOMON, F. T.: Urol. & Cutan. Rev., *49*, 742, 1945 (Plastic Induration).

CHEN, C. H., *et al.*: Arch. Dermat. & Syph., *58*, 703, 1948 (Granuloma Inguinale).

D'AUNOY, R., and vonHAAM, E.: Am. J. Trop. Med., *17*, 747, 1937 (Granuloma Inguinale).

FARRINGTON, J., and GARVEY, F. K.: Urol. & Cutan. Rev., *51*, 96, 1947 (Balanitis Xerotica Obliterans).

FREEMAN, C., and LAYMON, C. W.: A. M. A. Arch. Dermat. & Syph., *44*, 547, 1941 (Balanitis Xerotica Obliterans).

KLINGER, M. E., and NORTHRIP, R. U.: J. Urol., *63*, 173, 1950 (Erythroplasia of Queyrat).

KOTEEN, H.: Medicine, *24*, 1, 1945 (Lymphogranuloma Venereum).

LEWIS, E. L.: J. Urol., *56*, 737, 1946 (Tuberculosis).

MADDEN, J. F.: J. A. M. A., *105*, 420, 1935 (Balanitides).

MARSHAK, L., *et al.*: A. M. A. Arch. Dermat. & Syph., *57*, 858, 1948 (Granuloma Inguinale).

McCREA, L. E.: Clinics, *4*, 796, 1945 (Gangrene).

ORMSBY, O. S., and MONTGOMERY, H.: *Diseases of the Skin*, 8th Ed., Philadelphia, Lea & Febiger, 1954.

PUND, E. R., and DICK, F., JR.: Urol. & Cutan. Rev., *51*, 345, 1947 (Lymphogranuloma Venereum).

PUND, E. R., and GREENBLATT, R. B.: A. M. A. Arch. Path., *23*, 224, 1937 (Granuloma Inguinale).

SATULSKY, E. M.: J. A. M. A., *127*, 259, 1945 (Chancroid).

SCOTT, W. W., and SCARDINO, P. L.: South. M. J., *41*, 173, 1948 (Plastic Induration).

SMITH, E. B., and CUSTER, R. P.: J. Urol., *63*, 546, 1950 (Lymphogranuloma Venereum).

SULLIVAN, M.: Am. J. Syph., *24*, 482, 1940 (Chancroid).

vonHAAM, E.: Am. J. Trop. Med., *18*, 595, 1938 (Fusospirochaetosis).

Physical Disturbances

CAVE, W. H.: Am. J. Surg., *61*, 305, 1943 (Priapism).

CURR, J. F.: Brit. J. Urol., *18*, 66, 1946 (Dislocation).

DAVIS, A. D., and BERNER, R. E.: Plast. & Reconstruct. Surg, *3*, 417, 1948 (Avulsion).

FETTER, T., and GARTMAN, E.: Am. J. Surg., *32*, 371, 1936 (Rupture).

GLAZIER, M.: Ann. West. Med. & Surg., *1*, 381, 1947 (Priapism).

HOFFMAN, H. A., and COLBY, F.: J. Urol., *54*, 391, 1954 (Incarceration).

INGRAHAM, N. R., JR.: J. A. M. A., *105*, 106, 1935 (Preputial Calculus).

JUDD, E. S., JR., and HAVENS, F. Z.: Am. J. Surg., *62*, 246, 1943 (Traumatic Avulsion).

O'CONNOR, G. B.: U. S. Nav. M. Bull., *45*, 147, 1945 (Rupture).

Tumors

COLON, J. E.: J. Urol., *67*, 702, 1952 (Carcinoma).

CULP, O. S., and KAPLAN, I. W.: Ann. Surg., *120*, 251, 1944 (Condyloma Acuminatum).

Dean, A. L., Jr.:J. Urol., *33*, 252, 1935 (Carcinoma).
Gersh, I.: Urol. & Cutan. Rev., *49*, 432, 1945 (Condyloma Acuminatum).
Harlin, H. C.: J. Urol., *67*, 326, 1952 (Carcinoma).
Hudson, P. B., *et al.:* South. M. J., *41*, 761, 1948 (Carcinoma).
Lenowitz, H., and Graham, A. P.: J. Urol., *56*, 458, 1946 (Carcinoma).
Winterhoff, E., and Sparks, A. J.: J. Urol., *66*, 704, 1951 (Penile Horn).

PROSTATE

Congenital Anomalies

Dees, J. E.: J. Urol., *57*, 304, 1947 (Congenital Cysts).
Emmett, J. L., and Braasch, W. F.: J. Urol., *36*, 236, 1936 (Cysts).
Hock, E.: J. Urol., *56*, 353, 1946 (Diverticula).
Lazarus, J. A.: Urol. & Cutan. Rev., *40*, 178, 1936 (Retention Cysts).
Senger, F. L., and Morgan, E. K.: J. Urol., *51*, 162, 1944 (Congenital Diverticulum).

Degenerations

Baird, H. H., *et al.:* South. M. J., *43*, 234, 1950 (Infarction and Metaplasia).
Mostofi, F. K., and Morse, W. H.: A. M. A. Arch. Path., *51*, 340, 1951 (Squamous Metaplasia).
Nanson, E. M.: Brit. J. Urol., *22*, 394, 1950 (Squamous Metaplasia).

Inflammations

Auerbach, O.: New Internat. Clinics, *3*, 21, 1940 (Urogenital Tuberculosis).
Baker, W. J., and Graf, E. C.: J. Urol., *66*, 254, 1951 (Tuberculosis).
Buchert, W. I.: Pennsylvania M. J., *46*, 910, 1943 (Chronic Prostatitis).
Crowley, E., and Thomas, E.: J. Urol., *58*, 367, 1947 (Syphilis).
Cumming, R. E., and Chittenden, G. E.: J. Urol., *39*, 118, 1938 (Pyogenic Prostatitis).
de la Pena, A., and de la Pena, E.: Brit. J. Urol., *16*, 125, 1944 (Tuberculosis).
Fetter, T. R.: Pennsylvania M. J., *50*, 812, 1947 (Prostatitis).
Forsythe, W. E.: Urol. & Cutan. Rev., *46*, 613, 1942 (Abscess).
Nesbit, R. M., and Lynn, J. M.: J. Urol., *61*, 766, 1949 (Tuberculosis).
Peterson, A. P., and Mast, W. H.: S. Clin. North America, *20*, 367, 1940 (Chronic Prostatitis).
Schwartz, J.: J. Urol., *43*, 108, 1940 (Abscess).
Tanner, F. H., and McDonald, J. R.: A. M. A. Arch. Path., *36*, 358, 1943 (Granulomatous Prostatitis).

Physical Disturbances

Baird, H. H., *et al.:* South. M. J., *43*, 234, 1950 (Infarction).
Gentile, A.: J. Urol., *57*, 746, 1947 (Calculi).
Henline, R. B.: J. Urol., *44*, 146, 1940 (Calculi).
Jacobs, A.: Lancet, *1*, 1088, 1951 (Retropubic Prostatectomy).
Mostofi, F. K., and Morse, W. H.: A. M. A. Arch. Path., *51*, 340, 1951 (Prostatic Infarction).
Rogers, W. G.: J. Urol., *57*, 481, 1947 (Infarction).
Ward, R. O.: Brit. J. Urol., *23*, 97, 1951 (Calculi).

Tumors

Baron, E., and Angrist, A.: A. M. A. Arch. Path., *32*, 787, 1941 (Occult Carcinoma).
Cancer Mortality in United States According to Site by Sex and Age, 1938, Pub. Health Reports, *55*, 731, 1940.
Colby, F. H., and Suby, H. I.: New England J. Med., *223*, 85, 1940 (Cystourethrogram).
Creevy, C. D.: J. A. M. A., *138*, 412, 1948 (Carcinoma).
Deming, C.: J. Urol., *61*, 281, 1949 (Heterologous Growth of Human Cancer).
Dixon, F. J., and Moore, R. A.: *Tumors of the Male Sex Organs*, Washington, Armed Forces Institute of Pathology, 1952.
Harrison, H. T., *et al.:* New England J. Med., *248*, 86, 1953 (Adrenalectomy for Carcinoma).
Herbut, P. A., and Lubin, E. N.: J. Urol., *57*, 542, 1947 (Cytologic Diagnosis Cancer).

HIGGINS, C. C.: Cleveland Clin. Quart., *14*, 181, 1947 (Prostatic Obstruction).
HUDSON, T. B.: Surg., Gynec. & Obst., *93*, 233, 1953 (Treatment Carcinoma).
HUGGINS, C.: Bull. New York Acad. Med., *23*, 696, 1947 (Etiology Prostatic Hypertrophy).
HUGGINS, C., and JOHNSON, M. A.: J. A. M. A., *135*, 1146, 1947 (Carcinoma).
HUGGINS, C., and STEVENS, R. A.: J. Urol., *43*, 704, 1940 (Castration in Benign Hypertrophy).
KAHLER, J. E.: J. Urol., *41*, 557, 1939 (Carcinoma).
LIPSCHUTZ, A., *et al.*: Cancer Research, *5*, 515, 1945 (Experimental Hypertrophy).
MOORE, R. A.: J. Urol., *33*, 224, 1935 (Carcinoma).
————: J. Urol., *50*, 680, 1943 (Benign Hypertrophy).
OCKERBLAD, N. F.: J. Urol., *56*, 81, 1946 (Giant Prostate).
RICH, A. R.: J. Urol., *33*, 215, 1935 (Occult Carcinoma).

SEMINAL VESICLES

AUERBACH, O.: Internat. Clinics, *3*, 21, 1940 (Tuberculosis).
FETTER, T. R.: Pennsylvania M. J., *50*, 812, 1947 (Seminal Vesiculitis).
HARLIN, H. C.: J. A. M. A., *143*, 880, 1950 (Seminal Vesiculitis).
HUGGINS, C., and MCDONALD, D. F.: J. Clin. Endocrinol., *5*, 226, 1945 (Hemospermia).
LAZARUS, J. A.: J. Urol., *55*, 190, 1946 (Malignant Tumors).
LUND, A. J., and CUMMINGS, M. M.: J. Urol., *56*, 383, 1946 (Cysts).
MCCREA, L. E.: J. A. M. A., *136*, 679, 1948 (Carcinoma).
PLAUT, A., and STANDARD, S.: Ann. Surg., *119*, 253, 1944 (Cystomyoma).
SCARDINO, P. L., *et al.*: J. Urol., *63*, 698, 1950 (Tuberculosis).
SHEA, J. D., and SCHWARTZ, J. W.: J. Urol., *58*, 132, 1947 (Calcification).
VALENTINE, J. J., and ROGERS, J. W.: J. A. M. A., *104*, 43, 1935 (Fistula).

SPERMATIC CORD

CAMPBELL, M. F.: J. Pediat., *33*, 323, 1948 (Torsion).
————: Surg., Gynec. & Obst., *47*, 558, 1928 (Varicocele).
COE, H. E.: Northwestern Med., *27*, 300, 1928 (Atresia Vas Deferens).
HECKEL, N. J., and DE PEYSTER, F. A.: J. Urol., *52*, 586, 1944 (Tuberculoma).
IBRAHIM ,A. B.: Lancet, *2*, 272, 1927 (Funiculitis).
MATHE, C. P., and DUNN, G.: J. Urol., *59*, 461, 1948 (Duplication Vas Deferens).
NELSON, R. E.: J. Urol., *63*, 176, 1950 (Absence Vas Deferens).
O'CONOR, V. J.: J. Urol., *59*, 229, 1948 (Severance Vas Deferens).
OECONOMOS, S. N.: Urol. & Cutan. Rev., *52*, 388, 1948 (Deferentitis).
PALOMO, A.: J. Urol., *61*, 604, 1949 (Varicocele).
PECK, S.: J. Urol., *62*, 701, 1949 (Torsion).
POWER, S.: Lancet, *1*, 572, 1946 (Funiculitis).
SCHULTE, T. L., *et al.*: J. A. M. A., *112*, 2405, 1939 (Tumors).
SKINNER, H. L.: Ann. Surg., *113*, 123, 1941 (Varicocele).
STRONG, G. H.: J. Urol., *48*, 527, 1942 (Lipomyxoma).
THOMPSON, G. J.: Surg., Gynec. & Obst., *62*, 712, 1936 (Tumors).

EPIDIDYMIDES

AUERBACH, O.: New Internat. Clin., *3*, 21, 1940 (Tuberculosis).
BORTHWICK, W. M.: Edinburgh M. J., *53*, 55, 1946 (Tuberculosis).
CAMPBELL, M. F.: J. Urol., *20*, 485, 1928 (Spermatocele).
COKELY, H. J.: U. S. Nav. M. Bull., *40*, 139, 1942 (Syphilis).
FALK, D., and KONWALER, B. E.: J. Urol., *66*, 603, 1951 (Adenomatoid Tumor).
FREEMAN, A.: A. M. A. Arch. Path., *39*, 336, 1945 (Adrenal Rests).
GIBSON, T. E.: Brit. J. Urol., *24*, 209, 1952 (Cholesteatoma).
GLASER, B. S.: Brit. J. Urol., *22*, 178, 1950 (Tumors).
HALPERT, B.: Am. J. Obst. & Gynec., *43*, 1028, 1942 (Hemorrhage).
HANDLEY, R. S.: Lancet, *1*, 779, 1946 (Nonspecific Epididymitis).
HENLINE, R. B., and YUNCK, W.: New York State J. Med., *43*, 1325, 1943 (Epididymitis).
JACOBSON, C. E., JR., and DOCKERTY, M. B.: J. Urol., *50*, 237, 1943 (Blastomycosis).
LAZARUS, J. A., and MARKS, M. S.: J. Urol., *57*, 567, 1947 (Anomalies Epididymis).
LONGO, V. J., *et al.*: J. A. M. A., *147*, 937, 1951 (Primary Tumors).
MASON, A., and REIFENSTEIN, G. H.: J. Urol., *52*, 338, 1944 (Epididymo-orchitis).
MCCREA, E. D.: Brit. J. Urol., *7*, 152, 1935 (Cysts).
ROBERTSON, J. P., and LEE, A. B.: Am. J. Surg., *30*, 462, 1935 (Acute Epididymitis).

SEIDEL, R. F., and YEAW, R. C.: J. Urol., *63*, 714, 1950 (Torsion Appendix Testis and Epididymis).
TUNBRIDGE, R. E., and GAVEY, C. J.: Lancet, *1*, 775, 1946 (Epididymo-orchitis).
WADDY, S. H.: Brit. J. Urol., *18*, 24, 1946 (Anterior Epididymis).
WAKELEY, C. P. G.: Brit. J. Surg., *31*, 165, 1943 (Cysts).

TESTES

Congenital Anomalies

HANDLEY, R. S., and CRAWFORD, T.: Brit. J. Surg., *31*, 300, 1944 (Polyorchidism).
HEPBURN, R. H.: J. Urol., *62*, 65, 1949 (Anorchism).
HUNT, R. W.: J. Urol., *44*, 325, 1940 (Ectopic).
KAWAICHI, G. K., et al.: New England J. Med., *240*, 334, 1949 (Monorchism).
LEWIS, L. G.: J. Urol., *60*, 345, 1948 (Cryptorchidism).

Degenerations

ENGLE, E. T.: J. Urol., *62*, 694, 1949 (Atrophy).
POLLAK, O. J.: Am. J. Clin. Path., *18*, 542, 1948 (Atrophy).
RATHER, L. J.: A. M. A. Arch. Int. Med., *80*, 397, 1947 (Atrophy).
WERNER, S. C.: Am. J. Med., *3*, 52, 1947 (Atrophy).

Inflammations

AUERBACH, O.: New Internat. Clin., *3*, 21, 1940 (Tuberculosis).
CAMPBELL, M. F.: Med. J. & Record, *129*, 147, 1929 (Suppurative Orchitis).
CHARNY, C. W., and MERANZE, D. R.: J. Urol., *60*, 140, 1948 (Mumps Orchitis).
CLEM, J. G.: Urol. & Cutan. Rev., *34*, 159, 1930 (Epididymo-orchitis).
GALL, E. A.: Am. J. Path., *23*, 637, 1947 (Mumps Orchitis).
GRABSTALD, H., and SWAN, L. L.: J. A. M. A., *149*, 1287, 1952 (Leprosy).
LONDON, M. Z.: J. Urol., *57*, 564, 1947 (Syphilis).
MENNINGER, W. C.: Am. J. Syph., *12*, 221, 1928 (Syphilis).
SANBORN, E.: Am. J. Surg., *63*, 131, 1944 (Brucellosis).
THOMAS, G. J., et al.: J. Urol., *44*, 67, 1940 (Tuberculosis).
WERNER, C. A.: Ann. Int. Med., *32*, 1066, and 1075, 1950 (Mumps Orchitis).

Physical Disturbances

BRUSKEWITZ, H., and EWELL, G. H.: J. Urol., *59*, 67, 1948 (Hydrocele).
NELIGAN, G. E.: Practitioner, *136*, 496, 1936 (Hematocele).
OCKULY, E. A.: Am. J. Surg., *71*, 93, 1946 (Luxation).
PRATHER, G. C.: New England J. Med., *226*, 255, 1942 (Hydrocele).
SENGER, F. L., et al.: J. Urol., *58*, 451, 1947 (Traumatic Rupture).
WILSON, W. W.: Lancet, *1*, 1048, 1949 (Hydrocele).

Tumors

CHRISTESON, W. W., and NETTLESHIP, A.: J. Urol., *67*, 350, 1950 (Interstitial Cell Tumors)
DEAN, A. L.: New York State J. Med., *51*, 485, 1951 (Diagnosis and Treatment).
DIXON, F. J., and MOORE, R. A.: *Tumors of the Male Sex Organs*, Washington, Armed Forces Institute of Pathology, 1952.
FRIEDMAN, M.: Tumors of the Testis and Their Treatment, Portmann, U. V.; *Clinical Therapeutic Radiology*, New York, Thomas Nelson & Sons, pp. 276–308, 1950.
FRIEDMAN, N. B., and MOORE, R. A.: Military Surgeon, *99*, 573, 1946 (Tumors).
GRAY, C. P., et al.: J. Urol., *64*, 690, 1950 (Teratoma).
JENSEN, O. J., JR.: J. A. M. A., *149*, 109, 1952 (Tumors).
KAPLAN, G., et al.: Am. J. Roentgenol., *66*, 405, 1951 (158 Malignant Tumors).
MELICOW, M. M.: J. Urol., *44*, 333, 1940 (Embryoma).
O'CONNELL, H. V., and GESCHICKTER, C. F.: U. S. Armed Forces M. J., *1*, 719, 1950 (Tumors).
SAUER, H. R., and BURKE, E. M.: J. Urol., *62*, 69, 1949 (Prognosis).

SCROTUM

Congenital Anomalies

ANDREWS, S. E., and ETTER, E. F.: J. Urol., *55*, 545, 1946 (Splenic Rests).
MACKENZIE, K.: Surg., Gynec. & Obst., *35*, 603, 1922 (Duplication).

Degenerations and Inflammations

BROWN, A. F., and JOERGENSON, E. J.: Ann. West. Med. & Surg., *1*, 301, 1947 (Paraffinoma).

Physical Disturbances

BESSESEN, D. H.: Urol. & Cutan. Rev., *36*, 432, 1932 (Fistula).
HINMAN, F., and JOHNSON, C. M.: J. Urol., *41*, 726, 1939 (Fat Necrosis).
SPEED, K.: S. Clin. North America, *11*, 29, 1931 (Aerocele).
VERNON, S.: Am. J. Surg., *78*, 131, 1949 (Hematoma).
WYNN-WILLIAMS, N.: Brit. M. J., *2*, 318, 1949 (Pneumocele).

Tumors

BROCKBANK, E. M.: Brit. M. J., *1*, 622, 1941 (Mule Spinner's Cancer).
DEAN, A. L.: J. Urol., *60*, 508, 1948 (Carcinoma).
HENRY, S. A.: Am. J. Cancer, *31*, 28, 1937 (Occupational Cancer).
HIGGINS, C. C., and WARDEN, J. G.: J. Urol., *62*, 250, 1949 (Carcinoma).
KENNAWAY, E. L., and KENNAWAY, M. M.: Cancer Research, *6*, 49, 1946 (Social Distribution Cancer).

33

Female Generative System

PATHOLOGIC PHYSIOLOGY

A. E. RAKOFF

THE *physiology* of the female reproductive system is primarily under hormonal regulation. The ovaries are stimulated by the gonadotropic hormones of the pituitary and, in turn, the ovaries secrete hormones which produce various physiologic and anatomic changes in the entire genital tract. It is generally believed that the *pituitary* secretes three gonadotropic substances, the release of which is regulated through the hypothalamus: (1) *follicle-stimulating hromone* (FSH), which causes growth and maturation of immature follicles and secretion of estrogen by their granulosa and theca cells, (2) luteinizing hormone (LH), which, acting in synergism with FSH, is responsible for ovulation, after which LH causes growth of the corpus luteum, and (3) *luteotropic hormone* (LTH), a term applied to lactogenic hormone to indicate its synergistic action with LH in maintaining the functional activity of the corpus luteum in secreting estrogen and progesterone and possibly also a protein hormone, relaxin. The normal human ovary secretes very little *androgen*, which in the female comes primarily from the adrenal cortex.

The *estrogens* secreted by the ovary are chiefly estrone and estradiol. They cause *growth* of the entire female genital tract, particularly the epithelium of the uterus and vagina. The rise in the secretion of estrogen in the pubertal years stimulates the maturation of the Mullerian derivatives, also growth of the breasts, appearance of pubic hair, and development of the other secondary female sex characters. During the reproductive years, estrogens are secreted in cyclic fashion. Soon after menstruation, the titer of estrogen (as indicated by vaginal smears and bioassay of the urine) rises progressively to reach a peak at about the time of ovulation. After this it drops moderately, then rises to reach a second peak about 4 or 5 days before menstruation, and finally is followed by a marked premenstrual fall.

Progesterone secretion begins promptly after ovulation and continues throughout the corpus luteum phase, which is quite regularly two weeks in duration. The level of progesterone (as indicated by the urinary titers of its excretion product pregnandiol) reaches a peak a few days before the expected menses, after which it drops abruptly along with estrogen. Progesterone is responsible for inducing secretory changes in the endometrium favorable for the nidation of a fertilized ovum and inhibiting motility of the myometrium. Progesterone also moderately increases basal metabolism and is responsible for the rise in basal temperature following ovulation.

Relaxin is believed to favor relaxation of the uterine ligaments and, during pregnancy, softening of the symphysis pubis and relaxation of the uterine muscle.

(1142)

The *cyclic changes* in *estrogen* produce corresponding functional and histologic changes in the reproductive organs, which are most clearly demonstrable in the first half of the cycle when estrogen is acting alone. After ovulation, its action is modified by progesterone. On the *endometrium* its actions are particularly striking in causing growth of the endometrium termed the *proliferative* (follicular or interval) *phase*. Morphologically the

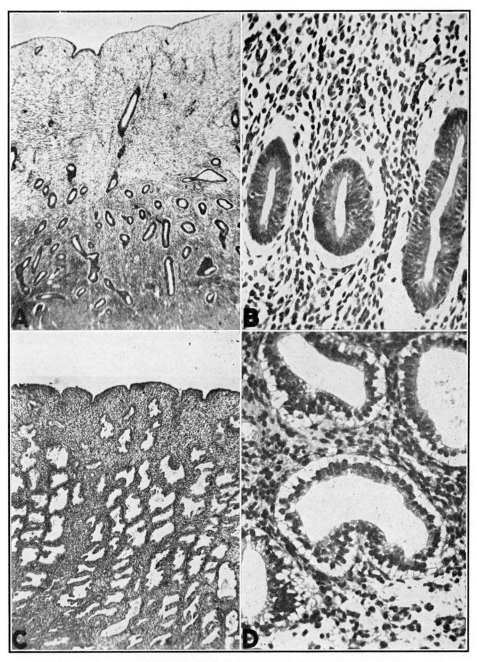

FIG. 559.—Endometrium showing *A* and *B*, early proliferative phase. × 17.5 and 200, and *C* and *D*, early secretory phase. × 17.5 and 200.

proliferative stage lasts from about the fourth to the fourteenth day from
the onset of the menstrual period in a normal 28 day cycle. Following
menstruation, the basilar layer and a portion of the spongiosa that remains
are covered with a single layer of columnar cells originating in the glands.
The tubular glands are few in number at first but gradually proliferate until
at 14 days they are aligned in parallel rows at right angles to the surface and
show beginning tortuosity (Fig. 559 *A* and *B*). They are lined by columnar
epithelial cells that have sharp borders, nonsecreting cytoplasm, and oval
basilar nuclei. Meanwhile the stroma remains abundant in amount and
dense. The *secretory* (corpus luteum, progesteronic, progestational, differentiative) *phase* (Fig. 559 *C* and *D*) begins immediately after ovulation and
lasts from the fifteenth to the twenty-sixth day of a 28 day cycle. Such
endometrium reflects the combined action of estrogen and progesterone. It
is characterized by (1) increasing tortuosity of the glands, (2) appearance
of first subnuclear and then general cytoplasmic glycogen positive droplets
of secretion, (3) blurring of the cell borders, especially those adjacent to the
lumen, (4) presence of secretion within the glandular lumens, which is then
resorbed, and (5) edema and decidual-like transformation of the stroma in
which the cells become larger, their cytoplasm more abundant and eosinophilic, and their nuclei more plump or rounded and vesicular. About *two
days before menstruation* the spiral arterioles which have grown and become
more coiled under hormonal stimulation, undergo marked vasoconstriction
and produce ischemia. The change is characterized by shrinking of the
endometrium as a whole, increased denseness of the stroma, collapse of the
glands, and appearance of luekocytes. *Menstrual endometrium* shows simply
an enhancement of the premenstrual changes with, in addition, disruption
of the architecture by massive hemorrhage (Fig. 560). These changes,
leading to menstrual bleeding, are believed to be mediated through the rapip
withdrawal of estrogen and progesterone, with vascular changes being influenced by biochemical changes in the enodmetrium, particularly an increase
in acetylcholine concentration. Similar changes leading to uterine bleeding
may occur also in an anovulatory cycle if sufficient estrogen has been
secreted by a growing follicle to produce a proliferative endometrium and
then regresses. This is spoken of as estrogen withdrawal bleeding, *anovulatory bleeding*, or *pseudomenstruation*.

The effect of the *ovarian hormones* on the *vaginal epithelium* is also quite
evident and of considerable clinical significance. In the castrate, the vaginal
epithelium is thin consisting of only a few rows of small cells. Under the
influence of estrogen, the epithelium proliferates rapidly to a thick epithelium
consisting of three distinct layers—a basal layer of small cuboidal or round
cells, an intermediate layer of transitional cells, and a superficial layer of
squamous cells. The superficial cells undergo increasing cornification as the
estrogen level reaches its peak. These changes can be readily followed by
examining the shed cells on stained vaginal smears (Papanicolaou), thus
providing the clinician with a simple method for evaluating estrogenic
function. During the corpus luteum phase there is increased desquamation,
folding, and twisting of the cells and regression of the estrogenic effect.
Glycogen is also deposited in high concentration in the vaginal epithelium
under estrogen stimulation. This is broken down to simpler carbohydrates
and utilized by the lactobacilli of the vagina with the production of lactic
acid to create a normal vaginal pH of about 4.0. In states of estrogen
deficiency this normal protective mechanism is altered; the pH may rise to
6.0 or more, and the normal flora may be replaced by various saphrophytes
or pathogens.

In most instances, *disturbances* in the *physiology* of the female generative system exert their influence by disturbing the function of the ovaries, either directly or by way of the pituitary. Less frequently, these physiologic changes are attributable to congenital abnormalities, acquired diseases, or functional irresponsiveness of the target organs (uterus, cervix, and vagina).

Hypofunction of the ovaries may (1) result from inadequate pituitary gonadotropic stimulation caused by an organic or functional disturbance affecting the pituitary or hypothalamus or (2) be caused by organic lesions or functional disturbances affecting the ovary itself. In the first category there is an absence of FSH in the urine, while in the latter group FSH excretion will be excessively high. The clinical manifestations depend not only upon the etiologic factor but also upon the period of life in which the condition occurs.

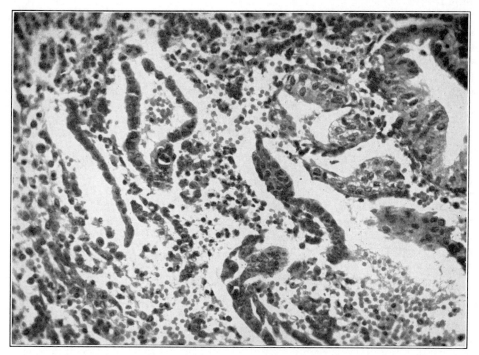

Fig. 560.—Menstrual endometrium demonstrating disruption of tissue by hemorrhage and leukocytic extravasation and collapse of the glands. × 200.

Congenital absence of functioning *ovarian tissue* results in *Turner's syndrome* (ovarian agenesis, gonadal dysgenesis, *etc.*) characterized by failure of sexual maturation, primary amenorrhea, dwarfism and sometimes other congenital defects, and high urinary gonadotropins. Chromosomal sex determinations (skin biopsy, or buccal or blood smears) indicate that many of these "girls" are really males in whom the embryonic absence of testicular tissue permitted the maternal estrogens to cause development of the Müllerian system and regression of the Wolffian system. *Impairment* of *ovarian function* during *childhood*, resulting from surgical castration, irradiation, mumps oophoritis, or gonococcal peri-oophoritis, produces the syndrome of *ovarian eunuchoidism* characterized by lack of development of the breasts and sex characters, infantile external genitalia, thin vaginal mucosa, and marked hypoplasia of the uterus. The epiphyses are late in closing causing tallness with relatively long limbs (eunuchoid proportions). These patients also have primary amenorrhea and anovulatory infertility.

In some *children* with *pituitary dwarfism* there is an associated deficiency in gonadotropic hormones causing sexual infantilism. The onset of gonadotropic and ovarian function may also be delayed in cretins, in untreated diabetics, and in children with other metabolic disturbances such as celiac disease.

The onset of ovarian *hypofunction* during the *early reproductive years* is more often the result of a functional disturbance than organic disease. The most common chief complaints are secondary amenorrhea or other irregularities of menstruation and infertility due to anovulation. There may be other endocrine stigmata such as hirsutism or obesity, depending upon the underlying cause. The most frequent functional cause is a decrease in gonadotropic hormone secretion (hypogonadotropism) resulting from nervous and emotional upsets, nutritional disturbances, obesity, infections, or systemic illness. The gonadotropins can also be inhibited by excessive androgen production by the adrenal cortex such as in *Cushing's syndrome* or the *adrenogenital syndrome*. Intracranial lesions such as pituitary tumors, craniopharyngioma, or lesions in the region of the hypothalamus may not only inhibit gonadotropin secretion but may, in addition, also inhibit other hormones of the pituitary to produce manifestations of *panhypopituitarism*. In the latter condition, laboratory studies show not only a decrease in gonadotropins but also diminished urinary 17-ketosteroids and corticoids, and low basal metabolic rate (BMR) and protein bound iodine (PBI).

Conditions which affect the ovary directly during the reproductive years will not only cause *menstrual dysfunction* and *anovulatory infertility*, but, in addition, if the estrogen secretion is markedly impaired, will also be associated with symptoms similar to those of the *menopausal syndrome*, such as hot flashes, headaches, increased nervousness, *etc.*, which are thought to be associated with hyperactivity of the pituitary, as indicated by a high urinary FSH level. Some of the conditions which may adversely affect the ovaries include pelvic inflammatory disease caused by gonorrhea, postabortal streptococcal infections, and pelvic tuberculosis. Endometriosis (page 1166) or other tumors or cysts which have destroyed much functioning tissue of the ovary may also be responsible. Rarely, neurogenic factors or systemic illness may cause a functional inhibition in ovarian responsiveness to gonadotropic stimulation. The type of menstrual irregularity which develops in patients with ovarian dysfunction depends chiefly upon the rise and fall in the estrogen level. Amenorrhea may result from a normal or high estrogen level which has been sustained or it may be associated with a complete absence of estrogen. *Polymenorrhea, hypermenorrhea,* or *irregular bleeding*, not associated with any organic lesion (so called "dysfunctional uterine bleeding"), is the result of an irregular rise and fall in estrogen secretion.

Polycystic disease of the *ovary* is generally associated with ovarian dysfunction. It may result in some instances from inflammatory thickening of the ovary inhibiting normal ovulation while in other instances it seems to be the result of a dysfunction in the endocrine mechanism controlling the growth and development of the follicles. Polycystic disease of the *Stein-Leventhal type* (page 1184) is associated with hirsutism as well as anovulatory infertility and secondary amenorrhea. It has been suggested that the hyperplastic theca which often surrounds the small cysts may be secreting an abnormal steroid which is mildly androgenic but not excreted as a 17-

ketosteroid. In this syndrome, the latter usually are in the top normal or slightly elevated range, gonadotropins are usually decreased, and estrogens are generally low or normal. Other investigators believe this condition may be secondary to adrenal dysfunction.

At the *menopause* ovarian hypofunction is the result of a progressive loss of functioning ovarian epithelium. Despite progressive gonadotropic stimulation, the ovary is no longer able to secrete adequate amounts of estrogen. The resulting physiologic changes of the menopasual syndrome may be attributable to estrogen deficiency and gonadotropic hyperfunction. The former is responsible for the menstrual irregularity and subsequent amenorrhea, atrophic changes of the vagina and external genitalia, and trophic changes in skin and bones (such as osteoporosis). The pituitary hyperfunction appears to be related in some fashion to the hot flashes and vasomotor instability. Undoubtedly, psychogenic factors at the climacteric also play an important role in the symptomatology.

Hyperfunction of the ovaries can be caused by functional disturbances or organic lesions which may make their appearance at various periods of life. When it has its onset during childhood, hyperfunction of the ovary causes *precocious puberty* characterized by the development of breasts, secondary sex characteristics, and sometimes menstrual bleeding. In about 90 per cent of the cases, this condition is classified as "*functional*"or "constitutional" in that no organic lesion can be demonstrated. In such instances, there has been premature awakening of the pituitary-ovarian-mechanism so that the child goes though all the pubertal changes at an early age. Early ovulation occurs and even pregnancy as early as the age of five has been reported. In rare instances, true precocious puberty may be caused by an intracranial lesion.

Granulosa-cell tumors of the ovary (page 1191) account for feminizing precocious puberty in about 10 per cent of the cases. This is a *pseudoprecocious puberty* since it is not associated with ovulation but rather by excessive estrogen secretion as can be demonstrated by vaginal smears and urine hormone assays. Roentgen studies show an advanced bone age. Differential diagnosis depends upon the pelvic findings of a unilateral ovarian enlargement.

Early pregnancy represents a perfect example of *functional overactivity* of the *ovary* in the reproductive years. The corpus luteum of pregnancy is maintained and stimulated by the rising titer of chorionic gonadotropin produced by the cytotrophoblast. The increasing estrogen and progesterone level thus secreted is responsible for the hyperhormonal amenorrhea, stimulation of breast growth, pigmentation of nipples, and many of the other early manifestations of pregnancy. A persistent corpus luteum in a nonpregnant woman can produce somewhat similar clinical and hormonal findings. This may occur in association with a corpus luteum cyst or there may be a functional persistence of the corpus luteum of psychogenic origin, most strikingly seen in patients with the *pseudocyesis syndrome*.

Hyperplasia of the *endometrium* (page 1165) results from (1) a relative or absolute increase in estrogen alone, such as may occur in prolonged anovulatory cycles of dysfunctional origin or associated with cystic disease of the ovaries, (2) estrogen producing tumors of the ovary, or (3) after exogenous administration of estrogens. This condition may also occur in patients in whom there is inadequate inactivation of endogenous estrogens because of liver diseases or dysfunction, causing an increase in the free (nonconjugated) estrogen level in the urine. Simple or cystic endometrium is a frequent finding at curettage in patients with menstrual disorders.

Functioning tumors of the *ovary* (page 1184) may secrete a variety of hormones. The granulosa cell tumors and thecomas secrete *estrogens*. Some granulosa cell tumors may be functionally inactive and others may secrete *progesterone* as well as estrogen. As indicated above, granulosa cell tumors occurring in childhood cause feminizing precocious puberty. In the reproductive years, the granulosa cell tumor or thecoma may produce hyperestrogenism characterized by irregular bleeding with endometrial hyperplasia, mastalgia, and hyperhormonal leukorrhea, while in the post menopausal woman, these tumors cause a striking "rejuvenation" with symptoms of returning ovarian function. The rare chorionepithelioma of the ovary is also a feminizing tumor since the high titers of chorionic *gonadotropin*, which it secretes, stimulates estrogen and progesterone production by the ovary.

Androgens are secreted by the arrhenoblastoma and various other tumors which have been grouped under the term of "adrenocorticoid tumors" (page 1193). When these tumors occur in childhood they produce masculinizing precocious puberty, whereas in the adult there is first loss of ovarian function and determinization followed by progressive virilism, including acne, hirsutism, deepening of the voice, and enlargement of the clitoris. There is usually a slight to moderate increase in the urinary 17-ketosteroids, usually much less than occurs in adrenal cortical tumors. Evidence of progesteronic activity, as indicated by the endometrial findings or steroid metabolites in the urine, have also been found in some of these tumors. In very rare instances, a Cushing's syndrome may be produced by an adrenocorticoid tumor of the ovary with secretion of *glucocorticosteroids* as well as androgens.

Thyroid hormone is secreted by the struma ovarii (page 1191), occasionally in amounts sufficient to produce hyperthyroidism.

GENERAL CONSIDERATIONS

In conformance with the organization of other portions of the book, this section on the Female Generative System will be considered from a regional point of view under the headings of Vulva, Vagina, Cervix, Body of Uterus, Fallopian Tubes, Ovaries, and Fetal Membranes.

VULVA

CONGENITAL ANOMALIES

Developmental malformations of the vulva may be enumerated as follows: (1) *hypoplasia*, (2) *hyperplasia*, (3) *common hymenal urethral opening* — due to a defect in the terminal portion of the septum between the vagina and urethra (Elden), (4) *rectum opening into fourchet*, (5) *absence of mons pubis*, (6) *duplication*, (7) *vulvar fusion* — also known as atresia or synechia vulva, occurring at all ages, consisting of adherence of the labia minora, probably being more on an acquired than on a developmental basis, caused by friction of clothing, complicated by urinary tract obstruction and infection, asymptomatic until complications arise, and treated by blunt digital separation of the labia (Nowlin and Bowles), (8) *imperforate hymen* — consisting of a hymen that completely closes the vaginal orifice, being rather uncommon, complicated by (*a*) retention of serous (serocolpos), watery (hydrocolpos), mucoid (mucocolpos), or purulent (pyocolpos) secretions in the vagina before menstruation sets in, (*b*) retention of menstrual secretions in the vagina (hematocolpos), cervix and uterus (hematometria), fallopian tubes (hematosalpinx), and peritoneal cavity (hematoperitoneum) after menstruation sets in, (*c*) urethrovaginal fistula, and (*d*) sterility, characterized clinically by (*a*) absence of menstruation, (*b*) pain in the pelvis and lower abdomen, and (*c*) abdominal pelvic mass, diagnosed by inspection and palpation, treated by surgical incision, and attended by a good prognosis (Doyle), and (9) *accessory mammary tissue*—rare, located in any portion of the vulva but most commonly affecting the labia, consisting of duplication of an entire or only a part of a breast, and complicated by swelling, discharge of milk, infection, or trauma (Fisher).

DEGENERATIONS AND INFLAMMATIONS

Since the vulva is covered with integument it is subjected to most of the degenerative and inflammatory diseases seen in the skin of other portions of the body. The more important conditions may be enumerated as follows: (1) *gonorrhea*—(p. 1025), (2) *acute ulcerative vulvitis*—also known as ulcus vulvæ acutum, cyclic ulcerative vulvitis and stomatitis, cyclic mucosal ulceration, recurrent buccal and genital ulceration, and (in the mouth) as aphthous stomatitis (p. 606) (Pappworth), (3) *gangrene*—rare and occurring in conjunction with massive edema of the vulva or debilitating diseases (Purdie), (4) *vulvitis* in *systemic disease*—characterized essentially by itching and edema and seen in connection with blood dyscrasias (agranulocytosis, hypoplastic anemia, leukemia, pernicious anemia, etc.), uremia, diabetes mellitus, vitamin deficiency (vitamin B complex), and allergy (Parks), (5) *bartholinitis*—inflammation of Bartholin's gland, often caused by *Neisseria gonorrhoeæ* but also by other pyogenic organisms (streptococci, staphylococci, and colon bacilli), being unilateral or bilateral, appearing as a reddened area permeated with pus, characterized clinically by painful swelling of the gland, and complicated by Bartholin's abscess and (when the infection dies out) cyst formation (Davies and Bland), (6) *chancroid*—(p. 1112), (7) *syphilis*—similar to syphilis of the penis (p. 1112), with (*a*) a chancre located on the cervix, labia, fourchet, urethra, clitoris, vagina, vestibule, anus, Bartholin's gland orifice, perineum, thigh, mons pubis, and buttocks, (*b*) syphilids located on the skin, (*c*) mucous patches located anywhere on the mucous membranes, (*d*) condyloma latum located in moist areas of the skin subjected to friction, and (*e*) tertiary lesions consisting of diffuse infiltrations, ulcerations, or gummas, located on the vulva or cervix, and being extremely rare (Davies), (8) *tuberculosis*—usually if not always secondary to tuberculosis in other organs of the body particularly the lower urogenital tract and the rectum, and affecting Bartholin's glands as a circumscribed swelling and the vulva as a hypertrophic or ulcerative lesion (Speiser, Barrow, and Schaeffer), (8) *senile vulvitis*—having no predilection for any race, generally seen in women beyond the menopause, probably caused by withdrawal of estrogens, affecting the entire vulva or limited to the labia minora and clitoris (Fig. 561), consisting initially of (*a*) *inflammation* characterized by itching, swelling, redness, and tenderness and later of (*b*) *atrophy* or *kraurosis* when the skin becomes thin and parchment-like with the epidermis disclosing atrophy and disappearance of the rete pegs and the underlying dermis revealing fibrosis and (*c*) *hypertrophy* or *leukoplakia* seen as thickened white areas with hyperkeratosis, hypertrophy of the rete pegs, and inflammation of the adjacent dermis, and complicated by (*a*) pruritus, (*b*) cracks associated with secondary inflammation, (*c*) narrowing of the vaginal orifice and dyspareunia, and (*d*) carcinoma (Mishell, Adair, and Miller), (9) *granuloma inguinale*—(p, 1112), (10) *lymphogranuloma venereum*—(p. 1112), (11) *herpes progenitalis*—(p. 607), and (12) *mycotic* and *yeast-like vulvovaginitis*—predisposed by pregnancy and diabetes, usually

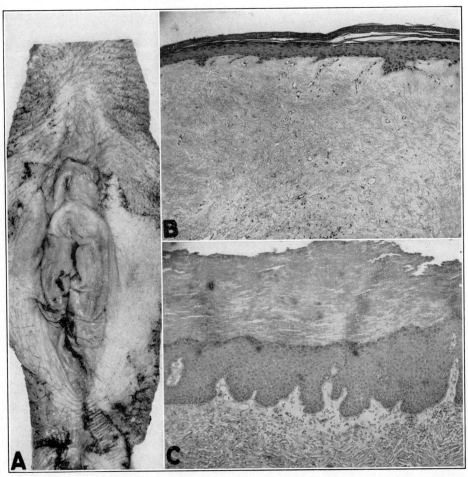

Fig. 561.—Senile vulvitis showing *A*, atrophy of especially the labia minora and clitoris, *B*, atrophy (kraurosis) of the epidermis and fibrosis of the dermis. × 50, and *C*, hypertrophy and hyperkeratosis (leukoplakia) of the epidermis. × 50.

caused by organisms belonging to the genus *Candida*, affecting not only the vulva but also the vagina and cervix, characterized in the acute stage by granulations that bleed readily upon manipulation, attended in the chronic stage by atrophy, fissuring, and inflammation, accompanied clinically by itching, discharge, and dyspareunia, diagnosed by isolating the causative organisms on Sabouraud's medium, and being refractory to treatment (Jones).

PHYSICAL DISTURBANCES

In this section, the following conditions of the vulva may be listed: (1) *edema*—part of a general process such as cardiac failure, nephrosis, or

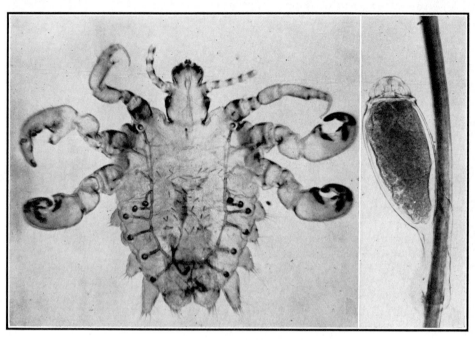

FIG. 562.—Pediculosis pubis illustrating the *Phthirus pubis* (pubic louse) free and attached to a hair.

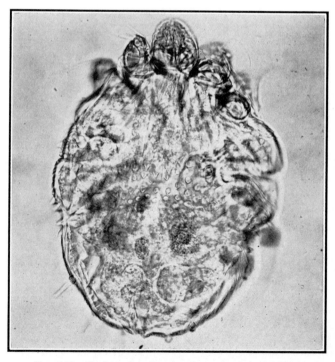

FIG. 563.—Scabies showing the *Acarus scabei.* × 200.

vitamin deficiency (p. 203) (Arnell), (2) *hematoma*—affecting the vagina as well as the vulva, seen as a complication of labor, occurring approximately once in every 1,650 cases, and occasionally complicated by shock (from loss of blood) or infection (Hamilton), (3) *varicosities*—rare, usually caused by pregnancy, consisting of irregularly dilated and compressible veins, and sometimes complicated by hemorrhage, hematoma, or infection (Adler), (4) *hernia*—consisting of protrusion of a viscus into the labia and corresponding to scrotal hernia in the male (p. 225), (5) *pediculosis pubis*—caused by the crab or pubic louse which is found attached to hair (Fig. 562), contracted incidental to coitus, and consisting of superficial abrasions produced by the lice and by the fingers of the victim from scratching (Ormsby and Montgomery), and (6) *scabies*—known as the "itch," defined as a contagious disorder caused by the *Acarus scabei* (Fig. 563), localized to moist areas of the skin (between fingers and toes, about the wrist, in folds of the axillæ and breast, and about the external genitals), consisting of a cuniculus or burrow that harbors the parasite and ova, diagnosed by finding the parasite and ova, characterized by intense itching, and attended by papules, pustules, crusts, excoriations, and pigmentations (Ormsby and Montgomery).

TUMORS

Orientation.—Tumors of the vulva are similar to tumors of the skin in general. Histogenetically they may be listed as follows: papilloma, condyloma acuminatum (p. 1115), carcinoma, hidradenoma (sweat gland tumor), hidradenoid carcinoma, Paget's disease, sebaceous cysts, Bartholin's cysts (p. 1149), nevus, melanoblastoma, myxoma, fibroma, myxosarcoma, fibrosarcoma, hemangioma, hemangiosarcoma, lymphangioma, lipoma, liposarcoma, neurofibroma, neuroma, ganglioneuroma, leiomyoma, myoblastoma, chondroma, lymphoblastoma, mixed tumors, urethral caruncle (p. 1027), endometriosis, and secondary tumors. Most of the neoplasms are identical with similar growths in the skin, lymph nodes, etc., and are considered in appropriate places in the text. Carcinoma, however, is of special interest and deserves a few additional words.

Carcinoma.—Carcinoma is the most common malignant tumor of the vulva accounting for about 3 per cent of all malignant tumors of the female generative system and 0.1 per cent of all gynecologic admissions (Palmer and Lunin). It is usually seen in women over sixty years of age and is perhaps somewhat more frequent in white people than in Negresses (Diehl). The *cause* is unknown but senile vulvitis is often noted as a precursor.

Pathologically any portion of the vulva (including Bartholin's glands) may be affected, with the labia and fourchet being most commonly involved (Fig. 564). Grossly the tumor starts as a hyperkeratosis, crack, eczema, papilloma, or indurated elevation. As it ages, it develops into (*a*) a fungating, firm, friable, sessile or more pedunculated, superficially ulcerating mass that may measure as much as 15 cm. in diameter or (*b*) an ulcerating defect with elevated edges, a floor covered with purulent or sanguineous material, and a base composed of gray friable tissue. *Histologically* the tumor is usually of a well-differentiated squamous cell variety composed of polyhedral prickle cells and well-formed pearls (Fig. 564). Less frequently, it consists of basal cells (Siegler) and rarely of cuboidal or columnar cells in glandular formation. In connection with unusual growths it may also be stated that sometimes a tumor is composed of epithelial cells that have not broken through the basement membrane—a condition referred to as

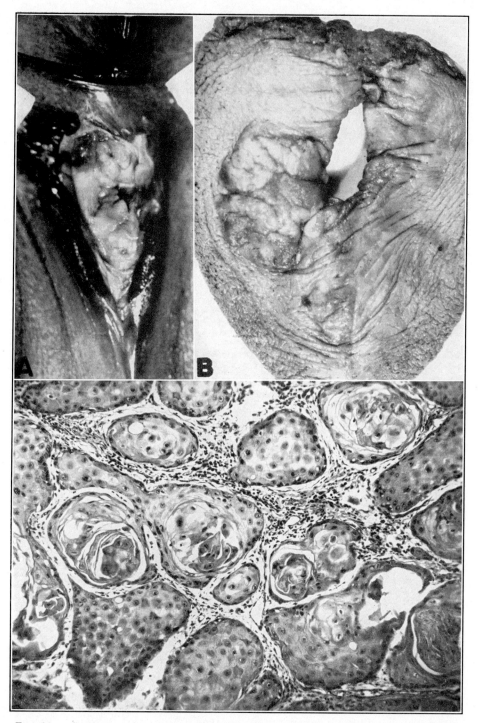

Fig. 564.—Carcinoma of the vulva demonstrating *A*, a fungating mass involving the upper portion of the right labium minus and clitoris, *B*, a superficially ulcerating lesion affecting the lower one-half of the right labium minus, and *C*, nests of squamous cells with well-formed pearls. × 100.

73

Bowen's disease or carcinoma-in-situ (Gardner). Sometmes, too, the neo-plastic cells originate in sweat glands and secondarily affect the skin—a condition called *Paget's disease* (Parsons and Huber). Each of these un-usual tumors, as well as basal cell carcinoma, is relatively benign and re-mains localized for long periods. Squamous cell carcinoma, however, is definitely malignant and *spreads* by (1) direct extension, (2) lymphatics to the inguinal, deep femoral, and obturator lymph nodes, and (3) blood vessels to the liver, lungs, and other organs.

Aside from extension and metastasis, the chief *complications* are secondary infection and cancer cachexia. The main *clinical manifestations* consist of a sore or a mass that later interferes with physical function and, as a result of infection, becomes painful and accompanied by a discharge. The final *diagnosis* is made by biopsy. *Treatment* of choice for squamous cell car-cinoma is radical vulvectomy (Cosby) while treatment for basal cell car-cinoma, Bowen's disease, and Paget's disease, is wide local excision. The *prognosis* in squamous cell carcinoma is fair, with the five-year survival being about 30 per cent (Newell). The outlook in basal cell carcinoma, Bowen's disease, and Paget's disease is considerably better.

VAGINA

CONGENITAL ANOMALIES

Developmental abnormalities of the vagina may be listed as follows: (1) *atresia*—connoting a failure of formation of a lumen, being extremely rare, and affecting the lower or upper portion (Maliphant and Thomas), (2) *absence*—complete lack of formation and usually associated with other genito-urinary anomalies (Counseller), (3) *transverse septa*—single or multiple, usually located in the upper portion, and generally consisting of a partial partition (Tritoftides), (4) *duplication*—also called double or septate vagina, characterized by a complete or incomplete longitudinal septum, and often associated with duplication of the upper portion of the generative tract (Mayer), and (5) *cysts*—occurring as often as once in every 500 gynecologic patients, usually arising from Gartner's (vestiges of wolf-fian) ducts and rarely from mullerian ductal epithelium, being unilateral or bilateral, located along the anterior or anterolateral surface of the vagina, measuring up to 10 cm. in diameter, and consisting of a connective tissue wall lined with cuboidal, columnar, or pseudostratified columnar epithelium (Lisenby, Sanders, and Wilder).

INFLAMMATIONS

Inflammation of the vagina is known as *vaginitis* or *colpitis*. The con-ditions in this category are generally associated with and are similar to corresponding inflammations of the vulva (p. 1149) and cervix. They may be listed as follows: (1) *gonorrhea*, (2) *acute ulcerative* (cyclic) *vaginitis*, (3) *nonspecific vaginitis*, (4) *emphysematous vaginitis*—presence of gas-filled cysts within the mucosa and submucosa, rare, and of unknown etiology (Bender), (5) *senile vaginitis*, (6) *fusospirochœtosis*, (7) *tuberculosis*, (8) *granuloma inguinale*, (9) *lymphogranuloma venereum*, (10) *mycotic vaginitis*, (11) *amebic vaginitis*, and (12) *trichomonal vaginitis*—acute to chronic recurring infection, caused by *Trichomonas vaginalis* (pear-shaped protozoa, measuring 10 to 30 by 5 to 15 microns, containing an oval nucleus near the blunt end and cytoplasmic granules throughout, and disclosing three to five anterior and one posterior flagella and an undulating membrane (Fig. 565), being the most common cause of leukorrhea in women, characterized clinically by a frothy discharge and considerable itching and burning pain, attended pathologically by a strawberry-like appearance grossly and a nonspecific inflammat on microscopically, and affecting not only the vagina but also the urethra and trigone of the urinary bladder in the female and the urethra, bladder, ureters, and prostate in the male (Brady and Allen).

PHYSICAL DISTURBANCES

Under the heading of Physical Disturbances the following vaginal conditions may be listed: (1) *trauma*—due to (*a*) delivery and located inferiorly, (*b*) coitus and located in the vault, or (*c*) surgery and located anywhere, consisting of (*a*) abrasion, (*b*) hematoma, (*c*) perforation, or (*d*) laceration, and complicated by (*a*) hemorrhage, (*b*) infection, or (*c*) trauma to adjacent organs (Diddle), (2) *accumulations* of *fluid*—(p. 1148), (3) *fistulas*—being caused by (*a*) congenital anomalies, (*b*) inflammations, (*c*) physical disturbances, and (*d*) tumors and resulting in communications of the vagina with the urethra, bladder, ureter, small or large intestine, uterine cervix, or uterine body (Bland), (4) *hernias*—encompassing (*a*) prolapse of the uterus or procidentia, (*b*) cystocele—protrusion of the urinary bladder and anterior vaginal wall, and (*c*) rectocele or proctocele—protrusion of the anterior wall of the rectum and posterior wall of the vagina, and caused (in the case of the uterus) by relaxation of the pelvic floor and stretching of the ligaments of the uterus and (in the case of bladder and rectum) by damage to and relaxation of the vaginal wall and the adjacent fibrous and muscle tissues, (5) *calculi*—rare, formed in the vagina or arriving there from the urinary tract, and resulting from vaginal obstruction and accumulation of urine (Stansfield), and (6) *foreign bodies*—relatively common, inserted from below, found mostly in youngsters but also seen in adults, consisting of virtually anything small enough to be inserted, and complicated by infection, ulceration, fibrosis, and fistulous tract formation (Hoge).

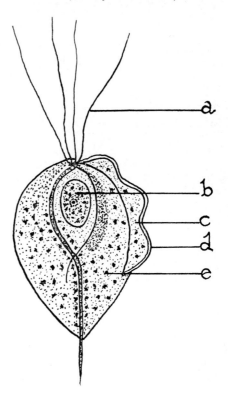

Fig. 565.—*Trichomonas vaginalis* showing *A*, anterior flagella, *B*, nucleus, *C*, undulating membrane, *D*, posterior flagellum, and *E*, cytoplasmic granules.

TUMORS

Orientation.—Histogenetically, tumors and tumor-like conditions of the vagina may be classified as follows: cyst, papilloma, adenosis, carcinoma, fibroma, leiomyoma, leiomyosarcoma, fibromyoma, neurofibroma, hemangioma, lymphangioma, deciduosis, mesodermal mixed tumor, teratoid tumor, melanoblastoma, endometriosis, and secondary tumors. Of these, carcinoma and mesodermal mixed tumor shall be commented on further.

Carcinoma.—Carcinoma of the vagina constitutes about 2 per cent of all primary carcinomas of the female generative tract (Bivens). It rarely occurs before the age of thirty years, is most common in the sixth decade of life, and has no predilection for any race. The precise *cause* is unknown but (1) irritation as in prolapsed uterus, especially in women who wear pessaries, (2) senile vaginitis, and (3) estrogenic stimulation are thought to act as precipitating factors (Geist and Bivens). *Pathologically* carcinoma may arise in any portion of the birth canal with the upper and posterior and the anterior and inferior portions being favored somewhat over other areas. In most instances, the growth is single. As in the vulva, it may be fungating or infiltrating and ulcerating. *Fungating* tumors are sessile or pedunculated, protrude and fill the vagina, are superficially ulcerated, and are composed of friable, rather soft, spongy tissue. Infiltrating growths exist as plaques or as cylindrical masses encircling part or all of the vagina and causing varying degrees of constriction. While the surface may be intact, more often it is granular or frankly ulcerating. *Histologically* carcinoma of the vagina is usually of a squamous cell variety of low or intermediate grade malignancy. As such, it exists as masses and nests of polyhedral prickle cells showing varying degrees of keratinization and pearl formation. Adenocarcinoma is extremely rare. Carcinoma of the vagina *spreads* by (1) direct extension to involve adjacent tissues and organs, (2) lymphatics to the iliac lymph nodes, and (3) blood vessels (rarely and terminally) to distant organs.

The most common *complications* are extension, metastasis, secondary infection, and fistulous tract formation. *Clinical manifestations* usually occur when the lesion is well established. They consist of vaginal bleeding, leukorrhea, pain, and dyspnea. The final *diagnosis* is made by biopsy. *Treatment* consists of surgical excision, irradiation, or a combination of these. The *prognosis* is guarded for the average five-year survival is in the neighborhood of 25 per cent.

Mesodermal Mixed Tumor.—This is a relatively rare tumor composed of mixed elements and called, among other things, *sarcoma botryoides* (Simpson). The tumor is about as *frequent* in the vagina as it is in the cervix and body of the uterus combined (Murphy, Schmidt, McElin and Fisher). The vaginal growths are generally found in children under three years of age while the uterine tumors occur in adults in the third and fourth decades of life. The tumor arises from pluripotent cells but the cause is unknown. *Pathologically* the vaginal, cervical, and sometimes corporal tumor exists as a large polypoid mass of tissue that has been likened to a bunch of fused grapes. In addition, the corporal tumor may appear as a flat pancake-like mass filling most of the uterine cavity. The pedicle is narrow or sessile. *Histologically* the growth is composed of mixtures of myxomatous tissue, connective tissue, striated and smooth muscle, myoblasts, cartilage, osteoid tissue, and squamous and glandular epithelial elements. The growths *spread* by local extension to all the pelvic tissues and by metastasis to the bones, lungs, and mediastinum (Amolsch). The *clinical manifestations* consist of vaginal discharge, passage or protrusion of the tumor through the vagina, and later pain. The *diagnosis* is made from the gross appearance of the lesion and biopsy. *Treatment* of choice is complete surgical removal.

The *prognosis* is poor with death generally occurring in from one to two years (Hardy).

CERVIX

CONGENITAL ANOMALIES

Developmental malformations of the cervix of the uterus consist of the following: (1) *rudimentary cervix*—diminutive in size or formed only in part, (2) *absence*—rare and resulting from a failure of differentiation of the lower portions of the mullerian ducts, (3) *duplication*—associated with duplication of the uterus, (4) *mesonephric remnants*—due to persistence of portions of the mesonephric (wolffian) ducts, existing in the lateral walls of the cervix and consisting of cysts, adenomatous proliferations, and adenocarcinoma (Huffman), and (5) *atresia*—absence of a normal opening, being congenital and due to abnormal canalization of mullerian ductal epithelium or acquired and due to trauma and/or infection, and complicated by sterility, hematometria, and hematosalpinx (Flemming, Maliphant, and Wanamaker).

INFLAMMATIONS

Orientation.—Inflammation of the cervix, as a whole, is known as *cervicitis*, of the vaginal portion only as *exocervicitis*, and of the canal portion as *endocervicitis*. The inflammations usually occur in connection with, and are similar to, those of the vulva and vagina. They may be listed as follows: gonorrhea, nonspecific cervicitis, chancroid, syphilis, leukoplakia, tuberculosis, granuloma inguinale, lymphogranuloma venereum, trichomoniasis, mycotic cervicitis, and actinomycosis. Of these, the most common and most important is nonspecific cervicitis.

Nonspecific Cervicitis.—Under this heading may be included those conditions that have been referred to as erosion, ectropion, eversion, laceration with infection, cystic cervicitis, etc. The condition *occurs* in as high as 80 per cent of all multiparous women, predominates in the fourth decade of life, and affects all races (Piper, Seaman, Findley, Fluhmann, Carmichael, and McIlrath). Predisposing *causes* consist of hyperestrinism, branching nature of the glands, alkaline mucus, and trauma incurred at childbirth. Precipitating causes are bacteria, especially gonococci, streptococci, staphylococci, and colon bacilli.

Pathologically the process may be (*a*) *acute*—seen most characteristically in the puerperium and during the first attack of gonorrhea, consisting grossly of swelling, redness, exudation, and laceration or ulceration, and exhibiting microscopically nonspecific denudation of the epithelium, hyperemia of the capillaries, edema, and leukocytic infiltration, or (*b*) *chronic*—charf acterized by destruction and repair (Fig. 566), showing varying degrees o-distortion from previous laceration and fibrosis, also exhibiting grossly large or small, single or multiple, reddened areas of superficial ulceration and exudation extending from the cervical canal onto the vaginal surface, and disclosing microscopically varying degrees of epithelial destruction, epithelial regeneration, glandular proliferation with (nabothian) cyst formation, fibrosis, and plasma cell, lymphocytic, and monocytic infiltration (Fig. 567). Of all these changes, the alterations affecting the columnar *epithelium* and called *squamous metaplasia* or *epidermidalization*, are the most spectacular. They occur at the junction of the covering squamous and columnar epithelium and within the racemose glands proper, and con-

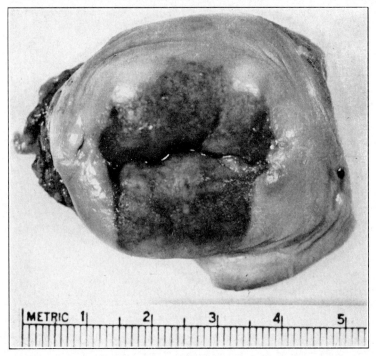

FIG. 566.—Nonspecific cervicitis illustrating a large, reddened, and granular area on each of the (anterior and posterior) lips.

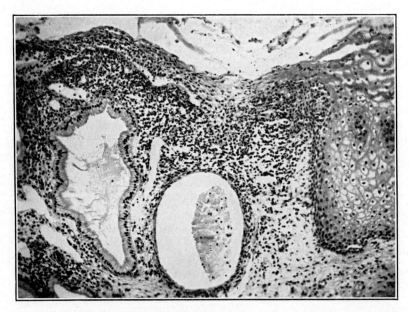

FIG. 567.—Nonspecific cervicitis demonstrating denudation of the epithelium, diffuse leukocytic infiltration, and nabothian cyst formation.   × 100. (Herbut's *Gynecological and Obstetrical Pathology.*)

sist of proliferations of basal cells with transformation into squamous cells (Fig. 568). The changes are usually multiple and characteristically disclose remnants of the secreting columnar cells covering the surface. The condition is important for it may readily be mistaken for intra-epithelial carcinoma (carcinoma-in-situ).

The *complications* of nonspecific cervicitis consist of (1) cervical atresia, (2) focus of infection for the urinary tract and rest of the body, and (3) carcinoma. While there is no doubt that carcinoma is more common in the presence of nonspecific cervicitis than it is in a noninflamed cervix, the relationship between the two still remains a moot question. The *clinical manifestations* consist of (1) leukorrhea—from the infection as such, (2) dysmenorrhea (and other pain) and sterility—from cervical obstruction,

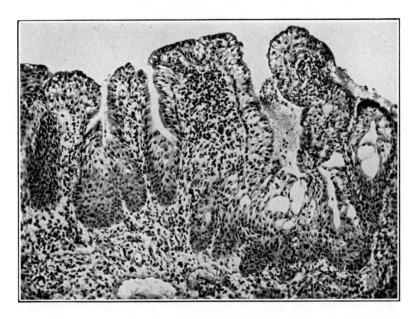

Fig. 568.—Nonspecific cervicitis with epidermidalization showing replacement of glandular epithelium with squamous epithelium at several points. × 100. (Herbut's *Gynecological and Obstetrical Pathology*.)

(3) pruritus of the vulva—from vaginal discharge, (4) vaginal bleeding—from ulceration, (5) frequency and urgency—from trigonitis, (6) arthritis and iritis—from secondary infection, and (7) mental distress—from fear of cancer (Zelezny-Baumrucker). The *diagnosis* is made from the history, direct visualization, and biopsy. *Treatment* is variable consisting essentially of cauterization, conization, or cervical amputation. The *prognosis* is good for cures can be expected in over 80 per cent of cases.

PHYSICAL DISTURBANCES

In this section the following lesions may be enumerated: (1) *atresia*—(p. 1157), (2) *prolapse*—(p. 1155), (3) *changes* in *pregnancy*—consisting of (*a*) the ordinary alterations encountered in nonspecific cervicitis with emphasis on hyperplasia of squamous epithelium and epidermidalization, and (*b*) decidual reaction in the stroma (called deciduosis or deciduoma) and important because it may be confused with carcinoma (Martin and Murphy), (4) *trauma*—incurred especially during delivery, consisting of irregular and usually multiple lacerations but sometimes also accompanied by detachment of the cervix and lacerations of the vagina and perineum, and complicated by hemorrhage, shock, and infection (Ingraham, Sheets, and Tollefson), (5) *cervical pregnancy*—(p. 1179), and (6) *irradiation changes*—encountered in connection with irradiation for uterine carcinoma, consisting (*a*) grossly of intense hyperemia followed by necrosis of tissue, profuse discharge, sloughing, and cicatrization and (*b*) microscopically of necrosis of epithelial and other cells, nonspecific leukocytic infiltration, fibroblastic proliferation, endarteritis obliterans, and collagenization, and complicated by (*a*) cervical occlusion, (*b*) irradiation changes in the bladder, ureter, rectum, and other adjacent tissues, and (*c*) fistulous tract formation (Waterman, Morton, and Farrar).

TUMORS

Orientation.—Tumors and tumor-like conditions of the cervix may be classified histogenetically as follows: papilloma, adenoma, carcinoma, fibroma, polyp, fibromyoma, fibroadenoma, sarcoma, mesodermal mixed tumor (p. 1156), hemangioma, hemangio-endothelioma, ganglioneuroma, leukemia, endometriosis, and secondary tumors. Of these, only polyps and carcinoma need be considered further.

Polyp.—Cervical polyps are common, being recorded as encountered in approximately 3.5 per cent of all adult women, 10 per cent of all gynecologic specimens, and 1.5 per cent of all gynecologic patients. While they may occur at any age, they are most common in women in the fifth and sixth decades of life (Serbin, Mezer, and Newgard). The *cause* is unknown but pregnancy (because of congestion and edema), chronic inflammation, trauma, and endocrine factors are thought to play contributory roles. *Pathologically* the lesions are usually single and, as a rule, originate within the cervical canal (Fig. 569). They may be long, bulbous, and attached by a narrow pedicle or they may be more squatty and sessile. The color varies from gray to red and the consistency is generally moderately firm. *Histologically* the external surface is usually covered with columnar epithelium which, however, may undergo focal epidermidalization. The core is composed of connective tissue disclosing varying degrees of congestion, edema, and leukocytic infiltration and containing regular, hyperplastic, or cystically dilated racemose glands (Fig. 569). The *complications* consist of infection and carcinomatous transformation. While some writers claim that carcinoma develops in as high as 6 per cent of all cervical polyps the incidence, in your author's opinion, is probably not any greater than it is in people showing only nonspecific cervicitis. *Clinically* cervical polyps are asymptomatic or are attended only by bleeding and cervical discharge. The *diagnosis* is made by inspection and biopsy. *Treatment* is surgical or electric excision. The *prognosis* is excellent.

Carcinoma.—Carcinoma of the cervix is commoner than any other malignant tumor of the female generative system and is said to account for about 20 per cent of deaths from all cancer in women (Morris). It constitutes about 5 per cent of all admissions to the gynecological service and is about four times as frequent as carcinoma of the endometrium (Raphael). While it may seen at all ages, from birth on, it is most common in the fifth and sixth decades of life (Scheffey and Baber). It affects all races but is more common in Negresses than in white women and is rare in Jewesses (Raphael). Although the precise *cause* is unknown, the following are considered to be of etiologic significance: syphilis, douching, race, hormonal imbalances, heredity, viruses, avitaminosis, and chronic cervicitis (Lombard and Bainborough).

Pathologically the lesion generally starts at the squamo-columnar junction. Grossly the earliest lesion (intra-epithelial carcinoma or carcinoma-in-situ) is not recognizable for the cervix appears normal or is merely that of chronic cervicitis. As the growth becomes macroscopically detectable it

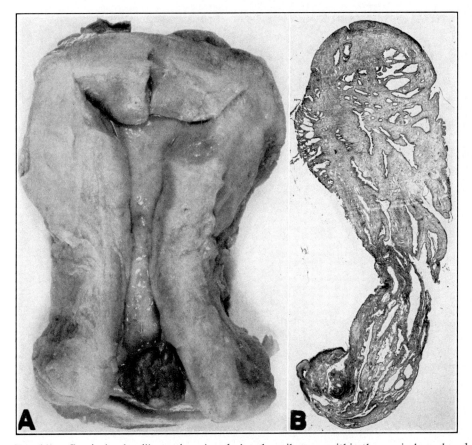

Fig. 569.—Cervical polyp illustrating *A*, a dark red sessile mass within the cervical canal and *B*, an elongated structure composed of connective tissue containing racemose glands and covered with columnar epithelium. × semigross.

assumes one of two forms—fungating or ulcerating (Figs. 570 and 571). A *fungating* tumor grows outwardly as a protruding, friable, grayish-white, superficially ulcerating mass that does not penetrate the cervix deeply and that ultimately may fill a good portion of the vagina. An *ulcerating* carcinoma grows in the reverse direction, permeating the cervical and adjacent tissues and ulcerating as it penetrates. Ultimately, not only may the entire cervix be dissipated but the adjacent tissues may be destroyed leaving fistulous tracts between the vagina and the uterus, bladder, and rectum (Fig. 571*B*).

Histologically the tumor is a squamous cell variety of carcinoma in about 95 per cent of cases (Fig. 568*B* and *C*). In its earliest form it exists as an *intra-epithelial carcinoma*, that is, an epithelial tumor composed of irregular prickle cells similar to those seen in invasive tumors but remaining confined by the basement membrane. As the lesion ages it infiltrates the underlying tissues in an irregular fashion just as does any other squamous cell carcinoma. As a rule, however, keratinization is minimal and while pearl formation may occur it is not as frequent as it is in cutaneous squamous

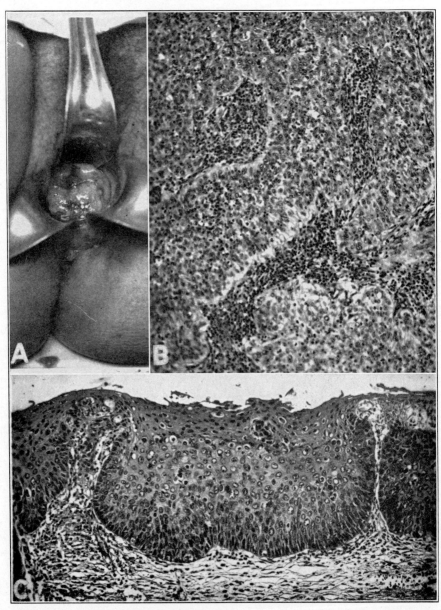

Fig. 570.—Carcinoma of the cervix showing *A*, a fungating lesion covering the posterior half of the cervix, *B*, an invasive growth of intermediate grade malignancy. × 100, and *C*, an intra-epithelial tumor confined by the basement membrane. × 100.

cell carcinoma. In about 5 per cent of cases the tumor is an adenocarcinoma and as such exists as cuboidal or columnar cells in acinar formation (Hepler). Although intra-epithelial carcinoma probably remains localized for years, invasive carcinoma *spreads* by (1) local extension (as indicated) to adjacent structures, (2) lymphatics to the lymph nodes adjacent to the cervix, in the broad ligaments, and along the iliac vessels and aorta, and (3) blood vessels (late in the course of the disease) to the organs of the abdominal cavity, lungs, bones, etc.

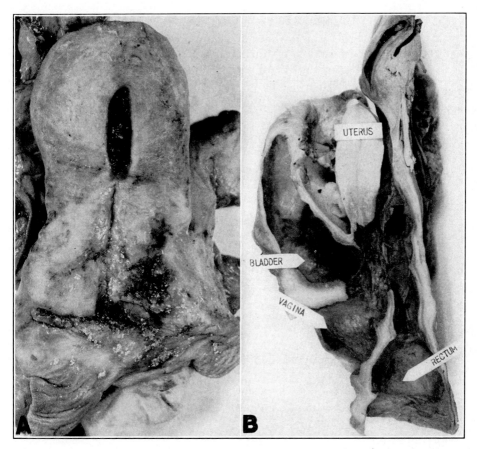

Fig. 571.—Carcinoma of the cervix illustrating *A*, invasion, ulceration, and destruction of the cervix and *B*, a similar lesion producing fistulas.

The chief *complications* are extension, metastasis, fistulous tract formation, obstruction of the ureter, infection, and hemorrhage. *Clinically* carcinoma of the cervix is asymptomatic until it ulcerates and becomes infected. At this stage, the earliest manifestations are intermenstrual vaginal bleeding or spotting and leukorrhea. As the lesion progresses and complications develop, pain, dysuria, urgency of urination, etc., become manifested. Bearing in mind the degree of localization or spread of the tumor, clinicians usually classify the lesion according to the criteria of Schmitz or League of Nations as follows (Galvin):

	Schmitz	*League of Nations*
Stage I	Clearly localized to the cervix with the cervix freely movable	Strictly confined to the cervix
Stage II	Doubtfully localized to the cervix with the mobility of the cervix impeded	Infiltrates the parametrium but does not invade the pelvic wall
Stage III	Invades parametrium or regional lymph node with the entire mass movable	Infiltrates the parametrium and invades the pelvic wall
Stage IV	Frozen pelvis with fixation of the tumor, extension to the bladder or rectum, and distant metastases	Extension to the bladder or rectum with spread outside of the true pelvis

The *diagnosis* of carcinoma of the cervix is made from the history, speculum examination of the cervix, Papanicolaou smears of vaginal secretions and cervical scrapings, and biopsy. *Treatment* of intra-epithelial carcinoma is still controversial (local excision, hysterectomy, or irradiation) while that of invasive carcinoma consists of radical hysterectomy or irradiation— each having its advocates. The *prognosis* varies. In intra-epithelial carcinoma the cure rate should be 100 per cent while in invasive carcinoma it is generally recorded as varying from 25 per cent to 40 per cent.

BODY OF UTERUS

CONGENITAL ANOMALIES

Developmental malformations of the uterus may be listed as follows: (1) *infantile uterus*—one that mimics a uterus during the prepuberal age and consists essentially of diminution in size, (2) *diverticulum*, and (3) *errors* in *fusion* of *mullerian ducts*—including all gradations from simple notching of the fundus to complete separation and partial development of the ducts, classified into (*a*) arcuate (notched) uterus, (*b*) double uterus with a single cervix, (*c*) septate uterus with a single or septate vagina, (*d*) double uterus with a double cervix, and (*e*) uterus with a rudimentary horn or absence of one horn, and complicated by sterility, inflammations, physical disturbances, and tumors (Taylor).

INFLAMMATIONS

Inflammation of the endometrium is known as *endometritis* and of the myometrium as *myometritis*. The more important lesions may be listed as follows: (1) *nonspecific endometritis*—uncommon, caused by the ordinary pyogenic organisms, and occurring in conjunction with partial obstruction of the cervix, tumors protruding into the uterine cavity, intra-uterine foreign bodies, and the puerperium, (2) *pyometria*—accumulation of pus in the uterine cavity, caused by the usual pyogenic organisms, occurring in the presence of complete obstruction of the cervical canal, and complicated by sterility and spread of the infection beyond the uterine cavity (De Voe), (3) *tuberculosis*—limited to the endometrium, almost always secondary to tuberculosis of the fallopian tubes, generally discovered histologically, and complicated (mostly as a result of tubal involvement) by infertility (O'Brien and Schaupp), (4) *blastomycosis*—rare and part of a systemic process, (5) *granuloma inguinale*—(p. 1112), and (6) *echinococcosis*—(p. 828).

PHYSICAL DISTURBANCES

Under this heading the following conditions may be enumerated: (1) *hematometria*—(p. 1149), (2) *displacement*—consisting of (*a*) anteposition—whole organ displaced forward, (*b*) retroposition—whole organ displaced backward, (*c*) lateral displacement, (*d*) ascent, (*e*) prolapse or procidentia—(p. 1155), (*f*) anteversion—rotation on its axis with the body tipping forward and the cervix backward, (*g*) anteflexion—forward bending of the body upon the cervix, (*h*) retroversion—rotation on its axis with the body tipping backward and the cervix forward, and (*i*) retroflexion—backward bending of the body upon the cervix, (3) *torsion*—axial rotation of the body on the cervix, generally caused by enlargement of the body by pregnancy or tumor along with thinning of the supracervical segment and characterized by congestion, edema, leukocytic infiltration, and focal necrosis in the superior segment with the changes depending upon the degree and tightness of the rotation (Siegler), (4) *inversion*—turning of the organ inside out, rare, usually seen after delivery but encountered also in nonpuerperal women when it is associated with submucous fibromyoma, and being complicated by shock, hemorrhage, anemia, infection, and sometimes death (Das), (5) *rupture*—being uncommon, usually seen in pregnancy, occurring in connection with (*a*) repeated pregnancies, (*b*) uterine cicatrices, (*c*) malposition (retroversion) of the uterus, (*d*) cervical stenosis, (*e*) congenital anomalies of the uterus, pelvis, and vagina, (*f*) prolonged labor, (*g*) destruction of the uterine wall by tumors, (*h*) overdistention of uterus (hydramnios), (*i*) fetal abnormalities (malposition, plural gestation, hydrocephalus, etc.), and (*j*) external injury, being complete or incomplete, and complicated by hemorrhage, shock, and death (Dugger and Beacham), (6) *wounds*—rare, usually seen in connection with pregnancy, and generally resulting from gunshot (Bost), (7) *fistulas*—uncommon, arising as a result of obstetrical or urological trauma or malignant tumor, and connecting the uterus with the urinary bladder, rectum, colon, small intestine, or vagina (Berlind), and (8) *irradiation changes*—seen in connection with irradiation for endometrial carcinoma and being similar to the changes in the cervix (p. 898).

TUMORS

Orientation.—Histogenetically tumors and tumor-like conditions of the body of the uterus may be classified as follows: endometrial hyperplasia, endometriosis, adenosis, endometrial polyp, endometrial carcinoma, fibroma, fibrosarcoma, uterine hypertrophy, myoma, myosarcoma, leiomyosarcoma, rhabdomyosarcoma, fibromyoma, carcinosarcoma, mesodermal mixed tumor (p. 1156), hemangioma, hemangio-endothelioma, lymphangioma, lymphangio-endothelioma, lymphoblastoma, lipoma, and secondary tumors. Of these, the following may be selected for separate discussion: endometrial hyperplasia, endometriosis, endometrial polyp, uterine hypertrophy, fibromyoma, endometrial carcinoma, and sarcoma.

Endometrial Hyperplasia.—Endometrial hyperplasia is *also known* as glandular hyperplasia, cystic glandular hyperplasia, and Swiss cheese endometrium. It is next in *frequency* to fibromyoma, affects women of all races, and is most common at or near the menopause (Geist, Novak, and Schwarz). The *cause* is probably excessive estrogenic stimulation occurring in conjunction with persistence of follicles, granulosa cell and theca cell tumors of the ovary, excessive adrenocortical hormone output, and therapeutic administration (Burch). *Pathologically* the endometrium throughout the uterine cavity is irregularly thickened (Fig. 572*A*). It is gray, soft, and velvety and may disclose foci of necrosis and hemorrhage and tiny cysts. *Histologically* it consists of an irregular hyperplasia of the glands (Fig. 572*B*). The glands may be small, large, or cystically dilated. They are often placed back to back and leave little intervening stroma. The lining epithelial cells are tall columnar and often several layers thick. They seldom show secretory droplets. The lumens of the cystically dilated glands often

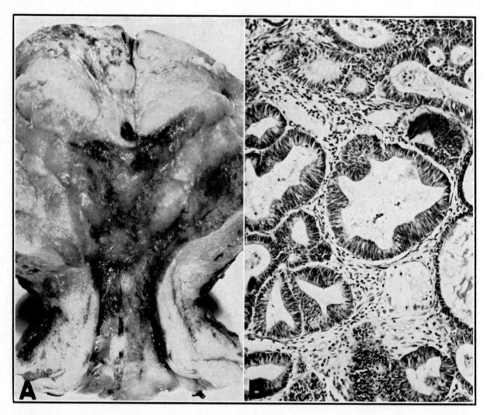

Fig. 572.—Endometrial hyperplasia illustrating *A*, diffuse but irregular thickening of the endometrium and *B*, irregular increase in number of glands lined by hyperplastic epithelium. × 100.

contain a pink precipitate. The most important *complication* of endometrial hyperplasia is transformation of the lesion into carcinoma. While the exact incidence of the two is difficult to determine, there is no question in your author's mind that a carcinomatous change occurs frequently enough to warrant close follow-ups on the patients. The most important *clinical manifestation* is uterine bleeding—irregular bleeding before the menopause and any bleeding after the menopause. The *diagnosis* is made by biopsy. *Treatment* has consisted of hormonal therapy, irradiation, curettage, or hysterectomy. The *prognosis* is generally good.

Endometriosis.—Endometriosis may be defined as the presence of endometrial tissue in abnormal locations. It is referred to as *internal* when it affects the myometrium and *external* when it affects extramyometrial tissues. Internal endometriosis is also called adenomyosis and is referred to as *endometrioma* or *adenomyoma* when it forms a discrete tumor mass.   The disorder is *common*, affects all races, and occurs during the reproductive period of life, especially the fourth and fifth decades (Meigs, Dockerty, Weeks, and Randall).   The condition has been considered to arise on the basis of (1) transportation of endometrium from the uterus to the areas concerned or (2) ectopic endometrium developing from local cells (Ranney). It is probable that both theories are correct, with the latter accounting for most cases.

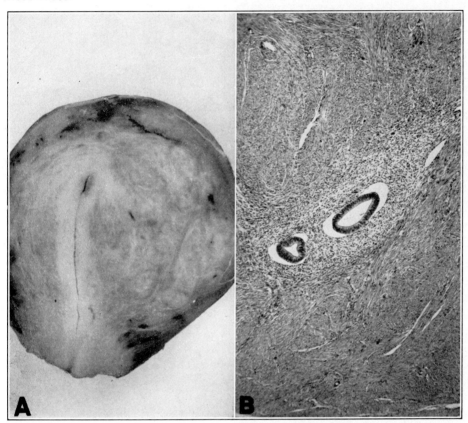

FIG. 573.—Endometriosis showing *A*, whorled myometrium dotted with hemorrhagic foci, and *B*, stroma and glands embedded within the myometrium.   × 50.

Pathologically, as far as the uterus is concerned, the organ is slightly or moderately enlarged and firm.   Cut surfaces disclose a whorling and bulging of the musculature with a smattering of deep red to brown irregular foci (Fig. 573*A*).   Sometimes the foci are larger and occasionally they consist of distinct tiny cysts filled with blood.   In organs other than the uterus the lesion is characterized by the presence of red to brown foci, larger cyst formations (up to 2 or 3 cm. in diameter), fibrosis, and adhesions.   The sites more commonly affected, in approximately decreasing order of frequency, may be listed as follows: surface of the uterus, *cul de sac*, surface of the ovary, rectosigmoid junction, ovary, urinary bladder, fallopian tubes, broad ligaments, round ligaments, parietal peritoneum, appendix, small bowel, abdominal scar, vulva, vagina, cervix, iliac lymph nodes, thigh, umbilicus, lungs, and muscles of the upper extremities (Kelly).

Histologically endometriosis is usually composed of endometrial tissue similar to that in the endometrium, undergoing (to a greater or lesser degree) the same cyclic changes (Fig. 573 *B*). When the lesion is on a surface the necrotic tissue and blood are shed with each menstruation, but when it is beneath the surface these degeneration products accumulate to form the chocolate-colored cysts already referred to. Occasionally, especially in the uterus, only endometrial stroma is present and the endometrial glands do not participate. Such a lesion is referred to as *stromal endometriosis* and, by the unwary, may be mistaken for sarcoma (Vesell).

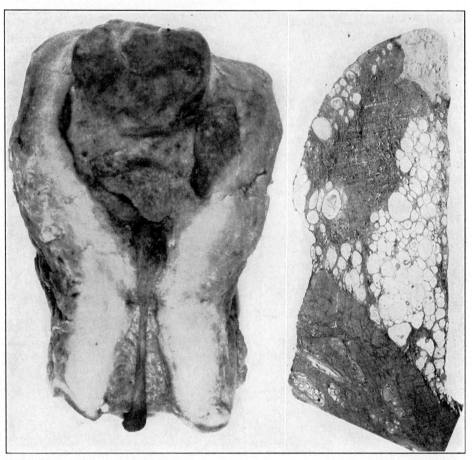

FIG. 574.—Endometrial polyp disclosing *A*, several sessile masses and a slender pedunculated structure and *B*, a sessile mass composed mostly of cystic spaces. × semigross.

The most common *complications* of endometriosis are menstrual disturbances, infertility, digestive disturbances, and urinary tract disturbances, depending upon which system or organ is affected. The *clinical manifestations* thus are extremely varied and range all the way from pain to uterine bleeding, dysuria, intestinal obstruction, and dyspareunia. The *diagnosis* is made by maintaining a high index of suspicion and by biopsy or examination of the specimen after surgical removal. *Treatment* has consisted of castration, irradiation, or surgical excision. The *prognosis*, as far as life is concerned, is excellent but the morbidity is often high.

Endometrial Polyp.—As in other areas of the body, an endometrial polyp may be defined as a finger-like projection of endometrial tissue above the surface of the endometrium. The condition is common, has no predilection for any race, and is most frequent in the fifth decade of life (Newgard). The *causes* are thought to be similar to those in cervical polyp (p. 1160). *Pathologically* any portion of the endometrium may be affected and there may be one polyp present, several polyps, or many polyps (polyposis). The size varies from a few to 6 or 8 cm. in greatest diameter and the lesion may be sessile or pedunculated (Fig. 574*A*). It is soft, gray to red, and occasionally superficially necrotic. Cut surfaces may disclose varisized cysts. *Histologically* the lesion is composed of endometrial tissue that appears similar to that in endometrial hyperplasia (Fig. 574*B*). The chief *complication* is a malignant transformation although such a change is extremely rare. *Clinical manifestations* are lacking in about one-third of the cases while in the rest they consist of uterine bleeding or discharge. The *diagnosis* is made upon curettage, unless the lesion protrudes through the cervix when it is made by direct visualization. *Treatment* consists of excision or hysterectomy. The *prognosis* is excellent.

Uterine Hypertrophy.—Uterine hypertrophy, known also as fibrosis uteri and myometrial hypertrophy, is characterized by diffuse enlargement of the uterus. It accounts for about 10 per cent of all uteri removed surgically, is more common in white women than in Negresses, and *occurs* between the ages of thirty and fifty years (Shoemaker). The *causes* have been thought to be inflammation, arteriosclerosis, chronic passive congestion, postpuerperal subinvolution, and an absolute or relative excess of estrogens (Truemner). *Grossly* the uterus is diffusely and uniformly enlarged, with the myometrium measuring as much as 4 cm. across (Fig. 575). The endometrium may be hyperplastic or it may show polyps. *Histologically* the myometrium may show combinations of the following: hypertrophy of the smooth muscle, increase of connective tissue, dilated and prominent vessels, and increase of elastic fibrils and collagen bundles in the media of arteries. The chief *clinical manifestations* consist of pelvic pain, menorrhagia, and leukorrhea. The *diagnosis* is made from the history and finding an enlarged uterus at the time of pelvic examination. *Treatment* consists of hysterectomy. The *prognosis* is excellent.

Fibromyoma.—As the name indicates, a fibromyoma of the uterus is a benign tumor composed of connective and muscle tissue. Commonly used synonyms are fibroma, fibroid, myoma, and leiomyoma. The lesion represents the most common tumor in females, *occurring* in about 30 per cent of all gynecologic patients and in from 4 to 11 per cent of all adult women. It is most prevalent between the ages of thirty and fifty years and is more common in Negresses than in white women. The *cause* is unknown but is thought to be estrogenic stimulation (Shute and Torpin). In support of this statement it has been shown that in humans (1) testosterone causes a decrease and estrogen causes an increase in size of tumor, (2) the tumor is frequently associated with endometrial hyperplasia, (3) it has a tendency to regress after the menopause, and (4) it develops only during the active reproductive life of the patient. *Experimental* evidence lies in the fact that administration of estrogen has resulted in the production of fibromyomas of the uterus in normal rabbits and mice and in spayed and unspayed guinea pigs.

Pathologically any portion of the uterus may be affected but the body is involved in over 95 per cent of cases (Fig. 576). The lesions are usually

74

multiple and although they start within the myometrium they may be located intramurally (within the wall), submucosally (protruding into the uterine cavity), or subserosally (protruding outwardly). In addition, some subserosal tumors may lose their attachment to the uterus and become attached to adjacent structures—a lesion known as a *parasitic fibroid.* Although the size may vary from barely detectable to that which fills the entire abdominal cavity, most tumors measure from 1 to 10 cm. in diameter.

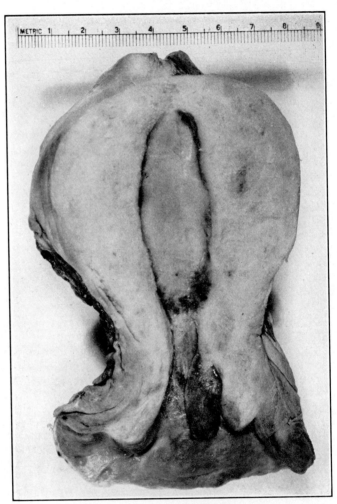

Fig. 575.—Hypertrophy of the uterus illustrating diffuse symmetrical enlargement. The cervical polyp is incidental.

Generally, the growths are sharply circumscribed, extremely firm, grayish white, whorled, and bulging. Degenerative changes, however, are frequent. They consist of hyalinization, necrosis, cyst formation, calcification, suppuration, torsion, red degeneration, and sarcomatous transformation. *Red degeneration* occurs in about 8 per cent of all fibromyomas, is characterized by a diffuse red to brown discoloration, and histologically discloses engorgement of blood space and/or degenerative changes with erythrocytic extravasation (Faulkner and Smith). A *sarcomatous transformation* is said to occur in up to 10 per cent of cases (McFarland). Although such tumors are similar to sarcomas arising directly from the myometrium they are somewhat less malignant. *Histologically* fibromyomas are composed of varying amounts of rather adult appearing fibrous and muscle tissue arranged in interlacing bundles (Fig. 577). Degenerative changes, as listed above, change the picture but are self-explanatory and need no further comment.

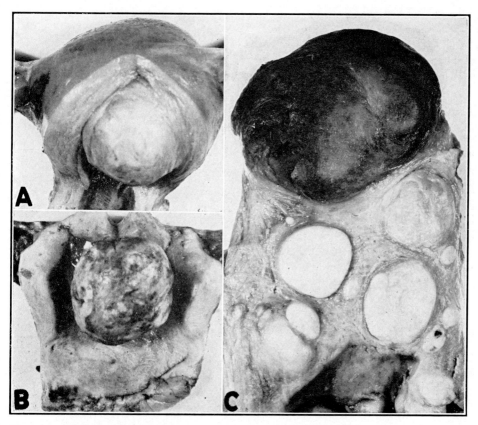

Fig. 576.—Fibromyomas of the uterus demonstrating *A*, an intramural lesion, *B*, a submucous growth, and *C*, several intramural tumors with red degeneration of one.

The *complications* of fibromyomas consist of the degeneration already referred to. The *clinical manifestations* result mainly from pressure upon adjacent structures. While they vary considerably, they may be listed as follows: vaginal bleeding, frequency of urination, dysuria, pains in the abdomen and pelvis, enlargement of the abdomen, constipation, etc. The *diagnosis* is generally made upon pelvic examination. *Treatment* consists of watchful waiting or hysterectomy. The *prognosis* is good.

Carcinoma.—Carcinoma of the endometrum is about one-quarter as *frequent* as carcinoma of the cervix and occurs about once in every 1,300 women (MacFarlane). It predominates in the sixth decade of life, is rare before the third decade, and, as compared with carcinoma of the cervix, is more common in nulliparas than multiparas (Scheffey, Hundley, Palmer, Diddle, Finn, Henriksen, and McGarvey). The *cause* is unknown although most authors believe that a hereditary predisposition and prolonged estrogenic stimulation account for most of the cases. Occasionally a purely extrinsic factor such as irradiation may act as a precipitating agent.

Pathologically carcinoma of the endometrium may arise in any part of the uterine cavity and is usually of unicentric origin. After a rather innocuous appearing start, the tumor usually develops into a polypoid mass or an infiltrating and ulcerating lesion (Fig. 578). A *polypoid* tumor protrudes into the uterine cavity. It is varisized, distends the uterine cavity as it enlarges, discloses a sessile or pedunculated attachment to the uterine wall, is pinkish gray, moderately firm and friable, and permeates the subjacent

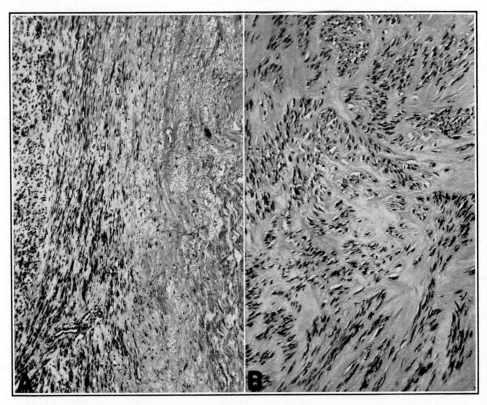

Fig. 577.—Fibromyomas of the uterus showing *A*, a typical appearance of spindle cells (to the left) and necrosis (to the right).   × 50, and *B*, hyaline degeneration in another tumor.   × 100.

myometrium for varying depths. An *infiltrating* tumor grows in the opposite direction and, as it does so, it generally ulcerates. *Histologically* carcinoma of the endometrium is usually of an adenomatous variety and fairly to moderately well differentiated (Fig. 579). It is composed of large or small glands lined by one or more layers of hyperchromatic, usually nonsecreting columnar cells. Sometimes, however, the tumor becomes quite anaplastic and rarely it is composed of a mixture of glands and squamous cells—*adenoacanthoma*. The tumor *spreads* by (1) local extension to involve the uterus and adjacent structures, (2) lymphatics to the iliac, aortic, hypogastric, and inguinal lymph nodes, and (3) blood vessels (late in the disease) to the lungs, liver, peritoneum, ovaries, adrenals, bones, etc.

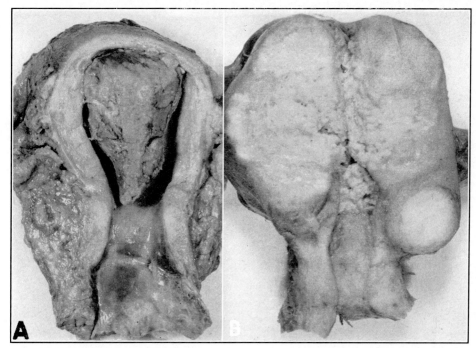

Fig. 578.—Carcinoma of the endometrium illustrating *A*, a fungating growth protruding into and filling the uterine cavity and *B*, an extensive infiltrating tumor permeating most of the myometrium.

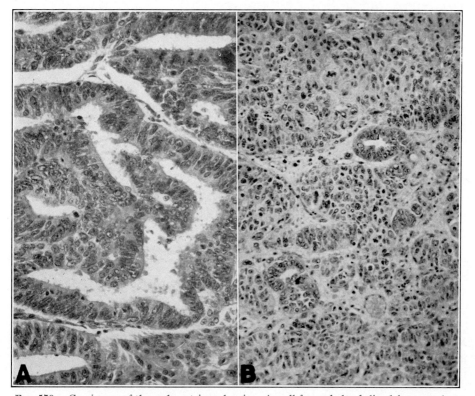

Fig. 579.—Carcinoma of the endometrium showing *A*, well-formed glands lined by several rows of irregular columnar cells. × 200 and *B*, a more malignant tumor with a diffuse arrangement of the cells and a poor attempt at glandular formation. × 100.

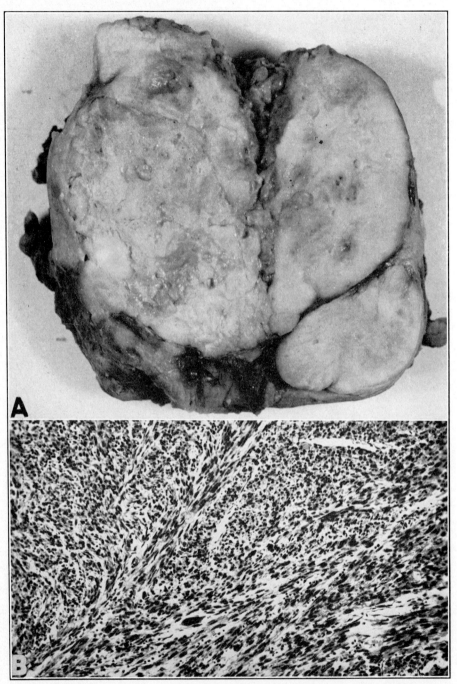

FIG. 580.—Sarcoma of the uterus demonstrating A, a leiomyosarcoma arising in a fibromyoma and B, a similar tumor composed of elongated and giant cells. × 100.

The *complications* consist of (1) spread of the tumor, (2) compression of the ureters and uremia, and (3) fistulous tract formation (usually with the bladder or large bowel). *Clinically* about 5 per cent of patients are asymptomatic, while the chief manifestations in the others consist of vaginal bleeding or spotting and/or leukorrhea. Pain occurs only late in the disease. The *diagnosis* is made from the history, Papanicolaou stained smears of vaginal secretions, and biopsy. *Treatment* consists of hysterectomy, irradiation, or a combination of the two. The *prognosis* in general is good, for if the patient is seen early and treated properly the five-year survival rate should be about 90 per cent.

Sarcoma.—Sarcoma of the uterus is considerably *less common* than the other tumors considered above, for it constitutes about 3 per cent of all malignant tumors in this organ. While it may occur at any age it is most frequent in the fifth and sixth decades of life (Randall, Cohen, Perry, Danforth, and McFarland). The *cause* is unknown but the factors operating are thought to be similar to those encountered in fibromyoma.

Pathologically sarcoma of the uterus generally arises in the myometrium and only rarely does it originate in the endometrium. The growth is usually single, appears fairly sharply circumscribed, is generally grayish white and brain-like, may disclose areas of necrosis and hemorrhage, and by the time it is discovered it measures 10 to 15 cm. in diameter (Fig. 580*A*). Depending upon its size and its precise point of origin, it may remain mostly intramural or it may protrude into the endometrial cavity or beneath the serosa. In any case, the uterus ultimately becomes enlarged and distorted. Histologically the most common tumors, in decreasing order of frequency, are leiomyosarcoma, fibrosarcoma, and rhabdomyosarcoma. Leiomyosarcoma consists of elongated, ill-defined, spindle cells with light staining, sometimes fibrillary, cytoplasm and evenly stained, elongated nuclei (Fig. 486*B*) while fibrosarcoma and rhabdomyosarcoma are identical with similar tumors in the skin and striated muscle.

Sarcoma of the uterus generally *spreads* by direct extension to adjacent structures and by blood vessels to the lungs, liver, and other organs. Lymphatic dissemination is *uncommon*. The *complications* consist of spread and ureteral obstruction. The *clinical manifestations* include vaginal bleeding, rapid enlargement of the abdomen, pain in the pelvis and abdomen, uterine mass, and general symptoms of tumor cachexia. The *diagnosis* is usually made at laparotomy or pathologically. *Treatment* consists of complete hysterectomy. The *prognosis* is generally poor with the five-year survival rate rarely exceeding 30 per cent.

FALLOPIAN TUBES

CONGENITAL ANOMALIES

Developmental malformations of the fallopian tube usually occur in association with developmental abnormalities of the uterus and may be unilateral or bilateral. They may consist of the following: (1) *agenesis*, (2) *incomplete development*, (3) *duplication*, (4) *multiple ostia*, (5) *diverticula*, (6) *displacement* (below usual point of attachment to the uterus), (7) *adrenal inclusions*—consisting of cortical tissue located in the free edge of the broad ligament, the ovary, and rarely the serosa of the uterus (Nelson), and (8) *Walthard cell rests*—consisting of solid or cystic nests of cuboidal or polyhedral cells located in the cortex or hilum of the ovary, tube, or broad ligament (Danforth).

INFLAMMATIONS

Orientation.—Inflammation of the fallopian tube (salpinx) is known as *salpingitis*. The lesions may be listed as follows: nonspecific salpingitis, salpingitis isthmica nodosa, tuberculosis, talcum powder granuloma, and actinomycosis. *Talcum powder granuloma* affects the serosal surfaces of the tubes and broad ligaments and has already been discussed (p. 899) while *actinomycosis* is rare and generally represents an extension from an infection at the ileocecal region. The other conditions merit brief separate consideration.

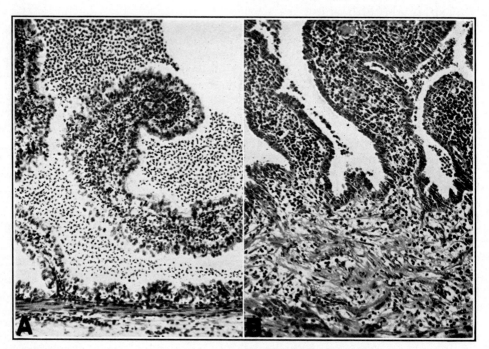

Fig. 581.—Salpingitis showing *A*, acute inflammation characterized by a diffuse permeation with neutrophils and *B*, chronic inflammation characterized by plasma cell infiltration and fibrosis. × 100.

Nonspecific Salpingitis.—Nonspecific salpingitis connotes inflammation of the fallopian tubes *caused* by gonococci, colon bacilli, streptococci, staphylococci, and other pyogenic organisms. The bacteria gain entrance by way of the lumen of the lower generative tract, interstitial tissues of the pelvis, or the bloodstream. The condition *occurs* at all ages but is most common in the third and fourth decades of life and prevails among the indigent (Mohler, Shaw, Hundley, and Black-Schaffer).

Pathologically the process is usually bilateral and affects not only the fallopian tubes but also the broad ligaments, ovaries, and all of the serosal surfaces of the pelvis. Thus, it is often referred to as pelvic inflammatory disease or P.I.D. In *acute salpingitis* the fallopian tubes are increased in size to three or four times normal. The serosal surfaces are hyperemic, dull, and roughened; the walls are thickened, edematous and rigid; the lumen is bathed by pus, and the fimbriæ show adhesions to each other and to adjacent structures. Histologically the villi are thickened, congested, edematous, and perfused with neutrophils; the epithelium shows degeneration and desquamation; the lumen is filled with pus, and the wall discloses a response similar to that in the villi (Fig. 581). In *chronic salpingitis* there is a progression of the process started in the acute phase together with reparation by fibrous tissue proliferation. Thus, there are usually combinations of pus formation, fibrosis, distortion, and adhesions with adjacent structures. Histologically plasma cells replace neutrophils and the other changes listed are self-evident.

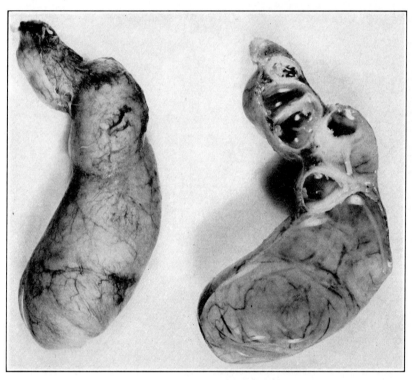

Fig. 582.—Hydrosalpinx illustrating the external and cut surface of a tube that had been distended by clear fluid.

The *complications* of salpingitis may be listed as follows: (1) *abscess formation*—occurring in about one-third of the cases, affecting (*a*) the tube itself and called *pyosalpinx*, (*b*) the tube and ovary and called *tubo-ovarian abscess*, and (*c*) the pelvis and called *pelvic abscess*, and conplicated by rupture with subsequent (*a*) peritonitis, (*b*) secondary abscesses, or (*c*) fistulous tracts involving the rectum, bladder, small intestine, vagina, and skin (Croce and Young), (2) *septicemia*—infrequent except when the salpingitis is due to puerperal infection, (3) *hydrosalpinx*—accumulation of watery fluid within a fallopian tube (Fig. 582) producing a retort-like structure and resulting (*a*) from a low grade inflammation sufficient to seal off the tube and allow secretion from the tubal epithelial cells to accumulate or (*b*) from conversion of a pyosalpinx by replacement with watery fluid, (4) *hemato-*

salpinx—distention of a fallopian tube with blood (Fig. 583) and resulting not only from hemorrhage into a hydrosalpinx but even more commonly from tubal gestation (Shaw), and (5) *bone formation*—probably resulting from metaplasia consequent to old inflammation (Kulka.)

The *clinical manifestations* of salpingitis may be divided into general and local. *General* manifestations are due to septicemia or absorption of toxic products. They consist of chills, nausea, vomiting, malaise, headache, fever, rapid pulse, leukocytosis, and increased sedimentation rate. *Local* manifestations are due to the inflammation as such, especially when it reaches the peritoneum. They consist of lower abdominal or pelvic pain,

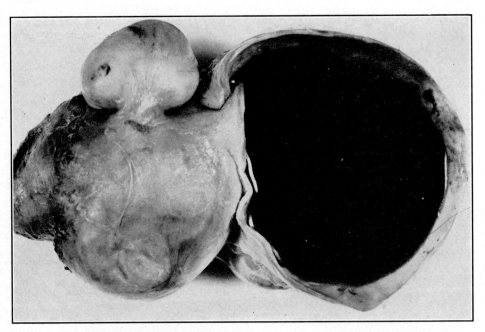

Fig. 583.—Hematosalpinx demonstrating blood in a portion of a greatly dilated tube.

abdominal rigidity, and (upon pelvic examination) exquisite tenderness with or without adnexal masses. In addition, infection of the lower genital tract accounts for vaginal discharge and infection of the urethra and trigone of the urinary bladder accounts for urinary symptoms. The *diagnosis* is made from the clinical manifestations and pelvic examination as listed. *Treatment* is medical in the form of bed rest, antibiotics, etc., and surgical (in chronic cases only) in the form of removal of the diseased organs or drainage of the abscesses. The *prognosis* depends upon the severity of the process, the complications, the promptness of effective treatment, etc. In general, it is good.

Salpingitis Isthmica Nodosa.—This condition, also known as endosalpingitis and adenosalpingitis, is characterized grossly by nodular thickenings of the wall of the tube at the isthmus and microscopically by the presence of glands lined by tubal epithelium and located in the musculature and serosa (Benjamin). The condition probably results from inflammation, muscular activity of the tube, and hormonal stimulation.

Tuberculosis.—Tuberculosis salpingitis *accounts* for from 2.7 to 11.6 per cent of all inflammations of the fallopian tubes (Greenberg). It is, however, less frequent now than formerly and is most common between the ages of eighteen and thirty-five years (Veprovsky). The condition is always *secondary* to some other focus of infection in the body and the most common route of contraction is hematogenous (Auerbach). *Grossly* the tubes may disclose small tubercles or may be filled with caseous material. *Histologically* they present typical tubercles or tuberculous granulation tissue. The *complications* consist of sterility, tubal pregnancy, fistulous tract formation, and peritonitis. The *clinical manifestations* consist of pain in the lower abdomen, dysmenorrhea, amenorrhea, and irregular menstruation. The *diagnosis* is usually made at operation. *Treatment* consists of salpingectomy—performed only when the process is localized and the extragenital tuberculosis is stabilized. The *prognosis*, as far as the fallopian tubes are concerned, is good.

PHYSICAL DISTURBANCES

Orientation.—Under this heading may be included the following disorders: (1) *obstruction*—due to (*a*) congenital anomalies such as agenesis, rudimentary formation, atresia, hypoplasia, and diverticula, (*b*) inflammations, (*c*) physical disturbances such as ligation, hemorrhage, and spasm, and (*d*) tumors, and complicated by sterility, (2) *ectopic pregnancy*, (3) *hernia*—into congenital or acquired defects in the broad ligaments or into the inguinal or femoral canal, (4) *torsion*—twisting, generally occurring in connection with some disease of the tubes, and attended by hematosalpinx and infarction (Shaw), and (5) *fistulas*—infrequent, connecting the fallopian tube with the colon, rectum, bladder, or skin and due to nonspecific salpingitis, tuberculosis, ectopic pregnancy, and pelvic abscess.

Ectopic Pregnancy.—By ectopic pregnancy is *meant* nidation occurring in other than the normal uterine position. In the United States the condition is said to *occur* once in every 100 pregnancies in Negresses and once in every 150 pregnancies in white women. Anything that delays the passage of the fertilized ovum down the fallopian tube *causes* nidation proximal to the uterine site and anything that accelerates its passage causes nidation below the usual uterine site.

Pathologically the localization, in decreasing order of frequency, is as follows: fallopian tube (over 95 per cent of all cases), ovary, abdominal cavity, and cervix (Jarcho, Frankel, Toplack, MacVine, and Ward). Regardless of the site of localization, the changes are similar. The embryo and fetal membranes initially develop as they do in the uterine cavity (Fig. 584). The placenta becomes attached to adjacent tissues which have undergone a decidual reaction. This reaction, however, is inadequate and sooner or later the blood vessels are destroyed, resulting in hemorrhage with extrusion and death of the developing ovum or embryo. The time at which this occurs varies from early in the course of gestation to almost at term. Early death of the fetus usually occurs and the products of conception are generally completely absorbed. Death occurring late in gestation is rare but when it does come about, the child, if not removed surgically, becomes calcified forming a *lithopedion*. Also, regardless of the site of nidation, the uterus is usually enlarged to the size of a two- to three-month uterine pregnancy. *Histologically* the site of nidation discloses fetal parts, chorionic villi, blood, and decidua. The endometrium reveals a decidual reaction in the stroma and either a proliferative or secretory type of endometrium (Rommey).

The *complications* of ectopic pregnancy are hemorrhage, shock, and (later) infection. The *clinical manifestations* consist of pain, faintness, and vaginal spotting occurring at any time after an amenorrhea of two weeks' duration. Pelvic examination discloses adnexal tenderness and a pelvic mass together with what appears to be an early pregnant uterus. The *diagnosis* is suspected from the clinical manifestations as listed and is confirmed at laparotomy. *Treatment* consists of surgical removal of all or of as much of the products of conception as possible. This generally means salpingectomy, as far as tubal pregnancy is concerned. The *prognosis* is good for the mortality rate should be less than 2 per cent.

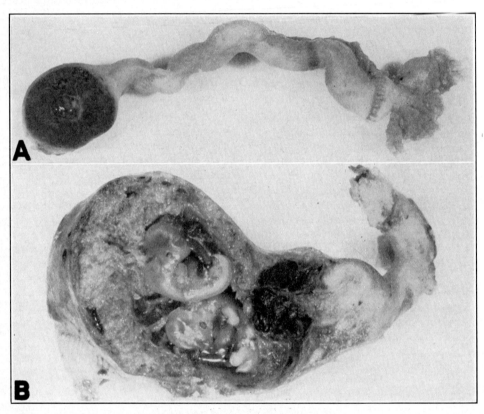

Fig. 584.—Ectopic tubal pregnancy showing *A*, an early nidation near the uterine end with extensive local hemorrhage and *B*, a later nidation with a well-formed placenta and two fetuses.

TUMORS

Orientation.—Tumors and tumor-like conditions (1) of the *round ligaments* consist of fibromyoma, endometriosis, epithelial-lined cysts, hemangioma, and cystadenocarcinoma, (2) of the *broad ligaments* of simple cysts, dermoid cysts, fibromyoma, and lipoma, and (3) of the *fallopian tubes* of dermoid cysts, adenomatoid tumors (p. 904), endometriosis (p. 1166), fibromyoma, hemangioma, lymphangioma, mesonephroma, granulosa cell tumor, carcinoma, sarcoma, and secondary tumors. Of these, simple cysts of the broad ligaments and carcinoma and sarcoma of the fallopian tubes only need be considered further.

Simple Cysts Broad Ligaments.—These cysts originate in remnants of the wolffian (mesonephric) body and among other things have been called para-ovarian cysts and hydatids of Morgagni (Gardner). They may be single or multiple, are found in the vicinity of the fallopian tube (usually the fimbriated end), vary in size from a few millimeters to many centimeters but usually measuring up to 2 cm. in diameter, possess a thin wall, are lined with cuboidal epithelial cells, and are filled with serous fluid. Aside from interfering with labor and being subjected to torsion, they are generally of little significance.

Carcinoma.—Carcinoma of the fallopian tube is rather *uncommon*, there being about 500 cases recorded in the literature up to 1950. It constitutes less than 0.5 per cent of all tumors of the female generative system, occurs at all ages beyond the second decade of life, and has no racial predilection

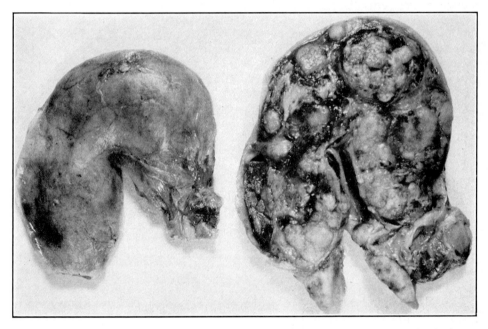

Fig. 585.—Carcinoma of a fallopian tube disclosing soft gray and somewhat hemorrhagic tissue distending the lumen of the organ with the external surface of the tube remaining smooth.

(Hu, Cruttenden, and Forbes). *Pathologically* the tumor is usually unilateral and generally located at the distal end of the tube. It may exist as a nodule, larger mass, or sausage-shaped structure filling the entire tube (Fig. 585). In most instances, the fimbriated end of the tube becomes sealed off while in a few it remains patent and the mass fungates into the peritoneal cavity. *Histologically* the tumor is either papillary or adenomatous, is composed of cuboidal or columnar cells, and shows varying degrees of differentiation. The tumor *spreads* by continuity to adjacent structures, by the lumen to the peritoneum or uterine cavity, by lymphatics to the iliac, para-aortic, and inguinal nodes, and by blood vessels to the lungs and other organs. The *clinical manifestations* are not specific and consist of vaginal discharge, pelvic pain, and pelvic mass. The *diagnosis* is usually made at operation. *Treatment* consists of removal of the ovaries, tubes, and entire uterus. The *prognosis* is only fair, with the five-year survival rate being less than 15 per cent.

Sarcoma.—Sarcoma of the fallopian tube is rare, there having been only 22 cases recorded up to 1946 (Scheffey). In general, the clinical picture and gross appearance are similar to those in carcinoma. Histologically the growths have been called spindle cell sarcoma, round cell sarcoma, myosarcoma, giant cell sarcoma, myxosarcoma, perithelioma, endothelioma, and periendothelioma. The five-year survival rate in the recorded cases has been about 25 per cent.

OVARIES

Developmental malformations of the ovaries may be listed as follows: (1) *variations* in *shape* and *size*, (2) *variations* in *position*—usually along the course of descent of the normal ovary and rarely in the inguinal canal (Mayer), (3) *absence*—fairly common when unilateral but rare when bilateral and usually associated with other abnormalities of the generative system, (4) *duplication*—recorded in as high as 4 per cent of autopsies and located anywhere along the course of descent of the normal ovary (Kriss), (5) *hermaphroditism*—rare and consisting of the presence of (*a*) both testicular and ovarian tissue (as a single organ or testis on one side and ovary on the other), (*b*) combinations of portions of the male and portions of the female generative systems, and (*c*) combinations of male and female habitus (Weed, Stirling, and van Campenhount), (6) *pseudohermaphroditism*—consisting of the presence of either testes or ovaries but with secondary sex characteristics and external genitals resembling those of the opposite sex, and including such conditions as congenital anomalies of the external genitals and adrenogenital syndrome (Bleyer and Kozoll), and (7) *precocious puberty*—puberty occurring before nine years of age, usually due simply to a constitutional hastening of activities, but sometimes due to adrenal tumors, pineal teratoma, ovarian (granulosa and theca cell) tumors, and cerebral lesions affecting the hypothalamus and floor of the third ventricle (Novak).

INFLAMMATIONS

Inflammation of the ovary is known as *oophoritis*. The condition almost always occurs in connection with salpingitis and the various types of inflammation are, therefore, similar to those in the fallopian tubes (p. 1176).

PHYSICAL DISTURBANCES

Ovarian conditions in this category may be listed as follows: (1) *ovarian pregnancy* (p. 1179), (2) *hernia*—through openings in the broad ligament or into the inguinal canal, (3) *torsion*—relatively common, occurring in connection with an abnormality, inflammation, or tumor of either the fallopian tube or ovary, and complicated by gangrene of the structures affected (Kelberg), and (4) *hemorrhage*—resulting from necrosis in a tumor, tearing of a pedunculated tumor, ectopic pregnancy, rupture of corpus luteum, and rupture of tubo-ovarian veins during pregnancy (Taniguchi and Hodgkinson).

TUMORS

Orientation.—Tumors and tumor-like conditions of the ovaries are *common*. While they occur at all ages they are most frequent beyond the third decade of life and they have no predilection for any particular race. The *causes* are unknown but histogenetically all cells that normally compose the ovaries are known to produce a benign and/or a malignant tumor. The more important *complications* consist of (1) pressure on adjacent structures and organs, (2) torsion about the pedicle with gangrene of the tumor, (3) obstruction to labor, (4) hemorrhage, (5) ascites and hydrothorax forming what has been called *Meigs' syndrome*, (6) rarely secondary infection, (7) endocrinologic manifestations (seen in some tumors only), (8) malignant transformation of benign tumors, and (9) spread or metastasis to the peritoneal cavity (producing hemorrhagic ascites) and abdominal and thoracic organs in cases of malignant tumors. The *clinical manifestations* are those of the complications. When the growths are small they are asymptomatic but as they increase in size they are attended by the following: pain (pelvic, abdominal, or renal), dysuria, frequency of urination, constipation, nausea, vomiting, enlargement of the abdomen, dyspnea, loss of weight, weakness, and anemia. In addition, hormonal tumors may be accompanied by amenorrhagia, masculinization (amenorrhea, hirsutism, atrophy of the breasts, loss of gluteal fat, change in voice, hypertrophy of the clitoris, increase in strength, increase in weight, and loss of libido), feminization (precosity in children, irregular menses during the reproductive age, and uterine bleeding after the menopause), and altered hormonal levels in the blood and urine. *Physical examination* reveals enlargement of the abdomen, ascites, and a pelvic or a pelvic and abdominal mass. The *diagnosis* is made from the history, physical examination, and laboratory studies including (in cases of malignant tumors with abdominal seeding) the finding of neoplastic cells in ascitic fluid. The only effective *treatment* is complete surgical removal. The *prognosis* depends upon the type of tumor and the completeness of its removal. It is excellent in benign growths, good in malignant tumors that are completely removed, and poor in malignant growths that have spread to the peritoneum or other tissues.

While the *classifications* of ovarian tumors are many (Barzilai, Novak, Schiller, Spencer, etc.) most tabulations differ only in minor details. On a hormonal and histogenetic basis, your author has found the following quite satisfactory:

NONFUNCTIONAL

Follicular Epithelium
  Follicular cyst
  Lutein cyst

Surface Epithelium
  Germinal inclusion cyst
  Surface papilloma
  Adenofibroma
  Serous cystadenoma
  Pseudomucinous cystadenoma

Urogenital Epithelium
  Brenner tumor
  Mesonephroma

Primitive Mesenchyme
  Dysgerminoma

Reticulum Cells
  Lymphoblastoma

Connective Tissue
  Fibroma
  Fibrosarcoma

Mesodermal Elements
  Chondroma
  Osteoma

Blood and Lymphatic Vessels
  Angioma
  Angiosarcoma
  Lymphangioma

Nerves and Nerve Cells
  Ganglioneuroma
  Neurofibroma
  Neurofibrosarcoma

Muscle (Lig. Ov.)
  Leiomyoma

Congenital Cell Rests
  Teratoid tumors
  Struma ovarii

Distant Areas
  Endometriosis
  Secondary tumors

FUNCTIONAL

Estrogenic or Feminizing   *Gonadotropic*
   Granulosa cell tumor   Chorionepithelioma
   Thecoma

Androgenic or Masculinizing   *Thyroxogenic*
   Arrhenoblastoma   Struma ovarii
   Adrenocorticoid tumors

In the ensuing pages only the more important lesions will be discussed for the majority of those omitted are identical pathologically to similar growths in other organs of the body.

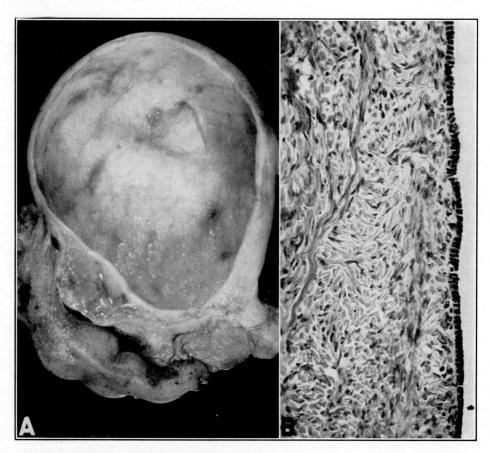

Fig. 586.—Serous cystadenoma of the ovary showing *A*, a solitary cyst filled with serous fluid and *B*, a fibrous tissue wall lined with cuboidal epithelium. × 200.

Follicular Cysts.—Follicular cysts originate from unruptured graafian follicles. They may be single or multiple. The former are referred to as *simple cysts* while the latter go under the caption of *polycystic disease* or the *Stein-Leventhal syndrome*. *Pathologically* the cysts usually measure up to 2 cm. in diameter, are filled with clear fluid, and are lined with granulosa cells. In polycystic disease there is generally amenorrhea clinically due to hyperestrogenism due to lack of progesterone.

Lutein Cysts.—In this group may be included (1) *corpus luteum cyst*—usually single, measuring up to 3 cm. in diameter, composed grossly of a cavity filled with bloody fluid and lined with an orange-yellow rim of tissue, and consisting histologically of a lining of lutein cells (Wheelan), (2) *corpus albicans cyst*—cystic dilatation of a corpus albicans, and (3) *theca lutein cyst*—multiple, arising from unruptured follicles, composed of varisized cysts lined with luteinized theca and granulosa cells, and associated with hydatidiform mole and chorionepithelioma (Novak).

Germinal Inclusion Cysts.—These cysts arise from surface epithelium, seldom measure more than 1 cm. in diameter, are lined by a single layer of cuboidal cells, and are of little clinical significance.

Surface Papilloma.—This lesion is uncommon. It consists of finger-like projections of connective tissue covered with mesothelial or cuboidal cells.

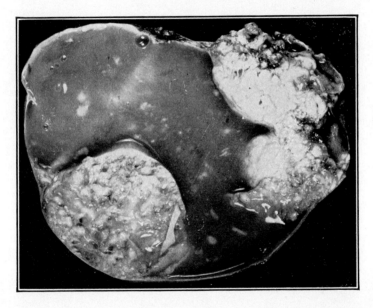

Fig. 587.—Pseudomucinous cystadenoma disclosing a cyst filled with mucoid material and containing two more solid masses of gray tissue. (Herbut's *Gynecological and Obstetrical Pathology.*)

Adenofibroma.—This is a benign tumor composed of varying proportions of connective tissue and epithelial elements (Scott). It has also been called serous adenofibroma, serous cystadenofibroma, cystic fibroma, etc. It is bilateral in 15 per cent of cases, may measure as much as 20 cm. in diameter, and is related to surface papilloma.

Serous Cystadenoma.—This tumor, also known as endosalpingioma and serous cystoma, is a benign cystic growth lined by cuboidal epithelium and containing serous fluid (Erdmann and MacLeod). It is one of the most common tumors of the ovary, constituting about one-quarter of all ovarian neoplasms. It is generally unilateral, varies from a few to 30 or 40 cm. in diameter, is rounded, discloses a smooth external surface, and is composed (*a*) of a single cavity—*simple serous cyst*, (*b*) of several cavities with papillary projections—*papillary serous cyst*, or (*c*) of several cavities, papillary projections, and epithelial tissue permeating the wall—*serous cystadenoma* (Fig. 586). Histologically, as already stated, the epithelial component

75

consists of cuboidal (and less often columnar) cells often containing droplets of secretion and sometimes covered with cilia. Serous cystadenoma, especially the papillary or more solid type, is prone to undergo a malignant transformation.

Pseudomucinous Cystadenoma.—This is a benign, multilocular or, less often, unilocular, cystic tumor lined by mucoid secreting, tall columnar epithelial cells, and filled with mucoid material (pseudomucin) that does not precipitate with dilute acetic and other acids (Figs. 587 and 588) (Selye,

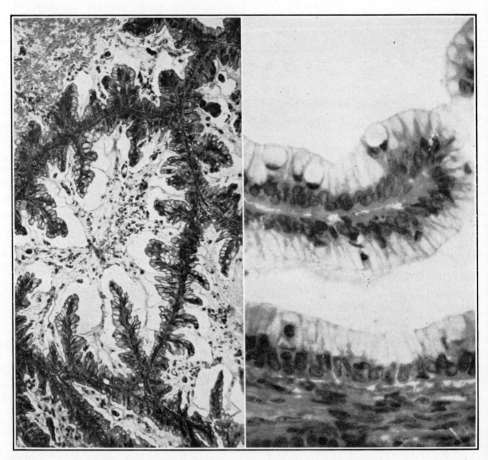

FIG. 588.—Pseudomucinous cystadenoma disclosing glands and papillæ lined by tall mucoid secreting cells. × 100 and 400.

Dockerty, and Buchanan). The tumor is less common than serous cystadenoma, is generally unilateral, measures up to 30 or 40 cm. in diameter, is smooth and glistening externally, may disclose papillary projections or more solid gray masses on cut surface, and may be complicated by a malignant transformation or (upon rupture) by pseudomyxoma of the peritoneum (p. 907).

Carcinoma.—Primary carcinoma of the ovary generally connotes a malignant tumor other than granulosa cell tumor, arrhenoblastoma, and other growths mentioned in subsequent paragraphs. Next to carcinoma of the cervix it is the most *common* malignant tumor of the female generative system (Montgomery, Allan, Speert, Wheelock, and Liber). When the tumor is recognized early it is usually *unilateral* but as it ages it has a tendency to be *bilateral* (Fig. 589). The size varies from a few to many centimeters in diameter; the shape is rounded or irregular; the external surface may be smooth or covered with irregular tumor projections and adhesions, and the cut surface may resemble serous or pseudomucinous cystadenoma or be composed of more or less solid, friable, gray tissue with foci of necrosis and hemorrhage. *Histologically* carcinoma of the ovary has been variously classified. Since most of the growths arise from serous cystadenoma or pseudomucinous cystadenoma they may be conveniently divided into serous carcinoma and pseudomucinous carcinoma and each

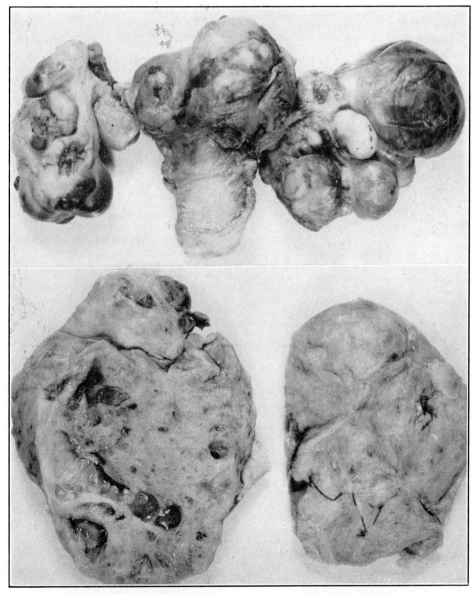

Fig. 589.—Carcinoma of the ovary showing (above) irregular, bilateral, ovarian masses and (below) cystic and solid cut surfaces of another bilateral carcinoma.

may be further divided into low, intermediate, or high grade malignancy. *Serous carcinoma* is fundamentally composed of well-defined cuboidal cells with a moderate amount of vacuolated cytoplasm and round or oval basal nuclei (Fig. 590). *Pseudomucinous carcinoma* is composed of tall columnar cells that have a propensity to secrete mucoid material (Fig. 590*B*). In either case, when the tumor is well differentiated, each forms glands with or without papillary projections, but as it becomes more malignant the pattern

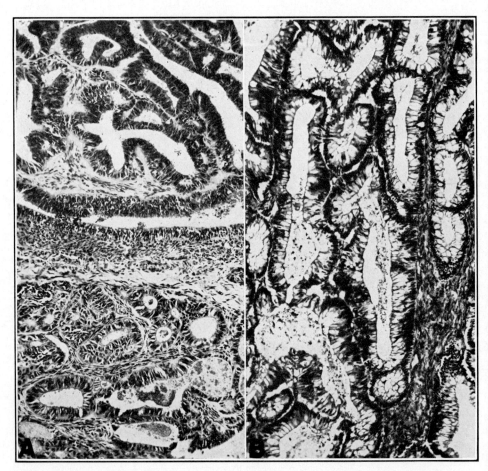

Fig. 590.—Carcinoma of the ovary illustrating *A*, a serous type of tumor with cuboidal and columnar cells and *B*, a pseudomucinous type of tumor with mucoid secreting columnar cells. × 100.

is less regular and the growth finally consists of sheets of individual cells aimlessly permeating the stroma. In addition, the more benign tumors of the serous type have a tendency to form irregular or concentrically laminated psammoma bodies.

Brenner Tumor.—This is a benign tumor and is said to constitute about 2 per cent of all ovarian neoplasms (Jondahl and Randall). It probably arises in Walthard cell rests (urogenital epithelium) (p. 1175), is generally unilateral, may measure up to 30 cm. in diameter, is solid grayish white in about two-thirds of the cases, is found in the wall of an ovarian cyst in the remaining cases, and is composed histologically of a stroma of dense fibrous tissue containing nests of polyhedral squamous-like cells with distinct borders, granular or reticulated cytoplasm, and elongated, lightly staining, folded nuclei (Fig. 591). The tumor rarely if ever undergoes a malignant change and is not hormone-producing.

Mesonephroma.—This tumor, also arising from urogenital epithelium, is a malignant growth that is indistinguishable grossly from other carcinomas and that is characterized histologically by arrangements of epithelial cells in clusters resembling renal glomeruli (Stromme).

Dysgerminoma.—A dysgerminoma, also known as ovarian seminoma, is generally a relatively benign epithelial tumor that histologically resembles seminoma of the testis (Pedowitz and Mueller). It is usually unilateral,

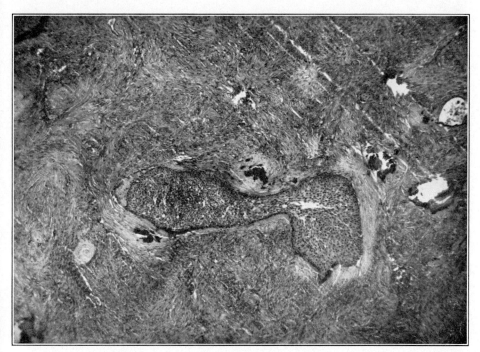

Fig. 591.—Brenner tumor disclosing a clump of regular epithelial cells surrounded by fibrous tissue that is partially calcified. × 50.

may be large enough to fill the entire abdominal cavity, is composed of moderately soft, brain-like tissue, and consists microscopically of nests or columns of sharply defined, polyhedral cells with clear cytoplasm and of foci of lymphocytes in the stroma.

Fibroma.—Fbroma of the ovary, as elsewhere, is a benign tumor. It is generally unilateral, is sharply circumscribed and encapsulated, consists of solid gray tissue, measures up to 27 cm. in diameter, and is composed of ill-defined spindle cells with a moderate amount of cytoplasm and elongated, evenly stained nuclei (Fig. 592). For some unknown reason, ovarian fibroma is prone to be associated with ascites and hydrothorax—a combination that is referred to as *Meigs' syndrome* (Dockerty and Woolridge).

Teratoid Tumors.—What has been said concerning teratoid tumors in the mediastinum (p. 548) applies also to the ovary. In this location, the cystic tumors (dermoid cysts) are said to constitute from 5 to 34 per cent of all tumors (Blackwell and Quinland) while the solid growths are much less common, constituting less than 1 per cent of all ovarian neoplasms (Curtis and Garrett). In the ovary, teratoid tumors arise in totipotent embryonal cells—perhaps by asexual reproduction (parthenogenesis). The tumors are bilateral in from 10 to 40 per cent of all cases, vary greatly in

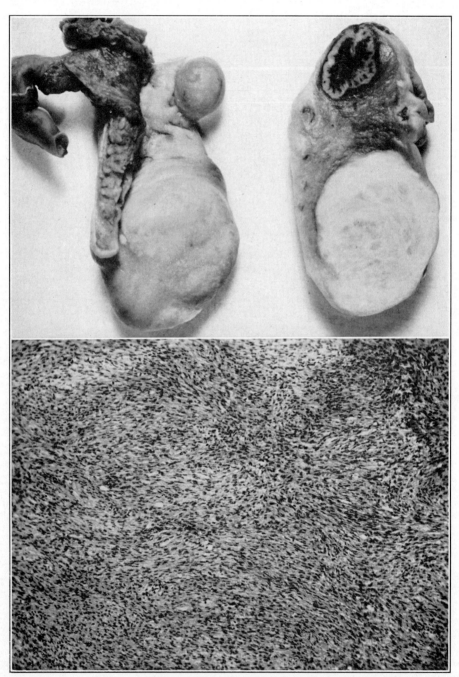

Fig. 592.—Fibroma of the ovary demonstrating the external and cut surface of a solid gray tumor and a histologic section of a growth showing rather regular spindle cells. $\times$ 100.

size, usually contain hair and sebaceous material, and can sometimes be diagnosed roentgenographically by demonstrating teeth or a portion of a jaw. The more solid tumors are prone to become malignant, with the epithelial cells usually being the culprits.

Struma Ovarii.—Struma ovarii is an ovarian tumor composed entirely or mostly of thyroid tissue (Fox and Baskin). The lesion represents a one-sided development of a teratoid tumor. Pathologically it may be solid or cystic and the thyroid tissue may resemble that seen in a normal thyroid, diffuse hyperplasia, adenomatous hyperplasia, or rarely carcinoma. About 5 per cent of patients with struma ovarii reveal evidence of thyrotoxicosis — that is, the tumor is actively hormone-producing.

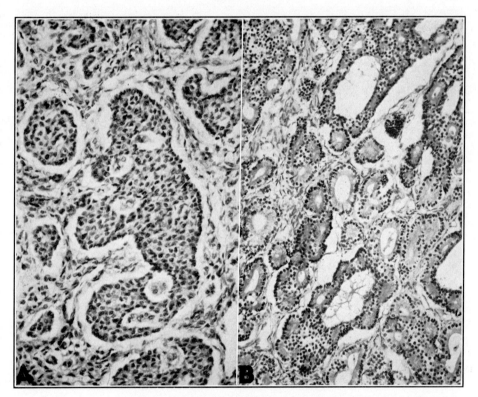

FIG. 593.—Granulosa cell tumor illustrating *A*, masses of regular polyhedral cells and *B*, glands of cuboidal cells. × 100.

Secondary Tumors.—Secondary tumors of the ovaries, also known as Krukenberg tumors, are common enough to warrant serious consideration in any case of ovarian enlargement (Leffel, Berens, and Karsh). The primary growth may be located in any organ of the body but the gastrointestinal tract and breast are most commonly affected. The route of metastasis is usually the blood vessels or lymphatics. It should also be noted that the primary tumor may be small enough to escape the closest scrutiny and the ovarian masses large enough to draw all the attention. In the ovaries the growth is generally bilateral, may be solid and/or cystic, and microscopically resembles the parent tumor.

Granulosa Cell Tumor.—Granulosa cell tumor is recorded as being the more common estrogenic or feminizing tumor (the other being thecoma) and is said to constitute from 0.9 to 3.0 per cent of all ovarian growths (Haines, Rhoads, Hodgson, Dockerty, and Jones). It is most common in the postmenopausal age and prevails in Negresses over white women. It is bilateral in about 17 per cent of cases, varies in size from microscopic to 40 cm. in diameter, is lobulated and well encapsulated, generally presents a solid grayish-white or yellowish cut surface but is sometimes partially cystic, and is composed of uniform-appearing cells with indistinct borders, moderate amount of granular cytoplasm and round or oval, uniformly stained nuclei. The cells are arranged to form follicle-like structures, glands, masses, cylinders, or diffuse sheets and the stroma varies from

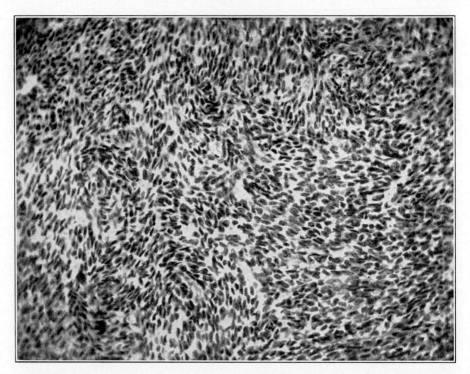

Fig. 594.—Thecoma composed of rather plump spindle cells forming interlacing bundles. × 200.

scanty to abundant (Fig. 593). Although granulosa cell tumor is ordinarily benign, a malignant transformation is recorded in from 10 to 55 per cent of cases. In addition, because of its estrogen-producing capacity, other complications consist of endometrial hyperplasia, endometrial carcinoma, fibromyoma of the uterus, and myometrial hypertrophy.

Thecoma.—A thecoma is recorded as occurring about one-third as frequently as granulosa cell tumor although, in your author's experience, the reverse is true (Gordon, Sternberg, and Sparling). It, too, is an estrogenic or feminizing tumor, rarely if ever becomes malignant, and is attended by complications similar to those in granulosa cell tumor. The growth prevails in women beyond the menopause, is almost always unilateral, is well encapsulated, measures up to 20 cm. or more in diameter, and resembles a fibromyoma of the uterus on cut surface. Histologically it is composed of ill-defined, spindle cells in interlacing, whorl, or "feather stitch" formation

(Fig. 594). The cells resemble those of fibroma and can be distinguished from the latter with certainty only because they take a positive fat stain.

Arrhenoblastoma.—Arrhenoblastoma is the more common of the androgenic or masculinizing tumors (Dockerty, Iverson, O'Connor, and Javert). It is unilateral in about 5 per cent of cases, varies in size up to 27 cm. in diameter, is well encapsulated, discloses solid grayish-white tissue with foci of necrosis and hemorrhage, and histologically presents a tubular, intermediate, and sarcomatoid arrangement. The cells may be cuboidal, columnar, spindle-shaped, rounded, or polyhedral with moderate to scanty eosinophilic cytoplasm and round or oval, evenly stained nuclei. A malignant transformation occurs in about one-fifth of all cases.

Adrenocorticoid Tumors.—This term has been coined to encompass all of the androgenic or masculinizing tumors that have been designated as *adrenocortical tumor, luteoma, luteinoma, masculinovoblastoma, virilizing lipoid cell tumors, interstitial cell tumor, Leydig cell tumor, sympathotropic cell tumor, hypernephroma, hypernephroid tumor, gynandroblastoma, andro-blastoma,* and *androgenic hilar cell tumors* (Herbut). The tumors are less common than arrhenoblastoma, are almost always unilateral, generally measure less than 3 cm. in diameter, are well encapsulated, present diffusely orange-yellow cut surfaces with occasional foci of necrosis and hemorrhage, and are composed of sheets or cords of cells that resemble those of the corpus luteum, liver, or adrenal cortex. Special stains generally disclose fat and glycogen-positive intracytoplasmic droplets. Adrenocorticoid tumors are benign, with a malignant transformation being only rarely recorded.

FETAL MEMBRANES

CONGENITAL ANOMALIES

Developmental malformations of the fetal membranes (chorion, placenta, amnion, and umbilical cord) may be listed as follows: (1) *variations* in *size* of *placenta*—increase (over 500 gm.) as seen in erythroblastosis fetalis and syphilis and decrease as seen in normal pregnancy with a small baby or in premature delivery, (2) *variations* in *configuration* of *placenta*—consisting of (*a*) *succenturiate* or *accessory* placenta—one or more masses of placental tissue connected to the main mass by vessels, (*b*) *placenta spuria*—accessory tissue with a separate vascular supply, (*c*) *duplex placenta*—placenta of two equal parts with vessels from each uniting to form the umbilical cord, and (*d*) *placenta membranacea*—placenta completely covering the chorion (Eastman), (3) *circumvallate placenta*—consisting of the presence of a hyalinized ring on the fetal surface at some point between the center and circumference of the organ (Hobbs), (4) *placenta* in *multiple pregnancies*—seen most often in twins and consisting of two fused placentas with two separate sacs (dizygotic with the partition consisting of amnion, chorion, chorion and amnion), a single placenta with two sacs (monozygotic with the partition consisting of amnion and amnion), or a single placenta with one sac (monoamniotic and no partition), and encountered less often in triple, quadruple, etc., pregnancies (Guttmacher and Quigley). (5) *placental cysts*—being common, of no known clinical significance, and classified as amniotic, chorionic, and decidual (Paddock), (6) *placenta* in *erythroblastosis fetalis*—characterized by increase in over-all size, thickening of the membranes, edema of the cord, deeply fissured maternal surface, bulky cotyledons, and (histologically) bulbous projections of edematous villi (Potter), (7) *variations* in *insertion* of *umbilical cord*—at margin of placenta (*marginal*) or into the membranes (*velamentous*), (8) *variations* in *length* of *umbilical cord*—shorter or longer than the normal 45 to 60 cm., (9) *variations* in *number* of *umbilical cords*—seen in connection with multiple pregnancies, (10) *varices*, (11) *cysts*—occurring near the abdominal end and consisting of extensions of the omphalomesenteric duct and urachus, (12) *incomplete formation* of amnion, (13) *amniotic bands*—of unknown cause but responsible occasionally for death of fetus or intra-uterine amputations (Lennon), and (14) *variations* in *amniotic fluid*—normal 1000 cc. and consisting of (*a*) increase—over 1500 cc., called polyhydramnios or hydramnios, seen in single or multiple pregnancies, and ascribed to transudation from exposed meninges as in spina bifida, increase secretion by increased amount of amniotic membrane, lack of swallowing of amniotic fluid, excess urinary secretion by fetus, and increase area of chorionic villi, and complicated by twistings of the umbilical cord, and (*b*) decrease—below 300 cc., called olighydramnios, thought to be due to a reverse of the conditions mentioned above, and complicated by fetal abnormalities.

DEGENERATIONS

Degenerative changes occur normally, to a certain extent, as the placenta ages. They consist of (1) *fibrin deposition*—replacement of trophoblastic cells, (2) *intervillous thrombosis*, (3) *infarction*—consisting of degenerated and necrotic villi deprived of their blood supply, and (4) *calcification*—focal and occurring in areas of infarction (Herbut). When these changes transgress the normal limits they become pathologic—but just where to draw the line between the two is sometimes difficult. Premature aging of the placenta is often seen in toxemia of pregnancy.

INFLAMMATIONS

Inflammation of the placenta is known as *placentitis*. The conditions may be listed as follows: (1) *acute placentitis*—arising as a result of ascending infection from the lower birth canal, caused by ordinary pyogenic organisms, characterized grossly by turbidity of the amniotic fluid, and histologically disclosing leukocytic infiltration in the amnion, placenta proper, and umbilical cord (Kobak), (2) *syphilis*—characterized by enlargement of the placenta as compared with the size of the fetus, enlarged bulbous villi, fibrosis of the villi, vascular thickening, and, rarely, plasma cell and lymphocytic infiltration (Montgomery and McCord), and (3) *tuberculosis*—infrequent, seen as a secondary infection in cases of active pulmonary tuberculosis, and consisting of areas of caseation or of miliary tubercles (Whitman and Schaefer).

PHYSICAL DISTURBANCES

Physical disturbances of the fetal membranes consist of the following: (1) *hematoma*—resulting from rupture of a placental vessel, (2) *abortion*—defined as termination of pregnancy before extra-uterine viability of the fetus is possible, generally occurring before the twenty-sixth week of gestation, said to constitute about 25 per cent of all pregnancies, being caused by (*a*) ovular factors such as pathologic ovum, fetal anomalies, and placental abnormalities, and (*b*) maternal factors such as uterine abnormalities, endometritis, toxemia of pregnancy, endocrine factors, trauma, etc., and characterized by uterine bleeding and the passage of the products of conception, that is, fetal parts and/or chorionic villi (Hertig, Javert, Collins, and Burge), (3) *retained placenta*—one that is not extruded from the uterus within the usual forty-five minutes allowable after delivery (Sewell), (4) *premature separation* of the *placenta*—separation of a normally implanted placenta during the last trimester of pregnancy, caused by hemorrhage which occurs as a result of necrosis at the trophoblastic decidual junction, and complicated by hemorrhage, shock, and death of the mother and/or fetus (Bysshe), (5) *placenta previa*—a placenta that has developed in the lower uterine segment encroaching upon or spanning the internal cervical os and complicated by hemorrhage, shock, and death of the mother and/or fetus (Johnson and Findley), (6) *placenta accreta*—one in which the chorionic villi become adherent to the myometrium with no line of cleavage between the two (McKeogh), and (7) *disturbances* of the *umbilical cord* consisting of coiling around various parts of the body, twisting on its axis knots, prolapse, rupture, hematoma, and hernia into the cord.

TUMORS

Orientation.—Tumors and tumor-like conditions of the placenta may be listed as follows: (1) *squamous metaplasia* of the *amnion*—of no known significance, (2) *placental polyp*—retained placental tissue maintaining its attachment to and nourishment from the uterine wall (Dorsey), (3) *chorioangioma*—benign growth composed essentially of thin-walled capillaries

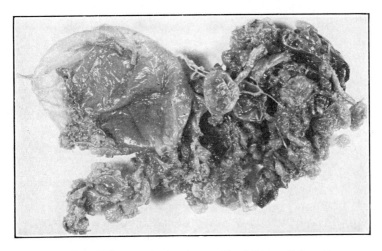

Fig. 595.—Hydatidiform mole showing varisized thin-walled cystic masses. (Herbut's *Gynecological and Obstetrical Pathology*.)

supported by a collagenous, myxomatous, or sarcomatous-like stroma, located on the fetal surface, measuring up to 22 cm. in diameter, and sometimes causing premature labor or dystocia (Marchetti and Fisher), (4) *hydatidiform mole*, (5) *chorionepithelioma*, and (6) *secondary tumors*. Of these, hydatidiform mole and chorionepithelioma only need be considered further.

Hydatidiform Mole.—This is a benign tumor composed of cystically dilated chorionic villi. It *occurs* about once in every 2,000 deliveries (Hertig, Payne, Holman, Novak). The condition *develops* as a result of deformity of the ovum or early death of the fetus. In a typical case, the embryo dies at about the fifth or sixth week of pregnancy. At this stage, the vessels of the chorionic villi are poorly developed and since the embryo dies they do not develop further. The chorion, however, continues to grow and function with the result that secretion products, instead of being removed by the vessels, accumulate within and distend the villi.

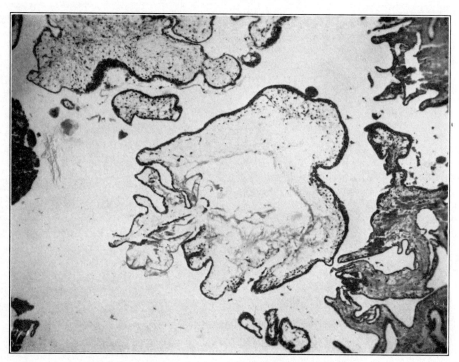

Fig. 596.—Hydatidiform mole illustrating edematous change and cyst formation in a villus. × 50.

Pathologically a hydatidiform mole may develop within the uterus as well as in ectopic sites. In a typical case, the uterus is enlarged to that of a three-month pregnancy. The placenta is partly or wholly converted into a cluster of thin-walled cystic spaces measuring up to 2 or 3 cm. in diameter (Fig. 595). *Histologically* the chorionic villi disclose a myxomatous change or cystic replacement of the cores and varying degrees of proliferation of the peripheral Langhans' and syncytial cells (Fig. 596).

The *complications* of hydatidiform mole are uterine bleeding, perforation of the uterus and peritonitis, and development of chorionepithelioma. The typical *clinical* story is simply early pregnancy complicated by vaginal bleeding and occasionally by vaginal passage of vesicles. Repeated quantitative determinations of *chorionic gonadotropic hormones* in the blood or urine show persistent high or increasing levels. The *diagnosis* is made from the history, the appearance of evacuated uterine contents, and gonadotropic determinations. *Treatment* consists of thorough uterine curettage.

The *prognosis* is good, although as high as 10 per cent of cases are said to develop a malignant transformation.

Chorionepithelioma.—Chorionepithelioma (chorion carcinoma) is a malignant tumor composed of chorionic epithelium. While the majority of cases arises on the basis of abortion and hydatidiform mole, the condition may also occur as a one-sided development of a teratoid tumor (Hertig, Novak, Freeth, Brews, Park, and Oliver). The *incidence* is difficult to determine because of the varying criteria used by the different authors, but it may be said that the tumor is uncommon.

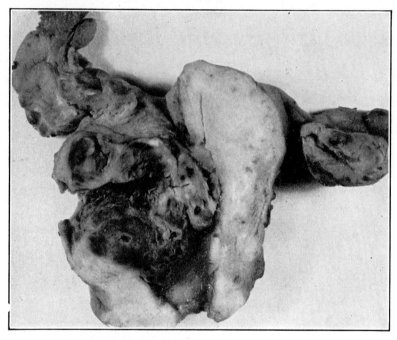

Fig. 597.—Chorionepithelioma demonstrating a hemorrhagic tumor mass penetrating the uterine wall. (Herbut's *Gynecological and Obstetrical Pathology*.)

Pathologically three lesions may be described—syncytial endometritis, chorionadenoma destruens, and chorionepithelioma. *Syncytial endometritis* (syncytioma or syncytial deciduitis) is actually not malignant. The condition consists of a permeation of the endometrium, decidua, and adjacent myometrium by syncytial cells found singly or in groups of twos and threes and penetrating between the host cells. In addition, there is always a leukocytic infiltration. *Chorionadenoma destruens* (invasive or destructive mole) is really a hydatidiform mole that invades and destroys the uterine wall all the way to and through the serosa. Grossly the lesion is accompanied by extensive necrosis and hemorrhage and is actually indistinguishable from chorionepithelioma. Histologically it consists of well-formed chorionic villi but with extensive proliferation of irregular trophoblastic (syncytial and Langhans') cells. The tumor, while being invasive, is only locally destructive and is not malignant in that it does not metastasize. *Chorionepithelioma* is the malignant counterpart of the lesions just referred to. Grossly, as already stated, it is indistinguishable from chorionadenoma destruens (Fig. 597). Histologically it differs from this lesion in that there are no chorionic villi present. The tumor is composed wholly of masses of irregular trophoblastic cells that penetrate and destroy all of the tissues they contact. Because of erosion of vessels, hemorrhage is the rule and metastases to the liver, lungs, etc., occur early.

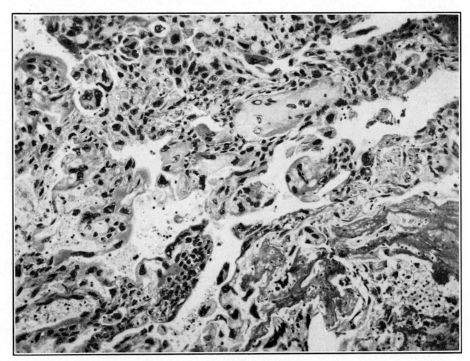

Fig. 598.—Chorionepithelioma illustrating masses of trophoblastic cells without villous formation. × 100.

The local *clinical manifestations* are similar to those in hydatidiform mole. The *diagnosis* is made from the history, appearance of the evacuated uterine contents, and increasing chorionic gonadotropic levels in the blood and urine. *Treatment* consists of hysterectomy and bilateral oophorectomy and salpingectomy. The *prognosis* is excellent in syncytial endometritis and chorionadenoma destruens but is poor in outright chorionepithelioma. When the lesion is truly malignant, death can be expected within six months.

REFERENCES

General

HERBUT, P. A.: *Gynecological and Obstetrical Pathology*, Philadelphia, Lea & Febiger, 1953.

Pathologic Physiology

ENGLE, E. T.: *Menstruation and Its Disorders*, Springfield, Ill., Charles C Thomas, 1950.
PASCHKIS, K. E., RAKOFF, A. E., and CANTAROW, A.: *Clinical Endocrinology*, 2nd Ed., New York, Hoeber-Harper, 1958.
PINCUS, G., and THIMANN, K. V.: *The Hormones*, Vol. III, New York, Academic Press, Inc., 1955.

PAPANICOLAOU, G. N., TRAUT, H. F., and MARCHETTI, A. H.:   *The Epithelia of Women's Reproductive Organs*, New York, The Commonwealth Fund, 1948.

RAKOFF, A. E.:   Hormone Assays in Cantarow and Trumper's *Clinical Biochemistry*, 5th Ed., Philadelphia, W. B. Saunders Co., 1955.

REYNOLD, S. R. M.:   *Physiology of the Uterus*, 2nd Ed., New York, Paul B. Hoeber, Inc., 1949.

SMITH, G. V.:   The Ovaries in Williams' *Textbook of Endocrinology*, 2nd Ed., H. Williams, Philadelphia, W. B. Saunders Co., 1955.

SOHVAL, A. R.:   Diseases of the Ovary in Soffer's *Diseases of the Endocrine Glands*, 2nd Ed., Philadelphia, Lea & Febiger, 1956.

WILKINS, L.:   *The Diagnosis and Treatment of Endocrine Disorders in Childhood and Adolescence*, 2nd Ed., Springfield, Ill., Charles C Thomas, 1957.

VULVA

Congenital Anomalies

BOWLES, H. E., and CHILDS, L. S.: Am. J. Dis. Child., *66*, 258, 1943 (Synechias of Vulva in Children).

DOYLE, J. C.: California and West. Med., *56*, 242, 1942 (Imperforate Hymen).

ELDEN, C. A.: Am. J. Obst. & Gynec., *36*, 507, 1938 (Aplasia).

FISHER, J. H.: Am. J. Obst. & Gynec., *53*, 335, 1947 (Mammary Tissue).

NOWLIN, P., *et al.:* J. Urol., *62*, 75, 1949 (Vulvar Fusion).

Degenerations and Inflammations

ADAIR, F. L., *et al.:* J. A. M. A., *114*, 296, 1940 (Atrophy).

BARROW, W., and MAXWELL, E. S.: Am. J. Obst. & Gynec., *44*, 145, 1942 (Tuberculosis).

BLAND, P. B.: *Gynecology, Medical and Surgical*, 3rd Ed., Philadelphia, F. A. Davis Co., 1939.

DAVIES, J. W.: Surg., Gynec. & Obst., *86*, 329, 1948 (Bartholin Cyst).

DAVIES, T. A.: *Primary Syphilis in the Female*, London, Oxford University Press, 1931.

JONES, C. P., *et al.:* Am. J. Obst. & Gynec., *54*, 738, 1947 (Mycotic Vulvovaginitis).

MILLER, N., *et al.:* Am. J. Obst. & Gynec., *64*, 768, 1952 (Leukoplakia).

MISHELL, D. R., and MOTYLOFF, L.: Am. J. Obst. & Gynec., *39*, 796, 1940 (Senile Vulvovaginitis).

PAPPWORTH, M. H.: Brit. M. J., *1*, 271, 1941 (Acute Ulcerative Vulvitis).

PARKS, J., and MARTIN, S.: Am. J. Obst. & Gynec., *55*, 117, 1948 (Systemic Vulvitis).

PURDIE, A. W.: J. Obst. & Gynaec. Brit. Emp., *48*, 495, 1941 (Gangrene).

SCHAEFER, G.: S. Clin. North America, *20*, 459, 1940 (Tuberculosis Bartholin's Gland).

SPEISER, M. D., and GUYER, H. B.: Am. J. Obst. & Gynec., *51*, 718, 1946 (Tuberculosis).

TORPIN, R., and CRICHTON, R. B.: Am. J. Obst. & Gynec., *36*, 703, 1938 (Gangrene).

Physical Disturbances

ADLER, S. S.: Am. J. Obst. & Gynec., *51*, 272, 1946 (Varicosities).

ARNELL, R. E., *et al.:* J. A. M. A., *127*, 1101, 1945 (Edema).

HAMILTON, H. G.: Am. J. Obst. & Gynec., *39*, 642, 1940 (Hematoma).

ORMSBY, O. S., and MONTGOMERY, H.: *Diseases of the Skin*, 8th Ed., Philadelphia, Lea & Febiger, 1954.

Tumors

COSBY, W. G.: Am. J. Obst. & Gynec., *63*, 251, 1952 (Carcinoma).

DEACON, A. L., and TAYLOR, C. W.: J. Obst. & Gynaec. Brit. Emp., *59*, 64, 1952 (Hydradenoma).

DIEHL, W. K., *et al.:* Am. J. Obst. & Gynec., *62*, 1209, 1951 (Carcinoma).

GARDNER, S. H., *et al.:* Am. J. Obst. & Gynec., *65*, 539, 1953 (Intra-epithelial Carcinoma).

HUBER, C. P., *et al.:* Am. J. Obst. & Gynec., *62*, 778, 1951 (Paget's Disease).

JEFFCOATE, T. N. A., *et al.:* J. Obst. & Gynaec. Brit. Emp., *51*, 377, 1944 (Bowen's Disease).

LUNIN, A. B.: Am. J. Obst. & Gynec., *57*, 742, 1949 (Carcinoma).

NEWELL, J. W., and McKAY, D. G.: West. J. Surg., *60*, 388, 1952 (Carcinoma).

PALMER, J. P., *et al.:* Surg., Gynec. & Obst., *88*, 435, 1949 (Carcinoma).

PARSONS, L., and LOHLEIN, H. E.: A. M. A. Arch. Path., *36*, 424, 1943 (Paget's Disease).

SIEGLER, A. M., and GREENE, H. J.: Am. J. Obst. & Gynec., *62*, 1219, 1951 (Basal Cell Carcinoma).

VAGINA

Congenital Anomalies

Counseller, V. S.: J. A. M. A., *136*, 861, 1948 (Absence).
Lisenby, J. O.: South. Surgeon, *10*, 554, 1941 (Cysts).
Maliphant, R. G.: Brit. M. J., *2*, 555, 1948 (Atresia).
Mayer, M. D.: Am. J. Obst. & Gynec., *42*, 899, 1941 (Duplication).
Sanders, R. L.: Ann. Surg., *107*, 863, 1938 (Cysts).
Thomas, G. B.: J. Obst. & Gynaec. Brit. Emp., *55*, 149, 1948 (Atresia).
Tritoftides, M.: J. Obst. & Gynaec. Brit. Emp., *54*, 861, 1947 (Transverse Septum).
Wilder, E. M.: West. J. Surg., *50*, 168, 1942 (Cysts).

Inflammations

Allen, E., and Butler, S.. Am. J. Obst. & Gynec., *51*, 387, 1946 (Trichomoniasis).
Bender, S., and Jeffcoate, T. N. A.: J. Obst. & Gynaec. Brit. Emp., *57*, 432, 1950 (Emphysematous Vaginitis).
Brady, L., and Reid, R. D.: Ann. Surg., *155*, 840, 1942 (Trichomoniasis).

Physical Disturbances

Bland, P. B.: *Gynecology, Medical and Surgical*, 3rd Ed., Philadelphia, F. A. Davis Co., 1939.
Diddle, A. W.: West. J. Surg., *56*, 414, 1948 (Rupture).
Hoge, R. H.: Virginia M. Monthly, *73*, 277, 1946 (Foreign Bodies).
Stansfield, F. R.: J. Obst. & Gynaec. Brit. Emp., *49*, 82, 1942 (Calculus).

Tumors

Amolsch, A. L.: Am. J. Cancer, *37*, 435, 1939 (Mixed Tumors Uterus and Vagina).
Bivins, M. D.: Am. J. Obst. & Gynec., *65*, 390, 1953 (Carcinoma).
Fischer, H. S., and Kantrowitz, A. R.: Am. J. Obst. & Gynec., *44*, 141, 1942 (Sarcoma Botryoides Cervix).
Geist, S. H., and Salmon, U. J.: Am. J. Obst. & Gynec., *41*, 29, 1941 (Carcinoma and Estrogens).
Hardy, J. A., Jr., and Moragues, V.: Am. J. Obst. & Gynec., *63*, 307, 1952 (Mesodermal Mixed Tumor Uterus).
McElin, T. W., and Davis, H., Jr.: Am. J. Obst. & Gynec., *63*, 605, 1952 (Mesodermal Mixed Tumor Uterus).
Murphy, G. H., and DuShane, J. W.: Am. J. Obst. & Gynec., *55*, 527, 1948 (Mesodermal Mixed Tumor Vagina).
Schmidt, E. C. H., and Schutz, R. B.: Am. J. Obst. & Gynec., *56*, 966, 1948 (Mesodermal Mixed Tumor Uterus).
Simpson, E. E.: A. M. A. Arch. Path., *35*, 535, 1943 (Botryoid Tumor Cervix).
Way, S.: J. Obst. & Gynaec. Brit. Emp., *55*, 739, 1948 (Carcinoma).

CERVIX

Congenital Anomalies

Flemming, E. A., and Kava, H. L.: Am. J. Obst. & Gynec., *40*, 296, 1940 (Congential Atresia).
Huffman, J. W.: Am. J. Obst. & Gynec., *56*, 23, 1948 (Mesonephric Remnants).
Maliphant, R. G.: Brit. M. J., *2*, 555, 1948 (Atresia).
Wanamaker, F. D.: Canad. M. A. J., *61*, 61, 1949 (Atresia).

Inflammations

Carmichael, R., and Jeaffreson, B. L.: J. Path. & Bact., *52*, 173, 1941 (Epidermidalization).
Findley, D.: Am. J. Obst. & Gynec., *49*, 614, 1945 (Cervicitis).
Fluhmann, C. F.: Am. J. Obst. & Gynec., *15*, 1, 1928 (Epidermidalization).
McIlrath, M. B., and Hellestrand, A. L.: J. Obst. & Gynaec. Brit. Emp., *54*, 746, 1947 (Cervicitis).

PIPER, M. C.: M. Clin. North America, *29*, 998, 1945 (Chronic Cervicitis).
SEAMAN, J. A.: South. M. J., *38*, 398, 1945 (Cervicitis and Urinary Tract Infection).
ZELEZNY-BAUMRUCKER, O., and BAUMRUCKER, G. O.: Surg., Gynec. & Obst., *67*, 17, 1938 (400 Cervical Erosions).

Physical Disturbances

FARRAR, L. K. P.: Am. J. Obst. & Gynec., *10*, 205, 1925 (Irradiation Changes).
INGRAHAM, H. A., *et al.*: Am. J. Obst. & Gynec., *57*, 730, 1949 (Lacerations).
MARTIN, R. T., and KENNY, M.: J. Obst. & Gynaec. Brit. Emp., *57*, 608, 1950 (Changes in Pregnancy).
MORTON, D. G., and KERNER, J. A.: Am. J. Obst. & Gynec., *57*, 625, 1949 (Irradiation Changes).
MURPHY, E. J., and HERBUT, P. A.: Am. J. Obst. & Gynec., *59*, 384, 1950 (Cervix in Pregnancy).
SHEETS, M. V.: West. J. Surg., *56*, 317, 1948 (Cervix after Delivery).
TOLLEFSON, D. G.: West. J. Surg., *56*, 285, 1948 (Postpartum Cervix).
WATERMAN, G. W., and TRACY, E. M.: Am. J. Roentgenol., *60*, 788, 1948. (Irradiation Changes).

Tumors

BABER, M. D., *et al.*: Brit. M. J., *1*, 392, 1951 (Carcinoma).
BAINBOROUGH, A. R.: Am. J. Obst. & Gynec., *61*, 330, 1951 (Histologic Carcinoma).
GALVIN, G. A.: Radiology, *54*, 815, 1950 (Clinical Classification Carcinoma).
HEPLER, T. K., *et al.*: Am. J. Obst. & Gynec., *63*, 800, 1952 (Adenocarcinoma).
HERTIG, A. T., and YOUNGE, P. A.: Am. J. Obst. & Gynec., *64*, 807, 1952 (Carcinoma-in-Situ).
HOFFMAN, J., *et al.*: J. A. M. A., *151*, 535, 1953 (Carcinoma-in-Situ).
LOMBARD, H. L., and POTTER, E. A.: Cancer, *3*, 960, 1950 (Carcinoma).
MORRIS, J. M., and MEIGS, J. V.: Surg., Gynec. & Obst., *90*, 135, 1950 (Carcinoma).
MORTON, D. G., and DIGNAM, W.: Am. J. Obst. & Gynec., *64*, 999, 1952 (Cause of Death in Carcinoma).
NOVAK, E. R., and GALVIN, G. A.: Am. J. Obst. & Gynec., *62*, 1079, 1951 (Intra-epithelial Carcinoma).
PERCIVAL, E.: Am. J. Obst. & Gynec., *65*, 386, 1953 (Results Treatment Carcinoma).
PETERSON, P., and HORNBROOK, F. E.: Am. J. Obst. & Gynec., *63*, 1290, 1952 (Surgical Treatment Carcinoma).
RAPHAEL, S. I., and WATERMAN, G. W.: New England J. Med., *245*, 281, 1951 (Carcinoma).
SCHEFFEY, L. C., *et al.*: Am. J. Obst. & Gynec., *64*, 233, 1952 (Irradiation Treatment Carcinoma).
WARD, S. V., *et al.*: Am. J. Obst. & Gynec., *63*, 989, 1952 (Causes of Death in Carcinoma).

BODY OF UTERUS

Congenital Anomalies

TAYLOR, H. C.: Am. J. Obst. & Gynec., *46*, 388, 1943 (Pregnancy and Double Uterus).

Inflammations

DEVOE, R. W., and RANDALL, L. M.: Am. J. Obst. & Gynec., *58*, 784, 1949 (Pyometra).
O'BRIEN, J. R., and LAWLOR, M. K.: J. Obst. & Gynaec. Brit. Emp., *54*, 636, 1947 (Tuberculosis).
SCHAUPP, K. L., JR.: West. J. Surg., *57*, 243, 1949 (Tuberculosis).

Physical Disturbances

BEACHAM, W. D., and BEACHAM, D. W.: Am. J. Obst. & Gynec., *61*, 824, 1951 (Rupture).
BERLIND, M.: Am. J. Surg., *52*, 384, 1941 (Fistulas).
BOST, T. C.: South. M. J., *34*, 1040, 1941 (Gunshot Wound Pregnant Uterus).
DAS, P.: J. Obst. & Gynaec. Brit. Emp., *47*, 525, 1940 (Inversion).
DUGGER, J. H.: S. Clin. North America, *25*, 1414, 1945 (Rupture).
SIEGLER, S. L., and SILVERSTEIN, L. M.: Am. J. Obst. & Gynec., *55*, 1053, 1948 (Torsion).

Tumors

BURCH, J. C., *et al.*: Arch. Path., *17*, 799, 1934 (Endometrial Hyperplasia).
COHEN, M., and CRAVOTTA, C. A.: Am. J. Obst. & Gynec., *56*, 997, 1948 (Sarcoma).
DANFORTH, W. C.: Am. J. Obst. & Gynec., *59*, 598, 1950 (Sarcoma).
DIDDLE, A. W.: West. J. Surg., *57*, 20, 1949 (Carcinoma).
DOCKERTY, M. B.: Minnesota Med., *32*, 806, 1949 (Endometriosis).
FAULKNER, R. L.: Am. J. Obst. & Gynec., *53*, 474, 1947 (Red Degeneration).
FINN, W. F.: Am. J. Obst. & Gynec., *62*, 1, 1951 (Carcinoma).
GEIST, S., and SALMON, U. J.: Am. J. Obst. & Gynec., *41*, 29, 1941 (Estrogens as Carcinogens).
HENRIKSEN, E., and MURRIETA, T.: West. J. Surg., *58*, 331, 1950 (Carcinoma).
HUNDLEY, J. M., JR., *et al.*: Am. J. Obst. & Gynec., *57*, 52, 1949 (Endometrial Carcinoma).
KELLY, F. J., and SCHLADEMAN, K. R.: Surg., Gynec. & Obst., *88*, 230, 1949 (Endometriosis).
MACFARLANE, C., *et al.*: J. A. M. A., *138*, 941, 1948 (Cancer Uterus).
MACFARLANE, K. T.: Am. J. Obst. & Gynec., *59*, 1304, 1950 (Sarcoma).
McFARLAND, J.: Am. J. Cancer, *25*, 530, 1935 (Malignant Myoma).
McGARVEY, R. N., and GIBSON, W. E.: Am. J. Obst. & Gynec., *63*, 836, 1952 (Endometrial Carcinoma).
MEIGS, J. V.: Ann. Surg., *127*, 795, 1948 (Endometriosis).
NEWGARD, K., and MORTON, D. G.: West. J. Surg., *53*, 268, 1945 (Endometrial Polyps).
NOVAK, E., and RUTLEDGE, F.: Am. J. Obst. & Gynec., *55*, 46, 1948 (Endometrial Hyperplasia).
PALMER, J. P., *et al.*: Am. J. Obst. & Gynec., *58*, 457, 1949 (Carcinoma).
PERRY, T., JR.: New England J. Med., *238*, 793, 1948 (Sarcoma).
RANDALL, C. L.: Am. J. Obst. & Gynec., *45*, 445, 1943 (Sarcoma).
————: J. A. M. A., *139*, 972, 1949 (Endometriosis).
RANNEY, B.: Internat. Abst. Surg., *86*, 313, 1948 (Etiology Endometriosis).
SCHEFFEY, L. C.: South. M. J., *42*, 44, 1949 (Fundal Carcinoma).
SHOEMAKER, R., and KAHLER, J. E.: A. M. A. Arch. Path., *44*, 621, 1947 (Fibrosis Uteri).
SHUTE, E.: Canad. M. A. J., *51*, 443, 1944 (Estrogens and Uterine Fibroids).
SMITH, J. L., and SHAW, W. F.: J. Obst. and Gynaec. Brit. Emp., *23*, 129, 1913 (Red Degeneration).
TORPIN, R., *et al.*: Am. J. Obst. & Gynec., *44*, 569, 1942 (Fibromyomas).
TRUEMNER, K. M., and KAUMP, D. H.: Am. J. Clin. Path., *19*, 544, 1949 (Uterine Hypertrophy).
VESELL, M.: West. J. Surg., *57*, 592, 1949 (Endometrial Sarcoma).
WICKS, M. J., and LARSON, C. P.: Northwestern Med., *48*, 611, 1949 (Endometriosis).

FALLOPIAN TUBES

Congenital Anomalies

DANFORTH, D. N.: Am. J. Obst. & Gynec., *43*, 984, 1942 (Walthard Cell Rests).
NELSON, A. A.: A. M. A. Arch. Path., *27*, 955, 1939 (Accessory Adrenal Tissue).

Inflammations

AUERBACH, O.: Surg., Gynec. & Obst., *75*, 712, 1942 (Tuberculosis).
BENJAMIN, C. L., and BEAVER, D. C.: Am. J. Clin. Path., *21*, 212, 1951 (Salpingitis Isthmica Nodosa).
BLACK-SCHAFFER, B.: Am. J. Obst. & Gynec., *48*, 374, 1944 (Postpartum Salpingitis).
CROCE, E. J.: Am. J. Surg., *73*, 618, 1947 (Pyosalpinx).
GREENBERG, J. P.: Bull. Johns Hopkins Hosp., *32*, 52, 1921 (Tuberculosis).
HUNDLEY, J. M., *et al.*: Am. J. Obst. & Gynec., *60*, 977, 1950 (Salpingitis).
KULKA, E. W.: Am. J. Obst. & Gynec., *44*, 384, 1942 (Bone Formation Fallopian Tube).
MOHLER, R. W.: Am. J. Obst. & Gynec., *57*, 1077, 1949 (Pelvic Inflammatory Disease).
SHAW, H. N., and GASPAR, J.: West. J. Surg., *55*, 81, 1947 (Chronic Salpingitis).
SHAW, R. E.: Brit. M. J., *2*, 421, 1949 (Hydrosalpinx).
VEPROVSKY, E. C., and ACHAEFER, G.: S. Clin. North America, *28*, 513, 1948 (Tuberculosis).
YOUNG, B. W., and BACCI, O. J.: J. Urol., *63*, 1057, 1950 (Tubo-ovarian Abscess).

Physical Disturbances

FRANKEL, A. N.: Am. J. Obst. & Gynec., *56*, 574, 1948 (Interstitial Pregnancy).
JARCHO, J.: Am. J. Surg., *77*, 273 and 423, 1949 (Ectopic Pregnancy).

MacVine, J. S., and Lees, D. H.: Brit. M. J., *1*, 263, 1949 (Ectopic Gestation).
Romney, S. L., *et al.:* Surg., Gynec. & Obst., *91*, 605, 1950 (Ectopic Pregnancy).
Shaw, R. E.: Brit. M. J., *2*, 421, 1949 (Hydrosalpinx and Torsion).
Toplack, N. J.: J. Obst. & Gynaec. Brit. Emp., *57*, 62, 1950 (Ovarian Pregnancy).
Word, B.: Surg., Gynec. & Obst., *92*, 333, 1951 (Ectopic Pregnancy).

Tumors

Cruttenden, L. A., and Taylor, C. W.: J. Obst. & Gynaec. Brit. Emp., *57*, 937, 1950 (Carcinoma).
Forbes, R. D., and Finlayson, B. L.: Northwestern Med., *50*, 429, 1951 (Carcinoma).
Gardner, G. H., *et al.:* Am. J. Obst. & Gynec., *55*, 917, 1948 (Cysts Broad Ligament).
Hu, C. Y., *et al.:* Am. J. Obst. & Gynec., *59*, 58, 1950 (Carcinoma).
Scheffey, L. C., *et al.:* Am. J. Obst. & Gynec., *52*, 904, 1946 (Sarcoma).

OVARIES

Congenital Anomalies

Bleyer, L. F.: Am. J. Surg., *76*, 448, 1948 (Pseudohermaphroditism).
Kozoll, D. D.: A. M. A. Arch. Surg., *45*, 578, 1942 (Pseudohermaphroditism).
Kriss, B. R.: J. Mt. Sinai Hosp., *14*, 798, 1948 (Supernumerary Ovary).
Mayer, V., and Templeton, F. G.: A. M. A. Arch Surg., *43*, 397, 1941 (Ectopic Ovary).
Novak, E.: Am. J. Obst. & Gynec., *47*, 20, 1944 (Precocious Puberty).
Stirling, W. C.: J. Urol., *56*, 720, 1946 (Hermaphroditism).
van Campenhout, E., and Witschi, E.: J. Clin. Endocrinol., *8*, 271, 1948 (Hermaphroditism).
Weed, J. C., *et al.:* J. Clin. Endocrinol., *7*, 741, 1947 (Hermaphroditism).

Physical Disturbances

Hodgkinson, C. P., and Christensen, R. C.: Am. J. Obst. & Gynec., *59*, 1112, 1950 (Ruptured Tubo-ovarian Vein).
Taniguchi, T., and Kilkenny, G. S.: J. A. M. A., *147*, 1420, 1951 (Rupture Corpus Luteum).

Tumors

Allan, M. S., and Hertig, A. T.: Am. J. Obst. & Gynec., *58*, 640, 1949 (Carcinoma).
Barzilai, G.: *Atlas of Ovarian Tumors*, New York, Grune & Stratton, 1949.
Baskin, R. H., Jr., and Counseller, V. S.: Proc. Staff Meet., Mayo Clin., *26*, 60, 1951 (Meigs' Syndrome).
Beecham, C. T.: Am. J. Obst. & Gynec., *61*, 755, 1951 (Pseudomucinous Cystadenoma).
Berens, J. J.: Am. J. Surg., *81*, 484, 1951 (Krukenberg Tumors).
Blackwell, W. J., *et al.:* Am. J. Obst. & Gynec., *51*, 151, 1946 (Dermoid Cyst).
Curtis, A. H.: Surg., Gynec. & Obst., *81*, 504, 1945 (Teratoid Tumors).
Dockerty, M. B.: Internat. Abst. Surg., *81*, 179, 1945 (Tumors).
Dockerty, M. B., and Masson, J. C.: Am. J. Obst. & Gynec., *47*, 741, 1944 (Fibroma).
Dockerty, M. B., and Mussey, E.: Am. J. Obst. & Gynec., *61*, 147, 1951 (Estrogen-producing Tumors).
Erdmann, J. F., and Spaulding, H. V.: Surg., Gynec. & Obst., *33*, 362, 1921 (Papillary Cystadenoma).
Fox, J. F., and Clement, K. W.: Ann. Surg., *133*, 253, 1951 (Struma Ovarii).
Garrett, S. S.: Am. J. Dis. Child., *79*, 321, 1950 (Teratoid Tumor).
Gordon, V. H., and Marvin, H. N.: J. Pediat., *39*, 133, 1951 (Theca Cell Tumor).
Haines, M., and Jackson, I.: J. Obst. & Gynaec. Brit. Emp., *57*, 737, 1950 (Granulosa Cell Tumor).
Hodgson, J. E., *et al.:* Surg., Gynec. & Obst., *81*, 631, 1945 (Granulosa Cell Tumor).
Iverson, L.: Surg., Gynec. & Obst., *84*, 213, 1947 (Masculinizing Tumors).
Javert, C. T., and Finn, W. F.: Cancer, *4*, 60, 1951 (Arrhenoblastoma).
Jondahl, W. H., *et al.:* Am. J. Obst. & Gynec., *60*, 160, 1950 (Brenner Tumor).
Jones, G. E. S., and TeLinde, R. W.: Am. J. Obst. & Gynec., *50*, 691, 1945 (Granulosa Cell Tumor).
Karsh, J.: Am. J. Obst. & Gynec., *61*, 154, 1951 (Secondary Tumors).
Leffel, J. M., Jr., *et al.:* Ann. Surg., *115*, 102, 1942 (Krukenberg's Tumor).

LEVENTHAL, M. L., and COHEN, M. R.: Am. J. Obst. & Gynec., *61*, 1034, 1951 (Polycystic Ovaries).
LIBER, A. F.: A. M. A. Arch. Path., *49*, 280, 1950 (Carcinoma).
MacLEOD, D. H.: J. Obst. & Gynaec. Brit. Emp., *41*, 385, 1934 (Cyst).
MONTGOMERY, J. B.: Am. J. Obst. & Gynec., *55*, 201, 1948 (Tumors).
MUELLER, C. W., *et al.*: Am. J. Obst. & Gynec., *60*, 153, 1950 (Dysgerminoma).
NOVAK, E.: *Gynecologic and Obstetric Pathology*, 3rd Ed., Philadelphia, W. B. Saunders Co., 1952.
O'CONNOR, K. A., and DIDDLE, A. W.: West. J. Surg., *57*, 235, 1949 (Arrhenoblastoma).
PEDOWITZ, P., and GRAYZEL, D. M.: Am. J. Obst. & Gynec., *61*, 1243, 1951 (Dysgerminoma).
QUINLAND, W. S., and ST. HILL, I. R.: South. M. J., *40*, 908, 1947 (Teratoid Tumors).
SAILER, S.: Am. J. Clin. Path., *13*, 271, 1943 (Struma Ovarii).
SCHILLER, W.: Surg., Gynec. & Obst., *70*, 773, 1940 (Classification).
SCOTT, R. B.: Am. J. Obst. & Gynec., *43*, 733, 1942 (Serous Cystadenoma).
SELYE, H.: *Encyclopedia of Endocrinology*, Montreal, Richardson, Bond, and Wright, 1946, 7, Sect. 4, pp. 98–142.
SPARLING, D. W.: Am. J. Obst. & Gynec., *59*, 1279, 1950 (Theca Cell Tumor).
SPEERT, H.: Ann. Surg., *129*, 468, 1949 (Cancer).
STEIN, I. F., *et al.*: Am. J. Obst. & Gynec., *58*, 267, 1949 (Polycystic Ovaries).
STERNBERG, W. H., and GASKILL, C. J.: Am. J. Obst. & Gynec., *59*, 575, 1950 (Theca Cell Tumor).
WHEELOCK, F. C., *et al.*: New England J. Med., *245*, 447, 1951 (Carcinoma).
WHEELON, H., and WILSON, G.: J. A. M. A., *112*, 2411, 1939 (Corpus Luteum Cysts).
WOOLRIDGE, W. E., and HAGEMANN, P. O.: Am. J. Med., *5*, 237, 1948 (Meigs' Syndrome).

FETAL MEMBRANES

Congenital Anomalies

EASTMAN, N. J.: *Williams' Obstetrics*, 10th Ed., New York, Appleton-Century-Crofts, Inc., 1950.
GUTTMACHER, A. F.: Am. J. Obst. & Gynec., *34*, 76, 1937 (Twins).
HOBBS, J. E., and PRICE, C. N.: Am. J. Obst. & Gynec., *39*, 39, 1940 (Circumvallate Placenta).
LENNON, G. G.: J. Obst. & Gynaec. Brit. Emp., *54*, 830, 1947 (Amniotic Bands).
PADDOCK, R., and GREER, E. D.: Am. J. Obst. & Gynec., *13*, 164, 1927 (Cysts).
POTTER, E. L.: *Pathology of Fetus and the Newborn*, Chicago, The Yearbook Publishers, Inc., 1952.
QUIGLEY, J. K.: Am. J. Obst. & Gynec., *29*, 354, 1935 (Monoamniotic Twins).

Inflammations

KOBAK, A. J.: Am. J. Obst. & Gynec., *19*, 299, 1930 (Placentitis).
McCORD, J. R.: Am. J. Obst. & Gynec., *28*, 743, 1934 (Syphilis).
MONTGOMERY, T. L.: Am. J. Obst. & Gynec., *31*, 253, 1936 (Fibrosis).
SCHAEFER, G.: Am. J. Obst. & Gynec., *38*, 1066, 1939 (Tuberculosis).
WHITMAN, R. C., and GREENE, L. W.: A. M. A. Arch. Int. Med., *29*, 261, 1922 (Tuberculosis).

Physical Disturbances

BURGE, E. S.: Am. J. Obst. & Gynec., *61*, 615, 1951 (Abortion).
BYSSHE, S. M.: Am. J. Obst. & Gynec., *62*, 38, 1951 (Premature Separation).
COLLINS, J. H.: Am. J. Obst. & Gynec., *62*, 548, 1951 (Abortion).
FINDLEY, D.: Am. J. Obst. & Gynec., *61*, 855, 1951 (Placenta Previa).
HERTIG, A. T., and LIVINGSTONE, R. G.: New England J. Med., *230*, 797, 1944 (Abortion).
JAVERT, C. T., and FINN, W. F.: Texas State J. M., *46*, 739, 1950 (Abortion).
JOHNSON, H. W.: Am. J. Obst. & Gynec., *59*, 1236, 1950 (Placenta Previa).
McKEOGH, R. P., and D'ERRICO, E.: New England J. Med., *245*, 159, 1951 (Placenta Accreta).
SEWALL, C. W., and COULTON, D.: Am. J. Obst. & Gynec., *52*, 564, 1946 (Retained Placenta).

Tumors

BREWS, A.: J. Obst. & Gynaec. Brit. Emp., *57*, 317, 1950 (Chorionepithelioma).
DORSEY, C. W.: Am. J. Obst. & Gynec., *44*, 591, 1942 (Placental Polyp).

FISHER, J. H.: Am. J. Obst. & Gynec., *40*, 493, 1940 (Chorio-angioma).

FREETH, D., and McCALL, A. J.: J. Obst. & Gynaec. Brit. Emp., *57*, 757, 1950 (Chorionepithelioma).

HERTIG, A. T., and EDMONDS, H. W.: A. M. A. Arch. Path., *30*, 260, 1940 (Hydatidiform Mole).

HERTIG, A. T., and SHELDON, W. H.: Am. J. Obst. & Gynec., *53*, 1, 1947 (Hydatidiform Mole).

HOLMAN, A. W., and SCHIRMER, E. H.: West. J. Surg., *55*, 525, 1947 (Hydatid Mole and Chorionepithelioma).

MARCHETTI, A. A.: Surg., Gynec. & Obst., *68*, 733, 1939 (Benign Tumors).

NOVAK, E.: Am. J. Obst. & Gynec., *59*, 1355, 1950 (Hydatidiform Mole and Choriocarcinoma).

OLIVER, H. M., and HORNE, E. O.: New England J. Med., *239*, 14, 1948 (Teratomatous Chorionepithelioma).

PARK, W., and LEES, J. C.: A. M. A. Arch. Path., *49*, 73 and 205, 1950 (Choriocarcinoma).

PAYNE, F. L.: Surg., Gynec. & Obst., *73*, 86, 1941 (Hydatidiform Mole).

Chapter

34

Breast

PATHOLOGIC PHYSIOLOGY

Joseph J. Rupp

The *growth* and *development* of the breast as well as its major function, lactation, are controlled by the female sex steroids and the pituitary lactogenic hormone. At the onset of puberty, the female breasts begin to enlarge in response to ovarian hormones. Ductule development is an estrogen effect while tubo-alveolar changes represent a response to progesterone. When puberty is completed and ovulatory menstruation is established, the breasts often increase in size and become tender premenstrually, with relief of the symptoms with the onset of vaginal bleeding. The fibrocytic changes which occur during the reproductive years result from cyclic hormonal stimulation of the breasts. Such changes usually regress at the menopause.

During *pregnancy*, enlargement and congestion of the breasts, as well as hyperpigmentation of the nipples, are constant findings. The hyperpigmentation is an estrogenic effect and may be induced in males or females by giving large amounts of estrogenic substances. Lactation does not occur during pregnancy because the pituitary release of lactogenic hormone is inhibited by the large amounts of estrogens produced by the placenta. Following delivery the estrogens decrease, lactogenic hormone production increases, and production of milk ensues. The antidiuretic hormone (vasopressin) plays an important part in milk delivery to the infant. In response to sucking, the antidiuretic hormone is secreted and alters the outflow tract of the breast. This action is referred to as the *milk let down function* of vasopressin.

Some breast *carcinomas* are hormone dependent, that is, their rate of growth is altered by hormonal factors. Of the various hormones incriminated as stimuli for the spread of mammary cancer, estrogens and pituitary growth and lactogenic hormones seem to fit the assigned roles best. There is, however, no evidence that these hormones cause breast cancer but they are considered rather to change the rate of growth of the tumor. Evidence in favor of this exists in the fact that regression of metastases and of the primary tumor may follow castration or adrenalectomy. In some patients castration produces an initial remission and a recurrence responds favorably to adrenalectomy only to be followed by recrudescence which, in turn, may again regress with hypophysectomy. The remission induced by adrenalectomy and castration results from the lowered estrogen production in the castrated adrenalectomized patient, while that induced by hypophysectomy is a reflection of the removal of the source of growth hormone and/or lactogenic hormone. Estrogen dependency of bone metastases can be assessed by measuring the changes in calcium metabolism produced by treatment with estrogens. Hypercalcemia, an increase in urinary excretion of calcium, and an increase in bone pain and tenderness follow estrogen treatment of patients with estrogen dependent tumors only. They do not occur in estrogen-treated patients with nondependent tumors. In about 20 per cent of postmenopausal women with metastasis from carcinoma of the breast, temporary improvement follows the use of androgens or estrogens. The doses required are large, and vaginal bleeding or virilization may occur. The mechanism responsible for the changes in tumor growth which follows the use of steroids is unknown. It should be stressed, however, that no amount of manipulation of the endocrine glands or treatment with hormones will result in cure of carcinoma of the breast. It results only in temporary abatement of symptoms and in decreased rate of growth of the cancers. All patients eventually die of the disease.

Gynecomastia is a common disorder that starts at or after puberty. In most patients the breast tissue regresses spontaneously but in some mammary enlargement, continues and well-developed breasts result. The exact mechanism responsible for gynecomastia is unknown although it may reflect the hormonal imbalance of puberty. Aside from spontaneously occurring enlargement of the mammæ, development of the male breast can be induced by estrogens, frequently by testosterone, and rarely by digitalis glucosides. Such enlargement is part of the clinical picture in choriocarcinoma, estrogen-producing adrenal tumors, cirrhosis of the liver, and during recovery from malnutrition.

GENERAL CONSIDERATIONS

The breast is a modified sudorific (sweat) gland that first makes its appearance in the six-week embryo as a bilateral thickening of the ectoderm along a line that extends from each axilla to each inguinal fold. Normally only the portions over the chest wall continue to develop to form the breasts while the remaining portions disappear. Normally, too, the breasts in the

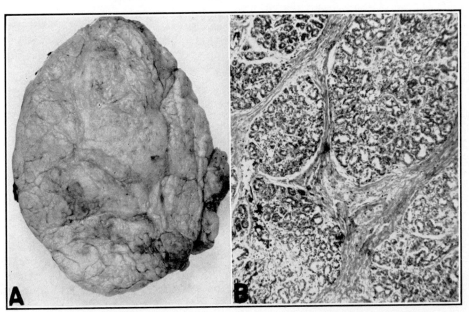

Fig. 599.—Prelactating breast showing *A*, a massive proliferation of pancreas-like tissue and *B*, numerous glands in lobular formation lined by cuboidal epithelium. × 50.

male remain rudimentary throughout life, while those in the female remain rudimentary until puberty when they increase substantially in size as a result of proliferation and accumulation of fat. Once menstruation is established, the breast undergoes cyclic changes as a result of action of hormones. In the premenstrual, as well as the prelactating and lactating stages, it becomes full, turgid, and painful. Grossly such an organ consists of solid masses of breast tissue that have the appearance of a normal pancreas (Fig. 599). Histologically it consists of numerous acini lined by cuboidal cells showing varying degrees of secretory activity and, by the unwary, may be mistaken for carcinoma. Pathologically, since the breasts are covered with integument, they are subjected to all the diseases that occur in the skin in general. Except for only a few conditions, however, these disorders will be omitted in the discussion in this Chapter and disturbances that affect the breast proper only will be considered.

CONGENITAL ANOMALIES

Developmental malformations of the breast may be listed as follows: (1) *inversion* of the *nipple,* (2) *microthelia*—decrease in size of nipple, (3) *athelia*—absence of nipple, (4) *polythelia*—more than one nipple, located anywhere along the embryonic milk line, and often associated with polymastia, (4) *polymastia*—accessory breasts, located anywhere along the milk line but most commonly found in the axilla, consisting of glandular tissue only or of glandular tissue and nipple, and subjected to the same physiologic vicissitudes and pathologic changes as a normal breast (Falk, Roberts, and de Cholnoky), (5) *amastia*—absence of breast, (6) *micromastia*—small breast, (7) *macromastia*—enlargement or hypertrophy of the breast, usually seen after puberty, and consisting of an increase of glandular, connective tissue, and fatty elements, and (8) *gynecomastia*—an enlargement of the breast in males not due to tumor, occurring at all ages but being most common in the third decade of life, occasionally due to a demonstrable excess of estrogens but generally being idiopathic, consisting of hypertrophy and hyperplasia of both the glandular and supporting tissue, usually bilateral, and treated by surgical excision in the presence of pain, anxiety neurosis, or failure to rule out tumor (Karsner).

DEGENERATIONS

Degenerative disorders in the breasts commonly occur in conjunction with most of the diseases. Three conditions, however, that may be singled out are (1) *atrophy*—seen after each menstrual period, after lactation, and after the menopause, (2) *mucoid degeneration*—encountered in connection with epithelial cells in mucinous carcinoma and in connective tissue cells in fibroadenoma and cystosarcoma phylloides, and (3) *calcification*—present not infrequently in fibroadenoma and in carcinoma (Gershon-Cohen).

INFLAMMATIONS

Orientation.—Inflammation of the nipple is known as *thelitis,* of the areola as *areolitis,* and of the breast as *mastitis.* The more important inflammations may be listed as follows: acute nonspecific mastitis, tuberculosis, plasma cell mastitis, syphilis, and actinomycosis. *Syphilis* of the breast usually attacks the skin or nipple area and may exist in the form of a chancre, syphilids, or condyloma latum. Rarely, the breast proper may disclose a gumma. *Actinomycosis* is uncommon and generally exists as an extension of an intrathoracic infection.

Acute Nonspecific Mastitis.—This lesion consists of a nonspecific inflammation of the breast *caused* by any of the ordinary pyogenic organisms but in most instances due to *Staphylococcus aureus*. The condition usually *occurs* within the first six weeks of the puerperium and the organisms generally gain entrance by way of cracked or fissured nipples (Hesseltine and Newton). Its incidence varies but it generally constitutes about 1 per cent of all maternity cases. Infrequently, acute mastitis may be nonpuerperal and may occur in conjunction with lesions of the skin overlying the breast, carcinoma of the breast, and other conditions. *Pathologically* the condition is usually unilateral (though it may be bilateral) and any portion of the breast may show the initial changes. The affected area is enlarged, ill defined, erythematous, firm, hot, and exquisitely tender. The inflammation either remains localized and regresses or it extends to involve most or all of the breast. The *histologic* changes consist of congestion, edema, and diffuse neutrophilic infiltration. If untreated, the condition may become *complicated* by abscess formation (Florey and Kilgore). The *clinical manifestations* consist of (1) pain, swelling, and tenderness in the breast — due to the inflammation and (2) chills, fever, and leukocytosis—due to absorption of toxic products or to septicemia. The *diagnosis* is made from the history, physical examination, and (when abscess forms) examination of aspirated pus. A differential diagnosis should include inflammatory carcinoma. *Treatment* consists of prevention (by proper care of the nipple) and of antibiotic (penicillin) therapy once infection has occurred. Surgical drainage may be necessary when abscesses form. The ultimate *prognosis* is good.

Tuberculosis.—Although tuberculosis of the breast is recorded as constituting as high as 1.87 per cent of all mammary lesions (Grausman) the actual over-all *incidence* is doubtlessly much less. The condition usually *occurs* in women between the ages of twenty and fifty years but in about 4 per cent of cases it affects males. While the *route* of invasion of the tubercle bacilli has been considered to be by way of the ducts, through the skin, directly through the chest wall, hematogenous, and lymphogenous it is the concensus that the lymphatic route from infections in adjacent lymph nodes is the most common. It is also the concensus that most cases are secondary and that only rarely is the lesion primary. *Pathologically* the process is generally unilateral and grossly may appear as a nodular caseating mass that measures as much as 10 cm. in diameter, as a more sclerosing lesion, or as a "cold" abscess. The histologic changes are typical of tuberculosis. The chief *complication* is extension of the lesion with sinus tract formation. The *clinical manifestations* consist of a painless lump in the breast, enlarged axillary lymph nodes, and occasionally a sinus tract. The *diagnosis* is generally made after removal of the lesion, for the condition is frequently mistaken for tumor. *Treatment* of choice is surgical excision. The *prognosis*, as far as the breast lesion is concerned, is good.

Plasma Cell Mastitis.—Plasma cell mastitis is a localized nonsuppurative condition of the breast of unknown *etiology* (Bynum). Bacteriologic studies are not significant and, although escaped lipid material is thought to be the irritant, there is no definite proof that it provides the necessary stimulus. The condition usually *occurs* in parous women between the ages of thirty and forty years and is dividable into an acute and residual phase. The *acute phase* consists of a sudden onset of pain, tenderness, and discomfort. The breast is swollen and hot and the axillary nodes are enlarged and tender. The *residual phase* consists of a painless lump in the breast associated with edema and attachment to the skin. The axillary lymph nodes remain enlarged and the condition thus resembles a carcinoma. *Grossly* the lesion consists of an ill-defined, firm, yellowish area of varying dimensions associated or unassociated with foci of necrosis (Halpert). The outstanding histologic change is a diffuse permeation with plasma cells. There are present in addition, however, giant cells, foam cells, and fatty acid crystals. *Treatment* consists of local excision. The *prognosis* is excellent.

PHYSICAL DISTURBANCES

Orientation.—Under this heading may be mentioned two unrelated conditions of the breast—discharge from the nipple and fat necrosis.

Discharge from the Nipple.—Discharge from the nipple is a *symptom* and not a disease. It may be seranguineous, sanguineous, serous, yellowish, greenish, milky, or brownish and it may be scanty or relatively copious (Donnelly). While it may occur as a result of failing ovarian function (Abramson) in over three-quarters of all cases it is *due to* cystic hyperplasia, intraductal papilloma, and carcinoma. In order to determine the underlying cause the following are employed: careful inspection and palpation, cytologic examination of the discharge for neoplastic and other cells (Saphir), mammography, and surgical exploration (Hollenberg). The *treatment* and *prognosis* depend upon the etiologic agent.

Fat Necrosis.—Fat necrosis of the breast is *infrequent*. It generally *occurs* in women with pendulous fatty breasts and frequently, but not always results from trauma (Adair). *Pathologically* the lesion exists as a sharply circumscribed, chalky area measuring as much as 2 to 3 cm. in diameter and often exhibiting foci of liquefaction and cyst formation. *Histologically* it exhibits opacities of some of the fat cells, necrosis of other fat cells, crystal formation, and a cellular reaction of foam cells, plasma cells, and foreign body giant cells. *Clinically* the chief presenting manifestation is a hard mass in the breast that is readily mistaken for carcinoma. *Treatment* consists of local excision. The *prognosis* is excellent.

TUMORS

Orientation.—Tumors and tumor-like conditions are much more *frequent* in females than in males, are similar in appearance and behavior in the two sexes, and while they may occur at any age, they prevail after the second decade of life. Although the precise *cause* of mammary tumors is unknown, there is considerable evidence that estrogens are at least of contributory significance (p. 151). *Pathologically* virtually all of the tissues that comprise the normal breast are capable of giving rise to a benign or a malignant tumor. The more important lesions may be listed as follows: Paget's disease (nipple), epidermal papilloma (nipple), sebaceous cyst (nipple), sweat gland tumor (nipple), duct papilloma, cystic hyperplasia, carcinoma, fibroma, fibrosarcoma, fibroadenoma, cystosarcoma phylloides, lipoma, liposarcoma, leiomyoma, leiomyosarcoma, neuroma, neurofibroma, neurofibrosarcoma, lymphangioma, hemangioma, hemangiosarcoma, lymphoblastoma, chondroma, chondrosarcoma, osteoma, osteosarcoma, and secondary tumors. The chief *complication* of benign tumors is a cancerous transformation while the chief complication of malignant tumors is spread to distant areas. The most important *clinical manifestation* is a painless lump in the breast. While the size of the lump in comparison with its duration, its location, its physical characteristics, etc., may be important in determining whether a tumor is benign or malignant, there are so many exceptions that the only sound principle to follow is to excise and examine pathologically every mass in the breast. The final *diagnosis* thus rests with the pathologist. *Treatment* consists of local excision in cases of benign

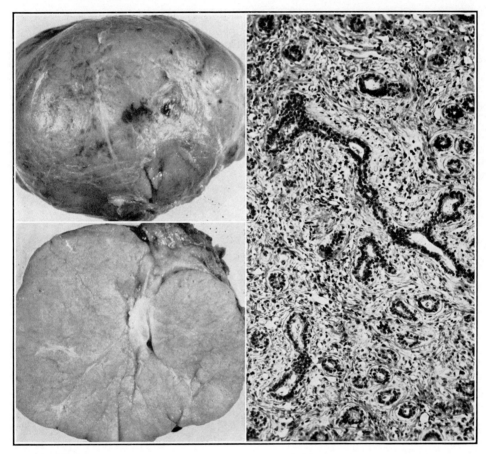

FIG. 600.—Pericanalicular fibroadenoma of the breast illustrating a well-encapsulated tumor with a flat cut surface and a loose connective tissue stroma containing small glands lined with cuboidal epithelium. × 100.

tumors and radical mastectomy in cases of malignant tumors. The *prognosis* varies with the type of growth. In general, it is excellent in cases of benign growths and fair in cases of malignant neoplasms. Aside from the above general remarks, a few separate remarks are warranted in each of the following: fibroadenoma, cystic hyperplasia, duct papilloma, carcinoma, Paget's disease, cystosarcoma phylloides, and sarcoma.

Fibroadenoma. — Fibroadenoma, also known as adenofibroma, is a common benign tumor of the breast that *occurs* predominantly in women of the childbearing age (Saltzstein and Warren). It is usually *single*, is most common in the upper and outer quadrant of the breast, varies from 1 to 20 cm. in diameter, is freely movable within the breast tissue, and is firm to palpation. *Pathologically* the tumor is well encapsulated, smooth externally, and bulges on cut surface. It is generally divided into two types—pericanalicular and intracanalicular. *Pericanalicular* fibroadenoma presents a smooth, gray, cut surface and microscopically consists of a stroma of loose connective tissue surrounding proliferated glands lined by cuboidal epithelial cells (Fig. 600). *Intracanalicular* fibroadenoma presents a rough or

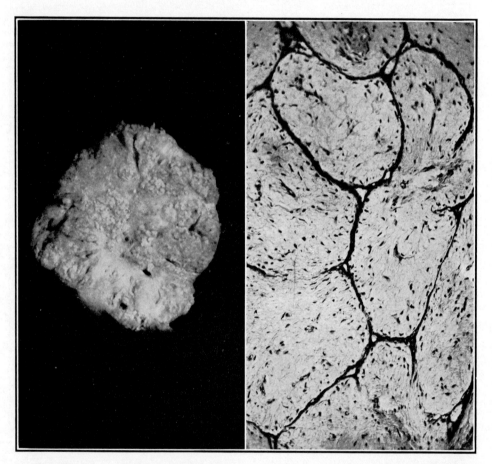

Fig. 601.—Intracanalicular fibroadenoma demonstrating a granular surface and a loose connective tissue stroma drawing the glands out into slit-like formations. × 100.

granular, gray cut surface and microscopically is composed of a stroma of loose connective tissue supporting glands that are drawn out into slit-like formations (Fig. 601). The division into the two types is largely academic although cystosarcoma phylloides (p. 601) is more prone to develop in the intracanalicular than in the pericanalicular variety.

Cystic Hyperplasia.—Cystic hyperplasia of the breast is a term that may be used to encompass lesions variously known as *cystic disease* of the breast, *chronic cystic mastitis, mammary dysplasia, Schimmelbusch's disease,* etc. The condition is the most common single disorder in the breast, generally *occurs* between the ages of twenty and forty-five years, is more common in parous than nonparous women, is not initiated in adolescence or after the menopause, and is manifested clinically by pain in the breasts, nodules in the breasts, and occasionally discharge from the nipples (Cole, Patey, and Copeland). *Grossly* the condition is almost always bilateral and multiple. It consists of numerous ill-defined areas of thickening measuring 3 to 4 cm. in over-all diameter and containing smaller, more circumscribed, solid or cystic areas usually measuring up to 1 cm. in diameter (Fig. 602). The cysts are rounded, bluish, or straw colored, and smooth walled. They contain clear fluid under tension and when they are incised they collapse. *Histologically* a typical case discloses the following: (1) cystic spaces lined

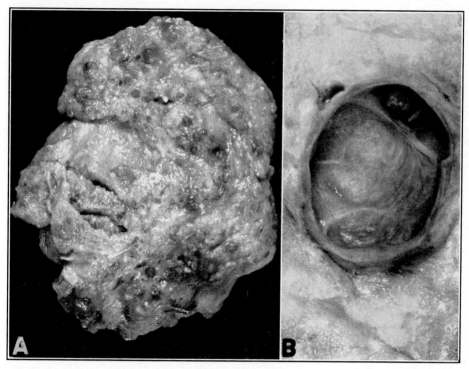

Fig. 602.—Cystic hyperplasia of the breast disclosing *A*, a mass of fibrous tissue containing numerous tiny cysts and *B*, a large cyst with evacuated fluid and a smooth lining.

with low cuboidal, columnar, or "pink" (sudorific) epithelium, (2) hyperplasia of the glands, (3) hyperplasia of the ductal epithelium, (4) connective tissue proliferation, and (5) focal lymphocytic and plasma cell infiltration. In some instances, cysts are not present and the lesion consists essentially of proliferation of acini and connective tissue. Such a combination may be referred to as *fibroglandular hyperplasia, sclerosing adenosis, adenofibromas, fibrosing adenomatosis,* or *fibroadenosis* (Heller and Atkins). *Treatment* is not standardized ranging from removal of "suspicious nodules" to aspiration of the cysts, hormonal therapy, and observation only. The *prognosis* is good. The question as to whether cystic hyperplasia predisposes to carcinoma is still a moot subject, although it is the consensus that cancer is slightly more common in such breasts than it is in normal organs.

Duct Papilloma.—Duct papilloma is a benign tumor usually affecting the main lacteal ducts. It may *occur* in an otherwise normal breast or in conjunction with cystic hyperplasia, is rare before the age of thirty years, and *clinically* is attended by combinations of discharge from the nipple, a palpable nodule within the nipple or beneath the areola, pain and tenderness, and retraction of the nipple (Estes, Chester, and Haagensen). *Pathologically* the lesion has been recorded as being multiple in as high as 37 per cent of cases. Grossly the ducts containing the tumors are generally dilated and contain deep brown to hemorrhagic fluid (Saphir). The ductal wall is thin and when sectioned retracts below the level of the tumor (Fig. 604).

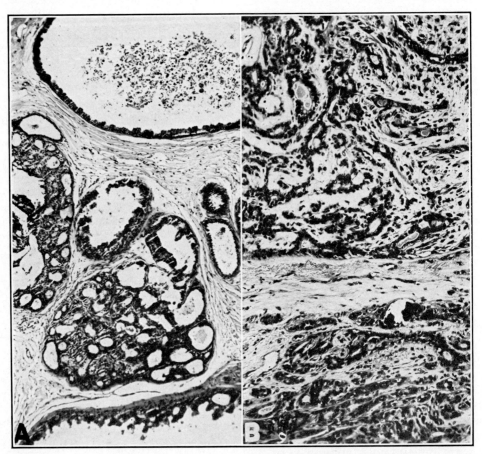

Fig. 603.—Cystic hyperplasia of the breast showing *A*, cysts lined with sudorific epithelium hyperplasia of the glands, slight lymphocytic infiltration, and deposition of collagenous tissue × 50 and *B*, (sclerosing adenosis) proliferation of collagenous tissue and glands. × 100.

The tumor is usually gray, serrated, friable, and attached to the wall of the duct by a thin delicate pedicle. It may measure as much as 4 or 5 cm. in diameter although usually it measures less than 1 cm. across. *Histologically* the growth arises from the wall of the duct and is composed of varying amounts of connective tissue and epithelium. At one extreme, it consists almost entirely of prongs or masses of edematous or more collagenous connective tissue covered by a single row of cuboidal epithelium which is pushed ahead of the tumor as it grows into the duct, while at the other extreme it consists almost entirely of epithelial cells arranged in glands or solid masses. Glandular tumors are composed of regular appearing cuboidal cells whereas the solid neoplasms are composed of uniform appearing polyhedral cells. *Treatment* consists of wide local excision or simple mastectomy. The *prognosis* is good. The solid epithelial tumors are prone to become malignant while the fibrous ones remain innocent.

Carcinoma.—Carcinoma of the breast usually *occurs* after the age of thirty years, has no predilection for any race, accounts for more than 60 per cent of all malignant tumors in females, affects males in about 1 per cent of cases and females in about 99 per cent of cases, and runs a similar course in both sexes (Ackerman, Shaw, Somerville, Guthorn, and Hunt).

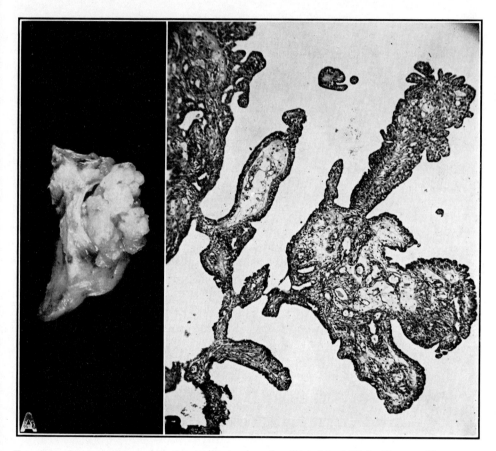

FIG. 604.—Duct papilloma of the breast illustrating *A*, a dilated duct filled with a papillary mass, and *B*, a core of edematous connective tissue covered with hyperplastic epithelium. × 50.

Pathologically any part of the breast may be affected but the most common location is the upper and outer quadrant. While the *classifications* of carcinomas of the breast are numerous, your author has found a division into the following five categories quite sufficient: scirrhous, medullary, duct or comedo, inflammatory, and mucinous. Each of these is considered briefly at the end of this general discussion. Regardless of the histologic type of tumor, carcinoma of the breasts *spreads* (1) by local extension to involve contiguous portions of the breast tissue, overlying skin, and chest wall, (2) by lymphatics primarily to the lymph nodes draining the quadrant

of the breast in which the tumor is located but also (in a retrograde manner) to other lymph nodes, and (3) by blood vessels to the lungs, liver,
bones, and other sites.

The earliest *clinical manifestations* consist of discharge from the nipple,
dermatitis of the nipple, shadow upon transillumination, thickening of the
skin or nipple, retraction of the skin, and an axillary nodule (Klopp and
Fitts). Later manifestations consist of (1) a lump or mass in the breast,
(2) stretched, ulcerated, or puckered (orange peel-like) skin covering the

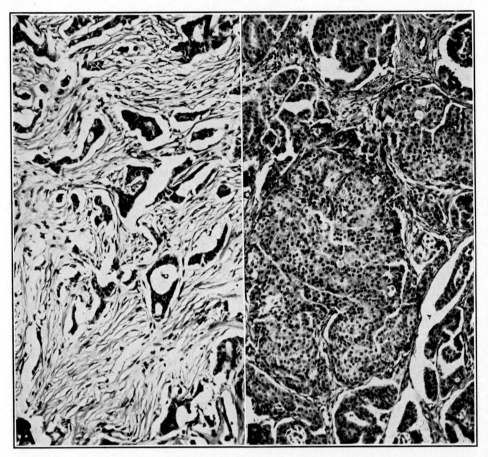

Fig. 605.—Carcinoma of the breast demonstrating *A*, a scirrhous type of lesion with a collagenous stroma enmeshing nests and glands of irregular epithelial cells and *B*, a medullary type with
large masses of irregular epithelial cells and a scanty stroma. × 100.

mass, (3) retraction of the nipple, (4) axillary and other masses, and (5)
symptoms and signs referable to distant metastases. As already stated,
the *diagnosis* is made from the history, careful physical examination,
microscopic examination of secretions from the nipple, and excisional
(frozen section) biopsy. The only curative *treatment* is complete surgical
excision which generally is accomplished only by radical mastectomy.
Irradiation and hormonal therapy (in the form of (1) oophorectomy, (2)
administration of androgens or estrogens, or (3) bilateral adrenalectomy)
are valuable but not curative adjuncts (Huggins, Segaloff, and Lewison).

PLATE VI

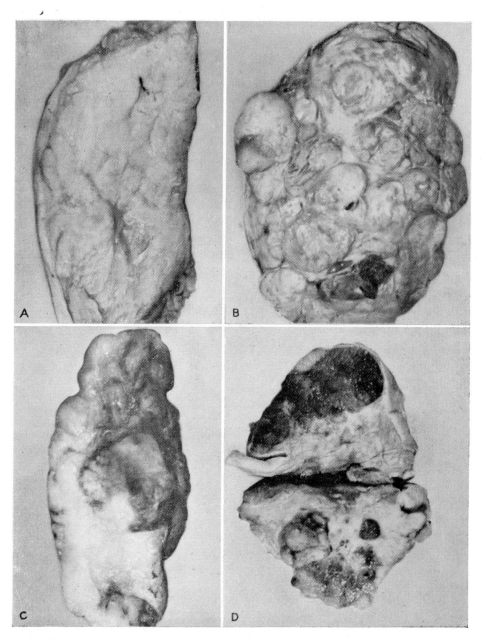

Malignant tumors of the breast showing A, a depressed, gray, irregularly circumscribed, scirrhous carcinoma. C, a rather large, more sharply delineated, brain-like medullary carcinoma, B, a large, bulky cystosarcoma phylloides, and D, hemisections of a gelatinous appearing mucinous carcinoma.

The *prognosis* depends upon many factors. It is (1) worse in early life as compared with old age, (2) worse when it occurs during pregnancy or lactation than in other physiologic states (Barker), (3) most grave in cases of inflammatory carcinoma, intermediate in cases of scirrhous, medullary or duct carcinoma, and best in mucinous carcinoma, and (4) better, of course, when the lesion is localized to the breast than when it has metastasized. The over-all five-year cure rates are generally in the neighborhood

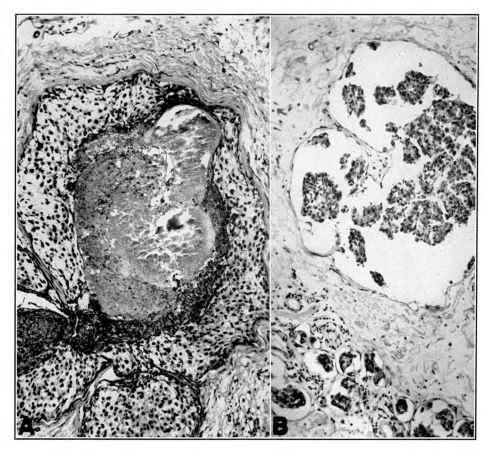

Fig. 606.—Carcinoma of the breast illustrating *A*, a duct type with a duct filled with a mass of irregular epithelial cells disclosing central necrosis and *B*, an inflammatory type with neoplastic cells filling capillary and lymphatic spaces. × 100.

of 75 per cent when the disease is localized to the breast, 40 per cent when metastasis has occurred to the axillary lymph nodes, and nil when metastasis has occurred to distant areas (Shimkin, Harrington, and Park).

Scirrhous (L. = hard) *carcinoma* usually measures not more than 2 cm. in diameter, appears fairly sharply defined but is definitely not encapsulated, is hard, cuts with a gritty sensation, consists of pearl gray tissue with yellowish foci, and retracts beneath the cut surface (Plate VI*A*). Histologically it is composed of an excessive amount of collagenous connective tissue enmeshing small collections, nests, or acini of irregular neoplastic cells (Fig. 605*A*).

77

Medullary carcinoma is the antithesis of scirrhous carcinoma. It is large and bulky, often measures 6 to 8 cm. in diameter, is sharply circumscribed but not encapsulated, and is composed of moderately firm brain-like tissue (Plate VI*C*). Histologically it consists of large masses or sheets of irregular epithelial cells generally with indistinct borders, moderate amounts of cytoplasm, and irregular hyperchromatic nuclei (Fig. 605*B*).

Duct carcinoma, also known as *comedo carcinoma*, receives the latter name from the gross appearance of the tumor for when the mass is slightly compressed the surface becomes dotted with yellowish foci that have a likeness to squeezed comedones (blackheads). In bulkiness, the tumor is usually between a scirrhous and a medullary carcinoma. Histologically the growth

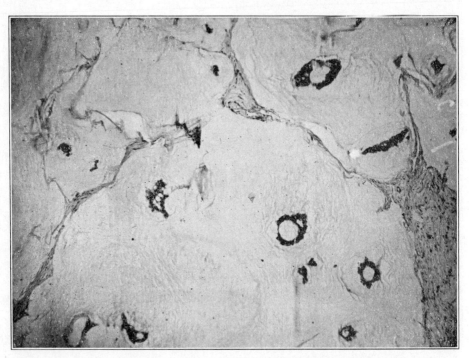

Fig. 607.—Mucinous carcinoma showing nests and glands of epithelial cells surrounded by an abundant amount of mucoid material.

consists for the most part of dilated ducts filled with masses of irregular neoplastic cells that have a tendency to undergo central degeneration and necrosis (Fig. 606*A*). As the lesion becomes more malignant it penetrates the ductal boundaries and then behaves like a scirrhous or medullary growth.

Inflammatory carcinoma is a clinical rather than a pathologic entity (Chris and Donnelly). It is a rapidly growing scirrhous or medullary carcinoma that permeates the lymphatic and capillary channels and produces stasis of blood (Fig. 606*B*). As a result of the blockage of the circulation, the breast becomes intensely hyperemic and clinically has the appearance of inflammation.

Mucinous carcinoma, also called colloid or gelatinous carcinoma, is a rather slowly growing tumor, is usually of years' duration, and occurs on an average of about a decade later than most other mammary tumors. The

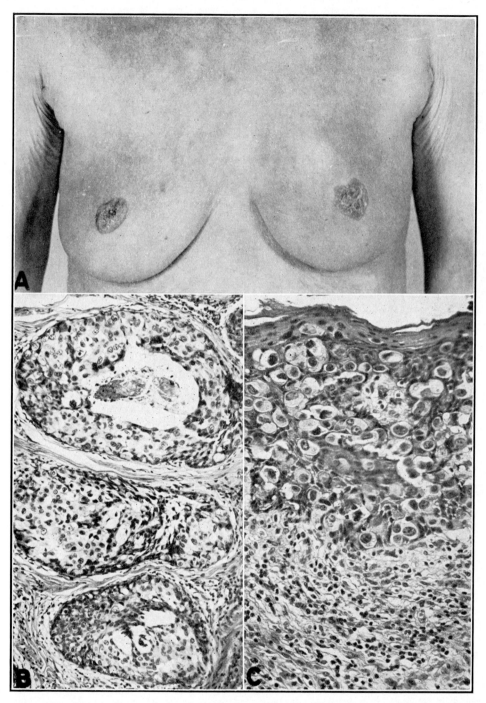

FIG. 608.—Paget's disease of the nipple demonstrating *A*, a bilateral eczematoid lesion of the nipple and areola, *B*, typical carcinoma of the underlying ducts. × 100, and *C*, similar type of large Paget cells in the epidermis of the nipple. × 200.

lesion is generally sharply circumscribed, varies from 2 to 20 cm. in diameter, is composed of varying amounts of gelatinous substance and gray tissue when small, and often becomes completely cystic and filled with a hemorrhagic or brownish fluid when large (Plate VI*D*) (Saphir).   Histologically the tumor consists of islands of irregular epithelial cells or of acini of cuboidal cells surrounded by an abundant amount of mucoid material (Fig. 607).

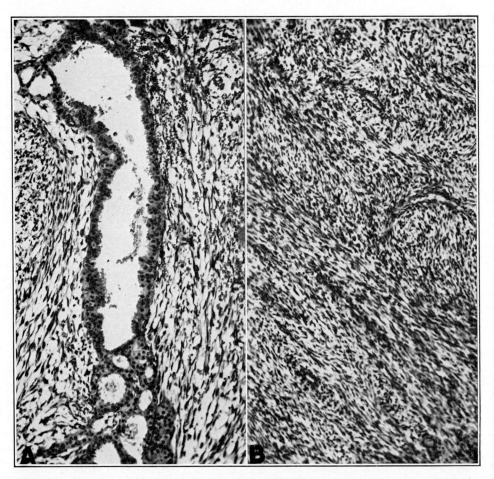

Fig. 609.—Sarcoma of the breast showing *A*, cystosarcoma phylloides with elongated hyperchromatic stromal cells supporting slit-like ducts lined with epithelium and *B*, fibrosarcoma with elongated, closely packed, hyperchromatic cells forming virtually the entire tumor.   × 100.

Paget's Disease.—The condition known as Paget's disease of the nipple was *first described* as an eczema of the nipple by Sir James Paget in 1874 (Sarason).   Since the cases which he described were not confirmed histologically, considerable controversy arose subsequently as to whether the lesion was inflammatory or neoplastic.   At present, however, the consensus is that the condition represents a carcinoma of the main ducts of the breast with an intra-epithelial spread of neoplastic cells to involve the nipple and/or areola (Inglis and Dockerty).   The disorder generally *occurs* in women beyond the fifth decade of life, is only rarely seen in males, is unilateral more often than bilateral, and is *characterized* by an excoriation of the nipple and/or areola that is preceded or succeeded by a lump in the underlying mammary tissue (Fig. 608). *Histologically* the mammary lesion is a typical duct carcinoma while the lesion in the nipple and areola consists of irregular neoplastic cells permeating the epidermal cells. The infiltrating cells (called Paget cells) are large and polyhedral or rounded, possess an abundant amount of light staining or vacuolated cytoplasm, and disclose irregular hyperchromatic nuclei. The prognosis is that of any mammary carcinoma arising in the main ducts.

Cystosarcoma Phylloides.—This tumor, also known as adenofibrosarcoma, *consists of* a sarcomatous transformation of a fibroadenoma (especially of the intracanalicular variety). It may *occur* at any age but is most common in the fourth and fifth decades of life (Trewes and Stephenson).

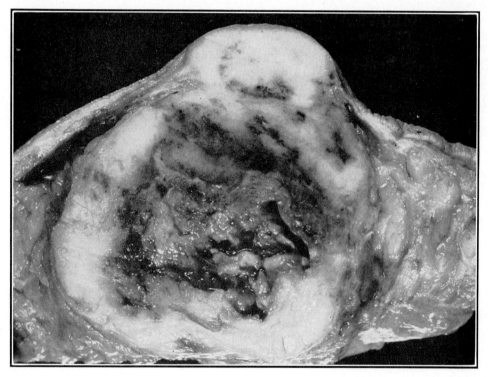

Fig. 610.—Fibrosarcoma of the breast disclosing a large, soft, brain-like tumor with a central area of necrosis and hemorrhage.

The usual history consists of the presence of a mass in the breast that has been present for years, that has gradually increased in size until pregnancy or trauma has supervened when the rapidity of growth increased greatly, and that has now become too heavy to carry around. *Pathologically* the lesion is generally unilateral and consists of an irregularly lobulated mass that may measure 20 to 30 cm. in diameter. Cut surfaces disclose a lobulated edematous structure with a tendency to irregular cyst formation often filled with edematous material (Plate VIB). *Histologically* the fundamental pattern of a fibroadenoma is still maintained but the connective tissue elements preponderate and assume a sarcomatous appearance (Fig. 609A). The *course* is usually benign although metastases to axillary lymph nodes and lungs occur occasionally.

Sarcoma.—Aside from cystosarcoma phylloides (which is a special type of sarcoma) the breast may be the seat of a variety of malignant tumors of mesodermal origin already mentioned under *Orientation* at the beginning of this section (Massie and Hill). Of all the lesions, *fibrosarcoma* is perhaps the most common. The tumor usually *occurs* after the third decade of life and is, as a rule, unilateral and single. It generally enlarges rather slowly and eventually may assume large proportions. *Pathologically* it consists of a circumscribed mass of grayish-white, brain-like tissue that has a tendency to undergo focal necrosis, hemorrhage, and cavitation (Fig. 610). *Histologically* it consists of sheets or interlacing masses of spindle cells with a moderate amount of ill-defined, light-staining cytoplasm and elongated hyperchromatic nuclei (Fig. 609*B*). *Metastasis* occurs by way of the bloodstream but is generally not found until late in the course of the disease.

REFERENCES

Pathologic Physiology

MARKEE, J. E.: *Glandular Physiology and Therapy*, 5th Ed., Philadelphia, J. B. Lippincott Co. 1954, p. 200.
NATHANSON, I. T.: *Glandular Physiology and Therapy*, 5th Ed., Philadelphia, J. B. Lippincott Co., 1954, p. 468.

Congenital Anomalies

DE CHOLNOKY, T.: New York State J. Med., *51*, 2245, 1951 (Accessory Breast).
FALK, V. S.: Wisconsin M. J., *49*, 1007, 1950 (Carcinoma in Aberrant Breast).
KARSNER, H. T.: Am. J. Path., *22*, 235, 1946 (Gynecomastia).
ROBERTS, J. M.: West. J. Surg., *60*, 175, 1952 (Aberrant Breast Tissue).

Degenerations

GERSHON-COHEN, J., et al.: J. A. M. A., *152*, 676, 1953 (Calcification).

Inflammations

BYNUM, G. A., and ROWE, E. B.: Am. Surgeon, *18*, 836, 1952 (Plasma Cell Mastitis).
FLOREY, M. E., et al.: Brit. M. J., *2*, 845, 1946 (Abscesses).
GRAUSMAN, R. I., and GOLDMAN, M. L.: Am. J. Surg., *67*, 48, 1945 (Tuberculosis).
HALPERT, B., et al.: A. M. A. Arch. Path., *4*, 313, 1948 (Plasma Cell Mastitis).
HESSELTINE, H. C., and PRIDDLE, H. D.: Am. J. Obst. & Gynec., *61*, 1370, 1951 (Puerperal Mastitis).
KILGORE, A. R., and FLEMING, R.: California Med., *77*, 190, 1952 (Abscesses).
NEWTON, M., and NEWTON, N. R.: Surg., Gynec. & Obst., *91*, 651, 1950 (Abscesses).

Physical Disturbances

ABRAMSON, P. B., and TUCKER, J. W.: Am. Surgeon, *18*, 1010, 1952 (Discharging Nipple).
ADAIR, F. E., and MUNZER, J. T.: Am. J. Surg., *74*, 117, 1947 (Fat Necrosis).
DONNELLY, B. A.: Ann. Surg., *131*, 342, 1950 (Discharge from the Nipple).
HOLLENBERG, H. G.: A. M. A. Arch. Surg., *64*, 159, 1952 (Bleeding from Nipple).
SAPHIR, O.: Am. J. Clin. Path., *20*, 1001, 1950 (Cytology Breast Secretions).

Tumors

ACKERMAN, L. V.: Am. Pract. & Digest. Treatment, *1*, 124, 1950 (Carcinoma).
ATKINS, H. J. B.: Brit. J. Surg., *38*, 147, 1950 (Fibroadenosis).
BARKER, J. M., and ALDREDGE, W. M.: South. Surgeon, *15*, 550, 1949 (Carcinoma During Pregnancy).
CHESTER, S. T., and BELL, H. G.: West. J. Surg., *59*, 603, 1951 (Papilloma).
CHRIS, S. M.: Brit. J. Surg., *38*, 163, 1950 (Inflammatory Carcinoma).
COLE, W. H., and ROSSITER, L. J.: Ann. Surg., *119*, 573, 1944 (Cystic Hyperplasia).
COPELAND, M. M.: Am. Surgeon, *18*, 992, 1952 (Cystic Hyperplasia).

DOCKERTY, M. B., and HARRINGTON, S. W.: Surg., Gynec. & Obst., *93*, 317, 1951 (Paget's Disease).

DONNELLY, B. A.: Ann. Surg., *128*, 918, 1948 (Inflammatory Carcinoma).

ESTES, A. C., and PHILLIPS, C.: Surg., Gynec. & Obst., *89*, 345, 1949 (Papilloma).

FITTS, W. T., JR., and HORN, R. C., JR.: J. A. M. A., *147*, 1429, 1951 (Occult Carcinoma).

GUTHORN, P. J.: Military Surg., *109*, 110, 1951 (Carcinoma in Males).

HAAGENSEN, C. D., *et al.:* Ann. Surg., *133*, 18, 1951 (Papillary Neoplasms).

HARRINGTON, S. W.: J. A. M. A., *148*, 1007, 1952 (Prognosis Carcinoma).

HELLER, E. L., and FLEMING, J. C.: Am. J. Clin. Path., *20*, 141, 1950 (Fibrosing Adenomatosis).

HILL, R. P., and STOUT, A. P.: A. M. A. Arch. Surg., *44*, 723, 1942 (Sarcoma).

HUGGINS, C., and DAO, T. L-Y.: J. A. M. A., *151*, 1388, 1953 (Adrenalectomy and Oophorectomy for Carcinoma).

HUNT, C. J., and KRAFT, J.: Am. J. Surg., *82*, 86, 1951 (Carcinoma in Males).

INGLIS, K.: Am. J. Path., *22*, 1, 1946 (Paget's Disease).

KLOPP, C. T., *et al.:* J. A. M. A., *150*, 856, 1952 (Diagnosis Early Cancer).

LEWISON, E. F., and CHAMBERS, R. G.: New England J. Med., *246*, 1, 1952 (Sex Hormones in Carcinoma).

MASSIE, F. M., and McCLELLAN, J. T.: South. M. J., *44*, 729, 1951 (Sarcoma).

PARK, W. W., and LEES, J. C.: Surg., Gynec. & Obst., *93*, 129, 1951 (Curability Carcinoma).

PATEY, D. H., and NURICK, A. W.: Brit. M. J., *1*, 15, 1953 (Cystic Hyperplasia).

SALTZSTEIN, H. C., and POLLACK, R. S.: J. A. M. A., *140*, 997, 1949 (Benign Tumors).

SAPHIR, O.: Surg., Gynec. & Obst., *72*, 908, 1941 (Mucinous Carcinoma).

SAPHIR, O., and PARKER, M. L.: Am. J. Path., *16*, 189, 1940 (Papilloma).

SARASON, E. L., and PRIOR, J. T.: Ann. Surg., *135*, 253, 1952 (Paget's Disease in Males).

SEGALOFF, A., *et al.:* Cancer, *5*, 1179, 1952 (Hormonal Therapy of Cancer).

SHAW, H. W.: Am. Surgeon, *18*, 1191, 1952 (Carcinoma).

SHIMKIN, M. B., *et al.:* Surg., Gynec. & Obst., *94*, 645, 1952 (Carcinoma).

SOMERVILLE, P.: Brit. J. Surg., *39*, 297, 1952 (Carcinoma in Males).

STEPHENSON, H. E., JR., *et al.:* Ann. Surg., *136*, 856, 1952 (Cytosarcoma Phylloides).

TREVES, N., and SUNDERLAND, D. A.: Cancer, *4*, 1286, 1951 (Cystosarcoma Phylloides).

WARREN, S.: Surgery, *19*, 32, 1946 (Benign Lesions).

Bones

PATHOLOGIC PHYSIOLOGY

ANTHONY F. DEPALMA

BONE is a highly specialized form of connective tissue comprising branching cells—the osteocytes, embedded in an intercellular substance—the ground substance. The most important *characteristic* of bone is its hardness which is the result of deposition within the organic matrix of a complex mineral substance composed chiefly of calcium, phosphate, and carbonate. This modification of connective tissue found in bone adapts it for the special *function* of providing a skeleton or framework for the body of most vertebrates. In addition, bone provides an encasement for the brain and for the thoracic viscera. The ground substance, in addition to being calcified, *comprises* a fibrilar structure, the fibers being mainly those of collagen. The essential material in the ground substance is mucopolysaccharide. The cellular constituents of bone comprise cells with specific function. These are (1) the osteoblasts, which are concerned with the formation of bone, (2) the osteocytes, which are concerned with the maintenance of bone as a living tissue, and (3) osteoclasts, which are primarily concerned with destruction or resorption of bone. It is generally conceded that all three of these cells have a common origin and are closely interrelated. During the process of growth, transformation of one cell to another, of the definitive morphologically different forms, is readily discernible. These transformations not only occur during the development and growth of bone but are also demonstrable in mature adult bone during certain abnormal conditions. In addition to providing a skeletal framework for the body, bone is the essential locus for the production of red and white blood cells and the repository for the storage of calcium.

That bone is not a nonviable, inorganic structure but a true, *living, specialized connective tissue* in which anabolic and catabolic processes are in constant equilibrium, cannot be overemphasized. Any disturbance in the normal physiologic processes of bone results in patho-physiologic processes which are readily discernible by the alterations that take place in the bone structure. The *normal physiologic processes* of bone may be *affected by* many factors. Some of these are (1) alterations in normal development as demonstrated by the numerous congenital anomalies of the skeleton, (2) local and general infections such as noted under the heading of inflammation in this chapter, (3) local physical and chemical disturbances such as noted under the heading of physical disturbance, (4) bone tumors, and perhaps most important, (4) generalized and systemic diseases which affect not only bone but also other tissues of the body. The osseous lesions which result from these systemic disorders are referred to as metabolic bone disorders.

Essentially, bone is *composed* of organic substances—30 per cent, inorganic substances—45 per cent, and water—25 per cent. Hardness of bone depends upon maintenance of the proportions between the organic and inorganic components. With increasing age, the water content of bone gradually diminishes and the bones become harder and more brittle. The inorganic portion of bone consists of calcium phosphate—85 per cent, magnesium phosphate—1.5 per cent, and calcium carbonate—10.5 per cent. For adult bone, the ratio of these substances is 1–6–10. According to Hari, analysis of the bone ash comprises calcium—37 per cent, magnesium—75 per cent, sodium—.7 per cent, potassium—.2 per cent, phosphorus—17.6 per cent, carbonate—.5 per cent, flouride—1.0 per cent, and chloride—1.0 per cent.

The most important factors which govern the *metabolism* of *caclium* are (1) the level of serum calcium and phosphorus, governed by the relationship between parathormone and vitamin D on the one hand and kidney function on the other and (2) absorption of calcium and phosphorus from the intestinal tract. In the *blood stream*, three calcium fractions are found: (1) *Ionized calcium*. This calcium fraction is combined with phosphorus, is active, and is ionized. It is found in the amount of 2.5 mg. per cent. (2) *Calcium phosphate*. This fraction is found in solution in the serum, it is nonionized, is active, and its level in the serum is governed by the action of the parathyroid glands. It equals 4 mg. per cent. (3) *Colloid*. This fraction is found in combination with the protein of the serum and constitutes 4 mg. per cent of the total serum calcium. It is inactive, nonionized, and nondiffusible. *Absorption* of *calcium* takes place in the upper third of the ileum. Absorption is enhanced by an acid chyme and adequate vitamin D. In the presence of an alkaline chyme and excessive phosphates, fatty acids, and carbonates, calcium is combined in the formation of soap and is lost from the intestinal tract. Also, excessive carbonates will result in the formation of calcium carbonate, hence the calcium is not absorbed by the intestinal tract. These factors have considerable bearing upon the amount of calcium which passes from the intestinal tract into the blood stream. Under normal conditions, about 10 per cent of the calcium is excreted from the lower bowel and 90 per cent is excreted from the urine. In the body as a whole, 99 per cent of the calcium is found in the skeleton and 1 per cent in the blood stream, muscles, and other tissues. Under normal conditions, there is a delicate balance between the calcium intake and the calcium output. When more calcium is absorbed than is excreted, a condition known as a *positive calcium balance* exists. This is normally found in childhood and in pregnancy. When more calcium is excreted than is absorbed, a *negative calcium balance* exists. This is commonly found during senility. Loss of calcium over a period of many years results in rarefaction of bone—a condition known as *osteoporosis*. The enzyme *phosphatase* is essential to *calcification* of bone. It breaks down phosphoric esters, liberates phosphorus ions, and, by disturbing the calcium-phosphorus balance, locally initiates participation of calcium salts. It is found in all areas in which active osteogenesis takes place and in those conditions characterized by active new bone formation. It is increased in amount, not only locally but also in the blood stream. A high phosphate content of the blood is found during the active periods of growth in von Recklinghausen's disease, in Paget's disease, and in some cases of cancer in which the process of new bone formation is profound. *Vitamin D* is essential in calcium metabolism. It promotes absorption of calcium from the intestinal tract and aids in its deposition in new bone. *Parathormone* is also essential in normal metabolism of calcium because it is concerned with the mobilization of calcium by acting on the ionizable clacium, and is thus an important factor in the maintenance of a normal calcium level in the blood. In diseases characterized by calcium deficiency, the parathyroid glands are responsible for increased calcium mobilization from the skeleton in order to maintain a normal calcium level. In certain pathologic states such as an adenoma or hyperplasia of the parathyroid glands, overactivity of this gland results in excessive mobilization of calcium from the skeleton, as demonstrated by the abnormally high calcium level of the blood.

Metabolic bone disorders may be grouped under two categories, according to Albright and Reifenstein—(1) those associated with too little calcified bone and (2) those associated with too much calcified bone. Under normal conditions, calcified bone is in a state of dynamic equilibrium whereby the net gain from the process of bone formation is equal to the net loss from the process of bone resorption. Hence, it becomes apparent that alteration of the total amount of calcified bone can be brought about in two ways—by changing the amount of bone formed or by altering the amount of bone resorbed. The formation of bone is dependent upon two processes—(1) the laying down of matrix by osteoblasts and (2) the deposition of calcium salts in matrix. For the *formation* of *matrix* normal body activity is essential because such activity stimulates osteoblasts to form this supporting substance. Hence, disuse of the body, which reduces the stress and strain of weight bearing, results in loss of the stimulus to osteoblasts and in a reduction in matrix formation. The laying down of matrix in sufficient quantities is also dependent upon adequate amounts of androgens, estrognes, protein substance, and ascorbic acid. A deficiency in any one of these substances will cause a decrease in osteoblastic activity and hence a diminution in matrix formation. Further, conversion of protein into energy is dependent upon adequate amounts of corticoid hormones. An excess of these hormones (as in Cushing's disease or syndrome) may interfere with normal matrix formation by decreasing the amount of protein present. Other disorders and factors depleting the availability of protein are hyperthyroidism, diabetes mellitus, malnutrition, avitaminosis C (scurvy), chronic corticoid therapy, and prolonged stress. The second factor concerned in the formation of bone, namely the *deposition* of *calcium*, has already been considered above. It, therefore, becomes apparent that too little bone formation may result from (1) a deficiency in the formation of matrix, (2) a deficiency in the calcification of matrix, or (3) a deficiency in both. When matrix formation is at fault, the metabolic disorder is known as *osteoporosis*. When the defect is in calcification of the matrix, the disorder is known as *osteomalacia*, or *adult rickets*. Too much resorption of bone may also produce a decrease in the amount of calcified bone. This disorder is known as *osteitis fibrosa cystica* or *von Recklinghausen's disease*. Too much calcified bone is either the result of too much bone formation or too little bone resoprtion. Too much bone formation may be the result of increased formation of bone matrix. The disorder is known as *hyperosteogenesis*. On the other hand, too much bone formation may be the result of excessive calcification of the matrix. This particular disorder does not occur clinically because the matrix cannot be supercalcified. The disorder due to too much calcified bone resulting from a defect in bone resorption is known as *osteosclerosis*.

GENERAL CONSIDERATIONS

While the bones are intimately connected with the hematopoietic system (bone marrow), joints, tendons, bursas, and skeletal muscles, this Chapter will be concerned only with disorders of osseous and cartilagenous tissues and with marrow cells exclusive of the conditions already discussed in connection with the Blood (Chapter 25, p. 926).

CONGENITAL ANOMALIES

Orientation.—Some developmental abnormalities of bones are common while others are rare. They may be readily apparent or they may be hidden but, in either case, they are generally easily discovered roentgenographically. A few of the more common conditions may be listed as follows (Mercer, Barsky, Adson, and Ross): (1) *agenesis* or *absence*—radius, ulna, humerus, forearm, tibia, fibula, femur, entire extremity, rib, clavicle, phalanx, etc., (2) *radio—ulnar synostosis*—fixation of forearm midway between pronation and supination as a result of fusion of the proximal ends of the radius and ulna, (3) *angulation* of *tibia*—consisting of unilateral or bilateral anterior bowing due to a pull by short calf muscles, (4) *pseudoarthrosis* of the *tibia*—consisting of (*a*) a gap in the midportion of the tibia, (*b*) sclerosis of the ends of the bones, and (*c*) a bridge of fibrous tissue and resulting from failure of development of a part of the bone, (5) *high scapula*—permanent elevation of the shoulder due to imperfect descent of the shoulder girdle, (6) *accessory rib*—occurring in the lumbar region and of little significance or in the cervical region and (as a result of pressure on nerves and arteries) producing (*a*) tingling and pain down the arm, (*b*) diminished cutaneous sensibility over areas supplied by the radial or ulna nerve, (*c*) weakness and wasting of the muscles of the hand, (*d*) dusky discoloration of the arm and hand, and (*e*) dull aching pain at the root of the neck, (7) *syndactylism*—(Gr. = together + digit), a binding together of two or more adjacent fingers or toes, (8) *polydactylism*—(Gr. = many + digit), duplication of phalanges of the hand or foot and usually being marginal in location, (9) *brachydactylism*—(Gr. = short + digit), shortening of the phalanges due to increase in length of the phalanges, decrease in number of phalanges, or shortening of the metacarpals, (10) *arachnodactylism*—(Gr. = spider + digit), long, thin, spider-like digits affecting the fingers and occasionally the toes, (11) *cleft* or *lobster-claw hand*—defect of the central portion of the hand with the digits divided into a radial and an ulnar group, (12) *megalodactylism* or *macrodactylism*—(Gr. = large + digit), unusual largeness or hypertrophy of the fingers or toes, (13) *short neck*—of varying degrees and consisting of a fusion of, and numerical decrease in, the cervical segments, (14) *spina bifida*—(L. = thorn + cleft), cleft of the vertebral arches with or without protrusion of the spinal cord and its meninges, (15) *scoliosis*—(Gr. = curvation), abnormal lateral curvature of the vertebral column, (16) *cranioschisis*—(Gr. = skull + fissure), congenital fissure of the cranium, (17) *craniorachischisis*—(Gr. = skull + spine + split), congenital fissure of the skull and spinal column, (18) *acephalus* or *anencephalus*—(Gr. = without + head), a headless or brainless monster, and (19) *cleidocranial dysostosis*—(Gr. = clavicle + head + bad + bone), aplasia of the clavicles, increase in transverse diameter of the cranium, and delay in closure of fontanelles. In addition to the above listed conditions, a few separate words should be said concerning achondroplasia, chondro-osteodystrophy, dyschondroplasia, hereditary multiple exostosis, osteogenesis imperfecta, osteopetrosis, gargoylism, and infantile cortical hyperostosis.

Achondroplasia.—Achondroplasia (Gr. = privation + cartilage + to form) is an inherited disturbance of bones laid down in cartilage resulting in the development of a *dwarf* (Mercer). *Pathologically* the most out-standing characteristics are (1) a great decrease in the rate and amount of cartilage proliferation at the ends of the bones thus impeding longitudinal growth of bones, (2) mucoid degeneration of cartilage cells that do form, thus further impeding longitudinal growth, and (3) normal deposition of subperiosteal bone resulting in maintenance of a normal diameter of the bones. *Clinically* the stature is stunted, the head is enlarged, the bridge of the nose is depressed, all long bones of the extremities are shortened, the hands are short and broad, the intelligence is above average, and the physical strength is greater than normal. *Roentgenographically* the epi-physes are expanded and the centers of ossification usually appear many years prematurely (Luck).

Chondro-osteodystrophy.—Chondro-osteodystrophy (Gr. = cartilage + bone + ill + to nourish) is also a type of dwarfism that differs from achon-droplasia in that the child is normal at birth and that subsequent skeletal development is at fault (Mercer). *Pathologically* the epiphyseal cartilage is increased in thickness, the articular cartilage is thicker than normal, ossification occurs from multiple foci and proceeds irregularly, and the epiphysis (as a result of pressure) becomes fragmented and distorted.

Dyschondroplasia.—Dyschondroplasia (Gr. = badly + cartilage + to form), also known as Ollier's disease, is a disorder beginning in infancy and characterized by the presence of masses of calcified or noncalcified cartilage in the metaphyses and diaphyses (Luck). When the masses are large they are responsible not only for expansion at the metaphyses (due to the tumor itself) but also for shortening of the bone and extremity (due to interference with growth). The cartilaginous masses may remain quiescent or they may gradually grow larger. The condition characteristically affects the long bones and may be unilateral or bilateral.

Hereditary Multiple Exostosis.—This condition, also known as multiple cartilaginous exostoses and diaphysial aclasis, is a congenital anomaly of skeletal development characterized by a tendency to bilateral and sym-metrical development of knobby bony protrusions, especially in the juxta-epiphyseal areas of the long bones (Jaffe and Rose). The tubular *bones* of the lower extremities are most commonly involved. When the protrusion is growing the lesion consists of a core of trabeculated bone capped by a zone of cartilage several millimeters thick. When it is no longer growing, most or all of the cartilage becomes replaced with bone. *Clinically* the condition is more common in males than in females and sooner or later is attended by deformity, discomfort, or inconvenience. The most important (but infrequent) *complication* is the development of a chondrosarcoma in one or more of the protuberances. *Treatment* is surgical excision of lesions that produce mechanical difficulty or that are suspected of being malignant.

Osteogenesis Imperfecta.—This condition, also known as *fragilitas ossium* is a congenital brittleness of bones that is accompanied by multiple frac-tures, often following slight and otherwise inconsequential trauma (Gain and Follis). The disorder is *seen* chiefly in infants but it may not be dis-covered until a later age, is as frequent in females as in males, and is often associated with blue scleras. The characteristic *changes* are found in the long *bones*. They consist of a thin cortex, thin periosteum, enlarged marrow space, soft shaft, degeneration of epiphysis, wide haversian canals, lack of bony lamella, and replacement of osteoblasts with fibroblasts, chondro-blasts, and transitional cells. *Roentgenograms* reveal thinning of the cortex, enlargement of the marrow cavity, osteoporosis, and angulations or bowings of the shaft.

Osteopetrosis.—Osteopetrosis (Gr. = bone + L. = stone), known also as *marble bones* and *Albers-Schönberg* disease, is a congenital disease affecting any or all of the bones of the body and characterized by a thick cortex, and encroachment upon or replacement of the marrow with medullary bone (Allman and Zawisch). The affected bones become hard, brittle, and chalk-like. The condition *occurs* with equal frequency in both sexes and is discovered at all ages. It is manifested *clinically* by (1) fractures after trivial trauma, (2) delayed dentition and dental caries, (3) severe anemia (from replacement of the marrow) associated with hepatosplenomegaly and lymphadenopathy, (4) optic atrophy, visual disturbances, deafness, and paralysis of muscles supplied by cranial nerves (due to narrowing of the cranial foramens), and (5) hydrocephalus in children. *Roentgenograms* reveal a marked increase in density of the bones, broadening of the cortex, and narrowing of the medulla.

Gargoylism.—The term gargoyle (L. = gullet) means a water spout often carved grotesquely. Medically, the term *gargoylism* connotes a congenital disorder consisting of chondrodystrophic changes in the skeleton and deposition of lipids in most tissues of the body, especially the brain (Cole and Henderson). The condition is also known as lipochondrodystrophy. It appears to be a combination of Niemann-Pick's disease (p. 915) and chondro-osteodystrophy (p. 1228). More specifically, it is *characterized* by dwarfism (especially with shortening of the trunk and neck), enlargement and distortion of the skull, depression of the bridge of the nose, coarse facies, stiffness of the joints, hump-back, hepatic and splenic enlargement with protrusion of the abdomen, cloudiness of the corneas, and mental abnormality.

Infantile Cortical Hyperostosis.—This condition consists of a hyperplasia of the cortex or periosteum of the tubular bones of the extremities, scapula, calvarium, ilium, ribs, and mandible (Bush). It is usually discovered by the third postnatal month. The cause is unknown. In addition to the bony changes, some patients also disclose pleurisy and fever. Laboratory studies reveal anemia, leukocytosis, increase in lymphocytes or neutrophils, elevated alkaline phosphatase in the serum, and increased sedimentation rate. The disorder is self-limited, with complete recovery usually ensuing within twelve months.

DEGENERATIONS

Orientation.—Degenerative disturbances in bone and cartilage are common associates of most skeletal disease processes. In addition, however, there are certain conditions that are wholly or almost wholly of a retrogressive nature. Some of these are (1) *lipoid storage diseases* (p. 913), (2) *ricketts* (p. 98), (3) *scurvy* (p. 96), (4) *myelofibrosis* and *osteosclerosis*, (5) *osteoporosis*, (6) *aseptic osseous necrosis*, (7) *chondromalacia* of the *patella*, and (8) *ainhum*. Some of these, as indicated, have already been considered, leaving the others to be discussed briefly in the order mentioned.

Myelofibrosis and Osteosclerosis.—This disorder, as the terms indicate, consists of a replacement of the bone marrow by fibrous tissue and/or endosteal bone (Erf and Cocchi). The condition may be focal or generalized and may be primary or secondary. *Primary* myelofibrosis and osteosclerosis is also called idiopathic for the cause remains unknown, while the *secondary* form of the disease usually develops consequent to replacement of the marrow by tumor cells or destruction of the marrow by chemicals. Of the two forms of the disorder, the *primary* or *idiopathic* type is the more spectacular. Because of the replacement of the bone marrow, extramedullary foci of hematopoiesis develop in the spleen, liver, and lymph nodes and these organs thus become progressively enlarged. In addition, the following are noted: (1) myeloid reaction in the blood consisting of erythroblasts, myeloblasts, and myelocytes, (2) progressive anemia, (3) moderate leukopenia, (4) weakness, (5) dyspnea, (6) intermittent bone and joint pains, (7) hemorrhagic diathesis (sometimes), and (8) increased density of the bones roentgenographically. The condition *occurs* more commonly in

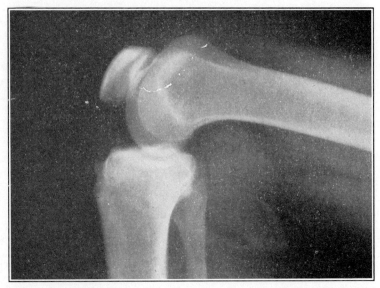

Fig. 611.—Aseptic necrosis of the tibial tuberosity showing irregular erosion in a lateral view of the bone.

men than in women, is usually found after the age of thirty years, is refractive to treatment, and terminates fatally on an average of five years. Because of the hematologic sequelæ, the condition has also been called *megakaryocytic myelosis* or *leukemia* and *leukoerythroblastic anemia*.

Osteoporosis.—The term *osteoporosis* (Gr. = bone + passage) signifies an abnormal porousness or rarefaction of bone brought about by diminished osteoblastic or increased osteoclastic activity and characterized by reduction in thickness of the cortex, thinning and disappearance of cancellous trabeculæ, widening of the marrow cavity, and (accordingly) increased fragility of bones. The condition is *seen in conjunction with* the following: disuse (bedfast), protein deficiency (malnutrition), basophilism (Cushing's syndrome), hyperthyroidism, postmenopausal syndrome, acromegaly, "alarm reaction" of Selye, osteogenesis imperfecta, chemical ingestion (strontium and magnesium), senility, and vitamin C deficiency (Luck).

Aseptic Osseous Necrosis.—This term indicates degeneration and necrosis of epiphyses, small bones, and articular osseocartilaginous tissues unattended by infection. *Pathologically* the process may be divided into three stages—(1) *early*—consisting of obliteration of vessels, necrosis of

osteoblasts, hyperemia and porosis of adjacent tissues, and influx of phagocytes to remove the dead tissue, (2) *regenerative*—consisting of an invasion
of capillaries, fibroblasts, osteoclasts, and osteoblasts and by gradual replacement of the dead tissue with osteoid tissue, and (3) *healed*—consisting
of regenerated bone but also of deformities that have resulted from stresses
and strains acting before ossification was complete (Luck). *Roentgenographically* the changes consist of decreased areas of density when the
process is active and of irregular areas of increased density when the process
is healed (Fig. 611). Depending upon the bone involved and the author
who first described the lesion, aseptic osseous necrosis has been *classified*
as follows: (1) tibial tubercle—*Osgood-Schlatter's*, (2) primary epiphysis
patella or tarsal navicular—*Kohler's*, (3) head of femur—*Legg-Perthe's*, (4)
os calcis—*Sever's*, (5) semilunar—*Kienback's*, (6) head second metatarsal—
Freiberg's, (7) secondary epiphysis patella—*Sinding-Larsen's*, (8) secondary
epiphyses vertebral bodies—*Scheurmann's*, (9) primary epiphysis vertebral
bodies—*Calve's*, and (10) head of humerus—*Lewin's* disease.

Chondromalacia of the Patella.—This condition represents softening and
fibrillary degeneration of the cartilaginous undercovering of the patella
(Carr). The disorder usually occurs in adults (of any age) and generally
follows trauma (Bronitsky). It is attended by pain and swelling and is best
treated by patellectomy.

Ainhum.—*Ainhum* or *dactylosis spontanea* is a chronic, slowly progressive
disease of unknown etiology, occurring in dark-skinned races (especially
the African Negro), characterized by annular constriction of the toes at
the digitoplantar level (especially the little toes), and proceeding in time to
spontaneous amputation of the digits (Jacobs).

INFLAMMATION

Orientation.—Inflammation of bone is known as *osteitis*, of bone marrow
as *myelitis*, of bone and bone marrow as *osteomyelitis*, of periosteum as
periostitis, of endosteum as *endostitis*, of cartilage as *chondritis*, of perichondrium as *perichondritis*, of epiphyses as *epiphysitis*, of metaphyses as
metaphysitis, and of diaphysis as *diaphysitis*. The more important inflammations may be listed as follows: hematogenous osteomyelitis, Brodie's
abscess, exogenous osteomyelitis, tuberculosis, syphilis, Boeck's sarcoid
(p. 501), brucellosis (p. 921), granuloma inguinale (p. 1112), leprosy (p. 415),
actinomycosis (p. 515), blastomycosis (p. 514), coccidioidomycosis (p.
514), and echinococcosis (p. 828). The first five of the conditions enumerated may now be considered in the order listed.

Hematogenous Osteomyelitis.—Hematogenous osteomyelitis connotes
inflammation of bone marrow and bone contracted by the hematogenous
route. The most common organism is the *Staphylococcus aureus* but other
bacteria such as streptococci, pneumococci, typhoid bacilli, influenza
bacilli, etc., may, on occasion, act as causative agents (Altemeier, Blanche,
and Jackson). A focus of infection in the skin (furuncle), tonsils, middle
ear, lungs, urinary tract, etc., is present in about one-third of the cases and
a history of trauma to the bone is elicited in from one-third to one-half
of the cases (White). The condition usually *occurs* in infants and children
who are active and robust but it may occasionally also be found in older
people (Dickson and Wear).

Pathologically any bone of the body may be affected (White) including the
spine (Wear) and small bones of the hands and feet but most infections are

found in the femur, tibia, and humerus (Blanche). The initial point of localization of the organisms is in the metaphysis of long bones. As the organisms multiply, they form a small abscess which presses upon the adjacent bone and extends into ramifying lacunæ. This results in necrosis of the osseous tissue and enlargement of the abscess. Ultimately the pus may extend into the medullary cavity, break through the cortex to the subperiosteum, or (less commonly) extend through the epiphysis into the joint cavity. In the medullary cavity and subperiosteum, the pus may trek for varying distances and then, at one or more points, re-enter the cortical bone or, from the subperiosteal space, it may break through the periosteum into the soft tissues or even onto the skin. As the lesion extends and a greater or lesser portion of bone becomes deprived from its blood supply, it dies and the dead bone is then known as a *sequestrum* (L. = to give up) (Fig. 612*A*). Concomitantly osteoblasts adjacent to the necrotic bone form new bone which invests the sequestrum resulting in the formation of an *involucrum* (L. = in + to wrap). In addition, new bone is ultimately formed throughout the affected area resulting in extensive dense sclerosis. *Histologically* two processes are apparent—destructive and reparative (Fig. 612*C*). The destructive process consists of vascular thrombosis, hyperemia, edema, leukocytic (neutrophilic in the acute stage and plasma cell and lymphocytic in the chronic stage) infiltration, and necrosis with osteoclastic activity. The reparative process consists of proliferation of fibroblasts and osteoblasts with the formation of fibrous, osteoid, and osseous tissue.

The *complications* of hematogenous osteomyelitis are (1) local extension with destruction of massive amounts of bone, sinus tract formation, and extension into adjacent joint cavities, (2) hematogenous dissemination of infection producing septicemia, endocarditis, and pyemic abscesses, (3) amyloidosis, and (4) formation of a malignant tumor (fibrosarcoma or carcinoma) in a draining sinus of years' duration (Wough and Devas). General *clinical manifestations*, consisting of a sudden onset of chills, fever, and leukocytosis, are due to septicemia and absorption of toxic products, while local manifestations, consisting of pain, tenderness, and swelling, are due to the infection as such affecting the periosteum. *Roentgenograms* disclose areas of rarefaction in the affected bone only after necrosis and destruction have occurred (Fig. 612*B*). Initially they are normal. The *diagnosis* is made from the history, clinical manifestations, culturing the causative organism from the bloodstream in the initial stages of the infection, and roentgenograms. *Treatment* consists of antibiotic therapy and, only if this fails, of surgical drainage. The *prognosis* is good. Most infections respond rapidly and completely to antibiotics. Thus, the complications listed above are now infrequently encountered.

Brodie's Abscess.—Brodie's abscess is in reality a hematogenous osteomyelitis that has become rapidly and effectively walled off (Luck). Thus, the process is usually caused by the *Staphylococcus aureus*—but a strain of such low virulence that the infection does not spread. Furthermore, as time goes on the organisms die off and the abscess becomes sterile. The infection occurs in the metaphysis and consists of a round or oval area of pus surrounded by dense sclerotic bone.

Exogenous Osteomyelitis.—Exogenous osteomyelitis, also known as chronic traumatic osteomyelitis, is a chronic infection of bone consequent to entrance of organisms from the outside. The condition *follows* a compound fracture or some form of external trauma and is thus common in

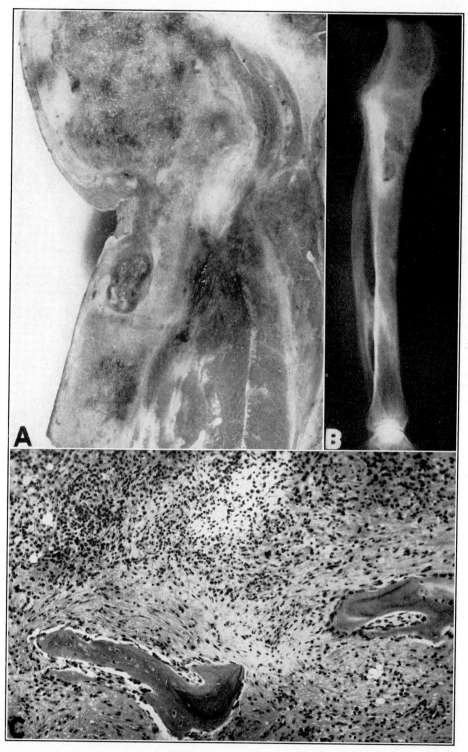

Fig. 612.—Hematogenous osteomyelitis illustrating *A*, a longitudinal section through a tibia with a sequestrum and with dense sclerosis of adjacent bone, *B*, a roentgenogram of the same tibia, and *C*, fibrosis and leukocytic infiltration from an affected area. × 100.

78

warfare (Smith and Fischer). In either case, the tissues covering the bone are lacerated and the bone is exposed directly to the exterior. Although many *organisms* may be the offending agents, the most common are proteus, pyocaneus, colon, and Friedländer's bacilli. The *pathologic* changes are similar to those seen in hematogenous osteomyelitis with the exception that the bone is usually damaged more extensively and that foreign material (pieces of clothing, dirt, shell fragments, etc.) is usually present. A special type of exogenous osteomyelitis is what has been termed *osteitis pubis*. It consists of a chronic inflammation of the anterior pelvic girdle and is seen following suprapubic or retropubic prostatectomy (Lavalle).

Tuberculosis.—Osseous tuberculosis is usually *caused* by tubercle bacilli of the human variety and only occasionally by organisms of the bovine type (Mercer). The condition is always *secondary* to tuberculosis in some other portion of the body (usually lungs or mediastinal lymph nodes), is generally contracted hematogenously and only rarely by direct extension, and is often preceded by a history of trauma. It affects both sexes with about equal frequency and while it usually *occurs* in children it may, on occasion, also occur in adults. *Pathologically* any of the bones of the body may be affected with the more common sites being skull, hands, feet, vertebræ, rib, tibia, ulna, femur, and humerus. The initial lesion may affect any portion of the bone although in long bones it is the metaphysis that is most commonly involved, in flat bones as the ribs—the periosteum, and in the phalanges—the diaphysis. As elsewhere in the body, the fundamental unit is the tubercle which increases in size, coalesces with adjacent tubercles, and elicits either a caseation and liquefying reaction or a fibrosing and proliferative process. Caseation and liquefaction bring about destruction and excavation while fibrosis and osseous proliferation bring about enlargement and sclerosis. According to which of these predominates, and in what proportion it predominates, the osseous lesions are generally divided into the following four varieties: encysted, infiltrating, atrophic, and hypertrophic (Fig. 613). The chief *complication* of osseous tuberculosis is extension of the process into a joint or through the periosteum into the soft tissues. Once it reaches such tissues, tuberculous pus accumulates locally (*cold abscess*) or treks along fascial planes for varied distances from the original site. Rupture of a cold abscess through the skin results in the formation of a draining sinus. The *clinical manifestations* consist of swelling, pain, and wasting of muscles. The *roentgenographic* changes correspond to those seen grossly. The *diagnosis* is made from the history, physical examination, and roentgenographic appearance. *Treatment* consists of general antituberculosis measures, antibiotic therapy, rest with immobilization, or operative interference (Ghormley and Allred). The *prognosis* in general is fair to good.

Syphilis.—Syphilis of bones may be congenital or acquired (Luck). *Congenital* syphilis is that which is contracted during intra-uterine life and is manifested at or shortly after birth or during childhood. It may be divided into three types—osteochondritis, osteomyelitis, and periostitis (Hill). *Osteochondritis* occurs principally in long bones at the junction of the metaphysis with the epiphysis. It consists of an irregular zone of calcification with an arrest of osteoblastic activity. The columns of cartilage cells are thinned and separated or destroyed by tissue composed of fibroblasts, capillaries, plasma cells, and lymphocytes with or without foci of necrosis (Fig. 614). When the process is severe the provisional zone of calcification may actually be split by the syphilitic granulations and may produce dislocation or slipping of the epiphysis. *Osteomyelitis* consists of one focus or several foci of destruction of bone marrow and bone by syphilitic granulation tissue or miliary gummas. The lesions are frequently located at the junction of the metaphysis and diaphysis but may be found in any portion of any bone. *Periostitis* involves any of the bones, especially the metaphysis and diaphysis of long bones such as the tibia and fibula. It consists first of an elevation of the periosteum by syphilitic granulation tissue and then a radial and longitudinal deposition of osseous tissue by stimulated osteoblasts. The changes are seen roentgenographically as a diffuse in-

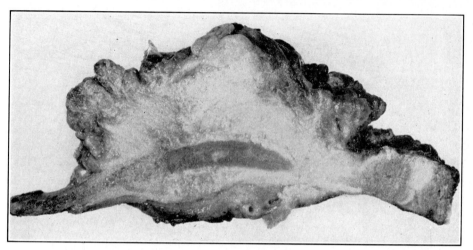

FIG. 613.—Tuberculosis of a rib, disclosing a hypertrophic type of lesion.

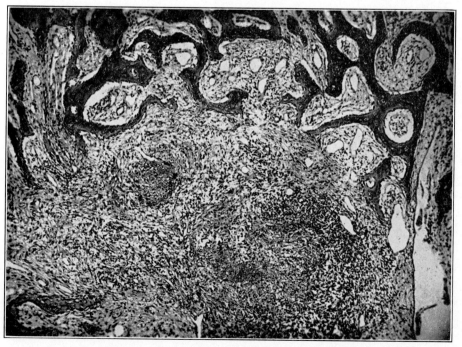

FIG. 614.—Syphilitic osteochondritis showing granulation tissue permeating and destroying the metaphyseal epiphyseal junction. × 50.

crease in density and thickness of the periosteum. Excessive thickening and osseous deposition of the tibia is prone to produce a deformity of the anterior and antero-medial aspects of the tibia that is referred to as *saber shin* (Fig. 615). *Acquired syphilis* is syphilis contracted in extra-uterine life. The lesions consist of *periostitis* and *osteomyelitis*. Each of these affects not only the long bones but also the skull and each is essentially similar to the corresponding lesion seen in infants and children.

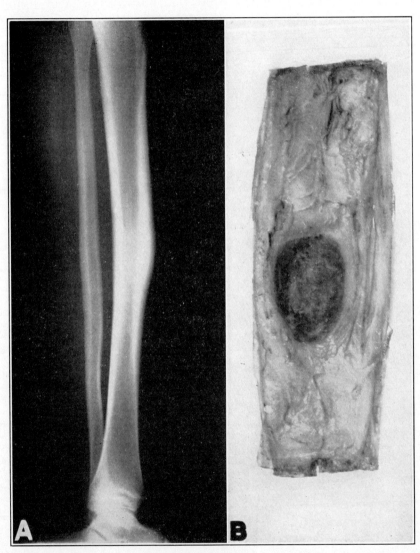

Fig. 615.—Syphilitic periostitis illustrating *A*, diffuse thickening and increase in density of the periosteum covering the tibia and fibula and *B*, the thickened periosteum from the tibia of the same case.

PHYSICAL DISTURBANCES

Orientation.—In this section the following unrelated conditions may be briefly considered: fracture, Milkman's syndrome, infarction, irradiation changes, and hypertrophic osteoarthropathy.

Fracture.—A fracture (L. = to break) may be defined as a break in continuity of a bone. It *occurs* at all ages (even during intra-uterine life) and, of course, affects both sexes and all races. The *cause* of a fracture is direct or indirect trauma. The former is brought about by a blow or a fall while the latter usually develops as a result of sudden muscular exertion. In either case, the bone may be entirely healthy before the injury or it may be previously weakened by infection, osteoporosis, tumor, or some other disease.

Fractures are *classified* according to (1) *time* in relation to birth and age as intra-uterine, extra-uterine, or senile, (2) *pre-existing pathologic process* as agenetic (imperfect formation), atrophic (atrophy of bone), dyscrasic (debilitating disease), endocrine, inflammatory, neoplastic, etc., (3) *causative agent* as automobile, march (bones of feet in soldiers carrying heavy packs), boxer's (first metacarpal), gunshot, paratrooper (jump), propeller, etc., (4) *type of injury* as direct (at point of injury), indirect (at some distance from point of injury or occurring by way of muscular contraction), or compression, (5) *bone affected* as tibial, fibular, etc., (6) *part of bone involved* as articular, intra-articular, condylar, extracapsular, intracapsular, intraperiosteal, etc., (7) *man first describing* the *lesion* as Colles' (distal end of radius), Bennett's (longitudinal of first metacarpal), Pott's (lower end of fibula), etc., and (8) *defect produced* as bending, butterfly, buttonhole (rounded perforation), closed (overlying tissue intact), comminuted (splintered), complete (entire diameter of bone), compound or open (external wound leading to a break), complicated (injury to adjacent tissue), greenstick (one side broken but the other side intact), impacted (one end driven into the other), linear, longitudinal, transverse, oblique, partial, spiral, silver fork (lower end of radius producing deformity like that of a silver fork), etc.

Pathologically the first thing that happens after a bone has been broken is hemorrhage from ruptured capillaries and larger vessels (Urist and Luck). Both the trauma and the extravasated blood induce a sterile inflammation at the junction of the injured and normal tissue so that, in from four to eight hours, the gap between the broken ends is filled with blood, fibrin, debris, and leukocytes. Within twenty-four hours, newly proliferated capillaries and fibroblasts begin to invade and organize the hematoma. Some of the fibroblasts remain as connective tissue cells but others form fibrocartilage and hyaline cartilage (Fig. 616). The newly formed mass, as a whole, is referred to as the *fibrocartilaginous callus* or *procallus*. Concomitantly new bone formation begins in the periosteum and endosteum near the line of fracture. Gradually it grows into and replaces the procallus resulting in increasing *ossification* and complete healing in from three to four weeks.

The *complications* of fracture are fat embolism (p. 221), osteomyelitis (especially when compound), and delayed or nonunion. Some of the causes of *improper union* are inadequate immobilization, distraction of fragments, displacement of fragments, changes in traction, infection, impairment of circulation, defective hematoma, and systemic diseases (Luck). The *clinical manifestations* are due to disruption of continuity, bleeding, and irritation of the sensitive periosteum. They consist of loss of normal function, deformity, swelling, and pain. *Roentgenograms* disclose the nature, location, and extent of the injury. The *diagnosis* of fracture is made from the history, clinical manifestations, and roentgenograms. *Treatment* consists essentially of re-alignment of the broken segments and immobilization of

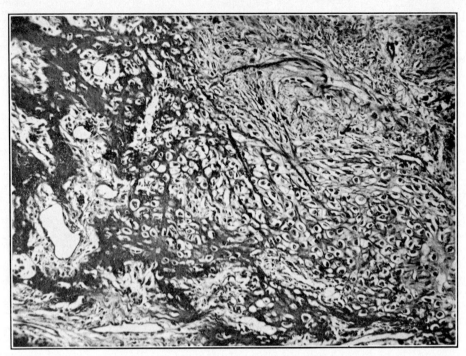

FIG. 616.—Healing fracture revealing fibrocartilage
being replaced with bony trabeculæ. × 100.

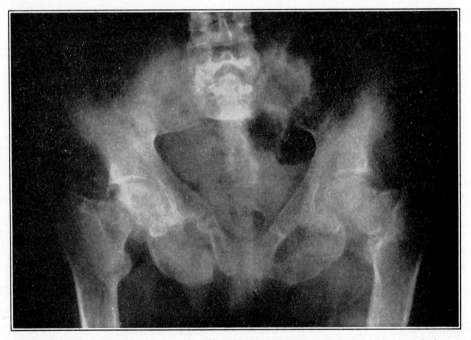

FIG. 617.—Milkman's syndrome disclosing multiple symmetrical fractures of the pelvic bones.

the bone for at least three to four weeks. The *prognosis* depends upon the age of the patient, the bone affected, the type of fracture, the presence or absence of previous osseous disease, the presence or absence of infection, etc. In general, however, it may be stated that the outlook is good to excellent.

Milkman's Syndrome.—This condition, also known as *multiple spontaneous idiopathic symmetrical fractures*, consists of the radiologic appearance of multiple, often symmetrical bands or zones in various bones (Fig. 617) that are interpreted as representing fractures (Edeiken). The process is accompanied by pain, disturbances of gait, and sometimes complete disability with bedfastness. The syndrome generally occurs in middle-aged women. The cause is unknown.

Infarction.—Osseous infarcts are usually *seen* in caisson disease (p. 222) and are thus more common in men, but sometimes they may be due to arteriosclerotic or other occlusion of the nutrient artery in which case they have no predilection for either sex (Kahlstrom). They generally *affect* long bones and may be single or multiple. When they arise in the head of a bone (humerus or femur) they ultimately bring about collapse of the bone, organization of dead tissue, and deforming arthritis. When they occur in the shaft of a bone they are replaced partly with new bone and partly with calcified material. *Roentgenographically* they are represented by dense blotchy shadows. *Clinically*, infarcts occurring in shafts are usually asymptomatic while those located at the ends of bones are asymptomatic only until collapse and arthritis supervene at which time they are attended by pain and limitation of motion.

Irradiation Changes.—Irradiation of bone may bring about leukemia, malignant tumors of bones, or osteoradionecrosis (DeYoung and Lawrence). Of these, *osteoradionecrosis* is the most frequent. It may be *defined* simply as a pathologic process (following heavy irradiation) characterized by pain, sequestration of bone, and permanent deformity. Its *incidence* is recorded in as high as 12 per cent of bones irradiated. Aside from the irradiation as such, added *causative* factors are infection and trauma. *Pathologically* any bone may be affected, but the mandible is especially vulnerable in patients treated for carcinoma of the mouth. As in other tissues of the body, damage occurs by direct action of the rays on the osseous cells and by indirect action through an obliterative endarteritis. The retrogressive changes consist of gradual irregular enlargement of the spaces about the bone cells, death of bone cells, formation of abnormal spaces between lamellæ, absorption and partial loss of calcium, complete necrosis of lesser or greater amounts of bone with sequestrum formation, and a foreign body giant cell reaction about fragments of dead bone. Osteoblasts are even more sensitive, are readily destroyed, and thus are incapable of replacing the necrotic bone with new osseous tissue or of forming an involucrum about the sequestrum. The *diagnosis* is made from the history and roentgenograms. The condition is *treated* conservatively, with removal of the sequestrum only after it has *completely* separated. The *prognosis* is guarded for the course is protracted and permanent damage frequently results.

Hypertrophic Osteoarthropathy.—Hypertrophic osteoarthropathy may be defined as clubbing of the fingers and/or toes (Mendlowitz). The condition is consequent to an increase in blood flow per unit of tissue brought about chiefly by increased digital arterial pressure. It consists of hypertrophy and hyperplasia of both the osseous tissue and the covering soft tissues, although the original bone also shows osteoclastic resorption. The disorder may be unilateral and unidigital but more commonly it is bilateral, multidigital, and symmetrical. The former cases occur congenitally or following some local disturbance of circulation while the latter cases are usually consequent to chronic pulmonary or cardiac disease.

TUMORS

Orientation.—Tumors and tumor-like conditions of bone constitute one of the most important and, at the same time, most fascinating fields of oncology. On a whole, they have no racial *susceptibility* but they do disclose certain age and sex predispositions (as indicated in succeeding paragraphs). The *cause* of bone tumors for the most part remains an enigma, although such factors as irradiation, irritation, and trauma are considered to be of predisposing importance in some instances. While *pathologic classifications* are numerous, a division of the growths according to their histogenesis is the most acceptable. Accordingly, the lesions may be tabulated as follows: osteoma, osteoid osteoma, infantile cortical hyperostosis (p. 1229), hereditary multiple exostosis (p. 1228), osteosarcoma, chondroma, benign chondroblastoma, chondromyxoid fibroma, chondrosarcoma, chordoma, fibroma, giant cell tumor, fibrosarcoma, hemangioma, hemangiopericytoma (p. 402), hemangioendothelioma (p. 399), myeloma, Ewing's tumor, lymphoblastoma (pp. 953 and 984), liposarcoma, neurofibroma, neurofibrosarcoma, adamantinoblastoma, unicameral bone cyst, aneurysmal bone cyst, osteitis fibrosa cystica, fibrous dsyplasia, osteitis deformans, and secondary tumors. The chief *complications* consist of (1) deformity from bulkiness of the tumor, (2) weakening of the bone with pathologic fracture, (3) anemia from replacement of the bone marrow with tumor, (4) malignant transformation in cases of benign tumor, and (5) metastasis in cases of malignant tumors. The *clinical manifestations* are due to the tumor as such and to the complications which occur. Among other things, they consist of pain (when the periosteum is affected), deformity, and disturbances in locomotion. The *diagnosis* is made from the history, physical examination, roentgenograms, and (open or aspiration) biopsy. The *treatment* varies with the type of lesion but consists essentially of local excision (benign tumors), radical excision or amputation (malignant tumors), or irradiation (malignant tumors). The *prognosis* varies with the type of growth and adequacy of therapy. Aside from the general considerations just concluded, a few additional remarks are merited concerning the more common conditions. In the ensuing paragraphs, benign lesions will be considered first.

Osteoma.—An *osteoma* is a benign tumor composed of adult-appearing cancellous or compact bone. The growth usually develops in membranous bones and is thus most common in the skull or bones of the face (Luck and Dowling). The tumor (1) has a broad base, (2) projects into the sinuses, base of skull, or externally, and (3) is characterized by an increased density roentgenographically. A *parosteal osteoma* is an unusual tumor that is most frequently seen in adults between twenty and forty years of age, that is most common in the upper end of the humerus and lower end of the femur, that consists of a mass of densely calcified bone lying outside the original bone but closely applied to it, and that has a tendency to become malignant (Geschickter). The most common tumor in the group of osteomas consists of adult-appearing cartilaginous and osseous elements and termed an *osteochondroma* (Luck). While this tumor is often composed of a core of osseous tissue capped by hyaline cartilage and a fibrous capsule, sometimes it consists of an irregular mixture of these elements (Fig. 618). The lesion occurs in any metaphysis but is most common in the lower end of the femur, upper end of the tibia, upper end of the femur, humerus, lower end of the tibia, pelvis, and vertebræ.

Osteoid Osteoma.—An osteoid osteoma is a benign tumor that (1) is located in the tibia, femur, feet, hands, vertebræ and other bones (Fig. 619), (2) usually measures not more than 1 cm. in diameter, (3) consists of a round or oval nidus composed of osteoid tissue and newly formed trabec-

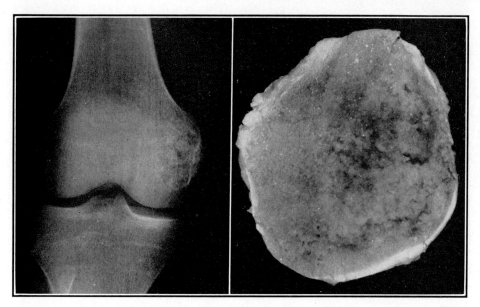

FIG. 618.—Osteochondroma of the lower end of the femur showing both the roentgen appearance and the excised tumor.

ulæ enmeshed in connective tissue and often evoking a peripheral rim of reactive sclerosis, (4) occurs in adolescents and young adults, (5) predominates in males, (6) is attended by pain that is not relieved by aspirin, (7) roentgenographically produces a central area of decreased density surrounded by a peripheral rim of increased density, and (8) responds well to complete surgical excision (Lichtenstein, Pines, and Dockerty).

Chondroma.—Chondromas are benign tumors *composed* both grossly and microscopically of relatively normal-appearing cartilage that is, however, abnormally arranged (Fig. 620). They are usually solitary and generally affect the phalanges, metacarpals, metatarsals, ribs, sternum, and vertebræ and, less commonly, the long bones (Luck and Coley). While they may be peripheral in location they are generally found in the central portion of the bone and hence are called *enchondromas*. The peak *incidence* is in the third decade of life and both sexes are equally affected. *Clinically* they are often symptomless although in time they are accompanied by deformity, pain, and pathologic fracture. *Radiologically* they appear as circumscribed areas of translucency. *Treatment* consists of complete surgical removal. The *prognosis* is good, although a malignant transformation is not rare.

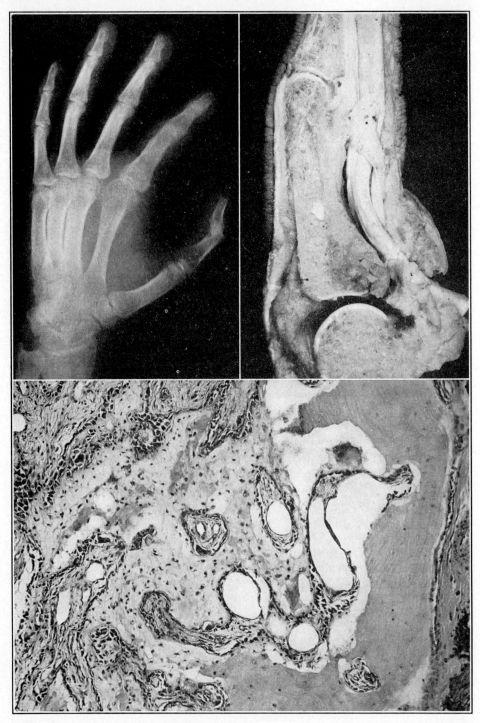

Fig. 619.—Osteoid osteoma disclosing a roentgenographic defect at the base of the proximal phalanx of the index finger, the tumor in the removed specimen, and the histologic appearance of a nidus of osteoid tissue supported by a connective tissue stroma and covered by sclerotic bone. × 100.

Benign Chondroblastoma.—This benign cartilaginous tumor was formerly considered a variant of a benign giant cell tumor (Lichtenstein and France). The lesion usually *occurs* in males in the second decade of life. It is generally single and located in the epiphysis of the femur, tibia, and humerus. *Grossly* the tumor is sharply circumscribed, partially destroys the epiphyseal cartilage, and consists of gray to brown tissue containing areas of calcification, cyst formation, and hemorrhage. *Histologically* it consists of (1) compact rounded cells of moderate sizes and containing a

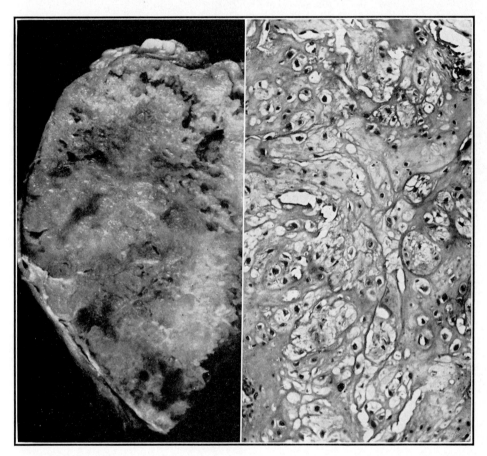

Fig. 620.—Chondroma illustrating a tumor mass composed of translucent gray lobulated substance and varisized cartilage cells irregularly arranged. × 100.

round nucleus (primitive cartilage cells), (2) focal areas of calcification, (3) scattered giant cells, (4) areas of fibrous tissue replacement, and (5) foci of degeneration and necrosis (Fig. 621). The chief *complaints* are swelling, pain, tenderness, and disturbance of locomotion. *Roentgenograms* disclose a fuzzy translucent focus encircled by well-defined, often sclerotic bone. *Treatment* consists of local excision. The *prognosis* is uniformly good.

Chondromyxoid Fibroma.—This condition is frequently mistaken for enchondroma, chondrosarcoma, or benign chondroblastoma (Lichtenstein). The lesion *occurs* most commonly in the second decade of life but is also seen in adults and it has no sex predilection. The *bones* most commonly involved are those of the lower extremities, especially the tibia, femur, and meta-tarsals. Unlike benign chondroblastoma the tumor is not related to the epiphysis. *Grossly* it is fairly sharply circumscribed, gray, rubbery, and resembles cartilage (Fig. 622). *Histologically* it is composed of spindle cells embedded in a myxomatous, cartilaginous, or collagenous matrix. Giant cells are not infrequent and foci of calcification and ossification may be noted. *Roentgenographically* the tumor is eccentric in position, is for the most part translucent, and is demarcated internally by a zone of sclerotic bone. The other features are similar to those in benign chondroblastoma.

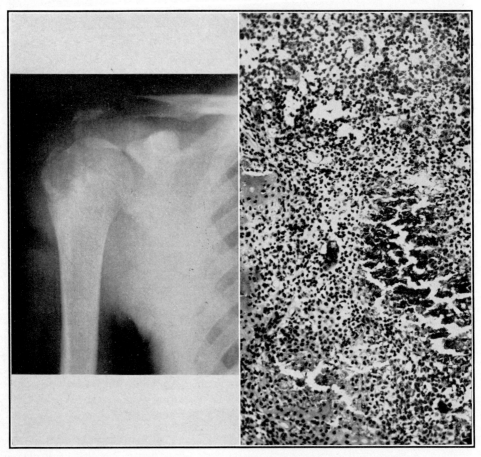

Fig. 621.—Benign chondroblastoma showing an osteolytic lesion in the humerus roentgeno-graphically and rounded (primitive cartilage) cells, giant cells, and focal necrosis and calcification microscopically. × 100. (Slide submitted by Dr. W. C. Herrick.)

Chordoma.—A chordoma is a rare tumor that arises in remnants of the primitive notochord (Dahlin). It *occurs* at all ages but prevails in the latter part of the fifth decade and it affects males more often than females. The growth is most common in the sacrococcygeal region, less common in the spheno-occipital area, and infrequent in the cervical, lumbar, and thoracic regions. *Grossly* it consists of a fairly well-encapsulated, lobulated mass of translucent, mucoid tissue and may measure up to 20 cm. in diameter (Fig. 623). *Histologically* it is composed of varisized, rounded or polyhedral,

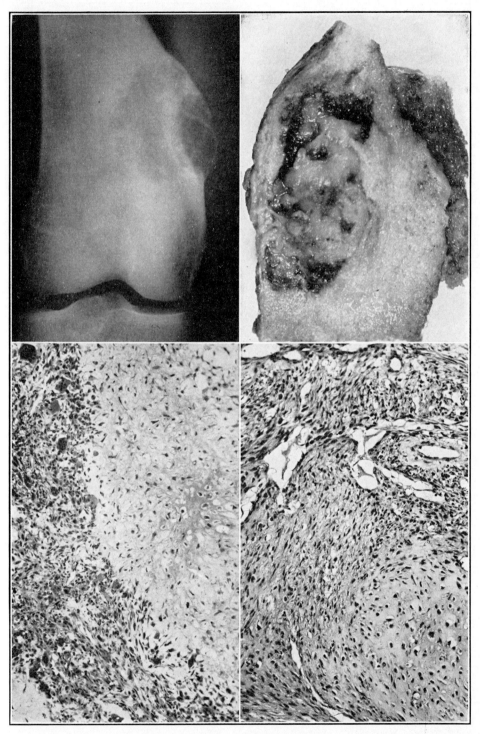

FIG. 622.—Chondromyxoid fibroma demonstrating a translucent area surrounded by sclerotic bone roentgenographically, the myxomatous appearance of the tumor grossly, and spindle cells embedded in a hyaline and myxomatous stroma microscopically. × 100.

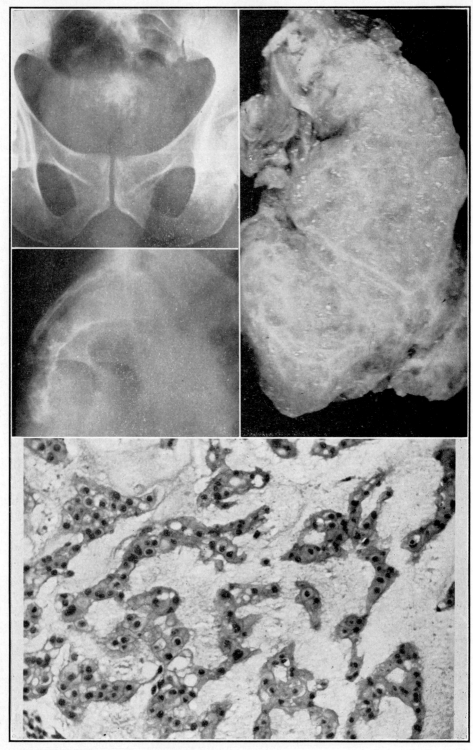

FIG. 623—Chordoma showing a soft tissue mass (with an area of calcification) and erosion of the coccyx and sacrum roentgenographically, the surgically removed mucoid mass, and well-defined polyhedral cells containing droplets of mucus and embedded in a mucoid matrix. × 200.

plant-like cells with distinct margins, rounded nuclei, and droplets of mucus within the cytoplasm. The matrix consists of mucoid material (Congdon). The *clinical manifestations* vary with the location of the tumor. They consist essentially of pain and pressure symptoms. Except for intracranial growths, the masses are often readily palpable. *Roentgenograms* disclose varying degrees of bony destruction by a translucent mass which may or may not show areas of calcification. The only effective *treatment* is wide excision. The *prognosis* is guarded for the lesion tends to recur and may become frankly malignant.

Fibroma.—Fibroma of bone may be ossifying or nonossifying. *Ossifying fibroma* is simply a fibroma that contains areas of ossification. The lesion is benign and is noted most commonly in the maxilla (p. 426) but is also seen in the mandible, other flat bones, vertebræ, and bones of the limbs (Lichtenstein and Smith). *Nonossifying fibroma* is a fibroma of bone that is devoid of osseous tissue. The tumor is usually seen in the shaft of a long bone (often of the lower extremity) and is located near an epiphysis. Pathologically it is eccentric in position, erodes the bone completely, is grayish white, and consists of spindle cells in whorl formation.

Giant Cell Tumor.—A benign giant cell tumor of bone is also known as *osteoclastoma* (Stewart, Windeyer, Willis, and Lichtenstein). It is a rather rare tumor that has, in the past, been confused with most of the other fibrous tumors of bones. The lesion usually *occurs* after the age of twenty years and has no predilection for either sex. The *bones* most commonly affected are lower end of the femur, upper end of the tibia, and lower end of the radius but jaw bones, upper end of the humerus, upper end of the femur, upper end of the fibula and the patella are also involved not infrequently. *Grossly* the end of the bone and adjacent metaphysis are usually affected (Fig. 624). The tumor is generally eccentric in location, expands the bone in all directions, destroys most of the bony substance leaving a mere shell peripherally and circumscribed trabeculæ centrally, and is composed of gray to brown, rather soft tissue that is permeated with blood and has a tendency to undergo small cyst formation. *Histologically* the fundamental structure consists of connective tissue cells that are either cellular or collagenous. In addition, the following elements are present in varying proportions: multinucleated giant cells, thin-walled capillaries, hemosiderin, foam cells, osteoid tissue, and foci of cartilage. The chief *clinical manifestations* consist of pain and swelling. *Roentgenograms* disclose expansion of the bone by translucent tissue with an over-all trabeculated or soap bubble-like effect. *Treatment* of choice consists of complete removal by curettage. The *prognosis* is good although recurrences and malignant transformations do occur.

Hemangioma.—Skeletal hemangioma is a rather uncommon tumor that usually *occurs* in patients beyond thirty years of age. Although the long *bones* of the body may be affected, the tumors are usually found in the skull (frontal and parietal bones) and vertebræ (Holmes, Manning, and Oosthuyzen). *Grossly* the growths appear hemorrhagic and sometimes spongy (Fig. 625). They are fairly sharply demarcated but are not encapsulated and may be accompanied by considerable bony reaction at the periphery. *Histologically* they are composed of cavernous spaces or of thin-walled capillaries filled with blood. The neoplasms are generally *asymptomatic* until they become large enough to cause pressure upon adjacent structures, pathologic fracture, or compression of vertebræ. *Roentgenograms* disclose an area of decreased density honeycombed with fine trabeculæ and surrounded at the periphery (when it reaches the periosteum) by new bone arranged at right angles to the surface. *Treatment* consists of local excision, cauterization, or irradiation. The *prognosis* is fair to good.

Neurofibroma.—Neurofibroma of bone is rare. The lesion may occur as a solitary mass or it may be present in conjunction with peripheral neurofibromatosis (von Recklinghausen's disease) (Mackenzie). Occas-

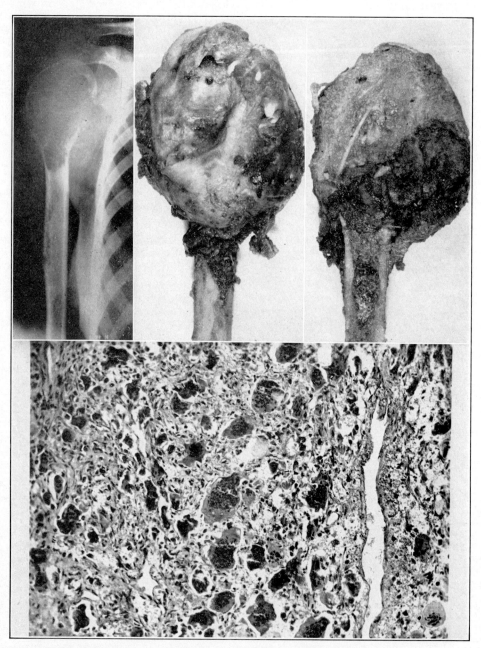

Fig. 624.—Giant cell tumor of the upper end of the humerus illustrating a typical soap bubble-like appearance roentgenographically, the external and cut surface of the tumor grossly, and the fibrous nature of the tumor with scattered giant cells microscopically. × 100.

ionally the tumor may undergo a sarcomatous transformation (Lichten-stein). Pathologically the tumors are the same as those in peripheral nerves (p. 1391).

Adamantinoblastoma.—Adamantinoblastoma (adamantinoma) usually occurs in the jaw (p. 617) but occasionally it may be located in the tibia (Mangalik). The tibial lesion probably arises on the basis of congenital or traumatic epithelial inclusions from the overlying skin.

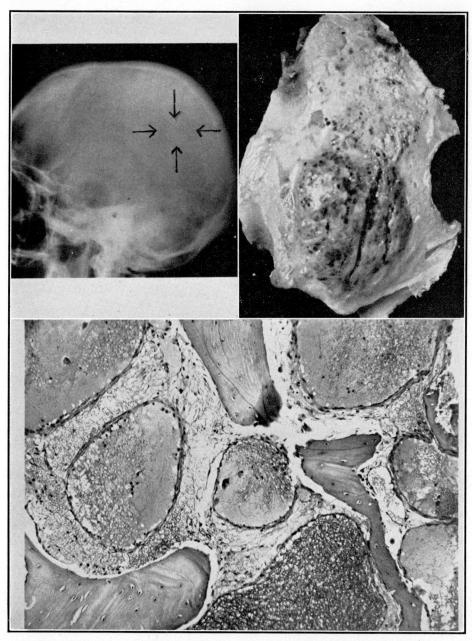

Fig. 625.—Hemangioma of the skull demonstrating a honeycombed area of translucency roentgenographically, a spongy tumor grossly, and cavernous spaces filled with blood microscopically. × 100.

Unicameral Bone Cyst.—A unicameral (L. = one + chamber) bone cyst is a solitary cyst that arises on the basis of an abnormality of development (Jaffe and James). The condition is *uncommon*, is almost always discovered in the first two decades of life, and predominates in males. In decreasing order of frequency, the bones involved are humerus, femur, tibia, ulna, and radius. The lesion starts in the metaphysis and, as the child ages, "grows away from" the epiphyseal line to occupy some portion of the diaphysis of the bone. *Roentgenographically* it exists as an expanding

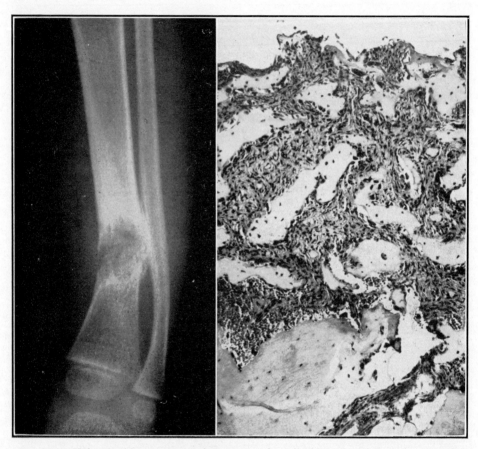

FIG. 626.—Unicameral bone cyst showing an area of rarefaction and pathologic fracture of the tibia roentgenographically and the wall composed of osteoid and osseous trabeculæ with scattered osteoclasts and a connective tissue stroma microscopically. × 100.

central area of rarefaction with gradual thinning of the cortex until the latter remains as a mere shell (Fig. 626). *Grossly* the cyst often produces a bluish sheen when seen through the periosteum. Cut surfaces disclose an extremely thin cortex and a solitary cyst. The latter is composed of a thin wall of gray to brown tissue and a lumen filled with yellow, brown, or hemorrhagic fluid. *Histologically* the wall is composed of loose-meshed osteoid and osseous trabeculæ disclosing scattered peripheral osteoclasts and embedded in varying amounts of well-vascularized connective tissue. The inner surface is lined with connective tissue which may contain hemosiderin deposits, a few trabeculæ, and foreign body giant cells. Attached to the lining are fibrin clots in various stages of disintegration and organization. *Clinically* the lesion is asymptomatic until pathologic fracture occurs. *Treatment* consists of thorough curettage and replacement with bone chips. The *prognosis* is good.

Aneurysmal Bone Cyst.—This is a relatively common benign osseous lesion that usually *occurs* in the second decade of life and appears to preponderate in males (Lichtenstein). The *bones* affected are vertebræ, pelvis, clavicles, ribs, and long bones of the upper and lower extremities.

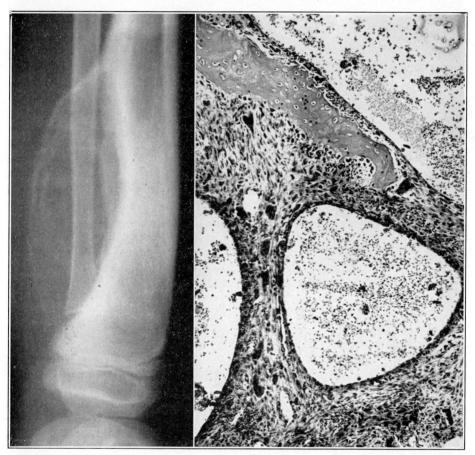

Fig. 627.—Aneurysmal bone cyst disclosing an expanding rarefied cortical lesion of the tibia roentgenographically and a connective tissue stroma containing cavernous spaces, giant cells and a reactive spicule of bone microscopically. × 100.

Roentgenographically the lesion consists of an eccentrically located, cystically expanded, ballooned area of rarefaction covered by a thin cortex (Fig. 627). *Histologically* it consists of a stroma of connective tissue containing numerous cavernous spaces filled with blood. Within the connective tissue are scattered foreign body giant cells, erythrocytes, some hemosiderin, and reparative new bone. The chief *clinical manifestations* are pain and bony deformity. *Treatment* consists of curettage or irradiation. The *prognosis* is good.

Osteitis Fibrosa Cystica.—Osteitis fibrosa cystica, also known as *von Recklinghausen's disease* of bone, represents the osseous lesions in primary

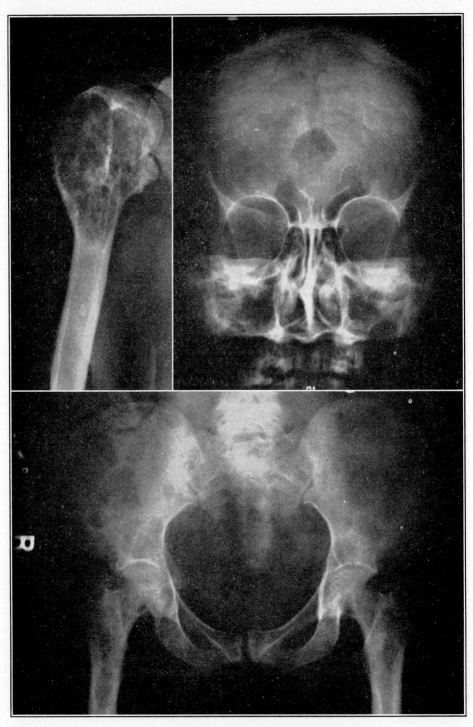

Fig. 628.—Osteitis fibrosa cystica illustrating widespread
areas of skeletal absorption and expansion.

or secondary hyperparathyroidism. The parathyroid lesions together with the chief characteristics of the disorder have already been discussed (p. 417) leaving only the osseous lesions to be considered here. Because calcium is withdrawn from the skeleton, *roentgenograms* of the bones disclose generalized demineralization, widespread deformities, and circumscribed, cystic areas of complete resorption that are similar to those seen in benign giant cell tumor (Fig. 628). The lesions occur in all bones of the body and

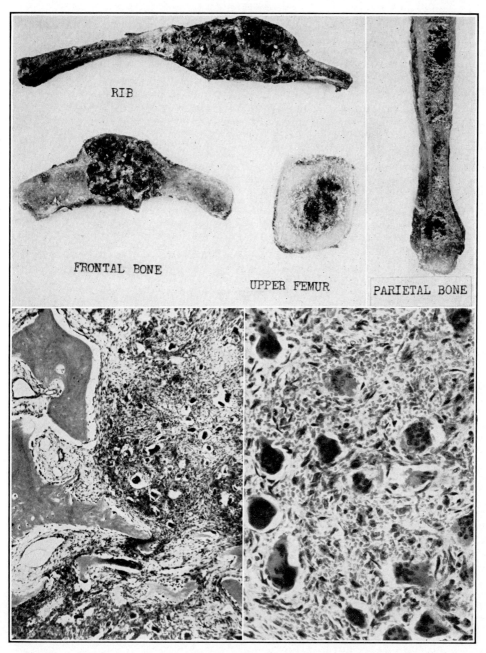

Fig. 629.—Osteitis fibrosa cystica demonstrating replacement of various bones by soft gray to brown tissue grossly and connective tissue containing giant cells microscopically. × 50 and × 200.

are always multiple. *Grossly* the bone is usually fusiformly or irregularly expanded, the cortex is thin, and the area of resorption is replaced with gritty, soft, reddish to yellowish, gelatinous substance containing varisized cysts (Fig. 629). *Histologically* the changes consist of complete or partial disappearance of bony trabeculæ and a replacement with connective tissue containing varying numbers of capillaries, foreign body giant cells, hemosiderin granules within and without phagocytes, extravasated erythrocytes, and foam cells.

Fibrous Dysplasia.—Fibrous dysplasia is a benign condition of bones that, among other names, has been called osteodystrophia fibrosa, juvenile Paget's disease, leontiasis ossea, etc. (Pritchard). It usually *occurs* near adolescence and is more common in females than in males. The *cause* is unknown. It is not related to hyperparathyroidism. The disorder may *affect* one bone (monostotic) or several or all bones (polyostotic) and it may consist of a single lesion or multiple lesions (Schlumberger). Long tubular bones are more commonly involved than other bones. *Roentgenographically* the affected areas are radiolucent, trabeculated, expanded, and somewhat "cystic" (Fig. 630). *Grossly* they are composed of grayish-white tissue that contains varying amounts of gritty material and bony trabeculæ. Small areas of degeneration may be present but well-formed cysts are not seen. *Histologically* the basic tissue is of a cellular fibrous nature. It contains varying numbers of osseous and osteoid trabeculæ and calcified islands of cartilage. The vessels are usually inconspicuous and osteoclasts, applied to the bony trabeculæ, are sparse. The *clinical manifestations* consist of pain, deformity, and pathologic fracture. In females (and rarely in males) with widespread disease, there may be associated brown pigmentation of the skin and precocious puberty—a combination referred to as *Albright's syndrome* (Hibbs, Vines, and Warrick). *Treatment* consists of excision or curettage and replacement with bone chips. The *prognosis* is good.

Osteitis Deformans.—Osteitis deformans, commonly known as *Paget's disease* of bone, is a benign condition that probably existed in ancient times but that was brought to the forefront by Paget in 1876 when he correlated the clinical and pathologic features (Rosenkrantz). The *incidence* has been recorded as varying from 1 in 170 to 1 in 15,000 admissions. The condition usually *occurs* in patients between the ages of forty and sixty years and is twice as common in males as it is in females. The *cause* is unknown. The *lesions* may be monostotic and localized or polyostotic and generalized. Of the two, the former are much more common. In decreasing order of frequency, the *bones* affected are pelvic bones, skull, femur, lumbar spine, thoracic spine, tibia, humerus, cervical spine, scapula, clavicle, sacrum, ribs, fibula, and mandible. *Roentgenograms* reveal an over-all thickening of the cortex of the bone with an irregular fuzzy mottling that is referred to as the "cotton-wool" appearance (Fig. 631).

Pathologically the process is one of softening and absorption of bone followed by replacement with connective tissue and new bone. *Grossly* the affected area is thickened, light in weight, and porous. Initially the lesion is quite soft and can be cut readily with a knife but later it becomes hard and calcified. During the soft stage, the usual stresses and strains result in the development of bone deformities. *Histologically* the new trabeculæ are irregularly formed. They consist of islands of osseous tissue separated by distinct basophilic lines resulting in what has been termed a "mosaic pattern." About the periphery of some of the spicules both osteoblasts

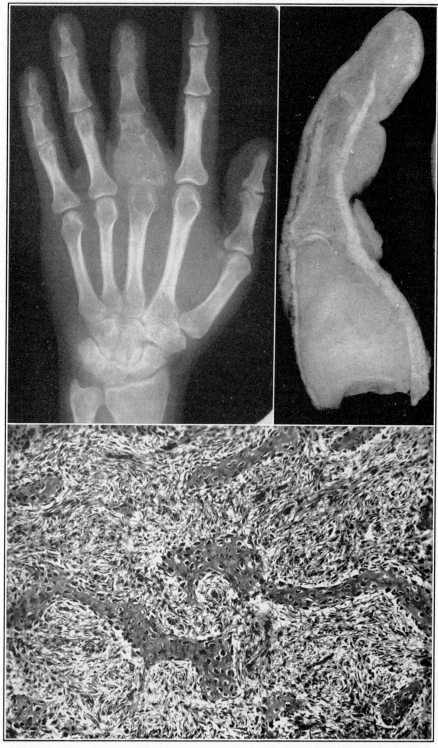

FIG. 630.—Fibrous dysplasia showing an expanding translucency of the proximal phalanx of the middle finger roentgenographically, replacement with grayish-white tissue grossly, and a stroma of dense cellular fibrous tissue containing osseous trabeculæ microscopically.   × 100.

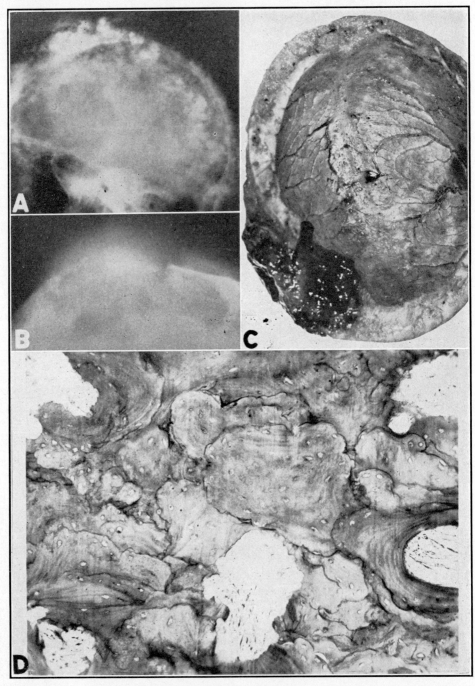

Fig. 631.—Osteitis deformans illustrating *A*, the typical "cotton-wool" appearance roentgenographically, *B*, a complicating osteolytic osteosarcoma roentgenographically, *C*, the thickened skull and osteolytic osteosarcoma grossly, and *D*, the typical mosaic structure microscopically. × 100.

and osteoclasts are occasionally present. The interstices between the bony trabeculæ are filled with well-vascularized, loose, connective tissue.

The *complications* of osteitis deformans consist of (1) bony deformities, (2) reduction in size of the cranial cavity with compression of the brain, (3) pathologic fractures, and (4) malignant transformation occurring in about 4 per cent of cases (Kirshbaum). The malignant lesions consist essentially of osteosarcoma (osteogenic sarcoma) and fibrosarcoma, although malignant giant cell tumor and multiple myeloma have also been recorded (Derman, Russell, and Gross). *Clinical manifestations* may be entirely absent. When present, they consist of pain in the various bones together with bony deformities, locomotive disturbances, increase in size of head, and (as a result of pressure) a variety of cranial disturbances (including headache, defective hearing, visual disturbances, tinnitus, etc.). Serum alkaline phosphatase is generally elevated. The *diagnosis* is made roentgenographically. *Treatment* is symptomatic unless sarcoma develops when it consists of surgical extirpation (when possible). In general, while the disease cannot be eradicated, the *prognosis* is fair to good, and the life span is not appreciably shortened.

Osteosarcoma.—Osteosarcoma is a malignant primary tumor of bone that is composed essentially of osteoblasts or their precursors. While the term *osteogenic sarcoma* is now generally more popular and is used synonymously with osteosarcoma it is probably better to drop it from the nomenclature entirely because the same caption has been (and often still is) used to encompass not only tumors composed of osteoblastic cells but also those composed of cartilaginous (chondrosarcoma) and fibrous (fibrosarcoma) elements (Coley). The tumor is next in *frequency* to multiple myeloma. It is more common in males than in females and *occurs* with greatest regularity between the ages of ten and twenty-five years (Lichtenstein). After the age of twenty-five years the tumor is generally encountered as a complication of osteitis deformans or some form of irradiation (Cahan). The *lesion* is usually single but rarely it may arise in multiple foci. In decreasing order of frequency, the *bones* affected are lower end of femur, upper end of tibia, upper end of humerus, upper end of fibula, iliac bone, vertebræ, jaw, and others. While any portion of the bone may be involved, the most frequent location is the metaphysis and adjacent epiphysis.

Pathologically osteosarcoma may be divided into two types—osteoblastic and osteolytic. *Osteoblastic osteosarcoma* is a solid tumor composed predominantly of osteoblastic tissue with formation of lesser or greater numbers of osseous trabeculæ. By the time a specimen is examined in the laboratory, the tumor is either fusiform in shape with the bulky end near the joint and the tapering end pointing toward the diaphysis or it is more irregular and bulky (Fig. 632). The periosteum is raised and may be penetrated. The space between the periosteum and bone is filled with gray tumor tissue that contains spicules of bone arranged at right angles to the shaft. The cortex of the old bone blends with the tumor and the medullary cavity is filled with similar tissue. The latter may extend for considerable distances within the bone beyond the external level of the growth. The *histologic* structure is variable. At one extreme, virtually the entire tumor is composed of trabeculæ of osseous and osteoid tissue. Such trabeculæ are usually small, irregular, and covered with and surrounded by neoplastic osteoblasts. At the other extreme, the tumor is composed only of osteoblasts with extremely little osteoid and osseous tissue. Neoplastic osteoblasts appear as diffuse infiltrations of irregular, varisized, polyhedral,

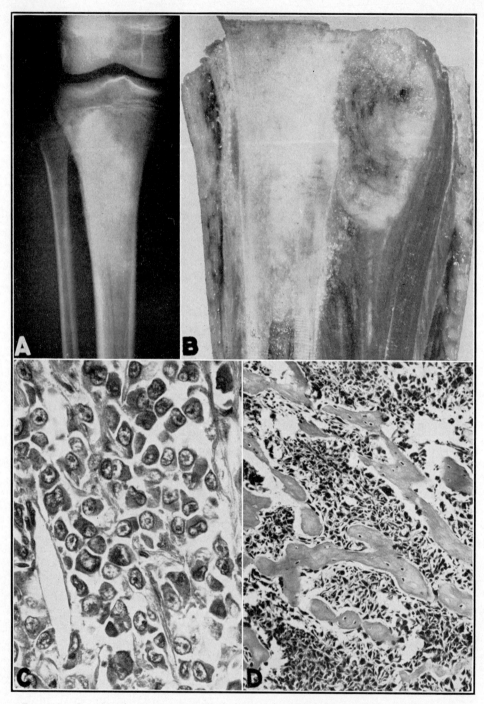

FIG. 632.—Osteoblastic osteosarcoma disclosing *A*, increased density of the upper end of the tibia along with a soft tissue mass on the fibular side, *B*, the amputated specimen (the joint was removed for another study after a mid-thigh amputation) with dense sclerotic tumor permeating the tibia and a soft tissue mass in the adjacent muscle, *C*, neoplastic osteoblasts with irregularity of cytoplasm and nuclei. × 400, and *D*, another tumor with greater irregularity of cells and new bone formation. × 100.

or spindle cells with varying amounts of slightly basophilic cytoplasm and irregular, single, or multiple hyperchromatic nuclei. Osteoclasts are seen but are, as a rule, few in number. *Osteolytic osteosarcoma* differs from the osteoblastic variety in that there is practically no bone formation and the bony trabeculæ that do form are destroyed by osteoclasts (McReynolds). The old bone is virtually completely destroyed by an expanding soft hemorrhagic and cystic mass that may bear some resemblance to that of a giant cell tumor (Fig. 633). *Histologically* viable tissue is found only at the

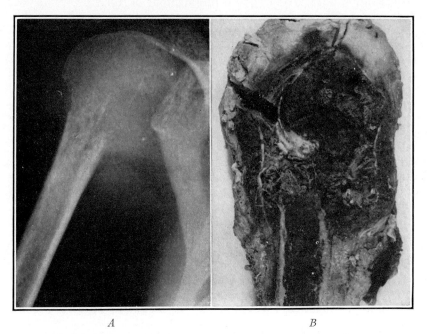

A   *B*

FIG. 633.—Osteolytic osteosarcoma showing *A*, complete destruction of the upper end of the humerus, and *B*, the hemorrhagic and cysti ctumor after removal of the entire extremity. (Herbut's *Surgical Pathology.*)

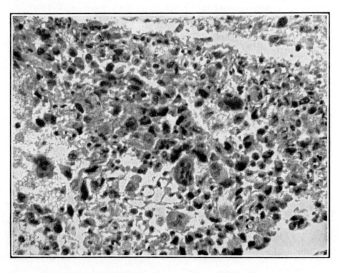

FIG. 634.—Osteolytic osteosarcoma illustrating osteoblasts, osteoclasts, necrosis, and erythrocytic extravasation. × 100. (Herbut's *Surgical Pathology.*)

periphery of the tumor. It consists of osteoblasts separated by numerous capillaries and extravasated erythrocytes (Fig. 634). Portions of bony spicules may be noted and osteoclasts are abundant. Most of the central portion of the neoplasm, however, is represented by completely necrotic tissue. *Osteosarcoma* spreads locally by extension and distantly by the bloodstream. The most common sites of metastasis are the lungs and liver. Other bones are rarely, if ever, secondarily involved.

The *complications* are metastasis and pathologic fracture. *Clinically* there are trauma, pain, swelling, and impairment of function. The trauma, however, serves only to direct attention to the growth and has nothing to do with its initiation. *Roentgenograms* are characteristic. In osteoblastic osteosarcoma they generally reveal a tapering tumor of increased opacity with the subperiosteal spicules of bone arranged at right angles to the shaft —producing what is referred to as a sunburst appearance. In osteolytic osteosarcoma the affected area shows complete dissolution of bone with no new osseous tissue demonstrable. The *diagnosis* is made chiefly from roentgenograms and biopsy. *Treatment* consists of complete surgical extirpation, removing the joint on either side of the affected bone whenever possible. Irradiation therapy has little effect. The *prognosis* is poor, with the five-year survival rate being less than 10 per cent.

Chondrosarcoma.—Chondrosarcoma represents the malignant counterpart of chondroma. It *accounts for* about 7.6 per cent of primary malignant bone tumors (O'Neal). The tumor *occurs* at any age but is most common after the third decade and it predominates slightly in males (Morton). The *cause* is unknown. Since the tumor is generally preceded by a benign cartilaginous growth, the *bones* most often affected are those involved by osteochondroma (p. 1240), chondroma (p. 1241), and hereditary multiple exostoses (p. 1228) (Monro). *Roentgenograms* disclose a small to large, fundamentally translucent mass replacing most or all of the bone in which it is located. Secondarily, varisized areas of calcification are generally present.

Grossly the tumor is fairly sharply circumscribed but is not encapsulated. By the time the pathologist examines the specimen, the growth is generally quite bulky and may measure 15 to 20 cm. in diameter. (Fig. 635) As a rule, most of the tumor appears gray, translucent, and cartilaginous. Bulkier growths have a tendency to undergo myxomatous changes with focal or massive areas of complete liquefaction and cyst formation. Calcification is often present in lesser or greater amounts. *Histologically* the neoplasms disclose a wide range from those composed of relatively normal-appearing cartilage cells to those composed of irregular polyhedral cells with abundant, slightly basophilic cytoplasm and rounded or irregular hyperchromatic nuclei and exhibiting no hyaline matrix whatsoever. (Fig. 635) In fact, it is the consensus that the lesions may appear so benign that they are frequently underdiagnosed. In an effort to overcome this error, Lichtenstein and Jaffe stated that a diagnosis of chondrosarcoma is justified when there are (1) many cells with plump nuclei, (2) more than an occasional cell with two such nuclei, or (3) any giant cartilage cells with large single or multiple nuclei or with clumps of chromatin. The growths *spread* by local extension, by bloodstream to the lungs, liver, and other organs, and rarely by lymphatics to draining lymph nodes.

The *complications* consist of metastasis and disturbances in locomotion from deformity or pathologic fracture. The *clinical manifestations* consist

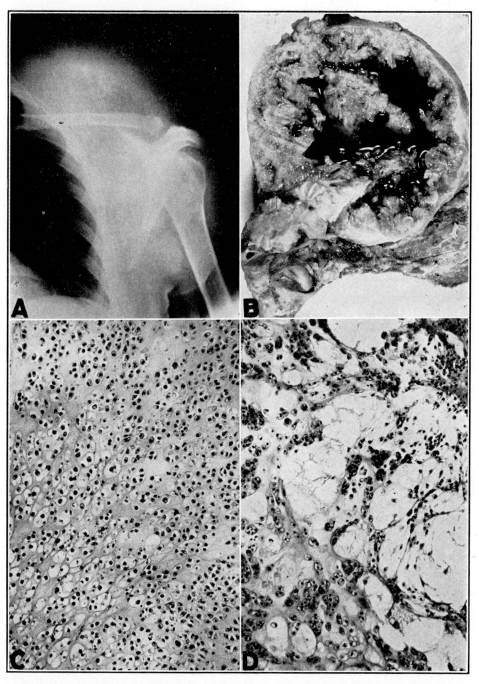

FIG. 635.—Chondrosarcoma disclosing *A*, a large translucent scapular mass, *B*, the removed tumor with typical cartilaginous tissue and a central area of liquefaction, *C*, fairly regular neoplastic cells embedded in a hyaline matrix, and *D*, irregular neoplastic cells with a hyaline and myxomatous matrix. × 100.

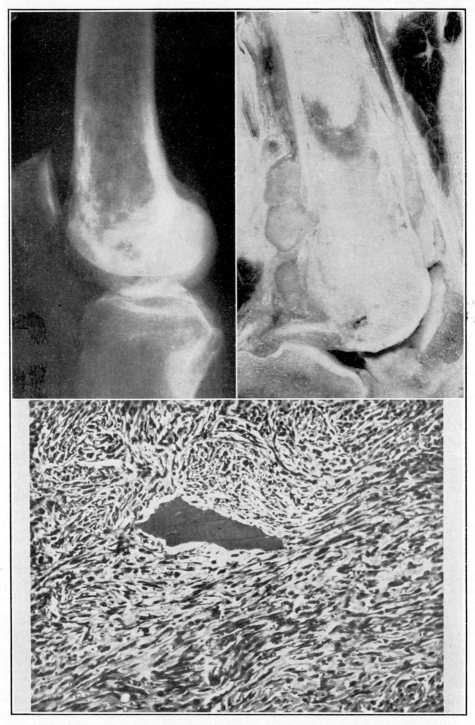

FIG. 636.—Fibrosarcoma demonstrating irregular radiolucency of the lower end of the femur, grayish-white tumor replacing bone and adjacent soft tissue in the removed specimen, and irregular spindle cells surrounding a spicule of old bone. × 100.

of pain, deformity, and functional disability. The *diagnosis* is made from a history of osseous tumor of long duration, roentgenograms, and biopsy. *Treatment* consists of wide local excision or of amputation (when the lesion is in an extremity) above the proximal joint. The *prognosis* is better than in any other malignant bone tumor. Over one-half of all cures of malignant bone tumors occur in cases with chondrosarcoma.

Fibrosarcoma.—Fibrosarcoma of bone represents the malignant counterpart of fibroma. The lesion usually *occurs* in patients beyond the third decade of life and is seen in both sexes with equal frequency. The *cause* is unknown although the lesion is sometimes encountered as a complication of a chronic draining sinus or of osteitis deformans. The *bones* most often affected are the tubular bones of the extremities, especially the femur (Lichtenstein). *Roentgenograms* reveal varisized radiolucent masses affecting primarily the endosteum, the medullary cavity, or the periosteum (Fig. 636). Eventually the tumor is also seen to extend into the soft tissues.

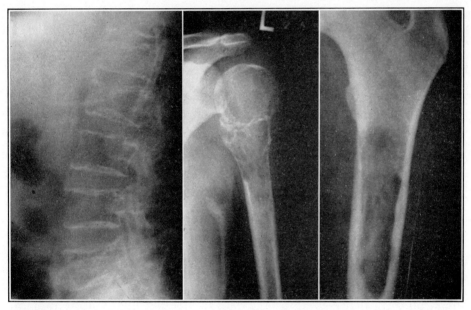

Fig. 637.—Multiple myeloma disclosing areas of rarefaction in the vertebræ, humerus, and femur.

Grossly the neoplasm exists as a solid mass of soft, gray, brain-like tissue primarily occupying the areas mentioned above but secondarily replacing most of the osseous tissue and later even extending into the adjacent fascias and muscles. *Histologically* it consists essentially of sheets or whorls of spindle cells with a moderate to scanty amount of ill-defined cytoplasm and elongated plump hyperchromatic nuclei. Mitoses may be numerous. The degree of vascularity varies but is generally not great. Bony spicules may be seen within the tumor but they represent inclusions of old bone for neither osseous or cartilaginous tissue is present as an integral part of the growth. Fibrosarcoma of bone remains localized for considerable periods of time but eventually *spreads*, chiefly by the bloodstream, to the lungs, liver, and other viscera. The *clinical manifestations* are not distinctive. The final *diagnosis* can be made only by biopsy. *Treatment* consists of wide resection or (if the tumor is in an extremity) amputation above the proximal

joint.   The *prognosis* is fair to good, with survival rates being second only
to those in cases of chondrosarcoma.

Myeloma.—A myeloma is a malignant tumor arising in bone marrow.   It
is referred to as *multiple myeloma* when the lesions affect more than one
bone and are multiple (Lichtenstein) and as *solitary myeloma* when the
lesion is confined to one bone and is solitary (Gootnick and Raven).   Of
the two, the multiple variety is more common.   The condition usually
occurs in patients over forty years of age, is practically unheard of before
the age of thirty years, and prevails slightly in males over females (Meacham
and Breitenbucher).   The *cause* is unknown.   Any of the *bones* of the body
may be involved with the vertebræ, sternum, ribs, skull, and long bones of
the extremities heading the list.   *Roentgenograms* usually reveal multiple,
fairly sharply circumscribed areas of marrow translucency encroaching
upon and destroying the adjacent cortex (Fig. 637).   In addition, there is
often general demineralization and widening of the medullary cavities—
sometimes to the exclusion of distinct tumor masses.

Grossly the tumors appear primarily within the medullary cavity.   They
are seen as gray to red, firm to mushy, ill-defined foci that are devoid of
bone and that irregularly erode the cortex (Fig. 638).   Sometimes the tumors
are bulkier and protrude as distinct masses beyond the regular limits of the
bones.   *Histologically* the tumors are regularly of a plasma cell type (plasmocytoma).   Although myelocytic, lymphocytic, erythrocytic, lipoblastic,
and megakaryocytoid varieties have been recorded (Herbut) some authors
doubt the existence of any but the plasmocytoma.   These growths consist
of diffuse sheets of rather regular-appearing plasma cells.   They are rounded,
possess an abundant amount of slightly basophilic cytoplasm, and disclose round, deeply staining, overhanging, usually single but occasionally
double nuclei.   Osseous or cartilaginous tissue is not formed.   Usually
myeloma is confined to bone; occasionally it (plasmocytoma) exists entirely
in extra-osseous foci, especially the respiratory tract, and sometimes the
osseous lesions *spread* to soft tissues such as lymph nodes, spleen, liver,
etc. (James).

The *complications* of multiple myeloma are fractures, hemorrhagic
phenomenon, amyloidosis, and renal insufficiency (Meacham).   The *clinical
manifestations* consist of pain in the bones, multiple bony lesions, elevated
serum protein, renal dysfunction, excessive rouleaux formation in peripheral
blood, anemia, Bence-Jones proteinuria (a globulin in the urine that precipitates out at 60° C. and redissolves upon boiling), myeloid immaturity,
osteoporosis, hypercalcemia, pathologic fracture, root pain, etc. (Bayrd).
The *diagnosis* is made from the history, roentgenograms, marrow aspiration,
and biopsy.   *Treatment* is unsatisfactory.   Solitary lesions can be controlled
for a while by irradiation or excision but ultimately the disease becomes
multiple and, in such cases, the *prognosis* is poor.   Chemotherapeutic
agents have been tried but are so far ineffective.

Ewing's Tumor.—Ewing's tumor is a malignant neoplasm of bone that
occurs in both sexes and prevails between the ages of five and twenty-five
years (Herrick and Breckenridge).   The *cause* of the growth is unknown
and, while a history of trauma is generally obtained, such a mechanical
disturbance probably plays no role in its genesis.   The tumor starts within
the marrow cavity and the *bones* affected, in decreasing order of frequency
are tibia, femur, pelvis, humerus, fibula, rib, clavicle, scapula, small
bones hands and feet, spine, radius, ulna, patella, skull, jaw, etc.   *Roentgenograms* are extremely variable but basically they show a lytic process

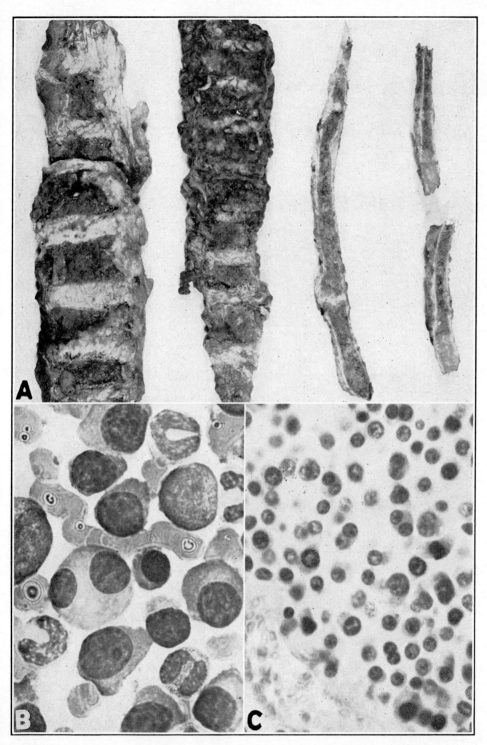

FIG. 638.—Multiple myeloma illustrating A, irregular small tumors in the vertebræ, sternum, and ribs, B, plasma cells in a smear of aspirated bone marrow. $\times$ 1380, and C, plasma cells in histologic sections of involved marrow. $\times$ 400.

that starts within the marrow cavity (Fig. 639). The changes may consist of mottled lysis, sclerosis, cystic loculation, and longitudinal (onion skin) periosteal bone formation (McCormack).

Pathologically the tumor varies greatly in size from a few to 20 cm. or more. Originally confined to the bone, it later breaks through the cortex and periosteum to form a bulky extra-osseous mass. Grossly the growth is primarily soft, gray, and brain-like but because of extensive necrosis it secondarily becomes mottled yellow and red. The tumor proper is devoid of all bone formation but the adjacent periosteum may be stimulated to new bone production. *Histologically* the lesion consists of a diffuse permeation of rounded cells with scanty cytoplasm and large, round, evenly

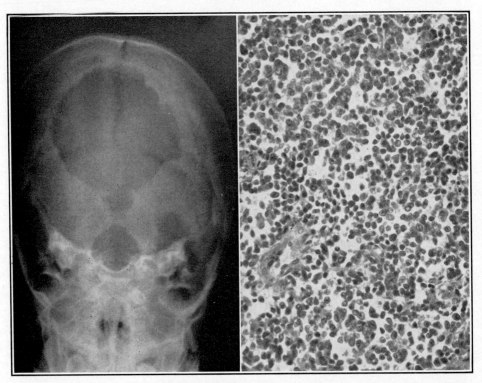

FIG. 639.—Ewing's tumor showing several osteolytic lesions in the skull roentgenographically and rounded cells with scanty cytoplasm and round, evenly staining nuclei microscopically. × 200.

stained nuclei (Fig. 639). Thin-walled capillaries are numerous and necrosis is conspicuous. Despite this constant microscopic appearance, the *histogenesis* of the tumor still remains in doubt with the following having been considered as progenitors at one time or another: endothelial or perithelial cells, lymphoblasts, myeloid cells, reticulum cells, and neuroblasts. Ewing's tumor *spreads* by local extension and by the bloodstream to the lungs and other organs. While originally the growth is generally solitary, it ultimately involves several or many bones. Whether such involvement indicates a multicentric origin or whether it represents metastases has not yet been settled.

The *complications* consist of pathologic fracture and metastasis. The *clinical manifestations* are pain, swelling, loss of function, slight fever, leukocytosis to 18,000, and slight anemia (McSwain). The *diagnosis* is made from the history, roentgenographic findings, and biopsy. A differential diagnosis should include osteomyelitis, neuroblastoma, and lymphoblastoma. *Treatment* has consisted of irradiation, wide local excision, amputation, and chemotherapy. The growth characteristically melts away with irradiation but it invariably returns and ultimately does not respond to further therapy. The *prognosis* is guarded for the five-year survival rate is extremely low.

Secondary Tumors.—Secondary growths of bone are much more common than primary neoplasms. Thus, in any osseous tumor it behooves one to first think of a primary lesion in some extra-osseous site. While the growths may reach the bone by direct extension they are most often metastatic. The osseous lesions may be solitary or multiple and, roentgenographically, they may be indistinguishable from primary bone tumors. While some growths are osteoblastic (carcinoma of the prostate) most are osteolytic. Virtually any malignant tumor in any organ of the body may secondarily affect bones but the more common type of tumor is carcinoma and the more common sites are in the prostate, thyroid, breasts, lung, gastrointestinal tract, and kidney.

REFERENCES

General

LICHTENSTEIN, L.: *Bone Tumors*, St. Louis, C. V. Mosby Co., 1952.
LUCK, J. V.: *Bone and Joint Diseases*, Springfield, Charles C Thomas, 1950.
MERCER, W.: *Orthopedic Surgery*, 4th Ed., Baltimore, Williams & Wilkins Co., 1950.

Congenital Anomalies

ADSON, A. W.: J. Internat. Coll. Surg., *16*, 546, 1951 (Cervical Rib).
BARSKY, A. J.: J. Bone & Joint Surg., *22A*, 35, 1951 (Anomalies of Hand).
BUSH, L. G., and MERRELL, O. E.: J. Pediat., *40*, 330, 1952 (Infantile Corticohyperostosis).
CASSIDY, W. J., *et al.*: A. M. A. Arch. Int. Med., *82*, 140, 1948 (Osteopetrosis).
COLE, H. N., JR., *et al.*: A. M. A. Arch. Dermat. & Syph., *66*, 371, 1952 (Gargoylism).
FOLLIS, R. H., JR.: J. Pediat., *41*, 713, 1952 (Osteogenesis Imperfecta).
GAIN, D. D., and LAWSON, D. E.: Radiology, *58*, 221, 1952 (Osteogenesis Imperfecta).
HENDERSON, J. L., *et al.*: A. M. A. Arch. Dis. Child., *27*, 230, 1952 (Gargoylism).
JAFFE, H. L.: A. M. A. Arch. Path., *36*, 335, 1943 (Hereditary Multiple Exostosis).
ROSE, J., and DOOLAN, P. D.: New England J. Med., *240*, 799, 1949 (Hereditary Multiple Exostosis).
ROSS, L. J.: Am. J. Dis. Child., *78*, 417, 1949 (Arachnodactyly).
ZAWISCH, C.: A. M. A. Arch. Path., *43*, 55, 1947 (Osteopetrosis).

Degenerations

BRONITSKY, J.: Bone & Joint Surg., *29*, 931, 1947 (Chondromalacia of the Patella).
CARR, C. R., and HOWARD, J. W.: U. S. Armed Forces M. J., *3*, 185, 1952 (Chondromalacia of the Patella).
COCCHI, U.: Am. J. Roentgenol., *68*, 570, 1952 (Myelosclerosis).
ERF, L. A., and HERBUT, P. A.: Ann. Int. Med., *21*, 863, 1944 (Myelofibrosis and Osteosclerosis).
JACOBS, E. C., *et al.*: Am. J. Clin. Path., *21*, 56, 1951 (Ainhum).

Inflammations

ALLRED, S. W., and MINEAR, W. L.: Am. Surgeon, *18*, 58, 1952 (Tuberculosis).
ALTEMEIER, W. A., and LARGEN, T.: J. A. M. A., *150*, 1462, 1952 (Antibiotics in Skeletal Infections).
BABER, M. D.: A. M. A. Arch. Dis. Child., *28*, 24, 1953 (Osteomyelitis Hands and Feet).

BLANCHE, D. W.: J. Bone & Joint Surg., *34*A, 71, 1952 (Osteomyelitis Infants).
DEVAS, M. B.: Brit. J. Surg., *40*, 140, 1952 (Cancer in Osteomyelitis).
DICKSON, F. D., *et al.*: A. M. A. Arch. Surg., *66*, 60, 1953 (Chronic Osteomyelitis).
FISCHER, K. A.: Surg., Gynec. & Obst., *83*, 507, 1946 (Osteomyelitis from War Wounds).
GHORMLEY, R. K.: J. Bone & Joint Surg., *34*A, 254–330, 1952 (Symposium Tuberculosis).
HILL, A. J., JR., *et al.*: J. Pediat., *30*, 547, 1947 (Syphilis).
JACKSON, H., *et al.*: A. M. A. Arch. Dis. Child., *28*, 19, 1953 (Typhoid Osteitis).
LAVALLE, L. L., and HAMM, F. C.: J. Urol., *66*, 418, 1951 (Osteitis Pubis).
SMITH, W. S., and GANEY, J. B.: A. M. A. Arch. Surg., *60*, 125, 1949 (Traumatic Osteomyelitis).
WAUGH, W.: J. Bone & Joint Surg., *34*B, 642, 1953 (Fibrosarcoma in Bone Sinus).
WEAR, J. E., *et al.*: Am. J. Roentgenol., *76*, 90, 1952 (Pyogenic Osteomyelitis Spine).
WHITE, M., and DENNISON, W. M.: J. Bone & Joint Surg., *34*B, 608, 1952 (Hematogenous Osteitis).

Physical Disturbances

BERNSTEIN, A., *et al.*: Am. J. Surg., *71*, 355, 1946 (692 March Fractures).
DE YOUNG, R.: Am. Surgeon, *18*, 816, 1952 (Sarcoma in Irradiated Bones).
DONALD, J. G., and FITTS, W. T., JR.: J. Bone & Joint Surg., *29*, 297, 1947 (March Fractures).
EDEIKEN, L., and SCHNEEBERG, N. G.: J. A. M. A., *122*, 865, 1943 (Milkman's Syndrome).
KAHLSTROM, S. C., and PHEMISTER, D. B.: Am. J. Path., *22*, 947, 1946 (Infarcts).
LAWRENCE, E. A.: Am. J. Roentgenol., *55*, 733, 1946 (Osteoradionecrosis).
MENDELOWITZ, M.: Medicine, *21*, 269, 1942 (Hypertrophic Osteoarthropathy).
URIST, M. R., and MCLEAN, F. C.: J. Bone & Joint Surg., *23*, 1, 1941 (Healing of Fractures).

Tumors

BAYRD, E. D., and HECK, F. J.: J. A. M. A., *133*, 147, 1947 (Myeloma).
BREITENBUCHER, R. B., and HERTZOG, A. J.: Minnesota Med., *32*, 986, 1949 (Myeloma).
CAHAN, W. G., *et al.*: Cancer, *1*, 3, 1948 (Sarcoma in Irradiated Bones).
COLEY, B. L.: *Neoplasms of Bone*, New York, Paul B. Hoeber, Inc., 1949.
COLEY, B. L., and HARROLD, C. C., JR.: J. Bone & Joint Surg., *32*A, 307, 1950 (Osteosarcoma).
COLEY, B. L., and SANTORO, A. J.: Surgery, *22*, 411, 1947 (Chondroma).
CONGDON, C. C.: Am. J. Path., *28*, 793, 1952 (Chordoma).
DAHLIN, D. C., and MACCARTY, C. S.: Cancer, *5*, 1170, 1952 (Chordoma).
DERMAN, H., *et al.*: Am. J. Roentgenol., *65*, 225, 1951 (Sarcoma in Osteitis Deformans).
DOCKERTY, M. B.: Ann. Surg., *133*, 77, 1951 (Osteoid Osteoma).
DOWLING, J. R.: A. M. A. Arch. Otolaryngol., *41*, 99, 1945 (Osteoma).
ERF, L. A., and HERBUT, P. A.: Am. J. Clin. Path., *16*, 1, 1946 (Wright Smears and Sections in Myeloma).
FRANCE, W. G.: Brit. J. Surg., *39*, 357, 1952 (Benign Chondroblastoma).
GESCHICKTER, C. F., and COPELAND, M. M.: Ann. Surg., *133*, 790, 1951 (Parosteal Osteoma).
——————: *Tumors of Bone*, 3rd Ed., Philadelphia, J. B. Lippincott Co., 1949.
GOOTNICK, L. T.: Radiology, *45*, 385, 1945 (Solitary Myeloma).
GROSS, R. J., and YELIN, G.: Am. J. Roentgenol., *65*, 585, 1951 (Multiple Myeloma in Osteitis Deformans).
HERBUT, P. A., and ERF, L. A.: Am. J. Clin. Path., *13*, 16, 1946 (Lipoblastic and Megakaryocytoid Myeloma).
HERRICK, W. C., and BRECKENRIDGE, R. L.: *Clinical Orthopedics*, Philadelphia, J. B. Lippincott Co., *1*, 161, 1953 (Ewing's Tumor).
HIBBS, R. E., and RUSH, H. P.: Ann. Int. Med., *37*, 587, 1952 (Albright's Syndrome).
HOLMES, E. M., *et al.*: Ann. Otol., Rhinol. & Laryngol., *61*, 45, 1952 (Hemangioma).
JAFFE, H. L., and LICHTENSTEIN, L.: A. M. A. Arch. Surg., *44*, 1004, 1942 (Unicameral Cyst).
JAMES, A. G., *et al.*: A. M. A. Arch. Surg., *57*, 137, 1948 (Unicameral Cyst).
JAMES, T. G. I., and TURNER, E. A.: Brit. J. Surg., *39*, 361, 1952 (Soft Tissue Involvement in Myeloma).
KIRSHBAUM, J. D.: A. M. A. Arch. Path., *36*, 74, 1943 (Fibrosarcoma in Osteitis Deformans).
LICHTENSTEIN, L.: *Bone Tumors*, St. Louis, C. V. Mosby Co., 1952.
——————: Cancer, *3*, 279, 1950 (Aneurysmal Bone Cyst).
LICHTENSTEIN, L., and JAFFE, H. L.: Am. J. Path., *19*, 553, 1943 (Chondrosarcoma).
——————: A. M. A. Arch. Path., *44*, 207, 1947 (Myeloma).
MACKENZIE, J.: Brit. J. Radiol., *23*, 667, 1950 (Neurofibromatosis).
MANGALIK, V. S., and MEHROTRA, R. M. L.: Brit. J. Surg., *39*, 429, 1952 (Adamantinoma Tibia).

MANNING, H. J.: Radiology, *56*, 58, 1951 (Hemangioma).

McCORMACK, L. J., *et al.*: Cancer, *5*, 85, 1952 (Ewing's Sarcoma).

McREYNOLDS, I. S.: Surg., Gynec. & Obst., *67*, 163, 1938 (Osteolytic Osteosarcoma).

McSWAIN, B., *et al.*: Surg., Gynec. & Obst., *89*, 209, 1949 (Ewing's Tumor).

MEACHAM, G. C.: Ann. Int. Med., *38*, 1035, 1953 (Plasma Cell Myeloma).

MONRO, R. S., and GOLDING, J. S. R.: Brit. J. Surg., *39*, 73, 1951 (Chondrosarcoma).

MORTON, J. J., and MIDER, G. B.: Ann. Surg., *126*, 895, 1947 (Chondrosarcoma).

O'NEAL, L. W., and ACKERMAN, L. V.: Cancer, *5*, 551, 1952 (Chondrosarcoma).

OOSTHUYZEN, S. F., and BARNETSON, J.: Radiology, *56*, 256, 1951 (Hemangioma).

PINES, B., *et al.*: J. Internat. Coll. Surg., *13*, 249, 1950 (Osteoid Osteoma).

PRITCHARD, J. E.: Am. J. M. Sci., *222*, 313, 1951 (Fibrous Dysplasia).

RAVEN, R. W., and WILLIS, R. A.: J. Bone & Joint Surg., *31*, 369, 1949 (Solitary Plasmo-cytoma).

ROSENKRANTZ, J. A., *et al.*: A. M. A. Arch. Int. Med., *90*, 610, 1952 (Osteitis Deformans).

RUSSELL, D. S.: J. Bone & Joint Surg., *31*, 281, 1949 (Malignant Giant Cell Tumor in Osteitis Deformans).

SCHLUMBERGER, H. G.: Military Surg., *99*, 504, 1946 (Fibrous Dysplasia).

SMITH, A. G., and ZAVALETA, A.: A. M. A. Arch. Path., *54*, 507, 1952 (Ossifying Fibroma).

STEWART, M. J., and RICHARDSON, T. R.: J. Bone & Joint Surg., *34*A, 372, 1952 (Giant Cell Tumor).

VINES, R. H.: A. M. A. Arch. Dis. Child., *27*, 351, 1952 (Fibrous Dysplasia).

WARRICK, C. K.: J. Bone & Joint Surg., *31*, 175, 1949 (Albright's Syndrome).

WILLIS, R. A.: J. Bone & Joint Surg., *31*, 236, 1949 (Giant Cell Tumor).

WINDEYER, B. W., and WOODYATT, P. W.: J. Bone & Joint Surg., *31*, 252, 1949 (Giant Cell Tumor).

36

Joints

PATHOLOGIC PHYSIOLOGY

Anthony F. DePalma

Joints loom forth as extremely important in the body, for disorders of these structures as a group are the greatest single cause of dysfunction and disability in man. From a more morphological viewpoint, there are five *types* of joints: (1) *Syndesmosis.* These are found as the sutures of the skull. They permit growth of the bones of the skull and are not concerned with motion. (2) *Synchondrosis.* These are found at the end of a long bone during growth and permit growth. Essentially, they comprise the epiphyseal disc and connect the bony epiphysis with the bony diathesis. (3) *Synostosis.* These comprise sutures of the skull and epiphyseal discs which have undergone ossification. The components on either side of the joint now become united with bone. (4) *Symphysis.* In these joints, the bone ends are capped with hyaline cartilage and are held firmly together by a band of fibrocartilage. These types of joints provide great strength and only a limited amount of mobility. An example is the symphysis pubis. (5) *Synovial joints.* These are the articulation joints with which we are primarily concerned. They represent a highly specialized type of joint designed to provide varying degrees of free motion. Essentially, they comprise bone ends capped with articular cartilage. Each joint is enclosed by a fibrous capsule lined by a synovial membrane and forms a closed space. In some specialized joints, such as the knee and the temporomandibular joint, intra-articular structures such as menisci are found which have specific functions necessary to the peculiarities of the individual joint.

The *synovial membrane* is a highly specialized connective tissue membrane composed of synovial cells and collagen fibers embedded in a gorund substance. This membrane, particularly at the periphery of the joint. has a rich capillary network and falls into folds and villi which project from the surface.

The *synovial fluid*, found in synovial joints, is essentially a dialysate of the blood. It contains hyaluronic acid which is a mucin and is responsible for the viscosity of the fluid. From a functional point of view, the synovial fluid plays an important role in the normal mechanics of synovial joints. Being in a closed space during motion, the synovial fluid forms a thin film over each articular surface and, inasmuch as fluid is incompressible, it protects the underlying articular cartilage. The formation of the film over the articular cartilage is brought about by the normal incongruity of the joint—in many instances by the presence of menisci and other intra-articular structures which favor the formation of an adequate film during motion. It becomes apparent that any disorder which impairs the formation of this important film of fluid predisposes the bone, particularly the cartilage, to degenerative changes. This is a common occurrence following ruptures and tears of the menisci in the knee joint and in the temporomandibular joint.

Inasmuch as the *ends* of the *bone*, in synovial joints, comprise cancellous bone which is vascular and supplied by end arteries, these areas are frequently the site of acute infection produced by organisms circulating in the blood stream and lodging in the terminal vessels. Such is the case in instances of suppurative arthritis and tuberculosis.

Finally, synovial joints are richly *innervated* by proprioceptive fibers and pain fibers. Hence, diseases of the central nervous system are frequently reflected in such joints. This is particularly true of those lesions which cause destruction of the proprioceptive and pain fibers subjecting the articulation to repeated abnormal stress and strain beyond the control of the patient. Such changes result in the so-called neurotrophic joint as described by Charcot and occur as a result of other lesions of the central nervous system.

CONGENITAL ANOMALIES

Developmental malformations of joints are often associated with developmental malformations of bones (Mercer). They may be listed as follows: (1) *absence*—seen in conjunction with absence of bones, (2) *genu varum*— knees abnormally separated (bowleg), usually acquired and due to rickets, (3) *genu valgum*—knees abnormally close together and commonly called knock-knee, (4) *genu recurvatum*—congenital hyperextension of the knee due to intra-uterine degeneration and contracture of the extensor quadriceps tendon, (5) *talipes equinovarus*—clubfoot or a foot which is turned inward to varying degrees, possibly due to imbalance between a strong anterior tibial muscle and subnormal or agenetic peroneals (Flinchum), and consisting of flexion of the ankle, inversion of the foot, adduction of the forefoot, and medial rotation of the tibia, (6) *dystrophy* of the *little finger*— lateral curvature of the distal phalanx of the fifth finger, (7) *symphalangism* —fusion of the interphalangeal joints (Barsky), and (8) *dislocations*. Congenital dislocations are found in the (*a*) *hip* occurring when the acetabulum retains its shallow embryonic composition and, less commonly, when the muscles of the proximal end of the femur become fibrosed, allowing the pelvis to "grow away" from the femoral head, consisting of varying degrees of anterior or posterior displacement of the head of the femur (Hart), and diagnosed by physical examination and roentgenographic studies (Kite), (*b*) *shoulder* occurring, in most instances, as a result of birth trauma and consisting of a posterior and subspinous displacement, and (*c*) *wrist* being rare, actually occurring as a result of postnatal trauma, and consisting of a forward displacement of the radius and more distal portions of the extremity leaving the ulna in the normal position.

DEGENERATIONS

Orientation.—As in other organs and tissues of the body, degenerations of joints are common in conjunction with every articular disease process. In addition, four predominantly degenerative disorders are gout, Charcot's joint, cysts of semilunar cartilages, and painful shoulder.

Gout.—Gout (L. = drop) is a hereditary disorder of purine (uric acid) metabolism characterized by increasingly more frequent, sudden, acute, extremely painful, nocturnal attacks of arthritis involving the big toe, other areas of the feet, the hands, and other joints (Weiss and Stecker). The condition *occurs* in both males and females but predominates in males and generally originates in the third to the sixth decades of life. Preceding and during an attack, the uric acid level of the blood is elevated. *Pathologically* the disorder consists of depositions of monosodium urate in various tissues of the body including the periarticular structures of the joints mentioned together with the ear, olecranon bursa, and even renal parenchyma. The deposits are referred to as *tophi*. *Grossly* they vary in size

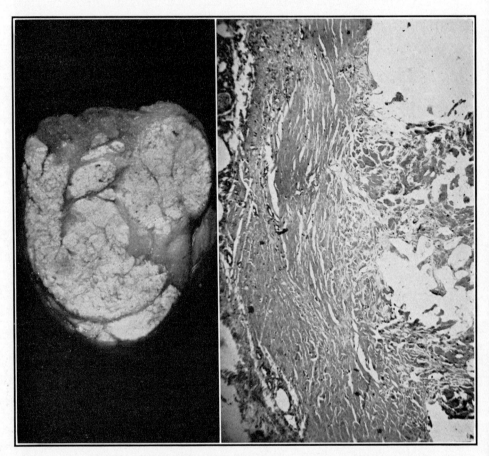

FIG. 640.—Gout showing a chalky deposit grossly and necrotic and crystalline material, collagenous fibrous tissue, and a peripheral inflammatory zone microscopically. × 50.

from a few millimeters to many centimeters. They consist of a conglomerate collection of cream-colored to gray, crumbly, chalky material embedded in and surrounded by dense collagenous fibrous tissue (Fig. 640). While the deposits are primarily periarticular they also extend into the joint by way of pannus (flat, apron-like mass of tissue) formation. *Histologically* the lesion is a granuloma consisting of (1) a central zone of urates, cholesterol, and necrotic debris, (2) a surrounding inflammatory zone of lymphocytes, plasma cells, and epithelioid cells, and (3) a peripheral zone of dense fibrous tissue (Rosenberg). As the lesion ages, the inflammatory cells tend to disappear, leaving a central crystalline and necrotic area and a peripheral sclerotic zone. The chief ultimate *complication* is renal impairment (Talbott). The *diagnosis* is made from the history, physical examination, increased uric acid level of the blood, and roentgenographic demonstration of osteoporosis adjacent to the deposits. *Treatment* consists of rest, low purine diet, and administration of drugs (colchicine, cortisone, phenylbutazone, etc.) (Smyth). The *prognosis* as to life is good but the morbidity is high.

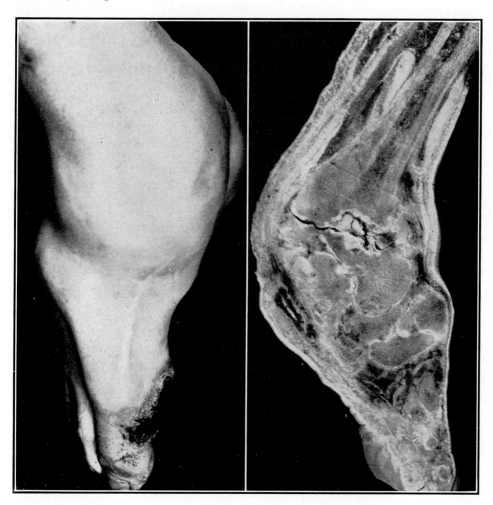

Fig. 641.—Charcot's joint illustrating the external and cut surface of an affected and markedly deformed ankle joint. Note the secondary traumatic ulcer of the great toe.

Charcot's Joint.—In 1868, Charcot described a degenerative condition of joints that accompanies central nervous system lesions to which his name has subsequently been attached (Steindler). While the lesion is usually an *accompaniment* of tabes dorsalis (syphilis of the spinal cord) it may also occur in conjunction with syringomyelia, trauma to the spinal cord, trauma to posterior nerve roots, tumors of the cord, spina bifida, tuberculosis of the spine, acute myelitis, diabetes mellitus, etc. (Delano and Sheppe). The condition usually *occurs* after the second decade of life and is somewhat more frequent in males than in females. It is probably *due to* trauma consequent to loss of sensitivity from disruption of the nervous reflex arc. The *joints* most commonly affected are the ankle, foot, knee, and hip.

Pathologically the process consists of extensive degeneration, necrosis, and destruction of the bones of the joint accompanied by exostosis, fragmentation, joint bodies, fractures, dislocations, and deformities (Fig. 641). The articular and periarticular tissues reveal degeneration, relaxation of ligaments, tears, secondary inflammation, and fibrosis. Ankylosis, however, does not occur. In fact, due to the destructive changes mentioned, the joint becomes hypermobile. The chief *complications* consist of secondary infection and dysfunction. The *clinical manifestations* consist of painless effusion and swelling, abnormal mobility, loss of sensation, and fractures. *Roentgenograms* disclose the retrogressive changes seen pathologically. *Treatment* is conservative by way of immobilization or operative by way of arthrodesis or amputation. The *prognosis* is fair to poor.

Cysts Semilunar Cartilages.—Cysts of the semilunar cartilages *represent* mucoid degeneration of the menisci and are probably of traumatic origin (Mercer). The condition usually *occurs* between the ages of twenty and thirty years and is more common in males. *Pathologically* the lateral meniscus is affected more frequently than the medial one and the changes are more pronounced in the lateral portions of the cartilaginous structures. The lesion consists of many small or one or more larger cysts filled with mucoid material. The *clinical manifestations* consist of swelling, pain, and limitation of motion of the affected knee. Although conservative measures may be employed, *surgical removal* alone effects a sure cure.

Painful Shoulder.—A painful shoulder is, of course, a symptom and not a disease. The *causes* of pain in the shoulder are numerous but since the most common single factor is degeneration within the shoulder and periarticular structures the more important conditions may be listed here (De Palma and Coventry). They include (1) *musculoskeletal* factors such as tendinitis, calcareous deposits, ruptured supraspinatus, ruptured cuff, tenosynovitis of biceps, arthritis, trauma, overuse, tumors, and immobilizing lesions, (2) *neurologic* factors such as syringomyelia, intramedullary tumors, and inflammation of, pressure on, or trauma to nerve roots, (3) *visceral* disturbances in the thorax or abdomen by way of reflex and referred stimuli, and (4) *peripheral vascular* lesions such as arteriosclerosis, Raynaud's disease, arterial aneurysm, phlebitis, lymphangiitis, etc.

INFLAMMATIONS

Orientation.—Inflammation of the synovial membrane is known as *synovitis* while inflammation of the joint as a whole is called *arthritis*. Although there are many *classifications* depending upon (1) the time of involvement as acute, subacute, or chronic, (2) the type of process as atrophic or hypertrophic, (3) the anatomic structures involved as osteo-arthritis, vertebral, navicular, etc., (4) the causative factor as allergic, tuberculous, pneumococcal, etc., (5) the number of joints affected as monarticular or polyarticular, (6) the author describing the process as Charcot's, Schüller's, etc., none is entirely satisfactory and, therefore, a combination of classifications must be used. The more inportant lesions are suppurative arthritis, tuberculosis, syphilis, rheumatic arthritis (p. 300), rheumatoid arthritis, ankylosing spondylitis, osteo-arthritis, hemophilic arthritis, Heberden's nodes, and villonodular synovitis.

Suppurative Arthritis.—Suppurative arthritis may be *defined* as infection of the joint by pus-producing *organisms*. The more common of these are pneumococci, staphylococci, and gonococci, although at times any organism may act as the causative agent (Blackford, Hench, and Robinson). Their *source* is often some other focus of infection in the body. The *route* of invasion is generally the bloodstream but direct extension from adjacent tissues (especially bone) or invasion from the outside (as a result of a penetrating wound) also happens occasionally. Suppurative arthritis

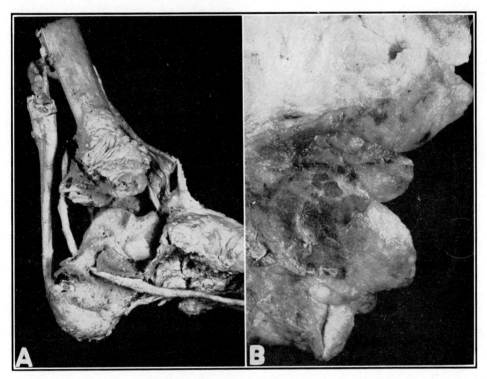

Fig. 642.—Tuberculous arthritis showing *A*, extensive destruction of the ankle joint and *B*, pannus formation.

occurs at all ages but is most common in the third and fourth decades of life. It has no predilection for either sex. Although any *joint* may be involved, those most frequently affected are knee, ankle, wrist, shoulder, hip, and elbow. The *pathologic* picture varies with the precise organism and the severity of involvement. In less severe cases, the synovial membrane discloses thickening, congestion, and edema and the joint space contains an excess of cloudy fluid. In more severe cases the synovial membrane reveals extensive thickening and ulceration with the latter also affecting not only the articular cartilages but also the adjacent bone. In such instances, the joint cavity is distended with pus. *Histologically* the entire process is nonspecific consisting essentially of neutrophilic infiltration in early stages and of plasma cell and lymphocytic infiltration in later stages. The chief *complications* are systemic spread of infection to distant areas and residual ankylosis. General *clinical manifesta-tions* consist of chills, fever, sweating, and leukocytosis while local mani-festations consist of pain, swelling, redness, tenderness, and limitation of motion. *Roentgenograms* reveal swelling of soft tissues, enlargement of the joint space, and destruction of articular surfaces. The *diagnosis* is made from the history, clinical manifestations, roentgenograms, and exam-ination of aspirated fluid. *Treatment* consists of administration of anti-biotics and of aspiration or surgical drainage when necessary. The *prognosis* is variable but the results are generally good.

Tuberculosis.—Tuberculous arthritis is always secondary to tubercu-losis elsewhere (lungs or lymph nodes) in the body (Balboni). The con-dition usually *occurs* in the first two decades of life but may be found at any age and affects both sexes with equal frequency. As a rule, the disease affects only one joint but occasionally several *joints* may be involved. The most common sites are spine (called Pott's disease or tuberculous spondy-litis), knee, hip, elbow, ankle, sacro-iliac, shoulder, and wrist. *Pathologically* the infection involves the synovial membrane, bone, and cartilage. The synovial membrane becomes thick, edematous, fibrous, and studded with tubercles (Fig. 642). As the process ages, a pannus of tuberculous granula-tion tissue covers and destroys the articular cartilage. When the articular surfaces are closely applied the granulation tissue erodes from the outside or penetrates behind the cartilage, resulting in its complete detachment. Secondarily, too, the underlying bone may be eroded, producing extensive destruction of all structures. Thus, the joint cavity may be converted into a pocket of tuberculous pus containing fragments of sequestrated cartilage and bone. The *complications* consist of progression of the process to form (cold) abscesses and sinuses in adjacent tissues, hematogenous dissemina-tion to distant areas, fibrous ankylosis of the joint, and amyloidosis. Gen-eral *clinical manifestations* consist of loss of weight with slight or no fever while local manifestations include doughy swelling of the joint, pain, stiffness, heat, limp on walking, spasm of muscles, limitation of motion, tenderness, and atrophy of muscles. *Roentgenograms* are not specific, dis-closing periarticular swelling, destruction of cartilage with narrowing of the joint space, and bony destruction with sequestration. The *diagnosis* is made from the history, clinical manifestations, roentgenograms, biopsy, and isolation of the tubercle bacillus. *Treatment* includes the usual anti-tuberculosis measures, antibiotic and chemotherapeutic agents, and some form of immobilization. The *prognosis*, as far as restoring joint function is concerned, is poor.

Syphilis.—With adequate early treatment of syphilis, syphilitic arthritis is now rare (Balboni). The condition may *occur* in any stage of either the congenital or acquired form of the disease. In *congenital syphilis* there may occur (1) *Parrot's syphilitic osteochondritis*—seen in about 5 per cent of syphilitic children, occurring in the first three weeks of life, affecting the upper extremity more often than the lower, and consisting of a gelat-inous degeneration in the bone and cartilage with a greenish effusion, (2) *symmetrical synovitis*—seen between the ages of eight and sixteen years, affecting the knees or elbows, and consisting of a symmetrical swelling of periarticular tissues and effusion of clear fluid into the joint cavities, and (3) *syphilitic dactylitis*—occurring at ages from one to three years, consisting of a spindle-shaped swelling of the fingers and toes, and affecting not only the joints but also the bones.

In *secondary syphilis* arthritic involvement may consist of (1) *arthralgia*—

occurring in about 10 per cent of cases and consisting simply of joint pains, (2) *syphilitic arthritis*—being rare, affecting several (and usually large) joints such as the knees, and consisting of fusiform swelling of the joints, thickening of the synovial membrane and periarticular tissue, and some muscle spasm, (3) *hydrarthrosis*—usually being polyarticular and consisting of transient watery effusion, (4) *tenosynovitis*, (4) *bursitis*, and (5) *spondylitis*—consisting of inflammation of the periosteum of the vertebræ, especially in the cervical area.

In *tertiary syphilis* arthritic involvement may consist of (1) *gummatous arthritis*—seen in early tertiary stages but also in some cases of congenital syphilis, affecting larger joints, characterized by swelling of the joint, effusion, and varying degrees of pain, and consisting of involvement of the synovial membrane, cartilage, and/or bone, (2) *juxta-articular gummas*—

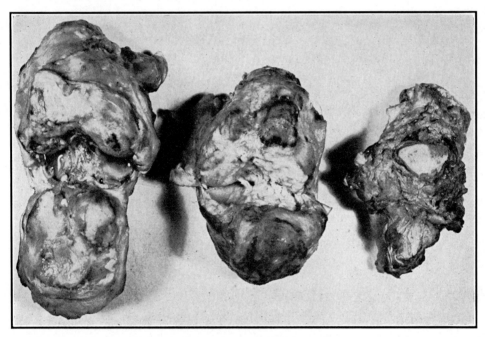

FIG. 643.—Rheumatoid arthritis disclosing villi, pannus formation, erosions, and distortion in several joints.

arising in tissues adjacent to joints but involving the latter by impingement, and (3) *Charcot's joint* (p. 1273). The *diagnosis* of syphilitic arthritis is made from the history, clinical manifestations, positive serologic tests, and response to penicillin therapy. The *prognosis*, except when there is extensive destruction of tissues, is good.

Rheumatoid Arthritis.—Rheumatoid arthritis is a chronic, destructive, nonsuppurative disease of joints that *occurs* most commonly during the second and third decades of life and affects females twice as often as males (Luck). The *cause* of the condition remains unknown but the *theories* may be listed as follows: (1) infection by streptococci—based not upon isolation of the organisms but upon positive agglutination tests, (2) allergy—to a variety of proteins including those of bacterial (streptococcic) origin, and (3) endocrine imbalances—embracing a number of hormones but having proof that only ACTH and cortisone produce an appreciable response in the disease (Bauer). The disease is characteristically *polyarticular* and the *sites* most commonly affected are hands, feet, wrists, knees, elbows, ankles, hips, spine, and temporomandibular joints.

Pathologically the disorder is primarily a synovitis (Gibson). Early in the course of the disease the synovial membrane is swollen, congested, and edematous. The lining cells proliferate to three or more layers in thickness and the underlying tissue is permeated with leukocytes. Gradually, villous processes project into the joint cavity and, with the advent of degeneration, the villi become necrotic and are extruded into the joint cavity either whole or as atheromatous material. The necrosis is of a fibrinoid nature and at its junction with living tissue fibroblasts and epithelioid cells become conspicuously arranged at right angles to the surface. The leukocytic cells are mostly plasma cells, lymphocytes, and monocytes. They invade not only the synovia but also the periarticular structures. Concomitantly there is usually an effusion of a turbid fluid. Aside from villous formation, the synovial membrane also responds by producing a pannus of similar (at first of granulation and later of fibrous) tissue. As the pannus forms it erodes both the articular cartilages from without and also the underlying bone resulting ultimately in extensive destruction and distortion of the entire joint (Fig. 643). Rheumatoid arthritis affects not only joints but also *extra-articular tissues*. The latter changes consist of (1) *subcutaneous nodules*—occurring in about one-quarter of all cases, resulting from trauma, found over bony prominences such as the olecranon, and consisting of a central area of necrosis encircled by connective tissue and epithelioid cells arranged at right angles to the surface and surrounded more peripherally by a fibrous tissue capsule (Sokoloff), (2) *cardiac changes*—identical with or resembling those in rheumatic fever (p. 293) (Bradfield), (3) *muscle lesions*—consisting of degeneration, atrophy, fatty infiltration, spotty necrosis, increase in number of nuclei of the fibers, and perivascular infiltration with round cells (Traut), (4) *lymph node changes*—consisting of follicular hyperplasia, increased reticulo-endothelial activity, proliferation of connective tissue, and lymphocytic invasion of the capsule (Motulsky), and (5) *nerve lesions*—occurring in the perineural connective tissue and consisting of focal necrosis, epithelioid reaction, and leukocytic infiltration (Gibson).

The chief *complications* of rheumatoid arthritis are crippling deformities, locomotor disability, and (occasionally) amyloidosis (Unger). *Clinically* the onset may be acute or insidious with wave after wave of attacks (Mercer). The manifestations consist of stiffness, localized sweating, decreased surface temperature, deformity with flexion or subluxation, pain, crepitus, increasing ankylosis, general lassitude, atrophy of muscles, feeble circulation, sallow skin, etc. *Roentgenograms* disclose diminution in size of the joint space, erosions of bone, and juxta-articular osteoporosis (Fletcher). The *diagnosis* is made from the history, clinical manifestations, and roentgenographic appearance. Aside from general medical care and physiotherapy, *treatment* consists of administration of cortisone, ACTH, and gold compounds (Levin, Ward, and Batterman). The *prognosis* is always guarded for the condition recurs and at least some degree of ankylosis is inevitable.

Ankylosing Spondylitis.—Ankylosing spondylitis (also known as Marie-Strümpell and rheumatoid spondylitis) is a chronic nonsuppurative inflammation of the spine that is usually classed in the group of rheumatoid diseases. The condition generally *starts* in patients between the ages of fifteen and thirty-five years and is about nine times as common in males as it is in females (Polley). The *cause* of the disorder is unknown but foci of infection, infectious diseases, trauma, and endocrine imbalances have all been held to play etiologic roles (Crenshaw). The process generally begins in the *lumbar* segment of the spine and then spreads inferiorly and superiorly but involvement of the hip, sternoclavicular, and other peripheral joints also occurs not infrequently.

Pathologically the disorder is similar to that in rheumatoid arthritis (Crenshaw). The changes consist of synovitis, chondritis, and juxta-articular osteitis. The leukocytic infiltration is of a plasma cell, lympho-cytic, and monocytic variety. Villi and granulation tissue grow from the synovial membrane destroying the cartilage and bone, filling the joint space, and ultimately causing calcific and bony ankylosis. The subchondral osseous tissue of juxta-articular bones becomes osteoporotic. In the spine, the paraspinal ligaments become calcified and ossified.

The *clinical manifestations* consist of periodic attacks of excruciating root pain distributed, of course, along the course of the nerves that emerge from the vertebral segments involved. Since the lumbar segment is often affected, sciatica is frequently an initial complaint. Other manifestations consist of swelling, redness, and tenderness of the area affected. The only pertinent laboratory findings are leukocytosis and an increase in sedimenta-tion rate. Ultimately, complete bony ankylosis results. Since the flexor muscles of the spine are stronger than the extensor muscles, their spasm (during the acute stage) causes kyphosis and, if care is not taken, the spine is ultimately fixed in this position. *Roentgenographically* there are no demon-strable changes early in the course of the disease but as the process ages the following develop: loss of sharp outline of the joint boundaries, juxta-articular osteosclerosis, osteoporosis, and calcification of the paraspinous ligaments. The *diagnosis* is made from the history, clinical manifestations, and roentgenograms. *Treatment* consists of maintenance of correct posture, relief of pain by aspirin, administration of cortisone and ACTH, roentgen therapy, and (when deformities have developed) corrective surgical pro-cedures (Hart and Potter). The *prognosis* as far as life is concerned is good but the morbidity is often great. Usually the disorder "burns itself out" in from ten to fifteen years.

Osteo-arthritis.—Osteo-arthritis is really a degenerative condition that is *found* to greater or lesser degree in all persons over the age of fifty years (Kuhns). The *causes* remain unknown but aging, obesity, and trauma seem to play leading roles. The larger *joints* are most commonly involved with those of the hands, feet, and other areas also often affected (Mercer). *Pathologically* the initial change consists of irregular degeneration, soften-ing, and erosion of the articular cartilage, leaving at first patchy and later complete denudation of the underlying bone. Simultaneously the periph-eral perichondrium and periosteum are stimulated producing irregular cartilaginous and osseous lipping about the circumference of the articular surface. The synovial membrane too is stimulated to proliferation, result-ing in the formation of irregular villi and adhesions. Ultimately, separation of fibrous, cartilaginous, and osseous tissues occurs, producing loose bodies (joint mice) within the joints. *Clinical manifestations* are present only in a minority of patients. They consist essentially of pain, swelling, and limitation of motion. *Roentgenograms* reveal normal bony texture, reduction in joint space, irregularity of articular surfaces, and spurs or

lipping about the periphery. The *diagnosis* is made from the clinical manifestations and roentgenograms. *Treatment* is symptomatic (with avoidance
of undue stresses and strains), physiotherapeutic, and occasionally surgical.
The *prognosis* on the whole is good.

Hemophilic Arthritis.—This condition occurs in hemophiliacs and stems
from bleeding into a joint (Luck). The *joints* affected are usually the
knees, hips, elbows, and shoulders. *Pathologically* the joint capsule thick-

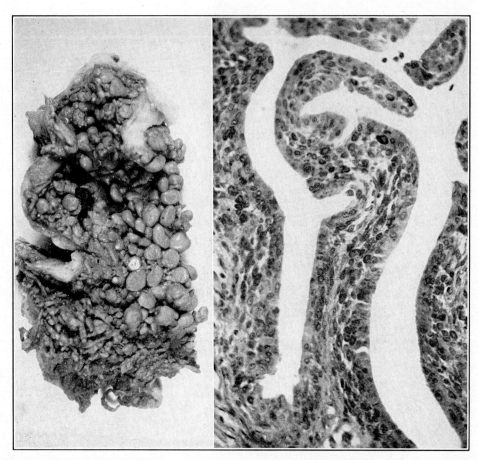

Fig. 644.—Villonodular synovitis illustrating numerous slender and bulbous villi studding the
synovia and a villus covered with hyperplastic synovial cells and containing a core of cellular
connective tissue permeated with hemosiderin granules. × 200.

ens, the synovial membrane becomes villous, the articular cartilage undergoes degeneration and erosion, and the subchondral bone becomes porotic.
Clinically the disorder starts in childhood and consists of repeated attacks
of effusion with pain, swelling, and tenderness. Ultimately the joint becomes permanently swollen and motion is generally impaired. *Treatment*
is prophylactic and symptomatic. The *prognosis* is guarded for the process
tends to recur.

Heberden's Nodes.—Heberden's nodes consist of small (usually up to
1 cm. in diameter) extra-articular nodules that occur opposite interphalangeal joints in osteo-arthritis and less commonly in other chronic arthritic

conditions (Stecher and Kellgren). They are more common in women than men, are often associated with trauma, and consist of either non-specific soft tissue swellings or of actual bony excrescences.

Villonodular Synovitis.—Villonodular synovitis is a benign hyperplastic condition of the synovial membrane of usually the knee joint that predominates in young male adults (Jaffe). The lesion probably develops on an inflammatory basis but the precise *cause* remains undetermined. *Pathologically* it exists as a diffuse and a localized form. In either case, the synovial membrane is thickened by numerous slender or bulbous, yellow to brown villi of varying sizes (Fig. 644). *Histologically* the surface is covered with one or several layers of hyperplastic synovial cells and the core is composed of well-vascularized, cellular, connective tissue containing lymphocytes, plasma cells, monocytes, foam cells, occasional giant cells, and varying amounts of hemosiderin. *Clinically* the only important manifestations are intermittent pain and swelling and occasional locking of the joint. *Roentgenograms* show only soft tissue swelling. *Treatment* consists of surgical excision. The *prognosis* is good.

PHYSICAL DISTURBANCES

Orientation.—The more important physical disturbances affecting joints are hydrarthrosis, dislocation, sprain, and Baker's cyst.

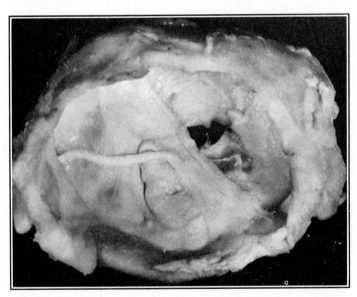

Fig. 645.—Baker's cyst disclosing a smooth-walled semipartitioned sac composed of dense sclerotic fibrous tissue.

Hydrarthrosis.—Hydrarthrosis (Gr. = water + joint) means simply an effusion of serous fluid into a joint cavity. While the condition may occur in conjunction with any low-grade mild inflammation, there is an entity known as *Clutton's joints* or *symmetrical hydrarthrosis* (Mercer). The disorder is found in children from eight to sixteen years of age, is of unknown cause, affects both knees, is insidious in onset, is not accompanied by pain or fever, and disappears spontaneously.

Dislocation.—As the term indicates, a dislocation (L. = apart + to place) or *luxation* of a joint connotes a displacement or disalignment of apposing bones. The condition may be congenital or acquired. The former usually occurs as a result of some maldevelopment in or around a joint while the latter is consequent to an acquired disease and/or trauma. The apposing bones may be only partly misplaced with portions of the articular surfaces still in partial apposition or they may be completely misplaced with one bone overriding the other. In either case, the capsule and ligaments of the joint are generally disrupted and the bones may be fractured.

Sprain.—A sprain may be defined as a wrenching of a joint with disruption of the surrounding capsule, ligaments, and other tissues but without dislocation of the apposing articular surfaces. The condition results from sudden twisting or trauma and, due to rupture of vessels, is characterized by hemorrhagic extravasation, rapid swelling, and discoloration. Clinically it is accompanied by severe pain and disability.

Baker's Cyst.—A Baker's cyst is a herniation of the synovial membrane through the posterior capsule of the knee joint (Meyerding). The condition *develops* because of a congenital weakness in the fibers of the oblique posterior ligament and enlarges as a result of motion of the knee. The *hernial sac* may measure as much as 10 cm. in diameter and, following the path of least resistance, may extend all the way to the heel (Fig. 645). The protrusion is usually unilocular and partially trabeculated, contains clear watery or mucoid fluid, and communicates with the joint by a narrow or wide ostium. Its wall is composed of dense fibrous tissue permeated with lymphocytes and lined by synovial cells. The *clinical manifestations* consist of aching and stiffness of the knee together with a fluctuant swelling in the popliteal area. *Treatment* consists of surgical excision. The *prognosis* is good.

TUMORS

Orientation.—Tumors of the joints are infrequent and not extremely varied. They may consist of lipoma, hemangioma, chondroma, giant cell tumor, and synovioma. Of these, the last mentioned only need be considered further.

Synovioma.—As the term indicates, a synovioma may be *defined* as a tumor arising in synovial tissue. It has *also* been *called* synovial sarcoma, synoviolosarcoma, synovioloma, and synovial fibrosarcoma (Sherman). From the synonyms listed, it is apparent that the lesion is malignant. It *occurs* at all ages but is most common in the second, third, and fourth decades of life and it has no predilection for either sex (Hale). The *cause* is unknown but trauma has been considered of etiologic importance in about one-quarter of the recorded cases. The precise *site* of origin is a joint or a tendon or bursa associated with a joint (Wright) and the most commonly affected joints are the knee, foot, wrist, hand, shoulder, ankle, and elbow. *Pathologically* the tumor grows slowly and may even appear encapsulated. It may measure from a few to 15 cm. in diameter and is composed of soft to firm, gray to mottled yellow and red, solid tissue that has a tendency to undergo focal necrosis, cyst formation, and even calcification (Fig. 646). While it invariably arises adjacent to bone, the growth sooner or later invades the cartilage, bone itself, and joint space causing extensive destruction and ultimately pathologic fracture. *Histologically* the lesion is usually composed of an intermingling of varying amounts of two types of neoplastic

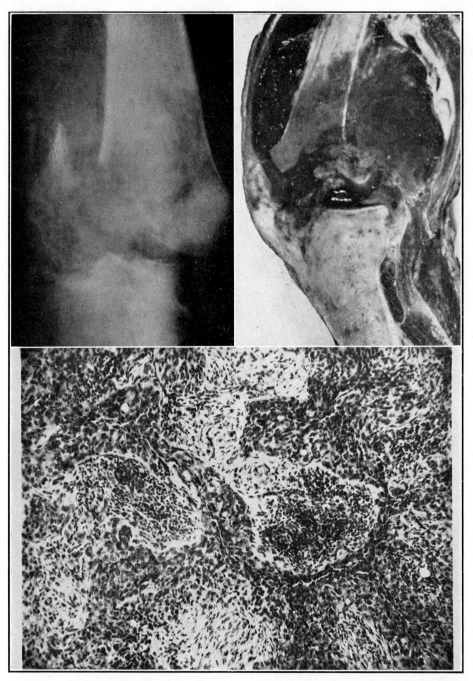

FIG. 646.—Synovioma showing a soft tissue mass eroding a femur and causing a pathologic fracture, a sagittal section of the amputated specimen, and a microscopic pattern of sarcomatous connective tissue and of irregular synovial (epithelial-like) cells. × 100.

cells—synovial and connective tissue (Bennett). The former exist as nests, strands, sheets, or glands of irregular, polyhedral, or cuboidal cells with a moderate amount of cytoplasm and irregular hyperchromatic nuclei. The connective tissue cells are identical with those of a fibrosarcoma and thus are most commonly elongated and ill defined, disclosing a moderate to scanty cytoplasm and elongated but hyperchromatic nuclei. The tumor *spreads* by local extension to surrounding structures and by metastasis to the lungs and other organs. The *clinical manifestations* consist of pain, swelling, tenderness, and disability. *Roentgenograms* reveal a more or less spherical soft tissue mass pressing upon and eroding bone. Calcification and periosteal reaction occur but are infrequent. The *diagnosis* is made from the history, clinical manifestations, roentgenograms, and biopsy. The only effective *treatment* is amputation or radical excision. The *prognosis* is fair to poor, with the recorded five-year survival rate being less than 10 per cent.

REFERENCES

General

LUCK, J. V.: *Bone and Joint Diseases*, Springfield, Charles C Thomas, 1950.
MERCER, W.: *Orthopedic Surgery*, 4th Ed., Baltimore, Williams & Wilkins Co., 1950.

Congenital Anomalies

BARSKY, A. J.: J. Bone & Joint Surg., *33*A, 35, 1951 (Anomalies of Hands).
FLINCHUM, D.: J. Bone & Joint Surg., *35*A, 111, 1953 (Talipes Equinovarus).
HART, V. L.: J. Bone & Joint Surg., *31*A, 357, 1949 (Dislocation Hip).
KITE, J. H., and KING, R. E.: Georgia M. A. J., *41*, 291, 1952 (Dislocation Hip).

Degenerations

COVENTRY, M. B.: J. A. M. A., *151*, 177, 1953 (Painful Shoulder).
DELANO, P. J.: Am. J. Roentgenol., *56*, 189, 1946 (Charcot's Joint).
DePALMA, A. F.: *Surgery of the Shoulder*, Philadelphia, J. B. Lippincott Co., 1950.
ROSENBERG, E. F., and ARENS, R. A.: Radiology, *49*, 169, 1947 (Gout).
SHEPPE, W. M.: Ann. Int. Med., *39*, 625, 1953 (Charcot's Joint in Diabetes).
SMYTH, C. J.: J. A. M. A., *152*, 1106, 1953 (Treatment Gout).
STECHER, R. M., *et al.*: Ann. Int. Med., *31*, 595, 1949 (Heredity of Gout).
STEINDLER, A., *et al.*: Urol. & Cutan. Rev., *46*, 633, 1942 (Charcot's Joint).
TALBOTT, J. H.: Ann. Int. Med., *31*, 555, 1949 (Complications Gout).
WEISS, T. E.: Am. Practitioner, *4*, 89, 1953 (Concepts in Gout).

Inflammations

BALBONI, V. G.: In Hollander—"*Comroe's Arthritis*," 5th Ed., Philadelphia, Lea & Febiger, 1953, p. 813 (Tuberculous Arthritis) and p. 831 (Syphilitic Arthritis).
BATTERMAN, R. C.: J. A. M. A., *152*, 1013, 1953 (Gold Treatment in Rheumatoid Arthritis).
BAUER, W., *et al.*: Practitioner, *166*, 5, 1951 (Etiology Rheumatoid Arthritis).
BLACHFORD, R. D.: Lancet, *1*, 26, 1953 (Suppurative Arthritis).
BRADFIELD, J. Y., and HEJTAMCIK, M. R.: A. M. A. Arch. Int. Med., *86*, 1, 1950 (Heart in Rheumatoid Arthritis).
CRENSHAW, A. H., and HAMILTON, J. F.: South. M. J., *45*, 1055, 1952 (Rheumatoid Spondylitis).
FLETCHER, D. E., and ROWLEY, K. A.: Brit. J. Radiol., *25*, 282, 1952 (Rheumatoid Arthritis).
GIBSON, H. J.: Practitioner, *166*, 54, 1951 (Pathology Rheumatoid Arthritis).
HART, F. D.: Brit. M. J., *1*, 188, 1952 (Cortisone and ACTH in Ankylosing Spondylitis).
HENCH, P. S., *et al.*: Ann. Int. Med., *28*, 66 and 309, 1948 (Arthritis).
JAFFE, H. L., *et al.*: A. M. A. Arch. Path., *31*, 731, 1941 (Villonodular Synovitis).
KELLGREN, J. H., and MOORE, R.: Brit. M. J., *1*, 181, 1952 (Osteo-arthritis and Heberden's Nodes).
KUHNS, J. G.: J. A. M. A., *151*, 98, 1953, (Osteo-arthritis).

LEVIN, M. H., *et al.;* Am. J. Med., *14*, 265, 1953, (Cortisone and ACTH in Rheumatoid Arthritis).
MOTULSKY, A. G., *et al.;* A. M. A. Arch. Int. Med., *90*, 660, 1952, (Lymph Nodes Rheumatoid Arthritis).
POLLEY, H. F., and SLOCUMB, C. H.: Ann. Int. Med., *26*, 240, 1947, (Rheumatoid Spondylitis).
POTTER, T. A.: Am. Practitioner, *1*, 1129, 1950, (Rheumatoid Spondylitis).
ROBINSON, J. A., *et al.;* Ann. Int. Med., *30*, 1212, 1949, (Gonococcal Arthritis).
SOKOLOFF, L., *et al.;* A. M. A. Arch. Path., *55*, 475, 1953, (Subcutaneous Nodule in Rheumatoid Arthritis).
STECHER, R. M.: Am. J. Roentgenol., *59*, 326, 1948, (Heberden's Nodes).
TRAUT, E. F., and CAMPIONE, K. M.: A. M. A. Arch. Int. Med., *89*, 724, 1952, (Muscle in Rheumatoid Arthritis).
UNGER, P. N., *et al.;* Am. J. M. Sc., *216*, 51, 1948, (Amyloidosis in Rheumatoid Arthritis).
WARD, L. E., *et al.;* J. A. M. A., *152*, 119, 1953, (Cortisone in Rheumatoid Arthritis).

Physical Disturbances

MEYERDING, H. W., and VAN DEMARK, R. E.: J. A. M. A., *122*, 858, 1943, (Baker's Cyst).

Tumors

BENNETT, G. A.: J. Bone & Joint Surg., *29*, 259, 1947, (Synovioma).
HALE, D. E.: Am. J. Roentgenol., *65*, 769, 1951, (Synovioma).
SHERMAN, R. S., and CHU, F. C. H.: Am. J. Roentgenol., *67*, 80, 1952, (Synovioma).
WRIGHT, C. J. E.: J. Path. & Bact., *64*, 585, 1952, (Synovioma).

Chapter

37

Fascias, Tendons, and Bursas

PATHOLOGIC PHYSIOLOGY

Anthony F. DePalma

Numerous *fascias* are found throughout the body. They comprise collagenous fibers forming a structure of varying thickness depending upon its location and function. In general, fascias are primarily concerned with enclosing muscle masses and separating muscle groups. By so doing, the direction of function of the muscle mass is determined. In addition, fascias are found in the region of joints where they provide support to the articulation. It becomes apparent that (1) these structures may be severely injured by trauma whereby the fascial coverings are ruptured allowing herniation of muscle masses or (2) they may be the site of an inflammatory process called fasciitis, either due to trauma such as excessive friction or infection. This results in adhesions of the fascia to the surrounding tissue, thereby affecting the function of the underlying structure, particularly if it is a muscle of a joint.

Tendons comprise collagen fibers and, in many instances, are surrounded by synovial sheaths encountered, for example, in the tendons of the hand and foot. A tendon usually inserts in bone and through the action of its muscle, activates the joint that it traverses. The most important disorder involving a tendon is an infection implicating its synovial sheath. This usually results in a hyperplastic reaction of the covering thereby restricting the tendon's range of motion and obliterating its gliding mechanism. This may have serious consequences because, being motorized by the tendons, it results in dysfunction of the joints. Tendons are also very vulnerable to serious trauma. As a rule, they are in an exposed position such as in the hand and foot and, hence, may be severed or lacerated. Severance of a tendon, of course, means complete loss of the function of the joint motorized by that tendon. Other disorders noted in tendons are those that implicate connective tissue in general, particularly disturbances involving primarily the collagen fibers. Tendons also exhibit the consequences of excessive stress and strain incident to function. The synovial sheath becomes hyperplastic and the tendon becomes shredded. The biceps tendon is a frequent site of such alterations. Also tendons may be the site of calcareous deposits secondary to local degenerative processes in the tendon fibers.

Bursas are closed spaces enclosed by a fibrous capsule and lined by a synovial membrane. These structures are usually located at points of maximum friction or pressure. As a rule, they are found between bone and the origins and insertions of tendons or between tendons. Occasionally, they comprise herniation of synovial membranes of a joint, such as occurs on the porterior aspect of the knee joint. Adventitious bursas may be formed in abnormal situations resulting from excessive pressure and friction. These are usually subcutaneous in position and are frequently found in the region of the prepatellar area or the olecranon area. The infections that implicate the bursas are the same as those implicating any synovial cavity. Since many of the bursas are found in vulnerable places they are often the site of infection as a result of direct continuity of the process from surrounding tissues.

GENERAL CONSIDERATIONS

Although the disorders of fascias, tendons, and bursas are many and although they involve widely separated regions of the body, the more important lesions may be considered under the following headings: fasciitis, bursitis, tenosynovitis, Dupuytren's contracture, ganglion, fibromatosis, and giant cell tumor.

Fasciitis.—Fasciitis is simply an inflammation of fascias. The disorder is seen in connection with a variety of inflammations of the subcutaneous tissues, muscles, and joints. Of special interest, perhaps, is the condition referred to as *necrotizing fasciitis* (Wilson). Some of the *synonyms* are gangrenous erysipelas, necrotizing erysipelas, and hospital gangrene. The *cause* of the infection is bacterial invasion, usually by hemolytic streptococci or staphylococci, and the condition may occur spontaneously or be preceded by an operative wound or an injury of one type or another. Once the *infection* is established it may progress extremely rapidly, may progress slowly, or may be dormant and then flare up. *Pathologically* the disorder consists essentially of widespread necrosis and gangrene of fascias often accompanied by cellulitis, diffuse hyperemia, ecchymoses, blisters, and gangrene of the overlying subcutaneous tissues and skin. The vastness of the process is due not only to the organisms as such but also to a concomitant venous thrombosis. The *clinical manifestations* are those of the local disturbances as outlined along with a systemic reaction of varying intensity. *Treatment* consists of surgical incision of the entire extent of involvement together with administration of antibiotics. The *prognosis* is generally good with an over-all mortality rate under 10 per cent.

Bursitis.—The term bursitis connotes inflammation of a bursa (Adams). The condition may *result from* bacterial infection, trauma, or degenerative changes in the underlying tendon. Of these, the two mentioned last are the most important. Bursitis is more common in males than in females and *occurs* with increasing frequency as the years advance. The *bursas* most often affected, in decreasing order of involvement, are (1) subdeltoid or subcoracoid bursa of the shoulder, (2) olecranon bursa over the tip of the olecranon process, (3) prepatellar bursa between the patella and overlying skin, (4) radiohumeral bursa over the lateral radial head, and (5) miscellaneous as gluteal, subcutaneous tibial, trochanteric, and gluteal femoral. In bursas that overly tendons, such as in the shoulder, the *pathologic* process usually starts in the tendon itself. It consists first of fibrillation and then of the formation of rice-like bodies and pultaceous material which, upon reaching the bursa, produces the inflammation. In bursas not overlying tendons, the inflammation is generally brought about by repeated trauma and, as already stated, only rarely is bacterial invasion the initiating factor. At any rate, the bursal involvement may be acute, subacute, or chronic. The lumen of the bursa is distended with watery, gelatinous, purulent, or cheesy material. The inner surface is usually rough and the wall is thick, unyielding, and fibrotic (Fig. 647). Calcification often occurs in the wall and in the inspissated contents. *Histologically* the process consists of nonspecific plasma cell, lymphocytic, and monocytic infiltration and of collagenization. The *clinical manifestations* consist of pain, interference in motion, and disability. The *diagnosis* is made from the history, physical examination, and roentgenographic appearance. *Treatment* of acute bursitis consists of supportive measures, resting of the part, physiotherapy, and occasionally of aspirating and washing out the sac. Treatment of chronic bursitis is surgical. The ultimate *prognosis* is generally good.

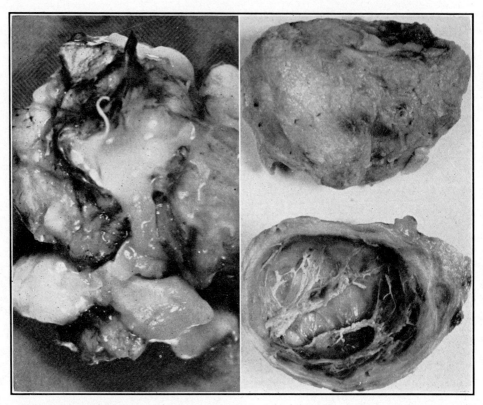

FIG. 647.—Bursitis showing (to the left) a greatly thickened fibrotic wall and a lumen filled with gelatinous material and (to the right) a fibrotic wall with a rough, partially trabeculated inner surface.

Tenosynovitis.—The term *tenosynovitis* means inflammation of a tendon sheath but actually encompasses inflammation of both the sheath itself (synovitis) and the tendon (tendinitis). The condition *occurs* at all ages and in both sexes but is perhaps more common after the third decade of life and in males. The *sites* of involvement are wherever there are tendons encased by synovial membranes but with the hands, shoulders, forearms, and ankles being most commonly affected. The *pathologic* appearance varies with the type of infection. The most common is *traumatic* tenosynovitis (Lapidus, Rhodes, Lipscomb, and Steen). In its simplest form this arises as a result of trauma as from rubbing of an unyielding shoe. Because of exudation of fibrin the area grates upon moving, unless the sheath becomes distended with fluid. If the trauma persists, such as in mechanics and other occupations, the sterile inflammation is attended by organization, thickening of the sheath, adhesion formation, and degeneration and disruption of the corresponding tendon. The next most common type of tenosynovitis is the *suppurative* variety caused by ordinary pyogenic organisms (Flynn). This type usually affects the tendons and sheaths of the hands, with the organisms gaining entrance by traumatic penetration from without or by extension from adjacent structures. Lesions in this

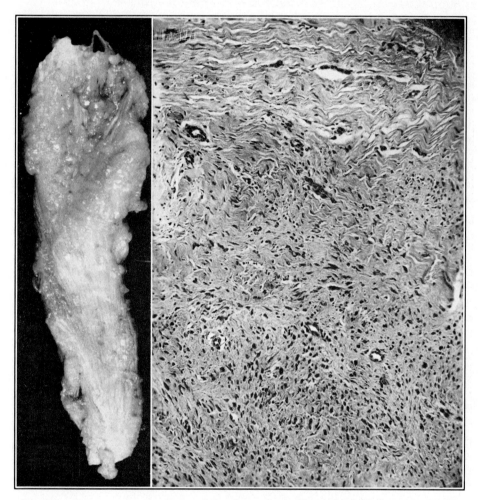

FIG. 648.—Dupuytren's contracture of the plantar fascia illustrating nodular thickening of the fascia grossly and both cellular and collagenous fibrous tissue microscopically. × 100.

category consist of nonspecific reactions attended by varying amounts of pus formation. The least common type of tenosynovitis is the *tuberculous* variety (Bickel). The infection may arise as a result of inoculation of bovine bacilli from the outside, as in butchers and farmers, but like other forms of tuberculosis is generally secondary to tuberculosis in other areas of the body. The tendons of the wrist are most commonly affected and the pathologic changes are similar to those in other tuberculous infections. The *clinical manifestations* of tenosynovitis are swelling, pain, stiffness, and crepitation or grating. The *diagnosis* is made from the history and careful physical examination. *Treatment* is removal of the cause in the traumatic variety and administration of antibiotics, surgical drainage, or synovectomy in the infectious type. The *prognosis* is fair to good.

Dupuytren's Contracture. — Dupuytren's contracture may be defined as fibrosis and contracture of the palmar and rarely the plantar fascias (Mason, Ross, Matthews, and Meyerding). The condition was first described by Dupuytren in 1832. It is much more common in males than in females, *occurs* after the second decade of life with an average in the fifth decade,

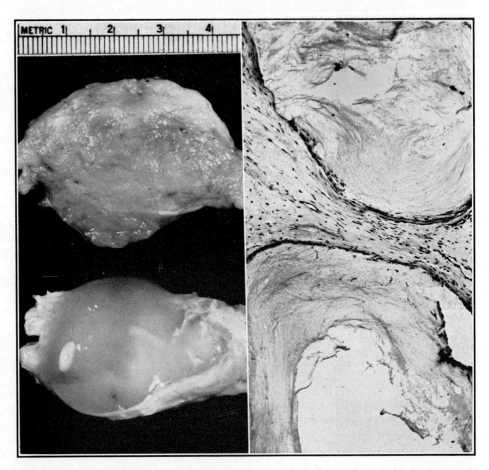

Fig. 649.—Ganglion disclosing the external and cut surface of a cystic mass filled with mucoid material and a multicystic structure composed of a collagenous wall and a lumen filled with slightly basophilic material. × 100.

and has a definite familial incidence. Aside from a hereditary factor, the most important causative factor is repeated minor trauma. *Pathologically* the lesion is characterized by diffuse or nodular fibrous thickening and shortening of the palmar and/or plantar fascias (Fig. 648). It has a tendency to be bilateral. *Histologically* the initial changes consist of cellular proliferations of fibroblastic tissue that may readily be mistaken for sarcoma. In such lesions, the vessels may be prominent and may disclose perivascular accumulations of lymphocytes, monocytes, and plasma cells. As the condition ages, the vessels become less conspicuous, the leukocytes disappear, and ever increasing amounts of collagen are deposited within the affected structures. The *complications* consist of flexion of the digits and increasing immobility of the joints. The *clinical manifestations* are those of the complications. The initial complaint is stiffness of the joints and this is followed after varied intervals of time by contraction deformities of the fingers and/or toes. Tingling sensations and pain may occur but are not prominent features. The *diagnosis* is made from the history and physical findings of a shortened, taut, nodular fascia causing flexion deformities of the digits. *Treatment* of choice is complete surgical excision. The *prognosis* is good.

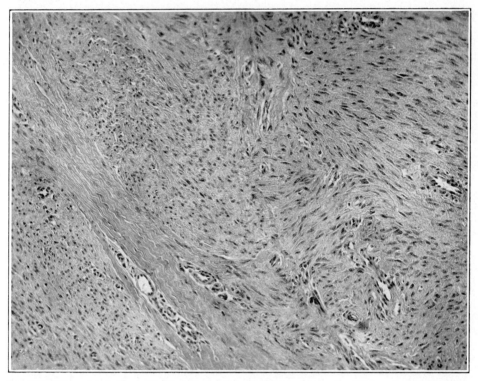

Fig. 650. Fibromatosis illustrating interlacing bundles of elongated cells with an abundant amount of cytoplasm and elongated rather large nuclei. × 100.

Ganglion.—A ganglion may be defined as a cystic swelling near a joint or tendon sheath with special predilection for the wrist, foot, or knee (Mercer). The condition is more common in women than in men and usually *occurs* in the second to the fourth decades of life inclusive. The *cause* is probably constitutional and traumatic. *Pathologically* the process is one of cellular proliferation and mucoid degeneration (Fig. 649). The lesion consists of a soft cystic mass that usually measures 1 to 2 cm. in over-all diameter. Cut surfaces disclose a fibrous wall of varying thickness enclosing a unilocular or multilocular cavity filled with stringy mucoid material. *Histologically* the wall is composed of collagenous fibrous tissue with varying degrees (but usually scanty) of lymphocytic and monocytic infiltration. Its inner surface may contain scattered giant cells and is

directly applied to a central collection of slightly basophilic mucoid substance. The *clinical manifestations* consist of swelling, pain, and some impairment of function. The *diagnosis* is made from the location of the swelling and its gross appearance. *Treatment* consists of surgical excision. The
prognosis is excellent.

Fibromatosis.—This lesion, also *referred to* as pseudosarcomatous fibromatosis, progressive fibromatosis, fascial fibromatosis, plantar (when occurring in the plantar region) fibromatosis, and infiltrative fasciitis, is a benign

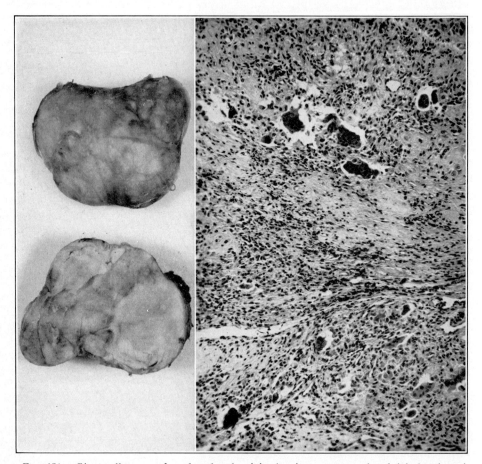

FIG. 651.—Giant cell tumor of tendon sheath origin showing an encapsulated, lobulated, variegated mass grossly, and cellular and collagenous fibrous tissue with giant cells and hemosiderin
granules microscopically. × 100.

tumor arising in fascias or tendon sheaths (Konwaler and Prior). The
lesion is relatively common, usually *occurs* between the ages of 10 to 40
years, and has no predilection for either sex. The *cause* is unknown. Even
its nature is not agreed upon—some people considering it to be inflammatory
rather than neoplastic. *Grossly* the tumor is usually found on an extremity
although occasionally it is situated on the trunk. It is generally single but
may be multiple and nodular, is located deep in the skin, and measures up
to 2 cm. in diameter. Cut surfaces are homogeneously gray. *Histologic*
section reveal sheets and bundles of elongated cells with varying amounts

of cytoplasm and usually elongated but plump hyperchromatic nuclei (Fig. 650). Mitoses are common and giant cells are occasionally seen. Interspersed throughout the tumor are moderate numbers of thin- and thick-walled blood vessels. In some areas there are, in addition, hemorrhagic extravasations. The only noteworthy, but rare, *complication* is a malignant transformation. The *clinical manifestations* consist of the presence of a nodule or a more diffuse nodular thickening that grows with varying degrees of rapidity, that may be tender, and that is not attached to the overlying skin but is attached to the underlying structures. The *diganosis* is made from the location of the tumor and its histologic appearance. *Treatment* consists of surgical incision. The *prognosis* regarding morbidity is guarded for recurrences, occurring within 3 to 6 months, are frequent. The tumor rarely undergoes a sarcomatous transformation.

Giant Cell Tumor.—A giant cell tumor is a benign lesion arising in a tendon sheath (Fletcher). Some of the many *synonyms* are benign giant cell synovioma, benign synovioma, myeloid tumor, xanthomatous giant cell tumor, and xanthoma (Wright). The disorder *occurs* more frequently in women than in men and, while it may be found at any age, its peak incidence is in the fourth decade of life. The *cause* is unknown. The *sites* of predilection are the digits, with three-quarters of the cases occurring in the upper extremities. *Pathologically* the tumors usually measure 1 to 2 cm. in diameter although they may measure as much as 6 or 8 cm. across (Fig. 651). They are generally well encapsulated, lobulated, firm, and solid. Cut surfaces disclose mottled gray, yellow, and brown tissue. *Histologically* the tumors consist fundamentally of cellular or collagenous fibrous tissue containing varying numbers of foreign body giant cells and foam cells and sprinkled with varying amounts of hemosiderin. The main *clinical manifestations* consist of tumor, disturbance in motion, and pain. *Roentgenograms* of adjacent bones frequently reveal a peripheral area of radiolucency from erosion by the adjacent nodule. The *diagnosis* is based primarily on physical examination. *Treatment* consists of surgical excision. The *prognosis* is excellent.

REFERENCES

Adams, J. D., and Coonse, G. K.: Occupat. Med., *4*, 137, 1947 (Bursitis).

Bickel, W. H., *et al.*: J. A. M. A., *151*, 31, 1953 (Tuberculous Tenosynovitis).

Fletcher, A. G., Jr., and Horn, R. C.: Ann. Surg., *133*, 374, 1951 (Giant Cell Tumor).

Flynn, J. E.: New England J. Med., *242*, 241, 1950 (Suppurative Tenosynovitis).

Henderson, R. G. and Main, R. G.: Br. J. Surg., *42*, 268, 1954 (Fibromatosis).

Lapidus, P. W., and Fenton, R.: A. M. A. Arch. Surg., *64*, 475, 1952 (Stenosing Tenovaginitis)

Lipscomb, P. R.: Ann. Surg., *134*, 110, 1951 (Stenosing Tenosynovitis Radial Styloid).

Mason, M. L.: A. M. A. Arch. Surg., *65*, 457, 1952 (Dupuytren's Contracture).

Mathews, D. N.: Practitioner, *169*, 641, 1952 (Dupuytren's Contracture).

Mercer, W.: *Orthopedic Surgery*, 4th Ed., Baltimore, The Williams & Wilkins Co., 1950.

Meyerding, H. W., and Schellito, J. G.: J. Internat. Coll. Surg., *11*, 595, 1948 (Dupuytren's Contracture Foot).

Prior, J. T. and Sessin, B. J.: Ann. Surg., *139*, 453, 1954 (Fibromatosis).

Rhodes, R. L.: Am. J. Surg., *73*, 248, 1947 (Tenosynovitis of Forearm).

Ross, J. A., and Annan, J. H.: Ann. Surg., *134*, 186, 1951 (Dupuytren's Contracture).

Steen, O. T., and McCullough, J. A. L.: Am. J. Roentgenol., *65*, 245, 1951 (Supraspinatus Tendinitis).

Wilson, B.: Am. Surgeon, *18*, 416, 1952 (Necrotizing Fasciitis).

Wright, C. J. E.: Brit. J. Surg., *37*, 17, 1951 (Giant Cell Tumor).

Chapter

38

Skeletal Muscle

PATHOLOGIC PHYSIOLOGY

J. C. E. Dorchester

THE *functional unit* of *muscular activity* is the motor unit composed of the anterior horn cell, the motor nerve fiber, and the group of muscle cells it innervates. The number of muscle fibers in each motor unit varies from as little as 5 to 10 where fine control is needed, to as many as 200 or more where power rather than precision is important. Recent evidence suggests that *in situ*, all the muscle fibers of the group do not necessarily respond in unison, but under certain conditions individual muscle cells may contract independently of the others in the unit. However, the muscle fibers included in the motor unit do rely on their innervation not only for their functional activity, but also for their morphological integrity. It has been demonstrated repeatedly that denervation atrophy is not prevented by electrically induced contractions of the paralyzed muscles. It, therefore, differs from disuse atrophy, which may be prevented by as brief a period of electrical stimulation as ten seconds per day. Obviously, a more fundamental and intimate relationship exists between the lower motor neuron and its attached muscles than that of a purely conducting pathway between the central nervous system and the skeletal muscles.

Gradation of *muscular contraction* in the motor unit is dependent on the frequency of impulses reaching the muscle fibers from the anterior horn cell. A single impulse produces a muscle twitch while a series of closely spaced impulses produce varying degrees of *tetanus*. The completeness of tetanic contraction is a function of the frequency of impulse formation and the type of muscle fiber. Thus, 200 stimulations per second may be required to produce complete tetanus of the pale muscles of the eye, while twenty or thirty per second will suffice for the dark muscles in the soleus. Under normal conditions, in the intact animal, tetanic contractions are the exception rather than the rule, and occur only under conditions of maximum effort. Instead, gradations of muscular effort are achieved by the asynchronous discharge of motor units, and variations in the numbers of units involved.

Motor loss and *denervation atrophy* result from lesions involving the anterior horn cells such as occur with poliomyelitis, trauma, syringomyelia myelitis, tumor, progressive muscular atrophy, or amyotrophic lateral sclerosis. The degree of disability depends on the number and location of the anterior horn cells involved, and ranges from muscular weakness to complete paralysis. A prominent feature of conditions involving slow degeneration of the lower motor neuron is *fasiculation*, which is a coarse twitching of the muscle cells comprising the motor unit. The exact mechanism of the phenomenon is unknown but it is apparently associated with abnormal activity of the anterior horn cells. Occasionally, fasiculations occur in normal individuals, but when they occur in combination with muscular weakness and wasting, they are to be regarded as signs of progressive degeneration of the cranial motor nuclei or the anterior horn cells.

Typical symptoms of loss of motor function also result from *damage* to the *motor nerves* such as occurs with ischemia as in Volkmann's contracture, or peripheral neuritis. However, since the afferent fibers running in the nerve are often involved, loss of sensation occurs as well. Providing that the cuase of injury is remedied early enough, most of the effects are reversible.

Within five days to a few weeks of the occurrence of any lesion which produces a rapid destruction of the nerve fibers, such as poliomyelitis or nerve section, spontaneous contractions of the denervated muscle fibers occur. These contractions are called *fibrillations*. In contrast to fasiculations they are rarely visible through the skin, except in the region of the tongue, and do not represent contractions of entire motor units, but rather, the asynchronous activity of individual fibers. Since fibrillations are not abolished by aneasthesia or curare, they are considered to be myogenic in origin and represent a sensitization through denervation being due to an increased sensitivity to acetylcholine reaching the muscle fibers through the blood or perhaps being produced locally.

Another feature of denervation is the *reaction* of *degeneration* in which the effectiveness of faradic stimulation of the muscle is decreased while that of galvanic stimulation is increased. This is simply due to the fact that activation of a normal muscle by means of electrodes applied to the overlying skin is the result of nerve and end plate sitmulation rather than direct stimulation of the muscle itself. After degeneration of the nerve fibers, activation through the overlying skin results in direct stimulation of the muscle tissue. Having a longer chronaxie than nerve, the muscle is refractory to brief pulses of current but responsive to currents of longer duration.

It is generally believed that the nerve endings at the *myoneural junction* release *acetylcholine* which depolarizes the end plate region thereby generating the nonpropagated end plate potential. The end plate potential in turn depolarizes the adjacent area of the muscle membrane resulting in the production of the muscle action potential. The acetylcholine released at the nerve endings is rapidly hydrolyzed through the action of cholinesterase. It can be seen that *disturbances* of the *myoneural junction* with consequent muscular weakness or paralysis may be due to (1) interference with the release of acetylcholine by the nerve endings, (2) interference with the activity of acetylcholine on the end plates, or (3) interference with the repolarization process. *Botulinus toxin* blocks neuromuscular transmission by preventing the release of acetylcholine from the nerve terminals. Although the exact mechanism is a matter for speculation, there is evidence that hyperpolarization or decreased permeability to potassium and sodium of the nerve membrane is a factor. *Curare* and its derivatives act directly on the myoneural junction without affecting either the nerve or the muscle tissue. They no not, apparently, inhibit the release of acetylcholine but compete with it for active groups on the end plate. Once the muscle membrane has been depolarized, it must be repolarized before the muscle is able to respond to another nerve impulse. Excess acetylcholine, or cathodal currents, block neuromuscular transmission by maintaining the depolarized state of the muscle membrane. The anticholinesterases also effect depolarization through their destruction of cholinesterase, which thus prolongs the action of the neurally released acetylcholine. *Myasthenia gravis* is a disease of neuromuscular transmission. However, study of the affected muscles reveals no abnormality of either the muscle cells or the end plates. Furthermore, there are no indications of central nervous system involvement. The similarity between the action of curare and the symptoms of myasthenia gravis, as well as the marked, if transitory, restoration of muscular function induced by neostigmine and other anticholinesterase drugs, has led to a number of conjectures as to the mechanism of the transmission defect. These hypotheses include (1) faulty synthesis of acetylcholine or its too rapid destruction by cholinesterase, (2) reduced sensitivity of the muscle fiber or end plate to the action of acetylcholine, and (3) the existence of a curare-like substance. However, none of these is entirely satisfactory and the manner in which the disease produces its effects is unknown.

The muscle cell membrane or *sarcolemma* serves two important functions —(1) the spread of excitation throughout the cell and (2) the maintenance of electrical and chemical potential differences between the exterior and the interior of the cell.

Potassium is concentrated inside the cell, while *sodium* is concentrated outside. This unequal distribution of ions results in a resting membrane potential of about 50 to 100 m.v.—the inside being negative with respect to the outside. Stimulation of the muscle results in a transitory breakdown of membrane permeability during which a rapid influx of sodium and an equivalent outflow of potassium occurs. This produces a reversal of the membrane potential and provides the energy for the generation of the muscle action potential. The muscle action potential differs from the end plate potential in that its propagation is away from the point of stimulation and spreading to all parts of the sracolemma. In some as yet unexplained manner, the muscle action potential triggers off the contractile elements of the muscle fiber causing them to contract.

Dysfunction of the *cell membrane*, or *disturbances* of *ionic equilibrium*, leads to muscular disability. Thus, *periodic familial paralysis* is characterized by low serum potassium and increased muscle potassium. Whether this is due to faulty carbohydrate metabolism in the muscle cell, or to an abnormality of the membrane itself, is not known, but the result is a defective conduction by the sarcolemma leading to paralysis of the muscle. Both *increases* and *decreases* in serum *potassium, calcium, magnesium,* and *sodium* result in muscular dysfunction. Since both sodium and potassium are intimately related to the maintenance of the resting membrane potential and the generation of the action potential, it is to be expected that disturbances involving their ionic equilibrium have their muscular effects mainly on the sarcolemma. The muscular weakness induced by large doses of magnesium is attributable to its action in preventing the release of acetylcholine by the nerve endings. The tetany of low calcium and magnesium is due to increased neuromuscular excitability.

It is realized that a great many diseases of muscle, both primary and secondary, have been omitted in this brief review. But space does not permit discussion of the large number of muscular disabilities which result from primary defects in metabolism or of the central nervous system. The smaller group of primary diseases of the muscle tissue itself have not been included because although much valuable work has been done on the morphological aspects of these disturbances, little is known of their physiology.

CONGENITAL ANOMALIES

Orientation.—Developmental malformations of skeletal muscles are comparatively infrequent. The more important lesions may be discussed

briefly under the following headings: absence, amyotonia congenita, torticollis, and scalenus anticus syndrome.

Absence.—Failure of development of muscles in different parts of the
body is not common. It is usually associated with obvious derangement of
bony development as, for example, absence of a portion or of an entire
limb. In addition, a not too infrequent site, as far as the anomaly itself is
concerned, is in the *abdominal wall* (Mathieu). In this condition, the
muscles may be partially or completely absent and there may be associated
maldevelopments of the genito-urinary and gastrointestinal tracts. The
lesion is usually discovered in infancy and is characterized by undue thinness and protrusion of the abdomen.

Amyotonia Congenita.—Amyotonia congenita, as the caption implies,
may be *defined* as a congenital lack of tone and lack of full development of
striated muscles (Mercer). The disorder is generally discovered at birth,
or certainly during infancy, and is thought to be *due to* intrinsic disease of
muscle or to a disturbance in the excitability of motor end plates which
results in abnormal transmission of impulses (Gordon). *Clinically* it is
characterized by undue weakness and flaccidity of the muscles of especially
the lower extremities but also, to a lesser extent, of those of the upper extremities, trunk, and face. Paralysis, however, does not occur but the
muscular tone is generally of insufficient degree to permit normal posture
let alone locomotion. As a result of the flaccidity, the joints are unduly
mobile and because of prolonged maintenance of abnormal positions,
secondary contractions of muscles are common. *Pathologically*, in uncomplicated cases, the muscles are diminutive in size and disclose varying
numbers of embryonal muscle fibers mixed with normal muscle bundles
(Cunningham).

Torticollis.—Torticollis (L. = twisted + neck) may be defined as contraction of the cervical muscles resulting in twisting of the head to the
opposite side and its inclination to the same side. It is also known as
wryneck. The condition may be congenital or acquired (Mercer). *Congenital torticollis* has been thought to be due to heredity, ischemia, defect
in central nervous system, intrauterine infection, and trauma during delivery (Charlewood). Of these theories, trauma during parturition with
ischemia of muscles appears to be the most logical explanation. The initial
change consists of acute venous obstruction, intravascular clotting, and
hemorrhagic extravasation. The resulting swelling is noted in the sterno-
cleidomastoid area for a period of two to three weeks. Gradually the tumor
disappears and is replaced with fibrous tissue which contracts, produces
shortening of the muscle and adjacent fascia, and thus causes the deformity
(Fig. 652*A*). *Acquired torticollis*, also known as spasmodic wryneck, occurs
in adults and is consequent to spasm of the sternocleidomastoid muscle and
homolateral trapezius muscle (Fig. 652*B*). The cause of the spasm is
unknown although neurosis, encephalitis, chorea, and arteriosclerosis have
been considered of etiologic significance.

Scalenus Anticus Syndrome.—This syndrome consists of a painful
symptom complex that affects the shoulder girdle, neck, chest, arm, and
hand and that is associated with numbness, tingling, weakness, and muscular atrophy of the arm (Judovich). It results from irritation of the radial
plexus and subclavian vessels by the scalenus anticus muscle in a manner
similar to that seen in conjunction with a cervical rib (p. 1227). The precise
reasons for the irritation are unknown for certain, although they are thought
to be due to bulging of the scaline muscles as a sequel to good muscular

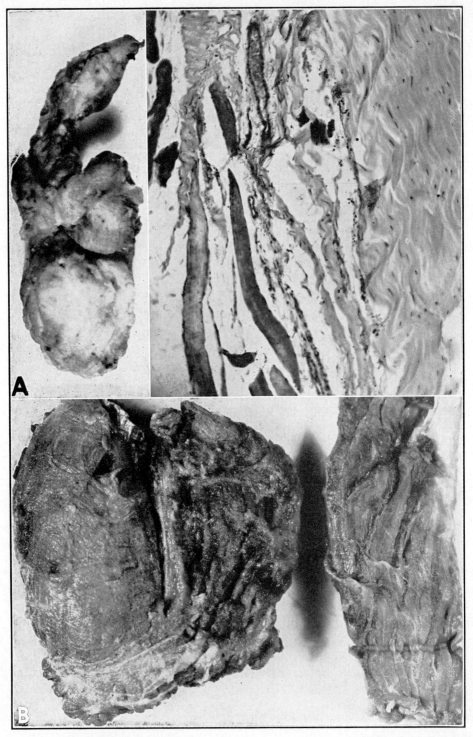

Fig. 652.—Torticollis showing *A*, the congenital variety with extensive fibrosis of the sterno-cleidomastoid muscle both grossly (to the left) and microscopically (to the right). × 100 and *B*, the acquired variety with spastic contraction and broadening of the affected muscle (to the left) as compared with a normal muscle (to the right).

development in the young or to relaxation of the musculature with sagging of the shoulder girdle in the older person (Tanna). Other theories are spasm of the scalene muscles, trauma, and faulty development.

DEGENERATIONS

Orientation.—Degenerative changes in muscle are frequently seen in conjunction with other disease processes. The most important retrogressive alterations are *atrophy* (p. 29) and *Zenker's degeneration* (p. 39), both of which have been referred to in Chapter 4. Aside from these, the disorder known as muscular dystrophy may be conveniently placed in this section.

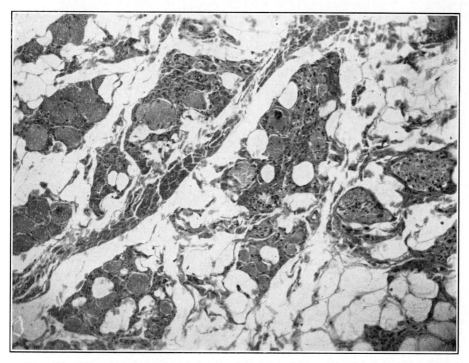

Fig. 653.—Muscular dystrophy of the pseudohypertrophic variety showing atrophy of muscle bundles and extensive permeation with fat tissue. × 100.

Muscular Dystrophy.—Muscular dystrophy (L. = muscular + Gr. = ill + nourish) is a hereditary disorder of creatinine, glycine, and amino-acid metabolism characterized by atrophy of striated muscles and disturbed physiologic function resulting therefrom (Mercer and Brown). When the atrophic muscle bundles are replaced with fat the muscle appears larger than normal but, since the enlargement is not due to hypertrophy of the muscle bundles as such, the change is referred to as of a *pseudohypertrophic type* (Fig. 653). The condition *occurs* in both males and females and usually makes its appearance in childhood or adolescence. Depending upon the muscles affected and the presence or absence of pseudohypertrophy, the condition is variously *classified*. Thus, it is referred to as (1) *pseudohypertrophic muscular dystrophy* or *paralysis* when there is (*a*) pseudohypertrophy of the calf and infraspinatus muscles, (*b*) atrophy of the biceps, latissimus dorsi, and lower portion of the pectoralis major muscles, (c) flexion deformities, and (d) a waddling gait, (2) *facioscapulohumeral muscular dystrophy* when there is atrophy of the facial muscles (especially orbicularis oris and orbicularis palpebrarum) followed by atrophy of muscles of the shoulder girdles, arms, and pelvic girdle and (3) *myotonia atrophica* when there is atrophy of the facial, sternomastoid, vasti, dorsiflexor of the ankle, forearm, masseter, and temporal muscles associated with slow relaxation of the muscles of the extremities (especially flexor muscles of the hands) after voluntary contraction. In general, *treatment* is ineffective and the patients usually *die* of general debility or cardiac involvement (Weisenfeld).

INFLAMMATIONS

Orientation.—Inflammation of muscle is known as *myositis*. The more important inflammations may be listed as follows: relapsing myositis, fibromyositis, myositis fibrosa generalisata, myositis in rheumatoid arthritis (p. 1277), Boeck's sarcoid, clostridial myositis, and trichinosis.

Relapsing Myositis.—This condition was described in 1952 by McLetchie and Aikens. It consists of an abrupt onset of muscular swellings, pains, stiffness, fever, leukocytosis, and complete functional restoration but with a tendency to relapse. The cause is unknown. Pathologically the changes consist of an acute hyaline and patchy necrosis of muscle fibers accompanied by an intense histiocytic reaction with rapid removal of the damaged tissue.

Fibromyositis.—This caption encompasses a group of nonspecific inflammations of muscle attended or followed by fibrosis (Slobe). The *acute stage* comprises hemorrhage, serofibrinous exudation between muscle bundles, degeneration of muscle fibers, and lymphocytic permeation. The *chronic stage* discloses more extensive hyalinization and degeneration of the muscle fibers and separation of muscle bundles by fibrous tissue. The *muscles* most commonly involved are those of the posterior portion of the body, that is, neck, shoulder, girdle, back, and gluteal regions. The usual *causes* are considered to be metabolic disturbance (joint), nutritional deficiency, endocrine imbalances, anemia, fatigue, lowered resistance in general, faulty posture, and strain or trauma. The *clinical manifestations* consist of pain, tenderness, and limitation of normal motion. *Treatment* is prophylactic and empirical. The *prognosis* is variable.

Myositis Fibrosa Generalisata.—Generalized myositis followed by fibrosis is a syndrome that usually occurs in infants or children but occasionally may start in adults (Stewart). The *cause* is unknown. *Pathologically* the muscles disclose hyalinization, loss of cross striations, atrophy, round cell infiltration, and an increase of fibrous tissue that surrounds and invades the muscle fibers. *Clinically* the disorder is insidious in onset, first affects an extremity (usually a lower one), and finally spreads to other muscles but generally spares the muscles of the face and the sphincters. The lesion starts as a small, painless, indurated area in the belly of a muscle which then spreads to involve most of its substance. In time, the muscle becomes atrophic and contracts, producing marked and varied deformities. There is no accompanying pain or fever. *Treatment* is unsatisfactory. The *prognosis* is poor.

Boeck's Sarcoid.—Boeck's sarcoid, as a disease, has already been described in Chapter 12 (p. 501). Involvement of muscle is considered to be rare yet Powell collected 18 recorded cases of the lesion and added 6 cases of his own. The *pathologic* changes are similar to those in other organs and tissues (p. 501). *Clinically* the disorder is characterized by the presence of nodules in the muscles (particularly those of the extremities) sometimes associated with weakness, soreness, actual pain, or atrophy. The *course* is that of the disorder in general.

Clostridial Myositis.—Clostridial myositis is inflammation of muscle by clostridial organisms. The condition generally *affects* an extremity and constitutes one of the most important types of gangrene (p. 60). It is

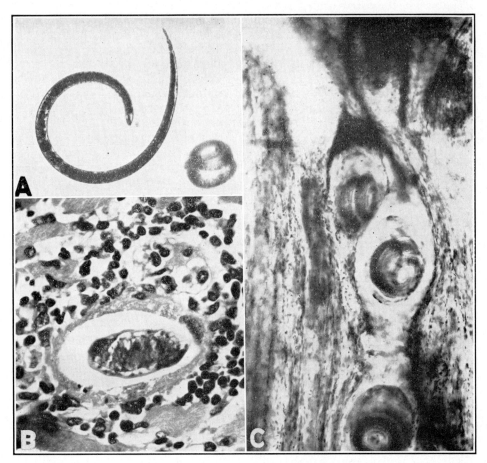

Fig. 654.—Trichinosis illustrating *A*, larvæ. × 100, *B*, leukocytic reaction at the point of lodgment of a larva in striated muscle. × 400, and *C*, encysted coiled larvæ in striated muscle. × 100.

brought about by a perforating trauma and is initiated only in the presence of necrotic muscle tissue and/or blood clot (Lowry). *Pathologically* it consists of rapid destruction of muscle tissue (which is rich in glycogen) that spreads along the entire length of the muscle and that is accompanied by gas-bubble formation. *Clinically* the infection is associated systemically with severe toxemia, fever, rapid pulse, apprehension, delerium, anemia, and reduced blood volume. Locally, it is characterized by pain and a sense of heaviness in the involved tissue. Gas bubbles can be felt in the affected muscles as crepitations and can be seen roentgenographically as areas of increased translucency. *Treatment* consists of surgical relief of tension, excision of necrotic tissue, and establishment of adequate drainage. The *prognosis* depends on the rapidity and adequacy of the treatment.

Trichinosis.—Trichinosis, also known as trichiniasis and trichinellosis, is an infection by the round worm *Trichinella spiralis* (Sawitz and Craig and Faust). The condition *prevails* in temperate zones and is particularly common in the United States. The disease is *transmitted* to man by eating insufficiently cooked pork that is infected with encysted *Trichinella spiralis* larvæ. The ingested organisms are liberated in the stomach and, within a week, grow into adult worms in the small intestine. The *adult* male worm is about 1.5 mm. in length, is round, and discloses two tail papillæ used to hold the female. The female worm is about 4 mm. long, is also round, and possesses a vulva at its anterior third. The entire life of the adult worm is spent in the small intestine and spans a maximum of about six weeks. During this time, the female (after copulation) produces about 1,500 larvæ (Fig. 654*A*). The *larvæ* measure approximately 100 × 6 microns, penetrate the mucosa of the small intestine, enter the small capillaries, pass through the liver, and, by way of the heart and lungs, reach the systemic circulation. Ultimately they become arrested in the heart, brain, lungs, liver, pancreas, bone marrow, kidneys, muscles, and almost any tissue of the body. At points of lodgment, they evoke a cellular reaction characterized by necrosis, edema, and leukocytic (especially eosinophilic) reaction (Fig. 654*B*). Eventually, however, the larvæ completely disintegrate and disappear except in skeletal muscle where they become encysted and calcified (Fig. 654*C*) (Gould). *Clinically* the condition is characterized by intestinal disorders during the intestinal phase and by fever, leukocytosis, eosinophilia, swelling about the face, muscle tenderness, and a variety of other manifestations (depending upon the organs affected) during the migratory and lodgment phase. The *diagnosis* is made by finding (1) the organism in duodenal aspirates, (2) the larvæ in circulating blood and other fluids, and (3) the larvæ in muscle biopsies. *Treatment* is symptomatic and prophylactic. The *prognosis* is good but death may occur from the fourth to the sixth weeks from overwhelming general infection or from myocarditis or encephalitis.

PHYSICAL DISTURBANCES

Orientation.—In this group the following unrelated conditions may be considered briefly: trauma, Volkmann's ischemic contracture, myositis ossificans, thermal disturbances, muscle cramps, tetanus, and myasthenia gravis.

Trauma.—Trauma to muscle may occur as a result of abnormal muscular activity or external injury. *Abnormal muscular activity* consists of violent contraction or of sudden relaxation or elongation when in a state of contraction (Mercer). It usually produces *rupture* of the muscle, either in its belly or at the musculotendinous insertion. Although any striated muscles may be affected, those usually involved are rectus abdominis, pectoralis major, adductors of the thighs, short extensors of the toes, gastrocnemius, plantaris, posterior tibial, rectus femoris, biceps, deltoid, trapezius, and sternomastoid (Adam, Hayes, Pearson, and Mercer). *Pathologically* the continuity of the muscle fibers is lost, hemorrhage occurs, and the defect ultimately heals by fibrosis. *Clinically* there is *sharp* pain, loss of function, swelling, and bulging upon contraction. *Treatment* consists of immobilization when the rupture is incomplete and upon operation and suture when it is complete. The *prognosis* varies with the degree of damage and the promptness of treatment.

External injury may be single or multiple, slight or severe, and penetrating or blunt. Thus, it may be responsible for (1) *focal necrosis* with leukocytic extravasation (Fig. 655), (2) *contusion* (p. 223), (3) *ecchymosis* (p. 196), (4) *hematoma* (p. 196), (5) *laceration* (p. 223), (6) *rupture*, or (7) *extensive maceration*. The *pathologic* changes vary according to the type of lesion and are self-evident. The *clinical manifestations* also vary from slight dysfunction to complete incapacity and from scarcely detectable signs to extensive swelling, obvious penetrating defect, etc. A common complication of extensive injury is the crush syndrome (p. 224). *Treatment* ranges from observation to surgical debridement suturing, or excision. The *prognosis* is also obviously variable.

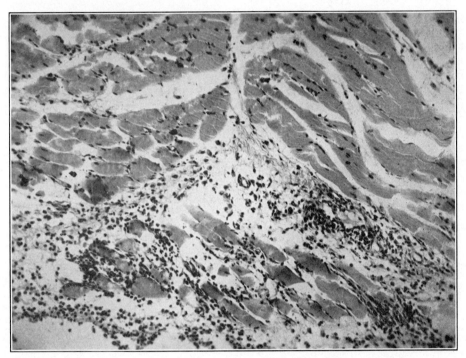

FIG. 655.—Focal traumatic necrosis and leukocytic extravasation in striated muscle. × 100.

Volkmann's Ischemic Contracture.—Contracture of muscles of the wrist and fingers following tight bandaging of the arm for treatment of fracture above the elbow was first described by Volkmann in 1875 (Mercer). The condition usually *occurs* in children in the first decade of life, is more frequent in the upper than in the lower extremity, is *due* to spasm of the main artery of the limb, and is generally an accompaniment of fracture (Thompson and Meyerding). *Experimentally* the condition has been produced in dogs and rabbits by inducing ischemia of a limb by means of a blood pressure cuff, tourniquet, or ligating the iliac arteries (Clarke). *Pathologically* the disorder consists of (1) degeneration, loss of striations and nuclei, and hyaline fusion of the bellies of the muscles and (2) fibroblastic proliferation and contracture at the peripheries of the muscles. Gradually the degenerated muscle disappears and is replaced by the fibrous tissue invading from without. The *clinical manifestations* begin shortly after the injury and consist of coldness, pain, swelling, cyanosis, and loss of function of the digits beyond the lesion. The acute symptoms subside within forty-eight hours following which the characteristic deformity of flexion of the wrist (or ankle), extension of the metacarpophalangeal (or metatarsophalangeal) joints, and flexion of the interphalangeal joints occurs. The *diagnosis* is made from the clinical manifestations. *Treatment* consists of restoring adequate circulation as soon as possible, including if necessary injection of sympathetic ganglia to interrupt reflex stimuli. The *prognosis* depends upon the stage of the process, being good when treated early (and adequately) and poor when treated late.

Myositis Ossificans. —As the caption indicates, myositis ossificans connotes a low-grade inflammation of muscles attended by its gradual conversion to bone. The disorders may be divided into two groups—myositis ossificans circumscripta and myositis ossificans progressiva (Mercer).

Myositis ossificans circumscripta is also known as traumatic ossifying myositis, ossifying hematoma, and calcified hematoma (Howard). It usually *occurs* between the ages of seventeen and twenty-five years and is more common in males than in females. The lesion may *arise* from osteoblasts of the adjacent periosteum, from reticulum cells within muscle, or from metaplasia of connective tissue or mesenchymal cells. The *cause* of the condition is trauma and the trauma may be in the nature of a single injury or of repeated injuries. The *muscles* most commonly involved are the adductors of the thighs (usually in horse-back riders), quadriceps of the thighs, and flexors of the elbows. *Pathologically* the lesion may be single or multiple, is usually sharply circumscribed, and may vary from a few to many centimeters in diameter (Fig. 656). It may be homogeneous gray or mottled gray to brown and solid or cystic. *Histologically* it is composed of varying amounts of bone, cartilage, muscle, and connective tissue. Aside from impairment of function an infrequent *complication* is a transformation into an osteosarcoma. *Clinically* the condition is attended by pain, swelling, and tenderness early after trauma and by persistence of a tumor with varying degrees of functional impairment later in the disease. *Roentgenograms* disclose an area or areas of increased density within the swelling. The *diagnosis* is made from the history, physical examination, and roentgenograms. *Treatment* consists of observation (with limitation of activity) in the early stages and of surgical excision after the process has become well localized. The *prognosis* is good.

Myositis ossificans progressiva is a rare, probably hereditary, chronic disease characterized by progressive replacement of muscles, tendons, and aponeuroses by bone (Vastine and Riley). The condition is more common in males than in females and usually makes its *appearance* in infancy or early childhood. Aside from heredity, specific *causative* agents are unknown. The first *manifestations* consist of a painful, tender, often reddened and hot, soft tissue swelling in the cervical or upper dorsal region. The swelling may then disappear or be replaced with bone. Subsequently other muscles are progressively affected, gradually resulting in increasing incapacity until the patient becomes bedridden. *Treatment* is unsatisfactory. The *prognosis* is poor with death ultimately occurring from respiratory failure.

Thermal Disturbances. —Exposure of muscle to heat or cold results in swelling, cyanosis, decrease in translucency, and increase in friability of the muscle grossly and coagulation necrosis and/or atrophy microscopically (Lewis). These changes are actually similar to the alterations caused by ischemia, although they are produced in a much shorter interval of time. The topics of hyperthermia and hypothermia have already been discussed in Chapter 6 (pp. 226 and 230).

Muscle Cramps.—Muscle cramps signify sudden, violent, usually prolonged, painful contractions of striated muscles attended by severe pain and lack of mobility. They are seen commonly in swimmers but are encountered also in other forms of muscular activity. While the exact mechanism involved is not entirely clear, local sodium chloride deficiency or alkalosis is thought to be the important initiating factors (Richardson).

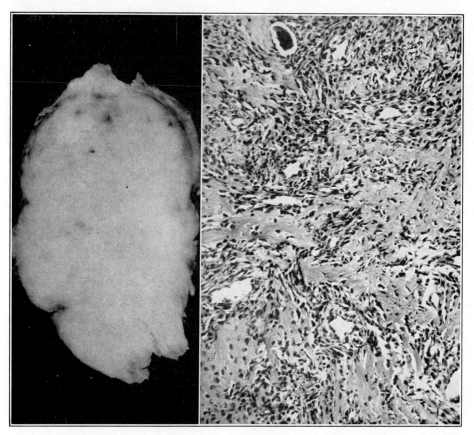

Fig. 656.—Myositis ossificans demonstrating complete replacement of a striated muscle by dense homogeneous gray tissue grossly and by newly formed osseous tissue microscopically. × 100.

Tetanus.—Tetanus (Gr. = to stretch), also known as *lockjaw*, is an acute infectious disease caused by the toxin of *Clostridium tetani* and characterized by spasm of the striated muscles of the jaw and other regions of the body. The causative organism is a gram-positive, anaerobic, bacillus that forms a terminal spore, that produces a powerful neurotropic toxin, and that is found in soil and in human, equine, or bovine feces. Human infection usually occurs as a result of contamination of a wound by *Clostridium tetani* in which there is necrosis of tissue or secondary pyogenic infection (Melnick). Sometimes a foreign body in the nose may act as a

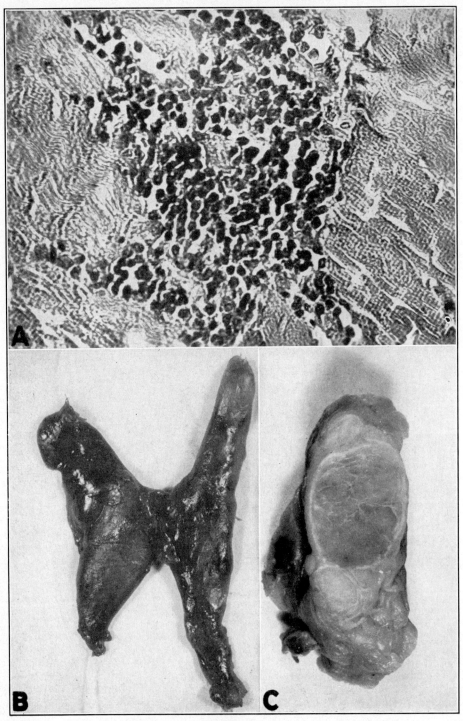

FIG. 657.—Myasthenia gravis showing *A*, lymphorrhages in striated
muscle. × 400, *B*, a persistent thymus, and *C*, a thymoma.

portal of entry (Tudor) while at other times the route of invasion remains undetected. At any rate, the organism grows locally and elaborates a toxin which is absorbed by the bloodstream. The toxin then acts upon the central nervous system with resulting spasm of muscles. The usual incubation period varies from two to twenty-one days. There is no natural immunity against tetanus but active immunization with tetanus toxoid does confer immunity for a limited period. Once the disease has developed, active treatment consists of sedation (with barbiturates, curare, etc.) and administration of tetanus antitoxin (Segar). If treatment is started early and is adequate the prognosis is good.

Myasthenia Gravis.—Myasthenia gravis is a neuromuscular disorder characterized by muscle fatigability on sustained effort (Schlezinger). It usually *occurs* in young adults but it has also been described at birth and in the ninth decade of life. The precise *cause* remains unknown although it has been determined that the disorder results from interference with transmission of nerve impulses across the neuromuscular junction (Katz). Whether this interference is due to a deficiency of acetylcholine, an overactivity of cholinesterase, the presence of a curariform substance, or some other metabolic or endocrine dysfunction is still uncertain. *Pathologically* the only noteworthy specific changes occur in striated muscle. They consist of focal necrosis with lymphocytic infiltration (lymphorrhages) in later stages (Russell). Of these, the latter is the more commonly encountered and more characteristic (Fig. 657). In addition, from 30 to 50 per cent of patients with myasthenia gravis are said to have a persistence or a tumor (thymoma) of the thymus gland and, conversely, about 75 per cent of cases of thymoma are said to have manifestations of myasthenia gravis (Katz). The chief *complication* consists of asthenia which ultimately *leads* to death from respiratory failure. The initial *manifestations* often appear in the extra-ocular muscles producing ptosis and diplopia. Subsequently, weakness develops in the muscles of the face, mastication, palate, pharynx, larynx, etc. The *diagnosis* is made from the history, clinical manifestations, and response to drug therapy. *Treatment* consists of administration of neostigmine bromide, tetraethylpyrophosphate, and/or octamethyl pyrophosphoramide or of thymectomy (Grob). The *prognosis* is guarded for the disorder is characterized by remissions and exacerbations. Of 202 patients followed at Johns Hopkins Hospital for periods of one to thirty-four years, 32 per cent died within an average of six years after the onset of the illness and 25 per cent had complete or nearly complete remission of an average duration of 4.6 years (Grob).

TUMORS

Orientation.—The important tumors of striated muscles consist of the following: desmoid, hemangioma, myoblastoma, and rhabdomyosarcoma.

Desmoid Tumor.—The term desmoid (Gr. = band + to form) literally signifies fibrous or fibroid and in connection with skeletal muscles connotes simply a hard fibroma within such mucsles. Actually the tumor arises from the musculo-aponeurotic structures. The *incidence* is difficult to determine but in large series of neoplasms, desmoid tumor accounts for about 0.03 per cent. The condition occurs at all ages from childhood on, is most common around the age of forty years, and affects females about three times as frequently as males (Booher and Musgrove).

The *cause* of the lesion is unknown although trauma and endocrine im-

balances are generally considered as of etiologic significance. The most
common *site* of involvement is the anterior abdominal wall, especially the
rectus abdominis muscles but almost every striated muscle of the body has
at one time or another been affected. *Pathologically* the tumor is usually
single. It generally measures from 6 to 8 cm. in greatest diameter, is
sharply demarcated but not encapsulated, discloses a homogeneously gray
cut surface, and is extremely firm (Fig. 658). *Histologically* the lesion is a

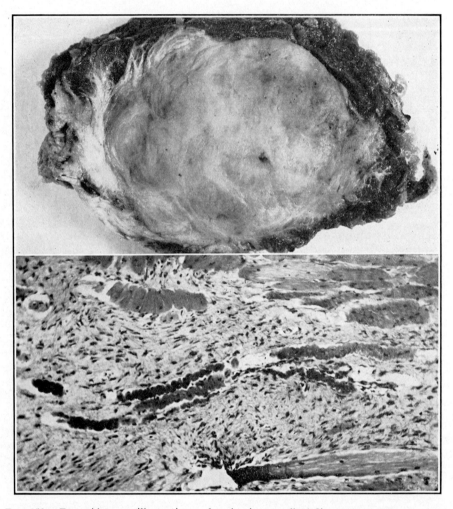

Fig. 658.—Desmoid tumor illustrating a sharply circumscribed fibromatous mass grossly and
rather cellular connective tissue cells surrounding and replacing muscle fibers microscopically.
× 100.

fibroma that encircles, separates, and replaces muscle fibers. It consists
of elongated, ill-defined, spindle-shaped cells that may be quite cellular or
that may be permeated with an abundance of collagen. The *clinical
manifestations* consist of tumor and pain. The *diagnosis* is made from the
history (slowly growing and of long duration), hardness on physical examination, and gross and microscopic appearance. *Treatment* consists of surgical
excision. The *prognosis* is good. Recurrences are due to incomplete ex-

cision for a sarcomatous transformation does not occur. The lesion, however, must be differentiated from a fibrosarcoma of muscle.

Hemangioma.—The general topic of hemangioma has been discussed in Chapter 9 (p. 393). The lesion, as far as striated muscle is concerned, is not uncommon for by 1948 a total of 335 cases had been recorded in the literature (Goeringer). The condition *occurs* with equal frequency in both sexes and predominates in the first three decades of life. Any *muscle* of the body may be involved with the most commonly affected sites being lower extremity, upper extremity, and trunk (Shallow). *Pathologically* the lesion is similar to that already described in connection with tumors of

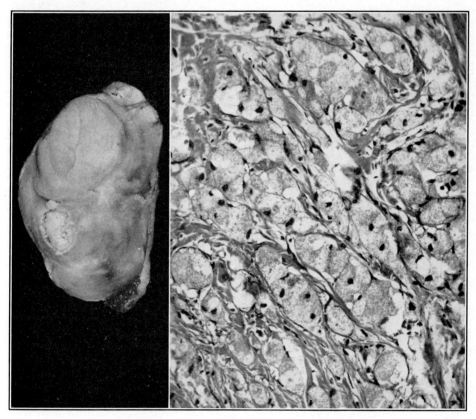

FIG. 659.—Myoblastoma disclosing a well-encapsulated tan tumor grossly and large, fat-negative, "foamy" cells microscopically. × 200.

vessels (p. 251). Grossly it exists as a varisized, ill-defined, spongy mass filled with blood, while histologically it is composed either of cavernous spaces or of capillaries. The *clinical manifestations* consist of mass, pain, pulsation, bruit, deformity, and disturbed function. The *diagnosis* is usually made after exposure of the mass although careful examination, roentgen demonstration of phleboliths, and angiograms do permit a correct preoperative evaluation. *Treatment* consists of surgical excision. The *prognosis* is good.

Myoblastoma.—A myoblastoma, commonly referred to as granular cell myoblastoma, is a benign tumor found most commonly in striated muscle but occurring also in areas where striated muscle normally does not exist

(Murphy). The lesion *prevails* in the third, fourth, and fifth decades of life and has no sex predilection (Rothchild). The *cause* is unknown. *Histogenetically* the tumor has been considered as arising from primitive muscle cells (myoblasts), from histiocytes with the foamy cytoplasm representing stored material, and from nerve sheath cells. Most authors have accepted the myoblastic origin but more recently the neurogenic theory appears to be gaining ground. In approximately decreasing order of frequency, the sites of involvement are tongue, skin, breast, subcutis, maxilla, other

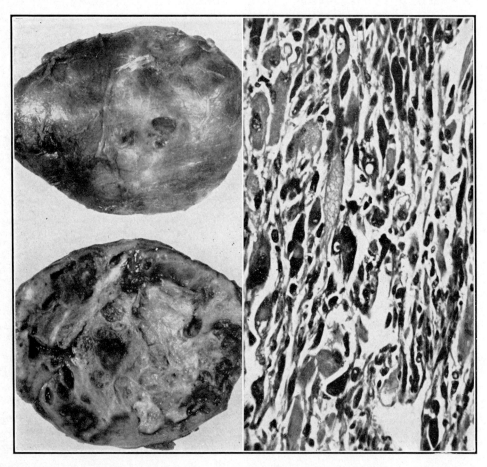

Fig. 660.—Rhabdomyosarcoma showing a fairly well-encapsulated variegated tumor grossly and irregular elongated cells with bizarre hyperchromatic nuclei microscopically. × 200.

striated muscles, vocal cords, etc. *Pathologically* the tumor may appear as a raised patch but more commonly it exists as a circumscribed tumor that measures up to 3 cm. in diameter (Fig. 659). Cut surfaces are homogeneously white to tan. *Histologically* it is usually composed of large, sharply defined, polyhedral cells, with granular cytoplasm and small, round, uniformly stained, central or slightly eccentric nuclei. Sometimes, however, the cells are considerably smaller and more pleomorphic. They can be differentiated from cells in a xanthoma in that they are negative for fat. The only important *complication* is a malignant transformation—a complication that occurs rarely, for by 1952 only 7 examples of such a change were noted (Ross). The most noteworthy *clinical manifestation* is a tumor mass. The *diagnosis* is generally made pathologically. *Treatment* consists of surgical excision. The *prognosis* is good.

Rhabdomyosarcoma.—A rhabdomyosarcoma is a malignant tumor of striated muscle. The neoplasm may *occur* at any age but is most common in the fifth and sixth decades of life (Stout). It has no predilection for either sex. The *cause* is unknown although trauma has often been considered as of etiologic significance. The *sites* of involvement in approximately decreasing order of frequency are lower extremities, trunk, head and neck, upper extremities, and diaphragm. *Pathologically* the tumors vary in size from a few to 15 or 20 cm. in diameter (Fig. 660). They may appear fairly well circumscribed or they are ill defined, merging intimately with the adjacent muscular tissue. The consistency is usually relatively soft. Cut surfaces disclose a variegated appearance composed of alternating areas of gray, pink, red, and orange-colored tissue. Cyst formation (from degeneration) may occur. *Histologically* the tumors are characterized by their variability and bizarreness. The cells (1) are small to large, (2) appear rounded, irregular, strap-like, or racquet-like, (3) disclose an abundant amount of intensely eosinophilic, occasionally cross-striated or longitudinally fibrillated cytoplasm, and (4) reveal rounded, irregular, hyperchromatic, single or multiple nuclei. Cross striations are particularly well demonstrated in sections stained with phosphotungstic acid. *Spread* occurs by local extension to surrounding structures and, in about one-third of the cases, by the bloodstream to distant organs, especially the lungs. The *clinical manifestations* consist of tumor, pain, and dysfunction. The *diagnosis* is generally not established until the lesion is examined pathologically. A differential diagnosis should include liposarcoma and fibrosarcoma. *Treatment* consists of wide excision, either locally or, if necessary, by amputation. The *prognosis* is poor with the five-year survival rate being less than 4 per cent.

REFERENCES

Pathologic Physiology

ADAMS, R. D., *et al.*: *Diseases of Muscle*, New York, Paul B. Hoeber, Inc., 1953.
GROLLMAN, A.: *Clinical Physiology*, New York, Blakiston Division, McGraw-Hill Book Co., Inc., 1957.
PATON, W. D. M.: Brit. Med. Bull., *12*, 161, 1956 (Symposium on Physiology of Voluntary Muscle).
SZENT-GEORGI, A.: *Chemical Physiology in Body and Heart Muscle*, New York, Academic Press, Inc., 1953.

Congenital Anomalies

CHARLEWOOD, G. P.: J. Obst. & Gynaec. Brit. Emp., *54*, 499, 1947 (Congenital Torticollis).
CUNNINGHAM, J. A.: South. M. J., *39*, 222, 1946 (Amyotonia Congenita).
GORDON, W. H., *et al.*: J. Michigan State M. Soc., *51*, 188, 1952 (Amyotonia Congenita).
JUDOVICH, B. D.: New York State J. Med., *48*, 2382, 1948 (Scalenus Anticus Syndrome).
MATHIEU, B. J., *et al.*: J. Pediat., *42*, 92, 1953 (Congenital Deficiency Abdominal Muscles).
MERCER, W.: *Orthopedic Surgery*, 4th Ed., Baltimore, The Williams & Wilkins Co., 1950.
TANNA, J. F.: Ann. Surg., *125*, 80, 1947 (Scalenus Anticus Syndrome).

Degenerations

BROWN, M. R.: New England J. Med., *244*, 88, 1951 (Muscular Dystrophy).
MERCER, W.: *Orthopedic Surgery*, 4th Ed., Baltimore, The Williams & Wilkins Co., 1950.
WEISENFELD, S., and MESSINGER, W. J.: Am. Heart J., *43*, 170, 1952 (Heart in Muscular Dystrophy).

Inflammations

CRAIG, C. F., and FAUST, E. C.: *Clinical Parasitology*, 5th Ed., Philadelphia, Lea & Febiger, 1951 (Trichinosis).
GOULD, S. E.: Am. J. Clin. Path., *13*, 627, 1943 (Trichinosis).
LOWRY, K. F., and CURTIS, G. M.: Am. J. Surg., *74*, 752, 1947 (Clostridial Myositis).
McLETCHIE, N. G. B., and AIKENS, R. L.: A. M. A. Arch. Path., *53*, 497, 1952 (Relapsing Myositis).
POWELL, L. W., JR.: Am. J. Clin. Path., *23*, 881, 1953 (Sarcoidosis).
SAWITZ, W. G.: *Medical Parasitology*, New York, The Blakiston Co., 1950 (Trichinosis).
SLOBE, F. W.: Occupat. Med., *2*, 329, 1946 (Fibromyositis).
STEWART, A. M., and MacGREGOR, A. R.: A. M. A. Arch. Dis. Child., *26*, 215, 1951 (Myositis Fibrosa Generalisata).

Physical Disturbances

ADAM, G. S.: J. Obst. & Gynaec. Brit. Emp., *54*, 358, 1947 (Rupture Rectus Abdominis Muscle).
CLARKE, W. T.: Canad. M. A. J., *54*, 339, 1946 (Volkmann's Ischemic Contracture).
GROB, D.: J. A. M. A., *153*, 529, 1953 (Myasthenia Gravis).
HAYES, W. M.: J. Internat. Coll. Surg., *14*, 82, 1950 (Rupture Pectoralis Major Muscle).
HOWARD, C.: U. S. Nav. M. Bull., *46*, 724, 1946 (Traumatic Myositis Ossificans).
KATZ, J. H.: New England J. Med., *248*, 1059, 1953 (Myasthenia Gravis).
LEWIS, R. B., and MOEN, P. W.: Surg., Gynec. & Obst., *95*, 543, 1952 (Thermal Changes).
MELNICK, T.: Pennsylvania M. J., *55*, 443, 1952 (Tetanus).
MERCER, W.: *Orthopedic Surgery*, 4th Ed., Baltimore, The Williams & Wilkins Co., 1950.
MEYERDING, H. W.: J. Internat. Coll. Surg., *19*, 675, 1953 (Volkmann's Ischemic Contracture).
PEARSON, C., *et al.*: New England J. Med., *239*, 213, 1948 (Traumatic Necrosis Muscles).
RICHARDSON, W.: New England J. Med., *247*, 811, 1952 (Muscle Cramps).
RILEY, H. D., JR., and CHRISTIE, A.: Pediatrics, *8*, 753, 1951 (Myositis Ossificans Progressiva).
RUSSELL, D. S.: J. Path. & Bact., *65*, 279, 1953 (Pathology Myasthenia Gravis).
SCHLEZINGER, N. S.: J. A. M. A., *148*, 508, 1952 (Myasthenia Gravis).
SEGAR, W. E., *et al.*: J. Pediat., *40*, 772, 1952 (Tetanus).
THOMSON, S. A., and MAHONEY, L. J.: J. Bone & Joint Surg., *33*B, 336, 1951 (Volkmann's Ischemic Contracture).
TUDOR, R. B.: J. A. M. A., *149*, 660, 1952 (Tetanus).
VASTINE II, J. H., *et al.*: Am. J. Roentgenol., *59*, 204, 1948 (Myositis Ossificans Progressiva).

Tumors

BOOHER, R. J., and PACK, G. T.: Cancer, *4*, 1052, 1951 (Desmoid Tumors).
GOERINGER, C. F.: Am. J. Surg., *76*, 58, 1948 (Hemangioma).
MURPHY, G. H., *et al.*: Am. J. Path., *25*, 1157, 1949 (Myoblastoma).
MUSGROVE, J. E., and McDONALD, J. R.: A. M. A. Arch. Path., *45*, 513, 1948 (Desmoid Tumors).
ROSS, R. C., *et al.*: Cancer, *5*, 112, 1952 (Malignant Myoblastoma).
ROTHCHILD, T. P. E., and CRARY, R. H.: Ann. Surg., *137*, 530, 1953 (Granular Cell Myoblastoma).
SHALLOW, T. A., *et al.*: Ann. Surg., *119*, 700, 1944 (Hemangioma).
STOUT, A. P.: Ann. Surg., *123*, 447, 1946 (Rhabdomyosarcoma).

39

Skin

PATHOLOGIC PHYSIOLOGY

EUGENE ASERINSKY

ENVELOPING the body is a complex membrane, the *skin*. This encasement *serves* to preserve the internal chemical composition and temperature within narrow limits. With extensive destruction of the skin as a result of *burns*, the water and *electrolytes* which constitute the internal medium ooze out and death may ensue. Furthermore, alien substances can easily invade and impair the interior. Nevertheless, the prinicpal role of the skin is not as a physical barrier but rather as one of the major mechanisms whereby the *internal temperature* may be stabilized to within a normal range of three or four Fahrenheit degrees in the face of environmental temperature fluctuations of one hundred degrees in temperate climates.

It is primarily for the *regulation* of body *heat* that elaborate appendageal organs of the skin such as sweat glands, hair, arrectores pilorum, and the arteriovenous anastomoses have developed. Ironically, this intricacy of structure has provided *additional features* which are subject to dysfunction as well as literal loopholes for penetration by foreign substances. Water and electrolytes are fairly well excluded by the skin. However, substances, especially those soluble in ether, which do gain entrance into the skin apparently do so by entering the orifice afforded by the hair follicle. Here the substances pass directly into the sebaceous gland and then through the thin wall of the gland into the corium.

Epidermis.—The epithelium of the skin is avascular and provides, in its uppermost layer, dead keratinized cells which act as a resilient shield to externally inflicted trauma. Although effective as a barrier to the entrance of water, the skin of the normal individual allows the passage outward of some 400 to 500 ml. of water per day as "insensible perspiration." This *water loss* is independent of sweat gland activity and accounts for about 10 per cent of body heat production. Most gases pass with relative ease through the stratum corneum. Indeed a significant amount of the skin's *oxygen* requirements may be met by the simple inward diffusion of atmospheric oxygen.

The *basal cells* (at least in the skin of the prepuce) undergo *mitosis* with a diurnal rhythmicity. At all times, however, the living cells of the epidermis utilize *glycogen* so rapidly that glycogen is infrequently found in normal skin. Trauma as gentle as the stripping of the stratum corneum with scotch tape inhibits the activity of the epidermal cells and glycogen can then be detected by histochemical means. Glycogen located in the basal cells is interpreted as an injury to the skin having occurred during the preceding 8 to 24 hours whereas glycogen in the midepidermis indicates injury some 3 to 5 days previously.

Malfunction of the skin epithelium is most frequently in the direction of overactivity with a consequent *hyperkeratinization*. Aside from corns and calluses, excessive keratinization may involve the epidermis lining the ducts of the sweat and sebaceous glands. Plugging of these ducts may lead to sweat retention symptoms and acne, respectively. The factors which initiate hyperkeratinization are inadequately understood. Irritation and pressure frequently stimulate epidermal cells. Thus, the frequent biting of a localized skin region by mental patients results in a thickening of the epidermis and hyperplasia of the sweat and sebaceous glands as well as growth of coarse hair in the area of trauma. The *hair growth* in this instance does not involve the development of new hair follicles nor the activation of resting hair follicles. Instead, growing hair follicles are stimulated to greater activity. In extreme cases of avitaminosis A there is likewise a thickening of the epidermis. The addition of *vitamin A* to a medium containing growing embryonic chick skin transforms the keratinized stratified squamous epithelium to a mucous-secreting type of epithelium. Nevertheless the role of vitamin A in skin function is yet to be elucidated inasmuch as administration of this vitamin has no obvious effect upon normal adult human skin.

Melanocyte.—*Sunlight*, especially ultraviolet rays, has a beneficial effect upon the skin by means of its bactericidal action and also through the conversion of the resident ergosterol to vitamin D which may then be absorbed. Still, the actinic radiation is capable of damaging the cells as well as casuing severe inflammatory reactions. As a partial *protection* against such harm, *melanocytes* in the basal layer of the epidermis produce a pigment, melanin, upon exposure to wavelengths primarily in the ultraviolet range of the light spectrum. This dark pigment is transported to the living cells of the epidermis presumably from the long, slender, dendritic processes of the melanocytes. Dark skin affords protection against ultraviolet light but, contrary to popular misconception, affords insignificant protection from infrared or heat radiation. *Heat rays*, which have wavelentghs longer than the visible spectrum, do not distinguish between light and dark skins. In the absence of melanin formation, as in *congenital albinism*, the skin is extremely photosensitive and subject to sunburn upon slight exposure.

Melanocytes are rarely absent from the skin. The principal difference in color of white and Negro skins is the amount of melanin produced rather than in the number of melanocytes present. A *decrease* in *melanogenesis* can be observed as a normal accompaniment of *aging*, especially with respect to the graying of hair. Abnormally, melanocytic hypofunction is seen in *vitiligo* and *leukoderma*. The basic fault underlying the failure of melanin production in the aforementioned conditions has not been determined. A clue, however, has been provided by the metabolic disorder, *phenylpyruvic oligophrenia*, which is manifested cutaneously by hypopigmentation. These patients have an abnormally high blood level of phenylalanine and a low level of tyrosine. Normally, phenylalanine is converted to tyrosine which is ultimately transformed into melanin. The phenylpyruvic oligophrenic person lacks an enzyme necessary for the hydroxylation of phenylalanine to tyrosine. The resultant high concentration of phenylalanine in itself also inhibits melanin formation. Patients provided with a special diet, low in phenylalanine content, exhibit a darkening of the skin.

An *increase* in *pigment* production is seen as *freckles* and as the dark skin patches (*chloasma*) of pregnancy. *Excessive numbers* of *melanocytes* are observed as noles (*nevi*) and in tumorous conditions. Local *trauma* and *irradiation* can stimulate melanogenesis. Furthermore, the process of pigment formation is unquestionably affected by *hormones*. *Hyperpigmentation* occurs prominently in such endocrine dysfunctions as Cushing's syndrome, Addison's disease and hyperthyroidism. Recently, a relatively high titer of melanocyte stimulating hormone (MSH) from the pars intermedia of the pituitary has been found in the blood during pregnancy. This, of course, would suggest a basis for the etiology of chloasma.

Dermis and Appendages.—Intimately attached to the epidermis by means of an amorphous, submicroscopic, intercellular cement is the dermis. This "true skin" consists essentially of a connective tissue matrix which is highly vascular and which supports the epidermis and cutaneous appendages. In this region of the skin occur the dynamic processes essential for *temperature regulation.*

An *elevation* of the *external temperature* provokes, by means of the central nervous system and axonal reflexes, a dilatation of the cutaneous arterioles. As a consequence, blood flows rapidly into the capillaries and into the wide-spread subpapillary venous plexuses. Heat from the blood is thereby lost to the skin surface through conduction and radiation. With still higher external temperatures, the sweat glands actively transfer portions of the extracellular fluid to the surface of the skin where it (sweat) is evaporated. In a hot, dry atmosphere about 1.5 liters per hour can be lost in this manner, accounting for a concomitant loss of over 800 calories. Of course, in a humid environment beads of sweat may form on the skin and roll off without evaporating and consequently not be accompanied by any significant cooling effect. Sweating, whether effective as a cooling mechanism or not, may cause serious dehydration and electrolyte imbalance.

Sweat Glands.—Sweat glands, concerned with *heat regulation*, are found over the entire skin but are most concentrated in the palms and soles as well as in certain facial areas. These *eccrine* glands are innervated by cholinergic sympathetic fibers and are therefore activated by acetylcholine and inhibited by atropine. When an individual is resting in a warm environment, the glands do not secrete continuously but rather in periodic bursts of activity. During the inactive periods, glycogen can be detected in the glands.

A peculiar attribute of the sweat glands of the skin of the palms and soles is there responsiveness to *emotional stimuli*. This outpouring of sweat lowers the electrical resistance of the skin and forms the basis for the lie detector test. To the dermatologist and psychiatrist, these areas are important as sites of *hyperhidrosis* or excessive sweating.

Sweat is generally hypotonic, containing from 0.2 per cent to 0.5 per cent sodium chloride. With acclimatization to hot climates, the excretion of sodium chloride decreases, probably as a result of secretion of adrenal *hormones*. In fact, the electrolyte pattern of sweat has been suggested as indicative of adrenal cortico-steroid production. Sweat gland dysfunction in which the sweat has an abnormally high sodium chloride concentration has been associated with *cystic fibrosis* of the *pancreas*. In conditions where the blood levels of urea, uric acid, and creatinine are high, the sweat glands act as *accessory kidneys* and excrete these substances. On the other hand, glucose is not secreted even when the blood glucose levels are high acutely or chronically.

Congenital absence of the *sweat glands*, or *hypofunction*, is disabling with respect to the toleration of high temperatures. In addition, absence of sweat or *hypohidrosis* aggravates such dry skin conditions as atopic dermatitis and erythroderma. *Obstruction* of the *sweat gland ducts* whether by hyperkeratinization or infection, a condition termed *miliaria*, can result in a "sweat retention syndrome" or *heat exhaustion*. An obvious treatment of these conditions is the avoidance of a hot external environment.

The *apocrine sweat glands* do not respond to heat. These glands are located in the axillary, pubic, and mammillary regions and respond to emotional or painful stimuli by extruding a *liquid* which is initially odorless but which, upon bacterial contamination, rapidly develops a characteristic *scent*. This peculiar sweat is continually secreted but is expelled only when the contractile myoepithelium which surrounds the tubules is activated by the adrenergic fibers which innervate the myoepithelium. The apocrine sweat glands represent the vestiges of scent organs which play a role in the sex activity in lower animals. In human beings, disorders of the apocrine sweat glands still point to their connection with sex. *Miliaria* of these glands (*Fox-Fordyce disease*) is seen frequently in females at the menopause. Furthermore, a carcinoma which affects the nipple (*Paget's disease*) is also occasionally seen in the skin regions which possess apocrine sweat glands (*extramammary Paget's disease*).

Sebaceous Glands.—A constant secretion of oily sebum by sebaceous glands onto the surface of the skin provides a physical barrier to water loss. At the same time, some of the fatty acids from the sebum may form emulsions which further aid in the retention of water. In the *absence* of sebum, the upper layers of the epidermis become dehydrated and flake off. Sebaceous secretion is not controlled neurally. Instead, the viscosity of the sebum itself may, to a degree, regulate the outpouring from the duct onto the skin. Thus, at low external temperatures (15 to 17°C.) the viscosity of sebum increases and its flow to the surface is thereby impeded.

Hormones undoubtedly have an effect on sebaceous gland activity. At *puberty* there is almost universally a seborrhea to some degree. A plugging of the sebaceous ducts frequently leads to *acne* in which inflammation and infection of the glands has occurred. Despite the obvious correlation of many cases of acne with sexual maturation, the effects of the gonadal hormones on the skin are still perplexing. *Sex hormones* administered topically, systemically, and locally to normal adult males do not produce any noticeable effect on the histology of the skin or sebaceous glands. The hair which is so closely associated histologically with the sebaceous gland is affected by various hormones but this depends too upon the location of the hair and upon *heredity*. For instance, *eunuchs* generally possess hair on the scalp. When androgens are administered to adult eunuchs, they develop a typical male type of baldness of the head, provided that there has been a noted familial tendency for baldness and that they are at an age when they would have been expected to become bald in the absence of the gonadal deficiency. The effects of hormones may also depend upon the condition of the target tissue. As an example, hair growth is not uniform but instead there are alternate periods of activity and rest. Irritants such as ether and benzene cause loss of hair (*alopecia*) only during the resting stage whereas x-irradiation is deleterious during the active stage of the growth cycle.

Blood and Vascular Conditions.—The *color* and *temperature* of the skin reflect many systemic disorders as well as conditions exclusively of cutaneous origin. *Decreased blood flow*, whether as a result of cutaneous arteriolar constriction, anemia, or mitral stenosis, causes pallor of the skin. A *bluish* or *cyanotic* hue appears when the concentration of reduced hemoglobin in cutaneous venules is greater than 5 gram per cent. This is seen in *polycythemia* and when the skin is exposed to *cold*. In the latter condition, the cutaneous arteriovenous anastomoses shut down and only a relatively small volume of blood reaches the venules after having passed through the capillaries. The blood entering the venules has had a great quantity of its oxygen removed, hence the blue color of the skin. The temperature of the skin is largely a function of arteriolar diameter or blood flow. It is thus possible to have a warm cyanotic skin as in polycythemia or exposure to cold and reddish skin as in carbon monoxide poisoning in which reduced hemoglobin is replaced by carbon monoxide hemoglobin.

Abnormal *spasms* of the cutaneous *arterioles* (Raynaud's disease) especially of the extremities upon exposure to cold cause a pale, cyanotic, cold skin. This disease has been treated surgically by sympathectomy but there is evidence that the abnormal response is conditioned by the environmental temperature prior to the exposure to cold. Thus, the disease may in reality be a central nervous system disorder. The counterpart of arteriolar spasms may be in the pathological arteriolar *vasodilatation* which occurs in *erythromelagia*.

Itching.—The most commonly distressing feature of skin disorders is the frequently concomitant itching (*pruritus*). The classical assignment of modality to a particular type of specialized nerve ending is no longer in favor. Be that as it may, the sensation of itching is believed to be *mediated* by fine, unmyelinated fibers which subserve pain. The stimulus for both pain and itching may very likely be the polypeptides which can be found in blister fluid and other exudates. Trauma to the skin involves damage to mast cells and to other cells which are known to release endopeptidases which can ultimately cause itching. Thus, it is not surprising that histological evidence is not always found to provide a cause for pruritus. To the predisposed skin, even slight mechanical pressure may be an adequate stimulus for itching.

GENERAL CONSIDERATIONS

Before proceeding with a discussion of specific diseases of the skin, it may be profitable—for purposes of orientation—to consider briefly (1) the anatomy of the skin, (2) a glossary of the more commonly used terms, and (3) a few over-all general aspects of dermatologic lesions.

Anatomy.—The skin is composed of three layers—epidermis, corium, and hypoderm. The *epidermis*, also called cuticle, is the outermost covering and is composed of stratified squamous epithelium (Fig. 661*A*). The external surface is more or less smooth while the inner surface is thrown into pyramidal projections called rete cones or pegs. From without in, the epidermis consists of four layers—(1) *stratum corneum*—composed of flat, dead, keratinized cells forming a layer of varying thickness, (2) *stratum lucidum*—consisting of several layers of flat but elongated cells with relatively clear cytoplasm and no nuclei, (3) *stratum granulosum*—composed of three to five layers of elongated flattened cells with elongated nuclei and fine basophilic cytoplasmic granules, and (4) *stratum germinativum*— also known as stratum spinosum and malphigian layer and consisting of a deep single layer of cuboidal or columnar cells and several superficial layers of large polyhedral cells with intercellular bridges, an abundant amount of eosinophilic cytoplasm, and round or oval, deeply staining nuclei. The basal cells of the stratum germinativum contain varying amounts of melanin pigment. The pigment is scanty in whites and abundant in Negroes.

The *corium*, also known as the cutis, derma, and true skin, is intermediate in location, being interposed between the epidermis and hypoderm. It is

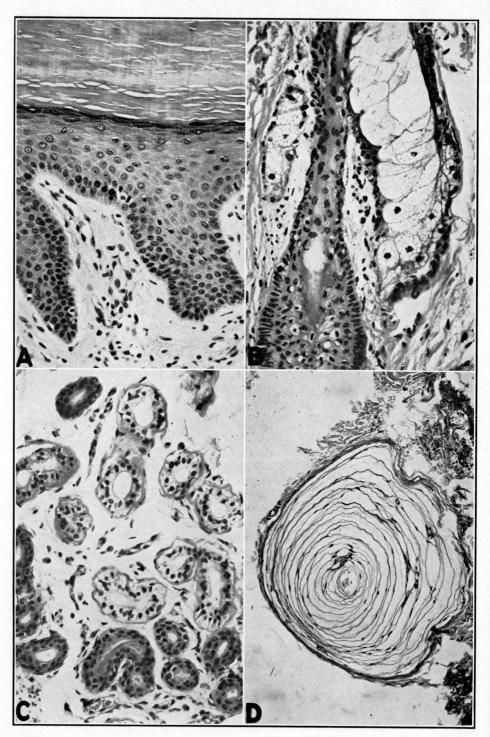

Fɪɢ. 661.—Normal skin showing *A*, a dermal papilla covered by epidermis which discloses from above down stratum corneum, stratum granulosum, and stratum germinativum (prickle cells above and basal cells below). × 200, *B*, hair sheath and shaft, and sebaceous gland. × 200, *C*, coiled sweat glands with several ducts. × 200, and *D*, a pacinian corpuscle. × 100.

composed essentially of collagenous and elastic fibers, forms papillæ that occupy the space between the rete cones, and contains blood vessels, nerves, pacinian (tactile) corpuscles, smooth muscle bundles (arrectores pilorum), and epidermal appendages (Fig. 661 *B*, *C* and *D*). *Pacinian corpuscles* are rounded or oval lamellated structures composed of concentrically arranged nerve fibrils. *Epidermal appendages* consist of nails, hairs, sebaceous glands, and sweat glands. *Nails* are composed of closely cemented, cornified, epithelial cells that grow from thickened epidermis at the level of the mid-portion of the distal phalanx. *Hairs* arise as downgrowths of the stratum germinativum. They consist of (1) the hair sheath which is composed of an outer layer of basal cells, and an inner zone of polyhedral prickle cells, (2) the root of the hair which consists of a bulbous expansion of the deepest portion of the sheath capping a papilla of connective tissue, and (3) the hair shaft which arises from the root, occupies the centralmost portion of the sheath, consists of cornified epithelium, and protrudes above the surface of the skin as the hair. *Sebaceous glands* (holocrine glands) are present in the skin of all parts of the body except the soles and palms. Most are attached to a hair sheath but some are connected directly with the epidermis. From without in they consist of a basement membrane, a single layer of flattened epithelial cells, and an inner mass of large, polyhedral, prickle-like cells that ultimately disintegrate, liberating sebum. *Sweat glands* are generally connected directly with the epidermis but sometimes they empty into hair sheaths. Each sweat gland consists of a duct which is lined by several layers of epidermal cells and a coiled secretory portion composed from without in of a basement membrane, a single layer of flat myoepithelial cells, and a single layer of cuboidal secretory cells. The *hypoderm*, also known as the stratum subcutaneum and the panniculus adiposus, is the innermost layer of the skin that is interposed between the dermis and the deeper structures. It is composed essentially of fat and loose connective tissue, supports vessels and nerves as they pass into the dermis, and contains pacinian corpuscles together with deeper portions of the hair apparatus and occasionally sweat glands.

Glossary of Common Terms.—Although pathologic processes in the skin are fundamentally similar to pathologic processes in other tissues and organs, certain terms have been developed to connote specific conditions, thus making dermatologic parlance rather unique. A few of the more commonly used terms may be listed as follows:

Acanthosis.—(Gr. = spine)—hypertrophy and hyperplasia of the prickle cells of the stratum germinativum.

Bulla.—(L.)—a large blister containing watery fluid.

Circinate.—(Gr. = circle)—having a circular or ring-like appearance.

Crust.—(L. = an outer layer)—an outer hard layer or scab composed of dried exudate or secretion.

Disseminated.—(L. = apart + to saw)—irregularly scattered over a considerable area.

Dyskeratosis.—(Gr. = ill + horn)—faulty development of the epidermis characterized by abnormal premature keratinization of the various layers with disarrangement of the cells.

Erosion.—(L. = to eat out)—a superficial defect resulting from destruction of the outer portion (but not all) of the epidermis with or without involvement of the tips of the subjacent papillæ.

Eruption.—(L. = to break out)—the act of breaking out, appearing, or becoming visible or the sum total of all cutaneous lesions appearing in one person.

Erythematous.—(L. = redness)—having a reddish blush.

Eschar.—(Gr. = scab)—a slough produced by burning or rapid necrosis of tissue.

Exfoliative.—(L. = out + leaf)—characterized by shedding of scales.

Foliaceous.—(L. = leaves)—pertaining to or resembling leaves or being scaly.

Fungoid.—(L. = fungus + Gr. = to form)—shaped like a toadstool or resembling a fungus.

Herpetiform.—(L. = herpes + to form)—vesicular or resembling herpes.

Hyperkeratosis.—(Gr. = over + horn)—hypertrophy of the stratum corneum or a condition characterized by excessive keratin formation.

Impetiginoid.—(L.)—resembling impetigo or characterized by the formation of pustules.

Lacuna.—(L.)—slit, defect, or gap.

Macule.—(L. = spot or stain)—a discolored varisized spot on the skin that is not elevated above the surface.

Multiformis.—(F. = many + shapes)—having many forms, shapes, or appearances.

Nigricans.—(L.)—blackish color.

Nodosus.—(L.)—having nodules or projections.

Nummular.—(L.)—coin-shaped or made up of round, flat discs.

Papillomatosis.—(L. and Gr. = papillary tumor)—formation of epithelial tumors in which the cells cover finger-like processes.

Papule.—(L. = pimple)—a circumscribed solid elevation of the skin that measures up to 0.5 cm. in diameter.

Parakeratosis.—retention of nuclei by the keratinizing cells of the stratum corneum.

Polymorphous.—(Gr. = many + form)—occurring in several or many forms.

Punctate.—(L. = point)—resembling or occurring in points or dots.

Pustule.—(L.)—a small (usually 1 to 5 mm.) elevation of the epidermis containing pus.

Rhagadiform.—(Gr. = rent + form)—fissured or containing cracks.

Rosaceous.—(L. = rose)—having a rosy or pinkish hue.

Scale.—(L. = squama)—a thin, plate-like mass of epithelial cells shed from the skin.

Senile.—(L.)—of or pertaining to old age.

Serpiginous.—(L. = to creep)—creeping or advancing in an irregular fashion.

Siccus.—(L.)—dry.

Spongiosis.—(Gr.)—intercellular edema of the prickle cell layer of the epidermis.

Ulcer.—(L.)—a local destruction of the entire thickness of the epidermis together with varying amounts of the dermis.

Versicolor.—(L. = to turn + color)—variegated or changing color.

Vesicle.—(L. = diminutive of bladder)—a circumscribed elevation of the skin measuring up to 0.5 cm. in diameter and containing serum, blood, or lymph.

Vulgaris.—(L.)—ordinary or common.

Wheal.—a whitish or pinkish elevation on the skin that usually arises rapidly as after the stroke of a whip.

General Aspects of Dermatologic Lesions. —Diseases of the skin are more *common* than diseases of any other single organ of the body. They *occur* at all ages from intra-uterine life to old age although many disorders have a predilection for certain age groups. The specific *causes* of the cutaneous lesions are the causes of diseases in general (p. 5), while predisposing factors range all the way from inherited defects to occupational exposure. *Pathologically* the disturbances may be classified according to (1) the specific anatomic structures affected such as the epidermis, epidermal appendages, dermis, and hypoderm, (2) the etiologic factor responsible, (3) the author who first described the condition adequately, or (4) the appearance of the lesion. Actually none of these classifications is entirely satisfactory and although an etiologic categorization is the best, the precise etiologic agent is not known in every disease and, therefore, a combination of the above listed classifications is usually used. As to a broader subdivision, the general outline of Congenital Anomalies, Degenerations, Inflammations, Physical Disturbances, and Tumors used in other portions of the text shall be employed here. The *complications*, as would be expected, are extremely varied. They may be local or systemic and they may be inconsequential or serious enough to cause death. The *clinical manifestations* are also local or local and systemic. Local manifestations consist essentially of the lesion itself, pain, tenderness, pruritus, and disability. Systemic manifestations may include malaise, fever, chills, nausea, vomiting, anorexia, loss of weight, anemia, leukocytosis, and eosinophilia. A correct *diagnosis* can only be made after a consideration of all the data available including a careful history, local and systemic physical examinations, cutaneous sensitivity tests, bacteriologic studies, serologic tests, roentgenographic findings (some instances), and biopsy. The importance of the pooling of all information on hand cannot be overemphasized in attaining a proper evaluation. Especially is this true in interpreting the histopathologic changes. *Treatment* is quite varied. In general, it consists of (1) internal measures including diets and various medications, (2) topical applications including cleansing with water and soap, oils, ointments, powders, solutions, pastes, plasters, specific drugs, etc., and (3) removing the lesion by surgical excision, electrical means, caustics, etc. The *prognosis* as would be expected, is also quite variable. Some conditions are readily curable, others tend to recur, and others still pursue a relentless downhill course, resulting in death.

Dermatology is a broad field concerning which volumes have been written. It is obvious, therefore, that only the highlights of some of the more important disorders can be touched upon in the space allotted in a text of this sort. Furthermore, while a few references to articles in various Journals are given, such standard works as Becker and Obermeyer, Lever, McCarthy, and Ormsby and Montgomery are highly recommended for supplementary reading for it is from these books that your author has gleaned much of the information that follows.

CONGENITAL ANOMALIES

Orientation.—In this section may be included not only the disorders in which there is an obvious physical defect of development, but also a few of the better known acquired lesions that result from defects inherent in the germ plasm. The latter are mostly degenerative and/or inflammatory disturbances that, however, develop on a congenital basis.

Cutaneous Defects.—Rarely, both the ectodermal and mesodermal derivatives of the entire skin are severely hypoplastic, forming a thin transparent external covering instead of the normal skin. More commonly, the different constituents are hypoplastic to various degrees, resulting in what has been termed *congenital ectodermal dysplasia*. Sometimes round, oval, or irregular areas of the epidermis, dermis, and hypoderm are completely defective or are replaced with gray scars. Such defects are present on the scalp (midline), trunk, and extremities.

Anomalies of Pigmentation.—Normally, melanin pigment is present in the basal layer of the epidermis and accounts for the degree of pigmentation of the skin in the various races. Thus, in the white race it is scanty in amount, in the yellow race moderate, and in the Negro race abundant. Abnormalities of pigmentation consist of either an increase or a decrease in the amount of melanin. The former is referred to as *hyperpigmentation* or *melasma* (Lerner). It occurs in connection with (1) *freckles* (ephelides), (2) *cholasma*—usually seen in pregnancy, sometimes referred to as the "mask of pregnancy," and consisting of yellowish to deep brownish macules scattered symmetrically over the forehead and face, (3) *suntan*, (4) *nevus* (p. 1393), (5) *Addison's disease* (p. 1002), and (6) *chronic malnutrition*. It should be remembered, however, that an increase in melanin does not account for all cases of increased pigmentation of the skin for such substances as iron (hemosiderosis and hemochromatosis), silver (argyria), bismuth, arsenic, etc., also produce cutaneous discolorations. A decreased amount of melanin pigment is referred to as *hypopigmentation*. It includes (1) *albinism*—consisting of a congenital absence of pigment not only in the skin but also in the hair and eyes, affecting either the entire body (complete) or only portions of the body (partial), and appearing white to pinkish (Cooke) and (2) *vitiligo*—being acquired rather than congenital, consisting of round, oval, or irregular areas of white depigmentation, and usually affecting the face, neck, and dorsal surfaces of the hands.

Anomalies of Hairs.—Developmental abnormalities of hairs consist of decreased or increased growth. The former is known as *hypotrichosis*. It may consist of complete lack of growth of hair or of poorly formed hair and it may affect the entire body or involve only the scalp (alopecia). Increased growth of hair is known as *hypertrichosis* or *hirsutism* (Callaway). The condition may be present at birth or develop at any time thereafter, is most common in females, and may consist of (1) abnormal growth in areas where only lanugo hair is found, (2) increase in length where normally only short hair grows (pubis, axilla, and face), (3) increase in density where hair is normally sparse, and (4) universal overgrowth producing what has been called "dog-men."

Anomalies of Nails.—The more important congenital and acquired abnormalities of the nails may be listed as follows: (1) *onychauxis* (Gr. = nail + increase) or *onychogryphosis* (Gr. = nail + bending)—defined as hypertrophy, affecting the fingers and/or toes, and consisting of increase in length, breadth, and thickness with varying degrees of horn-like twisting, (2) *anonychia* (Gr. = negative + nail)—indicating an absence of one or more nails of the fingers and/or toes, (3) *onychatrophy* (Gr. = nail + privation + food)—indicating atrophy, being acquired, and consisting of decrease in length, width, and thickness with varying degrees of furrowing and distortion, (4) *leukonychia* (Gr. = white + nail)—consisting of white streaks or spots beneath the nails, (5) *onychorrhexis* (Gr. = nail + split)—connoting longitudinal splitting or fracturing of one or more nails, (6) *koilonychia* (Gr. = hollow + nail) or spoon nails—indicating a central concave deformity of the nails with the production of a saucer-like depression, (7) *onychoschizea* (Gr. = nail + divide)—consisting of separation of the nail into two or three layers, (8) *onycholysis* (Gr. = nail + loosening)—connoting varying degrees of separation of the entire thickness of the nail from its bed, (9) *onychoclasis* (Gr. = nail + breaking)—indicating breaking of a nail, and (10) *onychocryptosis* (Gr. = nail + to conceal)—known also as ingrowing toenail and consisting of growth of the lateral portion of the tip of the nail (usually of the great toe) toward the adjacent skin producing pressure, pain, and sometimes infection.

Anhidrosis.—The term *anhidrosis* (Gr. = privation + sweating) may be defined as absence of sweating and should be differentiated from *oligo-*

hidrosis (Gr. = scanty + sweating) and *hypohidrosis* (Gr. = under + sweating) which means a partial or relative decrease in sweating. The condition is often part of congenital ectodermal dysplasia (Metson) but may also be acquired when it is idiopathic or secondary to a generalized skin disorder. The chief clinical manifestations are lack of perspiration and intolerance to heat.

Bromhidrosis.—The term *bromhidrosis* (Gr. = stench + sweat) connotes the presence of a highly unpleasant but characteristic odor to usually excessive perspiration. The areas affected are the axillæ, inframammary folds, groins, genital and anal areas, and feet. Although bromhidrosis is often congenital, local cleanliness helps greatly in minimizing the odor emitted.

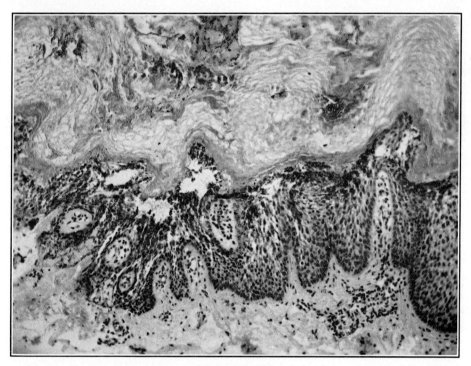

Fig. 662.—Ichthyosis disclosing extensive hyperkeratosis of the epidermis. × 100.

Xerosis.—Xerosis (Gr.) indicates unusual dryness of the skin and/or the eyes. It may be congenital or acquired. *Congenital* xerosis is due to insufficient activity of sebaceous and sweat (in the eye lacrimal) glands while *acquired* xerosis (chapping) results from exposure of the skin to alkalies, too frequent bathing, cold air, etc. The areas most commonly affected are those poor in perspiration normally. They appear dry, scaly, fissured, and erythematous.

Ichthyosis.—The term ichthyosis (Gr. = fish) denotes an unusual dryness, thickness, and scaliness of the skin that resembles the covering of an alligator or a fish. The condition begins in early fetal life, may be attended by death of the infant at the time of delivery, and is characterized by abnormal epidermal cornification or hyperkeratosis (especially marked about the hairs) together with absence of the stratum granulosum (Fig.

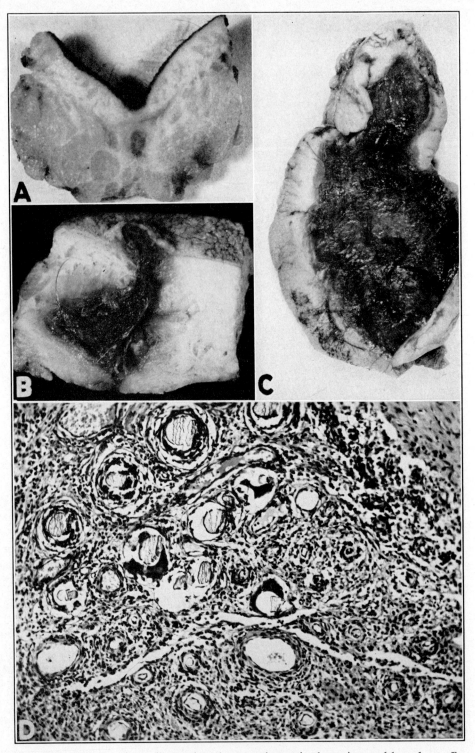

FIG. 663.—Pilonidal disease illustrating *A*, an oval tract in the corium and hypoderm, *B*, a sinus (containing hair) communicating with the epidermis, *C*, an opened cyst containing hair, and *D*, an infected sinus with hairs, chronic inflammation, and foreign body giant cells. × 100.

662) (Lattuada). Sometimes the disorder may be attended by the formation of intra-epithelial bullæ (Barker).

Seborrhea.—While the conditions included under the caption "seborrhea" are varied, the term (L. = sebum + flow) actually connotes a functional disturbance of sebaceous glands characterized by excessive secretion of sebum. The condition is particularly noticeable around puberty, is present in both sexes, and is thought to be due to androgenic substances. The areas of the body most commonly affected are the face, scalp, anterior and posterior portions of the chest, axillæ, and pubic area. The skin is shiny, oily, or actually scaly, discloses yellowish to black plugs in the pores, and is predisposed to seborrheic dermatitis, acne vulgaris, and alopecia.

Rubber Skin.—This condition, also known as cutis laxa, connotes a hyperelasticity of the skin that makes its appearance at or before puberty. It consists of an anomaly of connective tissue development. The collagenous tissue is loose and myxomatous but the elastic tissue is normal.

Ectodermal Cysts and Sinuses.—Ectodermal cysts and sinuses result from defective closure of embryonal clefts. They usually occur (1) about the *nose* (p. 409), (2) in the region of the *neck* both in the midline (p. 560) and laterally (p. 601), (3) in the *pre-auricular* area (p. 601), (4) along the *genitoperineal raphe* (p. 1111), and (5) along the spine at any point between the occipital and coccygeal regions (Mount). In the last mentioned category the most important are defects located opposite the *sacrococcygeal region* of the spine and termed (1) *pilonidal* (L. = hair + nest) *disease* including all types of lesions, (2) *pilonidal tract*—limited to a tubular tract beneath the epidermis, (3) *pilonidal cyst*—connoting a cystic dilatation of the tract, and (4) *pilonidal sinus*—indicating a tract communicating with the exterior (Donald, Palumbo, and Grau). Pilonidal disease *occurs* more commonly in males than in females, has its greatest incidence in the third decade of life, and is said to account for approximately one in every one thousand hospital admissions. The *pathogenesis* of the lesion has been explained on the basis of representing (1) a remnant of the medullary canal, (2) an invagination of surface epithelium in embryonic life, and (3) the preen gland found in some birds. Of these, the first mentioned is the most widely accepted. Regardless of its origin, the disorder remains quiescent until it is *traumatized* and secondarily *infected*. The usual invading organisms are streptococci, staphylococci, and colon bacilli. *Pathologically* the defect exists as a tract, cyst, or sinus located in the corium and hypoderm (Fig. 663). It usually measures up to 3 or 4 cm. in greatest diameter, consists of a single or branched cavity, and generally contains sebum, hair, and debris. The overlying epidermis contains a longitudinal midline depression which contains the ostium in cases developing a sinus. The *histologic* changes are similar regardless of the type of defect. Originally the lining consists of squamous epithelium with epidermal appendages in the underlying tissue. With supervening infection, however, all of these structures may be destroyed and the lining may consist only of nonspecific granulation tissue. Because of the presence of hairs and sebum, foreign body giant cells, cholesterol crystals, and foam cells may be quite conspicuous. The *complications* consist of infection, extension of the infection to adjacent structures, and (rarely) development of carcinoma. The *clinical manifestations* consist of pain, tumor, and discharge. The *diagnosis* is made from the appearance and location of the lesion. *Treatment* of choice is complete surgical excision. The *prognosis* is good.

Hydroa.—Hydroa is a papular and vesicular eruption that is prone to occur on the exposed parts of the skin in boys in summer. It is dividable into two types—hydroa vacciniforme and hydroa æstivale. *Hydroa vacciniforme* is more serious, exists throughout life, is characterized by epidermal vesicles and dermal inflammation, and heals by scarring. *Hydroa æstivale* is less serious, terminates at puberty, discloses minimal inflammation of the corium, and heals without scarring.

Epidermolysis Bullosa.—Epidermolysis bullosa consists of the formation of vesicles and bullæ, often at points of trauma. *Histologically* the accumulations of fluid may be found within the epidermis (simple form) in which case healing occurs by scarring. The former subsides at puberty while the latter continues throughout life and is associated with similar lesions in the mouth and with dystrophy of nails.

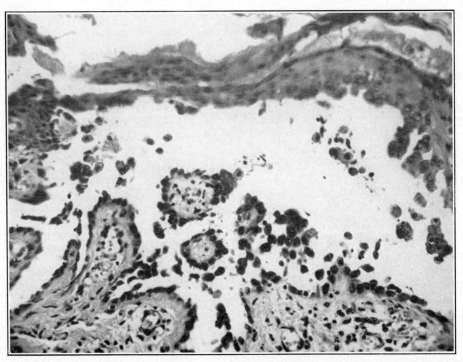

Fig. 664.—Darier's disease showing a lacuna between the basal and prickle cells, several corps ronds, a few grains, and hyperkeratosis. × 200.

Darier's Disease.—Darier's disease, also known as *keratosis follicularis*, is characterized by an extensive papular eruption occurring first about the head and face and then affecting other parts of the body from above down (including sometimes the oral, pharyngeal, and vulvar mucosas). As the lesions age, they become crusted, papillomatous, and even tumor-like. *Histologically* the epidermis discloses dyskeratosis, hyperkeratosis, and papillomatosis. At the junction of the basal and prickle cells are elongated lacunæ (Fig. 664). Adjacent to the lacunæ are degenerating cells called corps ronds—consisting of pyknotic nuclei and dense eosinophilic cytoplasm, and in the superficial layers are grains—consisting of parakeratotic cells with prominent elongated nuclei.

Sclerema Adiposum Neonatorum.—This condition consists of hardening of adipose tissue in the subcutaneous areas and less commonly within the body of newborn infants (Zeek). The *cause* is unknown although the following have been considered: (1) obstetrical trauma, (2) low body temperature, (3) deficiency of olein, (4) presence of a lipolytic ferment, and (5) glandular dyscrasia. *Grossly* the fat of the skin (and affected organs) is indurated, thickened, congealed, and firm. *Histologically* it discloses varying degrees of degeneration, necrosis, and crystallization of fat along with a granulomatous reaction in which foreign body giant cells may be prominent (Fig. 665).

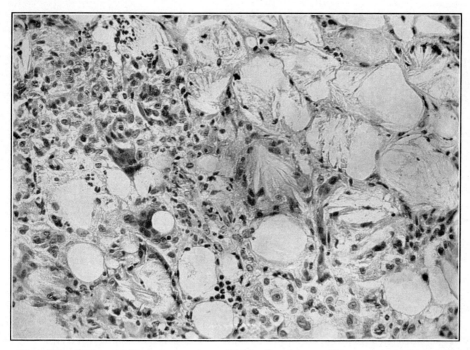

Fig. 665.—Sclerema adiposum neonatorum illustrating degeneration, necrosis, and crystallization of fat as well as foreign body giant cell formation and infiltration with plasma cells, lymphocytes, monocytes, and a few neutrophils. × 200.

Congenital Nodular Calcification.—The general topic of dystrophic calcification, metastatic calcification, and calcinosis has already been considered (p. 61). Congenital nodular calcification of the skin is a form of dystrophic calcification that usually occurs in a hamartoma of sweat gland origin but that may also be superimposed upon epidermal, dermal, or sebaceous cysts (Winer). The lesion is generally solitary, measures 4 to 6 mm. in diameter, and consists of collections of calcific deposits in the papillæ or in sites normally occupied by epidermal appendages.

Milroy's Disease.—Milroy's disease, also known as *chronic hereditary lymphedema*, is a hereditary edema of the lower extremities that affects several members of the same family in several generations (Cook). The condition consists of a firm, indolent, symmetrical swelling of both extremities, usually involving the ankles and legs as far up as the knees but sometimes extending to the thighs. The *histologic* changes in the corium and hypoderm consist of edema fluid permeating and separating the tissues, condensation of papillæ, hyaline degeneration of the collagen, absence of elastic fibers, and slight perivascular collection of lymphocytes. Other than heredity, the cause of the condition remains unknown.

DEGENERATIONS AND INFLAMMATIONS

Orientation.—Since degenerative and inflammatory disorders of the skin are intimately blended, a strict division of the two processes is impossible and, therefore, they may be considered together. In connection with inflammation, *epidermitis* (Gr. = on + the skin + inflammation) indicates inflammation of the epidermis and *dermitis* or *dermatitis* (Gr. = skin + inflammation) means inflammation of the derm or corium. Dermatitis, however, is generally used to encompass inflammation of the entire skin or any of its layers. Because afflictions of the skin are often associated with similar disturbances in other tissues and organs, many cutaneous diseases have already been discussed in previous Chapters of the book. Most of these may be listed as follows: *plague* (p. 504), *Waterhouse-Friderichsen syndrome* (p. 1005), *cellulitis* (p. 135), *phlegmon* (p. 135), *rheumatic nodule* (p. 300), *Osler's nodes* (p. 309), *chancroid* (p. 1112), *tularemia* (p. 491), *glanders* (p. 417), *leprosy* (p. 415), *Boeck's sarcoid* (p. 501), *rickettsia* (p. 153), *herpes simplex* and *progenitalis* (p. 606), *foot* and *mouth disease* (p. 607), *cat scratch disease* (p. 984), *lymphogranuloma venereum* (p. 1112), *granuloma inguinale* (p. 1112), *fungi* in *general* (p. 157), *nocardiosis* (p. 516), *blastomycosis* (p. 514), *histoplasmosis* (p. 513), *actinomycosis* (p. 515), *scabies* (p. 1152), *filariasis* (p. 379), *elephantiasis* (p. 381), *leishmaniasis* (p. 923), *pellagra* (p. 94), *disseminated lupus erythematosus* (p. 309), *myxedema* (pp. 204 and 571), *leukoplakia* (p. 607), *dermatopathic lymphadenitis* (p. 980), *Heberden's nodes* (p. 1280), *berylliosis* (p. 468), and *paraffinoma* (p. 470). Some of the more important remaining conditions may now be discussed in the general order of bacterial infections, spirochetal diseases, viral disturbances, fungous disorders, parasitic involvements, and other degenerative, allergic, etc., states.

Impetigo.—Impetigo (L. = to attack) is an acute contagious infection of the skin characterized by the formation of papules, vesicles, and pustules, and generally occurring in the face and hands. The *cause* is direct cutaneous inoculation (often by way of finger nails) of streptococci and/or staphylococci. The *source* of infection in children is usually the nose, in women contact from children, and in men towels, razor, etc., in the barber shop. *Histologically* the changes are essentially intra-epithelial in location. The process heals by crust formation and leaves no sequela.

Furuncle.—A *furuncle* (L. = petty thief) or *boil* is an acute infection of a hair follicle and sebaceous gland or less often a sweat gland by the *Staphylococcus aureus*. The presence of several boils simultaneously or in succession is referred to as *furunculosis*. In many cases, *predisposing factors* are not apparent while in some cases diabetes, leukemia, anemia, malnutrition, low basal metabolism, humid atmosphere, perspiration, rubbing of clothing, uncleanliness, etc., definitely act as contributory agents (Gant and Barnes). The *lesion begins* as a painful, tender, erythematous, raised induration of the skin that measures up to 1 or 2 cm. in diameter (Fig. 666*A*). Within two to three days, the center becomes necrotic, points to a summit, perforates, and discharges creamy pus. The process then heals in from a few days to a week or two by collapse of the walls, filling in with granulation tissue, and often residual scar formation. *Histologically* the lesion is an acute nonspecific abscess (Fig. 666B). While any part of the body may be affected, the most common locations are face, neck, anogenital region, buttocks, wrists, and axillæ. *Treatment* consists of surgical incision to promote drainage and of eliminating predisposing causes. The *prognosis* is good.

Carbuncle.—A carbuncle (L. = little coal) is similar to a furuncle except that the lesion consists of an inflammation of several adjacent epidermal

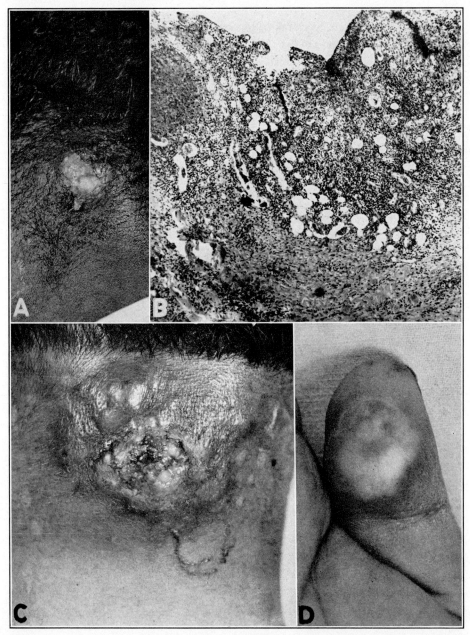

Fig. 666.—Pyogenic cutaneous infections illustrating *A*, a furuncle, *B*, a furuncle at the back of the neck with the usual changes of an acute abscess. × 50, *C*, a carbuncle at the back of the neck with multiple areas of pus formation, a large area of necrosis, and extensive surrounding hyperemia, and *D*, a felon in the pulp of the thumb.

84

appendages, that the area of involvement usually measures several centimeters in diameter, that it is characterized by multiple discharging sinuses and later by extensive sloughing, that it heals by obvious scar tissue replacement, and that it is attended by constitutional symptoms (chills, fever, malaise, and leukocytosis) in addition to local manifestations (McLaughlin and Dale). Most carbuncles are *located* on the back of the neck (Fig. 666C). The causative factors are the same as those in furuncle. *Treatment* consists of eliminating the causes, of surgical incision, and of antibiotic therapy. The *prognosis* is good.

Paronychia.—A paronychia (Gr. = near + nail) is an acute pyogenic infection near a nail generally caused by staphylococci or streptococci (Robins and Scott). The process may *start* in the subepithelial tissue adjacent to the nail or it may begin along the edge of a "hangnail" (Kanavel). It is *attended by* pain, swelling, redness, and pus formation. If untreated (by surgical incision) the infection spreads around the nail sulcus and under the eponychium, ultimately destroying the entire nail bed and nail.

Felon.—A *felon* (ME = villain) or *whitlow* (Old Norse = flaw or sore at the quick of the nail) is an acute streptococcic or staphylococcic infection of the pulp of the distal phalanx of a finger. The *source* of the infection is often a pin prick or another unnoticed trauma (Kanavel). The infection is *characterized by* severe throbbing pain and a tender, red swelling of the pulp of the finger (Fig. 666D). In a day or two the area becomes purulent and unless the pus is evacuated, the subcutaneous tension may become severe enough to cause ischemia and necrosis of the adjacent bone. *Treatment* consists of surgical incision and drainage. The *prognosis* is good.

Erysipelas.—Erysipelas (Gr. = red + skin) is an acute infectious disease of the skin usually *caused* by streptococci. The organisms gain entrance by way of an epidermal appendage or a break in the epidermis. Any *portion* of the *body* may be affected with the face and neck being most commonly involved. The *lesion* starts as a small, raised, irregular, sharply circumscribed, erythematous plaque which spreads rapidly to involve larger portions of adjacent skin. In most cases, the inflammation reaches its intensity within a week and then gradually subsides. In some instances, however, it may progress to form vesicles, bullæ, pustules, and even gangrene. *Histologically* the lesion discloses marked congestion, edema, and neutrophilic infiltration of the corium and hypoderm. The local *manifestations* consist of redness, swelling, pain, itching, and tenderness while the general manifestations encompass malaise, chills, fever, anorexia, nausea, vomiting, headache, and occasionally delirium.

Anthrax.—Anthrax (Gr. = coal or carbuncle) is an acute infectious disease *caused* by the *Bacillus anthracis*. This is a gram-positive, nonmotile, spore bearing, ærobic and facultative anærobic, encapsulated bacillus that grows readily on artificial media and that usually infects cattle, sheep, hogs, and goats. Occasionally the organisms are transmitted to *man* by way of handling infected animals and the disorder is thus seen in cattlemen, butchers, tanners, and woolsorters. The *route* of infection is usually by way of the skin, uncommonly by way of the respiratory tract, and rarely by way of the intestines. The *cutaneous* lesion is contracted through a break in the epidermis and is generally located on the face, neck, or arms. It consists of a papule which in twenty-four to forty-eight hours is transformed into a bulla filled with pus or bloody material (malignant pustule). Upon rupture, a dark eschar is exposed. Meanwhile the surrounding skin is intensely swollen and edematous and maybe affected with secondary bullæ (Fig. 667).   The draining lymph nodes enlarge and often suppurate. *Histologically* the process is a nonspecific acute inflammation which abounds in *Bacillus anthracis*.   Local manifestations consist of the lesion as described with accompanying burning and itching.   Systemic manifestations consist of malaise, chills, fever, headaches, prostration, and delirium.   In patients who recover, the lesion heals by granulation while in those who die the local process generally extends, producing extensive gangrene.   *Respiratory* lesions consist of a hemorrhagic pneumonia and *intestinal* lesions are composed of a hemorrhagic enteritis.   Both the respiratory and the intestinal diseases are much more serious than the cutaneous disorder.

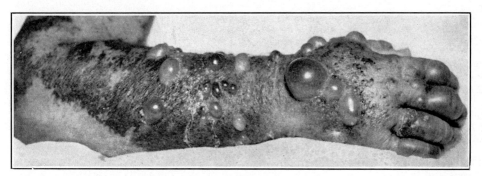

FIG. 667.—Anthrax showing varisized bullæ and marked edema of the skin of the forearm and hand.

Tuberculosis.—Tuberculosis of the skin is relatively uncommon in the United States.   It *occurs* at all ages, affects both sexes, and (in some forms) is more common in Negroes than in the white population.   The *cause* is, of course, *Mycobacterium tuberculosis*.   The disease may be contracted by direct cutaneous inoculation or by the hematogenous route.   According to Ormsby and Montgomery, *inoculation tuberculosis* may be divided into the primary tuberculous complex and secondary inoculation disease.   The *primary tuberculous complex* is analogous to the Ghon complex in the lungs.   It represents an initial infection of the host and thus commonly occurs in children.   The cutaneous lesion may be located on the face as a result of kissing or it may affect any other portion of the body in an area previously traumatized by an abrasion, cut, etc.   The sore becomes evident two to three weeks after inoculation as a nodule, ulcer, or even a furuncle. This is followed in several weeks by lymphangiitis and lymphadenitis and in time both lesions usually resolve or heal by scar tissue formation.   Occasionally the cutaneous sore extends to produce lesions similar to those in the secondary inoculation type.

Secondary inoculation form of tuberculosis represents a direct cutaneous infection in a person who has already had or still has tuberculosis.   Any part of the body surface may be affected; the lesion appears within a few days after inoculation, and a break in the epidermis usually predisposes to the lesion.   Grossly the disorder is manifested in many forms and in equally many combinations.   Some of the more common *types* may be listed as follows: (1) *tuberculosis verrucosa cutis*—consisting of warty elevations, often existing as a single nodule, usually disclosing hyperkeratosis and ulceration, and frequently located on the fingers, (2) *lupus vulgaris*—being the most common form of cutaneous tuberculosis, affecting the face and extremities more commonly than other portions of the body, initiating as a small nodule in the corium which coalesces with other nodules to form larger patches which then break down, ulcerate, scale, heal, fibrose, become hyperpigmented, extend, break down again, etc., and being complicated by tuberculosis of other organs and (in from 0.5 to 2 per cent of cases) by local carcinoma, (3) *scrofuloderma*—consisting of secondary involvement of the skin by tuberculous lesions in subjacent tissues as bones and lymph nodes, occurring most frequently in the neck and over bony prominences, and disclosing nodules which ulcerate and produce draining sinuses, and (4) *tuberculosis cutis orificialis*—consisting of tuberculosis of the mucous membranes of the nose, mouth, anus, and genital regions and encompassing

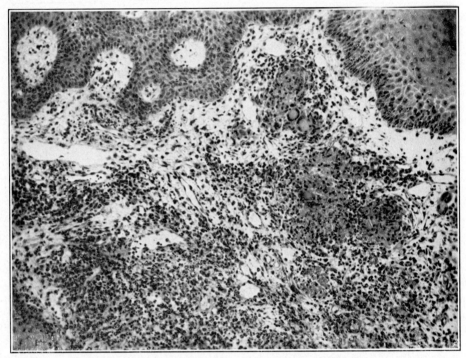

Fig. 668.—Tuberculosis of the skin showing several hard tubercles in the outer portion of the corium.

nodules and/or various types of ulcerations. *Hematogenous tuberculosis* of the skin is always secondary to tuberculosis in other organs and tissues of the body and is usually more widely disseminated than the inoculation variety. The more important lesions may be listed as follows: (1) *disseminated miliary tuberculosis*—usually occurring in children and consisting of a variety of nonspecific macules, papules, and vesicles, (2) *lichenoid tuberculosis*—consisting of small collections of follicular, indolent papules, (3) *disseminated follicular tuberculosis*—consisting of follicular lesions composed of papules or papulopustules, (4) *papulonecrotic tuberculosis*—consisting of acne-like lesions that break down, caseate, ulcerate, and heal by scar tissue formation, and (5) *indurated cutaneous tuberculosis*—consisting of deeply located subcutaneous indurated nodules affecting the legs and referred to as erythema induratum or nodosum (p. 1346). Regardless of the gross appearance of the lesions, the *histologic* changes usually consist of hard or soft tubercles (Fig. 668) or of a more caseating type of necrosis (p. 167).

Syphilis.—Since syphilis is an extremely protean disease that affects all tissues and organs of the body, it has already been discussed or mentioned in most of the preceding Chapters. In this section, therefore, some of the more important facts will be consolidated and the disease as it pertains to the skin will be briefly discussed. The origin of the term *syphilis* is not known for certain. According to one explanation it is derived from the name of a shepherd who contracted the disease, while, according to another, it is derived from two Greek words meaning together and to love. It may be *defined* as a contagious venereal disease caused by the *Treponema pallidum*. This is a tightly coiled, thread-like organism possessing eight to fourteen spirals and pointed ends and measuring from 8 to 14 microns in length and from 0.25 to 0.3 microns in diameter. Syphilis is dividable into two types—acquired and congenital.

Acquired syphilis is the more common of the two. It is usually contracted by sexual intercourse, although rarely it is picked up by contact of other parts of the body with infected material. Traditionally, the disorder is divided into three stages—primary, secondary, and tertiary although modern syphilologists prefer two groupings—early syphilis (encompassing the primary and secondary stages) and late syphilis (encompassing the tertiary stage). The *primary stage* consists of the *chancre*. It occurs in from one to six weeks after inoculation of the organisms and is usually located on the external genitals (p. 178). Extragenital chancres, however, may occur at the following sites: lips, mouth, nose, face, nipples, etc. (Tucker). Grossly the chancre consists of a papule that enlarges to form a raised, painless, firm, superficially ulcerated, sharply circumscribed mass that measures about 1 cm. in diameter (p. 178). The draining lymph nodes are enlarged, firm, and nontender. The lesion disappears spontaneously in from two to eight weeks. The *secondary stage* usually becomes manifested up to three months after inoculation. It is characterized by (1) symmetrically distributed cutaneous macules, papules, vesicles, or pustules, (2) mucous patches in the mouth and other mucosal surfaces (p. 178), (3) acute pharyngitis, and (4) systemic manifestations consisting of malaise, headache, anemia, pains in the bones and joints, etc. The *tertiary stage* occurs at any time after the primary inoculation and may be found in any organ or tissue of the body. The cutaneous lesions are widely disseminated and protean in appearance. As a rule, they are asymmetrical in distribution, deeply infiltrative, nodular, ultimately ulcerative, and may measure from a few millimeters to many centimeters in diameter. They heal by resolution or by granulation tissue formation and fibrosis.

Congenital syphilis is that form of the disease that is contracted from the mother during intra-uterine life and that is apparent at birth or that becomes manifested during infancy or childhood. The cutaneous lesions are similar to those in the secondary and tertiary stages of the disease with the chancre not being encountered. The lesions in the nose (p. 413), mouth (p. 608), lungs (p. 503), spleen (p. 971), liver (p. 818), thymus (p. 994), and bones (p. 1234 have already been discussed.

The *histologic changes* in the various stages of syphilis have been considered in Chapter 5 (p. 178). The *diagnosis* of the disorder is made from the history, from the appearance of the lesions, by demonstration of *Treponema pallidum* by the dark field method, and by serologic tests on the blood (Beerman). *Treatment* consists of prophylaxis and administration of penicillin. The *prognosis* varies with the stage of the disease and the organ affected. Cutaneous lesions generally respond readily and completely to therapy.

Yaws.—Yaws is a nonvenereal, syphilitic-like, infectious disease caused by the *Treponema pertenue* which gains entrance by way of some break (cut, abrasion, insect bite, etc.) in the skin. The disorder *prevails* among the poorer classes of the colored race in the tropics. Both sexes are affected and all ages are represented. As in syphilis, there are three stages. The *primary* lesion (mother yaws) occurs at an extragenital site in from three to four weeks after inoculation. It consists of several papules which fuse, become covered with crust, and ulcerate. It may heal by scarring or it may go on to the second stage. *Secondary* manifestations are apparent from one to three months after the primary. They consist of constitutional symptoms of fever, headache, malaise, etc., and of disseminated cutaneous papules which disappear, leaving dandruff-like patches or which progress to form nodules with serrated surfaces that discharge serous fluid. The *tertiary stage* is characterized by gummatous-like nodules and deep ulcers. The *microscopic* changes are similar to those in syphilis.

Bejel.—Bejel is a spirochetal disease found among the Arabs of the Euphrates Valley. The condition is similar to (or a form of) syphilis or yaws.

Pinta.—Pinta (Sp. = painted) is a nonvenereal spirochetal disease particularly prevalent in dark-skinned races of Latin America and Mexico. It *occurs* among the poorer classes, affects children and young adults, and is caused by the *Treponema carateum*. The disorder is similar to syphilis and yaws. The *primary lesion* occurs at the point of inoculation and consists of a 5 to 10 cm. erythematous plaque surrounded by satellite nodules. *Secondary lesions* occur from six months to a year after inoculation and consist of generalized macules and papules called pintids. Both primary and secondary lesions reveal parakeratosis, hyperkeratosis, acanthosis, and intraepithelial abscesses. *Tertiary lesions* develop after months or years and consist of symmetrically distributed hyperpigmented patches alternating with hypopigmented areas. In addition, there are palmar and plantar hyperkeratosis and fissuring together with aortitis and juxta-articular or generalized lymphadenitis.

Exanthemata.—The term *exanthem* or *exanthema* (Gr. = eruption) signifies a cutaneous disorder characterized by the presence of an eruption, by contagiousness, and by fever. Diseases in this group (exanthemas or exanthemata) usually (but not always) occur in children and, as a rule, are accompanied by life-long immunity following a single attack. Included in the category are scarlet fever, rubeola, rubella, varicella, and variola.

Scarlet Fever.—Scarlet fever (*scarlatina* from L. = red) is an acute contagious disease that is caused by a *Streptococcus hemolyticus*, transmitted by contact with secretions from the nose and throat, attended by an incubation period of from several hours to several days, and *characterized by* an eruption and constitutional symptoms. Systemic manifestations consist of vomiting, headache, sore throat, fever to 105° F., and rapid pulse. The throat is scarlet red; the cervical lymph nodes are enlarged, and the skin discloses a diffuse redness composed of minute red points in close apposition. The eruption appears within twenty-four hours after the onset, is first noted about the neck, and spreads rapidly to involve the face, trunk, and extremities. The lesions fade in from three to seven days and the areas affected then desquamate for periods of from two to six weeks. The *complica-*

tions of scarlet fever may consist of (1) profound intoxication with coma and death, (2) nephritis, (3) otitis media, (4) pneumonia, (5) pericarditis, and (6) pleuritis.

Rubeola.—Rubeola (L. = red) or *measles* is an acute contagious disease *caused* by a virus. The incubation period varies from ten to fourteen days, following which the disorder is ushered in by coryza, photophobia, chilliness, and fever. Examination at this stage discloses Koplick spots in the buccal mucosa (p. 607). In four days an eruption occurs on the neck or face and then spreads to the trunk and extremities. The *lesion* consists of slightly raised red macules that coalesce to produce large irregularly blotchy areas of cutaneous involvement. The zenith is reached in about four days

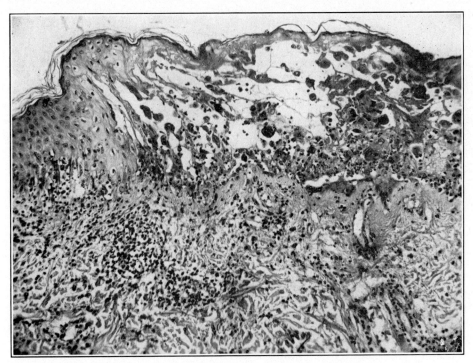

Fig. 669.—Varicella illustrating degeneration of epithelial cells and an intraepithelial vesicle. × 100.

after which the eruption begins to fade, leaving at first a yellowish-brown discoloration and then slight scaling before the skin is restored to normal. *Histologically* the deeper layers of the epidermis disclose vacuolic degeneration while the corium reveals nonspecific inflammation. The *complications* of measles may consist of (1) pneumonia, (2) encephalitis, (3) keratitis, (4) otitis media, and (5) nephritis.

Rubella.—Rubella (L. = reddish) or *German measles* is an acute contagious disease *caused* by a virus. After an incubation period of from seven to twenty-one days mild headache, malaise, and fever are followed by a pink to red, macular *eruption* which begins on the face and scalp, reaches a maximum within twenty-four hours, and disappears by the fifth day. The disorder is accompanied by posterior cervical lymphadenopathy, which incidentally aids in arriving at a correct diagnosis. Complete recovery is the rule. Although it has been suggested that the incidence of developmental abnormalities is increased in infants born of mothers who had rubella during their pregnancy, such contentions are not left unchallenged (Beswick).

Varicella.—Varicella (L. = dim. variola) or *chickenpox* is an acute contagious disease *caused* by a virus. After an incubation period of about fourteen days the disease is ushered in with mild malaise and slight fever and these are followed by an eruption on the trunk, head, and later the extremities. The *eruption* consists of successive crops of discrete papules that pass through the stages of vesicles and (sometimes) pustules and, within three to four days, heal by crust formation. *Histologically* the vesicle is intra-epidermal and multilocular and the adjacent epithelial cells disclose intranuclear inclusions (Fig. 669).

Variola.—Variola (L. = various) or *smallpox* is an acute, contagious disease *caused* by a virus. After an incubation period of from one to two weeks the disease is ushered in suddenly with malaise, chills, headache, fever, epigastric pain, and (sometimes) nausea and vomiting. The *eruption,* occurring on the third or fourth day, is first noted on the scalp and face and then spreads to involve the rest of the body. Unlike in varicella, where successive crops of eruptions are noted, variola is characterized by an approximately similar stage in all lesions. The initial lesion is a papule. This is followed by a vesicle in two to three days, by a pustule about the sixth day, by drying and crusting about the twelfth day, and (often) permanent scar formation upon healing. Sometimes the eruptions are more confluent and at other times (more severe cases) they may be distinctly hemorrhagic. *Histologically* the vesicles and pustules are intra-epithelial and the adjacent degenerating cells disclose both intracytoplasmic and intranuclear inclusion (Wolman) bodies. The *complications* of variola are (1) cutaneous—furuncles, abscesses, erysipelas, and gangrene, (2) encephalitis, (3) otitis media, (4) conjunctivitis, (5) tracheobronchitis and pneumonia, (6) nephritis, and (7) occasionally arthritis.

Vaccinia.—Vaccinia (L. = cow) or *cowpox* is an acute infectious disease *caused* by a virus, ordinarily seen in cows, and occurring in man as a result of vaccination against variola (Mustard). Sometimes, however, the disorder in man becomes generalized. Regardless of which type of lesion is present, the eruption passes through the stages of papules, vesicles, pustules, crusting, and healing by scarring. It is thus similar to that seen in variola. *Histologically,* however, the inclusion (Guanieri) bodies are found only intracytoplasmically.

Milkers' Nodules.—Milkers' nodules are erythematous papules occurring on the exposed surfaces of the hands and sometimes the face and neck (Cawley and Nomland). They develop slowly, persist for a few weeks or months, are *caused* by the natural cowpox, and are contracted by milking cows. *Histologically* the epidermis discloses parakeratosis, acanthosis, and tiny vesicles while the corium reveals nonspecific granulation tissue.

Kaposi's Varicelliform Eruption.—This condition is an acute contagious disorder *caused* by the virus of herpes simplex. It is generally grafted upon an eczema or atopic dermatitis and is thus seen at all ages (Miller). The *lesions* consist of groups of vesicles associated with local edema and pain, all appearing over a period of three to seven days. In addition, regional lymphadenopathy, leukopenia, fever, anorexia, and malaise are usually present. The pathologic changes are similar to those in herpes simplex (p. 606). Some of the *complications* are recurrences, pneumonia, conjunctivitis, otitis media, and encephalomyelitis.

Herpes Zoster.—Herpes zoster (L. = creep + L. or Gr. = girdle or zonal) or *shingles* is an acute cutaneous disorder that is usually *caused* by a neurotropic virus with an affinity for the posterior spinal root ganglia (Combes) but that is sometimes secondary to trauma (Feldman), other infection, chemicals, or tumors (p. 1458). The *lesions* are unilateral and segmentally distributed along the course of the affected nerves. Initially there are hyperesthesia, itching, and often intense pain. These are followed by successive crops of macules, pustules, and then vesicles mounted

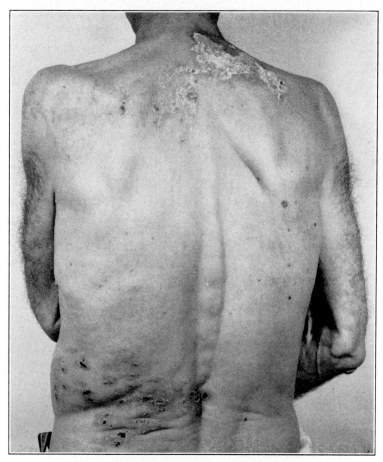

FIG. 670.—Herpes zoster disclosing segmental distribution (shoulder and lumbar) of vesicles that have crusted.

upon a hyperemic and edematous base (Fig. 670). The vesicles are followed by crusts which fall away in about a week, leaving hyperemic or pigmented areas. The *pathologic changes* consist of inflammation of the ganglia, sometimes peripheral neuritis (involving the segmental nerves), intra-epithelial vesicles in the epidermis, hemorrhagic necrosis of the corium, and intranuclear (epithelial cells and occasionally connective tissue cells) inclusion bodies of Lipschütz (Fig. 671). Herpes zoster is self-limited, terminating without complications in from one to three weeks.

Molluscum Contagiosum.—Molluscum contagiosum (L. = soft + contagious) is a slightly contagious auto-inocuable disorder *caused* by a virus. It *occurs* commonly in children that are housed in institutions but is also found in older individuals. The *sites* of predilection are the face, arms, and genitals. The *lesions* usually develop gradually, are generally multiple, and when fully formed consist of rounded, centrally umbilicated, firm nodules that measure up to 8 mm. in diameter and that exude (upon pressure) a gray milky or sebaceous-like material. *Histologically* the prickle cells proliferate, producing pear-shaped structures that extend into the corium and compress the papillæ. The deep cells of the proliferate are normal but the more superficial cells contain characteristic molluscum bodies (Fig. 672). These are conspicuous, round or oval, homogeneously eosinophilic intracytoplasmic structures that increase in size as the superficial cells are approached.

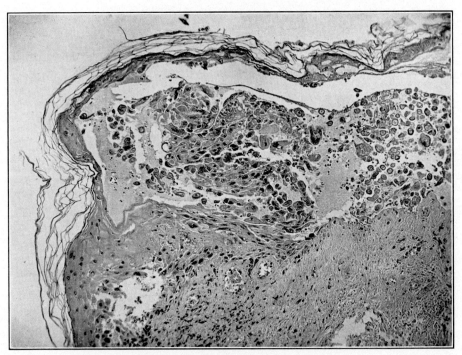

Fig. 671.—Herpes zoster illustrating an intra-epithelial vesicle containing fluid and degenerating epithelial cells with intranuclear inclusions. × 100.

Roseola Infantum.—Roseola (L. = rose-colored) infantum or *exanthem subitum* is an acute disorder occurring in infants and probably *caused* by a virus (Kempe). It is characterized by a sudden onset of fever, irritability, and maybe convulsions followed by a pale pink (rose) macular rash that appears behind the ears, over the trunk, and on the buttocks and thighs but spares the face. Other findings are suboccipital lymphadenitis, slight splenomegaly, and leukopenia. The entire illness lasts about a week.

Dermatomycoses.—By *dermatomycoses* (Gr. = skin + fungus) or *tineas* (L. = moth) is meant superficial fungous infections of the skin *caused* by a variety of closely related organisms and best classified according to the regions of the body affected. Included in the group are the following: (1) *tinea pedis*—also known as *epidermophytosis* and *athlete's foot*, transmitted by bath mats and the like, occurring more commonly in men than in women, usually affecting the feet but seen also on the hands, having a predilection for moist areas between the digits but involving also the soles and palms, and consisting essentially of (*a*) acute vesicular or bullous eruptions that coalesce, break down, and present a weeping itching surface, (*b*) chronic intertriginous lesions usually with fissures, maceration, and desquamation, and (*c*) chronic papules with hyperkeratosis, (2) *tinea unguium*—also known as *onychomycosis*, affecting the nails, and consisting of distortion of the nails by ridging, warping, hyperkeratosis, fragmentation, disintegration, and discoloration, (3) *tinea corporis*—also known as *ringworm* of the *body*, affecting any portion of the body (except areas specifically designated herein), and consisting of the following types of spread-

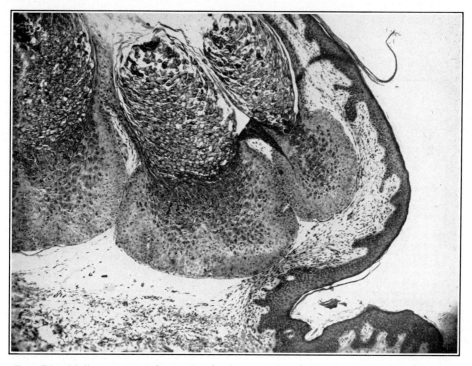

Fig. 672.—Molluscum contagiosum showing hypertrophy of the prickle cells, invasion of the corium, and numerous eosinophilic molluscum bodies within epithelial cells. × 50.

ing (by contiguity) lesions: herpetiform, circinate papular, circinate plaque-like, ulcerated granulomatous, and generalized encrusted, (4) *tinea cruris*— also known as *jockey itch* and *ringworm* of the *groin*, affecting moist areas of the anogenital region and sometimes the axilla, and consisting of a bilaterally symmetrical, sharply demarcated, scaly rash with marginal vesicles and pustules, (5) *tinea capitis*—also known as *ringworm* of the *scalp*, usually occurring in children, affecting primarily the hair, and consisting of coalescing erythematous areas attended by crusting, inflammation, ulceration, and loss of hair, (6) *tinea barbæ*—also known as *barber's itch* and *ringworm* of the *beard*, occurring on the face and neck, affecting the hair, consisting of circinate lesions with vesicles peripherally or pustules located deep in the follicles, and attended by loss of hair, (7) *tinea favosa*— also known simply as *favus*, occurring at all ages and in both sexes, affecting primarily the scalp but also involving other parts of the body including the nails, and consisting of small reddish or yellowish spots (at the exit of hairs) surrounded by vesicles that heal by crusting and atrophy or scar formation, and (8) *tinea versicolor*—also known as *pityriasis versicolor*, being essentially asymptomatic, and consisting of light brown, dark brown, reddish or even blackish desquamating macules involving the axillæ, groins, shoulders, thighs, and face.

Madura Foot.—Madura foot, also known as *maduromycosis* and *mycetoma*, is a chronic infection of the feet that is *caused* by a variety of fungi of the *Actinomycetaceæ* group, especially the genus *Nocardia*. The disorder *occurs* in tropical and subtropical climates in shoeless people of both sexes and all ages. It affects both the skin and underlying tissues and may even extend to bone. Early *lesions* consist of papules, nodules, or indurated areas and vesicles. Late lesions consist of large masses and abscesses that rupture and form sinuses. The lesions are progressive and the ultimate *prognosis* is poor.

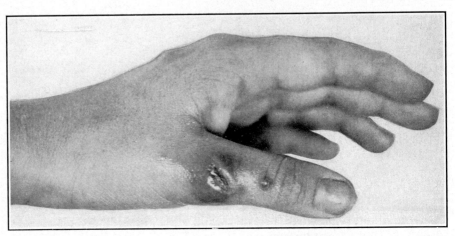

Fig. 673.—Sporotrichosis of the thumb illustrating a discharging abscess as well as two satellite (one distal and one proximal) abscesses.

Sporotrichosis.—Sporotrichosis is a chronic cutaneous lymphogenous and sometimes systemic disorder *caused* by the *Sporotrichum schenkii* (Singer and Cawley). The organism is a normal inhabitant of plants and is transmitted to man by direct inoculation. The disease is thus prevalent in the upper extremities of farmers, gardners, and the like. The initial *lesion* occurs at the site of trauma (abrasion, thorn prick, etc.) as a small abscess. This ultimately breaks down, discharges pus on the surface of the adjacent skin, and thus initiates satellite abscesses (Fig. 673). The infection enters the lymphatic channels and lymph nodes where it produces a chain of abscesses along the path of the lymphatic drainage. *Histologically* the lesion is a granuloma composed of tubercles (Fig. 674). These disclose a central abscess of nuclear fragments and neutrophils, a midzone of epithelioid cells and occasional giant cells, and a peripheral zone of lymphocytes, plasma cells, and monocytes. Short, cigar-shaped, causative organisms are rarely identified histologically but they can be isolated in the peritoneal pus of intraperitoneally inoculated white male rats.

Pediculosis.—Pediculosis (L. = louse) or lousiness is a cutaneous disorder *caused* by lice. The condition is called *pediculosis capitis* when it affects the scalp, *pediculosis corporis* when it affects the body, and *pediculosis pubis* when it affects the genital region. *Pediculosis capitis* affects the scalp in general but the occipital area in particular, is especially common in young girls, and the ova (nits) are attached to the hairs near the scalp. In *pediculosis corporis* the organisms lodge in seams of underwear and migrate to the body only for feeding purposes and deposition of ova. The latter are found attached to hairs. *Pediculosis pubis* has already been referred to in Chapter 33 (p. 1152). In any case, the parasites produce itching and the cutaneous lesions are mostly the result of scratching. In severe cases, secondary infection may complicate the picture.

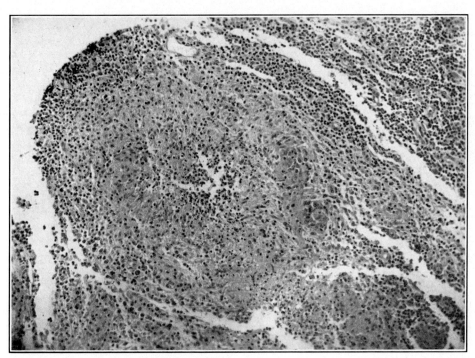

FIG. 674.—Sporotrichosis disclosing a tubercle composed of a central collection of neutrophils and nuclear fragments and of a peripheral zone of epithelioid cells.   × 100.

Demodex Folliculorum Infection. —The *Demodex folliculorum* is a microscopic mite that is commonly found alongside a hair with its head directed internally in the hair follicle (Breckenridge). It may cause fracture of the hair, hyperkeratosis, collection of sebum, and occasionally lymphocytic permeation. Grossly the lesion is represented as a small raised area or appears like a comedo.

Onchocerciasis. —Onchocerciasis (Gr. = tumor + tail) is a filarial infection of the skin caused by the *Onchocera volvulus* and prevailing in Central Africa, Venezuela, Guatemala, and Southern Mexico (Sawitz). The condition is characterized by the formation of fibrous cutaneous nodules containing coiled male and female worms and measuring up to 1 cm. in diameter (Fig. 675). Onchocerciasis is spread by the black gnat, *Simulium*, which sucks up microfilariæ that have wandered into the tissues adjacent to the main mass.

Myasis.—Myasis (Gr. = fly) is infection with, or simply the presence of, maggots on or within tissues. The larvæ may be found in cavities such as ears, eyes, mouth, gastrointestinal tract, genito-urinary tract, and especially ulcers of the skin. The condition results from contamination either by ova of flies or directly by the larvæ.

Arachnidism.—Arachnidism (Gr. = spider) is a condition produced by a bite of a poisonous spider—especially of the black widow variety. The spider's habitat is decomposing trees and seats of privies. The venom in-

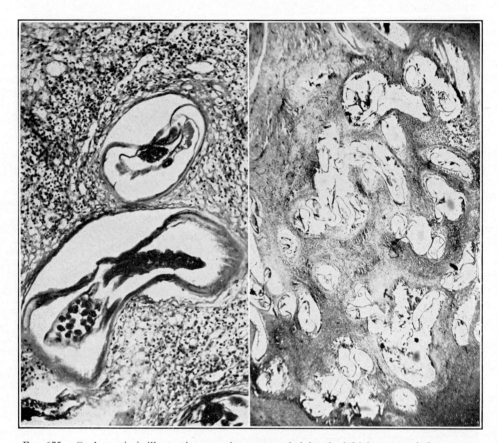

Fig. 675.—Onchocerciasis illustrating parasites surrounded (to the left) by recent inflammatory tissue and (to the right) by old collagenous tissue. × 100 and × 4.

troduced at the time of the bite is of a neurotropic variety and produces violent cramps in the abdomen, legs, thorax, and back together with nausea, perspiration, chills, and prostration. Death occurs in about 4 per cent of the victims.

Ophidism.—Ophidism (Gr. = snake) is poisoning by snake venom. Some of the venoms are neurotoxic while others are hemolytic. The condition may result from the bite of a poisonous snake or from artificial injection of the material.

Eczema.—Eczema (Gr. = to boil out) is a rather nonspecific term used to encompass a variety of cutaneous disorders characterized (1) clinically by redness, heat, burning sensations, itching, and occasionally constitutional manifestations of restlessness, fever, etc., (2) grossly by vesication, induration, watery discharge, scales, and crusts, (Fig. 676) and (3) histologically by parakeratosis, hyperkeratosis, acanthosis, and formation of vesicles in the epidermis and by vascular dilatation, edema, and leukocytic infiltration of the corium (Fig. 677). The disorder characteristically *occurs* in infants and young children, starts on the face, and spreads to involve most other portions of the body. Eczema is generally considered to be an expres-

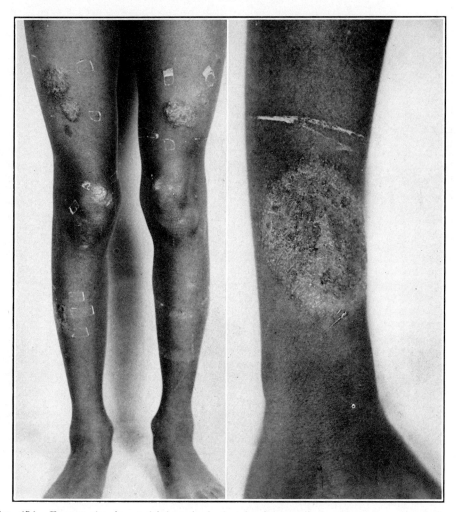

FIG. 676.—Eczema showing multiple, raised, sharply circumscribed, scaly and crusting lesions.

sion of *hypersensitivity* to a variety of inhaled, ingested, and cutaneously contacted allergens including dust, pollens, and proteins (Hill and Glaser).

Neurodermatitis.—Neurodermatitis (Gr. = nerve + skin + inflammation) may be defined as a disorder of the skin attributed primarily to *nerve stimuli*. It is held that commonly encountered emotions such as insecurity, anxiety, hostility, and guilt cause stimulation of the autonomic nervous system which results in flushing, sweating, itching, and excoriation (Frumess and Seitz). The disorder may be local or disseminated and the *lesions* are varisized. Initially the affected area is dusky pink and mottled. Later it becomes thickened, shows increased normal markings, and reveals furrowings that produce a mosaic pattern. Scaling, papule-like lesions are often present in the midzonal area. *Histologically* the epidermis reveals hyperkeratosis, parakeratosis, acanthosis, and hypertrophy of the rete cones while the corium discloses prominent papillæ together with superficial infiltration with lymphocytes and eosinophils (Fig. 678).

Exfoliative Dermatitis.—Exfoliative dermatitis is a cutaneous disorder characterized by varying degrees (usually severe) of scaling. It is a protean condition (1) that may result from toxemia, gout, tuberculosis, alcoholism, topical applications of various chemicals, and ingestion of

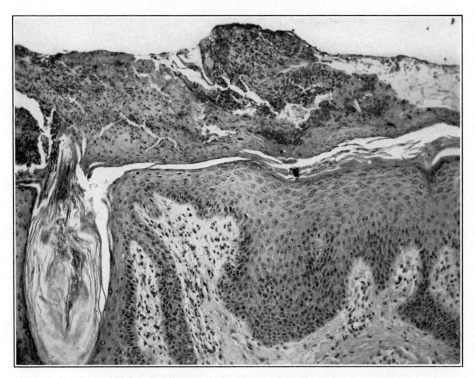

FIG. 677.—Eczema showing abundant parakeratosis, hyperkeratosis, and acanthosis of the epidermis and leukocytic permeation of the corium. × 100.

various medicines and (2) that is influenced by climate in that it is more prevalent in the fall. The disorder is more common in males than in females and *prevails* in the third and fourth decades of life. Usually large *areas* of the body (especially the extremities and back) disclose varying degrees of redness and are covered with conspicuous laminated scales that desquamate freely. *Histologically* the following are noted: hyperkeratosis, parakeratosis, acanthosis, intercellular edema, and superficial leukocytic infiltration of the corium.

Dermatitis Venenata.—Dermatitis venenata (L. = poison) or contact dermatitis is an acute to chronic inflammation of the skin *caused* by contact with chemical, animal, or vegetable (poison ivy) materials (Underwood). The condition often develops on an allergic basis. The area involved depends upon the site and extent of exposure and the *lesions* vary in severity from slight erythema to gangrene. As a rule, they develop within a few hours or at most a few days. The changes consist of combinations of erythema, papules, vesicles, bullæ, pustules, crusts, scales, and occasionally greater desquamations, abscesses, and gangrene. The *histologic* alterations are entirely nonspecific consisting of hypertrophy, vesicle formation, and ulceration of the epidermis together with varying degrees of inflammation of the corium. The condition generally resolves in from one to three weeks after removing the offending agent.

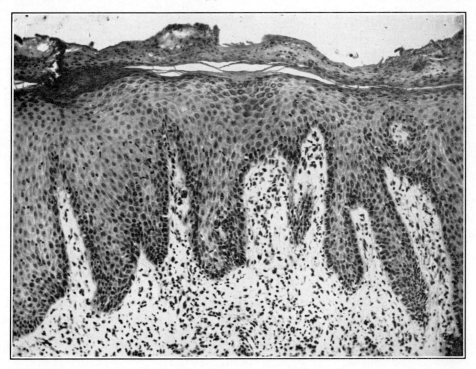

Fig. 678.—Neurodermatitis disclosing parakeratosis, acanthosis, and enlargement of the rete cones of the epidermis and prominence of the papillæ together with leukocytic infiltration of the corium. × 100.

Urticaria.—Urticaria, also known as *nettle rash* and *hives*, is an acute disorder of the skin resulting from the action of "toxic" substances in a sensitized person. The *causative* factors may consist of (1) ingested foods such as shellfish, strawberries, eggs, caviar, etc., (2) drugs either ingested or applied externally such as quinine, salicylates, sulfonamides, etc., (3) inhalants, (4) bites of mosquitoes, flies, and wasps, and (5) emotional stimuli (Graham). The condition may occur precipitously and without warning or it may be preceded by constitutional symptoms. The cutaneous *lesions* generally develop rapidly. They consist of flat but slightly raised, smooth, pinkish wheals that may measure up to 3 or 4 cm. in diameter. They may be few in number and discrete or they may be numerous and coalescing in which case they form large plaques. The surrounding skin is reddened for varying distances. Depending upon their figurative appearance, the lesions have been called *urticaria annularis* (ring-like), *vesiculosa* or *bulbosa* (vesical or bullous formation), *papulosa* (papillary), *solitaria* (single lesion), *factitia* (formed rapidly to desired configuration), etc. The main *histologic* changes are found in the corium and consist of capillary dilation, severe edema, and varying degrees of neutrophilic and eosinophilic infiltration. The lesions generally resolve within two days.

Erythema Multiforme. — Erythema multiforme is an acute cutaneous disorder that may occur as a *result of* drug ingestion, upper respiratory infection, gastrointestinal disturbances, pyogenic infection, bite of a wasp, or trauma, or that may be seen in conjunction with rheumatic fever, Sydenham's chorea, erysipelas, or vaccinia (Costello). The condition is prevalent in the autumn and spring and usually affects young people. The *eruption* is usually symmetrical and involves the following areas with decreasing frequency: lower extremities, upper extremities, face and vermilion border of the lips, neck, genitalia, trunk, palms, dorsum of the hands, soles, inner surfaces of the thighs, back, and chest. The lesions are attended by itching, burning, or tenderness. They consist of varisized erythemas, macules, papules, vesicles, and bullæ which coalesce, rupture (vesicles and bullæ), and crust. Depending upon the appearance of the lesions the disorder has been called *erythema annulare* or *circinatum* (depressed center and erythematous ring-like periphery) (Fig. 679), *figuratum* (peripheral coalescence of several rings), *marginatum* (well-formed marginal band remaining as a sequel), *papulatum* or *papulosum* (papular), *tuberculatum* or *tuberculosum* (nodular), *urticatum* (urticarial), *vesiculosum* (vesicular), *bullosum* (bullous), and *iris* (iris-like). The *histologic* changes consist of marked edema and moderate neutrophilic and eosinophilic infiltration of the corium as well as varying degrees of edema of the epidermis. Erythema multiforme is a self-limited disorder that resolves spontaneously within a few weeks.

Erythema Nodosum. — Erythema nodosum is an acute self-limited disease of the subcutaneous tissues overlying the tibias *caused* by a variety of bacterial, toxic, and chemical agents in a hypersensitive person (Wasserman and Doxiadis). Among others, it has been seen in connection with tuberculosis, streptococcic infection, rheumatic fever, coccidioidomycosis, Boeck's sarcoid, etc. The condition is more common in children than in adults. The *lesions* consist of bright red, shining, ill-defined, single or coalescing, round or oval areas of tender induration that may measure up to 5 cm. in greatest diameter. In four to ten days the color changes from red to purple after which it fades to brown and disappears. The *histologic* changes consist of capillary dilation, edema, and moderate leukocytic infiltration with occasional giant cell formation. The disorder may be accompanied by fever, arthralgia, sore throat, cervical lymphadenitis, slight leukocytosis, and increased sedimentation rate. All manifestations usually resolve completely in two to three weeks.

Acrodynia. — Acrodynia (Gr. = extremity + pain) is a mild to severe *symptom complex* that includes a cutaneous eruption, alopecia, salivation, loss of teeth, occasional loss of nails or phalanges, excessive perspiration, hypotonia, itching and burning or pains in the extremities, increased pulse rate and blood pressure, photophobia, insomnia, and apathy alternating with irritability (Warkany). The *eruption* starts as erythematous spots on the palms and soles associated with swelling, cyanosis, and ecchymosis. Vesicles or bullæ may precede or follow the erythema and, in time, the process spreads proximally to the limbs and trunk. Eventually the epidermis desquamates and the affected areas remain as brownish or blackish pigmentations. The *cause* is unknown with the following, however, being considered as of etiologic significance: virus, allergy, infection, endocrine disturbances, toxins, vitamin deficiency, neurosis, disturbances of the gastrointestinal tract, and hypersensitivity to mercury. The disorder is subjected to relapses with the over-all duration not extending over three months.

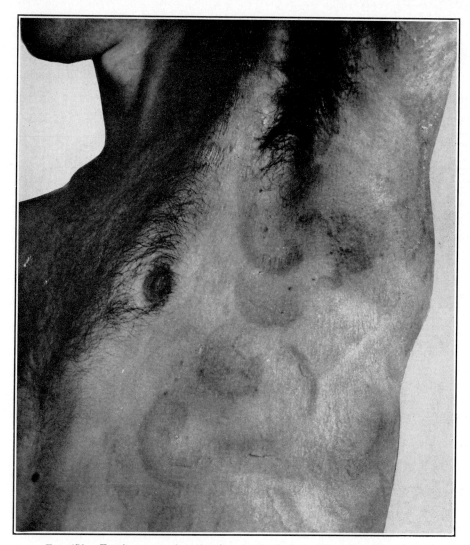

FIG. 679.—Erythema annulare showing circular lesions with depressed centers.

Granuloma Annulare.—Granuloma annulare is a chronic cutaneous disorder of unknown *etiology* characterized by the formation of deep-seated nodules or rings of pink to bluish-red color that measure up to 3 cm. in diameter. The *lesions* have a predilection for the dorsum of the fingers, wrists, elbows, neck, feet, ankles, and buttocks. *Histologically* the changes are those of a granuloma. They are located in the outer portion of the corium and consist of a focus of coagulation necrosis surrounded by radially arranged epithelioid cells and fibroblasts that are permeated with plasma cells and lymphocytes. The disorder is persistent and tends to recur.

Seborrheic Dermatitis.—Seborrheic dermatitis is a chronic inflammation of the skin occurring in patients with seborrhea (p. 1325). The predisposing *factor* is increased secretion of sebum and oil. This allows growth of saprophytic staphylococci and streptococci which, in turn, produce the infection. The *areas* of the body commonly affected are the face, scalp, chest, axillæ, and pubic region. The initial *lesions* consist of papules that develop around the follicles. With age, the papules coalesce and produce rounded, serpiginous, or irregular yellowish to pinkish, greasy, scale-covered plaques. In the scalp, minor degrees of inflammation are represented simply by the formation of dandruff. The *histologic* changes are not characteristic. The epidermis discloses hyperkeratosis, parakeratosis, slight acanthosis, and intercellular edema while the corium reveals moderate numbers of lymphocytes and neutrophils.

Acne Vulgaris.—Acne (Gr. = point) vulgaris, generally known as "pimples," is an extremely common chronic inflammation of the skin that usually becomes manifested at *puberty* but may appear in older people and even in infants (Giknis). Like in seborrheic dermatitis, excessive secretion of sebum and oil predisposes to growth of saprophytic staphylococci and streptococci which, in turn, cause the inflammation. The infection has a predilection for the face, neck, and upper part of the thorax. The *lesions* consist essentially of varying numbers of papules or larger nodules that are prone to develop pustules and, when the latter are severe, to heal by scar tissue formation. In addition, the skin is distinctly oily and comedones are prevalent. *Histologically* the follicles are initially distended with sebum and keratin and the perifollicular tissues are infiltrated with lymphocytes, plasma cells, and occasional giant cells. When pustules form, the changes are those of an acute abscess.

Acne Rosacea.—Acne rosacea is a chronic disorder of the nose, cheeks, and sometimes chin and forehead that is thought to be *due to* improper gastrointestinal elimination, imbibition of alcohol, and a variety of local irritants (including heat and cold). The condition *occurs* after the third decade of life and, in its severe form, is more common in men than in women. The initial *lesion* consists of varisized areas of erythema which at first are evanescent but later persist for longer and longer periods. Gradually the color becomes permanent, the skin becomes oily, the orifices of the sebaceous glands become plugged with dry sebum, and papules, nodules, and pustules appear. Exacerbations and remissions finally result in rhinophyma (p. 424). *Histologically* the changes consist of dilatation and prominence of the dermal capillaries, lymphocytic infiltration about epidermal appendages, and some hypertrophy of sebaceous glands (Fig. 680).

Pemphigus.—Pemphigus is an acute to chronic recurrent cutaneous disorder of adults characterized by the formation of bullæ. The *cause* is unknown although the condition has been thought to be the result of salt retention, unknown toxins, viral infection, and inhibition of an enzyme (Lever). Excluding *familial benign chronic pemphigus* (which is considered to be bullous Darier's disease (p. 1326) the disorder is generally dividable into four types—vulgaris malignus, vegetans, foliaceus, and erythematosus. *Pemphigus vulgaris malignus* is characterized by the formation of vari-sized bullæ in previously normal appearing skin on any or all parts of the body. The bullæ may resolve but usually rupture, leaving superficial erosions that show no tendency to healing. The condition is grave for the patient virtually always dies of the disorder within a year. *Pemphigus vegetans* differs from vulgaris malignus in that papillomatous proliferations develop upon the excoriations which follow rupture of the bullæ and that the course is more protracted. *Pemphigus foliaceus* is characterized by bullous formation followed later by generalized desquamation of the superficial layers of the epidermis. The course of the disease is usually chronic, extending over a period of years. Finally, *pemphigus erythematosus* discloses bullæ superimposed upon varisized areas of erythema. It probably represents a mild form of pemphigus foliaceus. *Histologically* the changes in pemphigus consist of the formation of vesicles or bullæ in the stratum germinativum or at the junction of the epidermis with the corium (Fig. 681). Early in the process there is no inflammatory reaction but after a

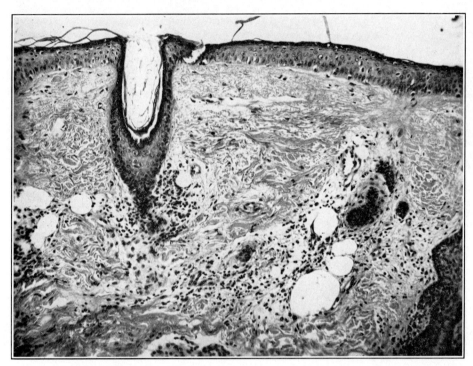

Fig. 680.—Acne rosacea illustrating prominence of the dermal capillaries and foci of leukocytic infiltration about epidermal appendages. × 100.

few days the corium and the bullous fluid are permeated with neutrophils and other leukocytes. In pemphigus vegetans the initial lesions are similar but the subsequent papillomatous proliferations consist first of branching papillæ covered with one to a few rows of epithelial cells and later of marked acanthosis of the epidermis with pseudo-epitheliomatous-like changes. In addition, intraepithelial abscesses are usually present.

Dermatitis Herpetiformis.—Dermatitis herpetiformis is a rare, acute to chronic, recurring, cutaneous disorder *occurring* in both sexes and at all ages and thought to be *due to* a "toxin" of undetermined origin. The initial *manifestations* may be of a mild constitutional type. These are followed by symmetrically distributed successive crops of erythematous patches, papules, vesicles, bullæ, or pustules (Fig. 682). *Histologically* the changes consist of (1) congestion, edema, and leukocytic infiltration of the outer part of the corium, (2) serum-filled vesicles at the junction of the corium and epidermis, and (3) edema between the prickle cells and increased pigmentation of the basal cells of the epidermis. The *prognosis* is fair to poor but recovery does occur.

Lichen Planus.—Lichen planus (Gr. = skin to L. = flat) is a relatively common chronic inflammatory disorder of the skin of unknown *etiology* but thought to be due to neurosis, toxemia, trauma, digestive disturbances, malnutrition, etc. The *eruption* is usually symmetrical and has a predilection for the flexor surfaces of the wrists and forearm and for the legs just above the ankles (Fig. 683). The *lesions* consist of single or coalescing,

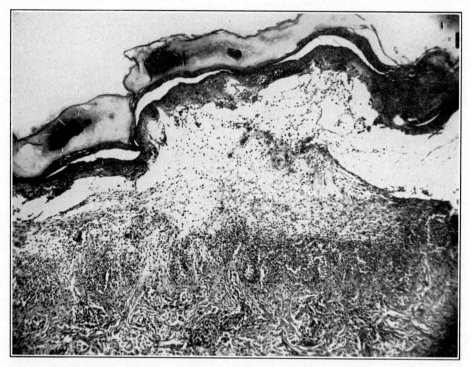

Fig. 681.—Pemphigus showing a vesicle at the junction of the epidermis with the corium crowded with neutrophils. × 50.

flat-topped or umbilicated, crimson colored, varishaped papules covered with a thin horny film. Itching is usually present and is of varying intensity. *Histologically* the following are noted: hyperkeratosis, acanthosis, liquefactive degeneration of basal cells, and an infiltration of the outer portion of the corium with neutrophils, lymphocytes, monocytes, and plasma cells. The *prognosis* in general is good.

Lichen Sclerosus et Atrophicus.—This is a chronic cutaneous disorder of unknown *etiology* that is similar to kraurosis of the vulva (p. 1149) and balanitis xerotica obliterans of the penis (p. 1114). It is more common in males than in females, usually appears in later life, and has a predilection for the trunk, neck, axillæ, and forearms. The *lesions* consist of discrete or aggregated, slightly raised, pearly-white papules, each of which discloses a smooth shining surface containing a central comedo-like plug of keratin. In later stages the plugs become more prominent and the entire area becomes parchment-like. The *histologic* changes consist of hyperkeratosis, keratotic plugging of the hair follicles and epidermal appendages, flattening of the rete cones, atrophy of the rest of the epidermis, and edema followed by hyalinization of the corium just beneath the epidermis (Fig. 684).

Psoriasis.—Psoriasis is a common chronic cutaneous disorder of unknown *etiology* that appears in both sexes and usually starts in the second and third decades of life. The *eruption* is generally symmetrical and in decreasing order of frequency involves the extensor surfaces of the extremities, scalp, sacrum, chest, face, abdomen, genitals, and palms and

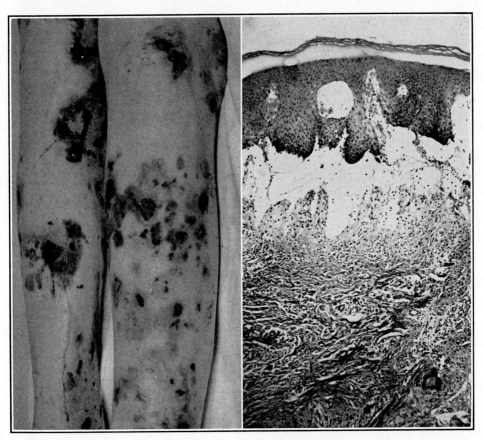

Fig. 682.—Dermatitis herpetiformis disclosing ruptured and unruptured vesicles grossly and a vesicle at the junction of the epidermis with the corium microscopically. × 50.

soles. The *lesions* first appear as papules and, over periods of weeks and months, extend and coalesce to form varisized, moderately elevated, irregularly shaped, sharply defined, reddish-brown plaques that may measure several centimeters in diameter (Fig. 685). The surface is covered with pearly-white scales which, when removed, leave a bright red base with or without bleeding points. The *histologic* changes consist of parakeratosis, micro-abscesses in the parakeratotic areas, acanthosis, club-shaped hypertrophy of the rete pegs, prominent papillæ, and leukocytic (lymphocytic, monocytic, and plasma cell) infiltration of the outer portion of the corium. The *course* of the disorder is protracted over a period of years and a cure is never certain for the disorder tends to recur.

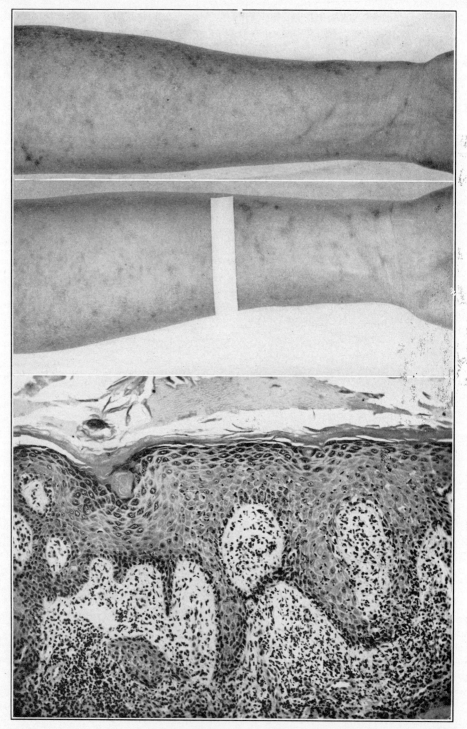

FIG. 683.—Lichen planus illustrating flat-topped, symmetrically distributed papules covering the flexor surfaces of both arms and, microscopically, hyperkeratosis, acanthosis, degeneration of the basal cells, and leukocytic infiltration at the junction of the epidermis with the dermis. × 100.

Scleroderma.—Scleroderma (Gr. = hand + skin) may be defined as a chronic sclerosing disorder of the collagenous tissue throughout the body but with special manifestations in the skin (Evans, Bergelman, and Beerman). While the *cause* remains uncertain, the condition has been known to develop after acute infections, exanthemata, pneumonia, influenza, exposure to dampness and cold, and even thyroid disease. It *occurs* in both sexes and at all ages. Three types of scleroderma are described—diffuse, circumscribed, and acrosclerosis. *Diffuse scleroderma* develops gradually, is attended by a feeling of stiffness, and initially affects the extremities,

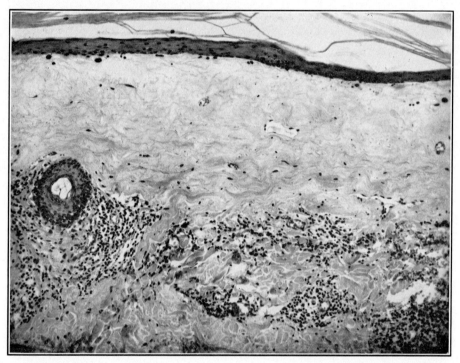

Fig. 684.—Lichen sclerosus et atrophicus disclosing hyperkeratosis, atrophy of the epidermis, disappearance of the rete cones, and hyalinization of the outer portion of the corium.

neck, face, or trunk (Fig. 686). The involved area discloses diffuse erythema along with gradually increasing edema and induration during which the normal markings become erased. Ultimately the skin and subcutaneous tissues become firmly united so that they cannot be moved over subjacent structures, atrophy may occur, and yellowish, ivory, or bronze pigmentation is noted. *Circumscribed scleroderma* is similar except that the process occurs in localized or circumscribed patches. *Acrosclerosis* is a syndrome combining Raynaud's phenomenon (p. 388) with sclerotic patches that affect the skin of the distal parts of the extremities, face, and neck. *Histologically* the essential changes in scleroderma consist of edema, slight leukocytic infiltration, and fibrinoid degeneration of the connective tissue of the corium followed by increasingly severe collagenization. In the process, the epidermal appendages become atrophic and disappear, the vessels become obliterated, brown pigment granules are found in the outer portion of the corium, and calcium is often deposited in focal areas. In

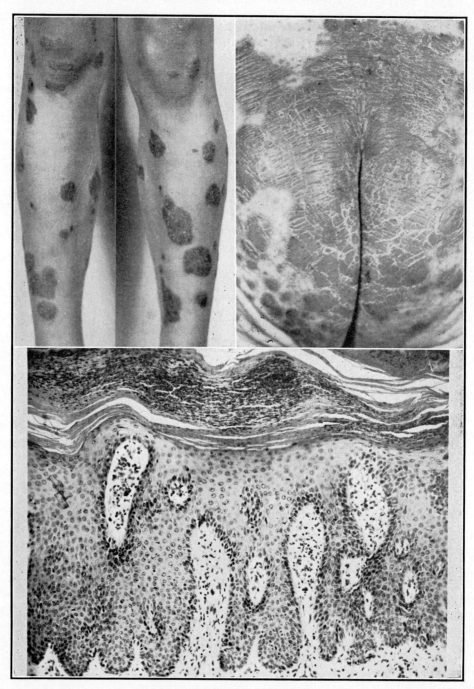

FIG. 685.—Psoriasis showing (above) typical plaque-like lesions on the extensor surfaces of the lower extremities and on the back and (below) parakeratosis, intraepithelial micro-abscess formation, acanthosis, clubbing of the rete pegs, prominence of papillæ, and leukocytic permeation of the outer portion of the corium. × 100.

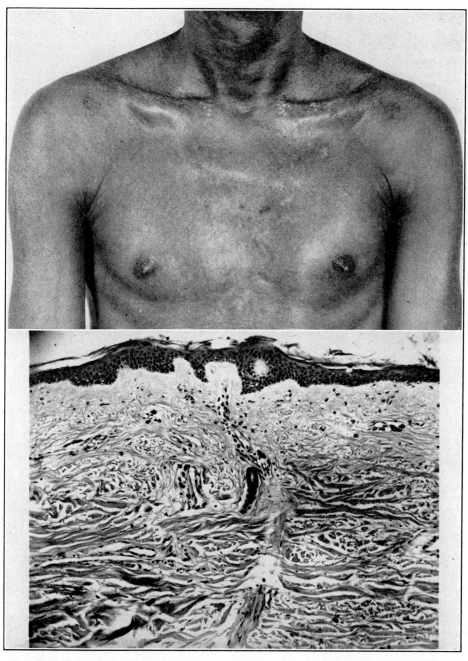

FIG. 686.—Scleroderma illustrating (above) thickened glistening skin covering the clavicles and sternum and (below) atrophy of the epidermis, pigmentation of the corium, and diffuse collagenization of the corium with atrophy of the epidermal appendages. × 100.

addition to the skin, *other organs* affected by the fibrosing process are lungs, esophagus, lower gastrointestinal tract, heart, vessels, endocrine glands, skeletal muscles, and joints.

Discoid Lupus Erythematosus.—This condition is a chronic disorder generally affecting the flush areas of the cheeks, occasionally involving the scalp and ears, and rarely implicating the skin of other parts of the body (Lever and Allen). The disease usually *occurs* in the third and fourth decades of life and is about 2 to 3 times as common in females as it is in males. While the *cause* is unknown, the same etiological factors prevailing in acute disseminated lupus erythematosus (page 309) must be considered, for it has

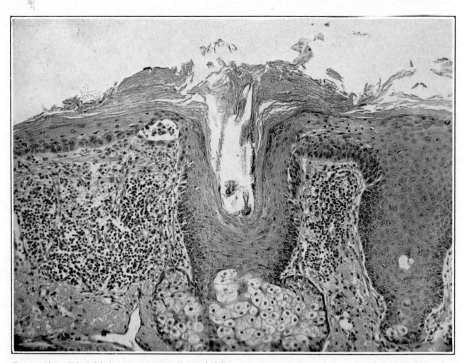

FIG. 687.—Discoid lupus erythematosus showing hyperkeratosis, keratotic plugging of the epidermal appendages, atrophy of the malpighian layer, liquifaction degeneration of the basal layer, basophilic degeneration of the outer portion of the dermis, and focal, mostly lymphocytic, infiltration of the dermis. × 100.

been shown that the two disorders are simply different stages of the same entity (Reiches and Dubois). *Grossly*, early lesions consist of slightly raised reddish-purple patches with adherent gray scales. They spread by peripheral advancement until, in the span of months or years, they form well-defined, erythematous, variform slightly infiltrative patches showing keratotic scales, follicular plugs, and occasionally atrophic scars. *Histologic* sections reveal (1) hyperkeratosis with keratotic plugging and atrophy of the epidermal appendages. (2) atrophy of the malpighian layer alternating with areas of acanthosis, (3) liquifaction degeneration of the basal cell layer, (4) patchy perivascular and peri-appendageal infiltration with mostly lymphocytes and fewer plasma cells and histiocytes, and (5) basophilic degeneration and edema of the outer dermis (Fig. 687). The only noteworthy *complication* is progression to the acute stage of the disease, which occurs in about one fifth of all cases. Generally, there are no readily detectable *clinical manifestations* but when careful study is performed most patients disclose some combination of the following: arthritis, fever, Raynaud's phenomenon, pleurisy, abdominal pain, lymphadenopathy, leukopenia, elevated sedimentation rate, hyperglobulinemia, or abnormal flocculation tests (Dubois). The *diagnosis* is made from the appearance of the lesions and biopsy. A differential diagnosis should include secondary syphilis and lymphoblastoma. *Treatment* consists of the administration of atabrine. The *prognosis* is guarded for, as already stated, about 20 per cent of the cases develop the acute disseminated form of the disease.

Dermatomyositis.—Dermatomyositis is an acute to chronic, often remittent inflammation of muscles and skin of unknown *etiology*. It *occurs* in both sexes and prevails in the fifth decade of life. The disorder is usually bilateral and symmetrical with involvement of the *muscles* of the upper extremities, shoulder girdles, neck, gluteal regions, and femoral areas in decreasing order of frequency. The affected muscles become weak, tender, painful, and at first soft but later firm. Because of the weakness, the head droops and the shoulders slope. *Histologically* the muscle fibers lose their striations, undergo vacuolic and hyaline degeneration, disclose lymphocytic and plasma cell infiltration, and ultimately are replaced with fibrous tissue. The cutaneous changes consist of erythema or urticaria or may simulate lesions of lupus erythematosus or scleroderma. The *prognosis* is variable although the outlook is not too good for death generally supervenes in an average of two years.

Chronic Atrophic Acrodermatitis.—Chronic atrophic acrodermatitis (Gr. = extremity + skin + inflammation) is, as the name suggests, a chronic atrophic dermatitis involving the extremities (especially the lower ones). The disease is generally *seen* after forty years of age and predominates in women. The *cause* is unknown although trauma, temperature, diet, occupation, endocrines, etc., have all been cited as of etiologic significance. Early *lesions* consist of soft, edematous, bluish-red, coalescing areas of induration on the extensor surfaces. Gradually (over a period of months) the skin assumes a bluish to brownish-red, thin, wrinkled or parchment-like appearance with a tendency to scaling. Because of the thinness, the superficial veins are readily visualized through the skin. Other features are (1) the presence of atrophic, fibrotic, or nodular linear bands that extend proximally from a finger or a toe and (2) occasionally the appearance of localized amyloid deposits. *Histologically* the early changes consist simply of slight parakeratosis of the epidermis and of edema and perivascular leukocytic infiltration of the corium. Later changes consist of hyperkeratosis, atrophy of the prickle cells, disappearance of the rete cones and papillæ, thin epidermis existing as a wavy line, diminution in the amount of connective and elastic tissue of the corium, diffuse lymphocytic permeation of the corium, and atrophy of all the epidermal appendages (Fig. 688). After reaching a certain point, the condition remains stationary and it appears to have no deleterious effect on the health of the person as a whole.

Relapsing Nodular Panniculitis.—Relapsing nodular panniculitis, also known as the *Weber-Christian syndrome*, may be defined as recurring attacks of nonsuppurative inflammation of the fat and connective tissue of the hypoderm. The condition is uncommon, prevails in females, and *occurs* at all ages (Beerman). The *cause* is unknown although the following have been considered as etiologic factors: iodides, bromides, bacteria and their toxins, trauma, metabolic disturbances, endocrine imbalances, etc. The condition is characterized by recurring attacks of fever and malaise together with the appearance of crops of hypodermal *nodules* distributed over the entire body but with a predilection for the extremities and especially the thighs (Koch). The nodules usually measure up to 1 cm. in diameter. The overlying portion of the skin is at first erythematous and occasionally may be ulcerated. Later, it forms a small depression over the healed nodule. The focus of involvement is ill defined, gray to light brown, and moderately firm. *Histologically* it discloses (1) an infiltration with mostly neutrophils but also with varying numbers of plasma cells, lymphocytes, monocytes, and eosinophils, (2) focal areas of fat necrosis, (3) a smattering of foam cells

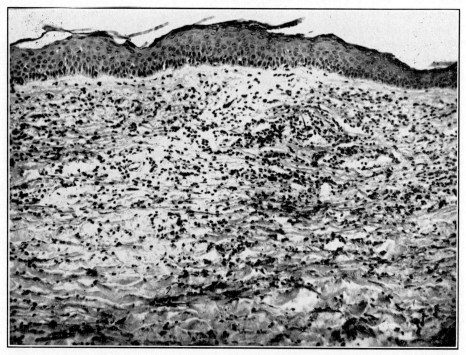

Fig. 688.—Chronic atrophic acrodermatitis revealing some keratin formation, atrophy of the epidermis, disappearance of the rete cones and intervening papillæ, atrophy and lymphocytic infiltration of the corium, and disappearance of the epidermal appendages. × 100.

and foreign body giant cells, (4) vascular changes consisting of thrombosis, intimal proliferation, medial thickening, and perivascular leukocytic permeation, (5) healing by fibrosis, and (6) lack of involvement of the corium and epidermis (Fig. 689). The *prognosis* in relapsing nodular panniculitis is guarded for death, apparently from cachexia, has occurred in about 15 per cent of the recorded cases.

Reticulohistiocytic Granuloma.—This condition is a nodular disorder of the skin that by some is regarded as a tumor but by most is looked upon as a granuloma (Purvis). By the former, it has been called a *reticulohistiocytoma*. It is of rather common *occurrence*, is acquired, and generally affects people of the younger age group. The *cause* is unknown, although on occasion a history of trauma is given as an inciting agent. *Grossly* the lesion is nodular, measures 1.5 to 2 cm. in diameter, is generally single but may be

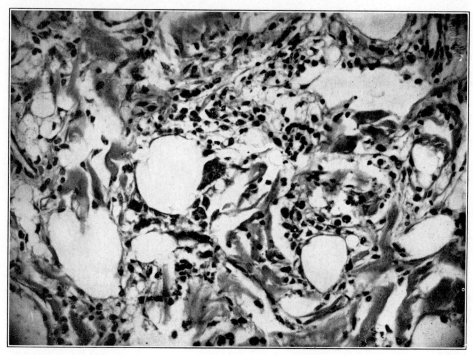

Fig. 689.—Relapsing nodular panniculitis showing an inflammatory focus of lymphocytes, plasma cells, and monocytes together with a foreign body giant cell and some deposition of collagen.   × 200.

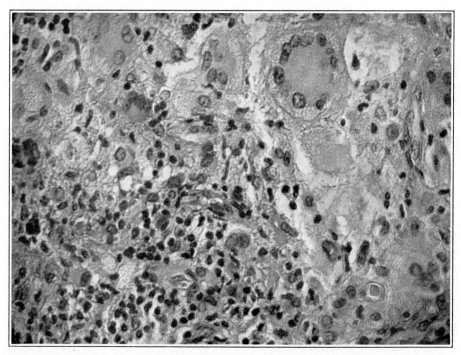

Fig. 690.—Reticulohistiocytic granuloma illustrating a stroma of spindle cells containing inflammatory cells, histiocytes, and giant cells.   × 400.

multiple, and is located in the skin of any portion of the body. Usually the
nodule is simply raised but it may be more sessile and, on occasion, even
pedunculated. The color varies from yellow to red to brown and the consistency from soft to hard. *Histologically* the lesion is usually located in the
outer portion of the dermis and is sharply delineated. The overlying epidermis is thinned and may even be ulcerated. The nodule is composed of a
stroma of spindle connective tissue cells showing varying degrees of collagenization. Within the stroma are present histiocytes, inflammatory cells
(mostly lymphocytes and neutrophils), and giant cells (Fig. 690). Of these,
the most characteristic are the giant cells. They vary in number from a few
to many but are always present. They are large, round, or irregular. Their
cytoplasm is abundant, eosinophilic, occasionally foamy about the periphery,
and often sprinkled with irregular basophilic material. Their nuclei vary
in number from 1 to 45 and are round, uniform, and vesicular. Fat is
demonstrable in the stroma and giant cells, both by appropriate staining
and polariscopic examination, and iron granules are frequently seen. The
only *complications* are irritation and trauma which result in bleeding. The
clinical manifestations consist of a slowly or rapidly growing nodule or nodules, occasionally associated with pain. The correct *diagnosis* is usually
made only upon microscopic examination. A differential diagnosis should
include xanthoma, xanthofibroma, dermatofibroma, sclerosing hemangioma,
and melanoblastoma. *Treatment* consists of surgical excision. The *prognosis*
is excellent for the lesion does not recur nor, since it is a granuloma, does it
metastasize.

PHYSICAL DISTURBANCES

Orientation.—Under this heading may be included a variety of unrelated
conditions of the skin that have as their basis destruction of cells caused
primarily by chemicals, heat, cold, light, electricity, and other physical
agents. Because of the nature of the causative factors, many of the disorders have already been mentioned in other portions of the text. They
may be listed as follows: *chemicals* such as acids, arsenic, barbiturates,
gold, silver, and sulfonamides (p. 242), *tattoo* (p. 83), *burns* (p. 226),
chilblains (p. 229), *trench foot* (p. 229), *immersion foot* (p. 229), *frostbite* (p.
229), *light* (p. 231), *electricity* (p. 232), *irradiation* (p. 233), *Raynaud's disease* (p. 388), *acrocyanosis* (p. 389), *livedo reticularis* (p. 389), *varicose veins*
(p. 389), *gangrene* (p. 89), *lymphedema* (p. 392), *purpura* (p. 943), and
trauma (p. 222). Left for further consideration are xeroderma pigmentosum and healing of wounds.

Xeroderma Pigmentosum.—Xeroderma (Gr. = dry + skin) pigmentosum is a rather rare type of hereditary skin disease characterized by
hypersensitivity of the skin to sunlight (Brockington). The condition
generally starts in *early life* and consists of erythema, hyperkeratosis, and
pigmentation of the exposed areas of the body together with varying degrees of conjunctivitis. In due course, *carcinoma* develops in the affected
areas and the patient generally dies from the new growth. The *histologic*
changes consist of hyperkeratosis, atrophy of the prickle cell layer, slender-
ization of the rete cones, proliferation of the basal cells, presence of lymphocytes and melanophores containing golden brown pigment in the outer
portion of the corium, and some degeneration of the midportion of the
corium. The complicating carcinomas are of a squamous and/or a basal
cell type.

Healing of Wounds.—The topic of trauma and consequent wounds has already been discussed in Chapter 6 (p. 222). The fundamental *cause* of wounds is violence of a sufficient degree to produce interruption of continuity of tissue. In the skin the more important specific causes are friction, blunt force or blow, and incision or puncture with a sharp object. Of these, incisional wounds are the most common for without them there could be no operations and no surgeons! Regardless of the causative factor or the type of wound present, *repair* is consequent to an inflammatory reaction (of lesser or greater magnitude), is brought about by primary or secondary healing, and is dependent upon ameboid movement, proliferation, and maturation of cells (Whipple).

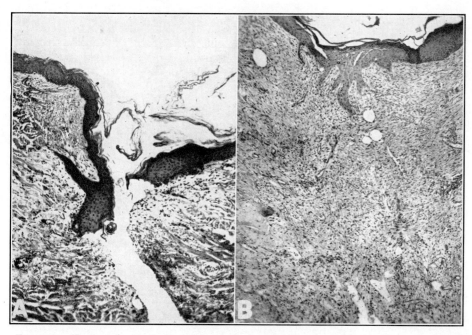

Fig. 691.—Healing of wounds disclosing *A*, a recent incision in which the edges contain some congestion, edema, and leukocytic infiltration. × 50 (the gap is an artifact) and *B*, an old incision that has been completely closed by regeneration of epidermis and corium. × 37.5.

Primary healing usually occurs in clean-cut wounds in which the severed surfaces are in close apposition, in which there is no superimposed infection, in which the blood supply is good, and in which foreign material is absent. The initiating trauma and/or products of destroyed cells are sufficient to induce a sterile inflammation of a slight degree. The immediate change consists of filling of the defect with blood, plasma, and fibrin (Fig. 691*A*.) Subsequently, capillaries and fibroblasts arise in adjacent tissues and replace the temporary elements. Concomitantly, the overlying epithelium proliferates and bridges the surface. In time, the cells and substances that are in excess resorb and the tissue is restored to normal (Fig. 691*B*). While the epidermis and corium regenerate, epidermal appendages do not reform. *Secondary healing* usually occurs in ragged or irregular wounds or in clean wounds in which the severed or disrupted surfaces are widely separated, in which there is superimposed infection, in which the blood supply is poor, and/or in which foreign material is present in varying amounts. Actually the repair is fundamentally similar to that seen in primary healing with the exception that the chronicity of the process and the amount of tissue destroyed induce the formation of an abundance of granulation tissue and this, in turn, is eventually converted into scar tissue.

Aside from *local factors* (listed above) having an effect on wound healing, *systemic factors* that may play an mportant role are as follows: (1) **age of the patient**—better in young than in old, (2) degree of hydration—both edema and dehydration having a deleterious effect, (3) diet—accelerated by a high protein or acid diet, and delayed by a high fat diet, (4) avitaminosis—delayed by deficiency of vitamins C (by way of interference in formation of intercellular substance, in maturation of fibroblasts, and in formation of collagen) and K (by way of promoting hemorrhage), (5) poor circulation and anemia—delayed, and (6) administration of ACTH and/or cortisone—delayed (Whipple, Bangham, Heifetz, Sandblom, and Marshall).

TUMORS

Orientation.—Tumors and tumor-like conditions of the skin are common. They may arise in the epidermis, epidermal appendages, corium, hypoderm, adjacent tissues, or distant areas (Beerman). Some of the lesions already mentioned in various portions of the text may be listed as follows: *leukoplakia* (p. 607), *erythroplasia* of *Queyrat* (p. 1115), *amyloid tumor* (p. 41), *hemangioma* (p. 393), *hemangioendothelium* or *hemangiosarcoma* (p. 399), *sclerosing hemangioma* (p. 395), *glomus tumor* (p. 396), *hemangiopericytoma* (p. 402), *Kaposi's sarcoma* (p. 401), *lymphangioma* (p. 398), *lymphangiosarcoma* (p. 403), *myoblastoma* (p. 1309), and *lymphoblastoma* or *mycosis fungoides* (pp. 984 and 990). Some of the more important remaining conditions (from without in) may now be considered in the balance of this Chapter.

Papilloma.—A papilloma (Gr. = papilla + tumor) is a sessile or pedunculated cutaneous tumor composed of finger-like cores of connective tissue covered with hyperplastic, often hyperkeratotic but otherwise regular-appearing, stratified squamous epithelium (Fig. 692*C*). The *tumors* affect any part of the body surface, are solitary or multiple, usually measure up to 1 or 2 cm. in diameter but may be larger, disclose a rough surface, occasionally contain pigment in the basal cells and thus may be confused with nevi (Fox), and are benign (Fig. 692*A*). Included in the group are (1) *condyloma acuminatum* (p. 1115), (2) *condyloma latum* (p. 1112), (3) *cutaneous horn* (Fig. 692*B*) (p. 1363), (4) *verruca vulgaris*—common wart, usually seen in the first two decades of life, probably of viral origin, most often located on the dorsum of the fingers or the hand, and frequently disappearing spontaneously, and (5) *verruca plantaris*—plantar wart, usually located over the metatarsophalangeal joints but occupying any of the plantar surface, composed of a central horny plate and a peripheral keratotic ring, attended (because of pressure) by exquisite pain, and being refractive to treatment (Robinson).

Clavus.—A clavus (L. = nail), commonly known as a *corn*, is a pyramidally-shaped mass of keratin located over pressure points on the foot, especially in the vicinity of the toes. A clavus is referred to as hard when it is located on the exposed surface and is dry and brittle, and it is called soft when it is located in moist areas as between toes and is soft and elastic. The size varies to as much as 6 to 10 mm. in diameter. *Histologically* the bulk of the lesion is composed of keratin (Fig. 693). This overrides atrophic or hyperplastic epithelium. Clinically the lesion is accompanied by considerable pain due to pressure upon the underlying papillæ.

Keratosis.—By keratosis is meant simply focal increase of keratin deposition. Generally, at least two types of keratoses are recognizable — senile and arsenical—and both of these are precancerous lesions (Ayres

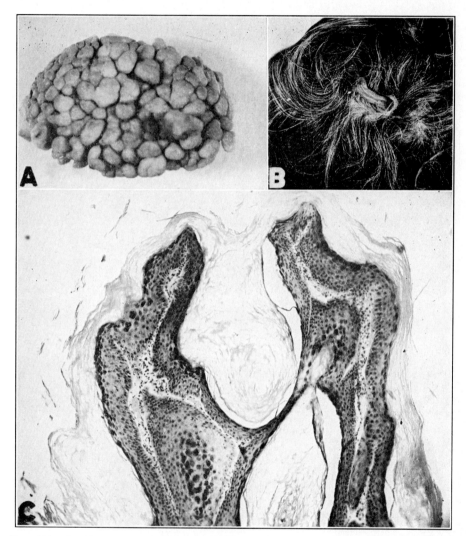

FIG. 692.—Papillomas illustrating *A*, a sessile tumor composed of innumerable pedunculated nodules, *B*, a cutaneous horn of the scalp, and *C*, cores of connective tissue covered with hyperplastic and hyperkeratotic but otherwise regular squamous epithelium. × 50.

and Sachs). *Senile keratosis*, as the term suggests, usually occurs in people beyond the age of fifty years. The *lesions* are generally multiple, are prone to occur on exposed parts of the body such as the face and dorsum of the hands, and result from a combination of a fair type of skin, excessive exposure to actinic (sun) rays, and age. Early changes consist of ill-defined, scarcely perceptible, gray, scaly areas that measure up to 6 or 8 mm. in diameter. As they age, they increase in size, undergo confluence, become thicker and even verrucal-like, and are thus more readily discernible. *Histologically* they disclose hyperkeratosis, acanthosis, and dyskeratosis with changes progressing to that of a frank squamous cell carcinoma (Fig. 694). The superficial part of the corium reveals leukocytic infiltration. *Arsenical keratosis* develops as a result of external or internal (ingestion) exposure to arsenic and may not occur until many years after contact. The lesions generally affect the palms and soles but may also involve other portions of the body. Pathologically they are similar to those in senile keratosis.

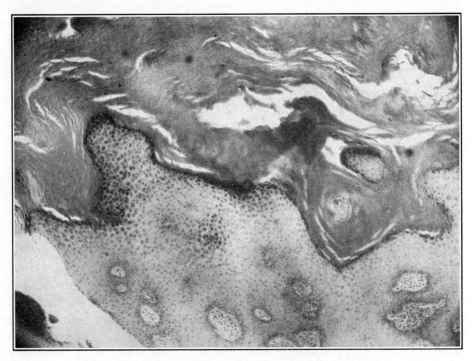

FIG. 693.—Clavus revealing severe hyperkeratosis and marked hyperplasia of the squamous epithelium. × 50.

Acanthosis Nigricans.—Acanthosis nigricans, also known as keratosis nigricans, is an uncommon disorder of the skin characterized by the formation of pigmented papillary nodules or masses. It is dividable into a juvenile and an adult form. The *lesions* are symmetrically distributed and affect most parts of the body, especially the axillæ, neck, external genitals, groins, and extremities. They vary in size from a few millimeters to several centimeters (the latter consisting of confluent aggregations) and are tan to deep brown or black. *Histologically* they reveal hyperkeratosis, acanthosis, atrophy of adjacent prickle cells, melanin pigmentation of the basal cells, similar pigment in the outer portion of the corium, and lymphocytic infiltration in the corium. While the juvenile disorder is benign, the adult type is frequently associated with cancer of the breast or an abdominal viscus and is thus referred to as malignant. The combination of lesions in adult acanthosis nigricans is unexplainable.

Keratoacanthoma.—This condition, also *called* verrucome, verrugoma, self-healing carcinoma, molluscum sebaceum, and psuedoepitheliomatous hyperplasia, is a benign, self-limited, proliferation of the epidermis (Monroe and McNulty). It is *dividable* into a solitary and a multiple variety (Epstein). The solitary variety is common, generally occurs in the sixth and seventh decades of life, and has no predilection for either sex. The multiple variety is rare, starts in adolescence or early life, and prevails in males. The *cause* is unknown. In the solitary form, infection, especially viral, has been suspected while sunlight and contact with tar and petroleum distillates as

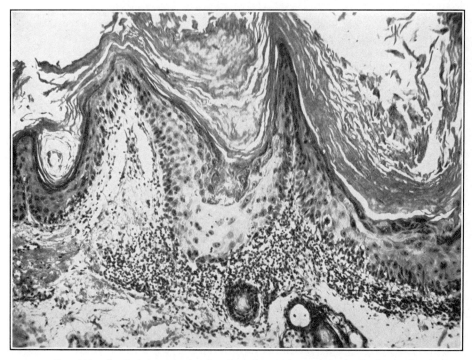

Fig. 694.—Senile keratosis showing hyperkeratosis, acanthosis, dyskeratosis, and leukocytic permeation of the corium. × 100.

well as focal trauma have been incriminated from time to time. In the generalized form none of the above listed etiologic factors appears to be of any significance but a familial tendency has been noted. *Grossly* the only differences in the lesions in the two varieties are number—single in the solitary and as many as thousands in the multiple, and location. Solitary lesions are usually found on the face, neck, ears, and arms. Multiple lesions are generally more common on the head, neck, and extremities but are also located on the trunk and genitals and in the mouth. Each lesion grows rapidly after its first appearance—reaching a maximum diameter of about 2 cm. in 4 to 6 weeks. It is elevated, indurated, and reddish. Its center forms a crater that is filled with keratin and surrounded by overhanging edges. *Histologically* the crater consists of a defect in the epidermis (Fig. 695). It is filled with keratin and is surrounded by acanthotic, dyskeratotic, stratified squamous epithelium that discloses papillary projections into the defect. The cells are large, bizarre, and hyperchromatic. The containing basement membrane, however, is always intact and the cells do not infiltrate the underlying structures. The adjacent epidermis discloses lymphocytes, plasma cells, eosinophils, and, as the lesion ages, giant cells of the foreign body type. The condition is not attended by any *complications*. Carcinoma does not develop. *Clinically* the lesion reaches its maximum growth in about 6 weeks and gradually regresses and disappears within about 12

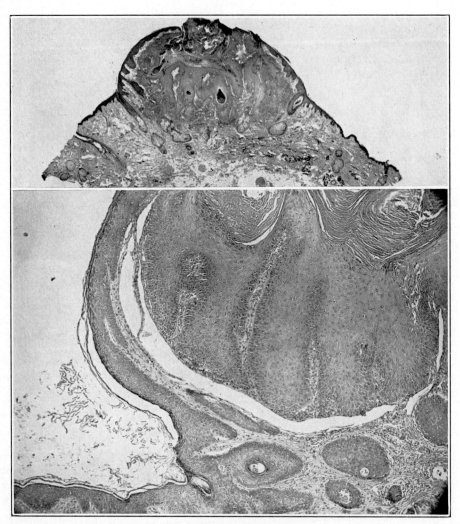

FIG. 695.—Keratoacanthoma showing a crater-like defect in the epidermis filled with keratin and lined with greatly hyperplastic, acanthotic epithelium. × 7 and × 50

months leaving only a fine scar. In solitary lesions, this constitutes the entire story but in multiple lesions new nodules continuously appear throughout the entire life of the patient. The *diagnosis* is made from the history, the gross appearance, and the microscopic examination. A differential diagnosis includes many epithelial lesions, especially squamous cell carcinoma. The usual *treatment* is surgical excision. The *prognosis* is good, for even without treatment the lesions spontaneously disappear by eversion and extrusion of the keratinous core. Continuous recurrences, however, account for high morbidity in the multiple variety.

Bowen's Disease.—Bowen's disease, often referred to as *intraepithelial carcinoma* or *carcinoma-in-situ*, is a chronic (years' duration) disorder of the skin characterized by the formation of keratin covered papules or nodules that usually measure up to 1 cm. in diameter (Beerman). The *lesions* are found in the skin of any region of the body, are slowly progressive, and (after years) may produce metastasis. The *histologic* changes consist of hyperkeratosis, acanthosis, dyskeratosis, irregularity and hyperchromatism of the prickle cells, increased numbers of mitoses, and leukocytic infiltra-

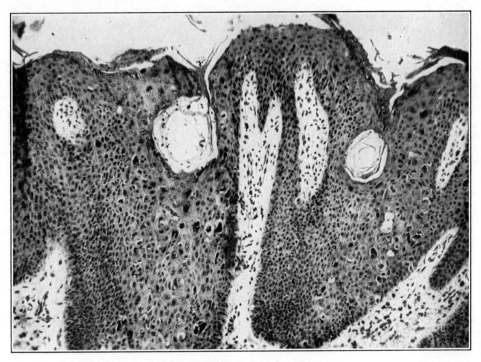

FIG. 696.—Bowen's disease disclosing hyperkeratosis, acanthosis, dyskeratosis, and irregularity of the epithelial cells together with leukocytic infiltration of the corium. × 100.

tion of the corium (Fig. 696). The epithelial basement membrane remains intact and the epithelial cells do not invade the corium. Local excision is generally curative.

Squamous Cell Carcinoma.—Squamous cell carcinoma of the skin is a malignant tumor composed of irregular epidermal prickle cells. The disorder can *occur* at any time after the first decade of life but is most common between the ages of fifty and seventy years and it affects both sexes with approximately equal frequency (Welton). While the exact *cause* of carcinoma of the skin remains undetermined it is known that trauma, heat, cold, ultraviolet and other rays, and chemical agents (hydrocarbons, aromatic amines, arsenic, etc.) may play an initiating role (p. 263) and that lesions such as keratoses, cutaneous horns, verrucæ, leukoplakia, kraurosis, erythroplasia, xeroderma pigmentosum, old burns, etc., are distinctly precancerous (Downing, Fisher, Arhelger, Ayers, and Lawrence)

Pathologically squamous cell carcinoma of the skin may affect any portion of the body but with involvement of the exposed portions (head, neck, and hands) occurring in over four-fifths of all cases (Welton and Roseberg). The lesions are usually single but may be multiple. The initial growth may appear as a small scaly area, a papule, an ulcer that fails to heal, or a small nodule. In any case, it gradually increases in size until it measures many centimeters in diameter and as it does so it becomes ulcerated, fungated, or both (Fig. 697). Once the tumor is well established

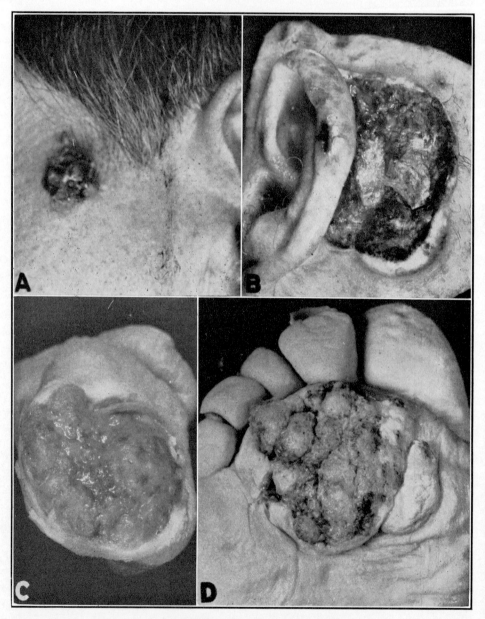

Fig. 697.—Squamous cell carcinoma illustrating *A*, a small raised nodular pre-auricular lesion, *B*, a postauricular ulcerating mass and senile keratosis of the ear, *C*, an ulcerating subungual tumor, and *D*, a fungating plantar growth.

it is fairly well circumscribed but is not encapsulated, assumes a grayish-white appearance, and is quite firm. *Histologically* squamous cell carcinoma is composed of prickle cells in varying degrees of differentiation (Fig. 698). When the lesion is examined early with sections at the correct level, finger-like projections and nests of neoplastic cells are seen to stream from the epidermis into the underlying corium. In better differentiated tumors the cells are large, sharply defined, and polyhedral. The cytoplasm is abundant and eosinophilic and the nuclei are large, rounded, or irregular and hyperchromatic. Keratin formation in the form of pearls or more diffuse masses may be abundant. In poorly differentiated tumors, the neoplastic cells invade the corium singly rather than in nests or clusters.

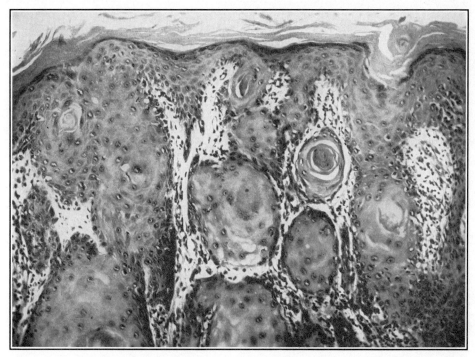

Fig. 698.—Squamous cell carcinoma revealing nests and strands of large irregular prickle cells invading the underlying corium. There are present several well-formed pearls and the stroma contains leukocytes. × 100.

The cells are small or large and sharply defined. The cytoplasm is variable in amount and the nuclei may be small or large, round or irregular, and watery or hyperchromatic. Between these two extremes are all gradations. In any case, the stroma may be of a loose or dense connective tissue variety, may be abundant or scanty, and is always permeated with plasma cells and lymphocytes. Carcinoma of the skin *spreads* by direct extension to involve adjacent structures, by lymphatics to the draining lymph nodes, and uncommonly (and usually late in the course of the disease) by blood vessels to the lungs, liver, and other organs (Mohs).

The *complications* of squamous cell carcinoma of the skin are extension to adjacent structures, metastases, secondary infection of the surrounding tissue and draining lymph nodes (all draining lymph node enlargements are not cancerous), and ulceration of vessels with hemorrhage. The *clinical manifestations* consist essentially of an indolent, painless "sore" that fails to heal. The *diagnosis* can be made with certainty only by biopsy. *Treatment* consists of local (but wide) surgical excision or irradiation. The *prognosis* is good for if the lesions are discovered early and treated adequately the cure rate should approach 100 per cent.

Basal Cell Carcinoma.—Basal cell carcinoma, also known as *rodent ulcer* (because it gradually eats away the adjacent tissues), is a locally malignant tumor that arises from the basal cells of the epidermis and/or

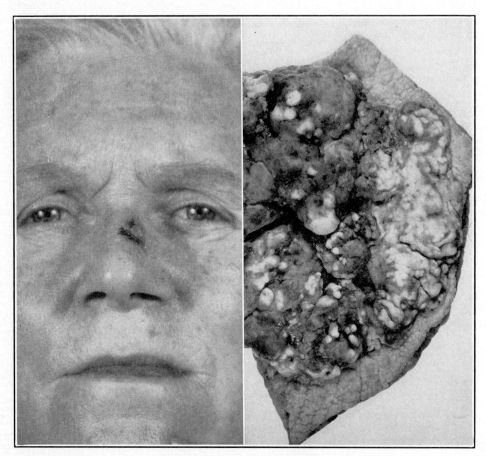

Fig. 699.—Basal cell carcinoma showing (to the left) an ulcerating lesion and (to the right) a fungating mass.

epidermal appendages and that reproduces cells that resemble the parent basal cells (Teloh). The neoplasm affects women about as frequently as men and usually *occurs* after the age of forty-five years. The precise *cause* is unknown but the predisposing factors are similar to those in squamous cell carcinoma (p. 1367).

Pathologically any part of the skin may be affected with, however, a marked predilection for the face above the level of the angle of the mouth. Most often the lesion is an ulcer (Fig. 699). It is irregular in outline, of varying depths, and slowly progressive. The edges are generally only slightly if at all elevated and induration of the infiltrated tissues is not great; the floor is covered with necrotic tissue, and the base is composed of gray tumor. The lesion is usually single but may be multiple and its size varies from several millimeters to that covering most of the face. Occasionally the growth is fungating, sessile or pedunculated, soft or cystic, superficially ulcerated, and as much as 3 to 4 cm. in diameter. Rarely, also there may be innumerable varisized fungating neoplasms covering the scalp in the form of a turban and thus being referred to as a *turban tumor* (Coloviras). *Histologically* most tumors are composed of varisized, sharply circumscribed, rounded masses of epithelial cells that may be attached to the structure from which they arose (Fig. 700). The cells are more or less of the basal type. They are of moderate sizes, are ill defined, possess a moderate amount of somewhat basophilic cytoplasm, and disclose large, round or oval, uniformly-appearing nuclei. Frequently the peripheral cells are somewhat elongated or distinctly cuboidal and are arranged at right angles to the main mass of cells. While the majority of the masses are solid, some disclose varying degrees of focal degeneration to complete disappearance of cells producing a cystic appearance. Basal cell carcinoma *spreads* by local extension—gradually eroding all structures that it contacts, even bone. It does not metastasize.

The *complications* consist of extension of the tumor, infection, and hemorrhage. *Clinical manifestations* consist simply of an ulcer or a mass. The *diagnosis* is made clinically from the appearance of the lesion and a history of long duration without metastases and pathologically by biopsy. *Treatment* consists of surgical excision or irradiation. The *prognosis* is good. All patients should be cured.

Extramammary Paget's Disease.—As already discussed (p. 1220), Paget's disease of the breast is a carcinoma of the larger ducts that spreads intraepithelially to produce an excoriating lesion of the nipple and areola. While there is still some controversy as to the nature of similar lesions found in the skin of other portions of the body (notably the anogenital region) it is generally conceded that the extramammary tumors represent carcinomas of sweat glands with involvement of the overlying epidermis (Dockerty).

Tumors of Epidermal Appendages.—Tumors of epidermal appendages may be considered together because of certain common gross pathologic and clinical manifestations. In general, they *occur* at all ages but are most prevalent beyond the third decade and they have no predilection for either sex (Warren, Gates, Warvi, and Beerman). The *cause* is unknown.

Pathologically (1) all appendageal structures are represented, (2) the lesions may be benign or malignant, and (3) only part of the body covering is usually involved with the greatest concentration occurring in areas possessing the greatest concentration of normal structures. Thus (1) tumors of sebaceous glands are most common about the face, eyelids, and scalp and are not seen in the palms or soles, (2) tumors of sweat glands prevail in the axillæ and anogenital region, (3) tumors of hairs are universally distributed except for the palms and soles, and (4) tumors of nails are found only about the terminal phalanges. *Grossly* there are no distinguishing characteristics. The tumors are primarily subepidermal and vary in size from a few millimeters to many centimeters in diameter (Fig. 701). Benign growths are generally comparatively small, sharply circumscribed and even encapsulated, solid or cystic, and covered with intact epidermis. Malignant tumors, on the other hand, are generally larger, less sharply circumscribed or distinctly invasive, usually solid, and often ulcerating. The color varies

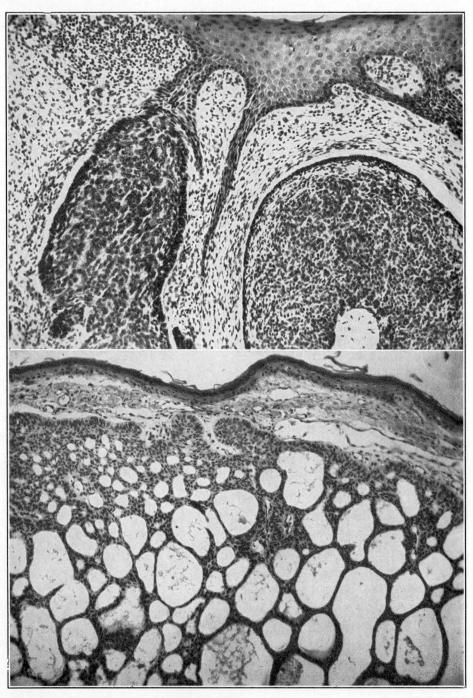

Fig. 700.—Basal cell carcinoma disclosing (above) masses of basal cells arising from the epidermis and (below) nests of basal cells with foci of liquefaction, thus producing a glandular appearance. × 100.

from gray to yellowish to brown. As a rule, the malignant tumors are locally destructive and seldom metastasize.

Histologically, as already stated, the lesions are benign or malignant but sometimes the gradation from one to the other is too subtle to be recognizable by our present microscopic techniques. In general, it may be stated that the more benign the growth the more it resembles its parent structure, and the more malignant the tumor the more it departs from its normal anatomic appearance. Regarding classification, the lesions are probably best referred to according to the parent structure and then further classified as to benign or malignant. Tumors of *sebaceous glands*

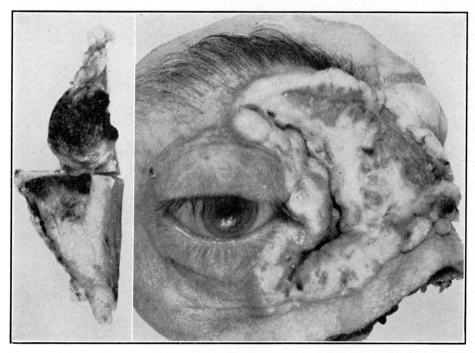

FIG. 701.—Tumors of sweat glands illustrating (to the left) a circumscribed subepidermal benign growth and (to the right) a large ulcerating tumor in the region of the inner canthus of the eye.

are usually divided into *hyperplasia* (as in rhinophyma, p. 424), *adenoma* and *carcinoma*. The more benign lesions consist of circumscribed nests of epithelial cells composed of polyhedral prickle-like cells peripherally and larger reticulated or vacuolated sebaceous-like cells centrally (Fig. 702). The more malignant tumors resemble basal or squamous cell carcinomas. Tumors of *sweat glands* are more variable. Among other names, they have been called *anhidroma, hidradenoma, spiradenoma, intracystic papilloma,* and *syringo-adenoma* when benign and *malignant anhidroma,* etc., or *anhidrocarcinoma,* etc., when malignant. The more benign growths approach the appearance of normal sweat glands. In general, growths arising in apocrine glands are composed of acini or larger glands with papillary infoldings, each lined with tall columnar cells exhibiting an abundant amount of eosinophilic cytoplasm and round or oval, relatively small, evenly stained nuclei (Fig. 703*A*). Growths arising in eccrine or exocrine glands are usually composed of small, rounded, acini lined with smaller cuboidal, columnar, or flattened cells with indistinct borders, a moderate amount of cytoplasm and round nuclei (Fig. 703 B). Myoepithelial cells may or may not be present at the periphery. The more malignant tumors appear as a basal cell carcinoma, squamous cell carcinoma, adenocarcinoma, or mixtures of these (Fig. 704). Tumors of *hairs* are either benign (*trichomas*) in which case they are composed of sharply circumscribed nests of squamous-

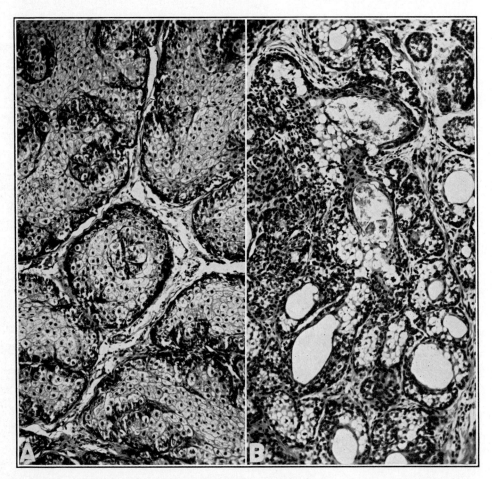

Fig. 702.—Tumors of sebaceous glands revealing *A*, a benign growth composed mostly of large sebaceous cells and *B*, a more malignant tumor resembling in part an ordinary squamous cell carcinoma. × 100.

like cells with or without central keratin (Fig. 705 *A*) or malignant (*trichoepitheliomas*) in which case they are composed of nests of irregular polyhedral cells indistinguishable from squamous cell carcinoma. Tumors of *finger nails* are usually carcinomas of a basal or squamous cell variety (Fig. 705 *B*).

Tuberous Sclerosis.—Tuberous sclerosis is a clinical syndrome consisting of the following: (1) sclerotic and calcified nodular areas of gliosis of the brain (p. 1453), (2) adenomas of sebaceous glands of especially the face, (3) fibromas of the head and back, (4) multiple fibromas and other benign

tumors of the kidneys, (5) retinal tumors (phacomas), (6) roentgenographically demonstrated sclerotic plaques in the cranial vault and cyst-like
areas of bone destruction in the phalanges, (7) mental deficiency, and (8)
convulsions (Holt).   The condition is hereditary, usually develops early
in life, and leads to death from involvement of the brain.

  Cysts.—Cysts of the skin are usually of three types—epidermal, traumatic, and dermoid (Warvi and Gross).   *Epidermal cysts* arise from any of
the epidermal appendages—hair follicles, sebaceous gland, or sweat glands.

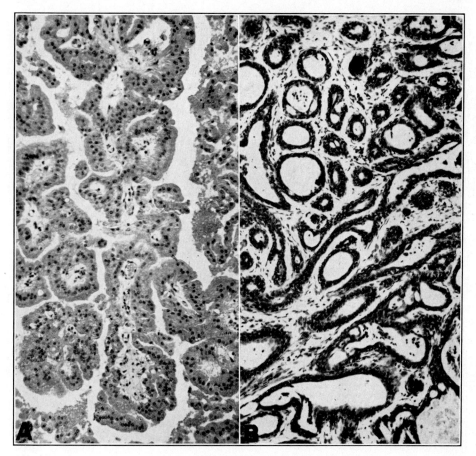

Fig. 703.—Tumors of sweat glands showing *A*, an apocrine growth composed of acini lined by
tall columnar cells with an abundance of eosinophilic cytoplasm and *B*, an eccrine growth composed of small glands lined with one to three layers of flattened cells.   × 100.

They may be found in the skin of any part of the body but are especially
common in the scalp, are located in the corium, are covered with intact
skin, are fairly sharply circumscribed, measure up to 2 cm. or more in
greatest diameter, disclose a gray wall, and are filled with gray sebaceous
material.   Histologically they are lined with stratified squamous epithelium
that may be hypertrophic or atrophic (Fig. 706).   Its inner surface is lined
with an abundance of keratin which, in turn, merges with and forms the
sebaceous material in the lumen.   *Traumatic cysts* arise as a result of (1)
displacement of epithelium, (2) alteration of epidermal appendages, or

(3) stimulation of epithelial growth. They usually occur at points of trauma in laborers (such as the hands) or in operative scars. Pathologically they are similar to epidermal cysts. *Dermoid cysts* occur along lines of closure of embryonic clefts. They have already been discussed in an earlier part of this Chapter (p. 1325).

Calcifying Epithelioma.—Calcifying epithelioma is a benign tumor of the skin probably arising from immature hair matrix. The condition *occurs* about once in every 2,000 surgical specimens, affects all races, is most common in the first two decades of life, and predominates in females (Lever

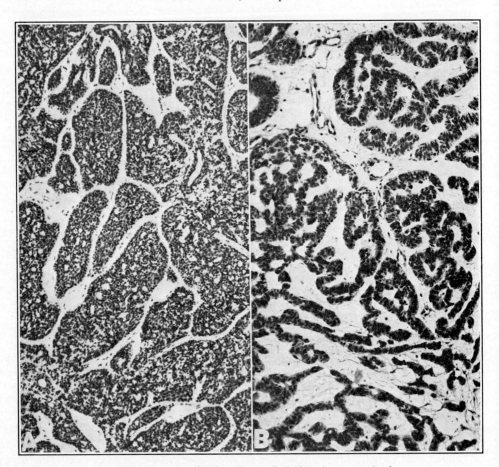

Fig. 704.—Tumors of sweat glands disclosing *A*, a growth of a basal cell variety and *B*, an adenocarcinoma. × 100.

and Tilden). *Pathologically* the lesions usually affect the face and upper extremities, are sharply circumscribed, measure up to 3 cm. in diameter, are firm to hard, and disclose varying amounts of calcium. *Histologically* they are composed of nests or masses of basal or squamous cells that show varying degrees of necrosis and calcification (Fig. 707). The necrotic cells are prone to elicit a foreign body giant cell response. The disorder is readily cured by excision. Metastasis does not occur.

Mixed Tumors.—Mixed tumors of the skin are rare (Morehead). They grow slowly and are usually recognized in adults. They are found mostly

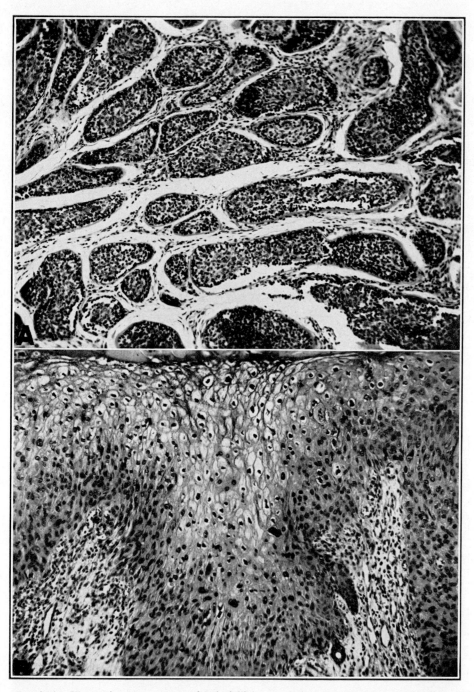

Fig. 705.—Illustrating *A*, a tumor of hair follicles consisting of nests of squamous-like cells surrounded by a distinct hyaline membrane and *B*, a squamous cell carcinoma of a nail with keratin on the surface and irregular cells that have not yet broken through the basement membrane. × 100.

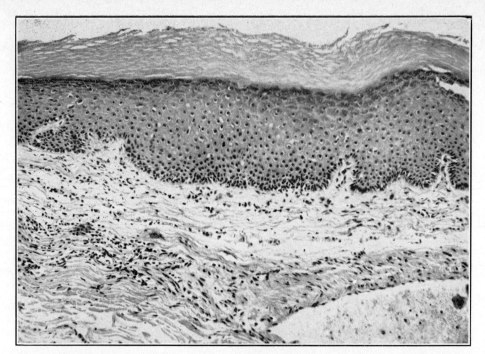

FIG. 706.—Sebaceous cyst revealing a wall of hyperplastic stratified squamous epithelium covered with an abundance of keratin. × 100.

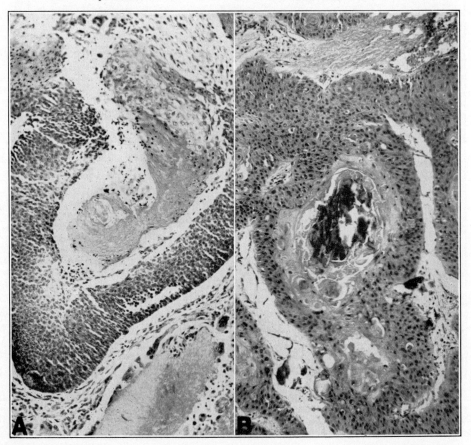

FIG. 707.—Calcifying epithelioma showing *A*, viable and necrotic basal cells with the latter eliciting a foreign body giant cell reaction and *B*, a nest of keratinizing squamous cells with a central area of calcification. × 100.

in the vicinity of *embryonic fissures* such as the lips, mouth, lacrimal glands, and palate but occasionally also affect the scalp, face, forehead, arms, hands, thighs, legs, and chest. The *tumors* may be single or multiple, measure up to 3 cm. in diameter, are located in the corium, are sharply circumscribed, and are firm in consistency. *Histologically* they are composed of varying combinations of squamous epithelium and epidermal appendages intermixed with connective tissue, lymphoid tissue, and cartilage (Fig. 708*A*). The growths probably represent ectodermal proliferations with subsequent metaplastic changes in mesodermal elements.

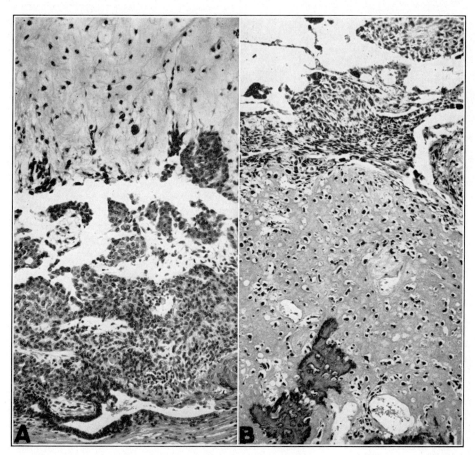

Fig. 708.—Illustrating *A*, a mixed tumor of the skin composed of cartilaginous and epithelial elements and *B*, an osteochondrosarcoma of the arm that metastasized to the lungs. × 100.

Osteoma.—Osteomas of the skin are usually multiple, measure 2 to 4 mm. in diameter, are located in the midcorium, and are composed of osseous tissue and fatty marrow (Carney). They generally *arise* on the basis of some previous scarring sclerodermatous disease and severe infections such as acne and syphilis.

Osteochondrosarcoma.—Osteochondrosarcoma or osteosarcoma of soft tissues is a malignant tumor that is akin to a similar lesion in bone and that probably arises on the basis of metaplasia of connective tissue cells or directly from reticulum cells. Such tumors have been *recorded in* the breast, thyroid, thigh, kidney, leg, upper arm, gluteal region, chest wall, mesentery, meninges, lip, urinary bladder, brachial plexus, and gallbladder (Shaffer). They *occur* at all ages, are more prevalent in females, and are of a few weeks to many years' duration. *Grossly* the growths are ill defined, moderately firm to hard, and measure from a few to many centimeters in diameter. *Histologically* they are composed of mixtures of irregular cartilaginous, osseous, and primitive cells (Fig. 708*B*). The lesions have a tendency to recur locally (after excision) and metastasize to the lungs, liver, and other tissues.

Sacrococcygeal Teratoma.—As the term indicates, a sacrococcygeal teratoma is a tumor that is located in the sacrococcygeal area and that is composed of tissues derived from the three germinal layers (Gross). Its *origin* is probably from pluripotent or totipotent cells that come from the "primitive knot" which is located near the coccyx. The tumors usually *occur* in infants or children and are more common in females than in males. *Grossly* the growths may measure up to 20 cm. or more in diameter (Fig. 709*A*). They are covered with skin, are sharply circumscribed, and are composed of solid and/or cystic tissue that may or may not disclose recognizable organoid (teeth, jaw, etc.) structures. As the lesions increase in size they tend to grow into the hollow of the sacrum and to replace and infiltrate the pelvic and perineal structures. *Histologically* skin, lining of the alimentary tract, salivary glands, respiratory epithelium, renal tissue, cartilage, bone, muscle, and nerve tissues have all been recognized (Fig. 709*B*). In general, the more cystic the growths the more benign the course. A frank *malignant transformation* (usually carcinoma) is seen in about 25 per cent of cases with metastasis occurring in the lymph nodes, liver, lungs, and bones. *Treatment* is surgical excision. If this is done early the *prognosis* is good.

Xanthoma.—Xanthoma (Gr. = yellow + tumor) is a varisized, yellow to brown, sharply circumscribed, moderately firm tumor that arises on the basis of abnormal metabolism of lipids. Histologically it is composed of large polyhedral cells with an abundant amount of lipid-positive foamy cytoplasm and small, round, evenly stained nuclei (Fig. 710). The lesions may be classified as follows: (1) *xanthelasma* or *xanthoma palpebrarum* (p. 876), (2) *xanthoma diabeticorum* (p. 876), and (3) *xanthoma tuberosum.* Of these, xanthoma tuberosum is perhaps the most important. The condition is frequently seen in the first three decades of life; the tumors are usually found in the subcutaneous tissues around the elbows, knees, and buttocks and attached to tendon sheaths, and there is often an associated severe arteriosclerosis which may cause coronary occlusion and death (Rigdon).

Keloid.—A keloid (Gr. = scar + form) is a localized overgrowth of connective tissue of the corium arising as a *sequel* to *injury* (Solomons). Some of the more common types of injury are as follows: pinprick, site of vaccination, pressure, abrasion, postoperative scar, burn, etc. *Heredity* is distinctly a predisposing factor, as indicated by the high incidence in the Negro race. The disorder has no predilection for either sex and while it may *occur* at any age it is most common in the third decade of life. The *lesions* may be single or multiple, are raised above the cutaneous surface, may be sessile or pedunculated, are nodular or plaque-like, and produce a wide variety of configurations (Fig. 711). *Grossly* they consist of ill-defined, grayish-white, moderately firm, homogeneous tissue (Fig. 712). *Histologically* they are composed of connective tissue cells. Early lesions are quite cellular while older lesions disclose increasing deposition of collagen. *Treatment* has been varied although currently irradiation or surgical excision followed immediately by irradiation seems to be preferred. The *prognosis* is guarded for the lesion tends to recur. A sarcomatous change is exceedingly rare.

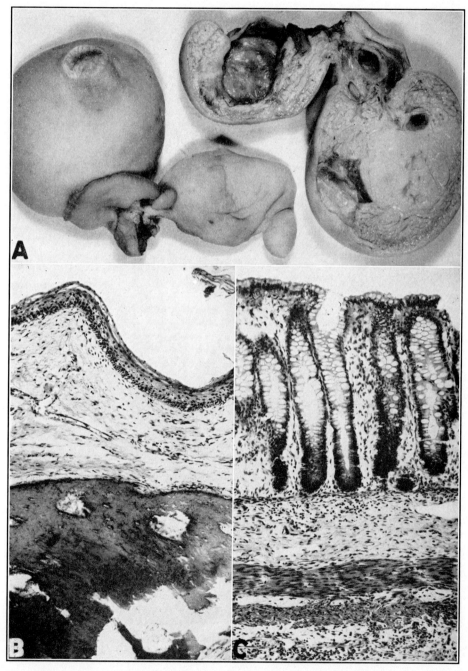

Fig. 709.—Sacrococcygeal teratoma demonstrating *A*, external and cut surface of a solid and cystic tumor, *B*, squamous epithelium, connective tissue, and bone. × 100, and *C*, intestinal mucosa, smooth muscle, and lymphocytic cells. × 100.

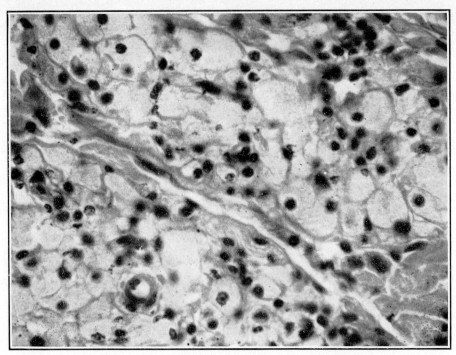

FIG. 710.—Xanthoma revealing large, sharply defined, polyhedral cells with an abundant foamy cytoplasm and small, round, evenly stained nuclei. × 400.

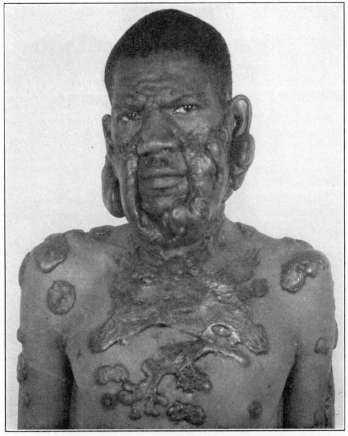

FIG. 711.—Keloids grotesquely disfiguring the body.

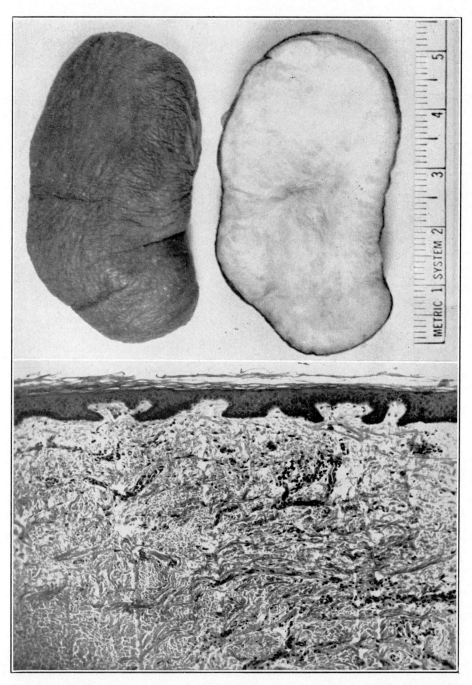

Fig. 712.—Keloid illustrating (above) the external and cut surface of a large solitary nodule and (below) thinning of the epidermis as a result of marked proliferation of subjacent connective tissue. × 100.

Fibroma.—A fibroma is a benign tumor originating in fibroblasts and occurring wherever connective tissue is present. Cutaneous fibromas are of two varieties (Stout). One is a soft, pedunculated or sessile mass while the other is an intradermal or subcutaneous, well-encapsulated growth (Fig. 713). Each consists of moderately firm to hard gray tissue. *Histologically* fibromas are composed of elongated, usually intertwining, ill-defined spindle cells with eosinophilic cytoplasm and elongated, evenly

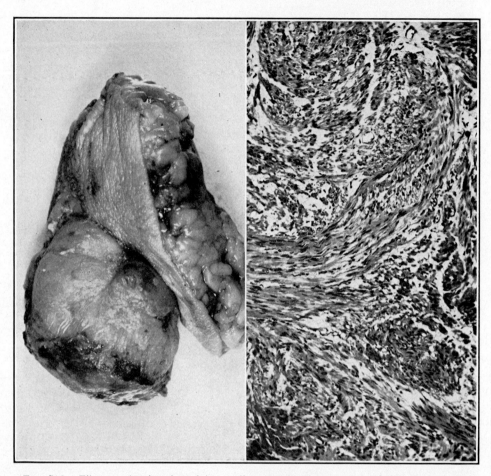

Fig. 713.—Fibroma showing (grossly) a well-encapsulated gray mass of fibrous tissue and (microscopically) interlacing bundles of spindle cells with a moderate amount of collagen deposition. × 100.

stained nuclei. The amount of collagen varies. When it is abundant the cellularity is decreased, while when it is scanty the cellularity is increased. In the latter instance, it is impossible to rule out a malignant tumor and many authors, therefore, refer to such growths as fibrosarcoma of low-grade malignancy.

Fibrosarcoma.—Fibrosarcoma arises from fibroblasts and is the malignant counterpart of fibroma (Stout). The condition *occurs* at all ages but is most common in the fifth to the seventh decades of life (Heller) and it prevails slightly in males over females. The *cause* is unknown although trauma and previous fibromas are often cited as predisposing factors. The tumors are *located* in the skin and subcutaneous tissues, retroperitoneum, and less commonly the various viscera. In the skin the condition is often referred to as *dermatofibrosarcoma protuberans* (Mopper and Hoffert) and any part of the cutaneous surface may be affected except the palms and soles but with the abdomen, back, and extremities being most often involved. *Grossly* the tumors vary in size from a few to many centimeters (Fig. 714). The cutaneous lesions are initially covered with skin but

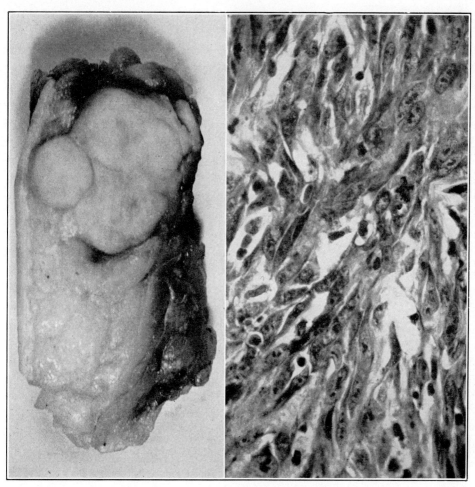

FIG. 714.—Fibrosarcoma disclosing (grossly) a lobulated pseudoencapsulated, diffusely gray, brain-like tumor and (microscopically) irregularly and elongated cells with hyperchromatic nuclei, one of which is in a state of bizarre mitosis. × 400.

secondarily may become ulcerated. Cut surfaces disclose an apparent encapsulation but with actual infiltration of the tumor into and beyond the false capsule. The growth is usually grayish white, is soft to moderately firm, and may disclose areas of degeneration or secondary cyst formation. *Histologically* the more benign growths are indistinguishable from cellular fibromas. The more malignant growths are composed of elongated, ill-defined, spindle cells with scanty cytoplasm and elongated large hyperchromatic nuclei. Mitoses are often numerous. As the tumors become more anaplastic the cells become even more irregular until they can scarcely be recognized as of connective tissue origin. The tumors *spread* by local extension and ultimately by vascular metastasis to distant organs. The chief *clinical manifestation* is the presence of a mass. The *diagnosis* is made histologically. *Treatment* consists of wide local excision or, if necessary and possible, of amputation. The *prognosis* is guarded, for recurrences are common and the over-all cure rate is less than 25 per cent.

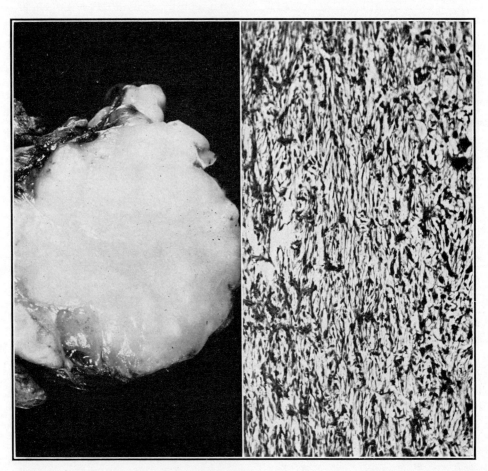

FIG. 715.—Myxosarcoma illustrating (grossly) a fairly sharply circumscribed, homogeneously gray, gelatinous tumor and (microscopically) hyperchromatic stellate cells separated by mucoid material. × 100.

Myxoma and Myxosarcoma.—A myxoma is a benign tumor and a myxosarcoma is a malignant tumor composed of neoplastic myxomatous tissue (Sponsel). Because the tumors parallel the age group, distribution, etc., of fibroma and fibrosarcoma, some authors say that they represent nothing more than variants of these connective tissue neoplasms. Since, however, they possess distinctive pathologic features, it is convenient to retain them in a separate category. *Grossly* the growths are generally bulky—usually measuring several centimeters in diameter (Fig. 715). They may appear fairly sharply circumscribed but just as often they are ill defined and permeate the adjacent tissues. They are usually soft and

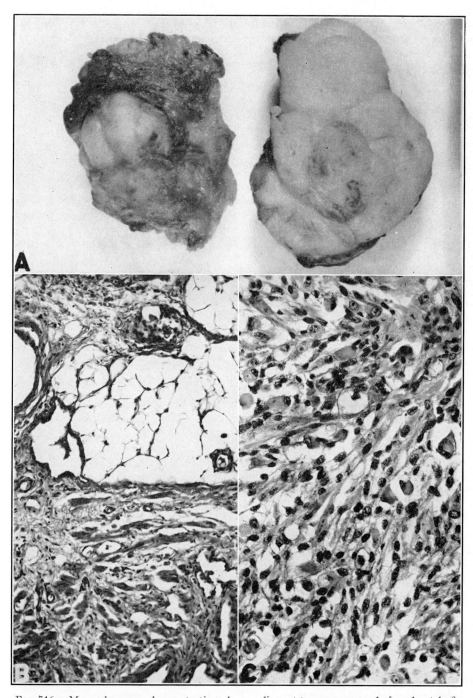

F ig. 716.—Mesenchymoma demonstrating *A*, a malignant tumor composed of moderately firm brain-like tissue, *B*, a benign growth consisting of connective tissue, fat, smooth muscle, and blood vessels. × 100, and *C*, a malignant growth composed essentially of connective tissue and fat tissue elements. × 200.

homogeneously gelatinous. *Histologically* they are composed of elongated stellate cells with long processes separated by varying amounts of mucoid material. In myxoma, the cells are more regular and uniform while in myxosarcoma they are more bizarre, showing greater irregularity in shape, size, and staining qualities of the nuclei. The transition, however, is subtle and often cannot be detected with certainty. The *diagnosis* is made pathologically. The *treatment* and *prognosis* parallel those in fibroma and fibrosarcoma.

Mesenchymoma.—A mesenchymoma is a tumor composed of a mixture of tissues of mesenchymal origin including connective tissue, fat, blood vessels, muscle, reticulum cell derivatives, cartilage, and bone (Stout). When the tissues are well differentiated they are readily recognizable and the tumor is called a *benign mesenchymoma* (Fig. 716*B*). When the tissues are poorly differentiated, primitive, or bizarre they may be recognized only with difficulty and the tumor is called a *malignant mesenchymoma* (Fig. 716*C*). The malignant growths may consist almost wholly of fibrosarcoma, leiomyosarcoma, liposarcoma, etc., of combinations of these, or of primitive cells that cannot be precisely tagged. *Grossly* there is nothing distinctive about the growths. The more benign neoplasms may appear similar to tumors of the most abundant element, that is, lipoma, fibroma, etc., while the more malignant tumors have a tendency to be composed of moderately firm, gray, brain-like tissue that may or may not disclose areas of necrosis, hemorrhage, and cyst formation (Fig. 716*A*). Mesenchymoma probably *arises* on a dysontogenic basis and may occur at any age. The usual *sites* of the body affected are legs, buttocks, other subcutaneous and striated muscle areas, perineum, and retroperitoneum. *Treatment* consists of surgical excision. The *prognosis* is good in benign tumors and parallels that of the most malignant element in malignant tumors.

Lipoma.—A lipoma is a benign tumor of fat tissue (Adair). The tumors *occur* more frequently in women than in men and are generally detected in patients around the age of forty years. They are *located* wherever there is fat tissue and may be classified as cutaneous, intermuscular, and visceral. Cutaneous lipomas are most common on the trunk, upper extremities, and upper portions of the legs. The *lesions* may measure from a few millimeters to 20 cm. or more in diameter and are generally single but in 6 to 8 per cent of cases are multiple (Fig. 717). The tumors are entirely subcutaneous, producing simply a varisized convex bulging or they protrude outwardly and are pedunculated. Cut surfaces usually disclose a sharply defined, well-encapsulated, lobulated mass of normal appearing fat tissue. *Histologic* sections reveal *lipocytes* supported by varying amounts of connective tissue stroma. The *diagnosis* is usually made pathologically. *Treatment* is surgical excision. The *prognosis* is good, for a sarcomatous transformation is rare. One should make certain, however, that the tumor is not initially a low-grade liposarcoma.

Liposarcoma.—Liposarcoma arises from lipoblasts and is the malignant counterpart of a lipoma (Stout). The tumor *occurs* somewhat more frequently in males than in females and while it may be found at all ages it is most common beyond the fourth decade of life. The *cause* is unknown despite the fact that trauma has often been incriminated. While the growths may be *located* anywhere in the body, they have a predilection for the retroperitoneum, mesentery, omentum, thigh, popliteal space, gluteal area, trunk, head, and neck. *Grossly* the tumors may attain large dimensions (20 to 30 cm. in diameter) for they grow slowly and are of long duration. The neoplasms are generally single but may be multiple, appear lobulated and fairly well encapsulated, are moderately firm, and on cut surface disclose fatty to gray tissue that is prone to degeneration, necrosis, and hemorrhage (Fig. 718*A*). *Histologic* sections reveal neoplastic cells that at one extreme resemble lipoblasts and at the other extreme resemble lipocytes (Fig. 718*B* and *C*). Between the two there are many gradations. Lipoblastic liposarcomas are composed essentially of relatively small

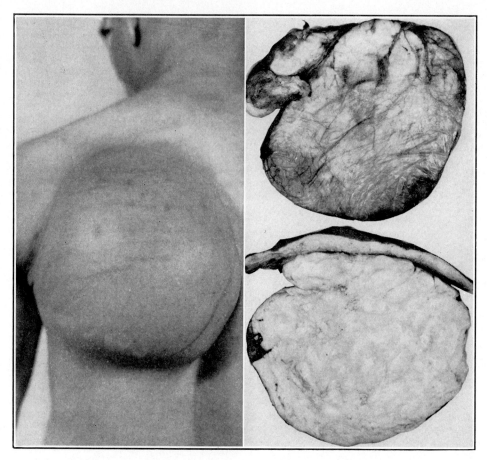

FIG. 717.—Lipoma over the left scapula showing (to the left) the intact tumor and (to the right) the external and cut surface of the excised mass.

rounded or polyhedral cells that resemble plasma cells, renal cortical cells, or hepatic cells. The cytoplasm is eosinophilic and contains only small, peppery, fat-positive droplets. Bizarre giant cells are present but are infrequent. Lipocytic liposarcomas are composed of sharply defined, large, polyhedral, neoplastic cells with abundant vacuolated, fat-positive cytoplasm and round, evenly stained, often peripherally located nuclei. Bizarre giant cells with multiple, hyperchromatic, irregular nuclei are common in the more malignant growths. The *diagnosis* of liposarcoma is made pathologically. *Treatment* consists of wide surgical excision for the lesion is locally invasive. If this is impossible, irradiation therapy offers good

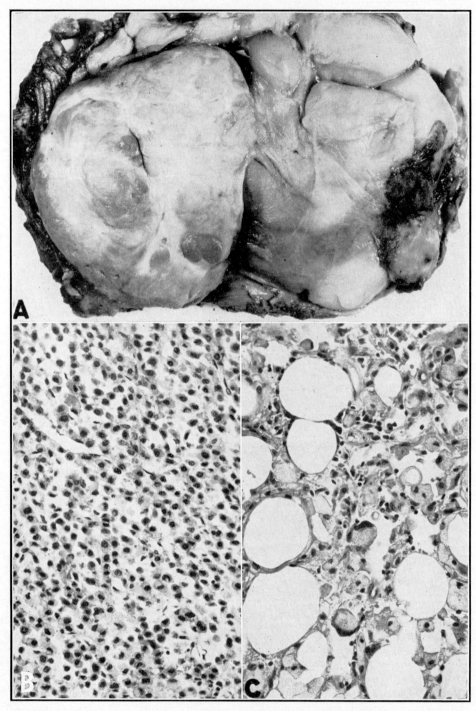

FIG. 718.—Liposarcoma revealing *A*, a hemisected, lobulated, apparently encapsulated mass of fatty tissue, *B*, a lipoblastic tumor composed of plasma cell-like or hepatic-like cells. × 200, and *C*, a lipocytic tumor composed of large polyhedral cells with reticulated or vacuolated cytoplasm. × 200.

palliation. The *prognosis* is variable. Unless treated radically, the usual story is repeated local recurrences followed ultimately by metastasis.

Leiomyoma.—A leiomyoma of the skin is a benign tumor of smooth muscle arising either from the media of vessels or from the arrectores pilorum muscles (Christopherson). The tumors usually occur in adults, are often painful, are widely distributed, generally measure as much as 1 cm. in diameter, and are composed of interlacing bundles of smooth muscle cells.

Neuroma.—A neuroma is a painful bulbous enlargement (usually measuring up to 1.5 cm. in diameter) of the terminal portion of the proximal segment of a severed nerve (Huber). The lesion is thus commonly seen in

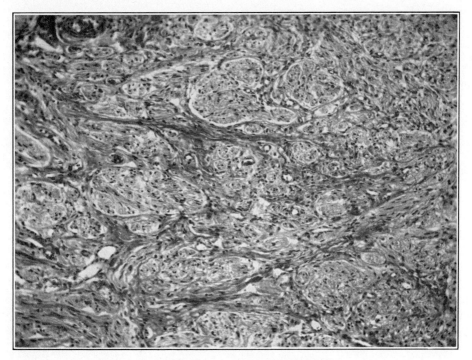

Fig. 719.—Neuroma showing bundles of nerve fibrils surrounded by sheaths of connective tissue. × 100.

the *stump* of an amputated extremity. It arises on the basis of irregular proliferation of the connective tissue sheaths with subsequent correspondingly irregular proliferation of axis cylinders. The result is a conglomerate mass of intermingling connective tissue and nerve fibrils (Fig. 719). The lesion is generally accompanied by pain that stems from the contraction of the connective tissue about the nerve fibers.

Neurofibroma.—A *neurofibroma* is a benign tumor that originates from, and is composed of, cells that cover the nerve fibrils of a peripheral nerve. Whether these cells are of mesodermal origin and therefore fibroblasts or whether they are of ectodermal origin and thus Schwann or neurilemma cells is still debatable (Tarlov and Murray). Proponents of the latter theory refer to the lesions as *neurilemmoma (neurilemoma), neurinoma,* or *schwannoma.* In your author's opinion, it matters little in precisely which

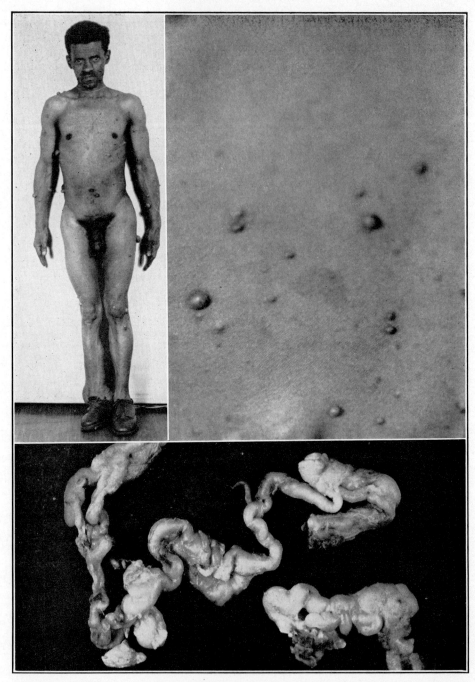

Fig. 720.—Neurofibromatosis illustrating (above) numerous, varisized, cutaneous nodules with a sarcomatous transformation of the lesion about the right ankle and (below) multiple excised nodules along the course of two nerves.

type of cell the tumor originates or what name is appended to it for pathologically and clinically they all have similar properties. The *tumors* may
arise in any peripheral nerve and may be single or multiple (Fig. 720). When
multiple (usually many to hundreds) the condition is referred to as *neurofibromatosis* or *von Recklinghausen's disease* (Wachstein, Inglis, and Preston). Neurofibromatosis is relatively rare *occurring* about once in every
two to four thousand hospital admissions. It is about two times as common
in males as in females, is seen in all races, and generally develops in adults.
Whether single or multiple, the *tumors* are located along the course of the
nerve (Fig. 721). They are well encapsulated, are moderately firm, measure
from a few to many centimeters in diameter, and are generally composed of
diffusely gray tissue. Some tumors have a tendency to undergo liquefaction
necrosis and cyst formation. *Histologically* they are composed of elongated,
ill-defined, evenly stained nuclei arranged in pallisade formation. The
chief complication is a transformation into a *neurofibrosarcoma*. Such a
change is said to occur in from 10 to 15 per cent of multiple lesions and in a
considerably lesser number of single lesions. A neurofibrosarcoma is
similar grossly, microscopically, and clinically to a fibrosarcoma (p. 1384).
The chief *clinical manifestations* are (1) visible and palpable tumors and
(2) symptoms and signs referable to any organ which may simultaneously
contain or be encroached upon by an identical growth. The *diagnosis* of
a single neurofibroma is generally made pathologically while that of neurofibromatosis is made from the gross appearance of the tumors. The latter
may be confused with multiple lipomas. *Treatment* of single tumors is
surgical excision while treatment of multiple lesions is removal of those
which are thought to be undergoing a malignant transformation. The
prognosis depends upon the location of the growth and the presence or
absence of a sarcomatous change.

Nevus.—A nevus, also known as a *pigmented nevus, mole,* and *nonvascular
birthmark,* is a benign lesion of the skin composed of nevus cells (Lewis).
The precise *origin* of nevus cells is still in doubt (Allen, Lund, and Masson).
In general, it has been maintained that they arise from epithelial cells,
connective tissue cells, and nerve tissue cells. Each of these theories has
its proponents and its opponents but it appears that most workers favor
the neurogenic theory. In your author's opinion, the evidence in favor of
this contention consists of (1) the frequent presence of nevus cells deep in
the hypoderm away from all epithelial structures, (2) the demonstration of
nerve elements in conjunction with nevus cells, (3) the complete lack of
response of malignant tumors of nevus cells (melanoblastomas) to irradiation therapy—a phenomenon that never occurs in any tumor of epithelial
origin, and (4) the clinical behavior of malignant tumors of nevus cells
being unlike that of malignant tumors of epithelial structures of the skin.
Regardless of their histogenesis, *nevi are* congenital in origin, are always
present at birth but (depending upon the amount of melanin present) may
not be apparent until later in life, increase in size with growth of the child,
affect both sexes with equal frequency, occur in all races, and affect almost
everybody.

Pathologically nevi are present in almost every part of the cutaneous
covering, including the palms and soles. They vary in number from one to
thousands and from a millimeter or less in diameter to that which covers
most of the body surface (Fig. 722). Some lesions are deep beneath the
integument (blue nevi), others are within the skin, and others still are raised
above the surface in a papillary fashion. They may or may not contain

88

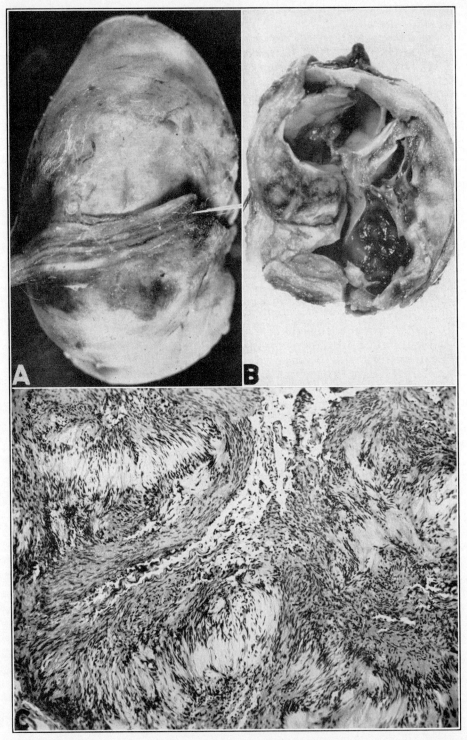

Fig. 721.—Neurofibroma disclosing *A*, the external surface of a well-encapsulated tumor with an attached nerve, *B*, the cut surface of a partly solid and partly cystic tumor, and *C*, elongated spindle cells with palisading of the nuclei. × 100.

hair. Depending upon the amount of melanin present, the color ranges from light tan to blue or black. *Histologically* nevus cells are quite variable in appearance (Fig. 723). At one extreme they are large, sharply defined, and polyhedral. The cytoplasm is abundant and lightly eosinophilic and the nuclei are large, round, and evenly stained. At the other extreme the cells are small, elongated or rounded, and ill defined. The cytoplasm is relatively scanty and the nuclei are elongated or rounded and evenly

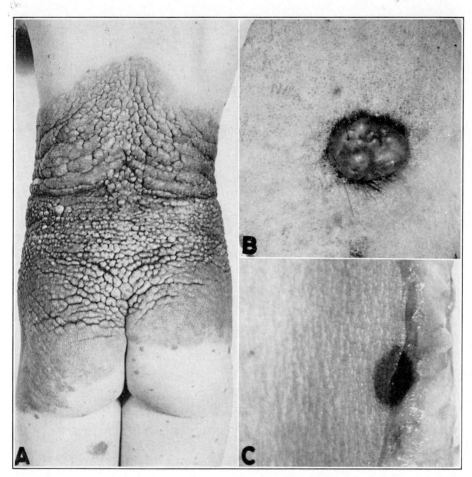

FIG. 722.—Nevi illustrating *A*, multiple brown lesions distributed in a bathing trunk fashion and singly, *B*, an elevated blue-black type containing hair, and *C*, a flat, deep blue type involving the epidermis, corium, and hypoderm.

stained. Between the two extremes are all gradations. In any case, the cytoplasm of some or many of the cells contains a variable amount of melanin. In cells that ordinarily do not contain melanin the pigment can be readily demonstrated by the "dopa" reaction (p. 79). Depending upon the location of the cells, nevi may be classified as follows: (1) *junction*— when nevus cells are found at the junction of the epidermis and corium. (2) *dermal*—when nevus cells are located in the corium, (3) *compound*— when nevus cells involve both the epidermis and corium, and (4) *blue*— when nevus cells are present in the hypoderm.

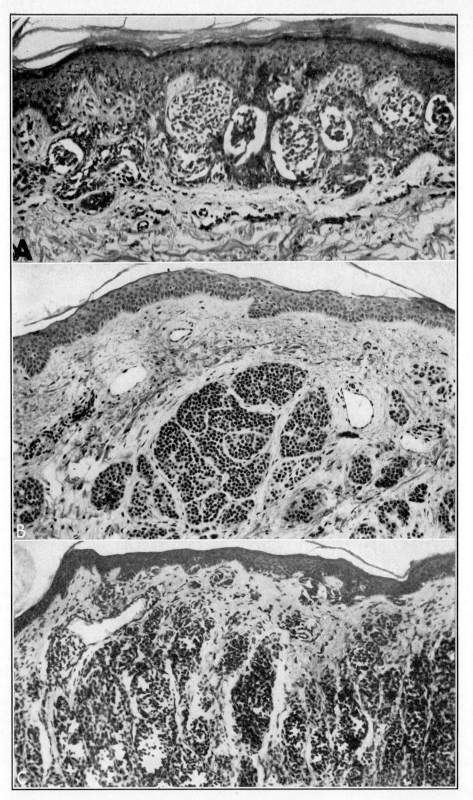

FIG. 723.—Nevi demonstrating *A*, a junctional type with nevus cells not only located at the junction of the epidermis and corium but also permeating the basal portion of the epithelium, *B*, a dermal type with polyhedral nevus cells scattered through the corium only, and *C*, a compound type with both the epidermis and corium affected. × 100.

The chief *complication* of a nevus is a malignant transformation (melanoblastoma). Since almost every person possesses nevi the relative incidence of such a change is low but, for the same reason, the absolute number of such cases is rather high. Although it is difficult to predict when a malignant change may occur, it has been shown that nevi located on the palms and soles are prone to such an alteration. Other significant factors are location at a point of irritation, deepening of the color, and increase in size.

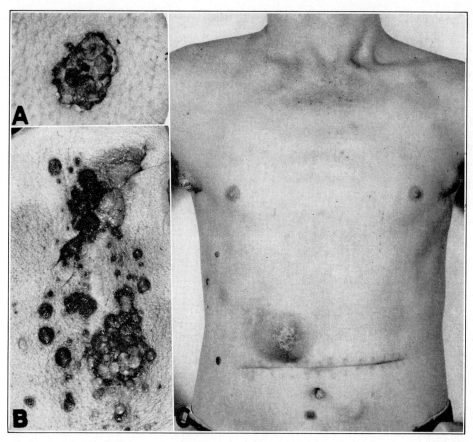

Fig. 724.—Melanoblastoma revealing *A*, a darkly pigmented primary tumor, *B*, many pigmented and apigmented local recurrences after excision, and *C*, scattered pigmented and apigmented cutaneous metastases.

The *diagnosis* of a nevus is made by inspection. *Treatment* consists of wide *surgical* excision of lesions exhibiting the location or characteristics listed above. The *prognosis* in general is good for, as already stated, the incidence of malignant transformation (percentagewise) is low.

Melanoblastoma.—Melanoblastoma (Gr. = black + germ + tumor) is a malignant tumor composed of melanin-producing cells (melanoblasts). It is the malignant counterpart of a nevus. Because the controversy concerning the histogenesis of melanoblasts (nevus cells) is yet unsettled the term melanoblastoma, in your author's opinion, appears to be the best for it is entirely noncommittal. Other designations are *melanoma, malignant melanoma, nevocarcinoma, melanoepithelioma, melanocarcinoma,* and *melano-*

sarcoma. The term *juvenile melanoma* is reserved for a tumor that (1) occurs in patients before the age of puberty, (2) has all the pathologic changes of a malignant tumor, but (3) is benign in that it remains localized (Truax). Melanoblastoma *occurs* with equal frequency in both sexes, affects all races, is usually found after the age of thirty years, is infrequent between puberty and thirty years of age, and is rare before puberty (Hall, Pack, and Morris).

Pathologically melanoblastoma usually starts in a nevus (frequently of the junction type and less often of other varieties) but may also arise in melanoblasts of the retina. Primary cutaneous lesions may involve any portion of the skin but predominate in the lower extremities (especially soles and around the nails), trunk, and head and neck (Pack). The growths vary greatly in appearance. When seen early they differ little from an ordinary nevus with the exception that, according to the patient's story, the lesion has increased in size and/or has become more deeply pigmented. As the tumors age they usually protrude above the surface, are generally sessile, measure not more than 2 to 3 cm. in diameter, may contain an abundant amount of pigment or be completely apigmented, and often ulcerate (Fig. 724). *Histologically* melanoblastoma is extremely variable (Fig. 725). In some instances it is virtually indistinguishable from a nevus. In other instances it appears like a squamous cell carcinoma, being composed of large, polyhedral, sharply defined cells with an abundant amount of cytoplasm and round to irregular, single or multiple, hyperchromatic nuclei. In other instances still it consists of elongated spindle cells with ill-defined borders, variable amounts of cytoplasm, and elongated hyperchromatic nuclei. Between these extremities are all gradations and combinations. Melanin pigment may be abundant or absent. It is always, however, demonstrable by the "dopa" method. Melanoblastoma *spreads* by lymphatic channels to the draining lymph nodes and by the bloodstream to the skin and to distant organs such as the lungs, liver, etc. Cutaneous metastasis is common and may consist of a few seedings in the vicinity of the primary tumor or may consist of thousands of small nodules scattered throughout the entire skin.

The chief *complication* of melanoblastoma is spread to local and distant tissues and organs. The *clinical manifestations* are simply those of a vari-sized and varicolored tumor. The *diagnosis* is made from the history, gross appearance, and histologic examination. *Treatment* consists of wide local excision together with dissection of the regional lymph nodes. The *prognosis* in general is poor. The outlook, however, is not always hopeless for even with metastasis to regional lymph nodes, Pack recorded a five-year cure rate of approximately 14 per cent.

Secondary Tumors.—Secondary tumors of the skin are infrequent. They arise either as local extensions of growths in adjacent tissues such as liposarcoma, fibrosarcoma, rhabdomyosarcoma, etc., or as metastasis from distant sites such as melanoblastoma, and carcinoma of the breast, kidney, lung, gastrointestinal tract, etc. Whether lymphoblastoma of the skin (mycosis fungoides) should be put in the category of secondary tumors or whether it should be considered as a lesion with multiple primary foci is still debatable. Cutaneous lesions arising on the basis of extension from adjacent tissues are usually single and may be quite bulky, while those arising on the basis of metastasis are generally multiple and, as a rule, do not measure more than 1 or 2 cm. in diameter. As would be expected, the histologic appearance varies and is identical with the primary focus.

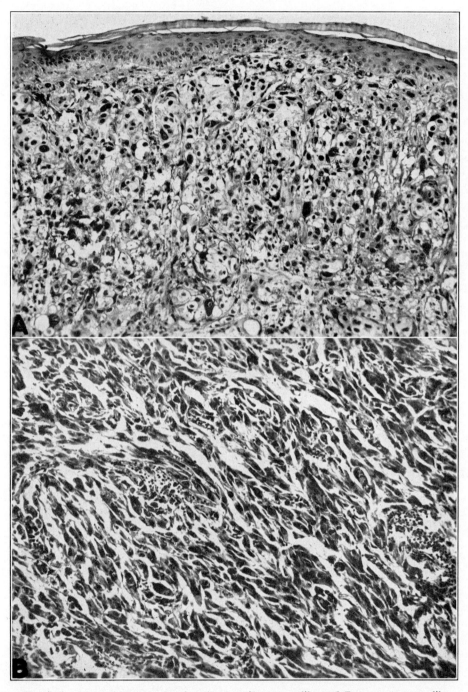

FIG. 725.—Melanoblastoma showing *A*, a carcinomatous-like and *B*, a sarcomatous-like tumor each with a moderate amount of melanin pigment. × 100.

REFERENCES

Pathologic Physiology

MONTAGNA, W.: *The Structure and Function of Skin*, New York, Academic Press, Inc., 1954.
PILLSBURY, D. M., *et al*: *Dermatology*, Philadelphia, W. B. Saunders Co., 1956.
ROTHMAN, S.: *Physiology and Biochemistry of Skin*, Chicago, University of Chicago Press, 1954.
SHELLEY, W. B., and ARTHUR, R. P.: Ann. Rev. Physiol., *20*, 179, 1958 (Physiology).
WIENER, K.: *Skin Manifestations of Internal Disorders*, St. Louis, C. V. Mosby Co., 1947.

General

ALLEN, A. C.: *The Skin*, St. Louis, C. V. Mosby Co., 1954.
BECKER, S. W., and OBERMAYER, M. E.: *Modern Dermatology and Syphilology*, 2nd Ed Philadelphia, J. B. Lippincott Co., 1947.
LEVER, W. F.: *Histopathology of the Skin*, 2nd Ed, Philadelphia, J. B. Lippincott Co., 1954.
McCARTHY, L.: *Histopathology of Skin Diseases*, St. Louis, C. V. Mosby Co., 1931.
ORMSBY, O. S., and MONTGOMERY, H.: *Diseases of the Skin*, 8th Ed., Philadelphia, Lea & Febiger, 1954.

Congenital Anomalies

BARKER, L. P., and SACHS, W.: A. M. A. Arch. Dermat. & Syph., *67*, 443, 1953 (Bullous Ichthyosis).
CALLAWAY, J. L., *et al.*: A. M. A. Arch. Dermat. & Syph., *60*, 528, 1949 (Hirsutism).
COOK, W., and MOORE, A. T.: J. A. M. A., *147*, 650, 1951 (Milroy's Disease).
COOKE, J. V.: J. Pediat., *41*, 1, 1952 (White Skin Spotting).
DONALD, D. C.: Am. J. Surg., *85*, 152, 1953 (Pilonidal Disease).
GRAU, H. R.: J. Internat. Coll. Surg., *15*, 591, 1951 (Pilonidal Sinus).
LATTUADA, H. P., and PARKER, M. S.: Am. J. Surg., *82*, 236, 1951 (Congenital Ichthyosis).
LERNER, A. B., and FITZPATRICK, T. B.: J. A. M. A., *152*, 577, 1953 (Melanin Hyperpigmentation).
METSON, B. F., and WILLIAMS, B. K.: J. Pediat., *40*, 303, 1952 (Ectodermal Dysplasia and Anhidrosis).
MOUNT, L. A.: J. A. M. A., *139*, 1263, 1949 (Dermal Sinuses).
PALUMBO, L. T., *et al.*: A. M. A. Arch. Surg., *63*, 852, 1951 (Pilonidal Cysts and Sinuses).
WINER, L. H.: A. M. A. Arch. Dermat. & Syph., *66*, 204, 1952 (Congenital Nodular Calcifications).
ZEEK, P., and MADDEN, E. M.: A. M. A. Arch. Path., *41*, 166, 1946 (Sclerema Adiposum Neonatorum).

Degenerations and Inflammations

BARNES, B.: J. Clin. Endocrinol., *3*, 243, 1943 (Furunculosis).
BEERMAN, H.: Am. J. M. Sci., *216*, 458, 1948 (Scleroderma).
————: Am. J. M. Sci., *225*, 446, 1953 (Relapsing Nodular Panniculitis).
BEERMAN, H., *et al.*: A. M. A. Arch. Int. Med., *91*, 493 and 633, 1953 (Recent Review Syphilis).
BEIGELMAN, P. M., *et al.*: New England J. Med., *249*, 45, 1953 (Scleroderma).
BESWICK, R. C., *et al.*: Am. J. Dis. Child., *78*, 334, 1949 (Rubella).
BRECKENRIDGE, R. L.: Am. J. Clin. Path., *23*, 348, 1953 (Demodex Folliculorum).
CAWLEY, E. P., *et al.*: South. M. J., *46*, 21, 1953 (Milker's Nodules).
CAWLEY, E. P.: Ann. Int. Med., *30*, 1287, 1949 (Sporotrichosis).
COCH, L. C.: Am. Pract. & Dig. Treat., *2*, 1013, 1951 (Relapsing Nodular Panniculitis).
COMBES, F. C., and CANIZARES, O.: New York State J. Med., *52*, 706, 1952 (Herpes Zoster).
COSTELLO, M. J., and VANDOW, J. E.: New York State J. Med., *48*, 2481, 1948 (Erythema Multiforme).
DALE, W. A., and HAUG, C. A.: J. A. M. A., *149*, 527, 1952 (Carbuncles).
DOXIADIS, S. A.: Medicine, *30*, 283, 1951 (Erythema Nodosum).
DUBOIS, E. L. and MARTEL S.: Ann. Int. Med., *44*. 482, 1956 (Discoid Lupus Erythematosus).
EVANS, J. A., *et al.*: J. A. M. A., *151*, 891, 1953 (Scleroderma).
FELDMAN, G. V.: A. M. A. Arch. Dis. Child., *27*, 126, 1952 (Herpes Zoster).
FRUMESS, G. M.: J. A. M. A., *152*, 1417, 1953 (Emotions in Dermatoses).
GANT, J. Q., *et al.*: Pub. Health Reports, *57*, 612, 1942 (Boils).
GIKNIS, F. L., *et al.*: A. M. A. Arch. Dermat. & Syph., *66*, 717, 1952 (Acne Neonatorum).
GLASER, J.: J. A. M. A., *137*, 527, 1948 (Eczema).

GRAHAM, D. T., and WOLF, S.: J. A. M. A., *143*, 1396, 1950 (Urticaria).
HILL, L. W.: A. M. A. Arch. Dermat. & Syph., *66*, 212, 1952 (Eczema).
KANAVEL, A. B.: *Infections of the Hand*, 7th Ed., Philadelphia, Lea & Febiger, 1939.
KEMPE, C. H., *et al.*: J. Pediat., *37*, 561, 1950 (Roseola Infantum).
LEVER, W. F.: Medicine, *32*, 1, 1953 (Pemphigus).
MCLAUGHLIN, C. W., JR.: Surgery, *11*, 797, 1942 (Carbuncles).
MILLER, O. B., *et al.*: A. M. A. Arch. Dermat. & Syph., *62*, 477, 1950 (Kaposi's Varicelliform Eruption).
MUSTARD, H. S., JR., and HENDRICK, P. W.: J. Pediat., *33*, 281, 1948 (Vaccinia).
NOMLAND, R., and MCKEE, A. P.: A. M. A. Arch. Dermat. & Syph., *65*, 663, 1952 (Milker's Nodules).
PURVIS, W. E. and HELWIG, E. B.: Am. J. Cl. Path., *25*, 1005, 1954 (Reticulohistiocytic Granuloma).
REICHES, A. J.: Ann. Int. Med., *46*, 678, 1957 (Discoid Lupus Erythematosus).
ROBINS, R. H. C.: J. Bone & Joint Surg., *34*B, 567, 1952 (Infections of Hands).
SAWITZ, W. G.: *Medical Parasitology*, New York, The Blakiston Co., 1950.
SCOTT, J. C., and JONES, B. V.: J. Bone & Joint Surg., *34*B, 581, 1952 (Infections of Hand).
SEITZ, P. F. D., *et al.*: J. Invest. Dermat., *20*, 263, 1953 (Neurodermatitis).
SINGER, J. I., and MUNCIE, J. E.: New York State J. Med., *52*, 2147, 1952 (Sporotrichosis).
TUCKER, H. A., *et al.*: Am. J. Syph., *32*, 345, 1948 (Extragenital Chancre).
UNDERWOOD, G. B., and GAUL, L. E.: J. A. M. A., *138*, 570, 1948 (Dermatitis Venenata).
WARKANY, J., and HUBBARD, D. M.: Am. J. Dis. Child., *81*, 335, 1951 (Acrodynia).
WASSERMAN, E., and YULES, J.: Am. Pract. & Dig. Treat., *2*, 772, 1951 (Erythema Nodosum).
WOLMAN, M.: Am. J. Clin. Path., *21*, 1127, 1951 (Variola).

Physical Disturbances

BANGHAM, A. D.: Brit. J. Exp. Path., *32*, 77, 1951 (Wound Healing).
HEIFETZ, C. J., *et al.*: A. M. A. Arch. Surg., *65*, 746, 1952 (Wound Healing)
MARSHALL, W.: Am. J. Surg., *84*, 675, 1952 (Wound Healing).
POSTLETHWAIT, R. W.: Am. Surgeon, *18*, 50, 1952 (Xeroderma Pigmentosum).
SANDBLOM, P.: Ann. Surg., *129*, 305, 1949 (Wound Healing).
WHIPPLE, A. O.: Ann. Surg., *112*, 481, 1940 (Wound Healing).

Tumors

ADAIR, F. E., *et al.*: Am. J. Cancer, *16*, 1104, 1932 (Lipoma).
ALLEN, A. C.: Cancer, *2*, 28, 1949 (Nevi and Melanomas).
ALLEN, A. C., and SPITZ, S.: Cancer, *6*, 1, 1953 (Malignant Melanoma).
ARHELGER, S. W., and KREMEN, A. J.: Surgery, *30*, 977, 1951 (Arsenical Carcinomas).
AYRES, S., JR.: California Med., *73*, 254, 1950 (Precancerous Dermatoses).
BEERMAN, H.: Am. J. M. Sci., *211*, 212 and 480, 1946 (Tumors).
CARNEY, R. G., and RADCLIFFE, C. E.: A. M. A. Arch. Dermat. & Syph., *64*, 483, 1951 (Osteomas).
CHRISTOPHERSON, W. M.: A. M. A. Arch. Surg., *60*, 779, 1950 (Leiomyoma).
COLOVIRAS, G. J., JR., and GARY, R. E.: J. A. M. A., *147*, 756, 1951 (Turban Tumors).
DOCKERTY, M. B., and PRATT, J. H.: Cancer, *5*, 1161, 1952 (Paget's Disease).
DOWNING, J. G.: J. A. M. A., *148*, 245, 1952 (Occupational Cancer).
EPSTEIN, N. N., *et al.*: A.M.A. Arch. Derm., *75*, 210, 1957 (Keratoacanthoma).
FISHER, R. E. W.: Arch. Ind. Hyg. & Occupat. Med., *7*, 12, 1953 (Occupational Skin Cancer).
FOX, R. A.: Arch. Path., *36*, 195, 1943 (Papilloma).
GATES, O., *et al.*: Am. J. Path., *19*, 591, 1943 (Tumors in Sweat Glands).
GODWIN, J. T.: Cancer, *5*, 708, 1952 (Neurilemoma).
GROSS, R. E., *et al.*: Surg., Gynec. & Obst., *92*, 341, 1951 (Sacrococcygeal Teratomas).
GROSS, S.: J. A. M. A., *152*, 813, 1953 (Sebaceous Cysts).
HALL, J. R., *et al.*: Surg., Gynec. & Obst., *95*, 184, 1952 (222 Cases Melanoma).
HELLER, E. L., and SIEBER, W. K.: Surgery, *27*, 539, 1950 (Fibrosarcoma).
HOFFERT, P. W.: Surgery, *31*, 705, 1952 (Dermatofibrosarcoma Protuberans).
HOLT, J. F., and DICKERSON, W. W.: Radiology, *58*, 1, 1952 (Tuberous Sclerosis).
HUBER, G. C., and LEWIS, D.: A. M. A. Arch. Surg., *1*, 85, 1920 (Neuroma).
INGLIS, K.: J. Path. & Bact., *62*, 519, 1950 (Neurofibromatosis).
LAWRENCE, E. A.: Surg., Gynec. & Obst., *95*, 579, 1952 (Carcinoma in Burns).
LEVER, W. F.: A. M. A. Arch. Dermat. & Syph., *56*, 157, 1947 (Carcinoma Sweat Glands).

Lever, W. F., and Griesemer, R. D.: A. M. A. Arch. Dermat. & Syph., *59*, 506, 1949 (Calcifying Epithelioma).

Lewis, G. M.: New York State J. Med., *53*, 1654, 1953 (Nevi and Melanomas).

Lund, H. Z., and Stobbe, G. D.: Am. J. Path., *25*, 1117, 1949 (Nevus).

Masson, P.: Cancer, *4*, 9, 1951 (Nevi).

McNulty, J. R. and Semmers, S. C.: Surg. Gyn. & Obst., *104*, 663, 1957 (Keratoacanthoma).

Mohs, F. E., and Lathrop, T. G.: A. M. A. Arch. Dermat. & Syph., *66*, 427, 1952 (Spread of Cutaneous Carcinoma).

Monroe, W. M.: South. M. J., *50*, 852, 1957 (Keratoacanthoma).

Mopper, C.: J. A. M. A., *152*, 570, 1953 (Fibrosarcoma).

Morehead, R. P.: A. M. A. Arch. Path., *40*, 107, 1945 (Mixed Tumors).

Morris, G. C., Jr., and Horn, R. C., Jr.: Surgery, *29*, 223, 1951 (Melanoma in Negroes).

Murray, M. R., et al.: Am. J. Path., *16*, 41, 1940 (Neurilemoma).

Pack, G. T., et al.: 136, 905, 1952 (1,190 Cases Melanoma).

Peden, J. C., Jr.: Ann. Surg., *128*, 1136, 1948 (Carcinoma Sebaceous Cysts).

Preston, F. W., et al.: A. M. A. Arch. Surg., *64*, 813, 1952 (Neurofibromatosis).

Rigdon, R. H., and Willeford, G.: J. A. M. A., *142*, 1268, 1950 (Xanthoma Tuberosum).

Robinson, D. W.: A. M. A. Arch. Surg., *66*, 434, 1953 (Plantar Warts).

Roseberg, B.: Am. J. Roentgenol., *69*, 196, 1953 (Carcinoma Eyelids).

Russell, L. W.: J. A. M. A., *144*, 19, 1950 (Carcinoma of Nail).

Sachs, W., et al.: A. M. A. Arch. Dermat. & Syph., *59*, 179, 1949 (Keratosis).

Shaffer, L. W., Jr.: Am. Surgeon, *18*, 739, 1952 (Osteochondrosarcoma).

Solomons, B., Jr.: Practitioner, *168*, 465, 1952 (Keloids).

Sponsel, K. H., et al.: J. Bone & Joint Surg., *34A*, 820, 1952 (Myxoma and Myxosarcoma).

Stout, A. P.: Ann. Surg., *119*, 86, 1944 (Liposarcoma).

—————: Ann. Surg., *127*, 278, 1948 (Mesenchymoma).

—————: Cancer, *1*, 30, 1948 (Fibrosarcoma).

Tarlov, I. M.: Am. J. Path., *16*, 33, 1940 (Neurofibroma).

Teloh, H. A., and Wheelock, M. C.: A. M. A. Arch. Path., *48*, 447, 1949 (Basal Cell Carcinoma).

Tilden, I. L.: A. M. A. Arch. Dermat. & Syph., *66*, 728, 1952 (Calcifying Epithelioma).

Truax, R. F., and Page, H. G.: Ann. Surg., *137*, 253, 1953 (Juvenile Melanoma).

Wachtstein, M., and Wolf, E.: A. M. A. Arch. Path., *37*, 331, 1944 (Neurofibromatosis).

Wallace, S. W., and Halpert, B.: A. M. A. Arch. Path., *50*, 199, 1950 (Tumors of Hair).

Warren, S., and Warvi, W. N.: Am. J. Path., *19*, 441, 1943 (Tumors Sebaceous Gland).

Warvi, W. N., and Gates, O.: Am. J. Path., *19*, 765, 1943 (Cysts).

Welton, D. G., et al.: A. M. A. Arch. Dermat. & Syph., *60*, 277, 1949 (Epithelioma).

Chapter

40

Central Nervous System

By Bernard J. Alpers

BRAIN

GENERAL PRINCIPLES

IT IS customary to regard the brain and other parts of the central nervous system almost as separate organs within the body, with diseases not only peculiar to them, but without connection with other body structures. A clear understanding of the brain and its diseases can be realized only through recognition of the fact that these represent an integral part of the bodily structure and are affected by bodily reactions and systemic diseases, just as are other organs in the body. In a broad sense, it is hardly possible to speak of diseases confined to the nervous system. For example, central nervous system syphilis is often accompanied by evidences of syphilis in other organs; meningococcal meningitis, poliomyelitis and encephalitis are associated with systemic disorders, and arteriosclerosis and senile changes involving the brain are associated with similar processes in other organs.

Despite these associations, however, there are characteristics peculiar to the brain and these must be recognized within the setting of the general bodily structure. The chief considerations are: (1) The brain is enclosed in a rigid case with little opportunity for expansion. This becomes important in many conditions causing a crowding of the brain and its structures, as for example, in extradural or subdural hemorrhage, in brain tumor, and in many conditions associated with edema or swelling of the brain. Because of its confinement, pressure by hemorrhage, tumor, or other localized processes may cause reactions in parts of the brain widely separated from the diseased portion, as by pressure against bony structures or the incisura of the tentorium, by excitation of long tracts in the brain, or by other mechanisms. (2) The brain is dependent for the maintenance of its blood supply as no other organ in the body. Though it constitutes only 2 per cent of the body weight it receives 17 per cent of the cardiac output. Anastomoses are present in the pia between areas of supply of adjacent arteries, and compensation for deficiency in blood supply can be established through the Circle of Willis and by extracranial arteries. After penetration into the brain, vessels of supply become end arteries, and after their occlusion the brain tissue depends on collaterals for survival. The brain is also greatly dependent on the condition of the systemic circulation reflecting accurately failure in this circulation by anoxic changes in the various constituents of the brain tissue. A heart which is unable to maintain adequate blood supply to the brain will cause ischemic-anoxic brain reactions. Hypertension will often be associated with brain hemorrhage, and endocarditis, coronary thrombosis, or mural thrombi may give rise to emboli involving one of the cerebral vessels. (3) The brain is surrounded by the cerebrospinal fluid. Normally it serves as a protection but in disease it may be responsible for injury to the nervous tissue. This may occur under many circumstances: by obstruction, with resulting hydrocephalus; by the presence of abnormal elements such as blood in subarachnoid hemorrhage; or by toxins circulating within it. (4) The cells of the brain depend heavily on carbohydrate and oxygen for their activity and have no power of regeneration when destroyed. (5) The brain is affected by systemic diseases of many sorts. Its constituents reveal changes with fever, metallic and other toxins, and with other diseases. (6) Despite the close relationship of systemic and nervous system disorders, there are diseases such as multiple sclerosis in which the nervous system alone seems involved, or if systemic involvement is present it has not been disclosed as yet. In other disorders such as hepatolenticular degeneration and the subacute combined degeneration of pernicious anemia the relationship of systemic and nervous system disease is close. In still others, as in senile dementia, the disease changes affect predominantly the brain, though other evidences of them are present elsewhere in the body.

REACTION OF BRAIN TO DISEASE

The brain reacts in a specific manner to many diseases—general paresis, tuberculous meningitis, multiple sclerosis, to select only a few random examples. Though the diseases which involve the brain evoke a specific type of pathologic reaction, the reaction is not so distinctive in many instances that a precise diagnosis can be made on the basis of histologic studies alone. To arrive at a definitive diagnosis requires a correlation of gross characteristics, microscopic study, and often of clinical features as well. Tuberculous meningitis as seen under the microscope is a lymphocytic meningoencephalitis, the diagnosis of which can be inferred if it is known that the exudate is chiefly over the base of the brain, and established only if tubercle bacilli have been found in the spinal fluid. Microscopically, it may resemble other forms of meningoencephalitis. The same holds true for other forms of meningitis. It is impossible to distinguish meningococcal meningitis from other forms of purulent meningitis without knowledge of the extent and heaviness of the exudate in the gross brain, the results of bacteriological studies, as well as other pertinent clinical facts. Similarly, it is impossible to separate one form of encephalitis from another merely by the microscopic features. Poliomyelitis involving the brainstem is histologically indistinguishable from encephalitis lethargica. Other examples could be mustered to emphasize the fact that the reaction of the brain to specific diseases is specific only in a limited sense and that understanding of the brain responses requires a correlation of systemic reactions of many sorts.

When the brain becomes diseased, responses develop in the nerve cells, the neuroglia, and often in the blood vessels, axis cylinders, and myelin sheaths. The *nerve cells* respond to disease usually in a nonspecific fashion. This is true of their reaction to diseases involving the brain primarily and in instances of reaction to systemic disease. There are several types of reactions of the nerve cells in disease but very few of these are specific and the nature of the disorder can usually not be determined from the appearance of the diseased nerve cells alone. The changes associated with deprivation of oxygen may be associated with many causes and vary with the duration of the anoxia. The nerve cell damage in general paresis, paralysis agitans, poliomyelitis, and many other disorders is nonspecific in nature. Nonspecific reactions occur also in many systemic diseases with fever and are equivalent to the cloudy swelling of other organs. In a few instances, however, specific reactions are encountered as in the fibrillary changes of senile dementia and presenile dementia (Alzheimer's disease), the lipoid changes in amaurotic family idiocy, and the distortions in tuberous sclerosis.

The chief interstitial tissue of the nervous system is represented by the *neuroglia* which responds to disease in various ways, either by proliferation or by reactions of other types. Scar formation is formed chiefly by special forms of neuroglia, the astrocytes. Proliferation of the microglia, microgliosis, is seen in general paresis. The *connective tissue* reactions in the nervous system are much less prominent than in other organs. Connective tissue response is weak in the brain itself since there is very little tissue of this sort within the brain substance, chiefly in and around the blood vessels. Consequently, connective tissue response is not prominent in diseases of the brain except in those wherein the meninges are primarily involved, causing a thickening of the dura or pia-arachnoid or in instances of trauma, in penetrating wounds of the skull.

The *axis cylinders* and *myelin sheaths* may be affected in diseases of the brain, either primarily or secondarily. In some instances, as in multiple sclerosis, the myelin sheaths are diseased primarily and predominantly, while in other conditions, as in destruction of the pyramidal tract, by disease, the myelin sheaths and axis cylinders undergo changes that are secondary to the cause of the pyramidal tract disorder.

There appears to be evidence of a selective passage of substances from the blood to the brain. This is referred to as the *blood-brain barrier*. Acid dyes do not penetrate the brain while basic dyes injected intravenously stain the nervous tissue. The blood-brain barrier serves in the capacity of selective inhibition of transfer of certain ions from the blood into the brain. The barrier is believed to be in the intima of the cerebral blood vessels. Despite this barrier, there are numerous instances of involvement of the brain in systemic disease. Nonspecific changes are found in the nerve cells in fevers of many sorts, in infections, and in intoxications. These serve only to emphasize the fact that most brain diseases must be understood as part of general system disease.

Disorders involving the brain and other parts of the nervous system are characterized also by a tendency to *localization* within specific parts of the brain. Some diseases involve only the meninges and, of these, some are associated with an encephalitis while others are confined to the meninges. Poliomyelitis involves the anterior horn cell system whether in the spinal cord, brain stem, or cerebral cortex. Encephalitis lethargica settles primarily in the brainstem. Methyl alcohol has a special affinity for the optic nerves. Hepatolenticular degeneration affects predominantly the lenticular nucleus. Many other examples could be cited. The reason for this localization or special affinity is not clear. It has been suggested that there may be a specific vulnerability of the nerve cells in certain brain areas and that this may, in turn, be dependent on peculiarities of blood supply, either a scanty blood supply leading readily to anoxia or a rich blood supply affording rich access of toxins and other noxious agents to the vulnerable areas. This does not explain the demyelination of multiple sclerosis or the posterior root and column selectivity in tabes dorsalis, as well as many other conditions. There are undoubtedly other mechanisms of local selectivity in nervous system disease but their nature is not clear at present.

The *nature* of the disease process affecting brain tissue is often known but in many instances remains obscure. In vascular diseases anoxia plays a significant role. Infection accounts for many disorders, reaching the brain by direct penetration, retrograde phlebitis, and by the blood stream. Intoxications of many sorts also cause brain disorders of various types. Tumors account for others. Many disturbances result from brain injuries of varied sorts. Others are due to hereditary and congenital influences, and still others result from causes which are not known.

NERVE CELLS

Nerve cells of the brain react in many different fashions, very few of which are specific in nature. Ganglion cell changes depend on the nature of the noxious agent but it should be emphasized that many different agents may produce a similar type of response.

Toxic Cell Disease.—This is one of the most common types of reaction found in the ganglion cells of the brain. It is equivalent to the cloudy swelling of other organs and is found in intoxications, infections, and systemic diseases with and without fever (Fig. 726A). It is characterized by a swelling of the cytoplasm, cell processes, nucleus, and nucleolus, and by a pulverization of the Nissl substance with a resulting obliteration of the angulation between cell body and the axones and dendrites. The total effect is that of a swollen ganglion cell.

Chronic Cell Disease.—This is also frequently encountered. It is seen in long-standing disease of ganglion cells, resulting from various causes. It is often found in cerebral arteriosclerosis or arteriolosclerosis, due probably to anoxia. It is found also after old infections, as in poliomyelitis, or in degenerative processes such as amyotrophic lateral sclerosis. It is characterized by a diminution in size of the entire cell (Fig. 726B). The cytoplasm is shrunken and darkly stained; the axone is often tortuous and may be visible for a longer distance than normally; the Nissl substance is often destroyed and cannot be seen; the nucleus is small and dark, and the entire cell is pyknotic.

Axonal Chromatolysis.—This type of cell reaction is much more common in spinal cord disease but rarely may be seen in brain disorders. It results from interruption of the axone by injury or disease with resulting retrograde degeneration of the ganglion cell. The cytoplasm becomes swollen; the axone and dendrites are swollen; the cytoplasm becomes filled with refractile globules which stain for fat; the nucleus is eccentric and becomes smaller, and the eventual appearance is that of a swollen, fat-laden cell with an eccentric nucleus. The process is reversible but if it persists the cells do not survive.

Anoxic Cell Disease.—This is a common type of cell reaction occurring as a result of ischemic-anoxic processes. It is difficult to describe since the appearance of the ganglion cells is not uniform due, in part, to the duration of the anoxic process. It is characterized by a shrinkage of the cytoplasm with pulverization and loss of Nissl substance and with shrinkage of the nucleus (Fig. 727A). If the anoxic process is prolonged, only a cell shadow may remain. In less severe injury the cell has the features described and stains less intensely than normal.

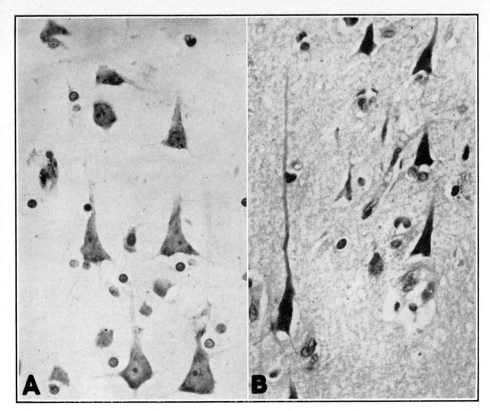

Fig. 726.—*A*, Toxic ganglion cell disease showing the swollen nerve cells and the pulverzied Nissl substance. × 400. *B*, Chronic cell disease showing the elongated apical dendrite and the dark shrunken cytoplasm. × 400.

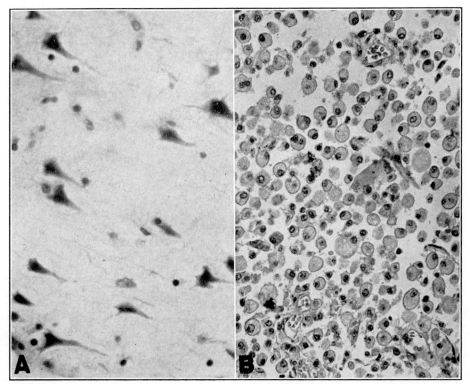

Fig. 727.—*A*, Ischemic cell disease showing the shrunken cytoplasm with pale staining properties and the pulverized Nissl substance. × 400. *B*, Gitter cells from an area of softening showing the typical round cells with eccentric nuclei and cytoplasm filled with fat. × 200.

(1407)

Fatty Degeneration.—Accumulations of fat are sometimes encountered in ganglion cells, either mild or severe. This is seen as a degenerative process in a variety of conditions. Fat droplets are seen in the cytoplasm and (in some types of degenerative change) lipoids may fill the cell body.

NEUROGLIA

Disorders of the neuroglia usually develop in response to diseases of other elements in the brain, either the ganglion cells or their processes or both. In some instances, however, disease may affect the neuroglia alone as in some forms of gliosis.

Astrocytes.—These elements may respond to disease in many ways. Their most common method of response is by proliferation with the production of an increase of cells and fibers referred to as *gliosis*. This is the process of scarring in the nervous system and is akin to the connective tissue response of other organs. This may be local or widespread, depending on the nature of the cause. It is characterized by an increase in the number of astrocytes seen in cell stains as an increase in astrocytic nuclei. This is associated with an increase in the number of neuroglia fibrils and the deposit of a heavy glial carpet which can be seen by special stains. By such stains also, the entire cell body of the astrocyte can be seen and may sometimes be found to be hypertrophied. Local increases in the number of astrocytes are seen in the responses to cell loss in the cerebral cortex where accumulations of glial cells are found replacing the destroyed ganglion cells. Diffuse increases in glia may affect the cortex and the white matter. Such gliosis develops under many circumstances such as, following the cell ravages of poliomyelitis or encephalitis, in plaques of multiple sclerosis, in areas of contusion and laceration due to head injury, in replacement of punctate hemorrhages, along tracks of penetrating wounds, and in a wide variety of conditions.

Astrocytes respond to disease in other fashions as well. These vary under many circumstances. Hypertrophy of astrocytes occurs in the vicinity of tumors, under the ependyma in advancing age, and at times in gliosis. *Plump* astrocytes with voluminous homogeneous cytoplasm and eccentric nucleus are found in the region of arteriosclerotic scars and in areas of degeneration. *Swelling* of astrocytes occurs as a degenerative process in brain edema, softening, abscess, and a variety of other toxic conditions. The changes in the cells are characterized by the occurrence of ameboid forms with large cytoplasm and irregular swellings. The changes are acute and degenerative.

Oligodendroglia.—Oligodendroglia increase in number under some conditions. The most common of these is an increase in the satellite cells when the nerve cells become diseased. This process is known as *neuronophagia*. It occurs in a wide variety of conditions when nerve cells are diseased and may result in the formation of a small knot of glial cells replacing the diseased ganglion cell. Degenerative changes develop in oligodendroglia in a disorder referred to as *acute swelling of oligodendroglia*. During this process the cytoplasm swells; spot-like processes spread from nucleus to the cell membrane, and the processes disappear. The end result is a swollen, hydropic cell which has lost its processes. The disorder is usually irreversible but may be reversible. It is associated with a variety of toxic conditions involving the brain. *Mucoid degeneration* of the oligodendroglia is found rarely. There is difference of opinion regarding its relationship to acute swelling, some regarding the processes as identical.

Microglia.—Microglia respond to disease in several ways. *Hypertrophy* and increase in numbers, producing in a microgliosis, occurs in the cerebral cortex of general paresis, and results in the typical rod cells found in this disease. The cytoplasm is increased in size; the processes become thickened and reduced in number, and the entire cell becomes enlarged. The end result is a bipolar type of cell with large projections at either pole and with small hypertrophied side branches. All stages from the normal cell to the rod cell can be seen in silver stains. In general paresis iron granules can be demonstrated in the cytoplasm of the rod cells. The process is irreversible.

When degeneration of nervous tissue develops, the microglia respond quickly by the formation of *compound granular corpuscles* or *gitter cells* (Fig. 727*B*). These are the chief phagocytic cells of the nervous system. By a relatively simple process the microglia cells become converted into gitter cells by means of loss of the cell processes and increase in the cytoplasm. The final result is a large round cell filled with phagocytic material, fat, and other catabolic products. The process is reversible. Gitter cells are found in great abundance in the region of areas of softening and in all destructive processes involving brain tissue. They make their appearance quickly (within a matter of hours) after injury of any sort. Early in the process, silver stains reveal all stages of transition between the gitter cells and the microglia. As the destruction of the tissues becomes more complete only large collections of gitter cells are seen, replacing the tissue which has undergone destruction. Under some circumstances, the microglia respond by swelling of their processes and cytoplasm to toxic processes of various sorts.

MENINGITIS

Meningitis may affect primarily the dura (pachymeningitis) or the pia-arachnoid (leptomeningitis). The latter is much the more frequent form. Meningitis may affect the entire brain (covering the cerebral hemisphere as well as the base of the brain) or it may be primarily basilar in type, as in tuberculous meningitis and in some forms of syphilitic meningitis. Along with the meningitis there is an associated reaction in the nervous tissue consisting essentially of edema of the brain and toxic changes in the ganglion cells and neuroglia. These changes vary with the severity of the meningitis and are more pronounced in some forms than in others. While most forms of meningitis (meningococcal, pneumococcal, streptococcal, influenzal) do not penetrate the pia-arachnoid barrier, other forms such as tuberculous meningitis are associated with an encephalitis. An associated encephalitis is found also in lymphocytic choriomeningitis and in syphilitic meningitis. Blood vessel changes in the infected meninges are not common but are regularly seen in tuberculous meningitis and are sometimes found in syphilitic meninigtis. The blood vessels over the brain are distended in varying degree in all forms of meningitis. The ependyma of the ventricles may be thickened and the ventricles themselves contain varying amounts of purulent material in some forms of meningitis. The choroid plexus may be infiltrated. In some forms of meningitis (syphilitic) the sheaths of the cranial nerves are infiltrated. Hydrocephalus may develop due to blockage of the cerebrospinal fluid.

Pachymeningitis.—This is seen in two forms—extradural abscess and subdural abscess. *Extradural abscess* results from extension of sinus or mastoid infection. It is characterized by a layer of neutrophils of varying thickness covering the dura, usually in the frontal region from infected sinuses but at times in the temporal region from mastoid infection. Initially the neutrophils are well preserved but later they become necrotic and the exudate becomes adherent to the underlying dura. There are often perivascular infiltration in the brain tissue underlying the meningeal infection and toxic ganglion cell changes in the cortex. *Subdural abscess* is found at times due to infection in the sinuses and mastoids. It consists of a collection of neutrophils lying under the dura, confined to an area that varies in size. It is often associated with infiltration of the pia-arachnoid as well.

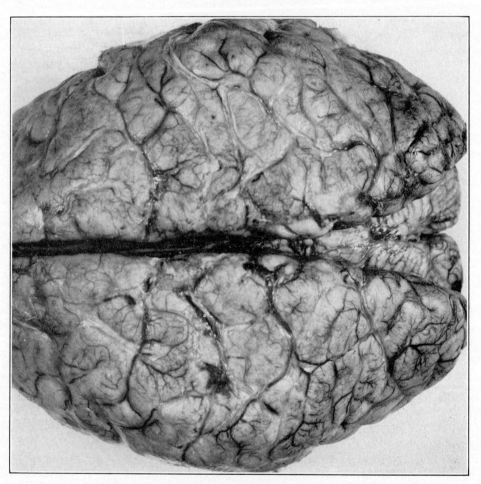

FIG. 728.—Purulent meningitis. Meningococcal meningitis showing the thin meningeal infiltration, especially prominent along the course of the vessels.

Leptomeningitis.—This is the term applied to most forms of meningitis with involvement of the pia-arachnoid membranes. It may be divided into two groups—purulent and lymphocytic.

Purulent Meningitis.—It appears in many forms. It is seen in meningococcal, pneumococcal, influenzal, staphylococcal, streptococcal, and other forms of infection. *Meningococcal meningitis* develops with a bacteremia (Fig. 728). The exudate may be chiefly over the hemispheres, the base of the brain, or generalized. It is usually not heavy and follows the course of the

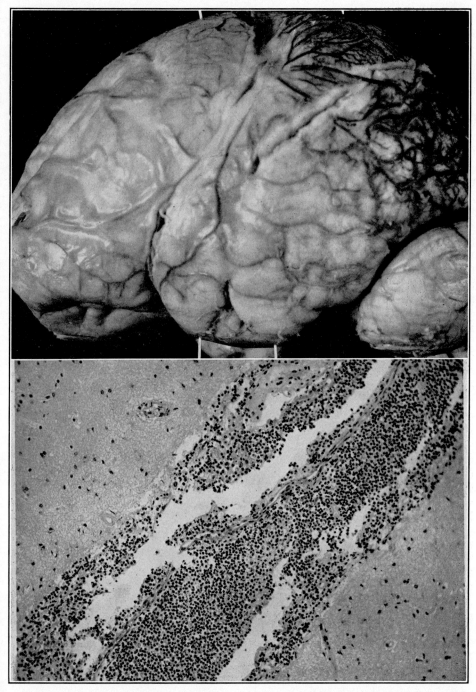

FIG. 729.—Purulent meningitis. Extensive pneumococcal meningitis covering the entire brain (above) and a heavy infiltration of neutrophils confined to the meninges and swelling of vascular endothelium (below). × 100.

vessels where it is seen as a thin, white exudate. When severe, it spreads to cover the brain tissue. The brain is swollen and edematous and the vessels are congested. Microscopic examination reveals a collection of neutrophils in varying states of preservation. There is usually no infiltration in the brain tissue but the ganglion cells show evidence of toxic ganglion cell disease. The exudate is resolved and the meninges are clean following treatment but, in instances of severe infection and heavy exudate, the exudate is replaced by fibrous tissue and is associated with adhesions between the pia-arachnoid and the underlying brain tissue, resulting in cortical or cerebellar atrophy and other sequelæ. *Pneumococcal meningitis* is secondary to sinus or mastoid infection. It usually consists of an exudate (Fig. 729) covering the entire brain but most pronounced over the cerebral hemispheres and obliterating all the brain markings when heavy. The vessels are greatly distended; the meninges are filled with neutrophils; the brain is edematous, and the ganglion cells show toxic changes. With treatment, large mononuclear cells and fibroblasts are found in varying degree among the exudate. *Influenzal meningitis* is usually severe, the entire brain being covered by a heavy exudate appearing as if it were cast in a mold of exudate. The vessels are greatly distended. The meninges are heavily packed with neutrophils. Despite the severity of the exudate, it seems to disappear after treatment. In *streptococcal meningitis* the exudate is not usually severe and follows along the blood vessels. *Staphylococcal meningitis* is associated with a heavy exudate which covers the brain and often involves the ventricles.

Lymphocytic Meningitis.—Many conditions give rise to lymphocytic meningitis but only a few can be described. One of the most important is *tuberculous meningitis*. This involves chiefly the base of the brain spreading out over the convexities in lesser degree (Fig. 730). It is seen as a fibrinous, translucent exudate covering the brain stem (especially the region from the optic chiasm to pons) but extending posteriorly as well and spreading by way of the Sylvian fissures over the cerebral hemispheres. Here it is found as a transparent exudate chiefly along the course of the vessels. On careful examination, minute tubercles may be seen as white dots here and there in the exudate along blood vessels. The exudate is not usually heavy and sometimes great care has to be exercised to see it. Sections of the brain may reveal tuberculomas in varying numbers and of various sizes in the brain substance. On microscopic examination varying numbers of lymphocytes are revealed in the pia-arachnoid membranes (Fig. 730). In addition, there are macrophages, plasma cells, and fibroblasts in varying degree. Tubercles may be found in the meninges. The blood vessels are always involved in tuberculous meningitis. Their walls are hyperplastic and are infiltrated with lymphocytes and plasma cells. The infiltration involves the entire structure of the blood vessel (intima, media, adventitia) but the lumen is almost always open. Rarely, there is occlusion of a blood vessel. In advanced cases, the walls of the blood vessels may become necrotic. The tuberculous exudate involves also the underlying brain tissue for varying depths. Usually the brain just under the meningeal exudate is affected but the parenchyma is not penetrated deeply. Perivascular infiltration with lymphocytes is seen and lymphocytes and plasma cells may be found free in the parenchyma. Tubercles may be found in the brain substance. *Lymphocytic choriomeningitis* is characterized by the occurrence of heavy infiltration with lymphocytes in the meninges, ependyma, and choroid plexus. Perivascular infiltration with lymphocytes is found in varying

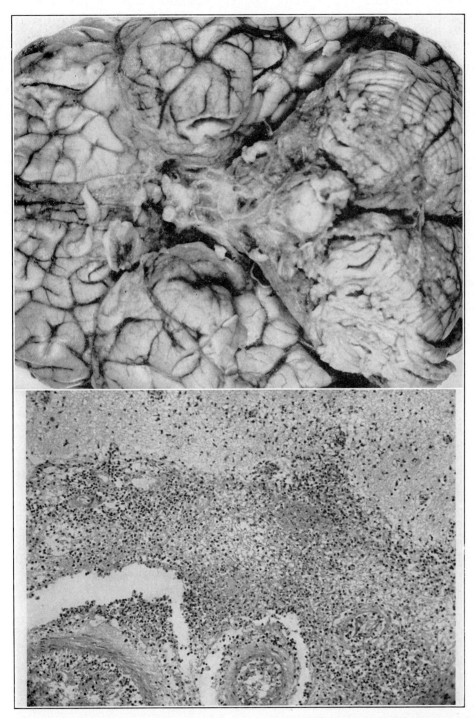

Fig. 730.—Tuberculous meningitis showing the typical fibrinous type of meningitis over the base of the brain (above) and lymphocytic infiltration in the meninges, meningeal vessels, and the underlying brain tissue (below). × 100.

degree in scattered brain areas. *Syphilitic meningitis* in the late stages of the disease is found chiefly over the base of the brain but may affect the convexities. It extends into the sheaths of any of the cranial nerves, particularly the second, third, and eighth. It may cause internal hydrocephalus. The pia-arachnoid is infiltrated with lymphocytes, plasma cells, macrophages, and fibroblasts. The blood vessel walls are infiltrated from adventitia to intima and there is usually intimal proliferation, often with occlusion of the lumen. Small gummas may be found at times. The brain tissue is infiltrated with varying numbers of lymphocytes and plasma cells and perivascular infiltration is found in the brain tissue just under the meningeal infiltration. Eventually the meningeal process becomes adherent to the underlying brain tissue.

Rare Forms of Meningitis.—Among the rare forms of meningitis, that of *Cryptococcus neoformans* (*Torula histolytica*) deserves special mention because of its clinical importance. It is characterized by a meningoencephalitis, with a heavy exudate over the brain, giving it a soapy appearance and feel. The meninges contain lymphocytes, giant cells, and organisms, and sometimes small granulomas. Small granulomas or cysts may also be found in the cortex.

ENCEPHALITIS

Encephalitis is a general term referring merely to inflammation of the brain. The disorder is caused by a wide variety of agents and may affect the gray matter alone (polioencephalitis), the white matter chiefly (leukencephalitis), or both gray and white substances (encephalomyelitis). In epidemic or viral encephalitis the gray matter is predominantly affected but the areas of involvement differ for the various forms of viral encephalitis, some affecting the brain stem almost exclusively and others both brain stem and cerebral hemispheres. The post-infectious forms (measles, varicella, vaccinia, etc.) implicate chiefly the white matter while still others involve gray and white matter (disseminated encephalomyelitis).

Viral Encephalitis.—In this group are included several forms of epidemic encephalitis caused by viruses. They involve chiefly the gray matter of the brain.

1. *Encephalitis Lethargica* (Von Economo's disease).—This involves chiefly the brain stem, especially the mesencephalon and diencephalon but it may extend into other parts of the brain stem and may rarely involve the cerebral hemispheres. Particularly vulnerable are the substantia nigra, the peri-aqueductal and periventricular gray matter, and the oculomotor nuclei. Microscopically, a thin infiltration of lymphocytes is seen in the meninges early in the disease. This disappears quickly and is not seen in later stages of the disease (Fig. 731*A*). In the affected areas the striking feature consists of infiltrations with lymphocytes and plasma cells in the sheaths of the vessels and the perivascular spaces, by the presence of lymphocytes free in the parenchyma, and by the presence of collections of glia cells, chiefly astrocytes. Punctate hemorrhages may be seen in the acute stages. Demyelination is not prominent. Degenerative changes of varying degree are seen in the ganglion cells with loss of Nissl substance, with loss of the pigment in the cells of the substantia nigra, and often with replacement of lost ganglion cells by glial cells that form typical glial rosettes. The destruction of ganglion cells may be mild or severe.

2. *St. Louis Encephalitis.*—The changes in this form of encephalitis differ from those of encephalitis lethargica in the following respects: the

meningeal reaction is more pronounced; the process is more widespread, involving the cerebral cortex as well as the brain stem but being more pronounced in the former, and the spinal cord is more frequently affected. Microscopically, the meninges are infiltrated with lymphocytes. The gray matter in the cortex and brain stem reveals dilatation of the blood vessels and perivascular infiltration with lymphocytes. The affected brain tissue contains diffuse infiltrations of lymphocytes, plasma cells, and neutrophils,

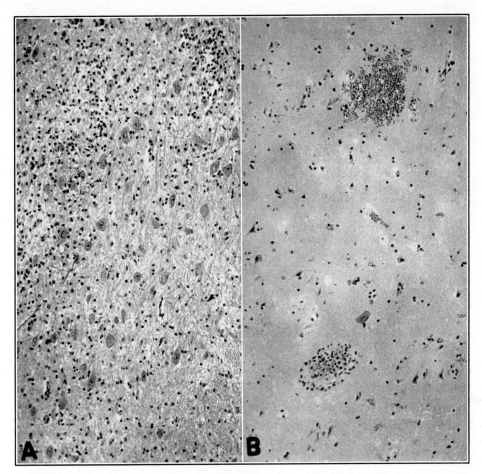

Fig. 731.—*A*, Epidemic encephalitis showing infiltration of lymphocytes in the oculomotor nucleus. × 100. *B*, Embolic encephalitis showing areas of neutrophil accumulations in subacute bacterial endocarditis. × 100.

with lymphocytes predominating. Small hemorrhages may be seen in the acute stages. The ganglion cells show marked evidence of disease with various stages of destruction and neuronophagia.

3. *Japanese B Encephalitis.*—Though caused by a virus similar to that of St. Louis encephalitis, the pathological picture of Japanese B encephalitis differs from that of the St. Louis type. It affects the cerebrum, the brain stem (especially the substantia nigra, red nucleus, and basal ganglia), the cerebellum, and the gray matter of the spinal cord. It involves particularly the Purkinje cells of the cerebellum which are destroyed in varying

degree.   Meningeal infiltration with lymphocytes is seen.   Perivascular infiltration with lymphocytes is prominent and there is degeneration of the ganglion cells in the affected areas.   Areas of softening are sometimes seen together with focal areas of destruction of the white matter and focal proliferation of microglial cells.

4. *Equine   Encephalitis.*—This   is   seen   in   two   forms—Western   and Eastern.   *Western equine encephalitis* resembles St. Louis encephalitis.   The lesions are widespread and involve both gray and white matter.   Meningeal infiltration with lymphocytes is mild as a rule.   Perivascular infiltrations are prominent and both lymphocytes and neutrophils are seen in the brain tissue.   Nerve cell damage is severe and glial proliferation with microglia and astrocytes is prominent.   Areas of softening and even thrombi may be seen in the white matter.   *Eastern equine encephalitis* is a severe form of encephalitis with widespread involvement of the brain, particularly the brain stem and basal ganglia and slight damage to the spinal cord.   The picture resembles that of the Western form but infiltration with neutrophils is prominent in the acute stages, being replaced later by lymphocytes. Endarteritis and thrombus formation in the small blood vessels is seen.

5. *Subacute encephalitis.*—Among the sporadic encephalitides there have evolved in the past few years a group of subacute infections which have a similar clinical and pathological picture.   On the continent these are called subactue sclerosing leukoencephalitis (Van Bogaert) related to the nodular panencephalitis of Pette and Döring.   There is a tendency in Great Britain and America to isolate a group of encephalitis cases under the term subacute inclusion body encephalitis of the Dawson type, since type A intranuclear inclusion bodies can be found in many such cases in the neurones and oligodendroglia.   Careful studies have demonstrated these inclusion bodies in the Van Bogaert type of subacute sclerosing leukoencephalitis.   In like manner a characteristic astroglial response in the white matter can be seen in many, if not all, of the cases of inclusion body encephalitis and in the nodular panencephalitis described by Pette and Döring—panencephalitis, because the white and gray matter are involved often with a sclerosing astroglial response.   Glial nodules are prominent especially in the cortex and brain stem as in Japanese "B" encephalitis.   An etiological factor has not been identified, but the virus origin of these closely related sporadic encephalitides is assumed by most authors.

The pathological picture in these subactue encephalitides is essentially that of a panencephalitis with involvement of cortex and subjacent white matter principally in the anterior half of the brain and decreasing in intensity as one proceeds caudally.   There is a motheaten, variable demyelination with corresponding astrogliosis.   The "U" fibers are not spared.   Damage to axones and myelin varies to the stage of neutral fat.   There are signs of subacute inflammation with lymphocytes and plasma cells perivascularly and in the parenchyma, with meningeal inflammation primarily over the more involved cortex. Type A intranuclear inclusion bodies are frequently observed in cortical neurones and in the oligodendroglia of the cortex and white matter.   In the involved cortex microglia proliferate to prominent red cells and fibrous porliferate to prominent red cells and fibrous glia are diffusely present.

In the acute necrotizing encephalitis of herpes simplex origin frank softening is found usually in the inferior temporal cortex and white matter, hippocampus and fornicate gyrus with signs of inflammation and eosinophilic intranuclear inclusions.

6. The pathological features of *other forms* of encephalitis in the epidemic group — Russian Far East, Venezuelan equine, and Australian X disease — are not sufficiently clear to warrant description.

Post-infectious Encephalitis. — This form of encephalitis follows infections of many types. It is seen chiefly after measles but it may develop after vaccination, variola, German measles, smallpox, yellow fever, varicella, mumps, and antirabic inoculation. It may be chiefly encephalitic (vaccinia), myelitic (antirabies inoculation), or encephalomyelitic (variola).

Measles encephalitis involves chiefly the white matter and may affect both brain and spinal cord but the gray substance may also be affected. It has no special predilections as to site, striking the cerebrum, basal ganglia, and brain stem indiscriminately. The meninges are not infiltrated. Perivascular infiltrations with lymphocytes and glia cells are prominent, especially around the veins of the white matter. Around the areas of infiltration perivascular demyelination is seen in myelin sheath stains. Gliosis may develop in the affected areas. Nerve cell degeneration is not prominent, the changes affecting chiefly the white matter. *Vaccinia encephalitis* is similar in its pathological features to that found in the encephalitis following measles.

Embolic Encephalitis. — Encephalitis may develop as a result of infective foci elsewhere in the body, particularly in disease of the heart valves, in mural thrombi in the auricular appendages or aorta, or after infection in the lungs or elsewhere. This is referred to as embolic or metastatic encephalitis. It may affect the gray or white matter or both and there may be few or many foci in the nervous system (Fig. 731*B*).

The brain in such cases reveals no evidence of meningeal infiltration. Within the brain are seen small areas of focal infiltration, characterized by areas of collections of neutrophils and associated with swelling of the vascular endothelium and perivascular edema. Because of the acuteness of the process there is no glial proliferation. If the foci involve gray matter the surrounding ganglion cells show evidence of toxic ganglion cell disease. The spinal cord is not affected.

Rare Forms. — Encephalitis occurs rarely during infection with trichinosis. The brain in *trichinosis encephalitis* reveals infiltration of meninges and brain substance with plasma cells, lymphocytes, neutrophils, and gitter cells. Trichinæ may be found in the dense foci of cells in areas under the cortex and in the cerebellum where they elicit a granulomatous reaction. Encephalitis is found at times during infection with *Torula*. It is characterized by cyst formation in the cerebrum and cerebellum with a typical soap-suds appearance of the brain tissue. Encephalitis is seen also in connection with *toxoplasmosis*.

BRAIN ABSCESS

Abscess of the brain almost always develops secondary to infection elsewhere in the body. The source of infection is usually in the sinuses and mastoid but metastatic brain abscess may develop following pulmonary infection (usually bronchiectasis and less commonly lung abscess) as well as infection elsewhere. Rarely, it may follow congenital heart disease giving rise to so-called paradoxical brain abscess.

Brain abscess may be solitary or multiple. Metastatic abscess is more often multiple than is abscess secondary to sinus or mastoid infection. The brain is edematous and at times there may be evidence of purulent meningitis. The vessels are congested (Fig. 732*A*).

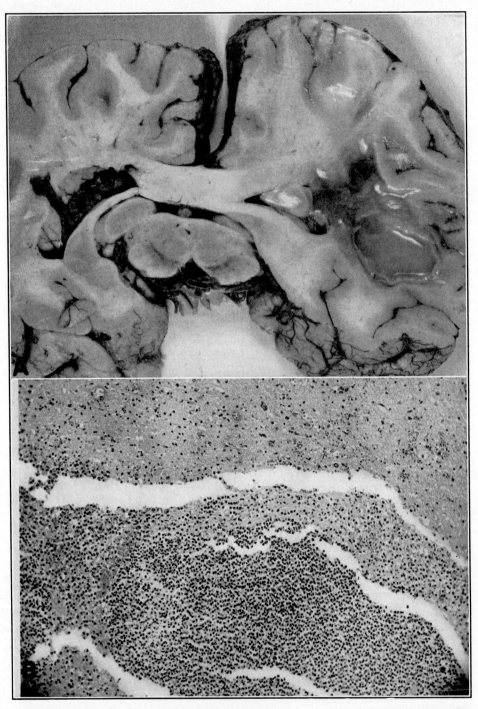

Fig. 732.—*A*, Brain abscess in the right temporal lobe secondary to mastoid infection. The abscess is sharply defined and capsule formation has begun. *B*, Brain abscess. The abscess is clearly seen with the encephalitic reaction in the surrounding brain tissue. Capsule formation is not seen. × 100.

The earliest evidence of an abscess, microscopically, is an encephalitis, characterized by a collection of neutrophils, the surrounding tissue showing evidence of perivascular edema, swelling of the endothelial cells of the blood vessels, and toxic ganglion cell disease. In abscesses associated with sinus or mastoid disease there is usually retrograde thrombophlebitis. As the abscess becomes more chronic, the brain tissue breaks down and a typical abscess forms with a core of neutrophils in varying stages of degeneration surrounded by a capsule which is well developed in some instances and poorly formed in others (Fig. 732B). This is composed of fibrous tissue which is more pronounced the closer the abscess lies to the surface of the brain. In the collagen meshes are neutrophils. The surrounding brain tissue shows evidence of toxic ganglion cell disease and there is usually perivascular infiltration with neutrophils which may also be seen lying free in the surrounding tissue. The overlying meninges often show infiltration with neutrophils in the acute stages of the process. In some instances the capsule of fibrous tissue is well formed while in others it is not. This is not entirely due to chronicity, the variability depending on time, resistance of the host, and character of the organism.

SYPHILIS OF THE NERVOUS SYSTEM

Syphilis may involve the meninges, blood vessels, or parenchyma alone, or in various combinations. Meningeal syphilis has been considered under meningitis.

Vascular Syphilis. —The most important form of vascular syphilis of the brain is the form referred to as *Heubner endarteritis*. This involves any of the large and medium-sized vessels of the brain, especially the vessels of the circle of Willis and their more proximal branches. The brain in such instances often reveals a thickening of the pia-arachnoid with a resultant fibrous appearance. Cortical atrophy, often localized, is present frequently. Because of the nature of the vascular process, areas of softening of varying extent are found in various parts of the brain. This type of syphilis gives rise to clinical pictures of focal cerebral symptoms such as hemiplegia, aphasia, etc.

The typical blood vessel changes in Heubner endarteritis are characterized by infiltration of the blood vessel wall with lymphocytes and plasma cells (Fig. 733). These infiltrate particularly the adventitia and to a much lesser degree the media, with eventual thinning of the media. There occurs also a splitting of the elastica and a proliferation of the intima often with occlusion of the blood vessel lumen. The intimal proliferation is composed chiefly of fibroblasts with varying numbers of lymphocytes and plasma cells present in the fibrous proliferation. Small gummatous infiltrations may at times be seen in the adventitia. In severe instances the entire blood vessel wall may be infiltrated with lymphocytes and plasma cells (panarteritis). In less severe cases, a periarteritis is present with the infiltration chiefly in the adventitia. Hyaline degeneration may be found at times involving the media.

General Paresis. —This is the most important form of brain syphilis. It is essentially a chronic meningoencephalitis resulting in breakdown of brain tissue.

The paretic process *involves* chiefly the cerebral hemispheres with particular involvement of the frontal lobes, the process fading off as it proceeds posteriorly in the brain. The basal ganglia are often involved and, to a much lesser extent, the brain stem and cerebellum. The spinal cord is often diseased.

Macroscopic inspection of the brain reveals a thickened dura and a thickened pia-arachnoid which appears white and fibrous and is often adherent to the brain. There is usually (but not always) atrophy of the cortical gyri with widening of the sulci. The ventricles are slightly or moderately widened due to shrinkage of the white matter (hydrocephalus *ex vacuo*). The ependyma of the fourth ventricle shows an ependymitis, visible as a sandy granular appearance due to proliferation of the ependyma cells and of the subependymal tissue.

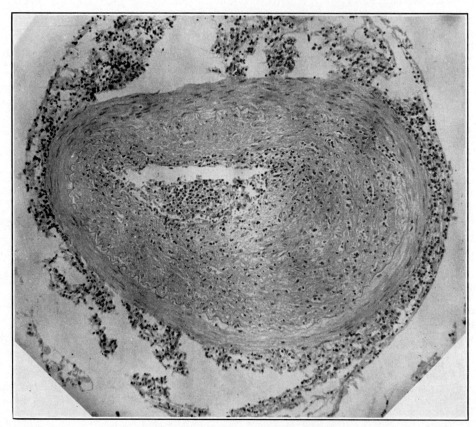

FIG. 733.—Vascular syphilis. Heubner endarteritis involving a pial vessel. × 100.

Microscopic study of the cortex reveals infiltration of the thickened pia-arachnoid with lymphocytes and plasma cells and numerous fibroblasts. The cortical architecture is disarranged. Delineation of the normal lamination of the cortex is difficult and the cells appear scrambled and arranged in disorderly fashion. The ganglion cells reveal degenerative changes of various types. Perivascular infiltration with lymphocytes and plasma cells is seen in active cases. It is slight in some instances and severe in others. The capillaries of the cortex are more than normally visible and there is increased capillary formation. Special silver stains reveal an increase of microglia (microgliosis), rod cell formation, and increase in number and size of the nuclei. Gold stains reveal an increase of astrocytes. Spirochetes may be demonstrated in the cortex but not in all instances. Myelin sheath stains reveal demyelination around the vessels of the white matter which are also the seat of perivascular infiltration. The spinal cord reveals demyelination of the posterior columns and often of the pyramidal tracts and infiltration of the meninges with lymphocytes.

Juvenile paresis is associated with changes similar to those of adult general paresis with the exception that perivascular infiltration is often not as severe and changes in the cerebellum are more extensive. The latter reveal special involvement of the Purkinje cells which show degeneration, hypertrophy, or even complete absence.

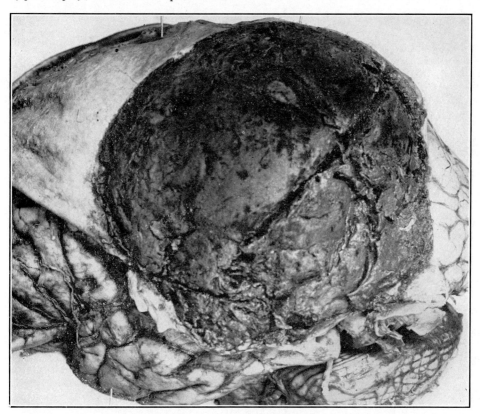

Fig. 734.—Extradural hemorrhage. A large extradural hemorrhage in the left fronto-temporo-parietal area due to rupture of the middle meningeal artery.

Histologic studies following treatment with malaria and arsenicals indicate that there is a decrease in the perivascular reaction and probably rearrangement of the cortical cells.

Gumma of the Brain.—Solitary gumma is rare and is found in any part of the cerebral hemispheres. Rarely it has been found to involve the pituitary gland. Miliary gummas are found in syphilitic meningitis, in association with vascular disease of the brain, and at times in the meninges in general paresis.

VASCULAR DISEASE OF THE BRAIN

Vascular disturbances may manifest themselves as meningeal hemorrhage, cerebral hemorrhage or softening, cerebral aneurysm, and vascular anomalies of various sorts.

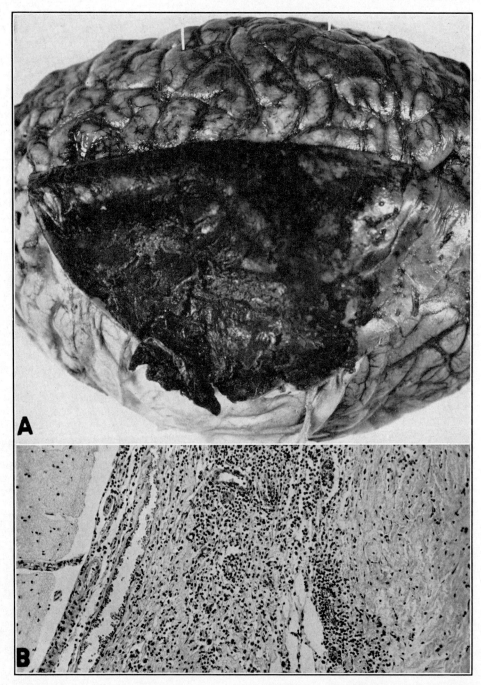

Fig. 735.—*A*, Subdural hemorrhage. A fresh subdural hemorrhage over the right cerebral hemisphere. The dura has been reflected to reveal the hemorrhage. The brain tissue is congested and a thin film of subarachnoid hemorrhage is visible over the right hemisphere. *B*, Subdural hematoma showing the thickened dura and the reaction under the dura in a chronic subdural hematoma. × 100.

Meningeal Hemorrhage.—This may involve the dura or pia-arachnoid. Extradural hemorrhage is almost always arterial due to bleeding from the middle meningeal artery. It is practically always due to trauma. It is seen as a collection of blood lying on the outer surface of the dura, usually in the fronto-parietal region but also in other areas (Fig. 734). The red cells comprising the clot are in various stages of disintegration and may be adherent to the surface of the dura. The underlying brain tissue is flattened and compressed.

Subdural Hematoma.—Subdural hematoma is one of the most important of the sequelæ of head injury. Bleeding occurs under the dura as a result of the trauma and is of venous origin. It develops from tears in blood vessels traversing or adjoining the subdural space or from the venous sinuses. Rupture is likely to occur at the point where the veins join the sinuses, as in the case of the superior cerebral veins and the longitudinal sinus (Fig. 735A).

The hemorrhage is usually unilateral but is bilateral in many instances. It is often located over the fronto-parietal area but it may cover any part of the brain and may be found in the posterior fossa, particularly in children. The size of the hemorrhage at the time of injury depends on the size of the ruptured vessel or vessels. Within a short time the hemorrhage becomes encapsulated and there results a chronic subdural hematoma or cyst. The hematoma or cyst varies in size from a small hemorrhage to one which may cover an entire cerebral hemisphere. The content varies from a fresh reddish-brown clot to clear fluid but is usually a coffee-colored fluid at the time of operation. Those containing clear fluid are usually referred to as *hygromas*. If the process has existed long enough the clot may become completely calcified.

Hemorrhage occurring under the dura becomes completely enclosed eventually in an envelope of fibrous tissue which begins to make its appearance about one week after the hemorrhage occurred (Fig. 735B). At this time fibroblastic proliferation from the under surface of the dura is seen on the dural surface of the clot and beginning envelopment occurs. In two to three weeks further envelopment has occurred, fibroblasts have penetrated the clot, and macrophages containing blood pigment are seen. The membrane on the dural side contains many large blood spaces and capillaries. Relatively few changes are seen in the dura itself. In many instances the blood clot becomes liquefied and the resulting cyst increases in size in the course of time, the cyst membrane acting as a semi-permeable membrane. The clot remains solid in other instances and becomes filled with fibroblasts. In old cases, calcification may occur but this is rare. The underlying brain tissue is slowly compressed by the hematoma or cyst and becomes somewhat flattened. There are few changes to be seen in the brain tissue itself. However, the pressure from the hematoma does not usually produce irreversible changes in the underlying brain.

Subarachnoid Hemorrhage.—Bleeding into the subarachnoid space may develop as a result of many conditions. It may be due to aneurysm, vascular anomalies, trauma, or to systemic disease such as hypertension (Fig. 736A). The hemorrhage is usually confined to the subarachnoid space but may be combined with subdural and even extradural hemorrhage in head injury. There may be only a few pools of blood visible to the naked eye or the entire brain may be covered by a sheet of blood. The bleeding may be chiefly over the base of the brain or over the vertex and it varies greatly in thickness. The blood may appear fresh or old, depending on

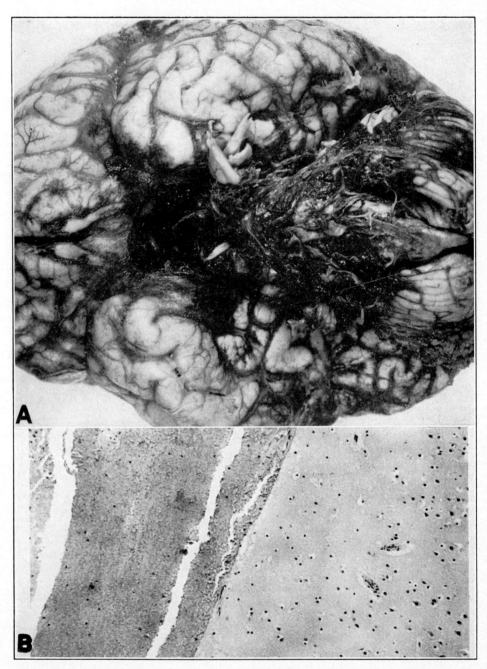

FIG. 736.—*A*, Subarachnoid hemorrhage. A moderately extensive hemorrhage chiefly over the base of the brain. A thin film of hemorrhage may be seen over parts of the left hemisphere. *B*, Subarachnoid hemorrhage showing the extensive bleeding in the subarachnoid space. × 100.

the duration of the symptoms. Microscopically, the subarachnoid space is filled with red cells, usually poorly preserved (Fig. 736B). Among them are scattered neutrophils and macrophages. Fibroblastic response is weak, even in prolonged cases, but there may be fibroblastic proliferation with resulting pia-arachnoid adhesions to the underlying brain.

Cerebral Hemorrhage.—Cerebral hemorrhage occurs usually as a result of hypertension but it may develop from rupture of an aneurysm and other causes. Bleeding may result from rupture of any vessel but occurs most often in the distribution of the middle cerebral artery. It may be small or

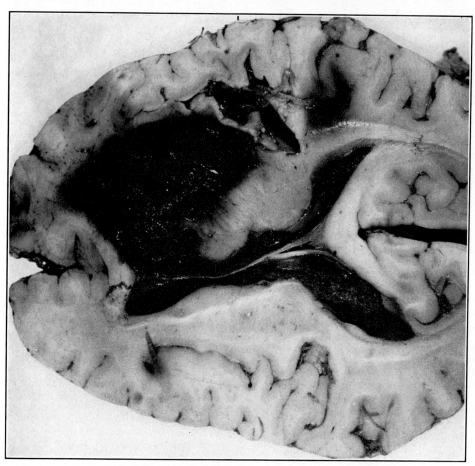

Fig. 737.—Cerebral hemorrhage. The hemorrhage involves the right frontal area and has ruptured into the lateral ventricles.

massive and occupy most of a cerebral hemisphere. It may also affect the pons and other parts of the brain stem. The brain is swollen, soft, and edematous. Arteriosclerosis of varying degree is seen in the larger vessels of the circle of Willis. The tissue overlying the hemorrhage is fluctuant and the hemorrhage may have ruptured through the surface. The subarachnoid space often contains blood and at times the ventricles are filled with blood. The hemorrhage is usually fresh and partially clotted (Fig. 737). The surrounding tissue is torn. Microscopically, there is pronounced edema of the tissue with widening of the perineuronal and perivascular spaces. There

90

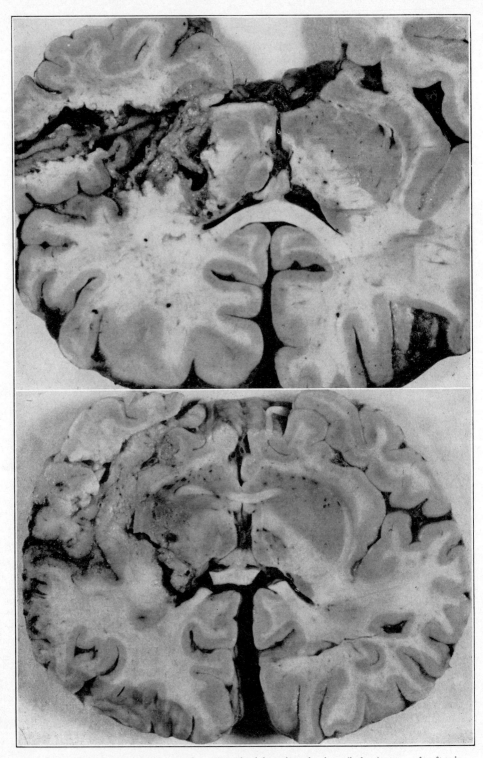

FIG. 738.—Encephalomalacia, showing an early (above) and a late (below) stage of softening in the temporal lobe due to thrombosis of the middle cerebral artery.

are often small hemorrhages in the tissue surrounding the hemorrhage and the ganglion cells show toxic or anoxic changes or evidence of chronic cell disease. Blood is often seen in the subarachnoid space microscopically and the larger blood vessels often show evidence of arteriosclerosis.

Cerebral Softening or Encephalomalacia.—This results from occlusion of a blood vessel by a thrombus or embolus and may be due to many causes. Thrombosis is usually associated with arteriosclerosis and the brain reveals sclerosis of the vessels of the circle of Willis in varying degree. The pia-arachnoid is often fibrotic and the brain generally shows evidence of cortical atrophy and also of edema if the thrombotic softening is fresh. The area of softening may involve any part of the brain but most often follows the distribution of the middle cerebral artery or one of its branches (Fig. 738). It

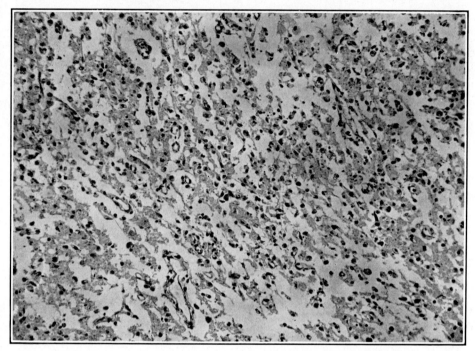

Fig. 739.—Encephalomalacia due to thrombosis of middle cerebral artery showing breakdown of tissue and numerous gitter cells.

may be extensive, involving a large part of a hemisphere if the main stem of the middle cerebral artery is occluded, or it may be seen as a small area of softening in the internal capsule, the basal ganglia, thalamus, cerebellum, or brain stem. In embolism, no evidence of vascular disease is seen. The brain, however, has the same characteristics as in occlusion due to thrombosis, except for the absence of pia-arachnoid fibrosis.

Regardless of the nature of the occlusion, the changes in the brain tissue are the same. Soon after the occlusion, the brain tissue grossly appears disintegrated and soft (white softening or infarct). There is breakdown of all elements of the nervous tissue with accumulation of large numbers of gitter cells filled with lipoid fat (Fig. 739). The nerve cells in the area surrounding the softening may show edematous changes or chronic cell disease and the astrocytes may be swollen. The capillaries in the surrounding brain tissue are increased. Eventually the softened tissue is completely disintegrated and a cyst is formed. In its wall may be seen astrocytes which are often large and hypertrophied and a dense layer of glia fibrils. Blood vessels are more numerous than normal but there is no appreciable increase in the number of fibroblasts. Incomplete softening is frequent in which case the

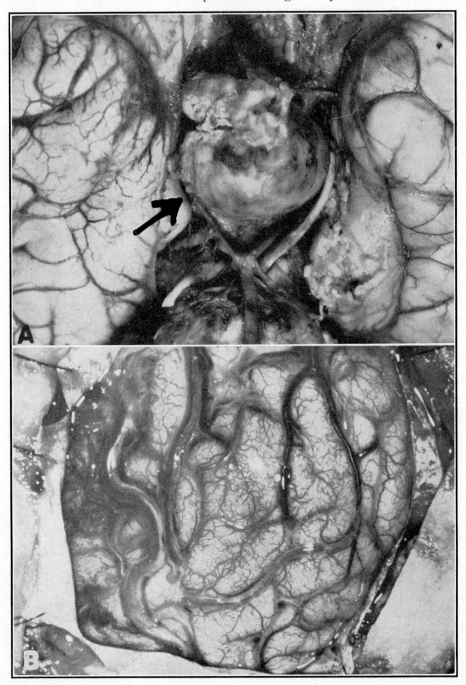

FIG. 740.—*A*, A large cerebral aneurysm of the internal carotid artery compressing the optic nerves and the right oculomotor nerve. *B*, Arteriovenous anomaly revealed at operation in a patient with seizures and subarachnoid hemorrhage.

tissue is not entirely disintegrated. The gangion cells show anoxic changes; the astrocytes are swollen, and gitter cells are present in varying degree depending on the severity of destruction of tissue.

Occlusion of a vein results in red softening or infarct. This is seen in the gross brain as a suffused, reddened area in which small hemorrhages may be visible. Punctate and coalescent hemorrhages are seen microscopically with evidence of changes in nerve cells and glia and with varying numbers of gitter cells. The disturbance is usually confined to the cortex and is more frequent in embolism but is found rarely in thrombosis of a cerebral vein.

Cerebral Ischemia Anoxia.—Under many circumstances of failure of the blood supply, the result falls short of complete breakdown of tissue, as in softening. The changes observed in the brain tissue in such instances, occur as a result of temporary interference with the circulation. Similar changes may be observed at the junctional zones of supply of two major cerebral vessels when one of them has been occluded. The nerve cells reveal evidence of ischemic cell damage. The astrocytes and oligoglia may show indications of swelling. Changes may occur in the myelin and axis cylinders. The brain changes in such cases may be reversible or irreversible, depending on the duration and degree of impairment of the circulation.

Cerebral Arteriolosclerosis.—Disease of the small blood vessels of the brain is associated with a clinical picture simulating senile deterioration. The brain is reduced in size and atrophy of the gyri may be seen, especially in the frontal areas. The pia-arachnoid is thickened and the ventricles are slightly enlarged. Microscopically, the ganglion cells are reduced in number in the cortex and areas of cell loss are visible. The remaining cells show evidence of chronic cell disease. Astrocytes may be increased in number. The arterioles are thickened and may show hyaline changes in their walls.

Cerebral Aneurysm.—Aneurysms are found usually in the circle of Willis at the junction of vessels. They are more common in the anterior portions, especially in relation to the internal carotid artery but may arise from any of the other vessels comprising the circle of Willis (Fig. 740*A*). They are saccular or fusiform. At times, arteriovenous communications are found, as in carotid-cavernous fistulas between the internal carotid artery and the cavernous sinus. They compress the cranial nerves lying in their vicinity, especially the oculomotor or optic nerves, and they may compress the underlying brain tissue. They may rupture and cause subarachnoid hemorrhage. Sometimes, as in the case of middle and anterior cerebral artery aneurysms, they cause cerebral hemorrhage. Microscopically, the aneurysm reveals a constant defect in the media with varying changes in the elastica. Cerebral aneurysms are due to congenital defects in the blood vessel wall, arteriosclerosis, and, rarely, to syphilis or trauma.

Vascular Anomalies.—These are found on the surface of the brain in the form of arteriovenous communications, and venous or arterial angiomas. The blood vessels in the adjacent brain tissue may be abnormal. The anomalies often rupture and cause subarachnoid hemorrhage (Fig. 740*B*).

BRAIN TUMORS

THE GLIOMAS

Gliomas of the brain *constitute* 42.6 per cent of brain tumors (Cushing). They represent the most frequent variety of tumor. They are infiltrating growths involving all parts of the brain but some occur more frequently in some locations than in others. Medulloblastoma occurs almost exclusively in the cerebellum, glioblastoma multiforme chiefly in the cerebral hemispheres, polar spongioblastoma in the brain stem, the rare neuro-epithelioma in the retina, and pinealoma in relation to the pineal gland and the pineal recess. The age of development of the glioma gives some clue as to its nature but this is by no means dependable in all instances. The cerebellar tumor of childhood is chiefly medulloblastoma but it may at times be cystic astrocytoma. The glioblastoma multiforme usually develops in adults but the same may be said of astrocytoma involving the cerebral hemispheres. The mode of onset of symptoms is of little help as a rule in distinguishing one glioma from another clinically. In a few instances, the onset is helpful in this connection but is not characteristic. The cerebellar medulloblastoma develops with symptoms of increased pressure, headache, and vomiting followed by signs of cerebellar involvement. The cerebellar astrocytoma may develop in similar fashion, the course of the disease, however, being slower in this case than in the case of medulloblastoma. The glioblastoma multiforme group is often characterized by an apoplectic onset. Apart from these few instances there are no distinguishing features of the clinical development of gliomas.

Pathologically, gliomas vary in size and appearance. They may occupy only a small part of the brain stem, cerebrum, or cerebellum; they may extend into most of a cerebral hemisphere as in some cases of glioblastoma multiforme, or they may spread across the corpus callosum. They are sometimes indistinguishable from the surrounding brain tissue as in solid astrocytomas or they may be clearly demarcated as in cystic astrocytomas. They are well preserved as in astrocytomas or degenerated and contain hemorrhage in varying quantities as in glioblastoma multiforme. For the most part they remain confined to one area but they may be multiple (glioblastoma multiforme) and they may extend beyond the confines of the main tumor. Medulloblastoma spreads at times through the subarachnoid space of the brain and spinal cord, as well as through the aqueduct and ventricular system. Other gliomas, such as oligodendroglioma and astrocytoma, have been found on rare occasions to spread into the subarachnoid space. Pinealoma has been found to spread into other parts of the brain and papilloma of the choroid plexus may seed into other parts. Gliomas are usually not adherent to the dura but such adherence may occur in the case of the glioblastoma multiforme. Calcium is seen in gliomas at times. Its appearance has no specific significance since it may be found in oligodendroglioma, astrocytoma, and glioblastoma.

The *clinical manifestations* produced by gliomas vary so greatly that no brief summary is possible. They depend on the location of the tumor and on the nature of the tumor itself. Since some parts of the brain respond more quickly by symptoms than do others, the location of the tumor is important. Gliomas involving the motor cortex will give rise to symptoms earlier as a rule than those of the frontal region or right temporal lobe. The development of increased intracranial pressure varies greatly but will occur earlier in gliomas which occlude the ventricular system. Gliomas, as well as other tumors of the brain, may at times be associated with an increase of the spinal fluid protein. This occurs most frequently in the case of gliomas encroaching on the subarachnoid space or the ventricular ependyma.

Medulloblastoma.—This is a tumor of childhood, *affecting* predominantly children of five to ten years but appearing at times in older subjects, even rarely in adults. It is almost exclusively a cerebellar tumor, involving the midline of the cerebellum, infiltrating the vermis, but extending at times into one or both cerebellar hemispheres (Fig. 741). It encroaches on and eventually occludes the fourth ventricle, producing internal hydrocephalus. It may extend into the aqueduct and third ventricle, and in some instances it spreads through the subarachnoid space of the spinal cord and cerebrum. The dissemination of the tumor may follow manipulation at operation or it may spread without handling.

Medulloblastoma infiltrates the cerebellar tissue. It may at times give a false impression of encapsulation. It is soft, with a gray or grayish-red appearance in the gross specimen. Cut surfaces are solid, have little or no tendency to break down, and contain no cysts or hemorrhage.

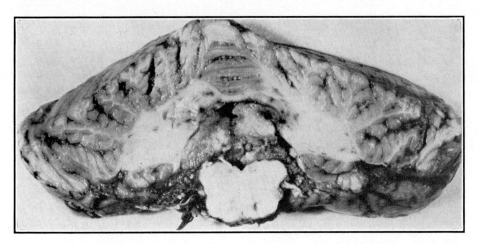

Fig. 741.—Medulloblastoma. The tumor involves the vermis and is seen projecting into the fourth ventricle which is almost completely occluded.

Microscopically, the neoplasm is rich in cells with the tumor cells arranged in no specific fashion though they tend at times to run in streams. Among the cells are thin-walled blood vessels and a fine reticulum. Collagen is not pronounced. The nuclei are oval, round, or carrot-shaped with a well-defined membrane, scattered fine chromatin material, and a nuclear dot. The cytoplasm is not seen in ordinary stains or even with special stains. Mitoses are seen in all cases and are numerous or relatively few in number. Irradiation of the tumor results in death of some of the tumor cells, with pyknosis and karyolysis of the nuclei.

Astrocytoma.—This is a slowly growing, benign glioma found in children and adults. It is almost always located in the cerebellum in children and is usually cystic in nature. In adults it is found both in the cerebrum and cerebellum and may even invade the brain stem. It is more commonly solid in adults but may occasionally be cystic. Astrocytomas are infiltrating, their rate of growth and extent varying widely. They may be confined to part of a single lobe of the cerebrum or involve almost a complete hemisphere with extension into the deep cerebral structures (Fig. 742).

Solid astrocytomas are usually firm and even hard, infiltrating imperceptibly into the surrounding brain tissue but they may at times be quite soft. They often have a white glistening appearance or may appear grayish, resembling the gray matter of the brain. The surface is avascular but

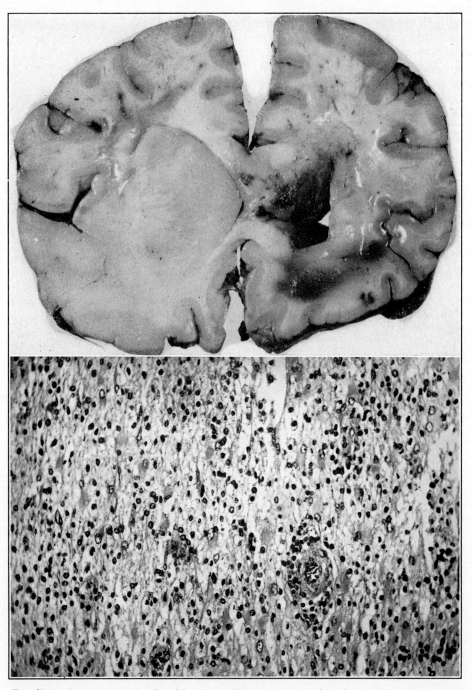

FIG. 742.—Astrocytoma showing (above) a solid tumor of the right frontal lobe with enlargement of the affected area, occlusion of the anterior horn of the ventricle, and diffuse infiltration by the neoplasm and (below) the characteristic nuclei and the fibrillar network of the tumor. Giant astrocytes are seen here and there. × 200.

degenerative areas and hemorrhages are not seen as a rule. Small cystic areas may be noted on cut surface.

Cystic astrocytomas consist of a central cystic space and contain within their walls a solid portion of neoplastic tissue. The amount of solid tumor varies from a small nubbin to a large tumor, the cyst varying in size with the amount of solid tumor. The solid portion of the tumor extends into the cyst cavity. Cystic astrocytomas are well delineated, have a distinct glistening cyst wall, and contain a straw-colored, yellowish fluid high in albumin and tending to clot on exposure to air. The cyst fluid is a transudate from the blood stream and reforms if the cyst is emptied.

Histologically, astrocytomas are moderately rich in cells but the cell population varies greatly (Fig. 742). The cells are round or oval with a fine deposit of chromatin and with nucleoli which are not very prominent. The cells are quite uniform in appearance. In some types of astrocytoma the nuclei tend to be somewhat more elongated. Large plump astrocytes are seen in some forms. Special stains (silver and gold stains) reveal typical astrocytic cytoplasm. Mitoses are rare. Among the cells is a carpet of neuroglia fibrils enmeshing the processes of the cells. The carpet of fibrils varies in density and is arranged in diffuse fashion, at times in parallel groups (piloid type). Blood vessels are not numerous but are sufficient to maintain tissue structure. Collagen is not prominent in the tumor except around blood vessels.

Glioblastoma Multiforme.—Tumors of this type *occur* chiefly in adults and are predominantly tumors of the cerebral hemispheres. They may occur in the brain stem and are rare in the cerebellum. They vary in size from tumors occupying part of a lobe and rarely appearing well defined to extensively infiltrating masses involving an entire hemisphere (Fig. 743). They frequently extend into the corpus callosum and they are sometimes multiple. They appear degenerated and necrotic to a large degree when sectioned; they contain hemorrhages of varying size and number, and they often have cystic areas of degeneration. The tumor is sometimes adherent to the overlying dura and the tumor surface is typically reddish and angry looking. Its gross appearance is unlike that of any other glioma.

Histologically, the tumor displays such a wide variety of forms that a specific cell type is hard to define (Fig. 743). Of the many types of cells seen, the most common is a small cell with oval or round nucleus and scanty cytoplasm. Spindle-like cells are also common and multinucleated cells are frequently seen. The latter are much more frequent in some types of glioblastomas than in others. The cell arrangement varies and follows no specific pattern. Pseudo-rosettes are common. Mitoses are frequently seen but are much more common in some tumors than in others. Blood vessels are numerous, are often arranged in glomerular-like patterns, and disclose adventitial proliferation. Thromboses are frequent. Collagen is seen in increased amounts, especially around vessels. Necrosis and hemorrhage are frequently present.

Oligodendroglioma.—This is an infiltrating tumor involving chiefly the cerebral hemispheres with extension at times into the lateral ventricles. It usually occurs in adults. The clinical course tends to be slow but is not as slow as it is in astrocytoma. The tumor gives at times a false impression of sharp demarcation (Fig. 744). It is grayish or grayish red on cut surface and is well preserved. Necroses, cysts, and hemorrhages are not usually seen in the gross specimen.

Histologically, the tumor is rich in cells, the cells being arranged roughly

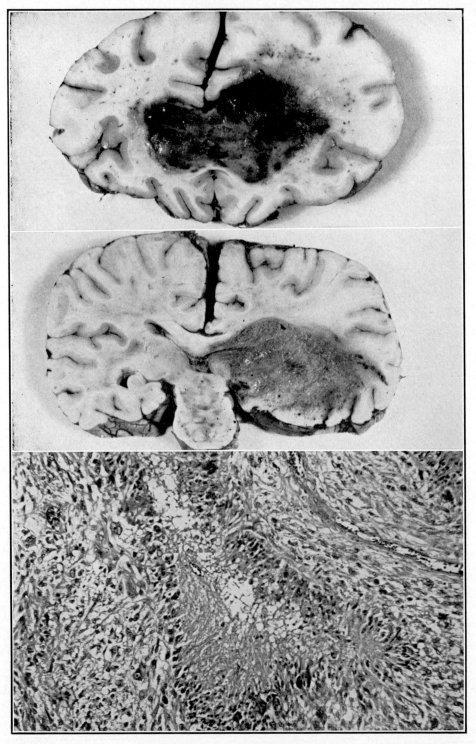

FIG. 743.—Glioblastoma multiforme involving (upper two) the fronto-temporal areas showing extensive infiltration, tendency to necrosis and hemorrhage, and spread across the midline through the corpus callosum and (lowest one) showing the pseudo-palisading, necrosis, and variability of cell types. × 100.

in rows resembling the normal arrangement of oligodendroglia cells in the normal white matter (Fig. 744). The nucleus is round and contains a coarse chromatin network. The cytoplasm is not visible by routine stains and is very difficult to disclose by silver stains. Mitoses are sometimes seen though the glioma tends to be benign. Blood vessels are moderate in number. Collagen is seen in the vicinity of the vessels. The tumor is thought to arise from the forerunners of the oligodendroglia cell in the adult.

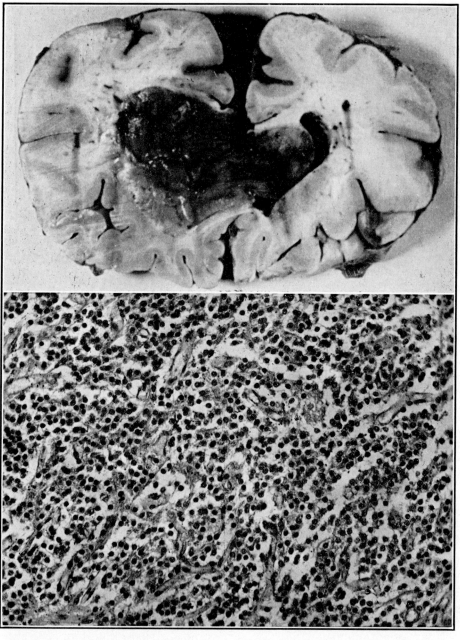

Fig. 744.—Oligodendroglioma involving (above) the right frontal lobe and extending into the ventricle and showing (below) the tendency to linear arrangement and the relative uniformity of the cell type. × 100.

Ependymoma.—Ependymomas arise in relationship to the ventricular system in any part of its course. They infiltrate and often attain large sizes. Their relationship to the ventricular system is often not apparent in the gross state and they may appear as infiltrating cerebral tumors. In other instances, they project into the ventricle, especially the third and fourth ventricle, and their relationship to the normal ependyma is more clearly apparent.

Histologically, they vary greatly in appearance. The nuclei are round, roomy, and contain a well-pronounced chromatin network. The cytoplasm is abundant and readily seen with conventional stains. Mitoses are common.

Pinealoma.—This tumor is found in the pineal recess and is associated usually with the clinical syndrome of macrogenitosomia praecox. The bulk of the tumor is usually encapsulated but it may infiltrate or compress the collicular plate region. It may also cause pressure on the mesencephalon and may as well produce increased intracranial pressure. It often attains a large size before it is recognized clinically. It has been found to spread from the pineal region on rare occasions, extending along the brain stem and burrowing under the ventricular ependyma. It is composed of two types of cells: (1) large epithelioid cells with large vesicular nuclei and (2) small round cells resembling lymphocytes. The latter are seen usually in groups. Blood vessels are moderate in number. Collagen is not prominent.

Spongioblastoma Polare.—Tumors of this variety differ from those of the glioblastoma multiforme group. They are much more benign than the latter, grow slowly, and are located chiefly in the brain stem, involving the pons, medulla, optic nerves, chiasms, and tracts. They are, however, not confined to the brain stem. They are found most often in the pons of children, adolescents, and young adults and are frequently referred to as pontile gliomas.

Histologically, the tumors are composed mainly of bipolar and unipolar cells resembling spongioblasts. The nuclei are oval with abundant chromatin. The tumors are benign in character and mitoses are rare. The cell cytoplasm is characterized by long processes extending into the tumor tissue, the processes lying in parallel arrangement.

Astroblastoma.—This type of glioma occurs chiefly in the cerebral hemispheres of adults. It is infiltrating and usually poorly defined and it grows relatively rapidly. It is a rare form of glioma. *Histologically*, the tumor is composed of cells with round nuclei containing coarse chromatin granules and roomy cytoplasm, the cells being arranged often around blood vessels. Special stains may reveal a long cytoplasmic extension often terminating as a perivascular foot around the blood vessel. The arrangement of the cells around vessels gives the tumor a characteristic appearance.

Ganglioneuroma.—This is a rare tumor which is found in the brain at times but occurs more frequently in the peripheral nervous system. It is infiltrating and slowly growing. *Histologically*, it is characterized by the presence of ganglion cells in varying stages of maturity and in varying numbers. The ganglion cells have typical nuclei and roomy cytoplasm. The normal cell processes may or may not be seen and Nissl substance may be present or absent. The rest of the tumor is composed of glial cells, usually astrocytes and axis-cylinders in varying numbers. Collagen is seen around the blood vessels but reticulum is absent. Areas of degeneration are frequent.

Neuro-epithelioma.—These are rare tumors, usually found in the retina but also in the brain and spinal cord. They are infiltrating and tend in their histologic appearance to resemble the primitive neural tube. The tumor cells are arranged in true rosettes surrounding a cavity, the cells being composed of an oval, heavily chromatinized nucleus and elongated cytoplasm resembling primitive spongioblasts. Cilia may be seen on some cells.

Papilloma of Choroid Plexus.—These tumors usually occur in children. They are found most often in the fourth ventricle and less frequently in the lateral and third ventricles and infiltrating the brain tissue. Grossly, they have a granular, cauliflower-like appearance and they usually attain large sizes before they are recognized clinically. Their cut surface is granular and they often contain cysts. They may seed into other parts of the brain. Histologically, they have the typical appearance of a papilloma. Mitoses are numerous.

MENINGIOMAS

(Meningeal Fibroblastoma, Arachnoidal Fibroblastoma, Endothelioma)

Meningiomas, the benign tumors of the nervous system, are found in 13.4 per cent of all brain tumors (Cushing). The term meningioma is nonspecific and indicates merely a tumor of meningeal origin. It represents a compromise because of lack of agreement concerning the precise *origin* of the tumors. The majority of investigators agree that meningiomas are derived from the fibroblastic cells of the arachnoid. They resemble the structure of the arachnoid villi and are found most abundantly over the cerebral hemispheres in areas where arachnoid villi are more frequent. Hence, they are particularly numerous near the superior longitudinal sinus. Their fibroblastic origin is derided by some investigators who regard them as of endothelial origin.

As already stated, they are *found* in relation to various parts of the brain and are most numerous over the cerebral hemispheres (Fig. 745). Here they may appear over any portion of the convexities from frontal to occipital regions. They are most frequently seen, however, in the parasagittal central region. In addition to their location over the cerebral hemispheres they are found in the following sites: (1) olfactory groove in relation to the base of the frontal lobe, (2) in the suprasellar area above the sella turcica, arising from the tuberculum sellæ, (3) in the parasellar region, lying on the lesser wing of the sphenoid bone adjacent to the sella turcica, and more laterally on the greater wing of the sphenoid bone, lying under the temporal lobe, and (4) in the posterior fossa where they are rare.

Meningiomas produce *symptoms* by compression of the underlying brain tissue, causing changes in the brain which are usually reversible but which may become irreversible if the compression has continued for a sufficiently long period of time. They may cause symptoms also by interference with blood supply. They almost never invade the brain tissue but rare instances have been recorded. They cause changes, usually hyperostosis, in the overlying bone in about 25 per cent of cases. Erosion of the bone may occur or there may be only great dilatation of the vascular channels in the bone seen roentgenographically. Hyperostosis is more frequently seen in the bones over the cerebral hemispheres and more rarely in the bones of the base of the skull. In rare instances, meningiomas in relation to the longitudinal sinus may invade the sinus and occlude it. The meningiomas at the base of the brain cause compression of cranial nerves—those of the olfactory groove compressing the optic nerves, those on the lesser wing of the sphenoid bone compressing not only the optic nerves but also the optic tracts and oculomotor nerve.

The *tumors* vary in size and appearance. They are usually global or bulbous but they may at times be flat—*meningiomes en plaques*. The global tumors have a well-defined capsule, are readily separated from the

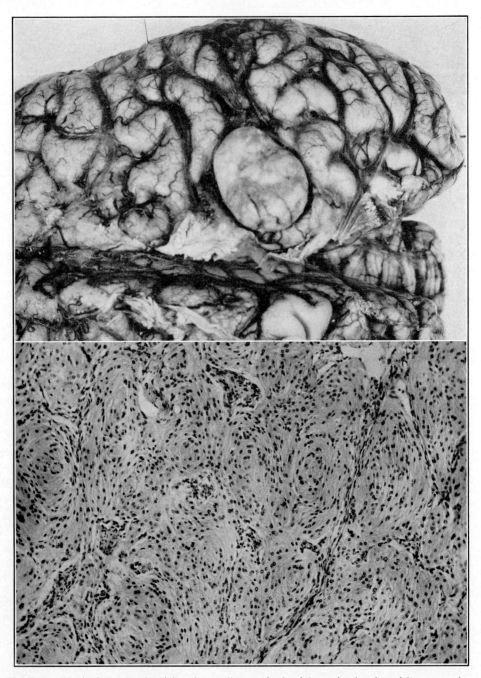

Fig. 745.—Meningioma showing (above) a small tumor in the right parietal region with compression of the underlying brain and (below) the typical whorl formation. × 100.

brain tissue, but are often intimately associated with the latter by a rich vascular supply which often makes their removal difficult and hazardous. The tumors are attached to the overlying dura, sometimes over a circular area, and they may be attached to a sinus wall. The surface appearance varies from smooth to lobulated. The cut surface is usually avascular and fibrous in appearance. They are well preserved as a rule with no evidence of degeneration. Hemorrhage within the tumor is not seen.

Histologically, meningiomas are characterized by sheets of cells among which are numerous blood vessels and abundant collagen, the latter most abundant around the vessels and penetrating into the tumor tissue (Fig. 745). The cells possess elongated nuclei with a moderate amount of chromatin. The cytoplasm merges with that of surrounding cells whose formations are frequently seen. Mitoses are not seen. Psammoma bodies are seen in some of the tumors. Calcium is sometimes present.

Several *types* of meningioma have been described histologically, among them the following: psammomatous, mesenchymal, angiomatous, osteoblastic, sarcomatous, lipomatous, and chondroblastic.

The dura overlying the meningioma is infiltrated with tumor cells in its lower layers and is adherent to the tumor.

TUMORS OF THE PITUITARY REGION

Tumors may involve the pituitary gland or the region in the vicinity of the pituitary.

Pituitary Tumors.—Tumors of the pituitary gland lie within the sella turcica. The vast majority consist of adenomas which constitute 13.2 to 17.8 per cent of all brain tumors. Rarely, a craniopharyngioma and very rarely a Rathke cleft cyst may be found within the sella turcica.

The *adenomas*, for all practical purposes, are the only primary pituitary tumors of significance. They are derived from elements of the pituitary gland and are of three types: (1) chomophobe, (2) chromophile, and (3) mixed. The chromophobe adenoma is derived from chromophobe cells of the anterior lobe of the pituitary gland. The chromophile adenoma may be (1) eosinophilic or (2) basophilic. Of these, the eosinophilic adenoma is derived from the eosinophilic cells of the anterior lobe and the basophilic from the basophilic cells. The mixed adenomas contain cells of the chromophobe and chromophile (eosinophilic) types.

Pituitary adenomas *grow* within the sella turcica causing enlargement of the pituitary fossa and encroachment on the surrounding tissues. This is true only of the chromophobe and eosinophilic adenomas. The *basopihilic adenomas* are microscopic in size and produce no symptoms of compresson. The *other adenomas* vary in size, depending upon the stage of their recognition but all are of sufficient dimensions to produce symptoms because of their presence. They expand within the sella turcica causing compression of the pituitary gland. This reaches a point eventually in which no trace of the pituitary gland can be found (Fig. 746). In pituitary adenomas which have existed for some time it becomes impossible to identify the pituitary gland at autopsy. Growth of the tumor may be chiefly upward against the diaphragma sellæ, downward against the floor of the sella turcica and the sphenoid sinus, or simultaneously in both directions. Upward growth of the tumor against the diaphragma sellæ brings it into contact eventually with the optic chiasm and optic nerves. The direction of compression varies. It may be directed evenly along the diaphragm or it may be more pronounced against anterior, posterior, or lateral portions. The tumor may at times escape through the opening of the infundibulum in the diaphragma sellæ or it may break through the lateral wall of the sella turcica. The manner in which the tumor compresses the optic nerves and chiasm depends on (1) the manner and direction of growth of the adenoma, (2) the position of the optic nerves and chiasm in relation to the pituitary gland, *i.e.*, whether it is prefixed or postfixed, and (3) the involvement of the blood vessels of the circle of Willis in the region of the sella turcica.

As already stated, the adenoma may *spread* out of the sella turcica into the base of the skull causing compression of other structures. They may, under these circumstances, attain large sizes and almost cover the brain stem. They may also compress the adjacent regions of the temporal lobes or extend into the cavernous sinus of one or both sides. Their downward growth causes depression of the floor of the sella turcica which encroaches on the sphenoid sinus. This may be greatly narrowed in full or part. In rare instances, the tumor may erode bone and may extend into the nasopharynx.

Histologically, the adenomas are characterized by sheets of cells among which are numerous thin-walled sinuses (Fig. 746). The nuclei are round and contain coarse chromatin granules. The cytoplasm is roomy and, by ordinary stains, reveals no specific granules. Special stains reveal no granules in the chromophobe adenoma, large eosinophilic granules in the eosinophilic type, and basophilic granules in the microscopic basophilic variety. Mitoses are not seen as a rule, except in the rare malignant types of adenoma.

The *clinical features* of the adenomas are characterized by optic atrophy, bitemporal hemianopsia, enlargement of the sella turcica, and endocrine disturbances. In addition, the chromophobe adenomas are associated with a hypopituitary syndrome while the eosinophilic adenomas are associated with acromegaly.

Suprasellar Tumors.—Tumors may lie above the sella turcica. They are of three main types: (1) adenomas, (2) meningiomas, and (3) craniopharyngiomas. The tumors in this area compress the straddling optic nerves and chiasm. The pituitary gland is not compressed. The *adenomas* are similar in structure to those within the sella turcica and are almost entirely of the chromophobe type. They are derived from cell rests above the sella turcica. The *meningiomas* are derived from cell rests above the sella turcica and originate probably from arachnoidal villi in the region of the cavernous sinus. Lying above the sella turcica and involving the third ventricle is sometimes found a *colloid cyst*. More precisely, it is situated at the anterior end of the third ventricle and is attached to the roof of the latter. It is round, smooth, and about 1 cm. in diameter. Its wall is composed of a layer of epithelial cells surrounded by a capsule of connective tissue. The cyst is filled with homogeneous colloid material. Such cysts develop from the paraphysis and are often referred to as *paraphyseal cysts*.

Craniopharyngiomas (hypophyseal stalk tumors, Rathke pouch tumors, adamantinomas, ameloblastomas) are found in the region above the sella turcica and, rarely, primarily within the sella turcica. They are derived from cell rests of the hypophyseal stalk lying on the infundibulum. They may extend into the third ventricle and practically occlude it. The tumors vary in size and appearance. They usually attain a large size before they are recognized (Fig. 747). They not only compress the optic nerves and chiasm, but they may grow downward to compress the pituitary gland and destroy

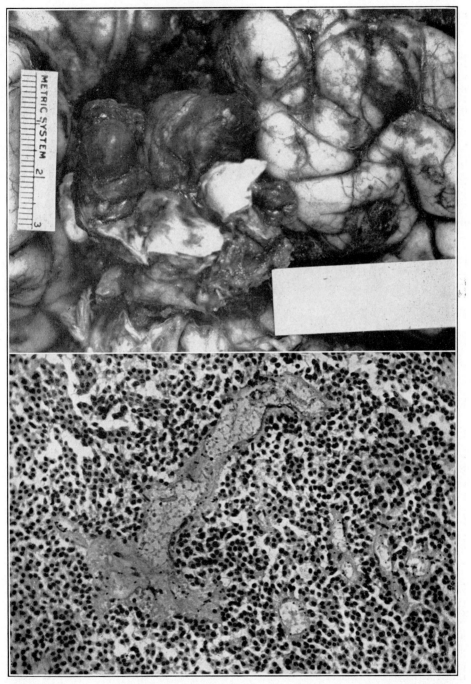

FIG. 746.—Chromophobe adenoma of the pituitary showing (above) a tumor compressing the optic nerve and chiasm and (below) uniform cellularity of the growth and numerous vascular spaces. × 200.

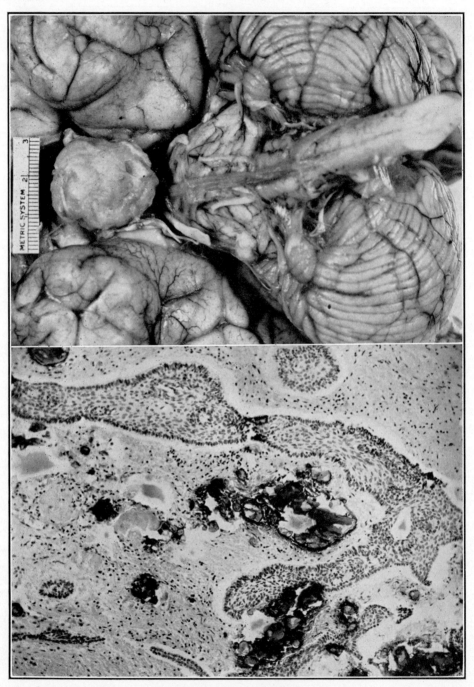

FIG. 747.—Craniopharyngioma showing (above) a tumor in the suprasellar area compressing the optic nerves and chiasm and (below) the epithelial nature of the tumor and calcification. × 100.

the sella turcica. They may also expand chiefly upward and obstruct the third ventricle and they may compress other parts of the brain stem and other cranial nerves. In rare instances, they may cover the entire brain stem and may extend into the posterior fossa. They become adherent to structures at the base of the brain in the course of their growth and they are difficult to remove surgically after they have attained a large size. The tumor grossly is encapsulated with the capsule being thin or thick. The growth is usually cystic. It is filled with greenish-yellow fluid that resembles motor oil, that does not clot on standing, and that contains cholesterol crystals. The majority of the tumors (75 to 85 per cent) are calcified, with sufficient calcium being present to be seen in the roentgenogram.

Histologically, the tumor has a characteristic appearance (Fig. 747). It is composed of epithelial cells in branching formation. There is a basement layer of columnar cells with heavily chromatinized nuclei; above this there may be seen an intermediate layer of cells, and more centrally there are stellate cells. Cornification of the epithelial cells occurs often. Cystic spaces and areas of degeneration are often seen. Connective tissue is present around vascular channels. Calcium is seen microscopically in the majority of tumors.

Parasellar Tumors. — Parasellar tumors are tumors lying adjacent to the sella turcica, usually along the lesser wing of the sphenoid bone. In the majority of instances they are meningiomas but may, in rare instances, be carcinomas. Meningiomas in this region straddle the lesser wing of the sphenoid bone, compressing the optic nerve and tract and often the oculomotor nerve. They may extend into the anterior and middle fossas if they become large.

NEURINOMAS

Neurinoma is *found* in the cerebellopontine angle. It arises from the auditory nerve in the internal auditory canal and lies in the angle between the pyramid, tentorium, and cerebellum. It is usually large when its presence is discovered. It is attached to the auditory nerve and may be attached also to the facial, glossopharyngeal, vagus, spinal accessory, and hypoglossal nerves. Seen at autopsy, the tumor is found to compress the cerebellum and pons, often attaining sufficient size to cause displacement and slight rotation of the brain stem. The growth is encapsulated and avascular in appearance. *Histologically* it is composed of streams of elongated bipolar cells, often with the nuclei arranged in parallel rows giving the impression of a palisade-like arrangement. The nuclei are elongated and the cytoplasm is scanty. Reticulin is abundant and collagen is seen around the blood vessels. Elsewhere in the tumor are numerous areas of degeneration and edematous spaces.

METASTATIC TUMORS

Metastatic tumors may reach the brain from various sources. They are found in 4.2 per cent of all brain tumors (Cushing). Carcinoma is the most frequent type of growth and chief among the sources of carcinoma metastasizing to the brain are lung and breast but other sources include the pharynx, larynx, uterus, rectum, prostate, skin, kidney, and generative organs. Sarcomas also metastasize to the brain. All parts of the brain may be involved by metastasis. No part is exempt nor are any parts of the brain especially vulnerable.

Carcinoma metastasis to the brain may appear in several forms (Fig. 748). These include the following: (1) *Multiple.* Such tumors involve various parts of the brain and are most common. They may appear anywhere in the cerebral hemispheres and brain stem. The tumors appear well defined and give a false sense of sharp definition from the surrounding tissue. Histologic study discloses, however, that carcinoma cells are found in the tissue surrounding the tumor. The tumors vary greatly in size. They are usually solid, their appearance varying with the original source of the carcinoma. They may at times be cystic. (2) *Solitary.* (3) *Encephalitic.* On rare occasions, carcinoma may involve the brain in an encephalitic form, characterized by small collections of carcinoma cells around blood vessels and in the parenchyma. In such instances, no gross tumors are apparent.

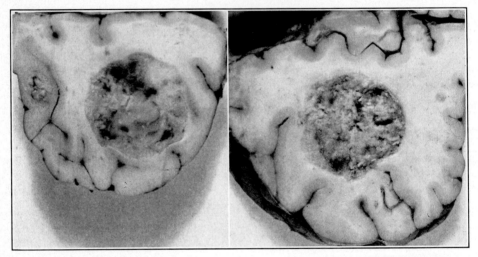

Fig. 748.—Multiple carcinomatous metastases in the brain from a bronchogenic carcinoma.

(4) *Meningeal.* Rarely, carcinoma may involve only the meninges, producing a true carcinomatous meningitis. This may be associated with generalized metastasis to the brain or it may be the sole manifestation of carcinomatous involvement. Carcinoma may also involve the dura either alone or in conjunction with metastasis to other portions of the brain. The dural tumor is usually seen as a diffuse adherent mass of tissue. Rarely, carcinoma to the brain may occlude a blood vessel giving rise to a typical picture of encephalomalacia. Rarely also, carcinoma cells may cause erosion of a blood vessel and produce massive cerebral hemorrhage.

The *histologic* appearance of carcinoma to the brain varies with the original source of the cancer. Despite the seemingly good definition from the surrounding tissue, masses of carcinoma in the brain are associated with infiltration of carcinoma cells in the parenchyma.

Sarcoma may metastasize to the brain. Primary sarcomas of the brain have been described, particularly the perithelioma.

CONGENITAL TUMORS

Congenital tumors of various types may be found in the brain (5.6 per cent, Cushing). These include craniopharyngiomas, cholesteatomas, dermoids, teratomas, and chordomas. *Craniopharyngiomas* have been discussed under the pituitary tumors. *Teratomas* of the brain are rare. They may be found in the region of the pineal gland, the third ventricle, the pituitary-hypothalamic region, and the cerebellum. Tumors derived from the three germ layers are less common than those derived from two layers, dermoids. *Dermoids* and *epidermoids* are found in the region of the pituitary and pineal glands, the third ventricle, in the region of the tuber cinereum, the cerebellopontine angle, and the posterior cistern. They, like the teratomas, are often associated with malformations in other parts of the body. *Cholesteatomas* are rare. They are found in relation to the cerebral hemispheres, in the suprasellar and parasellar regions, the cerebellopontine angle, and indeed anywhere along the subarachnoid spaces at the base of the brain from the optic chiasm to the posterior cistern. They arise from misplaced rests of epithelial cells in the leptomeninges. They have a typical mother-of-pearl appearance. Their shape varies since they often accommodate themselves to the surrounding tissue. They are encapsulated with tough outer layers and inner layers which are soft, cheesy, and avascular. Histologically, they possess a thin outer fibrous layer with flattened epithelial cells, sometimes containing granules of keratohyalin. Polygonal cells are found in the internal portions of the tumor and in the innermost portions are dead cells. *Chordomas* occur rarely. They arise in the basisphenoid as a remnant of the notochord. They expand within the sphenoid projecting upward into the sphenoid sinuses, nasopharynx, or even into the orbits and they often extend downward to the foramen magnum. Histologically, the tumors resemble notochord structures, being composed of chords or masses of large cells with many large vacuoles in the cytoplasm. The cells often contain more than one nucleus, the nuclei also being vacuolated (p. 1244).

GRANULOMAS

Granulomas of the brain are not common. They comprise 2.2 per cent of brain tumors (Cushing). They are chiefly tuberculomas and rarely gummas. *Tuberculomas* may occur in any part of the brain. They may be solitary or multiple and they may involve any portion of the cerebrum, cerebellum, pons, and basal ganglia. The cerebellum appears to be a favorite site both for solitary and multiple tuberculomas. The gross appearance of tuberculomas involving the brain is similar to that of tuberculoma elsewhere in the body. A false appearance of clean definition from the surrounding tissue is usually apparent. Microscopic study reveals, however, that in the surrounding tissue are areas of perivascular infiltration with lymphocytes, some of which may lie free in the tissue. Lymphocytic infiltration may be seen in the meninges overlying the tuberculoma, particularly if the latter lies near the surface. *Gummas* of the brain are rare. They may be found in the cerebrum, brain stem, basal ganglia region, and even in the pituitary gland. They are usually solitary but may be multiple. They are generally associated with gummas in other organs and are the result of acquired syphilis. Other rare types of granuloma may be found. One of these is coccidioidal granuloma.

BLOOD VESSEL TUMORS

Blood vessel tumors comprise 2.0 per cent (Cushing) of all brain tumors. The most clear-cut example is the *hemangioblastoma* of the cerebellum which is at times associated with *angiomatosis retinæ*. The tumors take their origin from a vascular primordium at the posterior end of the fourth ventricle. They vary in size but often occupy almost an entire cerebellar hemisphere. They lie within the cerebellum from which they are readily separated. The tumors are cystic and projecting into the cystic cavity is a neural nodule of solid tumor of variable size. It may be extremely small and may be difficult to discover or it may measure 1 to 3 cm. or more in diameter. The nodule has a reddish appearance. The cyst contains a yellowish or yellowish-orange fluid which coagulates on standing. Histologically, the neural nodule is composed of many capillary spaces lined with endothelial cells that disclose vesicular nuclei and dense cytoplasm. The vascular spaces vary in size and are often cavernous. They are surrounded by a network of reticulin and scattered collagen. Sheets of solid tissue lie among the vascular spaces. Their cytoplasm is filled with fat droplets. Cyst formation is common and hemorrhage is frequently seen.

Angiomas of *other types* occur in the brain and are of arterial, venous, or capillary nature. Hemangiomas of the skin are in many instances associated with vascular malformation of the brain. The latter may be seen as capillary telangiectases over the cerebral cortex or as venous malformations consisting of masses of large veins appearing like coiled snakes and lying on the surface of the brain. Arteriovenous malformations may also be seen.

EXTRAPYRAMIDAL DISEASES

Diseases of the extrapyramidal system involve chiefly the basal ganglia but the cerebral cortex and other parts of the nervous system may be affected.

Paralysis Agitans.—This is characterized by changes chiefly in the striatum and pallidum with involvement also of the corpus subthalamicum and the substantia nigra. The substantia nigra is said to be more affected in the postencephalitic variety and the striatum and pallidum in the senile type but this distinction is not sound. The disturbance consists chiefly of degenerative cell changes with eventual loss of ganglion cells and reactive gliosis in the basal ganglia. The large cells of the striatum, the ganglion cells of the pallidum, and the zona compacta of the substantia nigra are particularly affected. No changes are seen in the blood vessels except in the arteriosclerotic form when the usual sclerotic alterations are present. In the acute stages of encephalitis, perivascular infiltration with lymphocytes is seen in the substantia nigra. While most of this disappears, a focus is said to remain to account for postencephalitic paralysis agitans which develops at varying intervals after the acute encephalitis.

Sydenham's Chorea.—Very little is known regarding the brain changes in this disease in humans. In infectious chorea (diphtheria) and in chorea gravidarum changes have been reported in the striatum consisting chiefly of cell degeneration and, to a lesser extent, of perivascular infiltration.

Huntington's Chorea (Chronic Progressive Chorea).—This is characterized by a degenerative process involving the cerebral cortex and the corpus striatum. In the striatum there appears to be selective disease of the small ganglion cells, with loss of many cells, with relative preservation of the large ganglion cells, and with moderate gliosis. There are either no changes in the blood vessels or the vessels may show evidence of fibrous change if the patient lives long enough. Myelin sheath stains of the striatum reveal a status fibrosus. The cerebral cortex discloses changes in the frontal and temporal lobes in particular. In these locations, cell loss and chronic cell disease involves especially the lower three cortical layers with the myelin architecture remaining normal.

Progressive Lenticular Degeneration (Wilson's Disease).—This is characterized by cirrhosis of the liver and degeneration of the lenticular nucleus (putamen and pallidum) and the caudate. These areas in the brain appear shrunken and small on gross inspection (Fig. 749). In addition, there is degeneration of the ansa lenticularis, of the corpus subthalamicum, and of the strio-thalamic and strio-subthalamic fibers. The affected basa

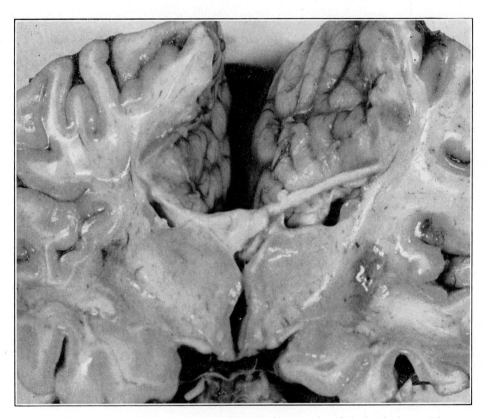

Fig. 749.—Hepato-lenticular degeneration showing atrophy of the lenticular nuclei.

ganglia show degeneration of the ganglion cells, astrocytic gliosis, and fat granule bodies. The cerebral cortex is usually normal. Vascular changes, if present, are secondary. Aminoaciduria is present and increased excretion of copper is found in the urine.

Status Marmoratus.—This condition, associated with congenital double athetosis, is characterized by excessive myelination of the striatum. Myelin sheath stains reveal a marbled appearance with dark areas of excessive myelination surrounding pale areas of nerve tissue. Astrocytes are increased in number and there is a heavy deposit of glia fibers in the affected areas. There may be similar areas of excessive myelination in the cortex. The appearance of the striatum in the myelin sheath stain gives a marbled appearance (status marmoratus) to the tissue.

Hemiballism (Hemichorea).—This disease, characterized by intense throwing movements of the limbs, is associated with a lesion in the opposite corpus subthalamicum. It is not clear whether the corpus subthalamicum alone is sufficient to produce the movements of hemiballism or whether injury to adjacent areas (Forel's fields) is also essential. The lesions have usually been vascular in character, softening or hemorrhage, but metastatic carcinoma and tuberculoma have also been found to cause the condition.

Other Extrapyramidal Diseases.—In addition to those listed, there are many other extrapyramidal diseases but they are not as well defined pathologically as those already mentioned. They include *status dysmyelinisatus*, consisting of demyelination involving chiefly the pallidum and the substantia nigra (zona reticulata); *progressive pallidal degeneration*, and *pseudosclerosis*, which is said by some to be similar to progressive lenticular degeneration.

MULTIPLE SCLEROSIS

This is a disease *characterized* by areas of demyelination scattered throughout the nervous system. The areas vary in number, size, age, and distribution. No part of the nervous system is immune to attack by the disorder but some parts are more frequently affected than others. The disorder involves chiefly the white matter but gray matter may be affected at times (Fig. 643).

In the *gross* specimen of the brain and spinal cord the areas of demyelination can be picked out readily with the naked eye, as grayish, translucent, sharply defined foci. They are seen in the spinal cord, often symmetrically involving posterior and lateral columns particularly but capable of affecting any part of the cord and even involving at times its entire cross section. In the brain stem the areas affect particularly the cerebellar peduncles, the pyramidal pathways, and the mesial fillet but the spinothalamic pathways and other long tracts may be involved. In the cerebral hemispheres, plaques are found in the internal capsule, under the ependyma of the lateral ventricles, and at times scattered through the white substance, especially just under the cortex and in the corpus callosum. One of the most frequent and often the earliest site of plaques is in the optic nerves and less often in the chiasm and in the optic tract and radiations. Rarely, plaques may be found in the cranial nerves, such as the trigeminal nerve or in the posterior roots of the spinal cord.

The size of the plaques and their number vary greatly from case to case. In some instances only a few small plaques are found and in others the entire brain, brain stem, and spinal cord may be affected.

Microscopically, the plaque of multiple sclerosis is characterized (in a myelin sheath stain) by loss of myelin sharply demarcated from the surrounding tissue and having a white or whitish-yellow appearance in contrast to the adjacent dark areas with normal myelin. The myelin in the plaques becomes broken up and eventually disappears. A glial scar is formed with a carpet of glial fibers of varying density. The axis cylinders show varying degrees of destruction and may disappear completely. In fresh plaques gitter cells may be seen, sometimes in large numbers. Lymphocytes may also be present, especially around the blood vessels. In such fresh plaques (acute multiple sclerosis) there is also present the demyelination found in older plaques with evidence of breakdown of myelin and the presence of myelin particles in macrophages.

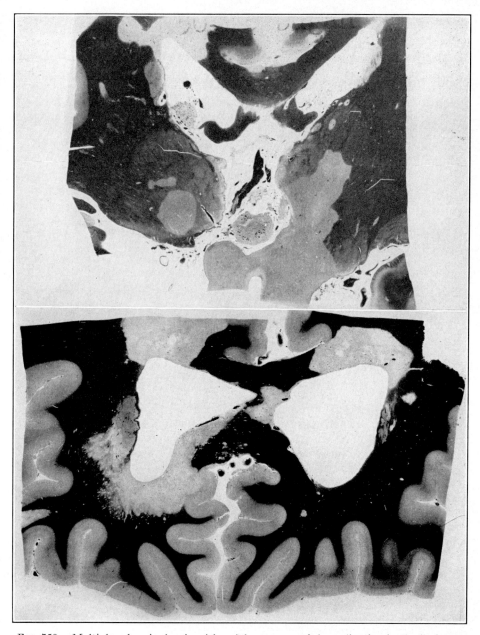

Fig. 750.—Multiple sclerosis showing (above) large areas of demyelination in the brain stem and (below) plaques of demyelination under the ependyma of the ventricle and in the corpus callosum. × semigross.

DIFFUSE SCLEROSIS

Under this term may be included a number of conditions which have little in common except that they involve the white matter to a large extent and are associated with sclerosis. For the most part they are quite rare.

Encephalitis Periaxialis Diffusa (Schilder's Disease).—This is characterized by extensive areas of sclerosis involving the white matter of the cerebral hemispheres, most often in the occipital lobes but found in the frontal as well. The process may extend into the internal capsule. Even in the gross specimen, the lesion can be seen as a breakdown of the white matter and appears as a softening of the tissue. In myelin sheath stains, the affected areas are white due to loss of myelin. Usually the arcuate fibers connecting adjacent gyri are spared. The axis cylinders escape for the most part. Astrocytes and glia fibrils are increased in number and large, plump glial cells are often seen in great numbers. Perivascular infiltration with lymphocytes is seen and gitter cells may be found in the tissue. The leukocytic reaction varies from one case to another since some cases are more acute than others.

Pelizaeus-Merzbacher Disease.—This is rare and occurs in families. It is characterized by demyelination around blood vessels involving the white matter of the brain, especially occipital and temporal areas and even brain stem. There is marked gliosis in the demyelinated areas.

Chronic Subcortical Encephalitis (Binswanger).—This is rare and is featured by degeneration of the white matter in the occipital and temporal lobes, occurring in foci and seen as areas of demyelination with pronounced gitter cell formation and with evidence of arteriosclerosis. It resembles Schilder's disease except that it is associated with disease of the blood vessels and occurs in advanced age.

CRANIAL TRAUMA

Many abnormalities may develop in the brain following head injury. They depend in a general way on whether there has been a closed or an open head injury, a penetrating wound, or a spinal fluid leak. Meningeal hemorrhage, which is common after head injury, has already been described. In addition to this, there may develop contusion and laceration of the brain, meningo-cerebral adhesions, cerebral scar, brain abscess, and meningitis. These give rise to a variety of symptoms, especially to epileptic seizures.

Contusion and Laceration.—Since these two conditions often occur together and merge into each other, they are best considered together. Areas of contusion and laceration may occur in both open and closed head injuries but are most common in the latter. They may be found anywhere in the brain substance, under the site of the injury and at some distance from it. They are often found on the basilar surface of the frontal lobes and on the mesial surface of the temporal lobes, from trauma against the incisura of the tentorium. The injured cortex appears swollen and bruised in the fresh state with bluish-red discoloration, often with a small pool of blood in the pia-arachnoid overlying the contused area and sometimes associated with extensive subarachnoid hemorrhage. The surface of the brain in the injured area may appear torn. In the fresh state, the contused areas show microscopically a film of red cells in the pia-arachnoid, punctate or confluent hemorrhages in the injured tissue, swollen ganglion cells with powdered Nissl substance and perineuronal edema, perivascular edema, swollen and distorted microglia which may develop into gitter cells if breakdown of tissue occurs, and swollen astrocytes and oligodendroglia. In most instances this is probably cleared away eventually with little change in the injured cortex but if the damage in the acute stage has been severe enough there will follow loss of nerve cells, deposit of glia fibrils, proliferation of astrocytes, and development of an *intracortical scar*. The latter may give rise to seizures in later life.

Meningocerebral Adhesions.—Adhesions may develop between the dura and pia-arachnoid and the underlying brain, or between pia-arachnoid alone and the brain tissue. They occur as a result of contusion to the dura by a missile which has not penetrated, by a depressed fragment of bone without penetration, or even in closed head injuries with severe contusions and lacerations, though this is not as common as in the other instances cited. The dura becomes adherent to the pia-arachnoid which is thickened and shows proliferation of fibroblasts. It, in turn, is adherent to the brain tissue which shows an increase of astrocytes in the superficial layers of the cortex. The underlying gyrus or gyri may become atrophied with loss of ganglion cells, with chronic cell disease of the remaining cells, and with an increase of astrocytes. Small pools of cerebrospinal fluid may be found in the adherent areas. The adhesions formed between the meninges and underlying cortex serve as stimuli for neuronal discharge.

Cerebral Scar.—Cortical scars may develop from penetrating skull wounds with penetration of the dura, resulting in an indriven segment of dura and pia-arachnoid into the underlying cortex. This serves as a core around which a scar develops. The injured brain tissue in the fresh state becomes the seat of an outpouring of microglia and gitter cells. Later, the debris is cleared and the area contains broken myelin, destroyed axis cylinders, and nerve cells. Later still, these are replaced by astrocytes with the formation of a firm glial scar in the tissue around the wedge of indriven dura. Gold chloride stains reveal a great proliferation of astrocytes and a heavy deposit of glia fibrils. The nerve cells in the surrounding cortex show varying evidences of degeneration. Fibroblasts are contributed by the indriven meninges and, due to proliferation of these, there develops a firm adherence between the core of meninges and the lacerated brain. The end result is a hard, firm scar. The ganglion cells in the adjacent brain tissue are stimulated to discharge by the tug of the adherent meninges.

Scars may develop in the brain as a result of a bullet wound which may leave a track of varying extent. Around the track there develops astrocytic gliosis and glial scar formation.

SENILE DISEASE

Advancing age brings with it scattered loss of ganglion cells in the cerebral cortex. This occurs in senescence and senile deterioration and is regarded as a normal development although not all subjects are affected. Senescence and senile deterioration are to be distinguished from senile dementia which is a disease of the senile period.

Senile Dementia.—This is a diffuse degenerative process affecting the entire brain but more pronounced in the frontal areas. The brain is small, often weighing 300 to 400 gm. less than the normal brain. The pia-arachnoid is thickened and whitish in appearance; the gyri are atrophied with increased spaces between them; there may be pools of cerebrospinal fluid over the atrophied gyri; the lateral ventricles are enlarged (hydrocephalus *ex vacuo*), and the white matter is reduced in size.

Microscopic examination of the brain reveals thinning of the cortical gray matter with loss of ganglion cells chiefly in the third cortical layer and with evidence of chronic cell disease in many of the cells (Fig. 751). Special silver stains reveal changes involving the neurofibrils of the ganglion cells. They appear thickened and form spirals, loops, or tangles at the base of the cell body (Alzheimer cell changes). By silver stain also, are seen the senile plaques which are characteristic of senile dementia. These are difficult to see in routine stains. They are found always in senile dementia but are not pathognomonic of this condition, since they are found in a form of presenile dementia (Alzheimer's disease) and have been described in senility and in a case of tabes. They vary in number from scattered to many. They are seen in the cortex as round or irregularly shaped areas in the midst of which is a dark-staining body surrounded by granular and fibrillar material and remnants of microglia or ganglion cells. Microglia appear to play an important role in their formation. They are not found in the cerebellum or brain stem and appear to be especially numerous in Ammon's horn in the temporal lobe. The blood vessels in senile dementia are often thickened.

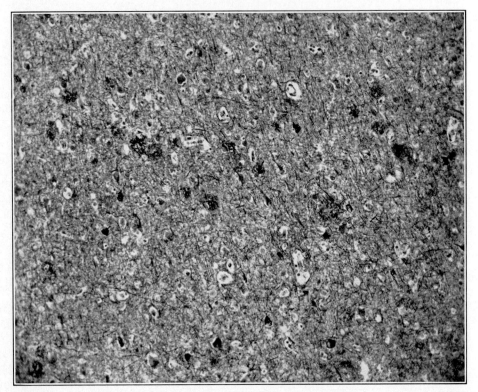

FIG. 751.—Senile dementia showing senile plaques in the cerebral cortex (silver stain). × 100.

PRESENILE DEMENTIA

This is a term applied to certain diseases in the presenium. Only two forms have a well-defined pathological substrate. These are Alzheimer's disease and Pick's disease.

Alzheimer's Disease.—The pathological changes in this disease are similar in all respects to those of senile dementia (see above) but they may be even more pronounced than in the latter. Rarely, the changes found in the brain in Alzheimer's disease have been described in young subjects.

Lobar Atrophy (Pick).—This is characterized by focal atrophy involving a single lobe of the brain or even a whole hemisphere. It affects the temporal lobe most often but it may involve the frontal lobe or any other part of the cerebrum. Grossly, the brain reveals striking atrophy and often increased firmness of the gyri in the affected area or areas with widening of the corresponding sulci.   The atrophy involves both gray and white matter and extends into the basal ganglia (striatum, pallidum, and s. nigra). Microscopic study reveals loss of ganglion cells especially in the upper three layers of the cortex, astrocytic gliosis in gray and white matter, and often argentophile inclusions in the ganglion cells.   The fibrillary changes in the ganglion cells and the senile plaques found in senile dementia and Alzheimer's disease are not found in Pick's lobar atrophy.

FAMILIAL, CONGENITAL, AND MISCELLANEOUS DISEASES

Amaurotic Family Idiocy (Tay-Sachs).—This is one of a group of diseases, the lipoidoses, which include amaurotic family idiocy, Niemann-Pick's disease, and Hand-Schüller-Christian disease.

Amaurotic family idiocy is a rare disease.   The infantile form is associated with generalized changes in the ganglion cells of the cortex but they are not always universal.   All parts of the brain may be affected, but in the juvenile form of the disease, the cerebellum is much more involved than in the infantile form.   Grossly, the brain is large and often firm and there is evidence of atrophy of the gyri, especially in the frontal lobes.

Microscopically, there is fibrous thickening of the pia-arachnoid and often an infiltration with lymphocytes and macrophages.   Changes in the ganglion cells are striking and cannot be confused with other processes.   These cells are swollen and ballooned; the nucleus is pushed to the periphery where it is surrounded by Nissl substance; the dendrites are not seen but the axis cylinder is usually visible, and the cytoplasm is honeycombed in appearance and is filled with round, refractile globules which represent lipoids and prelipoids.   They fail to stain with the usual methods used to demonstrate neutral fat.   Silver stains reveal clumping of the neurofibrils at the periphery of the cell.   Gitter cells are seen in the brain.   The astrocytic glia is proliferated.   There are no changes in the blood vessels.

Niemann-Pick' disease reveals changes similar to those of amaurotic family idiocy but is associated with changes in the viscera, especially the liver and spleen where foam cells are seen in abundance (p. 915).   Changes in the brain may be minimal while those in the viscera are severe or there may be severe changes in all organs.

Hand-Schüller-Christian's Disease.—This is characterized by the occurrence of firm, granulomatous masses in the dura, hypophysis, hypothalamus, and elsewhere in the brain stem.   Foam cells are seen in the affected areas as well as in lungs, spleen, liver, and lymph nodes (p. 917). The cells stain for neutral fat and cholesterol esters.

Tuberous Sclerosis.—This disease is associated with adenoma sebaceum and with visceral tumors in the heart, liver, kidney, and other organs (p. 1374).   In the brain, hard nodules are seen in the cortex and walls of the ventricles, often with a little depression or dimple and with widened convolutions.   Microscopically, they reveal abnormal ganglion and glial cells. The ganglion cells are large and distorted and assume many forms.   The glial cells particularly are abnormal.   They are large and may attain great sizes.   Dense networks of glia fibrils are seen in the cortical areas.   Many atypical glial cells are seen with single or, at times, multiple nuclei of many shapes.   Giant glia cells are also seen.

THE AMYOTROPHIES

The amyotrophies are characterized primarily by involvement of the anterior horn cell system of the spinal cord and brain stem and, at times, of the cerebral cortex (Betz cells). They include such diseases as amyotrophic lateral sclerosis, progressive bulbar paralysis, and progressive spinal muscular atrophy. There is disagreement whether these represent variants of a single disorder.

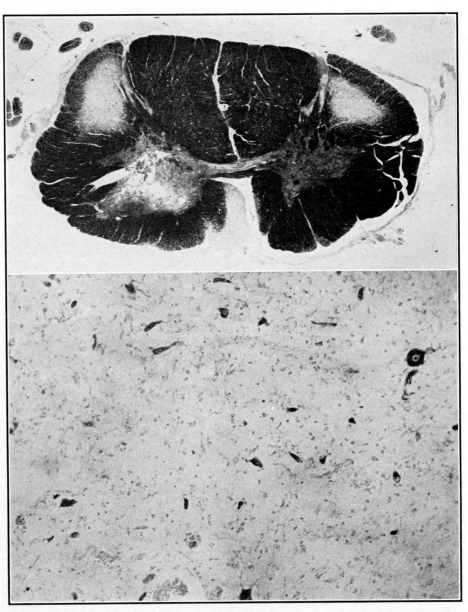

FIG. 752.—Amyotrophic lateral sclerosis (myelin sheath stain) showing (above) the demyelination of the pyramidal tracts in the cervical portion of the spinal cord and (below) decreased number of anterior horn cells and the various states of chronic cell disease of the remaining cells. × 100.

Amyotrophic Lateral Sclerosis.—This is a disease which affects the anterior horn cells of the spinal cord and brain stem and the pyramidal tracts. The degree of involvement varies. In some instances, the anterior horn cells are diffusely affected in the spinal cord and brain stem and the pyramidal tracts are severely affected. In other instances, there may be slight anterior horn cell involvement at a single level of the cord with pronounced pyramidal tract disease. In other instances still, there may be pronounced anterior horn cell disease with only minor pyramidal tract involvement. Also, the anterior horn cells of the brain stem may be severely diseased with only slight implication of those of the spinal cord or the converse may be true.

The *anterior horn cells* of the *spinal cord* may show, microscopically, severe disease at all levels or there may be spotty involvement at one or more levels (Fig. 752). The lesions are usually symmetrical but they may be predominantly unilateral. The cell changes are degenerative and consist of shrinkage with resulting chronic cell disease and with their eventual loss. No inflammatory changes are seen. Astrocytes are increased in number and there is an increase in the amount of neuroglia fibrils. If the process is sufficiently widespread in any segment, the anterior horn itself becomes shrunken and reduced in size.

The disease involves the anterior horn cells of the *brain stem* with some areas more prone to the disorder than others. The hypoglossal (XII) and vagus (X) nuclei are particularly affected but any of the motor nuclei may be involved although those of the oculomotor gray column are usually spared. The changes found in the brain stem nuclei are similar to those in the spinal cord.

The *pyramidal tracts* are also diseased in amyotrophic lateral sclerosis. They may be affected at the spinal cord level alone or at any level along the path of the pyramidal tract. The process, seen microscopically, is one of demyelination with breakdown and loss of myelin and of the pyramidal fibers. The large ganglion cells of the motor cortex are diseased but not in every instance. They become shrunken and often disappear.

No changes are seen in the posterior roots. The posterior columns may rarely show evidence of demyelination in the disease.

Progressive Spinal Muscular Atrophy.—This is a disease of the spinal cord but since it is one of the amyotrophies it is best included here. It is characterized by disease of the anterior horn cells, usually beginning in the cervical portion of the spinal cord but extending eventually to involve the entire cord. It is usually, but not always, symmetrical. The process consists of chronic cell disease involving the anterior horn cells with eventual loss of the affected cells, with overgrowth of astrocytes and neuroglia fibrils, and with shrinkage of the affected anterior horns. Inflammatory changes are not seen. The brain stem is not usually affected. Demyelination of the pyramidal tracts may be found at autopsy, giving rise to the contention that the disease is the same as amyotrophic lateral sclerosis. The anterior spinal roots become thin and the motor nerve fibers in the peripheral nerves degenerate. The muscles become atrophic with healthy and atrophic fibers mingling at first and later becoming completely involved. The sarcolemmal nuclei are increased in size and the interstitial tissue is increased in amount with progress of the disease.

A special form of progressive muscular atrophy (*Werdnig-Hoffman*) is seen in *infants*. The anterior horn cells are reduced in number and those remaining are shrunken. There is an increase of glia and decreased myelination of the anterior horns. Often the ganglion cells give the appearance seen in axonal chromatolysis. Changes have been observed rarely in the hypoglossal nuclei.

CONGENITAL MALFORMATIONS

There are many forms of malformations involving the skull, brain, and meninges. They may be single or multiple. *Cranioschisis* is a condition in which the base of the skull is more or less completely exposed due to improper development of the skull. The brain and meninges show defective development. *Cerebellar aplasia* is characterized by lack of development of the cerebellum. It may involve almost the entire cerebellum, leaving only remnants of it or it may implicate only one hemisphere. *Cerebellar hypoplasia* is characterized by impaired development of the entire cerebellum or only a single hemisphere, resulting in decreased size of the cerebellum. *Arnold-Chiari malformation* is characterized by downward elongation of the fourth ventricle, brain stem, and cerebellum into the upper portion of the spinal canal with displacement downward of the upper portion of the cervical cord and with associated hydrocephalus due to blockage in outflow of the cerebrospinal fluid from the fourth ventricle. The cranial nerves of the medulla and pons may be elongated by the malformation. The condition may be associated with spina bifida. *Congenital stenosis of the aqueduct of Sylvius* is associated with hydrocephalus. The tissue shows evidence of surrounding gliosis, hyperplasia of ependymal cells, and many diverticula of the aqueduct. *Platybasia* (basilar impression) is a deformity of the posterior portion of the base of the skull with a flattening of the inclined plane formed by the clivus. The foramen magnum is misshapen and often small. There may be associated deformities such as occipitalization of the atlas. The condition may be associated with syringomyelia or with other evidences of cranial nerve and medullary involvement due to interference with blood supply or to an associated arachnoiditis. *Porencephaly* consists of cavity formation within the brain. It may be congenital in origin or it may result from degenerations or softenings of the brain in adult life. The porencephaly varies in size from a small cavity to one which may occupy an entire lobe. It has no predilection regarding site but it occurs often in the region of the central gyri. Bilateral porencephalic cysts are not uncommon. The porencephaly usually communicates with the ventricle and often with the subarachnoid space. The gyri overlying the porencephaly are usually small and atrophic but the covering of cerebral tissue in the roof of the cyst varies in thickness. In advanced cases only a thin shell of cortex remains with pronounced loss of ganglion cells, destruction of the cell layers, chronic cell disease of the remaining cells, and overgrowth of astrocytes. The pia-arachnoid is usually adherent to the cortex. In other instances, the destruction of the cortex is less complete. The cortical lamination remains but there is chronic cell disease of many of the remaining ganglion cells. *Cyclopia* is featured by the presence of a single optic bulb in the midline and is associated with malformations of the optic nerves and pathways and other organs. *Arhinencephaly* consists of absence of the olfactory bulbs, tracts, and trigones and is usually associated with other malformations. *Absence of the corpus callosum* may be complete or may involve only the anterior or posterior parts. *Absence of the septum pellucidum* may be found as an isolated defect in an otherwise normal brain. *Agyria* is a condition characterized by a smooth brain surface with no gyral pattern. It is often associated with other anomalies. *Pachygyria* is characterized by the presence of gyri which are larger than normal. *Microgyria* is featured by small cortical gyri due either to congenital maldevelopment or to extrinsic factors.

THE SPINAL CORD

The fallacy of arbitrary division of diseases of the brain, spinal cord, and peripheral nerves is nowhere better illustrated than in disease of the cord itself. There are relatively few diseases confined to the spinal cord level, but since some are predominantly spinal cord disorders it seems desirable to consider them from the conventional approach.

INFLAMMATIONS

Poliomyelitis.—Anterior poliomyelitis is a systemic disease which *affects* the spinal cord, brain stem, and at times the brain. It is a polio-encephalitis with predominant spinal cord involvement. It may affect the *spinal cord* exclusively, as it does in most instances; it may involve with it the brain stem and even the brain; it may involve only the brain stem, or, in rare instances, it may affect only the cerebrum. It is a disease of the gray matter, involving the anterior horn cells of the spinal cord or their analogues, the motor nuclei of the brain stem, or the Betz cells of the motor cortex. The sensory portion of the nervous system is not affected. The degree of devastation at any given level varies considerably. There may be extensive disease in all levels of the spinal cord; only a single level may be involved (lumbar or cervical), or there may be implication of only isolated groups of cells within a single segment. Although the disease is often symmetrical it is as often asymmetrical and produces symptoms in only a single limb.

Nothing specific is seen in the *gross* specimen. Cut surfaces of the spinal cord or brain stem appear engorged in the region of the gray substance but apart from this there is nothing significant. *Microscopically*, the meninges of the spinal cord or brain stem are infiltrated with a thin layer of lymphocytes in the early stages of the disease. These disappear early but, while present, they give rise to signs of meningeal irritation (neck stiffness and Kernig's sign). The main changes are found within the nervous system tissue itself. These consist of devastation of the anterior horn cells which, in the early stages, appear swollen and their Nissl substance powdered or fragmented (Fig. 753). Lymphocytes are found free in the parenchyma and around vessels. There is a prompt reaction of microglia early and microglial nuclei are seen in abundance in these stages of the disease. The posterior horns of the cord and the white matter often show perivascular infiltrations in the acute stages. The infiltrations disappear in the later stages of the disease.

As the process grows *more chronic* the glial response predominates and there is an abundance of microglial nuclei with astrocytic response in varying amounts. The lymphocytic reaction in the tissue and around the vessels disappears in time. The ganglion cells of the anterior horns may recover and resume their normal structure or, if affected beyond the reversible stage, they show shrinkage and chronic cell disease and may disappear in varying numbers. Astrocytes appear in later stages and neuroglial fibrils are laid down. The anterior horn eventually shrinks and is smaller than normal.

The changes observed in the motor nuclei of the *brain stem* are similar to those observed in the spinal cord. They involve not only the medulla but also other parts of the brain stem. The pons has been found to be regularly involved and the hypothalamus has been affected in a high percentage of cases.

In the *cerebrum*, poliomyelitis affects the cells of the motor cortex. When this occurs the process is similar to that in the spinal cord with disease of the Betz cells and inflammatory reactions in the cortex itself.

Herpes Zoster (Posterior Poliomyelitis).—Herpes zoster is a disease characterized by skin eruptions in dermatomeric distribution and by pain (p. 1061). These are associated with changes in the spinal cord and, less

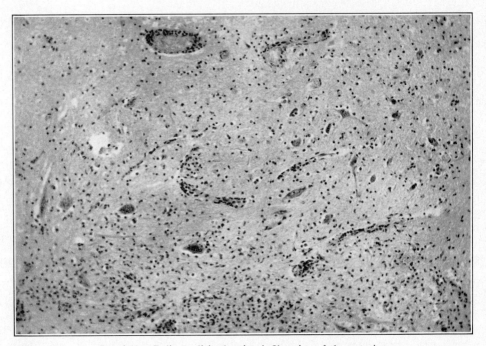

Fig. 753.—Poliomyelitis showing infiltration of the anterior horn and the loss of anterior horn cells. × 100.

often, in the brain stem, particularly in the distribution of the trigeminal nerve. The spinal cord changes are usually found at the same dermatomere level as the skin changes but at times they may be found at different levels.

The *pathological* changes are found in the posterior root ganglion, posterior root, and posterior horn. If the fifth nerve is affected, similar changes are found in the gasserian ganglion and its posterior root. The affected areas show infiltration with lymphocytes, disease of the posterior ganglion cells, and perivascular infiltration with lymphocytes. The posterior horns show perivascular infiltration. The acute changes may rarely affect the anterior horn cells and roots. The posterior roots show evidence of demyelination in the acute stages.

After the acute inflammation, there may be chronic changes characterized by astrocytic proliferation and a deposit of neuroglial fibrils. These may be associated with persistent pain (postherpetic neuralgia).

Myelitis.—The term myelitis refers to inflammation involving the spinal cord. The condition itself occurs under many circumstances and involves gray or white matter or both. Many of the forms of myelitis are well known, such as those in multiple sclerosis, syphilis, and subacute combined degeneration. There remain forms in which the cause is obscure, usually associated with infection or with toxic-infectious conditions. These probably do not all have the same cause or similar pathological features. They are characterized by patches of disease involving the white matter chiefly and varying in size and extent. There is breakdown of myelin, disease of the axis cylinders, and perivascular infiltration with lymphocytes. Myelin sheath stains reveal demyelination. Microglial and astrocytic reaction develops, the latter predominating as the disease becomes more chronic. The posterior and anterior roots are involved in some cases (myeloradiculitis). These show myelin destruction and evidence of demyelination with a myelin sheath stain. Meningeal reaction with lymphocytes may be found in some instances also.

A special form of myelitis, *subacute necrotic myelitis*, is found in rare instances. This is characterized by patchy areas of necrosis in the spinal cord with destruction of myelin and axis cylinders and with disease of the blood vessels in the meninges of the cord and within the cord itself. The changes consist of thickening of the vascular walls and occlusion of the lumens but are neither arteriosclerotic or syphilitic. The areas of necrosis are dependent on the changes in the blood vessels.

Still another unusual form is represented by *neuromyelitis optica*, characterized by disease of the spinal cord and optic nerves and resembling multiple sclerosis. Pathologically, it consists of the presence of multiple softenings in the spinal cord, chiefly in the cervical region. In the spinal cord are foci of varying size containing gitter cells and occasionally lymphocytes and plasma cells. Myelin is destroyed in the affected areas and axis cylinders show heavy damage as a rule. The blood vessels show no evidence of disease. Similar foci are found in the optic nerves.

Arachnoiditis.—Following infectious trauma, spinal anesthesia, and other conditions there may develop inflammation of the pia-arachnoid, resulting in arachnoiditis. This is usually localized but may involve the entire length of the spinal cord. The arachnoid becomes thickened and fibrous and adherent to the spinal cord with resulting interference with the flow of spinal fluid and with the circulation of the spinal cord (Fig. 754). The very early stages of the process have not been studied carefully for lack of material. The end process consists of a thickened arachnoid containing many fibroblasts and much fibrous tissue with macrophages in the earlier stages. There may be areas of demyelination in the spinal cord itself, due to ischemia resulting from compression of the vessels by the adherent arachnoiditis.

Extradural Abscess.—This usually results from a furuncle but may follow bloodstream infection. The condition is acute and is found in the same metamere as the skin infection. It consists of a collection of pus on the outer side of the spinal dura with thrombophlebitis of the extradural veins. The abscess has a typical picture with neutrophils, fibrin, and other features of an acute abscess. The spinal cord shows damage from the onset and is characterized by myelomalacia which may involve the entire cross section of the cord at the affected level. The myelin and axis cylinders are destroyed and the gray matter is similarly affected, the tissue being replaced by large numbers of gitter cells. Eventually, if the process persists long enough, only a rim of spinal cord is left.

Rabies.—Rabies may involve the entire central nervous system, particularly the spinal cord and brain stem. It affects the gray matter, especially the anterior horns which show evidence of severe damage. The anterior horn cells are swollen and their Nissl substance is pulverized and eventually the cells may disappear. Lymphocytes are abundant in the anterior horn cells and around the vessels. Microglial proliferation is prominent and later astrocytes become increased in number. Negri bodies may be demonstrated in the ganglion cells by special stain but are not always easy to find. Similar changes are found in the motor nuclei and gray matter of the brain stem. Perivascular infiltration with lymphocytes is seen in the affected areas of the spinal cord and brain stem and a mild lymphocytic reaction may be found in the meninges in the early stages.

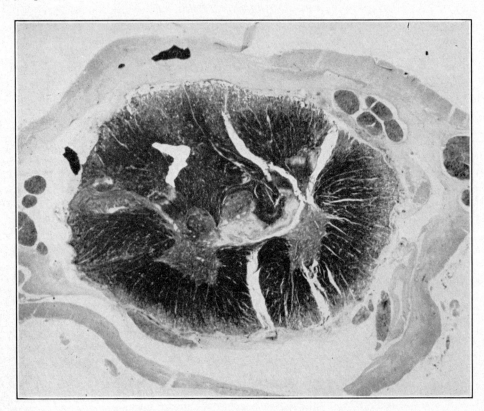

Fig. 754.—Arachnoiditis from a case of spinal anesthesia showing the thickened dura and the thickened and adherent pia-arachnoid.

TUMORS

The spinal cord is a relatively infrequent seat of tumors—being less often involved than the cranial cavity. Statistical studies indicate a predominance of brain over spinal cord tumors in a ratio of 6 to 1. In general, the types of tumor found in the spinal canal and spinal cord are similar to those encountered in the skull and brain. Tumors of various types involve the spinal cord but, unlike the brain, encapsulated tumors are more frequent. They are found in greatest numbers in the thoracic region, followed in frequency by the cervical and lumbar regions. They may be extradural, subdural, or, as the case of dumb-bell shaped tumors, both extra- and intradural. They are located most frequently on the lateral surface of the cord but they may be anterior or dorsal. The cord is compressed in the course of their growth, the tumor forming an excavation of varying depths and degree. In extreme instances only a thin ribbon of cord may be left. The spinal cord itself shows evidence of myelin destruction and nerve cell damage, resulting in clinical signs of spinal cord compression. The cord damage may be reversible or irreversible.

Perineurial Fibroblastoma (Neurinoma, Schwannoma, Neurilemmoma). —This is the most commonly encountered tumor in the spinal canal. It takes its origin from the perineurium of the nerve sheath. It is encapsulated and varies in size from 0.5 cm. to several centimeters, extending over several segments of spinal cord. The shape varies. As a rule, the tumors are oval but they may be fusiform, globular, or dumb-bell shaped (Fig. 755*A*). In

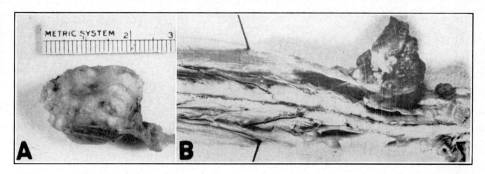

Fig. 755.—Tumors of the spinal cord showing (*A*), a perineurial fibroblastoma with the attached nerve root compressing the spinal cord and (*B*), a nodule of metastatic carcinoma lying extradurally and compressing the spinal cord.

the latter instance, part of the tumor lies extradurally while the rest is intradural. The surface is usually smooth but occasionally is nodular. The tumor is attached to one or more nerve roots which are firmly adherent to the capsule and are compressed by the tumor. The spinal cord is compressed and may be displaced to greater or lesser degree by the pressure of the tumor. Erosion of the bone may occur at times. The tumor, on its cut surface, is avascular, white or yellowish white, fibrous in appearance, and soft or relatively firm. Histologically, the cells are arranged in streams and palisading of the nuclei is often seen. The nuclei are elongated and contain coarse chromatin granules. The cytoplasm is elongated. Mitoses are rare. Collagen is abundant in the solid areas of tumor and blood vessels are adequate to maintain structure. Looser areas of tissue are seen as well as areas of degeneration.

Meningiomas.—These are not as numerous as the perineurial fibroblastomas. They are extramedullary in location and encapsulated. As in the case of their cranial counterparts they have a firm dural attachment. They vary in size, extending over one or more segments. Their shape may be oval, round, or flattened and their surface smooth or lobulated. The tumor capsule is well formed and fibrous. The cut surface is fibrous and soft and has a gray or grayish-red appearance. Calcium may be present in the capsule and in the body of the tumor. The histological appearance differs in no way from that of the cerebral type.

Gliomas.—Gliomas involve the spinal cord in an incidence of 10 to 17 per cent of all spinal cord tumors. Any of the types of glioma involving the brain may affect the spinal cord but the incidence of tumor types differs in the two locations. Gliomas may involve only a few segments of the spinal cord or may extend throughout almost the entire length of the cord. They result in enlargement of the cord and destruction of the spinal cord tissue. Some types such as the astrocytomas are less destructive than others. As the tumor grows, there follows encroachment on the subarachnoid space and the spinal canal with resultant filling of the entire canal in some instances. The growth of the tumor is not uniform. It may infiltrate the entire diameter of the spinal cord at one level, taper off at another, and expand at still another. As in the case of extramedullary tumors, the highest incidence of gliomas is at the thoracic level, with lesser frequency in the cervical region, and least in the lumbar area. Multiple gliomas are found in rare instances. Cavity formation is not an infrequent accompaniment of spinal cord tumors and may occur in astrocytomas and ependymomas.

Various *histologic types* of glioma may be found in the spinal cord. The most frequent type is the ependymoma. Astrocytomas are next in frequency but are much less numerous than ependymomas. The ependymomas of the spinal cord may appear at any level but are more frequent in the lumbosacral cord, the conus medullaris, and the filum terminale. Other gliomas found in the cord include the glioblastoma multiforme, oligodendroglioma, astroblastoma, spongioblastoma polare, ganglioneuroma, medulloblastoma, and neuroepithelioma. The histologic features of the spinal cord gliomas are similar to those of their cerebral counterparts.

Hemangioblastoma.—This type of tumor may be found in the spinal canal as an extension of a cerebellar hemangioblastoma into the cervical region; it may be found as an independent intramedullary tumor, or it may be encountered as an intramedullary tumor associated with a typical cerebellar medulloblastoma. The intramedullary hemangioblastomas appear as red or reddish-brown tumors that are soft to firm in consistency. They are usually well demarcated from the spinal cord tissue. Their histologic appearance is similar to that of the cerebellar hemangioblastoma.

Metastatic Carcinoma.—Carcinoma may involve the spinal canal from many sources, particularly from the prostate, breast, and lung. It is usually found as a discrete, flattened mass lying extradurally in the extradural fat but it may be subdural (Fig. 755*B*). It is attached to one or more nerve roots which may be infiltrated with carcinoma cells. The underlying spinal cord is softened and shows evidence of myelomalacia in greater or lesser degree. Histologically, the spinal cord is disintegrated, the myelin sheaths and axis cylinders are broken, and the area is filled with gitter cells.

Other Metastatic Tumors.—*Sarcomas* of various types may involve the spinal cord. These include lymphosarcoma, osteosarcoma, reticulum cell sarcoma, spindle cell sarcoma, giant cell sarcoma, Hodgkin's disease, myeloma, and others as well. *Hodgkin's disease* may involve the spinal canal. It may be found as an extradural mass compressing the spinal cord or it may involve the spinal cord by direct invasion. *Myeloma* may be found in the spinal canal as part of multiple myeloma. It may involve the extradural space as a discrete tumor mass or cause encroachment on the extradural space and compression of the cord by angulation of diseased vertebræ.

Congenital Tumors.—*Chordomas* may appear in the spinal canal just as they do in the cranial cavity (p. 1244). They occur predominantly in the sacrococcygeal region and rarely at other levels though they are found in the cervical region. *Cholesteatomas* are found rarely in the spinal canal. They have been found at various levels but seem to be more common in the thoracic region. *Dermoids* are rare and are usually intramedullary. They are more common in the lower portion of the spinal cord where they involve the conus and cauda equina. *Teratomas* are rare. They may be intramedullary or extramedullary, are chiefly cystic, and may be associated with syringomyelic cavities of the spinal cord. They may occur at any level. *Lipomas* are rare in the spinal canal. They are extramedullary tumors and may be either extradural or intradural. They are more commonly extradural and, under these conditions, are often associated with spina bifida. The intradural lipomas are usually found on the dorsal surface, may affect any level of the spinal cord, are subarachnoid in location, and often extend into the spinal cord. Histologically, they consist of typical large polygonal cells.

SYPHILIS OF THE SPINAL CORD

Syphilis may involve the spinal cord in various forms. Meningeal syphilis as such is rare and is seen in pachymeningitis. Vascular syphilis of the cord is also rare. The most common type of spinal cord syphilis is tabes dorsalis. Meningomyelitis and other forms are also seen.

Pachymeningitis.—This occurs chiefly in the cervical region. The dura is thickened to many times normal and surrounds the spinal cord, compressing it like a tumor. The pia-arachnoid underlying it is adherent to the dura and all the membranes are in turn adherent to the spinal cord. The dura shows great increase of fibrous tissue, collections of lymphocytes and plasma cells, and at times small gummas. The roots are infiltrated with lymphocytes and plasma cells and the spinal cord is invariably damaged. Areas of demyelination are seen together with focal infiltrations of lymphocytes and plasma cells in both gray and white matter.

Vascular Syphilis.—This is a rare form of spinal cord syphilis. When it occurs the anterior spinal artery is affected by the Heubner form of endarteritis previously described in cerebral vascular syphilis. The spinal cord in such cases reveals evidence of myelomalacia in the anterior portion of the cord with destruction of anterior horns and the white matter. The involvement of other arteries of the spinal cord is very rare.

Tabes Dorsalis.—This is the most frequent form of spinal cord syphilis. It is characterized by changes in the posterior roots and posterior columns of the spinal cord. The process involves the lower portions of the spinal cord—the lumbar and sacral areas—more frequently than other levels but the cervical cord may be affected. The brain stem is involved (Argyll-Robertson pupils) and at times the cerebrum is affected (taboparesis).

There is little to be seen on gross inspection of the spinal cord in tabes. On microscopic examination many characteristic features are revealed (Fig. 756). The pia-arachnoid in active tabes is thickened and reveals increased amounts of fibrous tissue, together with infiltrations with lymphocytes and plasma cells. The hematogenous elements may be absent in long standing cases of tabes. The meninges tend to be adherent to the underlying spinal cord. Cell stains reveal infiltration with lymphocytes and plasma cells in the posterior root ganglia and, in fresh cases, in the posterior roots. Myelin sheath stains show demyelination of the posterior roots and intact anterior roots. The axis cylinders are decreased in number. Demyelination of the posterior columns is clearly seen. Since the process is most common in the lower portions of the spinal cord, the columns of Goll (gracilis) are involved but in instances of cervical tabes, the columns of both Goll and Burdach (gracilis and cuneatus) are affected. They show evidence of demyelination with greater or lesser loss of axis cylinders. Astrocytic gliosis with the deposit of a heavy carpet of glial fibrils develops in the course of the process. Demyelination and decreased numbers of axis cylinders are found in the peripheral nerves. In some instances, tabes is associated with cerebral changes similar to those found in general paresis (taboparesis).

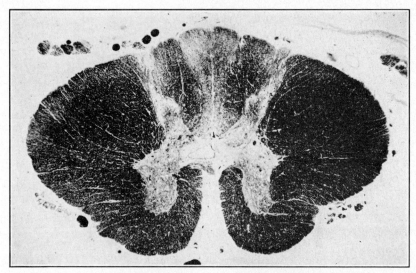

Fig. 756.—Tabes dorsalis. Myelin sheath stain showing the demyelination of the posterior roots and posterior columns.

The tabetic process is thought to result from changes primarily in the posterior roots or in the radicular nerves. The degeneration of the posterior columns follows as a result of the changes in the posterior roots. There are some who believe that the pathological changes in tabes develop primarily in the posterior columns, the other changes being secondary to this. Whatever the primary process, tabes dorsalis is a disease affecting the posterior columns and posterior roots and ganglia with no involvement of the other tracts in the spinal cord.

Meningomyelitis.—There are some forms of spinal cord syphilis which resemble tabes but in which the cord involvement is widespread. These forms, referred to as meningomyelitis, may involve both white and gray matter and may occur at all levels of the spinal cord, although they too are more frequent in the lower spinal cord levels.

The meninges are infiltrated with lymphocytes and plasma cells and the pia-arachnoid is thickened. Similar infiltrations are seen in the posterior roots but these are not consistently affected as in tabes. Within the spinal cord itself are infiltrations of lymphocytes and plasma cells and patchy areas of demyelination which may affect several areas of the cord, involving the posterior and lateral as well as other columns. In some instances, an entire cross section of spinal cord may be involved, giving rise to a transverse myelitis. The anterior horns may be infiltrated and, in rare instances, the resulting process resembles amyotrophic lateral sclerosis. Disease of the anterior horn cells is found in these cases with lymphocytic and plasma cell infiltration in the tissue and around the vessels and with disease of the pyramidal tracts.

Meningomyelitis differs from tabes in the less constant involvement of the posterior roots and the extension of the process in the spinal cord beyond the posterior column system.

MYELOMALACIA

Softening of the spinal cord results from obstruction to the blood supply and may develop from many causes. The most important primary cause is disease of the anterior spinal artery with resulting occlusion due usually to thrombosis. This may be due to syphilis or arteriosclerosis. The anterior half of the spinal cord is damaged as a result of the vascular occlusion with involvement of the anterior horns, the spino-thalamic tracts, and the ventral spinocerebellar pathways, as well as part of the lateral columns. Myelin sheath stains reveal demyelination of the affected areas. Cell stains disclose numerous gitter cells with breakdown of the tissue which may be so extensive as to leave no parts intact.

Myelomalacia occurs also with metastatic carcinoma involving the spinal cord. This is extradural or subdural and is associated with softening of the spinal cord. Similar softening is found in extradural abscess.

TRAUMA

Injury to the spinal cord may result from a direct blow to the spine and spinal cord in diving accidents or in fracture-dislocations, from a penetrating wound, from indirect transmission by a bullet ricocheting off the spine, or from a fall. Several types of disorder may develop, some much more frequently than others. These include hemorrhage, herniated intervertebral disc, and concussion.

Hemorrhage.—Extradural or subdural hemorrhage may occur in spinal cord injuries but is very rare. As in the case of similar hemorrhage in the cranial cavity it produces its symptoms by compression of the nervous tissue. Subarachnoid hemorrhage confined to the spinal cord may develop from cord injury. It is common also in subarachnoid bleeding in the cranial cavity.

Concussion.—The term spinal cord concussion has been given to spinal cord injury resulting from direct or indirect trauma to the cord. The process is in reality contusion and laceration of the cord. The damage is found not only beneath the point of impact of the blow to the vertebral column but usually at other levels as well. It is, therefore, usually diffuse in its distribution although it may be most pronounced at a single level. Gross inspection in the acute stages reveals a greatly swollen cord, especially at the level of injury. Hemorrhages may be seen within the cord substance. Microscopic study reveals swelling of the gray and white

matter.   Punctate and confluent hemorrhages are seen.   The ganglion cells
are swollen and the white matter is edematous.   Gitter cells are found in the
white matter and elsewhere and the neuroglia is swollen.   The process may
be reversible but when it is not it is followed by an increase of astrocytes
and glial scarring and by demyelination.

Herniated Intervertebral Disc.—This is associated with a history of
indirect (more commonly) or direct injury in 50 to 60 per cent of cases.   The
lesion is most common in the lumbar area (L5 and L4 discs) but is found
also in the cervical region and rarely in the thoracic area.   It is associated
with protrusion of a portion of the annulus fibrosus of the intervertebral
disc, or of the nucleus pulposus through a tear in the annulus.   The herniated tissue compresses one or more of the adjacent posterior roots thus
causing its symptoms.

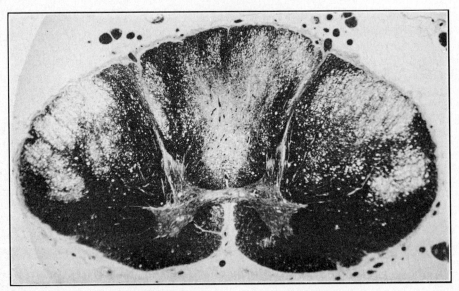

FIG. 757.—Subacute combined degeneration in pernicious anemia.   Myelin sheath stain
showing the postero-lateral demyelination and its spongy appearance.

Hematomyelia.—Hemorrhage within the spinal cord may occur as a
result of injury or other conditions.   It may be extensive and involve a
large part of the cord at a given level.

Subacute Combined Degeneration.—Subacute combined degeneration is
a disease of the spinal cord involving, in varying degrees, the posterior and
lateral columns.   It is found in *pernicious anemia* but many other diseases
may produce a similar type of syndrome (postero-lateral syndrome) although not with a similar pathological process.   The disorder is confined to
the spinal cord and does not affect the brain or brain stem.   It is most frequent in the thoracic and lumbar levels but may be found at all levels.

The *posterior* and *lateral columns* are chiefly affected and, of these, the
columns of Goll are more often involved than those of Burdach (Fig. 650).
There may be predominant involvement of the posterior columns with only
slight implication of the latter; the lateral columns may be predominantly
affected, or they may be involved with equal severity.   Besides the posterior
columns and the pyramidal tracts, the disorder may affect the spino-

cerebellar paths and the direct pyramidal columns, and, in rare instances, the entire cross section of the spinal cord.

Myelin sheath stains reveal *demyelination* in the areas described, particularly in the columns of Goll and the pyramidal tracts. The meninges, posterior roots, and posterior root ganglia show no evidence of disease and the root entrance zone medial to the posterior horn is unaffected. The demyelinated areas have a lacunar appearance (status spongiosus). The vacuoles in these areas are usually empty but may contain macrophages or gitter cells. The myelin is broken up and fat stains are positive. Macrophages may be present in great numbers. The axis cylinders show degenerative changes but may not be severely damaged and the process of myelin breakdown and axis cylinder damage may be reversible. Glial proliferation and glial scarring are not prominent.

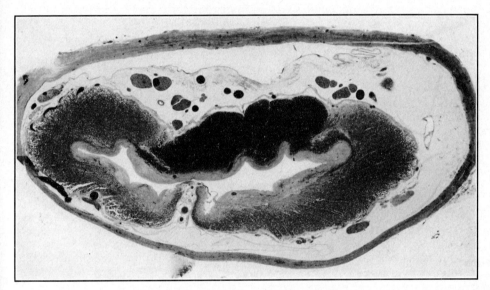

Fig. 758.—Syringomyelia. Myelin sheath stain to show the syringomyelic cavity in the center of the cord with destruction of cord tissue.

Degeneration of the posterior and lateral columns (postero-lateral sclerosis) is seen in many *other conditions* besides pernicious anemia. It is found in multiple sclerosis, syphilitic meningomyelitis, and even in spinal cord tumor. Although the distribution of the process resembles that of subacute combined degeneration, the pathological process differs from that found in pernicious anemia.

SYRINGOMYELIA

Syringomyelia is a condition characterized by cavity formation within the spinal cord. It *occurs* most frequently in the cervical portion. It may be confined to a single segment or a few segments; it may extend for almost the entire length of the spinal cord; it may extend upward into the brain stem, or it may involve only the brain stem (syringobulbia).

The *location*, form, and extent of the cavity vary. It is found commonly in the central gray matter. It may be seen as a slit-like cavity within a posterior horn or it may be found in the region of the posterior column. It may affect the entire spinal cord at a single level, leaving only a rim of cord while at other levels. Its shape, size, and location within the cord may vary greatly. Because of the irregularity of size and shape of the cavity a description of the spinal cord tissue involved in the process is difficult. From its original area in the gray commissure of the spinal cord the cavity may extend into the posterior columns, anterior horns, and lateral columns and may eventually involve an entire cross section of the cord. It may also involve any of the areas described alone.

The syringomyelic cavity is filled with fluid (Fig. 758). *Symptoms* are produced by distention of the cavity as well as by destruction of the tissue of the spinal cord. The rim surrounding the cavity is lined by a network of glia fibrils with a mixture of fibrous tissue and blood vessels, although the connective tissue element is not prominent. Adjacent to the cavity and the nervous tissue are homogeneous areas containing glia fibrils, nuclei, ameboid glia, and vascular islands. The meninges are thickened. Myelin sheath stains of the spinal cord reveal demyelination of varying extent, depending upon the size of the syringomyelic cavity.

The *nature* of syringomyelia is not clear. It is thought by some to be a neoplastic process. Cavities resembling syringomyelia may occur as a result of maldevelopment, in intramedullary tumors, in injuries, and in vascular occlusions.

CONGENITAL MALFORMATIONS

Malformations of the spinal cord are found involving various portions of the cord. *Meningocele* and *meningomyelocele* may occur in conjunction with spina bifida. These malformations are found in the sacral or cervical region, the lower portions of the spinal cord being the more frequently affected. The deformity is seen as a protruding, fluctuant, often translucent mass, covered with skin or a thin transparent membrane. In the case of the meningocele the sac contains meninges and spinal fluid. In a meningomyelocele spinal cord tissue is present and there are often cauda equina roots in the lower portions of the spinal cord. Hydrocephalus is usually present.

Rare malformations such as *diplomyelia*, a doubling of the spinal cord, may occur.

REFERENCES

ALEXANDER, L.: *Diseases of the Basal Ganglia*, Baltimore, Williams & Wilkins Co., 1942 (Paralysis Agitans).

ALPERS, B. J.: Arch. Otolaryngol., *29*, 199, 1939 (Abscess).

ALPERS, B. J., and FORSTER, F. M.: J. Neuropath. & Exp. Neurol., *4*, 262, 1945 (Subarachnoid Hemorrhage).

ALPERS, B. J., and GASKILL, H. S.: J. Neuropath. & Exp. Neurol., *3*, 210, 1944 (Embolic Encephalitis).

BAILEY, P.: Springfield, Charles C Thomas, 1948 (Brain Tumors).

BAILEY, P., and CUSHING, H.: Philadelphia, J. B. Lippincott Co., 1926 (Gliomas).

BAKER, A. B.: Am. J. Path., *11*, 185, 1935 (Hemorrhagic Encephalitis).

CUSHING, H., and EISENHARDT, L.: Springfield, Charles C Thomas, 1938 (Meningiomas).

DAVISON, C.: A. M. A. Arch. Neurol. & Psychiat., *46*, 1039, 1941 (Amyotrophic Lateral Sclerosis).

DONOHUE, W. L.: J. Pediat., *19*, 42, 1941 (Mumps).

FERRARO, A.: A. M. A. Arch. Neurol. & Psychiat., *52*, 443, 1944 (Multiple Sclerosis).

FERRARO, A., and SCHEFFER, I. H.: A. M. A. Arch. Neurol. & Psychiat., *25*, 748, 1931 (Measles).

References1469

FORSTER, F. M., and ALPERS, B. J.: J. Neuropath. & Exp. Neurol., *4*, 146, 1945, (Aneurysm).
GATES, E. M., and others: Medicine, *29*, 71, 1950 (Abscess, Metastatic).
GLOBUS, J. H., and STRAUSS, I.: A. M. A. Arch. Neurol. & Psychiat, *18*, 215, 1927 (Hemorrhage).
HASSIN, G. B.: A. M. A. Arch. Neurol. & Psychiat., *38*, 713, 1937 (Multiple Sclerosis).
HOWER, H. A., and BODIAN, D.: New York Commonwealth Fund, 1942 (Poliomyelitis).
KENNEDY, F., and others: Surg., Gynec. & Obst., *91*, 385, 1950 (Arachnoiditis).
PUTNAM, T. J., and CUSHING, H.: A. M. A. Arch. Surg., *11*, 329, 1925 (Subdural Hematoma).
VON ECONOMO, C.: London, Oxford University Press, 1931 (Encephalitis Lethargica).
WHITTIER, J. R.: A. M. A. Arch. Neurol. & Psychiat., *58*, 672, 1947 (Hemichorea).
WILSON, G., and WINKELMAN, N. W.: A. M. A. Arch. Neurol. & Psychiat., *9*, 170, 1923 (Chorea).
WILSON, S. A. K.: Brain, *34*, 295, 1912 (Progressive Lenticular Degeneration).

Index